Histology

HISTOLOGY

Arthur W. Ham, M.D., F.R.S.C., D.Sc.

Professor Emeritus, Department of Anatomy,
Division of Histology, Faculty of Medicine,
University of Toronto

David H. Cormack, Ph.D.

Associate Professor, Department of Anatomy,
Division of Histology, Faculty of Medicine,
University of Toronto

EIGHTH EDITION

J. B. Lippincott Company

Philadelphia and Toronto

EIGHTH EDITION

Copyright © 1979 by J. B. Lippincott Company
Copyright © 1974, 1969, 1965, 1961, 1957 by J. B. Lippincott Company
Copyright 1953, 1950 by J. B. Lippincott Company

ISBN-0-397-52089-1

Library of Congress Catalog Card Number 79-13185

Printed in the United States of America

5   7   6   4

Library of Congress Cataloging in Publication Data

Ham, Arthur Worth, 1902-
  Histology.

  Bibliography: p.
  Includes index.
  1. Histology.   I.   Cormack, David H., joint author.
II. Title. [DNLM: 1. Histology. QS504.3 H198h]
Qm551.H147 1979 611'.018   79-13185
ISBN 0-397-52089-1

Preface

The period over which the eight editions of this book have been published (1950–1979) coincides with the time during which the most rapid and exciting advances in knowledge in histology have been made. Over this period, authors of histology textbooks have been required not only to describe the new technics which have helped make these advances possible, but also to explain how their application has increased both the depth and breadth of the subject. For the most part, the new knowledge in histology, specifically, that related to the tissues and the organ systems (Parts 3 and 4 of this book), has not been of a sort that would substitute for that already available from light microscopy. The latter has provided a sound and essential foundation on which the new has readily fitted. As a result, for histology to serve its normal role as the link between gross anatomy and histophysiology and histopathology, both the old and the new histology must now be learned.

The situation with regard to the histology of the cell is somewhat different. The cell, of course, has always been the first component of body tissue to be considered in a histology course or textbook. But before the advent of electron microscopy in the 1950s, relatively little was known about the cell. It has been in connection with the cell that the greatest proliferation of biological knowledge has occurred over the past quarter century. As one consequence, the information on histology of the cell, which in the first edition required only a few pages, now requires an entire section (Part 2) consisting of five chapters in the present edition. It quite literally amounts to a small book in itself.

The new knowledge about the cell, however, has had another effect. The relatively rigid definitions and concerns of the various life-science disciplines are vaguer now. Biochemistry, physiology, genetics, and immunology, as well as histology and histopathology, have participated in the elaboration of this new knowledge which has in turn become part of the subject matter of all these disciplines. Moreover, the mass of information presently available about the cell is now often considered to constitute a discipline in its own right. Courses are now given in, and books written about, cell biology. Some students who enroll in histology courses may already have studied it, but many others have not. Our position is that, since the cell has always been the first and most important single tissue component considered in histology, all new knowledge about the cell pertinent to histology belongs in a histology text. In any event, we feel that students who have studied cell biology and subsequently come to use this book, although they may find some repetition, will nevertheless find much in Part 2 to interest them further and, in particular, to facilitate their reading of subsequent chapters.

It should be emphasized that, whereas traditionally a histology course or text has been expected to include such knowledge about the cell as was available and pertinent to histology, a course or text on cytology or cell biology has never been, and should never be, expected to be, or substitute for, a course or text on the much more comprehensive subject of histology.

A special problem associated with learning any anatomical subject is its language. This explains why there was a time when students were required to study the classic languages before beginning anatomy. It was Jamieson, in the preface to the second edition of Dixon's *Manual of Human Osteology*, who coined the term "small Latin and less Greek" to denote the language complement of his students (and others like us) after the language requirements were removed from the liberal arts curriculum. However, Jamieson also noted that many students were interested and enlightened to learn the original meanings of the terms. We, too, have noticed this, and therefore we have tried to give the derivation of each new word that is introduced. Furthermore, we have shown that if a student learns the meanings of some of the more important building blocks of these words, his medical vocabulary can grow very rapidly.

In our opinion, another function of a textbook should be to encourage students to become research-minded. One of the easiest ways to do this is to include in the text accounts of how various important discoveries came about. Some students, of course, may consider reading such information an unnecessary burden, but we hear from many that these accounts are a most interesting feature of the book.

Another way of making histology more interesting, particularly for medical and paramedical students, is to emphasize that what they are learning will have significant application to their later clinical work and to give examples. A glance at the index will show that we have done this. (Look, for example, over the words listed under *A* in the index and see the terms *Acromegaly, Addison's disease, Allergy, Allograft rejection, Anaphylaxis, Anemia, Anomalies (chromosomal), Asthma, Atherosclerosis,* and *Autoimmune disease* listed.) Anyone who reads the accounts of the relation of histology to understanding these clinical conditions will find that he has a substantial head start when he later studies the clinical aspects in depth.

It has been our aim to explain histology simply enough for undergraduate students to *learn* the subject, not merely to memorize bits and pieces of it. However, as Samuel Johnson wrote in the preface to his famous *Dictionary of the English Language* published in 1755, "To explain requires the use of words less abstruse than that which is explained." To do this in histology often takes a lot of simple words. The alternative, if brevity is one's goal, can lead to the use of terms even more abstruse than what is being "explained."

Dr. David H. Cormack, my coauthor, has brought to the present edition some special and previously lacking features. Because he has been using the previous editions of this book in his teaching, and because of his association with students who use it or who have used it in previous years, he has become well aware of both its merits and shortcomings. This has enabled us to remedy many of the latter. Some details of the changes in this edition follow.

Part 1 was almost completely rewritten. The special purpose of this *Introduction* is to alleviate a difficulty that commonly arises because the students who enter courses in histology often have very different backgrounds of basic instruction in biology. Accordingly, we have tried to provide information early in the first chapter, which would seem to be necessary for reading and understanding the material in the remainder of the book.

Part 2, *Cell Biology,* constitutes a small book in itself. These chapters have been altered from the previous edition. First, the order has been changed to facilitate continuity. Furthermore, since much new information has been added, large parts have been rewritten and a large number of new illustrations added. Chapter 6 in particular has been revised and deals with cell differentiation in more detail and particularly with how it could depend on the expression of inducible genes. It seemed, moreover, that a section dealing with cell biology would not

be complete unless it included at least an elementary discussion of both viruses and neoplasia. Both of these topics are introduced, together with some speculation which we hope may be stimulating. Moreover, we have considered concepts relating to the control of cell populations in somewhat greater detail before going on to describe briefly the embryonic development of the four basic tissues.

In Part 3, *The Tissues of the Body,* Chapters 7 and 8, on epithelium and on the intercellular substances of connective tissue and the formation and absorption of tissue fluid, have been modified. In Chapter 9, which deals with the cells of loose connective tissue, the topic of the relation of cells to immunological reactions is introduced and discussed in some detail. Chapter 10 contains new information on platelets. In Chapter 11, Leukocytes, the granulocytes and monocytes and their functions in inflammation are considered in detail. Only the morphology of lymphocytes is described here; they are dealt with in greater detail in Chapter 13. Chapter 12, Myeloid Tissue, has been almost completely rewritten in the process of updating the account of the formation of all blood cells. Chapter 13, Lymphatic Tissue, deals with the cellular basis for immunological reactions in such detail that it, too, had to be largely rewritten.

Chapters 14 through 16, which deal with the skeletal tissues, require special comment. The extent, breadth, and depth of research in this area over the last few years has been most impressive; one result has been that several previously held concepts have been discarded in favor of new ones more in accord with the evidence that has become available. Furthermore, the histology of the development, growth, and remodeling of bones, together with an understanding of how injuries to bone and joints heal and how bones serve as calcium storehouses, now constitutes too important an aspect of surgery and medicine to be treated lightly or briefly. Accordingly, the section on skeletal tissues has been rearranged to achieve a better order, rewritten so as to explain the new findings and their significance, and provided with many new illustrations, all of which have required that it be very considerably expanded.

Chapters 17 and 18, Nervous Tissue and Muscle Tissue, have been updated, and a considerable number of the illustrations are new.

In Part 4, *The Systems of the Body,* the original order has been retained. Chapter 19, The Circulatory System, has been altered in several ways to improve it and bring it up to date. The section on the peripheral circulation was rewritten and the illustrations improved. In response to the widespread interest in the impulse-conducting system of the heart that has been generated by the advent of artificial pacemakers, both it and the pacemaker cells in particular are considered in detail, and a brief description of pacemakers and their implantation is included to round out the account. The basic features of an electrocardiogram are also described, to explain how the system's function can be checked.

In Chapter 20, The Integumentary System, new concepts of the way the cells of stratified squamous keratinizing epithelium are stacked are described and illustrated. Features relating to clinical medicine and surgery, such as skin grafting and the vascularization of grafts, the healing of wounds, and fluid loss from burns and their healing have, of course, been retained.

My good friend Dr. C. P. Leblond, who was kind enough to revise Chapter 21, The Digestive System, for the seventh edition, happily agreed to do so again. That is really all we need to say about its quality.

Chapter 22, The Pancreas, Liver, and Gallbladder, presented a problem. Although it is now generally taught that the liver parenchyma exists in the form of perforated anastomosing plates of parenchymal wells, we think it easier for students to visualize its three-dimensional structure from the study of random sections by visualizing the parenchyma as being composed of a network of anastomosing perforated trabeculae of hepatocytes which radiate from the central vein areas to the peripheries of lobules, and thus we have described this concept. New information is also provided about the functions of hepatocytes and the structure of sinusoids.

The chapters on the respiratory system and the urinary system have been updated and expanded with new material. The Endocrine System, The Female Reproductive System, and the Male Reproductive System have likewise been revised. The most extensive changes were made in the chapter on endocrine glands.

The final chapter in this edition, Chapter 28, deals with the histology of the eye and the ear. It should be pointed out that the description and illustrations of afferent nerve endings have been moved to the chapters dealing with the tissues in which they are found. Our feeling was that, in this arrangement, their great importance might be more readily appreciated. New material has, of course, been added to the descriptions, and several new illustrations have been added to supplement them.

Finally, while the subject matter of histology continues to grow, the time allotted for its teaching does not; indeed, in many institutions it is being reduced. The time allotted for histology lectures and labs is no longer adequate to cover it fully. It seems inevitable that formal teaching must now be supplemented by student reading if important matters are not to be neglected. It is hoped, first, that this edition of *Histology* permits students to obtain a satisfactory grasp of the subject and, further, that any parts selected by teachers for supplementary reading will effectively provide full coverage of this very important subject. Furthermore, because of the relatively broad treatment of topics of medical, paramedical, and biological interest, and on the basis of comments from students who have used earlier editions, it is hoped that this book will prove useful not only in the particular term in which histology is studied but also that it will become a helpful "old friend" to be consulted again in connection with studies of related subjects.

A.W.H.

In the 13 years I have been teaching histology I have come to appreciate how very valuable a teaching-type of textbook can be to undergraduate students as an aid to their learning of the subject. This appreciation has been reinforced by opinions expressed by students, including those in later years of their medical studies who have been able to evaluate the usefulness of different types of textbooks in their learning of basic science subjects. The realization that a teaching-type of histology textbook can be a very efficient way of imparting not only basic knowledge of cells and tissues but also a general understanding of many other medical subjects on the cellular level had much to do with my joining Dr. Ham as a coauthor of this edition. Although the dual task of keeping abreast of recent developments and suitably incorporating them into the text has been a big undertaking, even for two, the productive association we have enjoyed in writing this edition has provided a constant stimulus for putting forward our best efforts in the time that was available.

Some of the revisions to be found in this edition are described in Dr. Ham's Preface. We have also added many new illustrations, brought the references up to date, and expanded the index. Bearing in mind, as always, the needs of undergraduate students, who seldom (if ever) have adequate time to devote to their studies, we have paid strict attention to the arrangement of the text under individual headings, and have provided cross-references and summaries where we thought they might be helpful in studying the subject. The portions of background material incorporated for interest and general information, but not considered essential core content for an abbreviated histology course, are recognizable (particularly in the latter part of the book), since they are set in smaller type. Previous experience in making histology teaching films has in some cases suggested to me alternative ways of illustrating some of the topics. The great majority of illustrations from the earlier editions, however, still have unique teaching value and, so, have been retained.

The aims of this book, of course, go beyond transmitting only "essential facts" about microscopic anatomy. We endeavor, for example, to explain many of the more difficult aspects of the functional morphology of cells and tissues — matters that are avoided in most core texts — and this, we feel, is important if a student is to understand the subject well, and not merely memorize the facts. In aiming for a balanced and comprehensive account of the subject with sufficient depth to meet the requirements of today's medical students, we have felt it a duty not only to organize and present the current knowledge in proper perspective, but also to provide some insight into how it all seems to be fitting together.

D.H.C.

Acknowledgments

Writing a section on acknowledgments is a somewhat hazardous undertaking. It is usually the last thing one does, and generally has to be done in a hurry. As a consequence, an author runs the risk of forgetting some of those whose help should have been acknowledged. Furthermore, since persons of considerable distinction in the scientific world are often kind enough to be of assistance, authors in thanking them adequately run the risk of being accused of name-dropping. Still another problem is that someone who has provided information about some topic may not like the way it was adapted in the book. Finally, there is the horrible thought that after reading extensive acknowledgments, a prospective reader might begin to wonder if the authors themselves knew enough to write a book. Nevertheless, we shall forthwith try to acknowledge the great deal of help we have received.

We shall first thank colleagues in our department. Dr. Arthur Axelrad, as well as being helpful in many areas, was responsible for much of the revision made in Chapters 12 and 13 which deal with one of his areas of special interest and one to which his research has made a substantial contribution. Dr. Vic Kalnins read, and helped greatly with the revision of, Chapters 2 through 5, and in addition, provided several original illustrations for these chapters. Dr. David McLeod provided special help on the section on platelets and atherosclerosis. Dr. J. Prchal provided information on blood cells, and Dr. John Duckworth and Dr. I. Taylor both contributed information and illustrations to the section on the impulse-conducting system of the heart. As in the past, our associates and friends of many years, Harry Whittaker and Bruce Smith, took much interest in the book and in particular helped with the preparation of suitable photomicrographs.

In addition to direct help from the members of our department we also received much support from members of other departments in our university and also from members of various departments elsewhere. In thanking those outside our department we must first describe the help provided by Dr. C. P. Leblond of McGill University. Dr. Leblond, who has given considerable assistance in the preparation of previous editions,

kindly consented again to revise the chapter on the digestive system. For this we are most grateful. Dr. Leblond furthermore participated in the revision of Chapter 27 and of the section on the Golgi apparatus in Chapter 5. Dr. J. Bergeron of the same department helped in the revision of the section dealing with the liver, and Dr. J. Brawer helped with the revision of the material on the origin of the hypothalamic hormones.

The most practical way to thank those of other departments in this university and those of various departments of other universities would seem to be by mentioning them in alphabetical order.

We are grateful to Dr. A. Angel for taking a great deal of trouble to help prepare and illustrate the section in Chapter 9 on adipose tissue. Dr. P. K. Basu read and commented on the chapter on the eye and provided several new illustrations for it. Dr. Earl Bogoch provided useful information about the intercellular substance of cartilage and other matters of interest with regard to joints. Dr. I. A. Boyd was of the greatest assistance with regard to the section dealing with muscle spindles. Dr. A. J. Collet responded to what was almost an emergency call for immediate help when we were behind schedule in preparing the chapter on the respiratory system, and he provided us with much interesting new material and some new illustrations. Dr. E. Farber kindly reviewed a chapter about which we were eager to have his expert comments. Dr. Brian Hall provided a great deal of information about cartilage and the development of the skeletal tissues. Dr. Daryl Harris was very helpful in providing information and illustrations about the repair of cartilage. Dr. W. S. Hartroft read much of the previous edition and made many notes on many matters, which we considered when preparing this edition and which led to considerable improvements in it. Dr. Marijke Holtrop provided us with several splendid electron micrographs for the chapter on bone and agreed to read the rough copy of the extensive section prepared for this edition on osteoclasts. Her comments were most helpful. We thank Drs. A. J. Kahn and D. J. Simmons for also reading the manuscript on osteoclasts, and for lending us one of their first illustrations that showed that the osteoclasts that develop in association with quail bone rudiments transplanted to chick embryos are of host origin. We thank Dr. S. C. Luk for helpful comments, and illustrations for the bone chapter. Dr. Alex Novikoff provided information and illustrations about lysosomes and also about the Golgi apparatus. Dr. Maureen Owen made our task in preparing certain parts of the chapter on bone much easier by providing us with material that facilitated our studies. Dr. R. B. Salter took enough time from his very busy life to read the three chapters that deal with cartilage, bone, and, joints and also provided us with the most recent data on and illustrations of the research work he and his colleagues have been doing on the repair of articular cartilage. Dr. G. T. Simon not only provided us with some splendid illustrations but was also very helpful in discussing relevant matters with us. Dr. A. H. Tinmouth kindly read the sections on the impulse-conducting system of the heart and artificial pacemakers. We had considerable and very helpful correspondence with Dr. Marshall Urist, particularly about bone induction and the cells from which induced bone develops, and we are grateful for the help which he so agreeably provided. Dr. Donald Walker kindly read the section on the formation of osteoclasts, which, of course, includes descriptions of the outstanding consecutive experiments he performed to establish their origin from cells that circulate in the blood.

We are most grateful to those who provided illustrations for this edition. All are acknowledged by name in the legends, so we shall not list them all again here. However, we wish to give special thanks to Dr. C. P. Leblond and Dr. M. Weinstock, who very kindly put at our disposal a collection of useful illustrations which appear in several chapters.

We also thank Rasa Skudra of the Art Section of the Instructional Media Services of the Faculty of Medicine, University of Toronto, for applying her special skills toward improving previous illustrations and making new ones for this edition.

We also thank June Pitter, Dr. Ham's next-door neighbor, who, though she holds a full-time position of considerable responsibility, again somehow found time to type most of the very large manuscript, often from rough copy that she alone could decipher.

Finally, it has been a pleasure to deal with Tina Rebane of the J. B. Lippincott Company, who so effectively edited our manuscript, and with Stuart Freeman, who was responsible for all other matters relating to the publication of this book.

A.W.H.
D.H.C.

Contents

PART THREE: THE TISSUES OF THE BODY

Histology

PART ONE

INTRODUCTION

1 Histology, Its Place in the Biological and Medical Sciences, and How It Is Studied

For those unacquainted with histology, this chapter is intended to serve the same sort of role that *Basic English* was designed to serve for those unfamiliar with the English language. *Basic English* is a list of 850 carefully selected words which, if learned by those unfamiliar with English, serve as a means for communicating in it. Moreover, knowing these particular words is believed to greatly facilitate the subsequent acquisition of a reasonably full command of the language. Likewise this first chapter is designed to provide a basic understanding of the subject matter of histology, including its language and the methods by which it is studied in the laboratory. We hope that by reading this chapter those who have little previous knowledge of the subject will quickly feel at home in it and will also be aided in subsequently acquiring a reasonably full command of it in the later chapters.

It has always been accepted that the understanding and potential usefulness of a new subject are better realized when a student is given a preliminary indication of its nature and scope. An appreciation of the relation of the particular subject to others that are being studied simultaneously, or will be studied in the immediate future, is also of value. Moreover, it now appears that providing a preview of what is to be learned is also a very important factor in increasing the reading speed with which the subsequent, more detailed text can be covered and assimilated. This first chapter is written with all these aims in mind. We shall first comment on the language used in histology.

THE VOCABULARY OF HISTOLOGY

The study of histology requires learning not only a new subject but also a new language. For it is in histology that one learns the names of everything that can be identified by microscopy in all the representative parts of the body. These names and those learned in gross anatomy provide a basis for the specialized language used in other subjects studied in the medical and paramedical sciences and in animal biology. Since learning what may seem an interminable number of new words can be both boring and time-consuming, one of our first tasks should be to explain that there is an interesting and relatively easy way to do it, that will now be described.

Perhaps because there was not so much science to learn in the past as there is today, those who contributed to its early development had enough time to become well-versed in the classical languages. Hence when something new was discovered for which a name was needed, scientists went back to their Latin or Greek to find suitable and meaningful building blocks for the new word that they wished to coin in their own language. To give a simple example, many decades ago a blue dye was commonly used to stain specimens removed from the body for microscopic study. Then, one day, someone happened to heat some of this dye before using it and found that instead of staining everything blue, it stained only some things blue, while coloring other things red and still others violet. Since a name was needed for this dye that possessed so many coloring properties, recourse to Latin and Greek led to its being called a *polychrome* dye (Gr. *polys,* many, and *chroma,* color). In itself this example is not very important, but if you examine a medical dictionary you will find there are six double-column pages of words that begin with *poly-* and over two pages of words that begin with *chromo-* or *chroma-.* Hence, by learning relatively few of the "building blocks" from Latin or Greek, which are used over and over again in various combinations, the student will find that the words used in histology and the subjects that follow it soon become increasingly meaningful. This is one of the reasons why a medical dictionary, which gives the derivation of each word that it defines, is often described as a medical or paramedical student's "best friend." However, in order to facilitate word-learning and save the student's time, we shall, in this book, attempt to give the derivation of each new word when it is first used.

THE ORIGIN AND SUBJECT MATTER OF HISTOLOGY

The Concept of the Body Being Composed of Different Tissues

From its derivation, the word *histology* (Gr. *histos,* tissues; *logia,* study or science of) means the *science of the tissues.* But what is a tissue? This word was derived from the French *tissu,* which means a weave or texture. It was introduced into the language of biology by Bichat, a brilliant young French anatomist and physiologist (1771–1802) who became so impressed with the different textures of the layers and structures of the body he encountered in gross dissections that he wrote a book on the tissues of the body in which he named more than twenty. However, he did not use the microscope to classify the tissues, for he considered that its use led to misconceptions, and indeed at that time microscopes were inferior instruments compared to what they became later. Furthermore, he did not devise the term *histology* even though, from the dictionary definition of the subject, he could be considered to have been the first histologist.

Histology Becomes a Microscopic Science

Seventeen years after Bichat's death, the term *histology* was coined by a microscopist, and since then it has been considered to be a subject studied by microscopy. Microscopy led to the devising of a new classification of the tissues, and eventually it became generally accepted that there were only four basic tissues, but that each had subdivisions. The elucidation of these thereafter constituted the subject matter of histology. But before giving their names, we must describe some other more or less coincidental developments.

The Concept of the Body Being Composed of Cells

In the 17th century Robert Hooke, an ingenious physicist and biologist, had built a compound microscope (a real achievement at that time), and with it he happened to examine a thin slice of cork and observed that it was composed of tiny empty compartments separated by thin walls of what we now know to be cellulose. He named the little compartments *cells,* a word that was already in use in England to denote small rooms. Subsequently, other biologists studied plant tissue with microscopes and it became obvious that in living plants the little compartments that Hooke had seen in dead, dried-out cork were not empty; instead, each contained a little jelly-like body. Furthermore, as animal tissue was studied with the microscope it became obvious that it too was composed of tiny jelly-like bodies, but here they were very seldom separated from one another by walls. So by 1839, the cell doctrine, that cells are the ultimate units out of which plants and animals are constructed, was postulated independently by Schleiden and Schwann. For a time there was still some confusion about the two meanings of the word *cell,* but eventually this term came to be used exclusively for minute, jelly-like bodies.

Relation Between Cells and Tissues

The use of the microscope thus established that cells were the ultimate living units out of which plants and animals were constructed, and also that the body was composed of several different tissues. It follows that the reason for these tissues differing from one another is that the cells of a given tissue differ from those of the other tissues by being structurally specialized to perform particular functions for the body. What are these functions?

Functions Are Based on the Physiological Properties of Cells

Physiology (Gr. *physis,* nature) is the science dealing with the functions of living creatures and their various parts. In order to compile a list of the physiological properties of living cells a great deal of study was devoted to unicellular creatures such as *Amoeba* and *Paramecium.* It could be reasoned that since unicellular animals are living creatures, each would possess the essential properties required to perform all the basic functions on which its life would depend. The time-honored list of the physiological properties of cells (originally considered to be properties that distinguish living creatures from inanimate objects) which follows will often be referred to in later chapters.

Irritability. This is a general term that indicates that when a stimulus of a physical, chemical, or electrical nature is applied to a living cell, it responds in some way that can be observed. What is termed *irritability* can be determined objectively only by observing that it leads to one or more of the following responses.

Conductivity. This physiological property of cells is manifested as a wave of excitation that originates at the site of the stimulus and passes along the surface of the cell to reach the other parts of the cell. The passage of a wave of excitation along a cell is associated with a measurable change in electrical potential along its course.

Contractility. This response to a stimulus is manifested by the cell shortening in some direction.

Absorption and Assimilation. All cells can take in food from their surface and utilize it.

Secretion. Cells are able to synthesize new useful products from what they absorb. Many of these products can be delivered (secreted) to the exterior of the cell for export.

Excretion. A cell must excrete through its surface the waste products that result from utilization of its food.

Respiration. Cells absorb oxygen, which is used to bring about the oxidation of food substances to provide energy, a process called *cell respiration.*

Growth and Reproduction. The growth of cells requires the synthesis of more cell substance. Cells become inefficient if they exceed a certain size, hence growth in multicellular organisms is generally achieved by cells remaining about the same size and increasing in number (instead of becoming larger). How this is done will be described in the next chapter.

THE EXPRESSION OF PHYSIOLOGICAL PROPERTIES IN THE CELLS OF THE VARIOUS TISSUES

The four basic tissues of the body are: *(1) epithelial tissue, (2) connective tissue, (3) nerve tissue,* and *(4) muscle tissue.* It requires many chapters (Chaps. 6–18) to deal with the specialized structure and functions of these tissues. All that needs to be stressed about them at this point is that the cells of each tissue are structurally specialized in order to express one or more of the physiological properties described above. For example, we shall find that although the cells of *epithelial tissue* (Gr. *epi,* upon) generally serve a protective function (because membranes made of epithelial cells cover external and line internal body surfaces), there is another division of this tissue which consists of groups of cells, situated more deeply in the body, that function to provide external or internal secretions important to the body.

Connective tissue plays many roles; one in particular will be mentioned here. When we say that the body is composed of cells we are not telling the whole truth, for if the body consisted only of cells it would be as soft as cells and hence would amount to no more than a big mound of jelly-like material. Actually the discovery of cells was preceded by the discovery of a nonliving component of tissue that provided structural strength for cell organizations, for it will be recalled that the plant material that Hooke saw under his microscope (the walls of compartments) was nonliving material. In the body the function of producing nonliving supportive materials is allotted almost entirely to certain of the cells of connective tissue that are specialized for this purpose. Such materials are called *intercellular substances* (L. *inter,* between). They sometimes lie between individual cells and sometimes between groups of cells. Some intercellular substances are delicate while others have great tensile strength or are weight-bearing. The intercellular substance lying between the cells of bone, for instance, is much like reinforced concrete. It is because of intercellular substances that the body can stand erect and that its various tissues stay intact. We shall find furthermore that connective tissue permeates all the other tissues of the body and thereby serves two purposes. First, its intercellular substances mechanically support the cells of the other tissues. Second, it ensheathes the blood vessels of the body, for they are all formed within connective tissue and thereafter travel through the body in it. Thus connective tissue holds the cells of other tissues in place and its blood vessels provide for their nourishment. However, not all the cells of connective tissue are specialized for producing intercellular substances; some have other functions, to be described later.

Nervous tissue is highly specialized with respect to irritability and conductivity. Thread-like extensions from nerve cells, in the form of nerves, lead from the brain and spinal cord to all the other parts of the body, providing a means for rapid communication between its different parts.

Finally, *muscle tissue* is highly specialized for contractility. It is, of course, because of our muscles that we can move our bones on one another at articulating joints and hence be mobile.

Cells and Tissues as Building Blocks of Two Different Orders

An analogy may be helpful here. There are two different orders of building blocks from which chemical compounds are assembled. Atoms of different kinds are the ultimate ones, and these are arranged together to form molecules. But when studying the composition of many chemical compounds it is often easier to visualize how they are built from molecules than from atoms. Likewise, in studying the organs (L. *organum,* a more or less independent part of the body that serves a special function), it is usually easier to appreciate how these are assembled from the four basic tissues than to understand their microscopic structure in terms of individual cells. For example, when it is understood why connective tissue (with its intercellular substances and blood vessels) would need to be present in an epithelial organ whose function was secretion, it is easy to understand why such an organ would be constructed of two different tissues, namely epithelium and connective tissue.

How Histology Came to Include the Subject of Microscopic Anatomy

There was an initial distinction between histology and microscopic anatomy. At first, histology dealt only with the basic tissues of the body, whereas microscopic anatomy dealt with the microscopic structure of organs and other body structures (which, of course, were all assembled from the four basic tissues). Hence early textbooks were usually called textbooks of "Histology and Microscopic Anatomy" and approximately half their contents were devoted to the microscopic study of tissues, while the second half covered the microscopic structure of the organs and organ systems of the body. The distinction was useful because a student would first learn about the tissues (the building blocks) and then learn how they were put together to form complicated organs. Indeed, this order is still followed in histology textbooks, including this one. However, over the years it became unnecessary to use both terms in the title, because the term *histology* came to include microscopic anatomy.

The Value of Histology and the Tissue Concept in Understanding Embryology and Pathology

The tissue concept was of great importance in the development of embryology. When the embryonic origins of the different tissues had been determined, it became much simpler to follow how they subsequently grew together to form organs. The tissue concept also was a great boon to the development of pathology (the study of disease). It was found, for example, that tumors differed because they originated from different tissues. They could then be classified on the basis of their origins; for example, one type of tumor developing from epithelium is termed an *epithelioma* (Gr. *oma*, a swelling). The tissue concept proved so helpful that the study of pathology of tissues with the microscope became established as a subject in its own right (histopathology).

The Relation of Histology to Physiology

As already explained, histology is concerned with studying how cells are arranged and structurally specialized to perform specific functions in different tissues. But histologists do not study the structure of cells as someone might, for example, take an interest in bric-a-brac. They study cells in order to determine how their microscopic structure enables them to perform their particular functions.

Thus histology is the study of the relation between cell structure and function. But since the science of function is physiology, it may seem difficult for the student to surmise how much function he should learn about in his study of histology. Because histology is concerned with establishing the structural basis for particular functions, histology necessarily has to deal with the existence of function. But physiology likewise has to deal with the structural basis for functions and, since it is generally assumed that the student will have studied histology before physiology, physiology deals with function more broadly and in greater depth, and in particular with measuring functions. Nevertheless, the relation between histology and physiology is very close—indeed, in some countries, histology is taught in departments of physiology instead of anatomy. Another indication of the close relation between these two subjects is that students who have studied histology will find many familiar illustrations in physiology texts.

The Relation of Histology to Cell Biology and Biochemistry

Before the early 1950s, the description of the microscopic structure of the cell did not take much space in a textbook. But during the second half of this century there was a colossal increase in knowledge about cell structure and its relation to function. Of the greatest importance in this regard was the fact that it became practicable for histologists to utilize the great resolving power of the electron microscope (described in detail at the end of this chapter) in their studies of cells and tissues. With the advent of the electron microscope, the cell stood revealed not only as the unit of structure in the body but as an entity in itself, with its own little organs (the organelles) functioning in an integrated manner to carry out its life processes. During this same period the chemical basis of the genetic code was discovered. Methods were rapidly developed by which various components of cells could be separated from one another by centrifugation of homogenates (disrupted cells) and collected in sufficient quantities for biochemical studies to reveal their functions. All this soon led to a marriage between the chemistry and structure of cells and the birth of an interrelated subject, *cell biology*. A valuable stage in the development of new knowledge in this area was the introduction of radioactive isotopes that could safely be given to animals and that became incorporated (like normal chemical building blocks) into cells and tissues. The sites of incorporation into cells could be determined not only in the biochemistry laboratory but also by light or electron microscopy by using the histological method known as radioautography, to be described in Chapter 3. Many of the findings grouped in cell biology were of course also retained in the subject matter of both biochemistry and histology. Since so many of these findings were of an interdisciplinary (L. *inter,* between; *disciplina,* a branch of learning or knowledge) nature, students may again find the same kinds of diagrams of cells in their biochemistry and histology textbooks. Furthermore, it now takes four chapters of the present edition of this textbook to cover the cell adequately (this subject occupied only a short preliminary chapter in the first edition in 1950).

The Relation of Histology to Genetics

The basis for inheritance through germ cells and the way in which hereditary material is consistently passed on by every cell of the body to its progeny will be discussed in subsequent chapters. We shall also consider how occasional accidents in the apportionment of the hereditary material can affect the tissues of the body and cause various kinds of anomalies. The detailed structure of the *chromosomes* (Gr. *chroma,* color; *soma,* body), the bearers of the genes of cells, and the mechanism underlying genetic expression in cells will also be described. There will also be examples of how blood-borne chemical messenger substances, known as hormones, can influence the expression of genes at the cellular level.

The Relation of Histology to Immunology

In recent years it has become evident that several different types of cells are involved in one way or another in immunological reactions (defined and described in Chaps. 9 and 13). We shall deal with the ways in which these cells are involved in combatting disease-causing organisms and describe the cellular basis for the body's reaction to sensitizing agents, such as pollens (a cause of hay fever), and to tissues that have been transplanted from one individual to another, a subject of great importance to those who may some day have to perform an organ transplant or receive a transplanted kidney from a donor.

THE TERMS USED FOR THE BASIC PARTS OF CELLS

After cells were discovered to be minute jelly-like bodies, the microscope revealed that they had two main parts. Living cells were seen to have a more or less central part that had a different refractive index from the rest of the cell. This central part was named its *nucleus* (L. *nux*, nut) because it reminded early investigators of a nut lying in the center of its shell. For the same reason the Greek prefix *kary-* (Gr. *karyon*, nut) may also be used in words with reference to the nucleus. For example, the dissolution of the nucleus as a cell dies is called *karyolysis* (Gr. *lysis*, dissolution).

The Parts of the Nucleus Seen After Staining

A membrane was seen to enclose the nucleus, so this was called the *nuclear membrane* or *envelope* (Fig. 1-1). One or more rounded, dark-staining bodies in the interior of the nucleus (Fig. 1-1) were each called a *nucleolus* (from the L. diminutive of nut; plural: *nucleoli*). Tiny granules or irregularly shaped clumps of dark-staining material scattered about in the nucleus were called *chromatin* (Gr. *chroma*, color) because of their affinity for certain dyes. The component in which the nucleoli and chromatin seemed to be suspended was termed the *nuclear sap* (Fig. 1-1). Details of the structure, chemical nature, and functions of the parts of the nucleus will be given in subsequent chapters.

Cytoplasm

The outer and generally larger part of the cell was called *cytoplasm* (Gr. *kytos*, something that is hollow or that covers; *plasma*, something molded), since it appeared to be molded so as to cover the nucleus. As we shall see, particular functions are performed by particular components of the cytoplasm, and its appearance varies in different types of cells, depending on the functions for

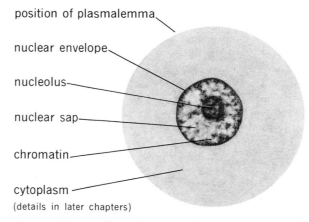

position of plasmalemma

nuclear envelope

nucleolus

nuclear sap

chromatin

cytoplasm
(details in later chapters)

Fig. 1-1. Diagram illustrating the basic structure of the cell.

which they are specialized. We should mention here, however, that while a few minute structures could be observed in the cytoplasm with the light microscope, it took the development of the electron microscope to reveal them all and disclose their structure. Now it is known that the cytoplasm contains a host of specialized components called *organelles* (*dim.* of organ). These are arranged so as to function in an integrated manner to bring about the chemical reactions necessary for life, which is therefore not the property of any single given substance. The cytoplasmic organelles lie suspended in what was in the past termed the *ground substance* or *cytoplasmic matrix*, but which is now more commonly called the *cytosol*.

Cytoplasmic Inclusions

The term *inclusion* originated when it was believed that cytoplasm was itself a "living" substance—a view no longer held—and it was used to denote such things as granules of pigment or globules of stored food (such as fat) that could have been of either internal or external origin. Because such materials were not considered to be part of the "living" cytoplasm, they were thought of as being substances that had somehow become *enclosed* by the supposedly living cytoplasm, but were not actually part of it, hence the term *inclusion*. What were termed *secretion granules* in cytoplasm were at one time also called inclusions, but as more was learned about them they came to be considered as just another component of cytoplasm, and indeed in the light of present-day knowledge the retention of the concept of a category of inclusions is of dubious value.

The Cell Membrane

Light microscopy could not demonstrate directly that the cytoplasm was enclosed by a limiting membrane (with properties different from those of cytoplasm itself) because the cell membrane is so extremely thin that cross sections of it could not be distinguished with this instrument. But the light microscope did indirectly help to establish its existence, for it was observed that when cells were immersed in either strong or weak salt solutions, something at the surface of the cell manifested the properties of a semipermeable membrane. Thus cells placed in weak solutions (or water) were seen to swell, while those in strong solutions would shrink and shrivel up. With the advent of the electron microscope, it was possible to observe the cell membrane itself, as will be described in Chapter 5. Because it once reminded someone of the bark around a tree, the cell membrane also received the name *plasmalemma* (Gr. *lemma*, bark).

Eukaryotic and Prokaryotic Cells

Although the kinds of cells with which this book deals all contain nuclei, it should be pointed out that in the general field of cell biology, two kinds of cells are recognized: those with nuclei, and those without. The former are known as *eukaryotic cells,* which term from its origin (Gr. *eu,* good; *karyon,* nut, nucleus) indicates that this kind of cell possesses a "good" nucleus consisting of material that is enclosed by a nuclear membrane or envelope (Fig. 1-1). Eukaryotic cells are the kind of cells of which all animals, plants, and microorganisms except bacteria and blue-green algae, are composed. In the two exceptions the nuclear material is not enclosed by a nuclear membrane. Cells of this type are termed *prokaryotic,* which term implies that they evolved before cells of the eukaryotic type.

The Size of Cells

Eukaryotic cells differ from prokaryotic cells in another way, for, as already mentioned, their cytoplasm contains a more varied range of specialized organelles than is found in prokaryotic cells. Hence they have to be larger than prokaryotic cells to house "good" nuclei and the variety and number of cytoplasmic organelles essential for the integrated chemical reactions on which their life depends. But since reactions in these cellular components must be fueled with nutrients and require oxygen, and because these substances have to reach the inside of cells from their surface, eukaryotic cells could not exist if they were very large—their innermost parts would be too far removed from the exterior to be adequately served. So although eukaryotic cells of different kinds differ somewhat in size there are upper and lower limits to their size; most are between 0.01 and 0.1 mm. in diameter. Prokaryotic cells (for example, bacteria), which lack nucleus and have fewer kinds of organelles, are thus smaller than eukary-

otic cells. It should be emphasized, however, that much of what is known about how eukaryotic cells work at the molecular level is based on the results of research performed on prokaryotic cells.

THE BASIC BIOCHEMICAL COMPOSITION OF BODY COMPONENTS

Three of the four basic tissues consist mainly of cells. However, most of the fourth kind, the connective tissues, contain both cells and substantial amounts of nonliving intercellular substances. Connective tissue permeates or lies close to structures composed of the other tissues and carries the blood vessels that nourish these tissues. Tissue cells receive their nutrient through the medium of a fluid called *tissue fluid* (or *extracellular fluid*), as will be described presently. Hence the three basic components of the body are (*1*) *cells,* (*2*) *intercellular substances,* and (*3*) *fluids.*

The chemistry of life, *biochemistry* (Gr. *bios,* life) is, of course, taught as a separate discipline. But a few aspects of the subject will be included here for three reasons. First, in a given curriculum, instruction in histology may precede formal instruction in biochemistry and hence it cannot be assumed that the reader will be familiar with those terms or concepts of biochemistry that are essential for the intelligent study of cell structure and function. Second, as already noted, electron microscopy has disclosed a whole new world of organized macromolecular structure within the cell, and the study of the form of these structures, together with the ways in which they participate in chemical reactions in cells, has become more or less common ground for histology and biochemistry. As already mentioned, this has had the desirable effect of helping to relate structure to both function and chemistry at the microscopic level and has led to the emergence of the new field of cell biology. Finally, there are certain aspects of the chemistry of cells, intercellular substances, and body fluids that should receive special emphasis in relation to microscopy because such aspects are necessary for understanding how biological materials are prepared for microscopic study.

The Composition of Cells

Four main types of chemical substances (aside from water, mineral salts and other substances present in very low concentration) enter into the composition of cells: these are proteins, nucleic acids (so named because they were first isolated from nuclei), carbohydrates, and lipids (fats). At this point we shall deal only with the proteins. The nucleic acids, carbohydrates, and lipids will all be dealt with in subsequent chapters.

Proteins. Of the four main substances, proteins, either by themselves or combined with other chemical entities, such as carbohydrate to form glycoproteins (Gr. *glykys,* sweet) or *lipid* (Gr. *lipos,* fat) to form lipoproteins, are the major components of cells. As Mulder wrote in 1838, "Without protein, life would be impossible on our planet." Proteins are of profound importance in histology because they are responsible not only for different appearances but also for diverse functions in cells. Thus proteins are implicated in the expression of the distinctive features, or *phenotypes* (Gr. *phainein,* to show; *typos,* type), of the various kinds of cells, features that permit histologists to distinguish one type of cell from another.

Proteins exist in the form of huge molecules (called *macromolecules*) assembled in linear fashion from building blocks called *amino acids.* There are 20 or so amino acids; each characteristically contains both an amino ($-NH_2$) and a carboxyl group ($-COOH$). Proteins thus contain nitrogen. Plant cells are able to synthesize amino acids (and hence proteins) from simple inorganic components: water, carbon dioxide, and nitrogen. Animal cells, however, cannot synthesize amino acids from these simple components, so they must acquire them by eating plants or milk, eggs, fish or meat, all of the latter group being obtained from animals that have eaten plants. In the digestive system proteins are broken down into amino acids and from the intestine the amino acids are absorbed into the blood, which carries them to the cells of the various parts of the body. In the body cells the amino acids are linked together to form various kinds of proteins. Our cells thus make their own proteins from amino acids. Curiously enough, each individual person, except identical twins, makes some protein different from that in everyone else.

Although proteins can also be used as fuel for cells, it is the carbohydrates and lipids that generate most of the energy. The chief role of the proteins is to provide cells with metabolic machinery and the material with which to build the diverse structures in which the chemical reactions of life proceed. To discuss these, we must first discuss *metabolism.*

The Role of Proteins in Metabolism. The sum total of all the chemical reactions that proceed in a cell, conferring on it the properties of life, constitute its *metabolism* (Gr. *metaballein,* to throw into a different position, change). Some of these metabolic reactions involve either destruction or production of cell substance. Those concerned with the breakdown of cell substance are termed *catabolic* (Gr. *kata,* down; *ballein,* to throw). Those concerned with the synthesis of new cell substance are termed *anabolic* (Gr. *anaballein,* to throw up). In some cells anabolic and catabolic activity remain in balance; such cells are said to be in a metabolically *steady state.*

Growth is dependent on the anabolic reactions' exceeding the catabolic reactions.

The chemical reactions involved in metabolism are catalyzed by *enzymes* (Gr. *en,* in; *zyme,* leaven), all of which are proteins. However, not all proteins are enzymes, for some, as previously mentioned, provide the structural material of the various cell components. For example, many of the cytoplasmic organelles are composed of *membranes,* which are made of lipids in association with proteins. Membranes also subdivide the cytoplasm into different compartments, each with different functions. Such membranes may serve to keep particular components apart in the cell and prevent them from interacting with each other with unhappy results. Moreover, enzymatic proteins are often incorporated into membranes, and many enzymatic reactions occur on the surface of such membranes. Enzymes in organelles or in the cytosol between them bring about the various reactions by which carbohydrates or lipids are metabolized to provide energy. Neither enzymatic nor structural proteins are permanent fixtures, for they are always being catabolized and new protein molecules must be synthesized to take their place. Life thus depends on the continuous synthesis of proteins.

A feature of protein molecules of particular interest in histology is that they have side chains possessing charged groups. These charges cause proteins to take up certain stains.

The Composition of Intercellular Substances

As already mentioned, were it not for the intercellular substances of the body, we would have remained mounds of jelly. Such intercellular substances are made almost entirely by certain cells in the connective tissue that permeates the other tissues of the body and provides them with support and nourishment. In order to provide both support and nourishment, there is a need for two different kinds of intercellular substances: *fibrous* and *amorphous* (Gr. *a,* without, *morphē,* form). These will now be described.

The Fibrous Intercellular Substances. The most abundant fibrous intercellular component is called *collagen* (Gr. *kolla,* glue; *gennan,* to produce) because boiling it down produces glue. The protein collagen consists of fibers of great tensile strength and is found, for example, in tendons, which must resist stretching as they transmit the pull of muscles on bones.

Another protein that can exist in the form of fibers is *elastin.* As well as forming fibers, this protein also forms layers, called *laminae* (L. *lamina,* flat layer), in the walls of arteries. Unlike collagen, elastin can be stretched. It is because of elastin stretching that the pulse can be felt

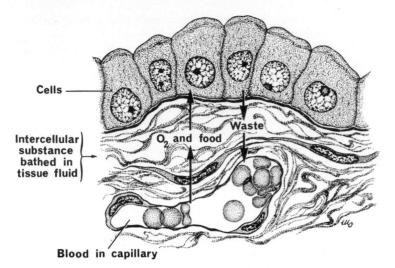

Fig. 1-2. Diagram to show the routes by which food and oxygen in blood capillaries reach cells that are not adjacent to capillaries, and how waste products from the metabolism of cells travel in the opposite direction. Both routes depend on the diffusion of substances through the tissue fluid that permeates the intercellular substances between capillaries and cells.

every time the heart pumps blood into an artery, and this stretching is the recoil mechanism that returns the artery to its former diameter between heartbeats. Elastin is a particularly sturdy substance, and some persists even to the present day in arteries of Egyptian mummies. In arteries most of the elastin is produced by muscle cells rather than cells of connective tissue, and this is discussed further in Chapter 19 (p. 597). Elsewhere, like collagen, it is produced by connective tissue cells.

The Amorphous Intercellular Substances. These substances, somewhat loosely referred to as *amorphous* or *ground substances*, contain carbohydrates, often bound to proteins. Here, the carbohydrates are in the form of polysaccharides in which hexuronic acids and amino sugars are alternately linked together to form long-chained molecules called *glycosaminoglycans,* a name that reflects how such molecules are made up of repeating disaccharide units. When glycosaminoglycans are covalently bound to proteins, they are called *proteoglycans.* Further details are given in Chapter 8 (p. 216).

As anyone knows who has thickened a sauce by adding cornstarch (which is a polysaccharide) and heating it, polysaccharides can exist in the form of viscous solutions, and this is the form they take in amorphous intercellular substances. As well as forming viscous solutions, often referred to as *sols*, polysaccharides can also exist in the form of semisolid (or virtually solid) *gels.* The sols in most parts of the body act as fillers between blood vessels and cells. Such gels as that in cartilage are solid enough to bear weight. Yet, whether they take the form of sols or gels, it is important to realize that the nonfibrous intercellular substances hold enough water to permit ready diffusion of dissolved substances (oxygen and nutrients) from sites of higher to those of lower concentration.

The Composition of Body Fluids. There are three main types of fluids in a body, (*1*) *blood,* (*2*) *tissue fluid,* and (*3*) *lymph.* The *blood* consists of two components: the *blood cells* and the slightly viscous fluid, called *plasma,* in which they are suspended. Throughout the body, the blood circulates in tubular *blood vessels,* and the smallest of these are so narrow that they are called *capillaries* (L. *capillaris,* hair). Capillaries pervade the intercellular substance so extensively that tissue cells are seldom far away from a capillary (Fig. 1-2).

Capillaries exude, through minute openings in their walls, a clear watery fluid called *tissue fluid* or *extracellular* (or *intercellular) fluid,* which is more or less a dialysate of blood plasma. This fluid permeates the amorphous intercellular substances lying between capillaries and cells (Fig. 1-2), being held there by their carbohydrate-containing macromolecules. The blood plasma within the capillaries contains both nutrients and oxygen (released from red blood cells) in simple solution. Since both of these are in greater concentration in the plasma than in tissue fluid, they diffuse out through the thin walls of the capillaries and into the tissue fluid and by this means reach the tissue cells (long arrows in Fig. 1-2). The cells in turn release waste products, and, since these become more concentrated in tissue fluid than in blood, they diffuse in the opposite direction (short arrows in Fig. 1-2) to enter and be carried away by the blood in the capillaries.

Sometimes more tissue fluid is produced than can be absorbed back into the capillaries; any excess is carried away by another series of small tubes called *lymphatics,* as will be described later (see Fig. 8-6, p. 218). The fluid they absorb (which is really tissue fluid) is called *lymph* (L. *lympha,* water) as soon as it lies within a lymphatic.

The lymphatics eventually connect with the bloodstream and empty into it.

WHAT IS STUDIED IN HISTOLOGY

Before considering the methods used in histology, it is useful at the outset to have a proper perspective about what these methods are really intended to disclose. Misconceptions are frequently met, and a common one is that histology is synonymous with microscopic anatomy and thus comprises a purely structural subject that should go no further than describing the parts of the body as seen under microscopes. We consider this to be an unimaginative and unjustifiably narrow point of view and suggest that if histology is to be considered as a structural subject, then "structure" should be used in the same sense as it is used in sociology, that is, to denote the structure of societies. For histology is really the study of the structure of cell societies. This is by no means a new concept, for over 100 years ago the great German pathologist Rudolf Virchow, who perhaps did more than anyone else to establish the nature of the tissues and initiate the science of histopathology, described the body as a cell state. (Perhaps it was because of such thinking that he turned to politics and entered a second career during which he was responsible for several reforms.)

The structure of a society of cells in the multicellular animal is similar in many respects to the structure of society in an industrialized state. As in states consisting of people, there is a profound division of labor (function) amongst the component members of cell societies. Unlike either primitive man or unicellular animals, the individuals of a highly developed society are no longer Jacks-of-all-trades that perform all the functions necessary for their continued survival. Specialization is bought at the price of independence, and, be it amongst people or cells, it demands a sacrifice of the ability to do everything in order to do a few things well. In a developed society, individuals must exchange with their fellows their respective services or the products of their work. Similarly, a continuous exchange between specialized cells must be effected for the body to live. The necessity for such an exchange becomes obvious with the realization that death of the whole body can rapidly follow the failure of an important group of cells to function properly. Rapid exchange between specialized cells is effected through an efficient transportation system, the bloodstream, into which specialized cells release their own particular products and from which they take the things they need to perform their work. The supply of these necessities is often kept up to demand by automatic regulatory mechanisms. In addition there are two communication systems that regulate the activities of specialized cells. First, there is the nervous system, which, much like a telephone system, supplies wire-like nerve fibers to parts of the body where nerve impulses can initiate or suppress cellular activities. Another system of regulation depends upon specialized cells sending appropriate chemical messages to different destinations via the transportation system. These chemical messages, called *hormones* (Gr. *hormaein,* to set in motion or spur on), may control the growth and activities of cells far distant from those cells that sent them.

The cell state, like a state of people, may be invaded by outside enemies: bacteria, viruses, or other parasites. Certain cells of the body are specialized to react to the invaders by moving through the bloodstream to where they are causing trouble in order to destroy them.

It is of interest too that, within the cell state, the population is constantly changing. Old cells die and must be replaced by new ones of the same kind. The cell population in each particular part of the body is carefully regulated by some means that is not yet clearly understood. As soon as there are enough cells to do the work, no more are formed until there is a further need for them. Thus the sizes of the various organs, such as the liver, kidney, stomach, and so on, are always kept in proper proportion.

There are more than 100 distinct types of cells in the human body, and the majority of these are specialized to perform one particular kind of task. As microscopic anatomists, histologists have to learn the characteristic structural features by which particular kinds of cells can be identified microscopically. They also seek to understand how these features relate to the ability of such cells to perform their distinctive functions. A further concern, however, is to determine how and why many different kinds of cells can arise within a cell community from a common ancestor and why, after various cell families have formed, the cells in a family thereafter reproduce only their own kind. This, of course, involves the study of the relative aspects of both heredity and environment at the cellular level, topics that will be considered as we proceed.

THE BASIC METHODS BY WHICH HISTOLOGY IS STUDIED

We may now begin to understand the nature and breadth of the subject matter of histology. First, histology is concerned with ascertaining and describing the structure revealed by all forms of microscopy and ancillary methods in every part of the body. But histology goes further than this because it is also concerned with the study of the structure of the cell society that inhabits the body, or to use Virchow's term, the study of the cell state. Some methods by which these two aspects of histology can be studied in the laboratory will now be described.

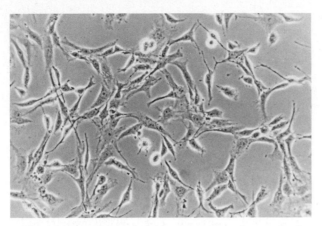

Fig. 1-3. Low-power phase contrast photomicrograph of a monolayer culture of glial cells isolated from a rat brain tumor. (Courtesy of L. Subrahmanyan)

The Study of Cells in Vitro

An approach that has provided much valuable information about cells is to isolate them from particular parts of the body and grow (or at least maintain) them in what are termed *cell cultures*, where they may be studied in detail by microscopy and other methods. Since the nutritive media in which the cells were grown were originally (and commonly still are) contained in glass receptacles, cell studies of this type were said to be done *in vitro* (L.*vitrum*, glass) and this term is still used even though cells are now commonly cultivated in plastic containers. In such cultures, cells can divide, move about, secrete various substances, and perform many of the functions that they would have carried out in the body. Cells may even become more specialized and express new characteristics and functions in vitro when they are provided with appropriate culture conditions. Furthermore, it is possible by using *microsurgical technics* to operate on cells in vitro and, for example, transplant the nucleus from one cell to another. Moreover cells from two different tissues or even two different species can be induced to fuse with one another in vitro. One of the many purposes for which in vitro methods are used is to determine the true sex of an athlete or patient. Another is to establish how toxic a particular substance might be to living cells. In vitro methods are also widely used in studying cell specialization and malignant changes in cells, and moreover they are the only ethically acceptable means available for experimenting with human tissues.

To prepare cell cultures, tissues are commonly dissociated with proteolytic enzymes, such as trypsin. The cells isolated from the tissues are then incubated at body temperature in a suitable medium, usually supplemented with serum. In a suitable medium the cells may grow either in suspension or, more commonly, in the form of a monolayer on the floor of the culture vessel (Fig. 1-3).

Few cells in a culture are able to continue dividing for more than a few months. However, some may persist and proliferate more or less indefinitely in the culture medium because of some change in their genetic constitution. Such cells form what are known as *continuous cell lines*; they can be stored in liquid nitrogen for considerable periods after carefully freezing with cryoprotective agents (that safeguard them against lethal damage by ice crystals). New cultures may then be started from thawed cells when required.

An important advantage of studying cells in vitro is that it permits their observation in a well-controlled environment that simulates that of the body, yet it avoids complex and variable influences that are known to affect the cells in the body. However, there is also a disadvantage, for the interrelationships that exist between the individual cells in a tissue are lost when they are displaced from their natural habitat. Because any transfer to a new and artificial environment is bound to affect the organization and functions of cells, it is not always clear how closely some in vitro findings reflect what really goes on in the body.

The Study of Cells in Histological Sections

In vitro methods that involve the isolation of the members of cell societies from their normal surroundings are not really designed for studying the lives and living arrangements of cell populations. Nor are they very suitable for observing changes in these arrangements with age or in disease conditions. However "cell sociology" can be studied by another method that does permit the lives and living arrangements of cells to be studied, at least to some extent. This involves cutting extremely thin slices of tissues (called *sections*) and preparing them so that they can be observed under the light or electron microscope. Since such a method necessitates the study of dead cells, it might at first be thought singularly inappropriate for studying the "sociology" of living cells. But it does preserve the structural relationships between cells in tissues, and it enables body parts to be observed at different ages and in different states of functional activity. With the use of tracer methods soon to be described, the life histories of cells labeled within living animals can also be investigated in samples of tissue obtained at various times after labeling. It is even possible to follow what happens to labeled molecules by such a procedure. Accordingly, just as we learn about societies of people by taking still pictures of their community life at particular times, so we can infer many things about societies of cells by looking at sections of tissues, taken from experimental animals of different ages, or after certain experimental procedures.

How Sections Are Studied by Light Microscopy. The cut surface of a piece of tissue, even under the microscope, reveals little of the internal structure of the tissue unless light can be transmitted through it, and this requires the tissue to be sliced very thinly. Furthermore, the slice must be extremely thin if superimposition of the various tissue components is to be avoided and individual cells are to be discerned clearly. Thus sections have to be thinner than the width of one cell. Each section, then, takes the form of a transparent shaving so fragile that it can only be handled by sticking it to the glass slide on which it will be stained (Fig. 1-4, *top*). The section is protected by a thin glass coverslip (Fig. 1-4, *bottom*) attached to the slide with a mounting medium of appropriate refractive index.

The term *section* is also now often used to denote the entire mounted preparation (slide, tissue slice, and coverslip) and we shall use the term indiscriminately. The student of histology will study sections prepared from all the important parts of the body.

How Sections Are Prepared. In order to study sections intelligently, it is helpful at the outset to know something about how they are prepared; we shall therefore briefly describe the steps by which this is done.

Obtaining the Tissue. The small piece of tissue from which the sections are to be cut must be obtained with the greatest care (we are using the term *tissue* here in a nonspecific way to denote a portion of body substance, instead of in its strict histological sense, meaning one of the four basic tissues). Any pinching or squeezing of the tissue with dull instruments will distort its appearance, so it must be cut with a very sharp scalpel, using little pressure. The small piece of tissue that is removed is called a *block* of tissue.

Fixation. The tissue block is immediately immersed in a solution known as a *fixative* because it fixes most of the tissue components in place so that they will not get lost during subsequent processing. The block of tissue should be no more than a few mm. thick, in order to permit quick penetration of the fixative.

Fixatives affect tissue in much the same way as boiling affects an egg and indeed, tissues can be fixed by boiling, but this method is not as good as chemical fixation. Chemical fixatives either crosslink proteins or denature and precipitate them by replacing the water associated with them. As a result, tissues become harder. Most fixatives also inactivate the enzymes of the cells. Unless there is prompt and thorough fixation, certain of the enzymes in cells continue to act so as to digest proteins and other macromolecular substances in the cells; this causes

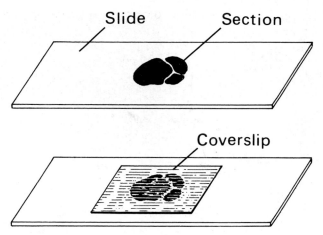

Fig. 1-4. (*Top*) A stained section on a glass slide. (*Bottom*) The same section with a coverslip on top.

what is called *postmortem* (L.*post*, after; *mors*, death) *degeneration* and it spoils the tissue for proper histological study.

Some fixatives are better than others for preserving polysaccharides and lipids although, by cross-linking the proteins with which these are usually associated, common fixatives do preserve some of the polysaccharides and even some fatty materials that might otherwise escape during the further processing of the material. Most fixatives are also good antiseptics and thus kill bacteria and other disease-causing agents present in infected tissues that might present a health hazard to those handling them. Appropriate fixatives can even enhance the uptake of stains by tissues. There are special fixatives for the preservation of specific cell or tissue components; these are listed in textbooks on histological technics. Probably the commonest one for routine work is a 4-per-cent solution of formaldehyde, buffered to neutral pH.

Preparing Sections by the Paraffin Technic. Dehydration. Possibly in the past some ingenious person, having noticed how easy it was to whittle thin shavings from a candle, may have conceived the idea of infiltrating tissue with wax so that it, like a candle, could be cut into thin slices. However, most tissues contain a great deal of water, which is not miscible with wax, particularly the paraffin wax which is routinely used. In order to introduce wax into tissues, the water must first be removed. The time-honored way of achieving this is by immersing the block of fixed tissue first into a weak solution of alcohol in water and then into progressively stronger solutions of alcohol until finally it is passed through two baths of absolute (100%) alcohol, after which no water remains in it. This completes its *dehydration.* Then another step called *clearing* is employed.

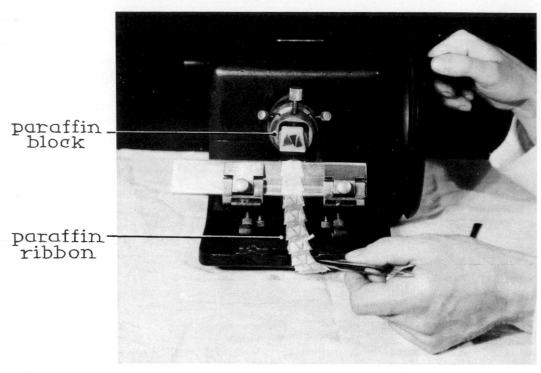

paraffin block

paraffin ribbon

Fig. 1-5. A microtome being used to cut a ribbon of paraffin sections. The paraffin block has three pieces of tissue embedded in it; the outline of these may be seen in each of the sections adhering to one another to form the ribbon.

Clearing and Infiltration. Clearing agents, for example, *xylol,* are soluble in both wax and alcohol. From absolute alcohol the block of tissue is passed through successive changes of xylol until all the alcohol is replaced by xylol. The block is then placed in melted paraffin and allowed to remain there until all the xylol has been replaced by paraffin; this step is called *infiltration.*

Embedding and Sectioning. After the block of tissue has become thoroughly infiltrated with paraffin, the latter is allowed to harden and then the excess wax is trimmed away. The *embedded* block is then mounted on a slicing instrument called a *microtome* (Fig. 1-5), which is equipped with an advance mechanism that can be adjusted to provide given different thicknesses of sections, and an extremely sharp and strong knife that resembles an old-fashioned (cut-throat) razor. The fixation and embedding procedures render tissues hard enough to be sliced sufficiently thinly to provide sections thin enough for microscopy. As can be seen in Figure 1-5, the sections that come off the knife are attached to one another in the form of a ribbon, for the edge of each section adheres to that of the next. Individual sections can be separated with forceps when the ribbon is floated on water.

Section Thickness. For routine light microscopy, sec-

tions should not exceed 5 to 8 micrometers in thickness. A *micrometer* is 0.001 mm. (10^{-6}m.) and is represented by the symbol $\mu m.$ (in the older literature it was referred to as a *micron* and the symbol used for it was μ). When a thinner section is required, the tissue is embedded in plastic or epoxy resin instead of paraffin. *Thin sections* for light microscopy are usually cut to a thickness of *1* $\mu m.$ When sections are cut from frozen tissues (see below), rather than embedded tissues, they cannot be prepared so thinly and are therefore usually cut about *10* $\mu m.$ thick.

Staining and Mounting. To stain sections cut by the paraffin technic there is a further problem, for stains are used in the form of alcoholic or aqueous solutions. So, before a section can be stained, the paraffin permeating it has to be removed and replaced by water. For this, the section is made to adhere to a glass slide and dipped first in xylol to remove the paraffin and then in absolute alcohol to remove the xylol. Then it is passed through alcohols of decreasing strength and finally water. After drying, the section (still on the slide) is ready for staining with dyes in alcoholic or aqueous solution. Following staining, the section is passed through alcohols of increasing strength to absolute alcohol and then into xylol. Now it can be *mounted* in a mounting medium soluble in xylol.

Finally, a coverslip is pressed down firmly on the section; this makes a permanent preparation (Fig. 1-4, *bottom*).

Preparing Sections by the Frozen Section Technic. The alternative method of preparing frozen sections is very much faster than the paraffin technic and hence is commonly used when, during an operation, a surgeon wants a microscopic examination to be made, for example, on a lump or mass of tissue which might possibly be cancerous. A block of tissue is removed from the lump and a frozen section is immediately prepared by a histopathologist who, on examining the stained section with the microscope, can, in a few minutes or less, tell the surgeon the exact nature of the diseased tissue. This enables the surgeon to finish the operation in the manner most appropriate for whatever disease is present.

Nowadays frozen sections are commonly cut in a *cryostat*, an apparatus that cools the entire microtome and block of tissue so that the whole cutting operation can be done at a subzero temperature.

As well as being quick, frozen sections have other advantages for special kinds of studies. But on the whole, because ice crystals damage tissue, frozen sections are not as satisfactory for general use as sections prepared by the paraffin technic. Also, for good preservation and staining the tissue should be fixed before freezing; this is usually done if time permits.

Why Sections Are Stained

Because the various components of living cells all have similar optical densities, they all reduce the amplitude of light waves passing through them to much the same extent, without any appearing lighter or darker than others. It should be mentioned, however, that cell components can alter the phase of light passing through them to different extents, and this property is used in the *phase contrast microscope* for observing unstained tissues and living cells, as will be described later in this chapter. Nevertheless, the time-honored and usual way to obtain enough contrast between the different components of cells and tissues to be able to distinguish them with the ordinary light microscope is to use dyes, which in histology are called *stains*. Stains are often taken up to different extents by various cell and tissue components and may act in two general ways to provide contrast. First, when a component absorbs a great deal of stain, its optical density increases, reducing the amplitude of light waves passing through it. It thus appears darker than components that absorb only a little stain. Second, absorbed stain imparts its color to the light emerging from the component that absorbed it. In this second respect, staining for the light microscope (LM) has an advantage over staining for the electron microscope (EM), for what is called *staining* in electron microscopy can increase the electron density of tissue components but cannot provide any color.

We will here mention a matter of interest to medical students. As more and more dyes were produced, some seemed to have very specific effects, leading to the hope that it might one day be possible to find a dye that would combine with and kill disease-causing microorganisms in the body, without the dye harming the body cells. Through the exploration of this possibility two great medical discoveries were made and the modern science of *chemotherapy* was initiated.

When Paul Ehrlich (1854–1915) was a medical student, he devised a method by which tissues from victims of tuberculosis could be stained so as to specifically color the bacteria responsible for the disease. He was so fascinated by his discovery that a dye could be so specific in its action that he spent many years testing one dye after another in animals infected with different disease-causing organisms to see if he could find one that would kill the organisms and yet leave the body cells unharmed. After years of work he had found only one (trypan red), and this had an effect only on a type of trypanosome. However, he then read in a journal how arsenic could be prepared as a drug, and so he turned to experiments with arsenicals. Eventually he found one that he called Compound 606; this later became known as the "magic bullet" because it seemed to have a profound and selective effect on the spirochete that caused syphilis, and this became the universal drug by which the disease was treated until it was superseded by penicillin. In 1932, Domagk took up the same kind of search for therapeutic dyes. Among others, he tested the effects of a red dye called Prontosil on mice infected with a virulent strain of bacteria (streptococci) and found that the mice recovered. The dye was then tested on patients with streptococcal or other bacterial infections and was found to have what seemed to be a wonderful curative effect. It was soon found, however, that the effect of Prontosil was due not to selective uptake of the dye by bacteria. Instead, it is converted in the body into another compound called sulfonamide that does, however, selectively interfere with the metabolism of certain bacteria. The sulfonamides were the first of the "wonder" drugs of the 20th century.

In the early days of light microscopy, sections were stained with a single dye. Later, it became more usual to use two dyes, first one that would color some components and then another that would stain the remaining ones a contrasting color. Many combinations were tried, but the one that stood the test of time and is now used routinely for staining sections used by students of histology and histopathology is *hematoxylin* and *eosin* (*H and E*).

Hematoxylin, as extracted from its natural source (the brownish-red wood of the logwood tree, indigenous to Central America), is only a weak dye. When extracts of hematoxylin are "ripened," another dye called *hematein*, which is the staining agent in hematoxylin solutions, is formed. However, not even hematein stains very effectively unless it is used in combination with what is known as a *mordant* (L. *mordere*, to bite), which in this case is a metallic ion. When the Al^{+++} ion is used, the complex formed is referred to as *alum hematoxylin* and has a deep purple-blue color. There are several types of alum hematoxylin, many of which bear the names of their originators. Hematein can also combine with other metallic ions to produce other types of hematoxylin stains, but an alum hematoxylin is the one usually used in "H and E" staining. The second stain used in the synthetic dye, *eosin*, imparts a pink to red color, usually to those components that do not stain very well with hematoxylin. Because there is an art as well as a science in good staining, experience is necessary in achieving the best colors and depth of staining.

Basophilia and Acidophilia. In H and E sections, substances colored blue by hematoxylin are said to be *basophilic*, while those that stain pink to red with eosin are called *acidophilic*. It is useful to know what these terms mean, for they are used frequently in histology. *Basophilia* means an *affinity for a basic stain*, and, conversely, *acidophilia* means an *affinity for an acidic stain*.

Basic and acidic stains are, in fact, neutral salts, each with its own acidic and basic radical. In *basic* stains, the color resides in the *basic radical*, while the color in *acidic* stains is in the *acidic radical*.

Nowadays these stains are more often referred to in terms of the charge that their molecules bear. The colored basic radical of a basic stain bears a positive charge and would therefore behave as a cation during electrolysis. *Basic* stains are thus *cationic* stains, and, conversely, *acidic* stains are often referred to as *anionic* stains. The color in the basic stain *alum hematoxylin* lies in the cationic complex of hematein with Al^{+++} ions of the mordant used (which have a positive charge). The color in *eosin*, on the other hand, resides in its anionic radical (which bears a negative charge).

Whether tissue components stain with basic or acidic stains depends on whether they bear enough charged sites to bind color-containing dye radicals of the opposite charge. Thus basophilic components have enough anionic (negative) charges to bind the colored cations of alum hematoxylin, while acidophilic components have sufficient cationic (positive) charges to bind the colored anions of eosin.

The Staining of Cells With Hematoxylin. In cells stained with H and E, certain nuclear components are stained with hematoxylin and hence are blue to purple in color. Their affinity for hematoxylin is due to their content of nucleic acids, of which there are two kinds, deoxyribonucleic acid (DNA) and ribonucleic acid (RNA). Both will be discussed in detail in Chapters 2 and 3. The two components of the nucleus that stain blue are the chromatin and the nucleoli. The *chromatin* usually appears as granules in the nuclear sap. The nuclear membrane also appears to stain, but this is due to the chromatin adhering to its inner surface, for, as can be seen in Figure 4-2 (on p. 86), if before staining the section is treated with the enzyme DNAase (which degrades DNA), there is no staining associated with the nuclear membrane. Second, the *nucleoli* also stain blue. As can be seen from Figure 4-2, part of their staining is due to DNA, for their staining also is reduced by pretreatment with DNAase. Some staining, however, is due to RNA (which, of course, is not removed by DNAase).

The cytoplasm of cells may also contain clumps of blue-staining material. As may be seen in Figure 4-2, these still stain after DNAase treatment, showing that they contain RNA. The functions of the DNA and RNA in their respective sites will constitute a main topic of the chapters that immediately follow.

The Staining of Cells With Eosin. In certain cells, to be described later, there are specific cytoplasmic granules that stain vividly with eosin. In most types of cells, however, it is structural proteins that stain pink to red. The extent to which such proteins are stained is affected somewhat by the pH of the solution in which they are stained. This is because under different physiological conditions proteins can act either as acids or bases in the body, thereby neutralizing excess base or acid; thus they are said to be *amphoteric* (Gr. *ampho*, both). So when the body's pH tends to become alkaline, proteins compensate for this by acting as acids and they restore the pH to neutral. Conversely, when the pH swings to the acid side, proteins act as bases and thereby restore the pH balance. Thus proteins constitute one of the buffer systems that maintain a neutral pH in the body. This also means that as far as staining is concerned, the number of anionic or cationic sites in protein molecules available to react with cationic or anionic stains will change with pH. When, for example, the pH of the staining solution is on the acid side, more cationic sites are available to bind the anionic stain, eosin. If, on the other hand, the staining solution is on the alkaline side, more anionic sites become available to bind cationic dyes. Furthermore, individual proteins can vary with regard to the number of sites available at any given pH to absorb such stains. For example, at the pH at which staining is usually done, there are sufficient cationic sites in the proteins of a liver cell to bind enough eosin to color the cytoplasm deep pink and to color the protein in red blood cells red. The cytoplasm of some other kinds of cells, however, is only colored a very light pink unless staining is done at a more acid pH.

Other Stains and Histochemistry. The chemical basis of staining is a complex subject and the foregoing account has been presented for the student not yet familiar with biochemistry. It should be stressed that not all staining methods depend on the binding of charged dye molecules to sites of opposite charge.

Known chemical reactions can sometimes be used to investigate the chemical nature of tissue components. In general either a colored product or an increase in optical density, indicating the presence of a specific chemical group, is generated at reacting sites. The science of such staining is called *histochemistry*, and a chemical reaction on which such staining is based is termed a *histochemical reaction*. Examples of other histochemical staining methods will be encountered from time to time throughout this textbook in places where they have contributed valuable information about cells and tissues.

Some Theoretical Considerations About the Light Microscope

The intelligent use of the light microscope is so important in histology that it is essential at the outset to have some idea of what the microscope can and cannot do. First, of course, it can make things appear larger. The compound microscope is, in effect, a two-stage magnifying system in which the specimen is magnified first by an elaborate lens system in the *objective* and then again by a second lens in the *ocular* (*eyepiece*). The position of these two optical parts on the microscope may be seen in Figure 1-6. The total magnification of the instrument is simply the product of the magnifications due to the objective and ocular, respectively.

The second feature of the compound microscope is that it enables its user to see more detail. The importance of this property can hardly be overemphasized, for unless clarity of detail stays hand-in-hand with an increase in size, the image becomes increasingly blurred and indistinct. Hence we must distinguish between the extent to which the size of an object appears increased in the image, which is called *magnification*, and the extent to which the details in the object are faithfully reproduced in the image, which is termed *resolution*. Resolution is the degree of separation that can be seen between adjacent points (details) in the specimen. The smaller the distance that can be distinguished between such points, the more detail there is in the image. It is likely that the reader has already encountered a problem of resolution in a lecture room while taking notes when an instructor who illustrates his lectures with diagrams draws two dots too close together on the blackboard. Although such dots can be seen clearly as separate entities by the students sitting in the front rows, the instructor is inclined to forget that those who sit at the back of the room will see them as only a single dot. At close range, points appear as different entities to the unaided eye only if they are separated by a distance of 0.2 mm. (200 μm.) or more; but if a good light microscope is used, points as close as 0.25 μm. can be distinguished from one another. This distance is the smallest that can be detected between any two details in an object using a light microscope and represents its *limit of resolution*. The fidelity with which a microscope can reproduce in its image the details present in a specimen is limited, because resolution is a function of the wavelength of the energy (light) employed for illumination. The only way around this particular limitation is to employ energy of shorter wavelength which, as we shall see, can be achieved if a stream of electrons is used in place of light rays.

The other optical parameter that determines how detailed the image will be is the proportion of the potential visual detail from the specimen that is able to enter the objective lens. Optically dense details in the specimen

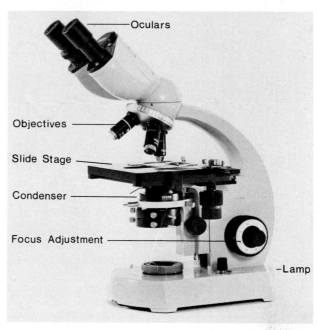

Fig. 1-6. A light microscope, showing its component parts. (Courtesy of Carl Zeiss Co.)

reduce the amplitude of all the light waves extending from them in every direction. However, not all of this potential visual information can be used to form the image, for only the light rays entering the optical pathway of the microscope can be used in building the image. The proportion of light rays put to good use in forming image details is determined by the aperture size of the objective lens, which depends on the angle of the cone of light rays accepted by the objective from the condenser. The wider the angle of this cone, the greater the proportion of potential detail reproduced in the image. The aperture size (fraction of wavefront admitted) is expressed as the *numerical aperture (NA)* of the lens* and its value is engraved on each objective, beside the magnification. Not only detail, but also the brightness of the image depends on NA. For maximum resolution and adequate illumination at any given magnification, it is important that the NA of the condenser lens be matched as closely as possible with the

---

*The *numerical aperture (NA)* of a lens is calculated from its *half angle of aperture,* that is, the angle between its optical axis and the most inclined rays of light it can accept. The angle is expressed as its sine value (to make it numerical) and multiplied by the refractive index of the medium (air or oil) between the specimen and the objective. The product gives the NA of the lens. The resolution that can be attained with an objective is directly proportional to the wavelength of the light used for illumination and inversely proportional to the NA of the objective lens. The brightness of the field is directly proportional to the square of the NA.

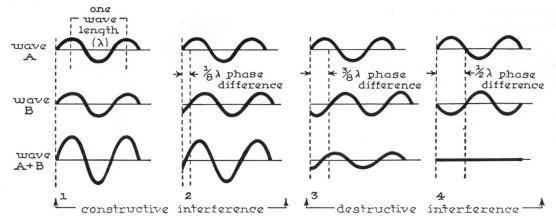

Fig. 1-7. Diagram showing how light waves can interfere with one another to increase or decrease the amplitude of the resultant waves.

NA of the objective. It turns out in practice that no more detail can be seen if the total magnification exceeds 1,000 × the NA of the objective. The maximum useful magnification of the LM is about 1,400 ×.

The Phase Contrast Microscope

As already noted, the components of cells are all of such similar optical density that, unless stained, the various components do not affect the amplitude of light passing through them sufficiently to allow them to be distinguished from one another with the ordinary light microscope. However, the various cell components do alter the phase of the light waves passing through them to different extents, but phase differences in light reaching the eye cannot be distinguished from one another. It is well known that light waves, like water waves, can interfere with each other so as to increase or decrease the amplitude of the resultant waves, as shown in Figure 1-7. Hence, if phase differences were converted into differences of amplitude, different cell components could be distinguished from one another in the microscope without any need for staining, enabling cells to be observed while still living. This is accomplished in both the *phase contrast microscope* and the *interference microscope*. In both types of instrument it is necessary to use two sets of waves, and these are combined with one another to create differences in amplitude in the light rays reaching the eye from different cell components. This is done in the phase contrast microscope (the more commonly used instrument) by using two sets of light waves, those of the light incident to the specimen and those diffracted by the specimen. These two sets of waves are recombined in the objective, where they interfere with each other to dif-

ferent extents so that the amplitude of light from the various cell components is different, and hence they are seen by the eye as light or dark objects, as may be seen in Figure 5-10.

General Advice on Looking at Sections

Before placing a section on the stage of the microscope, get in a comfortable position. Then hold the section up to the light and examine it with the unaided eye. First you will discover the side of the slide on which the coverslip is mounted and hence avoid placing the slide upside down on the stage. Second, you will notice if the coverslip is dirty or has any immersion oil on it and be able to clean it. Third, if the source of the section is unknown as, for example, in a practical examination, you often get a good hint about the structure or organ it was prepared from, especially when sections of many different tissues and organs have been studied.

Next, resist the temptation to use the greatest magnification as soon as possible. A famous histopathologist is said to have removed all the high-power objectives from the microscopes of his graduate students so that they would fully appreciate the great value of the low-power objective in diagnosing pathological conditions. One reason for using the lowest possible magnification is that it discloses a large area of the section so that, by moving the slide, it is possible to examine every part of the section. Often the most important clue about the part of the body the section was taken from (of importance in practical examinations even in normal histology), or the nature of a disease process (important in diagnostic histopathology) will be found in only one small place in the section, and this could easily be missed unless the whole section is initially investigated in a thorough manner with the lowest-power objective. Moreover, this preliminary inspection with the low-power objective often reveals the best area for further examination at higher magnification. Occasionally it is advantageous to use even less magnification than is obtainable with the lowest power objective, in order to bridge the gap between what can be seen with the unaided eye and the low-power appearance of a particular section. This can be achieved by using an ocular, carefully removed from the microscope and inverted, as a simple magnifying glass.

The High-Power Objective. There should be no problem in swinging the high-power objective into place to examine the area centered with the low-power objective. But if the high-power objective cannot be focused, the chances are that the slide is upside down and hence the slice of tissue is too far away to be focused under high power.

The Oil-Immersion Objective. This objective must approach the coverslip so closely that there is danger of its hitting the coverslip and breaking either the coverslip or the objective in focusing.

A way of focusing the oil-immersion objective safely is this: after centering the particular area to be examined with the high-power objective, the stage of the microscope is lowered with the coarse adjustment and the oil-immersion objective is swung into place. A small drop of oil is then applied to the slide over the center of the condenser. Watching the bottom of the oil-immersion objective from the side of the microscope, the stage is raised until the objective just enters the drop of oil. In this position, the oil-immersion lens is still *above* the plane of focus. Looking down the microscope, the stage is then slowly raised with the fine adjustment until the field comes into focus. If it does not come into focus within 1 or 2 turns of the fine adjustment, it is best to stop and question whether something might have gone wrong. Two possibilities should be considered: there may be no stained part of the section under the very small area visible with the oil-immersion objective, or the objective may already be *below* the level at which it is in focus. If some color can be seen on looking down the microscope, the first possibility can be ruled out, and if the color becomes better defined with further focusing, the chances are that the objective lens is still *above* the plane of focus and that the stage can be safely raised a bit farther. But if there is any reason to doubt this, the stage should be lowered, the oil wiped from the objective and the slide, the area centered again with the high-power objective, and the procedure repeated. It is always advisable to *proceed very cautiously* until experience has been gained.

Cleaning the Optical Parts. If the field under view seems irregularly clouded or covered with specks, (*1*) the coverslip of the section may be dirty, (*2*) the objective lens may have become smeared with oil, (*3*) the oculars

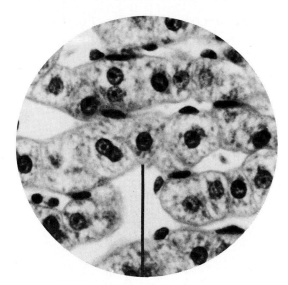

Fig. 1-8. A pointer in the eyepiece can be used to indicate a particular structure in the section under view.

may be dirty, or (*4*) the top lens of the condenser may be dirty. If the cloudy appearance or specks move when an ocular is turned, the trouble is a dirty ocular lens.

The top lens of an ocular can be cleaned by breathing on it and polishing it very gently with lens paper. However, specks of dirt often remain and should be blown off with a blast of dry air, such as that from a rubber bulb kept for this purpose. Any oil on a coverslip or objective lens can be wiped off gently with a tissue, using a trace of xylol.

Fitting a Pointer. The best way for an instructor to identify or demonstrate something in a section to a student is to use a pointer fitted into one of the oculars, as may be seen in Figure 1-8. In the type of ocular supplied with older microscopes, there was a diaphragm to which a short piece of hair could be cemented (Fig. 1-9). However, oculars in some of today's microscopes lack such a diaphragm. If yours are of the new type, it will help to have an ocular of the older type fitted with a pointer and use that instead, in order to be able to point to particular things in sections.

THE INTERPRETATION OF WHAT IS SEEN IN SECTIONS

There are two major difficulties in trying to interpret the appearance of sections. First, a section is obviously only one slice and a single slice is not really enough to enable an observer to visualize the sort of structure from which it was cut. In fact, it can even be quite misleading. Suppose, for instance, each person in a group of people

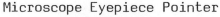

Microscope Eyepiece Pointer

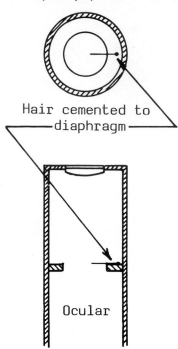

Hair cemented to
diaphragm

Ocular

Fig. 1-9. If the top lens mount is unscrewed from an eyepiece, it will appear as in the upper picture, and a hair can be cemented to the diaphragm with a small drop of mountant. The lower diagram shows the position of the hair in the eyepiece.

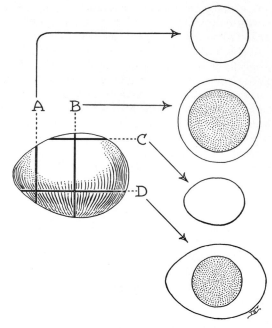

Fig. 1-10. Diagram showing how sections cut through an object in different planes may give different impressions about its structure. A hard-boiled egg is shown at the *left*. Note how cross sections cut at A and B would be different from one another and differ from longitudinal sections cut at C and D.

that had never before seen an egg was individually shown one different slice of a hard-boiled egg, as depicted in Figure 1-10. Would not each person have a rather different concept about the structure of an entire egg? Because of this difficulty of interpreting single sections, much time and effort has been devoted by histologists in establishing the microscopic structure of the various parts of the body. This was commonly done by making *reconstructions* of the part from sections, which is the counterpart of fitting the slices of an egg together again. It required sectioning of the whole structure. Each consecutive (*serial*) section was numbered, stained and projected so that a wax or plastic replica of correct thickness (and highly magnified) could be made. The replicas were then all fitted together in the right sequence so as to constitute a large scale model, in which the structure of parts of interest could be seen with the unaided eye. Cuts could even be made into the model to facilitate observation of its internal arrangements.

The second problem of interpretation is how to recognize various structures, whose gross anatomical shapes are known, from their appearance in single sections. We shall now give some examples.

Tubes

We know that the human body abounds in tubes of different kinds and sizes. Blood vessels are tubular and they are seen almost everywhere. In the lungs there are air tubes, and in many organs there are also tubes (called *ducts*) that carry secretions from one place to another. Lymph is carried along in tubes. The chief difficulty in recognizing tubes is that in any given section they may have been cut longitudinally, obliquely, or in cross section. Figure 1-11 shows how portions of a straight tube in a section can vary in appearance depending on how the tube was cut. The appearance of certain slices through a curving tube in a given section may be even more puzzling (Fig. 1-12).

Partitions

Many organs abound in partitions (termed *septa*, from L. *saeptum*, wall) that divide the organ into numerous smaller areas. Although such areas may all be of the same general size, they may not appear to be so in a section, as can be demonstrated by slicing an orange in various planes (Fig. 1-13).

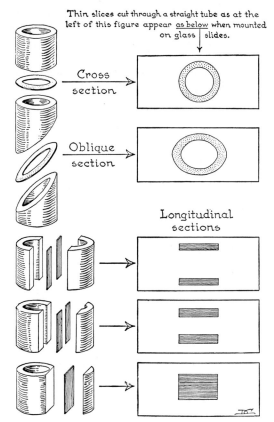

Fig. 1-11. Diagram showing how sections cut through straight tubes in different planes present different appearances. Note that it is even possible to cut a longitudinal section of a tube without having its lumen in the section.

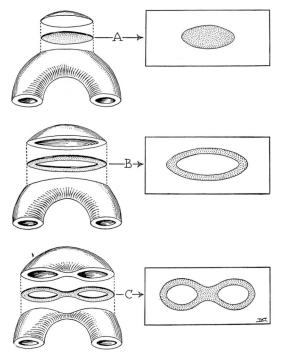

Fig. 1-12. Diagram showing the different appearances of sections cut through a curved tube at different levels.

Nerves

Nerves are often seen in sections and these, too, may be cut in various planes. Since they are much like cables containing many insulated wires, recalling the familiar appearances of cables, as seen by any amateur electrician who has cut them at different angles, will help in interpreting the different appearances of nerves cut in various planes (Fig. 1-14).

Cords

If in a section an observer were to see a row of cells stretching across the field of view, in the manner depicted in the top part of Figure 1-15, he might assume that it is a single row, or cord, of cells. But for all practical purposes what can be seen in a section has only negligible depth, and so the possibility exists that this might be just one slice through a whole plate of cells, as depicted in the bottom part of Figure 1-15, rather than just a single cord of

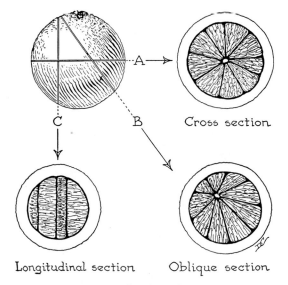

Fig. 1-13. Diagram showing the different appearances presented by sections cut in different planes through an object that contains partitions (an orange).

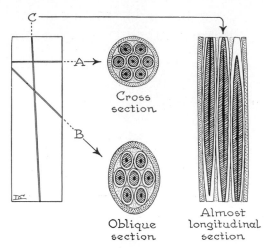

Fig. 1-14. Diagram showing how the appearance of sections cut through an electrical cable containing many insulated wires differs according to the plane in which the section is cut.

cells. The lesson to be learned here is that one always has to try to visualize what could have been present above and below the plane of section before arriving at any conclusion. Several of the structures we shall encounter in histology were mistakenly called cords for the very reason that people forgot to think in three dimensions.

The Sizes of Cells and Nuclei

It is very easy indeed to be misled by the apparent size of cells and nuclei in sections. To go back to our example

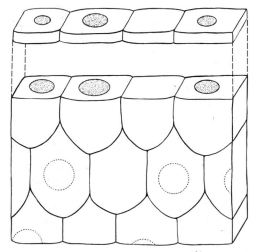

Fig. 1-15. Diagram showing how what at first glance might seem to be a row or cord of cells (as seen at the *top* of the diagram) could actually be a slice through an entire plate of cells (as seen at the *bottom*).

of the hard-boiled egg, it can be seen from Figure 1-10 that it is possible to obtain slices (A and C) that do not disclose its yolk. Similarly, sections cut at a thickness of about 7 μm. through cells with a diameter of about 15 μm. need not disclose their nuclei (Fig. 1-15). When the section does include the nucleus of a cell, it will often appear smaller than it really is, as can also be seen in Figure 1-15. Furthermore, the cell itself may also appear smaller than it really is, depending on which part of the cell is present in the section. Hence the cells in a section may seem to vary considerably in size when, in fact, they may be quite uniform in size.

Artifacts

An *artifact* (L. *ars*, art; *factum*, made) is something artificial. In histology, this term is used for unwanted features in sections that are the result of accident or poor technique. Every step in the preparation of a section provides a further opportunity for distorting the appearance of tissues. Since artifacts are sometimes seen in sections studied in the laboratory, it is helpful to learn how to recognize common ones now in order to disregard them later. The inexperienced student sometimes spends a lot of time worrying about a feature in a slide about which he has received no instruction, only to find out later that this feature does not exist in living tissue at all. We shall mention here a few common artifacts.

Postmortem Degeneration. Although this is the commonest cause of poor quality in sections, postmortem degeneration is, strictly speaking, not a true artifact. This is because, instead of being something inflicted on the tissue by human hands, it is the result of something's not being done properly. The importance of rapid and thorough fixation has already been emphasized. Unless tissues are fixed as soon as they are obtained, they suffer a prolonged period of *anoxia* (Gr. *an*, without) meaning without oxygen and this, as we shall see in Chapter 5 (p. 138), causes hydrolytic enzymes to be released from cytoplasmic vesicles known as lysosomes. The hydrolytic enzymes commence to literally digest the cells, so that details are lacking when seen under the microscope.

Shrinkage. The various reagents used in preparing sections, including hot paraffin, often cause shrinkage of tissues. As a result, tissues that lie attached in life may become pulled away from each other, leaving empty spaces, as indicated by the arrows in Figure 1-16A. This is a very common artifact, and the student should be forewarned that, with the exception of such true anatomical spaces as the peritoneum or pleural cavity, which are filled with tissue fluid, there are no such seemingly "empty" spaces in the living body.

Precipitate. Numerous particles of precipitate are fre-

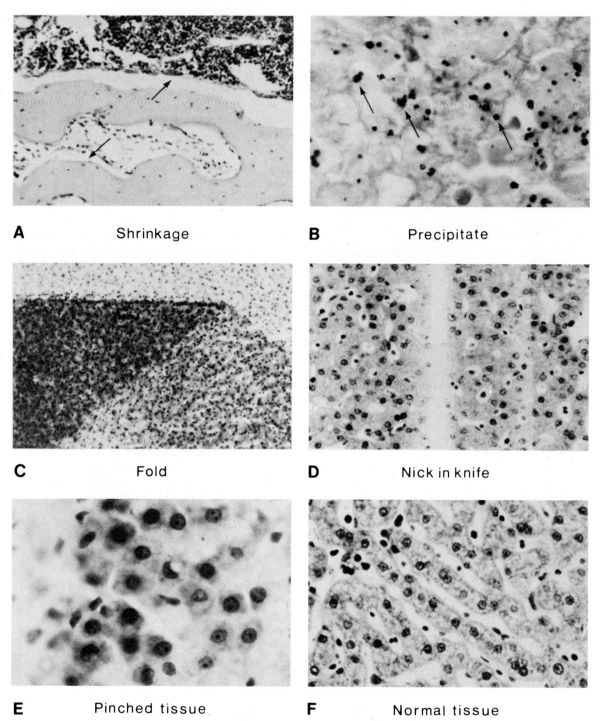

A   Shrinkage

B   Precipitate

C   Fold

D   Nick in knife

E   Pinched tissue

F   Normal tissue

Fig. 1-16. Photomicrographs illustrating some common kinds of artifacts (*A* to *E*) and the appearance of normal tissue (*F*). For details, *see* text. Note that the cells of pinched liver tissue (*E*) appear distorted compared with the cells of normal liver tissue (*F*). (Courtesy of B. Smith)

quently seen (Fig. 1-16B) in tissues fixed in formaldehyde solutions that are poorly buffered and therefore acidic. Where acidic formalin reacts with the red pigment *hemoglobin* of erythrocytes (or *myoglobin* in muscle cells), a brown granular pigment is also formed, called *formalin pigment*. These artifacts increase with the time the tissue is left in formaldehyde. Other fixatives, too, will form precipitates unless properly removed.

Precipitation can also occur during certain staining procedures, especially in the use of blood stains (page 261). It can be avoided by not allowing the stain to become too concentrated or dried out during staining.

Folds and Wrinkles. Paraffin sections are so thin that it is not unusual for them to become somewhat wrinkled or folded when prepared and sometimes these wrinkles or folds cannot be smoothed out entirely when the section is being mounted on a slide. They then appear in a section as shown in Figure 1-16C.

Nicks in the Knife. Microscopic nicks in the microtome knife cause a characteristic defect in sections. As the knife sweeps across a paraffin block in a straight plane, any nick in it creates a defect in the section that appears as a straight line across it (Fig. 1-16D). Thus any defect seen as a straight line passing across a section is likely to be an artifact of this type.

Rough Handling of Fresh Tissue. Another type of artifact often seen in sections, which may lead to the incorrect surmise that the tissue under view has been the site of some pathological change, is produced by rough handling of tissue as it is being cut from the body. Commonly, in obtaining tissue, forceps are used to hold the piece that is being cut away; sometimes the cutting is done with scissors (instead of a very sharp knife), and dull ones at that. The pinching caused by holding living tissue firmly with forceps and cutting it with dull scissors profoundly affects the appearance it presents in stained sections. This appearance is illustrated in Figure 1-16E. Figure 1-16F shows how the tissue would have appeared normally had it not been mistreated.

THE IDENTIFICATION OF CELLS IN H AND E SECTIONS

Choosing a Suitable Section

It is not as easy as might be thought for a beginner to identify cells in sections from a verbal description of their appearance. Sections from various parts of the body contain cells of different shapes, sizes, and appearances. Some have a great deal of cytoplasm while others seem to have hardly any. In some tissues the cells may vary greatly in shape. Furthermore, they may be confused very easily with intercellular substances or structures that

are only easy to identify after one has learned about their histological structure (and this, of course, comes after one has learned how to identify cells). The easiest way for a beginner to identify and learn the general appearance of cells in an H and E section is to choose a section of some organ composed chiefly of cells that are mostly of the same kind and in the same type of arrangement. This is the state of affairs in the liver, which is why we suggest that an H and E section of liver is eminently suitable for a beginner to commence studying.

Comparing What Is Seen With the Microscope With Illustrations

In order to learn how to recognize cells (or any other microscopic structures) in sections, it helps if the student is able to compare what is seen down the microscope with a labeled illustration of the material being studied. Since most photomicrographs of sections and all electron micrographs are in black and white and since colored sections are seen with the microscope, it is useful to realize that in black and white photomicrographs of H and E sections, the degree of *blackness* observed is generally an indication of the depth of staining with *hematoxylin*, while the *gray* tones are due either to staining with *eosin* or to *lighter* staining with *hematoxylin*.

The Size of Cells in Relation to the Field of View

How large might a comma on this page appear in the field of a microscope equipped with a 10× objective and a 10× eyepiece? As can be seen in Figure 1-17, a comma would just about stretch across the whole field. The printed comma is about 1.5 mm. long, so the field seen would have a diameter of about 1.5 millimeters. For light microscopy the unit of measurement usually used is the *micrometer* which, as previously mentioned, is 10^{-6} meter and given the symbol μm. A comma is thus 1500 μm. long. The magnifications and fields of view obtained with commonly used objectives are given in the following table.

Table 1-1. Magnification and Field of View in Low-Power, High-Power, and Oil-Immersion Microscopy

	Eye-piece	Objective	Magni-fication	Diameter of Area Under View
Low-power	10×	10×	100×	1,500 μm.
High-Power	10×	40×	400×	375μm.
Oil Immersion	10×	100×	1,000×	150μm.

If we now wished to distinguish a single liver cell in a section of liver, and we knew that each cell had a diameter of about 15 μm., we would expect that it would take about 100 of them to stretch across a field of view that was 1,500 μm. wide. At this magnification, individual cells are hard to distinguish, but their general arrangement can be seen to advantage (Fig. 1-18A). With the high-power objective it would take a row of about 25 cells to cross the field (Fig. 1-18B) and under oil-immersion there would be about 10 (Fig. 1-18C). Fortunately, in sections liver cells do commonly appear to be arranged in rows and these rows are separated from one another by blood spaces (empty looking spaces in Fig. 1-18, that need not concern us here).

We should now try to decide what portions of the rows seen under high-power (Fig. 1-18B) and oil-immersion objectives (Fig. 1-18C) would correspond to individual cells. This is not particularly easy as the cell borders between neighboring liver cells are seldom distinct; some borders are indicated by arrows in Figure 1-18B and C.

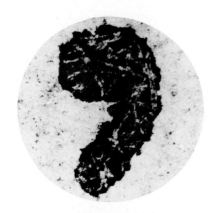

Fig. 1-17. Photomicrograph ($\times$ 100) of a printed comma, as seen with a microscope equipped with a 10$\times$ objective and a 10$\times$ eyepiece. Note that the comma, which is almost 1.5 mm. long, stretches across the entire field of view; hence the field seen at 100$\times$ magnification is about 1.5 mm. (1,500 μm.) in diameter.

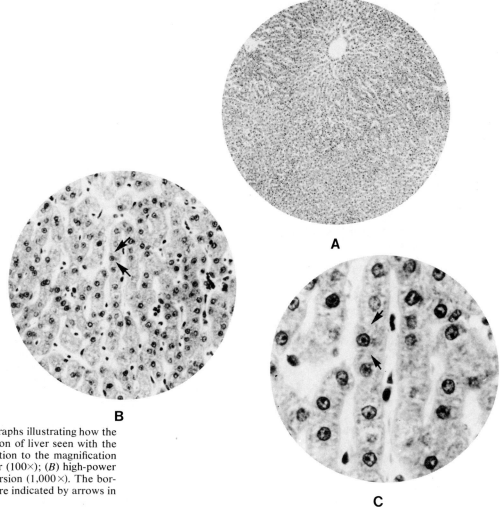

Fig. 1-18. Photomicrographs illustrating how the size of the area of a section of liver seen with the microscope varies in relation to the magnification employed. (*A*) Low-power (100$\times$); (*B*) high-power (400$\times$); and (*C*) oil-immersion (1,000$\times$). The borders of a single liver cell are indicated by arrows in (*B*) and (*C*).

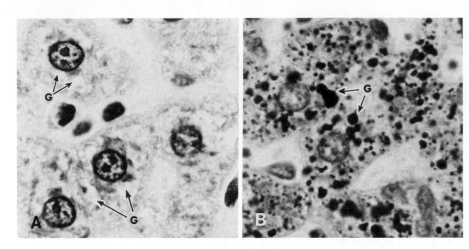

Fig. 1-19. Photomicrographs of sections of the liver of a well-fed rat. (*A*) An H and E section, in which the sites of glycogen in the cytoplasm appear as ragged-edged, clear areas (G). (*B*) A similar section stained by the PAS technic, which stains glycogen (G) a magenta color.

Furthermore, the beginner sometimes mistakes nuclei for whole cells. The nucleus of each cell stains darkly and one criterion that can be used in judging the size of a cell is that in liver cells the diameter of the nucleus is somewhat less than half the diameter of the cell it occupies. Within many nuclei, nucleoli and chromatin granules can be discerned. The proteins in the cytoplasm stain pink with eosin, and there are also patches of basophilic material, which appear slightly blue when stained with hematoxylin (see Plate 1-1, *top left*). The cytoplasm has an uneven appearance due to what seem to be empty spaces. Dark, ovoid nuclei seen occasionally along the sides of the rows of liver cells belong to cells lining the blood spaces between the rows.

Why the Cytoplasm of Liver Cells May Contain Empty Spaces

Liver cells play a very important role in regulating the level of sugar in the blood. Sugars are absorbed from the intestine, not at a constant rate but in relation to meals, and so it might be thought that the level of the blood sugar would go up just after meals and go down between meals. However, the liver cells regulate the level of the sugar in the blood by removing it when it goes up and storing it in their cytoplasm as a polysaccharide called *glycogen* which, like starch, is composed of a large number of interconnected glucose residues. Glycogen is *not stained* with either hematoxylin or eosin, so translucent deposits of it in the cytoplasm of a cell appear as irregularly shaped, ragged, seemingly empty spaces in the cytoplasm (see Plate 1-1, *left,* and G in Fig. 1-19A).

Spaces indicating the presence of glycogen are seen only in some livers. The reason for this is that if the liver tissue was taken (as often happens) from a person who

died after a lengthy illness in which his appetite had failed, his liver cells would not have been storing glycogen. However, if liver tissue was obtained surgically from a healthy person shortly after eating a hearty meal, the cells of his liver may be so riddled with seemingly empty spaces that the student hospital pathologist, who is accustomed to seeing the liver cells of people who have died after lengthy illnesses, can sometimes scarcely recognize it as liver. The liver cells in Plate 1-1 and Figure 1-19 were taken from a healthy, well-fed laboratory animal.

Example of a Histochemical Reaction

The Staining of Glycogen by the Periodic Acid-Schiff Technic. Glycogen is not very soluble in water; hence it is not readily dissolved in the preparation of a stained section. However, unless fixation is prompt, hydrolytic enzymes begin to operate in cells after death and rapidly convert glycogen to glucose, which, of course, is soluble and washed out as the section is prepared. Moreover, if fixation is less than perfect, the fixative, in penetrating cells slowly from one side to the other, coagulates protein progressively from one side of the cell to the other, and in doing so pushes the glycogen ahead of it to some extent; as a result, the glycogen is displaced toward one side of each cell, which position for it is, of course, abnormal.

The *periodic acid-Schiff (PAS) technic* is a two-step procedure based on the application to histology of two reactions well known to chemists. *Periodic acid* reacts with *1,2-glycol groups* (-CHOH-CHOH-), which occur in the glucose residues linked together in glycogen. On treating sections containing glycogen with periodic acid, both members of each glycol group yield an *aldehyde group* (-CHO), so that the polysaccharide chain of glycogen becomes converted into a polyaldehyde chain. The second step is to treat the sections with a well-known reagent for aldehydes; this is a dye known as *basic fuchsin*, which can be bleached with *sulfurous acid*, when it is then known as the *Schiff reagent*. Aldehydes combine with the bleached dye to produce a *magenta-* or *purple-*colored complex (such as that seen at the sites of glycogen in Plate 1-1, *top right* and Fig 1-19B), and this can readily be seen in the microscope. Accordingly, it is said that glycogen is a PAS-positive substance.

Glycogen is readily broken down by α-amylase, an enzyme present in saliva, and after treatment with this enzyme it can be washed out of sections. Hence when a PAS-positive substance is found in a cell, it is customary to incubate another unstained section in a solution of purified alpha amylase (or in saliva, which is rich in this amylase) to extract glycogen and then stain it by the PAS method. Disappearance of the purple-staining material proves that the material was glycogen.

The Staining of Fat. Another kind of seemingly empty space can be seen in the cytoplasm of the cells of some livers. Such spaces differ from those of glycogen by being round and having sharp edges (Fig. 1-20) instead of having irregular shapes and fuzzy edges. Round empty spaces are left by the dissolution of stored droplets of fat by the reagents employed in making paraffin sections. If the cells of liver contain a great many of these round holes or a single large one, as in Figure 1-20, the person is said to have a *fatty liver*. Commonly this condition is seen in individuals who have, for a lengthy period, omitted nourishing food from their diets in favor of considerable amounts of alcohol.

Since the fat in liver cells dissolves away during preparation of a paraffin section, frozen sections are used to demonstrate fat with such special stains as Scharlach R or Sudan III (compare bottom two illustrations in Plate 1-1).

The Use of Special Technics While many other special technics are also employed in studying histology, these are more meaningful to the student if they are described in connection with the particular information that their use has yielded. Special technics will therefore be described in this textbook where they are most appropriate, but anyone wishing information about particular technics at this point will find them in the Index.

ELECTRON MICROSCOPY

The Search for Greater Magnification

The usefulness of the light microscope, as already mentioned, is limited by the wavelength of visible light. Its maximum resolving power is about *0.2 μm*. A remarkable advance in microscopy was made in the 1920s when it

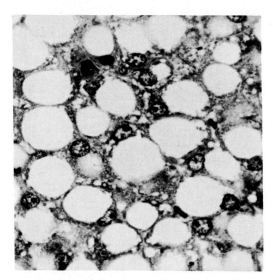

Fig. 1-20. Photomicrograph of a section of fatty liver (from a choline-deficient rat). The liver cells are distended with fat. Note the round, sharp edges of the spaces left by the large fat droplets in these cells being dissolved away during processing. (Hartroft, W. S.: Anat. Rec., *106*:61)

was discovered that suitably shaped electromagnetic fields could be used like lenses to shape and focus beams of electrons. Moreover, at high voltages a stream of electrons has a very short wavelength and is therefore capable of giving very much better resolution than visible light. These principles were incorporated into the design of a microscope that uses electrons in place of light and which now achieves a resolution approaching *0.2 nm*. in the best instruments available today.

The Development of the Electron Microscope. The first electron microscope was built in 1931 by Knoll and Ruska in Germany, and by 1933 they had made one that had a resolving power greater than the LM. The first EM built in North America (1932) was constructed in the Department of Physics at the University of Toronto by Prebus, Hillier, and Burton. Soon afterward commercial instruments became available and were steadily improved. But many years elapsed before it became possible to study tissue sections with this new instrument. It was not until around 1950 that means were evolved for preparing sections thin enough and otherwise suitable. Since then the stream of information that has flowed from EM studies of cells has opened up a new world of knowledge about the detailed structure of cells and tissues. Although the design of the EM need not be considered in great depth here, brief mention of the types of instruments used for biological work is in order so that the preparation and interpretation of electron micrographs may be understood.

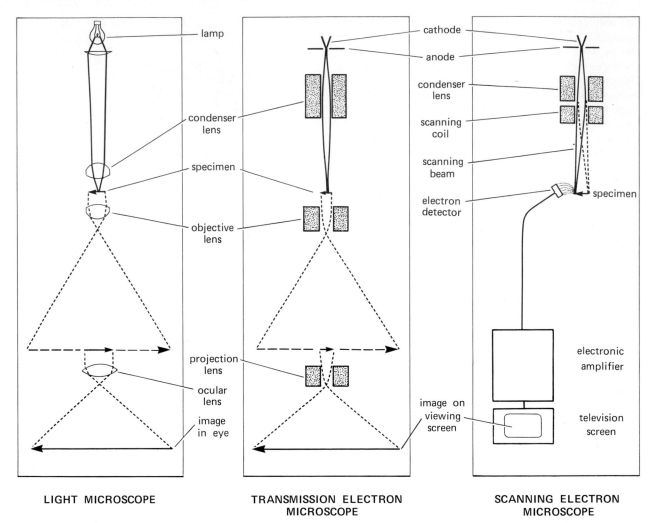

Fig. 1-21. Diagram comparing the optical paths of the light microscope (*left*), transmission electron microscope (*middle*), and scanning electron microscope (*right*).

A Comparison of the Light and Electron Microscope

The optical path of the EM is easily understood if it is compared with that of the LM. In the type of EM routinely employed for the study of tissues, the electron beam is used much like a beam of light and passes *right through* many parts of the specimen. This particular kind of EM is therefore called a *transmission electron microscope* and we shall describe the design and operation of this type of EM first. However, in order to compare its optical path with the LM, it is necessary first to consider how an image is produced in the LM.

The optics of the LM are shown on the left side of Figure 1-21 but, in order to compare them easily with those of the EM, the optical path of the LM is drawn upside down.

In the LM, light is focused with a *condenser lens* onto the object—for example, a stained specimen. The light passing through the object enters the *objective lens*, which brings an image of the object into focus somewhere between the objective lens and the *ocular lens;* the latter then further magnifies this image. Alternatively, the ocular lens can be used to bring the enlarged image into focus on *photographic film* placed at the site indicated by the bottom arrow (Fig. 1-21, *left*), so as to produce a *photomicrograph.*

The optics of the *transmission EM* are illustrated in the middle of Figure 1-21. The path of the electrons is influenced by electromagnetic fields just as light is influenced by glass lenses. The strength of these fields can be varied by changing the amount of current passing through the coils of wire in the electromagnetic lenses (stippled in Fig. 1-21). The whole instrument (Fig. 1-22) is, in essence, a cathode-ray tube in which a vacuum must be maintained by continuous pumping, for electrons can travel only for very short distances in air. From the electrically heated *cathode,* which is a V-shaped tungsten filament, electrons are emitted and accelerated toward the *anode* (usually by a potential difference of 50 to 100 kilovolts). The anode has an aperture so that the stream of electrons can pass through it and be focused by the *condenser lens* and directed at the specimen, which is generally a specially prepared and extremely thin slice of tissue.

As the electrons pass through the specimen, some are scattered out of the beam by the electron-dense parts of the specimen. Those electrons that are scattered by the specimen are removed from the beam by the blocking action of a very fine *aperture* (not shown on the diagram) positioned just above the objective lens. The role of this aperture (which is usually about 30 μm. in diameter) is to provide more contrast in the image. The remaining electrons (those not scattered by electron-dense parts of the specimen) are focused by the *objective lens,* and an enlarged image of the specimen is thereby obtained. This image is enlarged further, first by a lens known as an *intermediate lens* (not shown in diagram) and then by a *projection lens;* the latter projects the image onto a *fluorescent screen,* or *photographic film* for taking *electron micrographs.* The microscope is used as follows.

Very thin sections of tissue are placed in the specimen holder and inserted into the microscope. A high vacuum must be produced before the electron beam is switched on and the specimen examined. There are various controls for moving the specimen around, changing the magnification and brightness of the image, and so on. The magnification is changed by altering the current passing through the intermediate or projector lenses. Focusing of the image is accomplished by altering the current in the objective lens, while observing the image on the fluorescent screen through a low-power binocular microscope.

The Preparation of Sections for Transmission Electron Microscopy

Fixation. For many years the only fixative of any practical use to electron microscopists was *osmic acid.* This fixative, however, removed some of the proteins from tissues and did not preserve all cell components to the same extent. Furthermore, histochemical methods that required the activity of enzymes would not work after osmic acid fixation.

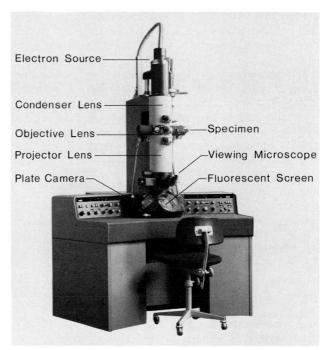

Fig. 1-22. A transmission electron microscope, showing its principal component parts. (Courtesy of Phillips Electronics Ltd.)

A procedure employing two fixatives was then introduced, in which initial fixation in an aldehyde was followed by postfixation in osmic acid. The aldehyde that gave the best results was *glutaraldehyde,* so glutaraldehyde fixation followed by osmic acid postfixation has come to be routinely used for electron microscopy. Recently, the addition of *tannic acid* to glutaraldehyde was found to reveal some previously undetected details. When the preservation of the activity of a particular enzyme is required, *formaldehyde* (a much poorer but milder fixative) is used in place of glutaraldehyde, and histochemical steps are done prior to osmic acid postfixation.

Dehydration. After fixation, the specimen is dehydrated in increasing concentrations of alcohol, which is then replaced by propylene oxide. The specimen is then infiltrated with unpolymerized embedding medium, as follows.

Embedding. Embedding media harder than wax are required to permit the cutting of very thin sections for the EM. The epoxy resins Epon, Araldite or Spur (which has a very low viscosity before polymerization) are most frequently used. To allow the epoxy resin to harden by polymerization, the embedded specimen is kept in an oven at 60° C. for several days before it is sectioned.

Sectioning. An electron beam does not penetrate very far into tissue, and it took a long time to find ways of cutting biological materials thinly enough for study in the EM.

EM sections are cut on a special instrument called an *ultramicrotome*, which advances the block of tissue by about 40 to 80 nm. between each cutting stroke. The fractured edge of a piece of plate *glass* or a *diamond* knife is used for cutting sections; the cutting edge of a diamond knife is so hard that it can be used much longer and can cut much harder tissues than glass knives. The cut sections are floated onto water located behind the knife edge and are picked up on small copper *grids*. These grids provide support for the fragile sections and yet permit the passage of electrons through their perforations. Grids are commonly first coated with a thin *supporting film* of plastic (Formvar) or carbon, so that the grid supports the film and the film in turn supports the section.

Staining. Although no colors are involved, the term *staining* is used in electron microscopy for procedures whereby sections are treated with solutions of salts of *heavy metals* that combine with various tissue components to different extents and hence make some components more electron-dense than others. This results in a greater contrast in the black-and-white images obtained on the fluorescent screen or photographic film. When osmic acid is used for fixation, it acts as a stain as well as a fixative, because osmium scatters electrons strongly and is taken up by certain cell components more than by others. Salts of other heavy metals commonly used as electron stains are *uranium (uranyl) acetate* and *lead hydroxide*. These are usually applied to sections after they have been placed on grids, and they act in a similar manner to increase contrast between cell components.

Electron Micrographs

Electrons are invisible, so the image formed by the electron beam passing through a specimen has to be rendered visible by focusing it on a fluorescent screen, where the energy of the electrons is converted into light. However, because electrons also cause *silver grains* to form in *photographic emulsions*, photographic film can be used in place of a fluorescent screen to obtain a photographic record (*negative*) of what is known as an *electron micrograph*. Because of the necessity for special training in EM technic, histology students seldom get the chance to use an EM and so must rely on seeing electron micrographs in order to learn about the *fine structure* (sometimes called the *ultrastructure*) of tissues. The electron micrographs most commonly used in illustrating textbooks of histology such as this one are obtained from *transmission* EMs and require that the electrons pass through the specimen in order to produce an image. In this respect, they are like photomicrographs taken with the LM. There is, however, another way in which an electron beam can be used to produce an image from a specimen: this is to use the electron beam to elicit the emission of other electrons from the surface of the specimen. These *secondary electrons* may then be assembled into an image of the surface of the specimen without any necessity for the electrons to pass through the specimen. This method, for reasons that will be apparent later, is called *scanning electron microscopy*.

The Interpretation of Transmission Electron Micrographs

The student should, at this stage, endeavor to become competent (if not expert) at interpreting transmission electron micrographs, for they are widely used as illustrations in lectures, books, and journals encountered not only in histology but also in almost all fields of medical and biological science. Lest there be any confusion, we should point out that in the following discussion we shall use the term *electron micrographs* to refer to those micrographs taken by electron microscopes of the *transmission* type. Where one has been taken with the EM of the *scanning* type, it will be so designated.

Why Electron Micrographs Are Enlarged. Enlarging a photomicrograph does not reveal very much more detail than can be resolved by eye with the light microscope; it tends to make everything larger, but at the same time fuzzier. However, because of the extremely short wavelength of an electron beam, an incredible amount of detail can be registered on suitable film. More detail is registered on such film than can be seen with the eye, and hence enlargements from negatives taken with the EM are routinely used to take full advantage of the resolving power of the instrument, which is about *1 nm.* for biological specimens in the transmission electron microscope.

Units of Measurement. The units now used for both the LM and the EM adhere strictly to the metric system. The *micrometer* (μm.) is 0.001 millimeter. The *nanometer* (*nm.*), derived from the Gr. *nanos*, dwarf, is 0.001 μm. (and hence one-millionth of a millimeter). The term *Angström unit* (Å) will also be met with, particularly in the older literature. Indeed, it was used almost exclusively for EM measurements until comparatively recently. The Angström unit is equivalent to 0.1 nm.; hence, 1 nm. = 10 Å.

Depth of Focus. The depth of focus of the oil-immersion objective of the LM is so short that it is impossible to have the whole thickness of a 7-μm. section in focus at the same time; the observer is thus obliged to focus up and down in order to see all parts of a section with this particular objective. This, however, may be an advantage as well as a disadvantage, for by focusing up and down the observer can generally tell whether a given part of a

Color Plate
1-1

Plate 1-1. This plate is designed to help the student interpret the colors he sees in stained sections. At *upper left* a single liver cell is shown as it appears in an H and E section. The nucleus has a blue rim, due to the nucleic acid, DNA, on the inner surface of the nuclear membrane. Within the nucleus there are granules of blue material (chromatin, containing DNA) and a larger rounded body called the nucleolus, which is blue because it contains another nucleic acid, RNA. The cytoplasm reveals some pink material; this is protein that stains with eosin. There are also patches of blue material in the cytoplasm; these are aggregations of RNA. Empty ragged-appearing spaces are also seen in the cytoplasm; these are due to deposits of glycogen, and appear empty because glycogen is not stained by either H or E. At *upper right* a similar cell stained by both the PAS technic (which colors carbohydrate containing macromolecules magenta) and hematoxylin is seen. The chief difference between it and the cell at the left is that the protein of the cytoplasm is not stained red (because no eosin was used), but the glycogen is colored magenta by the PAS technic. The *middle illustration* shows a layer of epithelial cells that lies on loose connective tissue. The staining here is PAS plus hematoxylin. Two of the epithelial cells are goblet cells which secrete a glycoprotein called mucus that is stained magenta by the PAS technic. The nuclei all stain blue with hematoxylin because of nucleic acids. In the loose connective tissue below the epithelial membrane there are some seemingly empty spaces; these contain glycosaminoglycans that do not stain sufficiently by the technic used here to be colored. The *lower* two pictures illustrate fat cells. The *left* one shows fat cells in an H and E section prepared by the usual paraffin technic in which the fat is dissolved away and leaves a rounded empty space in its place. At the *right,* fat cells are shown as they appear in a frozen section, in which the fat is retained so that it can be stained with a special stain for fat. In this case a red stain was used.

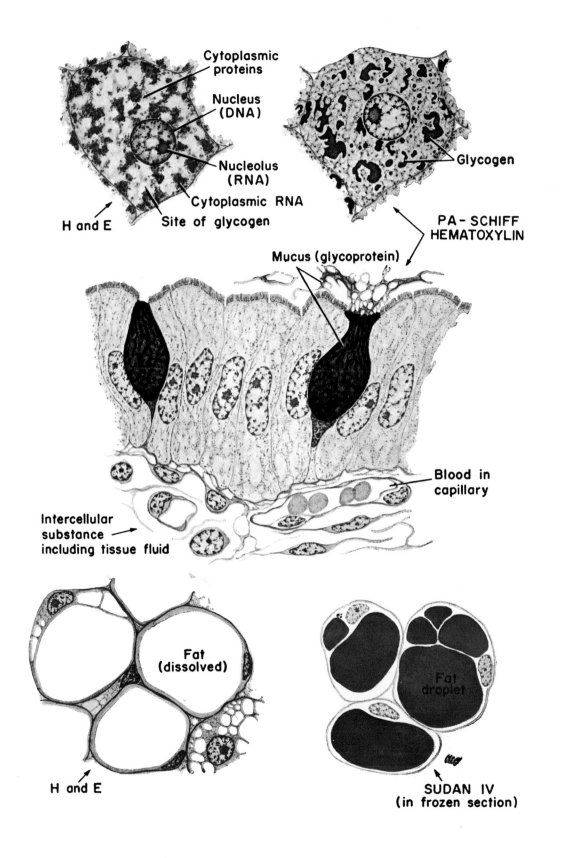

Cytoplasmic proteins

Nucleus (DNA)

Nucleolus (RNA)

Cytoplasmic RNA

Site of glycogen

H and E

Glycogen

PA-SCHIFF HEMATOXYLIN

Mucus (glycoprotein)

Blood in capillary

Intercellular substance including tissue fluid

Fat (dissolved)

H and E

Fat droplet

SUDAN IV (in frozen section)

Fig. 1-23. Micrograph (×8,000) of a cell in a culture of mouse embryo cells, taken with a scanning electron microscope. Note the three-dimensional appearance obtained with this type of electron microscope. (Courtesy of H. Yeger)

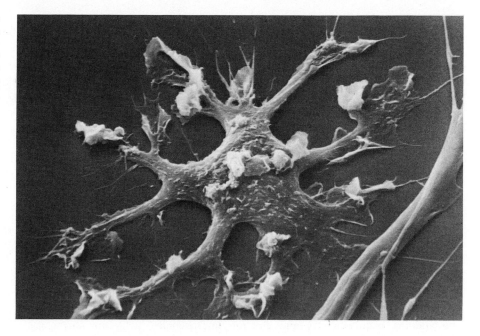

specimen is above or below an adjacent part. In the EM, such a distinction is not possible, for everything within the thickness of an EM section is in focus at the same time. For example, in the EM a tiny granule below a larger thin-walled sac would appear as if it were inside the sac.

Section Thickness. An important consideration in interpreting electron micrographs hinges on the fact that the sections used for the EM (60 to 80 nm.) are much thinner than those used for the LM (5 to 8 μm.); hence they are often called *ultrathin* (L. *ultra,* beyond) *sections.* Whereas only two or three sections are required to section a liver cell for the LM, about 400 are required to section a comparable cell for electron microscopy. This explains why, for example, a cell in an LM section may seem to be filled with granules, while in an EM section such a cell may show only very sparse granules. A series of such sections, cut thinly enough for the EM and stacked one upon another so as to achieve a thickness equivalent to that of an LM section would, of course, appear to be heavily granulated.

The interpretation of electron micrographs will be considered again in Chapter 5 on page 110, when we discuss the structure of the various cytoplasmic organelles.

Scanning Electron Microscopy

This is a relatively recent development that does not depend on electrons passing through the specimen and hence it differs somewhat in principle from routine (transmission) electron microscopy. The image obtained with

the scanning EM has the appearance of a three-dimensional picture (Fig. 1-23) and is assembled from the energy of electrons emitted from different parts of the surface of the specimen.

The general design of the scanning EM is illustrated in Figure 1-21 (*right*) on page 28. It resembles the transmission EM (see same figure) only in utilizing electromagnetic lenses to produce an electron beam, which thereafter is used in an entirely different manner. The *condenser lens* produces an extremely thin, pencil-like beam of electrons; this passes through a *scanning coil* that moves it back and forth over the surface of the specimen in a rapid scanning motion corresponding to the scanning pattern on a television screen. At each place the scanning beam strikes the specimen, secondary electrons are emitted from its surface coating (to be described shortly). These secondary electrons are collected by *electron detectors* (Fig. 1-21) and their energy is converted into an electrical signal, the intensity of which is displayed at the corresponding position of a *television screen.* The scanning beam follows the same path as the image-producing spot on the television screen and travels in synchrony with it so as to build up the image. Micrographs are obtained by photographing the image on the television screen.

A specimen has to be specially prepared for its surface features to be examined in the scanning EM; it does not need to be cut into sections. Following suitable fixation, the specimen is first *dehydrated* as gently as possible in order to avoid distortion. After it has been mounted on a small platform, the specimen is coated with a thin layer of metal, such as gold or platinum, that scatters electrons and thereby enables the surface features of the specimen to be observed.

Scanning electron micrographs are generally somewhat easier to interpret than micrographs taken with the transmission EM because we are so accustomed to seeing things in three dimensions. The scanning EM accomplishes this in considerable detail and its use helps a great deal in trying to reconstruct three-dimensional structure from the two-dimensional electron micrographs obtainable with the transmission EM.

REFERENCES AND OTHER READING

Since this chapter is of an introductory nature, few specific references need be given. However, the student should be aware that the science library of his or her college or university would be likely to have a selection of textbooks dealing with various aspects of light microscopy, phase contrast microscopy, tissue culture, the many kinds of histological preparative technics, stains and staining histochemistry and electron microscopic technics, should these be required for reference. Only a few of the many reference sources available are listed below. For atlases and books on the fine structure of cells, see references at the end of Chapter 5.

THE LIGHT MICROSCOPE AND TECHNICS EMPLOYED

Barer, R.: Lecture Notes on the Use of the Microscope. Oxford, Blackwell, 1968.

Dixon, K.: Principles of some tinctorial and cytochemical methods. Chap. 4 *In* Champion, R. H., Gilman, T., Rook, A. J., and Sims, R. T. (eds.): An Introduction to the Biology of the Skin. Oxford, Blackwell, 1970.

Parker, R. C.: Methods of Tissue Culture. ed. 3. New York, Harper & Row, 1961.

Paul, J.: Cell and Tissue Culture. ed. 2. Baltimore, Williams & Wilkins, 1960.

Pearse, A. G. E.: Histochemistry—Theoretical and Applied. ed. 3. vols. 1 and 2. Boston, Little, Brown, 1968.

Willmer, E. N. (ed.).: Cells and Tissues in Culture. Methods, Biology and Physiology. vols. 1 to 3. London, Academic Press, 1965.

THE ELECTRON MICROSCOPE AND TECHNICS EMPLOYED

History

Bradbury, S.: The Evolution of the Microscope. New York, Pergamon Press, 1967.

Technics

Agar, A. W., Alderson, R. H., and Chescoe, D.: Principles and practice of electron microscope operations. *In* Glauert, A. M. (ed.): Practical Methods in Electron Microscopy. vol 2. Amsterdam, North Holland, 1974.

Everhart, T. E., and Hayes, T. L.: The scanning electron microscope. Sci. Am., *226:*54, Jan. 1972.

Glauert, A. M.: Fixation, dehydration and embedding of biological specimens. *In* Glauert, A. M.: (ed.): Practical Methods in Electron Microscopy. vol. 3, part 1. Amsterdam, North Holland, 1975.

Hayat, M. A.: Basic Electron Microscopy Technics. New York, Van Nostrand Reinhold, 1972.

————: Principles and Techniques of Electron Microscopy. New York, Van Nostrand Reinhold, 1972.

————: Introduction to Scanning Electron Microscopy. Baltimore, University Park Press, 1978.

Koehlered, J. K.: Advanced Techniques in Biological Electron Microscopy. New York, Springer-Verlag, 1973.

Lewis, P. R., and Knight, D. P.: Staining methods for sectioned material. *In* Glauert, A. M. (ed.): Practical Methods in Electron Microscopy. vol. 5. Amsterdam, North Holland, 1977.

Reid, N.: Ultramicrotomy. *In* Glauert, A. M. (ed.): Practical Methods in Electron Microscopy. vol. 3, part 2. Amsterdam, North Holland, 1975.

Williams, M. A.: Autoradiography and immunocytochemistry. *In* Glauert, A. M. (ed.): Practical Methods in Electron Microscopy. vol. 6, part 1. Amsterdam, North Holland, 1978.

————: Quantitative methods in biology. *In* Glauert, A. M. (ed.): Practical Methods in Electron Microscopy. vol. 6, part 2. Amsterdam, North Holland, 1978.

Wischnitzer, S: Introduction to Electron Microscopy. ed. 2. New York, Pergamon Press, 1970.

PART TWO

CELL BIOLOGY

As was explained on page 6, modern cell biology is a relatively new subject. It was born in the second half of this century, when it became obvious that the knowledge being gained from new technics of microscopy was opening up further areas for biochemical studies of where and how in the cell the various chemical processes concerned in life occurred. Moreover, during this same period the chemical basis for genetic function was discovered, and the pathways through which genes direct protein synthesis were elucidated by combining biochemical and microscopic methods. Since the cell is the keystone around which the rest of histology is built, a comprehensive treatment of the cell is of fundamental importance in a histology textbook. Any adequate presentation of the cell now requires the interdisciplinary approach of cell biology, so this section of the book includes material from the other parent subjects of cell biology, biochemistry and genetics.

Those students who have studied cell biology before beginning histology will, it is hoped, find this part of the book a helpful review. Those who have not studied cell biology before beginning histology will find it an indispensible prelude to the study of the tissues in Part 3 and the systems in Part 4.

2 The Nucleus and Cell Division

It was realized long ago that there was a division of labor between the nucleus and the cytoplasm. For example, it was obvious from observing secretion granules in the cytoplasm of secretory cells and fibrils in the cytoplasm of muscle cells manifesting contractile properties, that the cytoplasm of cells was responsible for the specialized work performed by different kinds of cells. It was also noticed long ago that the nuclei of all kinds of specialized working cells, though of somewhat different sizes and shapes, all had a similar internal structure, with granules and clumps of chromatin and one or more nu-

cleoli (Fig. 2-1). The functions of the nucleus will be discussed in this and the next two chapters. In Chapter 5, we shall deal with the cytoplasm.

DEVELOPMENT OF KNOWLEDGE

In the late 1870s and early 1880s, the German biologist Walther Flemming made two very important contributions to knowledge about nuclei. First, he described and named *chromatin granules* in nuclei of working cells (Fig.

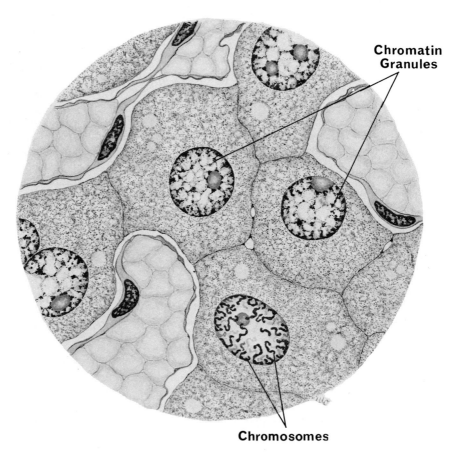

Chromatin Granules

Chromosomes

Fig. 2-1. Diagram of liver cells, showing the appearance of the nucleus in nondividing cells and in one that has just entered mitosis. The nuclei in the upper three cells are typical of the interphase and show chromatin granules. Chromosomes can be seen in the bottom cell, which has entered mitosis. It is in early prophase (*see* text) and still shows a nucleolus.

35

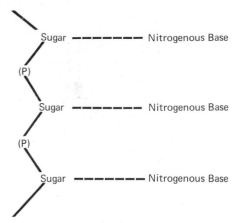

Fig. 2-2. The basic structure of nucleic acids.

2-1). Second, by staining and examining a great number of cells of the same kind but at different times, he was able to piece together in sequence a series of nuclear appearances that indicated that a nucleus could pass through a series of consecutive stages (to be described shortly) that terminate in the division of the nucleus and the cell into two daughter cells, each with a nucleus. A function for the nucleus was thus ascertained: it played a dominant role in cell division.

Flemming observed that when the series of events he had described occurred in a cell, the chromatin of the nucleus did not remain in its usual distribution of granules or clumps (Fig. 2-1, *Chromatin granules*) but instead were replaced by thread-like (or rod-like) bodies (Fig. 2-1, Chromosomes). Because of the appearance of these thread- or rod-like bodies, he called the process by which the nucleus and the cell divided *mitosis* (Gr. *mitos*, thread; *osis*, state or condition). About ten years later, Wilhelm von Waldeyer gave the name *chromosomes* (Gr. *chromo,* color; *soma,* body) to the deeply colored thread- or rod-like bodies seen in mitosis.

The Discovery of the Relation Between Chromosomes and Genes

Although Mendel had finished his now-famous studies on heredity before Flemming discovered mitosis, Mendel's work went relatively unnoticed for a long time. It was not until the beginning of this century that the concept of a relation between genes and chromosomes developed. Genes were at first defined as the self-reproducing, biologic units of heredity, but nothing about their physical basis was known. Later, however, it seemed that genes must have a physical basis of some kind and furthermore that they must be somehow strung along the chromosomes. The reason for the latter view was that since it

was already known that chromosomes split longitudinally in the process of mitosis (as will be described presently), so that each daughter cell receives one longitudinal half of each of the mother cell's chromosomes, genes, whatever they were, must be similarly split in mitosis so that each daughter cell obtains the same genetic heritage as the mother cell. But, as we shall see, no precise information about this matter was obtained until the 1950s. In the interval, other knowledge about nuclei came to light.

The Discovery and Characterization of Nucleic Acids

Nucleic acids were discovered in the last century. In those days there was no direct way of controlling bacterial infections in open wounds. Hence hospitals contained many patients with infected wounds, to which countless leukocytes (blood cells that serve in defense reactions) would migrate by way of the patient's bloodstream (as will be described on pp. 284–285) to combat the bacteria causing the infection; so many, in fact, that dead leukocytes commonly oozed from infected wounds in the form of *pus* which soaked into the covering bandages. Using the latter as a source of nuclei, the biochemist Friedrich Miescher, who knew that leukocytes exuding from the wound contained nuclei, was able to extract from them, not just another kind of protein, but a new type of biochemical substance that was soon named *nucleic acid.* Intensive research continued on nucleic acids into the 20th century, and it became established that a nucleic acid exists in the form of an enormously long unbranched macromolecule; indeed, nucleic acids were found to be the largest naturally occurring polymers known. The long macromolecule was shown to be made up of alternating units of sugar and phosphoric acid, with side chains consisting of nitrogenous bases attached to the sugars (Fig. 2-2). In due course it was shown that there are two kinds of nucleic acids: *deoxyribonucleic acid (DNA)* and *ribonucleic acid (RNA).* The two differ with regard to the kind of sugar their molecules contain. DNA contains 2-deoxy-D-ribose and RNA, D-ribose. The two nucleic acids also differ slightly with regard to their nitrogenous bases.

A Histological Test Developed for DNA Revealed Its Presence in Chromatin and Chromosomes

Since both DNA and RNA are acids, they are basophilic. But because other components of cells might be basophilic it became important to be able to distinguish histologically the two nucleic acids not only from each other, but also from other possible cellular components that might absorb basic stains. In 1924, a specific test for DNA, now termed the *Feulgen reaction*, was devised by Feulgen and Rossenbeck. Sections of fixed material are subjected to a strong acid to break the bond between the nitrogenous base purine and the deoxyribose in any DNA present; this releases the aldehyde group of the 2-deoxy-D-ribose and the released aldehyde is then detected by means of the Schiff reaction described in connection with the PAS technic (on page 26), by which the sites in which DNA is present in a section are colored magenta. This histochemical method showed that DNA was located in the chromatin of the nuclei of nondividing cells and in the chromosomes of dividing cells (Fig.2-3).

Since the process of mitosis could now be followed easily by the Feulgen staining method for DNA and since it showed that the DNA of each mitotic chromosome became divided in mitosis (Fig. 2-3), it was natural to question whether DNA might somehow serve as the genetic material. That it could act in this way was first established from studying certain bacteria.

The Discovery of Transformation

Two strains of a pneumonia-causing kind of bacteria (*Pneumococcus*) contributed in an important way to showing that DNA was indeed the hereditary material of cells. Briefly, the story began in 1928 with an experiment in which two strains of pneumococci were used, one type being lethal for mice and the other not lethal. An important difference between these two strains was that pneumococci of the first strain possessed a polysaccharide-containing capsule while those of the second lacked such a capsule. This difference accounted for the lethality of only the first strain because the capsule protected the bacteria of this strain from the defense mechanism of their hosts so that they could continue to multiply and kill their hosts. Bacteria of the nonencapsulated strain were unprotected and therefore destroyed by their hosts. It was shown, however, that a mixture of bacteria of the non-lethal strain and *heat-killed* bacteria of the lethal strain would also kill mice, and, when cultures were made of tissues from the dead mice, the bacteria recovered were found to be of the capsule-producing, lethal type. Something from the dead heat-killed bacteria of the lethal type had changed some nonlethal living bacteria into the lethal type in the mice. Although the results of this experiment did not attract much attention, others repeated the experiment and similarly concluded that some substance passed from one type of bacteria to the other and *transformed* the second type so that it gained certain characteristics of the first type. Furthermore, they showed that *these characteristics could be passed on to future generations* of bacteria. The substance that could transform the bacteria of one type into another was sought by chemical methods and finally was shown to be DNA. Since the bacteria that were transformed by the DNA that had been extracted from those of the lethal strain passed on

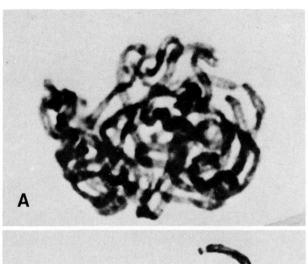

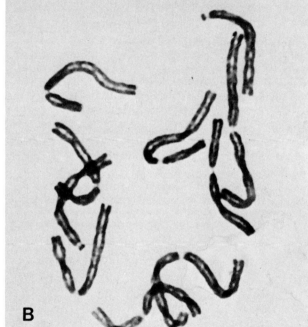

Fig. 2-3. Oil-immersion photomicrographs of plant chromosomes (*Trillium*), stained by the Feulgen reaction for DNA. (*A*) In prophase of mitosis. (*B*) In metaphase of mitosis. (For details of mitosis, *see* p. 46.) Note the double nature of the mitotic chromosomes; each half of any given chromosome will go to one of the daughter cells resulting from mitosis, so that the DNA of each mitotic chromosome will become divided between the two daughter cells. (Courtesy of K. Rothfels)

their new characteristics to subsequent generations, it was apparent that the DNA in this instance *acted as a gene.* From this beginning many further experiments were performed that showed eventually that all genes have their chemical basis in DNA.

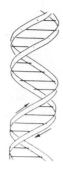

A

B

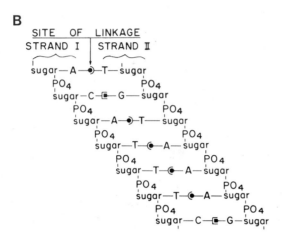

SITE   OF   LINKAGE

STRAND I | STRAND II

sugar—A—●—T—sugar
      PO₄   PO₄
     sugar—C—■—G—sugar
          PO₄   PO₄
         sugar—A—●—T—sugar
              PO₄   PO₄
             sugar—T—●—A—sugar
                  PO₄   PO₄
                 sugar—T—●—A—sugar
                      PO₄   PO₄
                     sugar—T—●—A—sugar
                          PO₄   PO₄
                         sugar—C—■—G—sugar

Fig. 2-4. (*A*) Diagram of a portion of a double-stranded DNA molecule according to the model of Watson and Crick. (*B*) Portion of a double-stranded DNA molecule showing how deoxyribonucleotides of one strand are joined to those of the other strand through their bases, by adenine being joined to thymine or cytosine being joined to guanine.

The Structure of the DNA Molecule Is Elucidated

Fundamental to the further development of knowledge about DNA was the elucidation in the early 1950s of the structure of the DNA molecule (Fig. 2-4) by Watson and Crick. According to their model, the DNA molecules of mammalian chromosomes each consist of two long strands wound together in the form of a double helix (Fig. 2-4A). Each strand has a backbone of alternating phosphoric acid and sugar units. A side chain (one of the four different nitrogenous bases represented in Fig. 2-4B by the letters A,T,C, or G) extends into the double helix from every sugar along each of its strands and each is attached to the nitrogenous base of the side chain of the other strand (Fig. 2-4B). There may be as many as 40 million of these base pairs in a single DNA molecule.

With this information at hand, it was inevitable that answers would be sought to such questions as: (*1*) How

could genetic information be stored in DNA? and (*2*) How could the huge macromolecule of DNA be duplicated so that it would allow a chromosome to split into two daughter chromosomes, each having precisely the same genetic information? We shall now attempt to answer these two questions in as simple a way as possible. (We shall deal with a further question, namely, how the information stored in the DNA of a working, functional cell is transmitted to the cytoplasm to direct the functions performed there, in Chap. 4.)

HOW INFORMATION IS STORED IN DNA

To help understand how information is stored in the DNA molecule, it is useful to consider briefly how information is contained in words. Words are composed of letters. However, words give different information not only because they are composed of different letters, but also because the same letters can be used in words in different sequences. When we consider the DNA molecule, we shall find that it has an alphabet of only four chemical "letters," with which "words" that convey different information are written and arranged into long sentences. We shall find, moreover, that this four-letter alphabet is used to write only three-letter words. With four letters, for example, a,e,p and r, it is possible to write several different three-letter words that convey different information, for example: ear, par, are, pea, per, ape, and pep. Were it not for the fact that words have to be pronounced (which requires that attention be paid to the placement of vowels and consonants) there would be 64 possible three-letter code words that could be written with a four-letter alphabet, and, of course, each of the 64 words could have a different meaning. As will be explained later, no more than 20 code words need be spelled out by the chemical letters of the DNA molecule, because, inconceivable as it may seem to anyone aware of the vast number of different attributes of living things explained by heredity, the only final path through which genes can act is by prescribing in each body cell which, and in what order, amino acids (of around 20) are to be linked together to form different proteins. How this is done will be described in Chapter 4. So all that is needed is that there be a different code word for each of the 20 or so amino acids. There are therefore enough extra words for some amino acids to have more than one code word, and this utilizes most of the possibilities.

The four chemical letters in the DNA alphabet are the four nitrogenous bases, *adenine, cytosine, guanine,* and *thymine.* These are represented in Figures 2-4B, 2-5, and 2-6 as A for adenine, C for cytosine, G for guanine, and T for thymine. The four bases are arranged in DNA molecules to code information, but in order to explain both this coding and how the three-letter code words are read and,

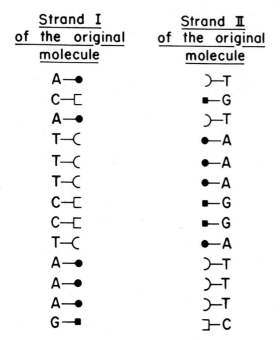

Fig. 2-5. The first step in the duplication of a DNA molecule, the separation of its two strands.

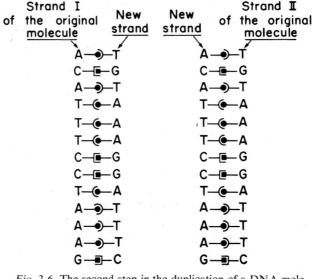

Fig. 2-6. The second step in the duplication of a DNA molecule. After the two strands of a DNA molecule have separated, as shown in Figure 2-5, a new strand is synthesized beside each of the two strands. An A always forms beside a T, and vice versa, and a C beside a G, and vice versa. As a result, each of the double-stranded molecules that are formed is identical with the one whose strands become separated. Compare both of these with each other and with one in Figure 2-4B.

further, how entire DNA molecules can be duplicated as a prelude to mitosis, we shall describe the DNA molecule in more detail.

WHEN DO DNA MOLECULES IMPART THEIR INFORMATION?

DNA molecules impart information under two different sets of circumstances. First, when the DNA of a cell is duplicated (which, as will be described later, occurs as an essential prelude to mitosis), the molecule must somehow impart its information to the mechanism that synthesizes the DNA required for the preexisting DNA to be duplicated. In this instance, every word of the DNA molecule must impart information. Second, in nondividing cells, DNA molecules must impart information to the mechanism that synthesizes the necessary proteins required by the cell for maintaining its normal protein constitution and for performing any function requiring the secretion of protein. In this instance only some of the words of the DNA molecule are read. Moreover, the words read in diverse kinds of functioning cells are sufficiently varied for these cells to synthesize different proteins and hence be dissimilar in both form and function. This will be explained in detail in Chapter 4.

INFORMATION COPYING IN DNA MOLECULES

How DNA Molecules Are Duplicated

As already noted, the information in DNA molecules takes the form of three-letter words composed from a four-letter alphabet (A,C,G,T). If we seek to copy information stored in the words in a book, we have to open the book to see the words printed on its pages. Likewise, for the three-letter words written along the course of a DNA molecule by various combinations of its four nitrogenous bases (A,C,G, and T) the molecule, like a book, has to be opened. As long as the nitrogenous bases on each strand of the two-stranded molecule are bonded to one another, the pages of the book, as it were, remain closed. This does not mean that in order for a DNA molecule to be copied its two strands have to come apart along their whole length at the same time, any more than a book, to be copied, has to be opened on all its pages simultaneously. A book is copied one page at a time. However, there are enough chemical "eyes" available to copy simultaneously all the different parts of the DNA molecule that are "open" at any given time.

With this introduction in mind we can now describe how the molecule imparts the information required for it to be duplicated in preparation for cell division. In this connection it is very important to appreciate that the nitrogenous bases of the two strands are not bonded together in a haphazard way but instead in a very specific way, by what is termed *complementary base pairing*, which requires that adenine bonds only with thymine and cytosine bonds only with guanine; the bases of each pair are thus complementary to each other. Accordingly, as shown in Figure 2-4B, wherever there is an A on one strand, there is always a T on the other strand, and wherever there is a C on one strand there is always a G on the other strand. Furthermore, when the two strands begin to come apart as the first step in the duplication of the two-stranded molecule (Fig. 2-5 shows them apart), each strand begins to have a new strand built beside it. Because of complementary base pairing, the information given by an A on an exposed old strand leads to the addition of a newly formed deoxyribonucleotide molecule of the T type in the newly formed strand (Fig. 2-6). Conversely, a T on an exposed strand of the original molecule leads to the addition of a new deoxyribonucleotide molecule of the A type on the newly forming strand. Complementary base pairing also occurs in connection with the Cs and Gs that become exposed as duplication proceeds along the length of the original molecule. As a result, two new double-stranded molecules are eventually formed, with half of each being new and the other half being one-half of the original molecule (Fig. 2-6). So, just as the two strands of the original double-stranded molecule were not identical (Fig. 2-5) but complementary to one another (because wherever there was, for example, an A on one, there was a T on the other), the two strands of each daughter molecule are likewise not identical but complementary (Fig. 2-6). Nevertheless, the two newly completed double-stranded molecules are identical not only to each other but also to the mother molecule from which one strand of each was derived (compare Figs. 2-5 and 2-6).

When Are DNA Molecules Duplicated?

It has already been mentioned that DNA molecules are duplicated before mitosis. Hence when mitosis begins, with thread-like chromosomes visible in the nucleus, each of the chromosomes already contains two complete DNA molecules. To be more precise about when DNA molecules are duplicated and the relation of this event to the beginning of mitosis requires that we explain what is termed the *cell cycle*.

THE CELL CYCLE

From its derivation (Gr. *kylos*, a circle), the word *cycle* is used to denote the repetition of a sequence of events during a given time period, with the final event terminating at the beginning of the first event of the next cycle. Circles are used to illustrate cycles because (for example) if a given point is marked on a circle with a pencil and the pencil is then moved (in one direction) around the circle, it will soon reach the starting point again, whereupon it is said to have completed one cycle. So if circles, segments of which are designated as different stages (or *phases*) of a process are drawn and marked with arrows to indicate direction, they provide a convenient way to illustrate how a series of changes or events can occur in sequence and be repeated over and over in the same sequence. For example, the way the four seasons follow in the same sequence year after year can be illustrated by a circle divided into four segments, each representing one of the four seasons, with the sequence of seasonal changes indicated by directional arrows (Fig. 2-7).

It should be mentioned here that the concept of cycles and cyclical behavior in the body is not limited to cells. Indeed there are many complex structures (particularly in the reproductive systems) that pass through cycles or exhibit cyclical behavior. This in general means that they regularly undergo a series of changes in structure and function that always ends with their return to the same structural and functional state that they were in before.

The concept of a cell cycle arose from the study of certain kinds of cells growing in vitro (page 12). Some kinds of cells under in-vitro conditions continue to divide at regular intervals. At the conclusion of each mitosis two daughter cells are formed and then, after a definite interval, each of these passes through another mitosis. After the same interval as before, each of these cells then undergoes mitosis, and so on. Cells that continue dividing regularly in this fashion (either in vitro or in vivo) are described as *cycling* cells.

Illustrating the cell cycle by a circle, however, is associated with a problem. The difficulty is that in passing through a cycle, the cell divides into two daughter cells; so in a diagram (Fig. 2-8A) the cell that returns to the starting point of the cycle is not the same cell that began the cycle; it is a daughter cell that begins the next cycle. But since two daughter cells are formed in each and every subsequent cycle, the diagram, to be accurate, should show these also (which would soon fill the page with circles). The problem is solved by forgetting about the other daughter cell in each cycle. This is justifiable because in cycling cells the one daughter cell we follow each time around the circle is taken to be identical with the parent cell we begin with.

The cell cycle is divided into two basic parts (*1*) *mitosis* and (*2*) the interval between the end of one mitosis and the beginning of the next; this interval is called the *interphase* (Fig. 2-8A) because it is the part of the cycle between consecutive phases of mitosis. At first the cell cycle was conceived of as having only these two phases.

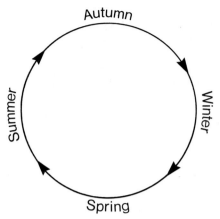

Fig. 2-7. The seasons of the year, a familiar example of a cyclic event.

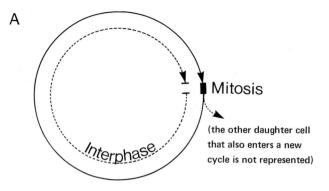

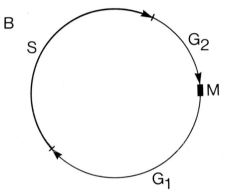

Fig. 2-8. The phases of the cell cycle, indicating (*A*) the two principal phases, the interphase and mitosis, (*B*) the three subdivisions of the interphase (G_1, S, and G_2), and mitosis (M). The relative duration of each phase of the interphase is indicated in (*B*) by the length of the arrow. There are considerable variations in the lengths of these phases between different cell types and also between cells of the same type but different species. However, some representative durations of the phases of the cell cycle for typical mouse cells in suspension cultures would be as follows: G_1: 8 hr., S: 7 or 8 hr., G_2: 4 hr., M: 1 hour.

Most body cells were normally seen in the interphase, and hence the interphase was commonly thought of as the phase in which a cell was either resting or performing its specialized work. And indeed it is still usual to refer to working, specialized cells, or any cells that are not in mitosis, as *interphase cells.*

Next, when the relation of DNA molecules to genes was established, it became obvious that DNA molecules would have to be duplicated sometime in the cell cycle if there were to be enough genes for two daughter cells. When a method was discovered by which new DNA undergoing synthesis could be labeled by radioautography, (described in Chap. 3 on p. 62), so that the new DNA could be detected microscopically, it was found that DNA molecules duplicated, not early in mitosis as might have been expected, but during the interphase, long before chromosomes could be detected with the LM as thread-like bodies. So the period in the interphase during which new DNA was synthesized was termed the *S phase* of the cell cycle (*S* for *synthesis*) (Fig. 2-8B). This stage was found to begin about 8 hours after the end of mitosis and took about 7 or 8 hours to complete. The *gap* in the cell cycle between the end of mitosis and the beginning of the S phase was then termed the G_1 (*G* for *gap*) *phase* and the *gap* between the end of the S phase and the beginning of mitosis was termed the G_2 *phase*. So the cell cycle came to have four stages: mitosis, G_1, S, and G_2, as shown in Figure 2-8B, where the relative time taken by each is indicated.

The finding that the DNA of the cell was duplicated during one portion of the interphase changed the widely held concept that the interphase was entirely occupied by a cell's performance of its specialized function. It now seemed logical to assume that during the S period, the energies of a cell would be directed toward duplicating its DNA instead of, for example, producing and elaborating secretions through its cell membrane. So it appeared that a cell would have to perform its specialized work in either the G_1 or G_2 phase of the cycle. The fact is, however, that continuously cycling cells do not have very much time in either of these two stages to specialize or perform specialized work. Furthermore, cells that continuously cycle in vitro are seldom highly specialized for particular functions, and during the 8 hours or so they spend in G_1 they are, generally speaking, fully occupied with building themselves up in content so that they will be large enough to produce two daughter cells. So for interphase cells to become highly specialized working cells, they leave the cycle, either temporarily or permanently, and commonly in the G_1 phase. A very few types of cells, however, can leave the cycle in G_2 to become specialized cells (and it is of interest that such cells are characterized by having double the customary content of DNA). Accordingly, the specialized functions performed by body cells are executed by cells that are, with few exceptions, in a prolonged G_1 stage, or by cells that have left the cycle in G_1 and will never enter it again.

When body cells remain in this prolonged G_1 stage, they are, of course, in an extended interphase, which justifies such highly specialized, functional cells being commonly referred to as *interphase cells*. Those cells that leave the cycle permanently in G_1, however, are not strictly speaking in interphase at all, since, if they are never to divide again, they cannot be regarded as being *between* two phases of mitosis. Nevertheless, they too are commonly called interphase cells because the term *interphase* has become so generally associated with cells that perform specialized functions.

Certain cells that leave the cell cycle in G_1 for a very extended period of time (and not necessarily to perform highly specialized functions) are sometimes said to have entered a G_0 *state*, which means that they are effectively *outside* the cell cycle. They can be triggered back from G_0 into the G_1 phase of the cycle by certain stimuli, and so they have not left the cell cycle permanently. Certain biochemical changes are characteristic of the G_0 state, making it possible to distinguish cells in the G_0 state from those in cycle. However, there are different opinions regarding the nature of the essential difference between the G_0 state and an extended G_1 stage.

The Significance of the Cell Cycle Concept in Histology

As far as the cell cycle concept is concerned, since most body cells are specialized functioning cells, they are either in a prolonged G_1 stage of the cell cycle or they have left the cell cycle permanently, to become what are termed *end cells*. But even in the fully grown body many cells must divide to replace those that wear our or that are being continuously lost from some surface. Injuries, moreover, commonly require the formation of new cells for their repair. Hence mitosis must occur among certain members of the cell population of the body throughout life. So if we accept that mitosis requires a cell to cycle, there must be cells of different kinds cycling in the body, even if only occasionally. Indeed in some tissues, as we shall see, cells cycle regularly and extensively. But not all body cells have the capacity to cycle. To explain what occurs in the body, it clarifies matters to divide the cells of the body into three categories and see how cell populations are, or are not, maintained in them.

HOW CELL POPULATIONS ARE MAINTAINED (OR NOT MAINTAINED) IN THE THREE CATEGORIES OF BODY CELLS

In considering maintenance of cell populations in the body, it helps to be aware of what is only a very general rule, to the effect that there is a more or less inverse relation between the degree to which a cell becomes specialized and its capacity for undergoing mitosis.

Category 1

By the time of birth, or at most after a very few years of postnatal life, there are some cells in the body in which a highly specialized state has been obtained only at the expense of a complete loss of reproductive capacity. Moreover, no provision is made at all for the replacement of these specialized cells if they wear out or are destroyed. Nerve cells are the classic example of cells of this category. After we are a few years old we have all the nerve cells that we shall ever possess. As they wear out and die, there is, throughout life, a continuous diminution of their number. To compensate for this discouraging thought, however, there is a comforting one: there is perhaps some advantage in their not being able to divide, for, if they did, it might upset our memories and other higher nervous functions.

Category 2

Many kinds of cells that become highly specialized to perform particular functions either wear out or become lost from body surfaces, often at a rapid rate. Furthermore, like nerve cells, highly specialized cells of this second category are unable to reproduce. However, there is provision for the replacement of the specialized cells of this category. This is accomplished by cells of the same lineage (family type) that have not yet become sufficiently specialized to have lost their ability to reproduce that continue to cycle. As a result, from this pool of cycling cells, new cells that can specialize are always available to take the place of those specialized cells that are lost. This means that in many parts of the body (described in detail later) there is a continuous and sometimes rapid turnover of the cell population, with relatively unspecialized cells that remain cycling often enough to yield daughter cells that can specialize to take the place of functioning cells that are lost. There thus exists a balance between cell production and cell loss in many parts of the adult body, so that the total number of cells remains the same although its individual members change. The cell populations of these parts of the body are thus referred to as *renewing cell populations* and they are maintained in what is called a *steady state*.

For example, we shall find that the cells lining most parts of the intestinal tract are continuously lost from its inner surface into its lumen. However, the cellular lining of the tract is kept intact because new cells of the same family type, but less specialized (and lying deeper in the wall of the tract) keep on cycling to yield daughter cells that leave the cycle in the G_1 phase to become specialized, and these move toward the surface to keep the lining layer of the intestine intact. As a result, the intestine has a new lining every few days. Certain of the cells of blood likewise live only a few days and so they must be replaced by cells that develop from less specialized cells of the same family type. These less specialized cells continue to cycle in the bone marrow or some other blood cell-forming tissue, where enough leave the cycle to become specialized and enter the bloodstream so as to keep the numbers of the different kinds of circulating blood cells relatively constant. Even in our bones, which we usually think of as being relatively permanent structures in adults, there is a slow turnover of the cell population, with the highly specialized bone cells living only for years or decades, instead of all through adult life as might be thought. But here also unspecialized cells of the bone cell lineage cycle often enough to maintain a pool of unspecialized cells on bone surfaces, where they can become specialized and form new bone when and where it is needed. They become particularly active, as we shall see, in the repair of bone fractures, where new bone forms rapidly to repair the break.

Several terms have been used to designate the unspecialized cells of a cell family that retain the ability to divide, an ability that is lost when the members of such families become highly specialized. For example, they have been termed the (*1*) *germinative*, (*2*) *mother*, (*3*) *progenitor* (L. for parent or ancestor), or (*4*) *stem cells* of the family. We shall comment further on this last term.

Stem Cells. Of the various terms mentioned above (and still others that might be included), the term *stem cell* has become very widely used in recent years and moreover has come to have a more or less special meaning. However, the semantic basis for this term and its meaning is somewhat obscure. For example, the word *stem* is not listed as an adjective in the dictionary. There are, however, a great many different meanings given for the noun and the verb. The meaning given for *stem* when used as an intransitive verb gives one clue to what might be implied if the word were to be used as an adjective, namely "to originate, derive or be descended." So if cells of some kind "stem" from an ancestor cell, the ancestral cell from which they originate or stem, could, if an adjective were to be coined, be logically termed a *stem cell*. But this is the same meaning that the terms *mother, germinative,* or *progenitor* cells have, and so there might

seem to be no good reason for coining yet another new term. However, the term *stem cell* implies something more. There are many examples of mother, germinative, and progenitor cells in the prenatal development of the body. However, different orders of these appear and some disappear prenatally in the body as it develops. The term *stem cell* has come to denote a cell of an ancestral type that persists as the same type of cell in postnatal life and hence remains able to cycle all through postnatal life, to provide cells that can become specialized and take the place of those that die or are lost. Furthermore, there is another connotation implied by the term *stem cell*, the only basis for which is to be found in one of the definitions of the noun *stem*, which is that it is the aboveground part of a plant from which leaves, flowers, and fruit are derived. This may be the reason for the term *stem* suggesting that several kinds of cells, but all belonging to the same family, may be derived from it in postnatal life. If the family of cells represents several somewhat different kinds of cells, but nevertheless all related, the stem cell is said to be *pluripotential*, which means that it has the potentiality to become specialized along several somewhat different routes; for example, in connection with the formation of blood cells, both red and white blood cells can be traced back to the same stem cell. But sometimes a cell is regarded as a stem cell even if only one kind of end cell can stem from it, but it is so regarded only if this involves the formation of a series of cells of an increasing order of specialization, with cells of one stage giving rise to those of the next, and so on until the end cell is formed. Stem cells of this type are sometimes said to be *unipotential* stem cells because although more than one form of cell is derived from them along the way, the final cell is an end cell of one particular kind. Later, examples will be given of both kinds of stem cells.

Next, as far as the cell cycle is concerned, although stem cells remain able to cycle all through life (Fig. 2-9, *top*) it should be pointed out that they do not have to be in continuous cycle. It would seem they cycle just often enough to maintain their population, from which some members are always leaving to become more specialized cells. Many stem cells thus remain in a prolonged G_1 phase without becoming specialized (Fig. 2-9, *middle*). Such cells are ready at any time to cycle again as stem cells to maintain their normal numbers. When stem cells leave the stem cell population, they do so in the G_1 stage and they then begin to become specialized (Fig. 2-9, *bottom*). However, in some kinds of stem cells, specialization occurs more or less in stages. When only partly specialized, a cell that left the stem cell pool may, in some instances, still be able to cycle in its new form. So there does not always have to be a division of the ancestral stem cell for every specialized cell that develops in a cell

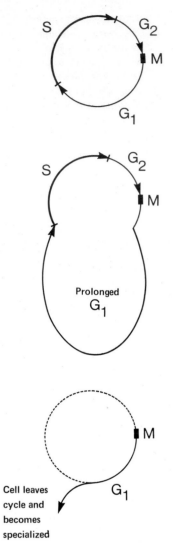

Fig. 2-9. Some examples of variation in the cell cycle of stem cells, in which the cells may be in cycle (*top*), remain in a prolonged G_1 without becoming specialized (*middle*), or leave the cycle in G_1 and begin to become specialized (*bottom*).

family. Indeed, the turnover of the stem cell population may be very slow. When fully specialized, however, it would seem that those (end) cells that finally develop from stem cells in postnatal life are unable to cycle.

The stem cell concept is important and will be easier to understand after we have described specific examples. The point to make here is that the maintenance of pools of stem cells of different kinds serves a vital function in the growth and maintenance of the cell populations of those tissues in which specialized functioning cells have lost their ability to cycle.

Category 3

Certain other kinds of cells in the body represent an exception to the generalization that specialized function interferes with reproductive capacity, for there are several examples of highly specialized cells that under certain circumstances seem able to go into cycle to bring their numbers back up to normal. However, the highly specialized cells in this category are not generally called upon to use their reproductive capacity once the growth of the organ to which they belong is completed. Cells of this category are found mostly in those organs where the functioning cells have a long life span and in which cell division seldom occurs after full growth of the organ has been attained. The cells of the liver (hepatocytes) are an example of this category. However, if up to two-thirds of the liver of an experimental animal is removed at an operation, the cells of the remaining portion will undergo division and reproduce themselves so rapidly that the liver is restored to its former size in less than two weeks. The cells that make hormones are also highly specialized. Under normal conditions few kinds need reproduce themselves to any extent, for they, like liver cells, live a long time; but under altered conditions most of these can undergo division indicating that, even though specialized, they have not entirely lost the ability to reproduce themselves.

Having now considered when, where, and why mitosis normally occurs, not only during growth but also in adult life, we shall deal with the physical aspects of mitosis after we briefly discuss chromatin and chromosomes.

CELL DIVISION

CHROMATIN AND CHROMOSOMES

What Is Chromatin?

Chromatin is not a chemical compound for which a formula can be written. As noted, its basophilia is due primarily to its content of DNA. We now know from EM studies that chromatin, although it appears with the LM to be in the form of granules or clumps in interphase (G_1) nuclei (Fig. 2-1) always exists in the form of very long fine threads, each of which, as will be explained shortly, is really a chromosome. The very long helical, two-stranded DNA molecule is itself coiled along its course so as to fit into the chromosomal thread. The DNA is associated with some RNA and also with histones and other basic proteins, and the possibility that some of these are involved in regulating the genetic expression of DNA is receiving much attention. To summarize: chromatin is the name given the complex material found in chromosomes.

How all these components of chromatin are structurally and functionally related to one another, and for what reasons, is not yet thoroughly understood.

What Are the Chromatin Granules Seen With the LM?

The chromatin in the nuclei of nondividing cells represents those sites where the chromosomal threads (which, when extended, are invisible with the LM) have become coiled, folded, or otherwise aggregated so as to become dense enough little masses to be visible with the LM as granules or clumps after staining. An easy way to visualize this is to take a long piece of very thin wire and then, here and there along its course, coil or crumple it into dense little masses. The wire would represent the chromosomal thread and the sites where it was coiled or crumpled into little masses would be the chromatin granules or clumps seen with the LM. With the LM the "wire," at sites where it was not coiled or crumpled, would be invisible.

The Condensed and Extended Chromatin of Nondividing Cells. The chromatin visible with the LM came to be referred to as *condensed chromatin* whereas the parts of the chromosomal thread invisible with the LM (but which can be seen with the EM, as will be described later) were termed *extended chromatin.* As is discussed in Chapter 4, it is very probable that only the DNA of the extended chromatin is active in providing information to direct protein synthesis in the nondividing cell. Hence the paradox that all the chromatin one can see with the LM in the nuclei of working cells of the body is probably not doing any work at all. This provides a reason for referring to the extended chromatin as *euchromatin,* good chromatin, because it works, and the condensed chromatin as *heterochromatin* (Gr. *heteros,* other), the other kind of chromatin.

Mitotic Chromosomes. When a cell enters mitosis, dark-staining thread-like bodies (Fig. 2-3) or rod-like bodies (Fig. 2-1) seem to have replaced the chromatin granules of the nondividing cell. Three events occur to cause this change. First, the DNA of each chromatin thread present in the cell in its G_1 phase is duplicated in the S phase, and the two DNA molecules thus formed separate from one another. Second, the proteins associated with a DNA molecule in a chromatin thread are synthesized either in the S and perhaps to some extent also in the G_2 phase, so that there are, by then, twice as many chromatin threads in the nucleus as there were in the G_1 phase. Third, each of these two chromatin threads becomes condensed in some fashion along its whole length so that by the time the cell enters mitosis what were single, only partly condensed, chromatin threads in the G_1 phase appear in the first stage of mitosis as double chromatin threads, with

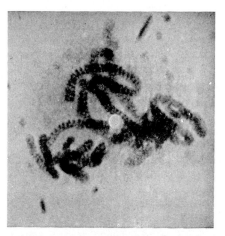

Fig. 2-10. Oil-immersion photomicrograph of chromosomes in mitotic plant cells (squash preparation), treated with sodium cyanide before staining by the Feulgen reaction for DNA. Their appearance after this treatment, which causes the chromosomes to extend slightly, suggests that the chromatin threads in them are coiled. (Courtesy of A. Gopal-Ayengar and L. Coleman)

the members of each pair lying side by side and joined at only one site, called the *centromere.* These double threads are seen (Fig. 2-3) because the DNA of each thread has become sufficiently condensed to be a stainable structure visible in the LM.

How chromatin threads become condensed to form the chromatin granules seen with the LM in nondividing cells and how they become condensed along their whole length in mitosis are unknown. At least in some plant cells, what is seen with the LM suggests that the chromatin threads may become coiled (Fig. 2-10). But EM studies of mammalian cells indicate that in mitosis the chromosomes become condensed by becoming folded, as will be described in the next chapter.

A Note on Terminology. It must be remembered that mitosis is a process described from studies made with the LM in the last century and that much of the terminology still used in describing the process was coined at that time. Hence it may be expected that some of the terms used now require some amplification and/or alteration if confusion is to be avoided.

After it was shown mitotic chromosomes were double structures, each strand of the double structure was called a *chromatid,* possibly because one meaning of *-id* is "the same," and certainly the two strands of a mitotic chromosome are the same, each having a full complement of the same genes. However, as we shall see at a later stage of mitosis, the two chromatids of each double chromosome separate from each other, with one chromatid of each chromosome going to what will become one daughter cell and the other chromatid going to the other cell. This, of course, is why the daughter cells are genetically identical. But here the original terminology becomes inadequate in the light of present knowledge. When the terminology was devised there was, of course, no reason to believe that each chromatid seen in mitosis would continue to exist as a long, extended thread during the interphase. Indeed, it was believed that at the end of mitosis the chromatids in each daughter cell broke up again into the chromatin granules seen in interphase cells, and that these granules somehow became reassembled into chromosomes when the daughter cell later began another phase of mitosis. However, we now know that chromosomes are the bearers of the genes and that each chromosomal thread persists as a single-stranded entity throughout the interphase and hence is still present (in its extended form) in cells in the G_1 phase and in cells that have ceased to cycle in order to function in some specialized way. It can therefore create confusion to designate both the single-stranded structures seen in interphase cells and the double-stranded structures seen in mitotic cells as chromosomes, without any kind of qualification.

Before the second half of this century it would have been fair in a histology examination to ask a student to describe a chromosome, because at that time a chromosome could be properly described only as a double-stranded, dark-staining body seen with the LM in cells undergoing mitosis. But since the same word is now also used for the single-stranded threads that are mostly invisible with the LM in the nuclei of nondividing cells (which, of course, constitute most of the cells of the body), to describe chromosomes only as double structures as they were originally defined, would now be an inadequate answer. Unfortunately, the association of the word *chromosome* with a double structure is constantly reinforced in students' minds because photomicrographs are frequently taken of mitotic chromosomes, since these are eminently suitable for studying chromosomal anomalies in the field of cytogenetics. So the photomicrographs a student sees of chromosomes are always ones of the double-stranded type. But in most body cells (which are in interphase) they are only single-stranded structures and their presence is indicated in the LM only by chromatin granules. The whole problem of describing chromosomes (which can become very confusing) would, in our opinion, be greatly simplified if single-stranded chromosomes were to be designated as *s-chromosomes* and double-stranded chromosomes (following the duplication of DNA in the S phase), as *d-chromosomes*. This practice will be followed hereafter in places where it might otherwise be unclear as to which type we mean. When asked to describe a chromosome, the student has the right to ask which kind, an s-chromosome or a d-chromosome.

THE PROCESS OF MITOSIS

THE MAIN EVENTS IN MITOSIS

When mitosis begins, there are 46 d-chromosomes in a human cell. During mitosis the two s-chromosomes (chromatids) comprising each d-chromosome separate from each other completely. The cell at this stage thus has 92 s-chromosomes. Half of these, corresponding to one of the two s-chromosomes (chromatids) from each of the original d-chromosomes, move toward one end of the cell (which in the meantime has usually become elongated) and the other half move toward the opposite end of the cell. In each of these two sites the s-chromosomes become reorganized into nuclei in the arrangement typical of the G_1 phase. The s-chromosomes become partly extended and hence capable of directing protein synthesis. The formation of two nuclei would lead to the cell's becoming binucleated were it not for the fact that in the meantime the cytoplasm becomes constricted at the midline to pinch the cell into halves. Each half thus constitutes a daughter cell complete with a nucleus that has a full complement of genes identical with those of the other daughter cell. The various stages in mitosis are illustrated diagrammatically in Figure 2-11 and in sectioned material in Figure 2-20; they will be described in detail shortly.

One of the more fascinating events observed in mitosis is the development of a delicate transient structure termed a *mitotic spindle.* This plays a most important part in bringing about (*1*) an alignment of the d-chromosomes in one plane in the middle of the cell (Fig. 2-11C) and (*2*) movement of the s-chromosomes (described above) toward each end of the elongated cell (Fig. 2-11C, D, and E).

Mitosis has four consecutive phases: *prophase,* (Gr. *pro,* before), *metaphase* (Gr. *meta,* after, beyond, hence a change or transformation), *anaphase* (Gr. *ana,* up, again) and *telophase* (Gr. *telos,* end). Mitosis is normally continuous, with each phase merging imperceptibly into the next. The whole process in animal cells takes from 1 to 1.5 hours, according to cell type.

Even though the formation of two daughter cells requires the division of both the nucleus and the cytoplasm, we tend to think of mitosis as being primarily a nuclear event in which the d-chromosomes in the mother cell are each split into two s-chromosomes, which are then distributed so as to provide a complete set of s-chromosomes for each daughter cell. However, as we shall see, this nuclear event only occurs as a result of the participation in the process of cytoplasmic organelles called *centrioles,* and upon which the formation of the all-important mitotic spindle is dependent. So before giving a detailed description of each of the four phases of mitosis,

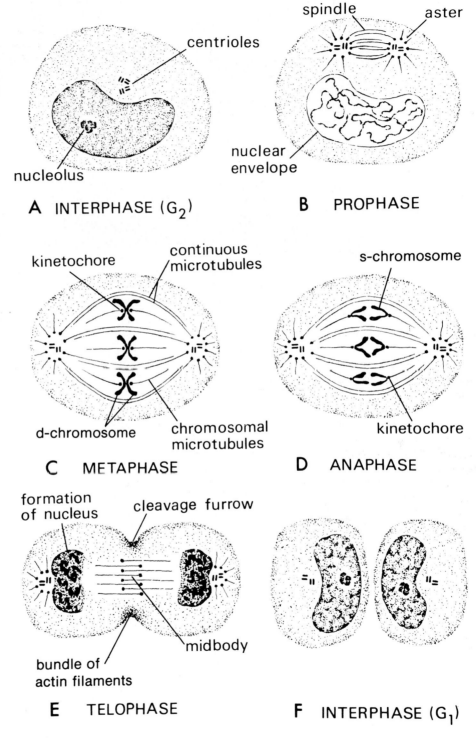

Fig. 2-11. Diagram illustrating the various stages in mitosis, including the condensation of chromatin into chromosomes, the formation of the mitotic spindle, and the separation of chromosomes and centrioles equally into the two daughter cells. (Courtesy of V. Kalnins)

centrioles

nucleolus

A INTERPHASE (G$_2$)

spindle   aster

nuclear envelope

B PROPHASE

kinetochore   continuous microtubules

d-chromosome   chromosomal microtubules

C METAPHASE

s-chromosome

kinetochore

D ANAPHASE

formation of nucleus   cleavage furrow

midbody

bundle of actin filaments

E TELOPHASE

F INTERPHASE (G$_1$)

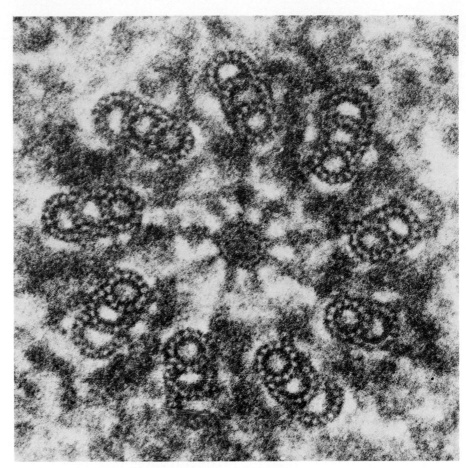

Fig. 2-12. Electron micrograph (×500,000) of a centriole in cross section. This is seen in a developing ciliated epithelial cell of chick trachea, fixed in the presence of tannic acid. Note the nine bundles of microtubules arranged in a characteristic radiating pattern in the wall of the centriole. Each bundle contains three microtubules embedded in a fine fibrillar material. The subunit structure of the microtubules (which is dealt with in Chap. 5) is shown to advantage by this technic. (Courtesy of M. Wassmann and V. Kalnins)

we must first describe the centrioles and their function in the stages of the cell cycle that precede mitosis.

Centrioles and the Formation of the Mitotic Spindle

Each body cell in the G_1 phase has in its cytoplasm two very small structures called *centrioles* (Gr. *kentron*, related to a center or central location) because they seemingly try to take up a position in the center of the cell (Fig. 2-11A). However, they generally cannot attain this position because of the usual shape and position of the nucleus. But they get as close to the cell center as possible, so that if, for example, the nucleus is indented on one of its sides, the centrioles commonly lie in the indentation (Fig. 2-11A).

With the LM and specially prepared material, it is sometimes just barely possible to see the centrioles in a cell in the G_1 phase as two little dots. With the EM, centrioles are revealed as cylindrical structures, each of which is 0.5 μm. long and has a diameter of 0.2 μm. The walls of a centriole consist of nine longitudinally disposed bundles of *microtubules* (Fig. 2-12). Microtubules are slender, rod-like structures, 24 nm. in diameter and, as seen in high-power electron micrographs, each resembles a tubule in that its central core is less dense than its periphery, which gives each microtubule a somewhat hollow appearance. Short sections of microtubules can be seen in longitudinal section in Figure 2-17 (where they are labeled *Mt*) and in cross section in Figure 2-16 (in the region indicated by *K*). Microtubules are formed in cytoplasm from a precursor protein called *tubulin*. In a centriole cut in cross section, microtubules (as already noted) can be seen to be arranged in bundles of three, and these bundles are embedded in a finely fibrillar material (Fig. 2-12) to form the wall of the cylindrical centriole.

A cell in the G_1 phase has two centrioles arranged at right angles to each other (Fig. 2-11F). However, if the cell is in cycle, it will enter the S phase of the cycle; by the time the G_2 phase is reached a small daughter centriole will have been assembled beside, and at right angles to, each of the two original centrioles (Fig. 2-11A). Each daughter centriole grows as a result of continued microtubule formation as is shown in the longitudinal sections of centrioles in Figure 2-13A and B. As a result of the duplication of the two centrioles, there are now two pairs of centrioles (that is, a total of four) in a cell during the G_2 phase of the cell cycle (Fig. 2-11A).

Prophase

When, or even just before, the prophase begins one pair of centrioles begins to move toward one pole of the cell and the other pair toward the other (Fig. 2-11B). More or less simultaneously with this movement, what appear with the LM to be delicate fibrils sometimes form and radiate out from the region of each pair of centrioles (Fig. 2-11B). These fibrils were first seen in dividing sea urchin eggs, where their appearance suggested the light that radiates from stars, so they were called *astral* (Gr. *astron*, star) *rays* or *asters* (Fig. 2-11B). However, asters are much less prominent in dividing mammalian cells. The EM discloses that a set of microtubules now begins to form from the side of each pair of centrioles facing the other pair (Fig. 2-11B). The precise small area to one side of each pair of centrioles from which the microtubules diverge is termed a *microtubule organizing center*. The microtubules, here as elsewhere, are assembled from the precursor protein *tubulin*. As shown in Figure 2-11B, the microtubules forming here soon extend from the microtubule organizing center of one pair of centrioles to meet the microtubules extending toward them from the other. Soon the microtubules diverging from the two sites are long enough to interdigitate with with one another. In order to distinguish these microtubules from another set that soon forms, they are termed *continuous* or *interpolar microtubules* because they extend (continue) from one pole to the other. As shown in Figure 2-11B, the arrangement of the continuous microtubules (which extend from the pair of centrioles at one pole of the cell to the pair of centrioles at the other pole) is widest in its midsection and tapers toward its ends. This must have reminded someone in the past of spindles used for weaving, which were rods tapered at each end, so the structure of microtubules that forms in mitosis was called a *spindle*. Very early in

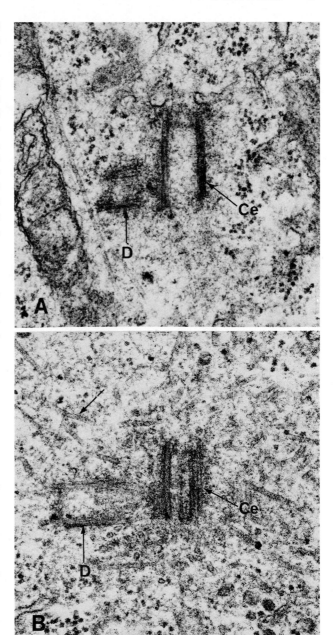

Fig. 2-13. Electron micrographs (×50,000) showing how new centrioles are formed (rat embryo ependymal cells). The cells are in interphase (*A*) and in metaphase (*B*). Two stages in the assembly of daughter centrioles (D) at right angles to mature parent centrioles (Ce) are shown. In both (*A*) and (*B*) the parent and daughter centrioles are cut in longitudinal section. The daughter centriole in (*A*) is much shorter than the parent centriole. In (*B*) the daughter centriole has grown to the same length as the parent centriole. Many microtubules (*arrow*) terminate in the region near the centrioles in (*B*). (Courtesy of J. Marshall and V. Kalnins)

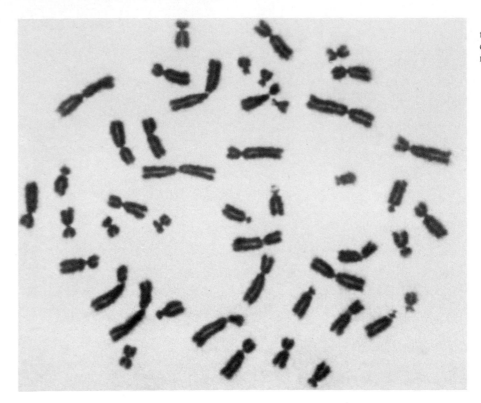

Fig. 2-14. Oil-immersion photomicrograph of the metaphase chromosomes of a normal human male. (Courtesy of C. Ford)

prophase the nuclear envelope is still intact (Fig. 2-11B) and so the spindle that is forming lies outside the nucleus (Fig. 2-11B).

But as the prophase proceeds, the nuclear envelope (the one seen with the EM) breaks up and the nucleolus or most of it, disappears as an entity (how this happens will be explained in Chap. 4). So there is now no structural barrier to prevent the developing spindle from moving into a central position in the cell, whereupon the d-chromosomes become more or less tangled in the microtubules of the spindle. Furthermore, as a result of the continuous elongation of the tubules, the two pairs of centrioles are pushed farther apart, and the cell itself also becomes elongated as a result.

At this late stage of the prophase the following situation thus pertains. The nucleus and nucleolus have both disappeared as visible entities. The cell is now more ovoid in shape, with a pair of centrioles near each of its ends. The continuous (interpolar) microtubules of the spindle now occupy the site formerly occupied by the nucleus, and the d-chromosomes of the nucleus lie in the intermicrotubular spaces of the spindle. But while this situation is developing another important event occurs, which results in the prophase giving way to the metaphase of mitosis. Describing this event requires that we discuss d-chromosomes in more detail.

Metaphase

In the prophase the d-chromosomes first become apparent in the LM as double thread-like structures (Fig. 2-3). As the prophase continues they become rod-like (Fig. 2-1, Chromosomes). The shortening and thickening of the d-chromosomes continues for a time in the metaphase so that metaphase d-chromosomes, when spread out on a slide and stained, are dense enough to be studied profitably with the LM. Spreads of human metaphase d-chromosomes can be prepared from ruptured cells (Fig. 2-14) and are much used clinically, as will be explained in Chapter 3 (page 71). As can be seen in Figure 2-14, there are differences between the various d-chromosomes in the cells of man; they show differences in length and with regard to the position of the *centromere* (Gr. *kentron* + *meros,* part). The centromere, however, is not usually in the center of the d-chromosomes. The portions of a metaphase chromosome between its centromere and its two ends are termed its *arms*. These, of course, are each double structures consisting of portions of two adjacent s-chromosomes (chromatids), as can be seen if the metaphase chromosomes in Figure 2-14 are inspected carefully. The arms of chromosomes differ in length.

The most striking feature seen with the LM in the

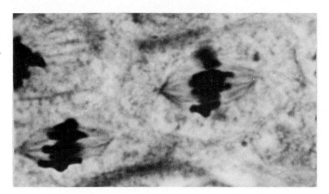

Fig. 2-15. Oil-immersion photomicrograph of cells in metaphase (rat testis, stained with iron hematoxylin). Note the mitotic spindle and the arrangement of the chromosomes in the equatorial plane of the cell. (Courtesy of Y. Clermont and C. P. Leblond)

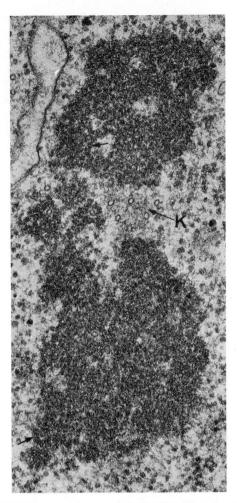

Fig. 2-16. Electron micrograph (×50,000) of a section through the centromere region of a mitotic chromosome, showing a kinetochore region (labeled K). The two dark masses represent parts of the same s-chromosome, bent around so that the two arms of the chromosome enter the plane of section. In the kinetochore region, which lies at the junction of the two arms, chromosomal microtubules cut in cross section may be seen. Note the granular appearance of the chromosome, due to its chromatin thread (visible at the two arrows as a curving thread) being sectioned innumerable times. (Courtesy of V. Kalnins)

metaphase is that all the d-chromosomes become arranged with their centromere regions in the same plane (Figs. 2-11C and 2-15). This plane is called the *equatorial plane* of the cell because, like the plane of the world's equator, it crosses from one side of the cell to the other at right angles to the longitudinal axis of the spindle. From the centromeres of the d-chromosomes arranged in this plane, the two s-chromosomes (chromatids) of each arm tend to diverge from one another and stick out to either side of the equatorial plane (Fig 2-11C). What causes the d-chromosomes to line up across the cell in this fashion? Studies with the EM disclosed a possible reason for the centromeres of d-chromosomes becoming arranged in the equatorial plane, but to describe this we have first to describe how the spindle gains a second set of microtubules.

The Fine Structure of Metaphase Chromosomes and the Development of Chromosomal Microtubules. When the LM showed the existence of a spindle during the metaphase of mitosis (as shown in Fig. 2-15), it was believed that the spindle was composed of fibrils of some sort. It was not until the spindle was studied with the EM that it was established that there were such things as microtubules and that the spindle was indeed composed of them. Furthermore, it was first assumed that all the microtubules of the spindle developed from the centrioles. However, we now know that the spindle consists of more than just the continuous microtubules, because it soon became apparent from EM studies that a second set of microtubules formed from the centromere regions of chromosomes.

As already noted, EM studies and other kinds of evidence indicate that s-chromosomes exist in the nuclei of nondividing cells in the form of long chromatin threads sufficiently condensed at intervals along their courses to

be obvious with the LM as chromatin granules (Fig 2-1). With the EM the condensed portions of s-chromosomes in working cells appear as dark granular irregularly shaped clumps of various sizes (Fig. 2-11F). When a metaphase chromosome is sectioned and examined in the EM, a slice cut through either of the two s-chromosomes of which it is composed appears as a dark fibrogranular mass with an irregular outline; two such dark masses are seen in Figure 2-16. It is believed that the granular appearance is due to the single thread-like s-chromosome

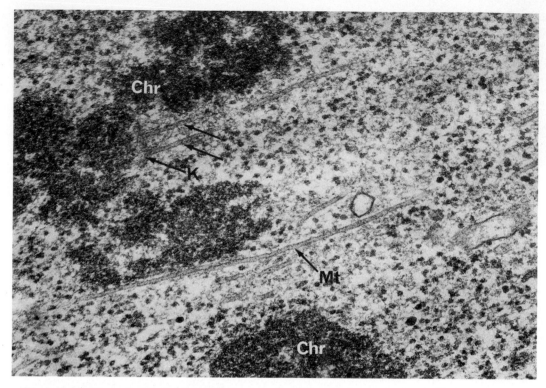

Fig. 2-17. Electron micrograph (×50,000) of a part of a cell in metaphase, showing continuous microtubules (Mt) between adjacent chromosomes (Chr) and chromosomal microtubules (*arrows*) attached to a kinetochore (K) of a chromosome. (Courtesy of V. Kalnins)

being tightly bundled and folded over its whole length in some manner so that a cut made through the mass of convoluted thread would account for its granular appearance. Further discussion about how the thread is bundled will be given in the next chapter.

In Figure 2-16, the section passed through the centromere region of the chromosome; this is seen between the two dark masses. It is labeled *K* because it shows a structure termed a *kinetochore*, one of which is present on each side of the centromere of a d-chromosome in the metaphase. The term *kinetochore* originally referred to the clear area, the centromere itself, where the two arms of each d-chromosome are joined. This was called a *kinetochore* (Gr. *kinetos*, movable; *chora*, space) because it may at first have been thought that since chromosomes had arms of different lengths it was the space that moved. But now the term is used to denote a small disk-like structure, one of which lies on each of the two sides of the centromere of a d-chromosome, where it can be seen only with the EM because it is so small. When activated, kinetochores act similarly to centrioles as microtubule-organizing centers and initiate the formation of

chromosomal (kinetochore) microtubules, some of which can be seen in cross section in Figure 2-16.

The reason for kinetochores only becoming active late in the prophase is that they cannot initiate microtubule formation until tubulin becomes available. The protein tubulin is produced in the cytoplasm, where a pool of it is present for the formation of continuous tubules. But tubulin does not become available to the kinetochores of chromosomes until the nuclear membrane disintegrates late in the prophase. So the assembly of chromosomal (kinetochore) tubules occurs later than the assembly of continuous microtubules.

The disintegration of the nuclear envelope has a second effect, for it permits the spindle consisting of continuous tubules to take up a central position in the cell (compare B and C in Fig. 2-11). At this point the d-chromosomes are enmeshed in the continuous microtubules, so that when the chromosomal microtubules grow out from each of the two kinetochores of each metaphase chromosome, they necessarily have to interdigitate with the continuous microtubules, and hence the spindle now becomes composed of two sets of microtubules (Figs. 2-17 and 2-18).

Fig. 2-18. Electron micrograph (×22,000) of part of a cell in anaphase, showing one of the poles of the mitotic spindle. A pair of centrioles (Ce), one cut in cross section and the other in oblique grazing section, are present at this pole and dense material surrounds them. Microtubules (*arrows*) of the spindle radiate out toward the densely staining chromosomes (Chr). The chromosomal microtubules are attached to the chromosomes at kinetochores (K). Rat embryo ependymal cells. (Courtesy of J. Marshall and V. Kalnins)

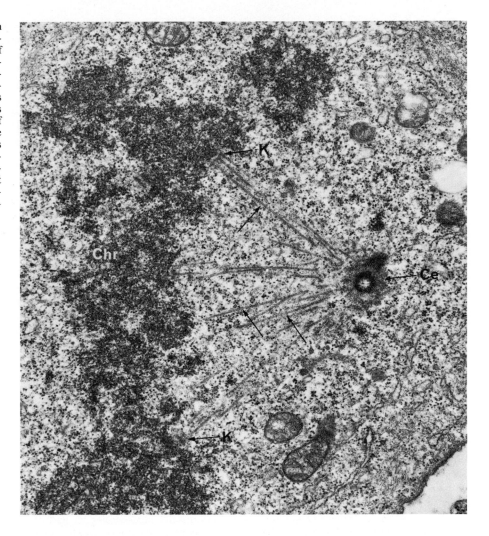

We can now theorize about how the formation and growth of chromosomal microtubules could cause the centromeres of the chromosomes to line up across the equatorial plane. The problem is perhaps similar to that of a man holding a two-part extension ladder in its middle and trying to open it in a narrow hallway. If he holds the ladder in the middle and then slides the two parts along each other to elongate the ladder, he soon finds that it has become too long to fit into the hallway any way except along its length. Furthermore, if he continues to stand in the middle of the extending ladder he finds that when the ladder is fully opened and reaches from one end of the hall to the other, he is positioned halfway between the two ends of the hall. Hence it might be thought that mechanical factors alone, due to the growth of chromosomal microtubules out from the kinetochores in opposite directions into a set (hallway) of virtually parallel continu-

ous microtubules (Figs. 2-11C and D) would tend to align the centromere regions of all the chromosomes at a position (the equatorial plane of the cell) halfway between the two ends of the spindle.

The s-chromosomes (chromatids) then begin to move from the equatorial plane toward the poles at the start of the anaphase.

Anaphase

The anaphase (Figs. 2-11D and 2-20D and E) begins with the centromere region of each of the chromosomes splitting so that the two s-chromosomes of each d-chromosome become completely separated from each other, whereupon, as already mentioned, each daughter cell will receive a set of 46 identical s-chromosomes. After the centromeres divide, half of the 92 s-

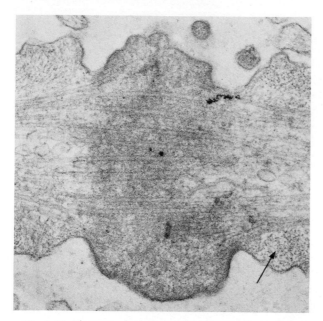

Fig. 2-19. Electron micrograph (×60,000) showing cell cleavage at the telophase stage of mitosis. A bundle of continuous microtubules, constituting the midbody, is seen here between the two daughter cells (which would lie to the left and right of the micrograph). Actin-containing filaments, cut in cross section, are indicated by the arrow; these were associated with the formation of the cleavage furrow. (Courtesy of S. Dales)

chromosomes begin to move toward one pole of the cell and the other half to the other pole. There has been much speculation through the years about how this movement occurs. The way the force for this movement toward the poles is generated is not yet understood. The recent discovery of actin-containing filaments and other muscle proteins in mitotic spindles suggests that the force pulling the chromosomes toward the poles via the chromosomal microtubules may be generated in the same way that the force for contraction is generated in muscle cells (which will be described later). As the s-chromosomes move toward the poles, the kinetochore microtubules become shorter, probably as a result of disassembly at the ends closest to the poles. One of the functions of the kinetochore microtubules may be to slow down and regulate the speed at which the chromosomes move toward the poles, so as to ensure an orderly, precisely directed separation of the chromosomes. It is interesting in this connection that chromosome movements are slow (about 1 μm. per min), compared with the faster movements characteristic of other motile systems.

It should perhaps be mentioned that mechanisms not requiring the participation of actin or other muscle protein-containing filaments have been postulated also. Here the movement of the chromosomes is thought to be brought about by sliding of the chromosomal microtubules past continuous microtubules with opposite polarity (microtubules undergo assembly at one end and disassembly from the other and hence possess a definite polarity). Models based on the concept that it is the microtubules that generate the force separating the s-chromosomes at anaphase have been proposed by McIntosh et al. (1969) and, more recently, Margolis et al.

As the chromosomes continue to separate in anaphase, there is also considerable further elongation of the mitotic spindle so that it becomes about twice as long as during metaphase. This elongation, which is thought to be the result of the continuous microtubules pushing the two ends of the spindle apart, also helps to separate the two sets of s-chromosomes.

Telophase

Toward the end of anaphase and at the beginning of telophase, a constriction begins to develop in the middle of the elongated cell (Figs. 2-11E and 2-20F and G). This constriction encircles the cell to form what is known as the *cleavage furrow*, because as it deepens it cleaves the cell into two daughter cells (Figs. 2-11F and 2-20H). At the time the cleavage furrow appears, an accumulation of actin-containing filaments also appears at this site, immediately beneath the cell membrane (Fig. 2-11E). As described when we discuss cytoplasm in Chapter 5 and muscle in Chapter 18, actin filaments are involved in contractile mechanisms but themselves are not contractile. However, it is probable that actin filaments in cooperation with other cytoplasmic components can institute a force that tightens the ring and thus makes the cleavage furrow deeper and deeper.

When the cleavage furrow deepens, a bundle of microtubules still connects the two cells that are about to separate; these constitute what is known as the *midbody* of the dividing cell (Figs. 2-11E and 2-19). Closer examination of the midbody has shown that it contains ends of microtubules embedded in a dense, fibrous type of material. Bundles of actin-containing filaments are also often seen in this region (Fig. 2-19). When cleavage is complete and the daughter cells have separated, a remnant of the midbody may remain attached to one of the two daughter cells, at the point where they separated, and persist well into the interphase.

Meanwhile, as shown in Figure 2-11F, the s-chromosomes in each daughter cell have become uncoiled to various extents to assume the form characteristic of s-chromosomes in interphase nuclei; hence they appear as chromatin granules, either packed together or dispersed. Nucleoli are re-formed as described in Chapter

4 and a new nuclear envelope is reconstituted in each daughter cell to surround the chromatin, nucleoli, and nuclear sap of the nucleus.

IDENTIFICATION WITH THE LM OF DIVIDING CELLS IN ROUTINE SECTIONS

Cells in any phase of mitosis encountered in sections are commonly said to be (or to contain) *mitotic figures.* Their presence in a section indicated that cell division was occurring in the tissue when it was obtained.

Mitotic figures are encountered in many normal body tissues until growth has been completed. Afterward they are seen in sites where cells must divide in order to maintain cell populations, as discussed earlier in this chapter. In addition, in abnormal conditions they appear in specific sites where repair of damage is in progress and also in abnormal cellular growths; such as cancer, where their prevalence is an aid to diagnosing the condition. The presence of mitotic figures in a section is so significant that learning to recognize them readily is imperative for the student of histology or histopathology.

Some Aids for Recognizing Mitotic Figures in Routine Sections

Important as it is to know the details of the mitotic process revealed by the EM and described above, one must approach the problem of identifying mitotic figures in H and E sections with the LM with the realization that only sizeable stainable structures will be obvious. Next, routine H and E sections slice through cells containing mitotic figures so they are cut in every conceivable plane; hence, it takes much hunting to find examples of the appearance commonly shown in diagrams and in which the section is cut perpendicular to the equatorial plane of the cell. Then, since in detecting mitotic figures great dependence must be placed on finding cells in which the ordinary arrangement of the chromatin of a cell in the G_1 phase is replaced by chromosomes, it must be realized that in routine sections the fixation of chromosomes is not as satisfactory as it is in spreads, and that in sections chromosomes are prone to clump together. This presents the problem of distinguishing between a mitotic figure and a nucleus of a dying or dead cell in which the chromatin commonly aggregates into a solid mass. Finally, the appearance depends on the stage of mitosis in which the cell was arrested when it was fixed.

The identification of most mitotic figures is made from seeing deeply staining chromosomes lying in the more central part of a cell (which is often pale) without their being enclosed by a nuclear envelope (*see* Fig. 2-20C, D, E and F). Furthermore, as noted above, in routine sec-

tions, the student cannot count on seeing the individual chromosomes clearly in mitotic figures, for they may be more or less clumped together to form an irregular, deeply basophilic conglomerate (Fig. 2-20C, D, E, and F). However, since either separated or clumped chromosomes stain deeply with hematoxylin, what should attract the eye as being a possible mitotic figure as one scans a section is material in a nucleus that is a deeper blue than the usual interphase nucleus in that section.

Metaphases, anaphases, and telophases are easiest to identify in cells sectioned approximately at right angles to their equatorial planes. In such sections, the appearances shown in Figure 2-20C, D, E, and F will approximately match those seen in the diagrams commonly used to illustrate mitosis. With special fixation and staining it is even possible to see a spindle in a metaphase figure (Fig. 2-15). It is easier to obtain sections of plant tissue in which dividing cells are all oriented in the same direction than it is to achieve this in animal tissues; hence sections of growing roots are commonly used for studying mitosis. But in most sections of human material, the cells of the tissue being examined are not all disposed in the same plane. Accordingly, the student has to be able to visualize how metaphases and anaphases would appear if the cells containing them were sectioned in some plane other than its long axis.

To be sure one is seeing mitotic figures, it helps to find some clear-cut example of anaphases, for an anaphase is the easiest kind of mitotic figure for the beginner (or anyone else) to identify, provided it is sectioned nearly perpendicular to the equatorial plane, as shown in Figure 2-20E. But since the chances of finding mitotic figures sectioned in this particular plane are much less than those of seeing them sectioned in other planes, it takes a lot of time and patience and the use of several sections to find mitotic figures illustrating all the stages of mitosis to good advantage. Nevertheless, if a clump of deep-staining material is seen lying in cytoplasm, often with a pale area around it and not surrounded by a nuclear membrane, and with a spiky appearance (Fig. 2-20C, D, or E) due to individual chromosomes that project from it at various angles, the chances are excellent that it is a mitotic figure. Since nuclei when they die often shrink to form a dark blue mass that might be mistaken for a mitotic figure, it should be remembered that a mass of clumped mitotic chromosomes tends to have a spiky outline (Fig. 2-20C and E) caused by individual chromosomes projecting from it.

A common mistake made by beginners is to think that two interphase nuclei lying close together could be a telophase and hence a mitotic figure. Unless good examples of earlier phases are evident in the same preparation, the presence of telophases would be unlikely.

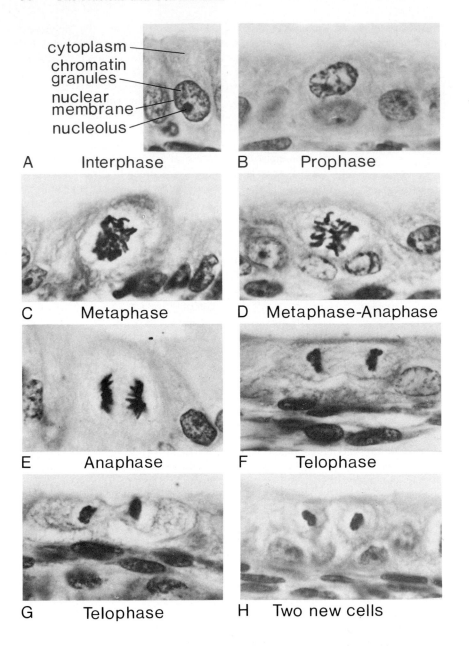

cytoplasm
chromatin
granules
nuclear
membrane
nucleolus

A   Interphase   B   Prophase

C   Metaphase   D   Metaphase-Anaphase

E   Anaphase   F   Telophase

G   Telophase   H   Two new cells

Fig. 2-20. Oil-immersion photomicrographs illustrating the various phases of mitosis. These are cells of the epithelial lining of the uterus of a rat that was injected two days previously with female sex hormone, one effect of which is to cause proliferation of these lining cells.

EFFECTS OF RADIATION ON CELL DIVISION

The manner in which radiation damages cells is very different from the way cells are injured by other kinds of physical agents. Indeed, knowing how damage results from a thermal burn or frostbite may hinder rather than help the student to understand radiation damage. For example, touching a hot stove causes local damage to skin and underlying tissue and this quickly becomes apparent. Furthermore, the damage done by heat to the skin is greatest at the surface and diminishes in relation to depth from the surface. The damage done by radiation, on the contrary, may not become apparent for a relatively long time and, furthermore, does not necessarily diminish in relation to depth from the surface; indeed, high-energy radiation may do considerably more damage below than at the skin surface.

The harmful effects of x-rays or gamma rays on living cells in their path are due to the high-energy photons of the radiation setting energetic electrons in motion in the nucleus and cytoplasm of the cells. These energetic electrons can knock other electrons out of atoms in the cell components, causing these atoms to become so intensely reactive that they immediately enter into new and generally inappropriate chemical combinations in their immediate environment, thus changing the chemical composition of the cell component with which they react.

We might now ask what effect this would have on the LM appearance of cells, such as those of the liver, with whose normal appearance we are now very familiar and which we know seldom undergo mitosis under ordinary circumstances. The answer is very little, if any at all. The same is even true of their appearance at the EM level. The reason that specialized functioning cells do not necessarily show evidence of damage from radiation that may actually have done considerable damage is explained, at least in part, as follows.

First, in a normal specialized cell only a small fraction of the genes are required to direct the synthesis of the special proteins that characterize that kind of cell. The chances of any of these particular genes being damaged would be much less than the chances of any of the more numerous unused genes in that cell being affected. Furthermore, if one or more of the active genes were damaged by the radiation, there could be undamaged duplicate genes to take over their work. Third, any chemical alterations due to intensely reactive atoms in the cytoplasm entering into new chemical combinations may be of only temporary significance if the genes directing the synthesis of new protein were unaffected, because new proteins are always being synthesized, and the altered material would soon be catabolized and replaced. So the cell could appear and continue to function very much as it did before.

The fact that cells in the interphase may appear normal but may, however, have suffered damage from radiation becomes apparent when the cells attempt to undergo mitosis, as has been shown experimentally. As previously mentioned, the cells of the liver of a normal adult animal seldom divide. But if a large portion of the liver is removed, the cells remaining soon divide actively and quickly restore the liver to its normal size. When this type operation is performed on an animal whose liver has previously been given sufficient radiation, instead of finding normal mitotic figures in the liver cells, many abnormal mitotic figures make their appearance. The same phenomenon is observed if cells proliferating in cultures are irradiated: the subsequent mitosis of cells is profoundly affected. The mitotic chromosomes may be altered in form, broken up, or joined together in abnormal ways, and fragments of them may become completely lost. The spindle, too, may show abnormalities—for example, it may have three poles instead of two, with the result that chromosomes are drawn in three ways instead of two (Fig. 2-21). The mitotic chromosomes act as if they were sticky, and in the anaphase the s-chromosomes (chroma-

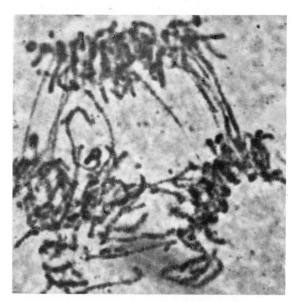

Fig. 2-21. Oil-immersion photomicrograph of an L cell in mitosis (squash preparation) following 5,000 rads of x-rays. The spindle in this cell has three poles instead of two, and many of the chromosomes are lagging, forming *chromosomal bridges.* Many of the chromosomes are of an abnormal form. (Till, J. E., and Whitmore, G. F.: Effects of x-rays on mammalian cells in tissue culture. *In* Proc. 3rd Canadian Cancer Res. Conf., New York, Academic Press, 1959)

tids) do not pull apart from one another evenly. Some may lag behind and form bridges between the two groups of chromosomes (Fig. 2-21).

The chromosomes may divide without the nucleus dividing; this gives rise to large nuclei with more than the normal number of chromosomes. In the last instance, the cells affected may become much larger than normal.

A possible reason why radiation damage to cells becomes apparent when cells attempt to undergo mitosis is that this is the first time that all the damage done to the chromatin of the interphase cell has the opportunity to manifest itself. As already described, the genes of cells have to be duplicated before a cell undergoes division, and, to accomplish this, the two strands of every DNA molecule have to separate, each strand thereupon serving as a template for the synthesis of a second strand. Two complete double-stranded molecules thereby become available to provide the double number of genes required for the two daughter cells that soon form (Figs. 2-5 and 2-6). To understand why undisclosed damage to DNA should become apparent at the time of mitosis, it should be reiterated that, in its ordinary work, a cell uses only a small fraction of its total number of genes—only those required to direct the protein synthesis required in that particular kind of cell. The great majority of the genes of most functioning cells are not used. But before a cell can divide, every molecule of the very large amount of DNA of the cell (only some of which was previously used in interphase) has to be duplicated in the S phase, and it is then that the changed portion of the DNA molecule prevents correct duplication in the complementary strands. If the damage is severe enough, it becomes apparent as broken chromosomes or abnormal mitotic figures. It can be so serious that all attempts at mitosis are unsuccessful and cell division ceases. Even a single chromosome break is considered potentially able to destroy the proliferative capacity of a cell.

This is part of the rationale for using radiation in the treatment of cancer. The aim is not primarily to kill cancer cells in the interphase but to damage them in such a way that they become unable to undergo successful mitosis, thereby slowing or stopping their further growth. Furthermore, radiation can be delivered in ingenious ways so that the site of a tumor receives more than the patient's surrounding or nearby tissues. This, of course, is desirable because radiation inhibits the proliferation of all the patient's cells (normal and cancer cells) in the irradiated area.

Mutagenic Effects

Sometimes radiation does not do enough damage to prevent a cell from undergoing mitosis. However, it may still affect the genetic material so that it becomes slightly altered. The altered gene or genes may not affect DNA duplication as a whole, so mitosis can be normal, but when the altered genes duplicate as a prelude to mitosis, their altered character is also duplicated. Thus the descendents of the affected cell will also have the qualities imparted by the altered genes that have duplicated. This is the way in which radiation, in doses that are not lethal to a cell, can induce cell *mutations*. A mutation in a body cell caused this way can initiate cancer, as occurred all too often in those who worked with x-rays before the danger of ionizing radiation was known. Moreover, a mutation resulting from the irradiation of germ cells can result in an anomaly in an offspring, which is then said to be a *mutant*.

What Is Meant by "Sensitivity to Radiation"

This term is often misunderstood for the following reasons.

First, under different environmental conditions the same kinds of cells receiving the same dose of radiation can suffer different amounts of damage to their DNA. A very important factor influencing the amount of damage done to cells by radiation is oxygen tension. Cells in sites of high tension are more sensitive to radiation than those in regions of low oxygen tension.

Second, it was once thought that cells were more sensitive to radiation when it was given while they were in mitosis. While this is occasionally true in certain cells of some species, it is not true of the same kinds of cells in other species. Therefore, no generalization should be made.

Third, it could be said that cells remaining in the interphase for long periods, or even for life, are less sensitive to radiation than those kinds of cells that divide frequently, because the former kind do not pass into the stage (mitosis) in which the lethal effects of radiation become operative. However, where the cell turnover rate is equal, all kinds of body cells in the same environment are about equally sensitive to radiation (at any phase of the cell cycle).

Finally, it could be said that tissues in which there is a very rapid turnover of the cell population are more sensitive to radiation than tissues in which there is a slow cell turnover. It is well known, for example, that in total body irradiation, much more damage is done to the lining of the small intestine and to the blood-cell-forming tissues than to tissues in which there is a slow or no cell turnover. However this is not because more cells are damaged due to their being in mitosis at the time of irradiation. More damage is done to cells with a high turnover rate because the population of cells in these tissues must be maintained through constant and rapid proliferation so as to produce new cells. Since radiation injures cells so that they cannot successfully negotiate mitosis, irradiation greatly slows the production of new cells to replace those with a short life span. Since the cells lining the intestine normally live for only a few days and certain white cells of the blood important in protecting the body from bacterial infections also live for only a few days, severe total body irradiation stops the lining of the intestine from being adequately maintained and causes the numbers of at least one kind of white cell in the blood to drop precipitously to almost zero. Hence tissues in which the cell turnover rate is high can be said to be more susceptible (sensitive) to radiation than tissues in which cell turnover is slow, but it should be clearly understood that the cells concerned are not more sensitive to radiation; rather, the tissues concerned are sensitive to anything that interferes with the constant production of new cells.

EFFECT OF COLCHICINE ON MITOSIS

An alkaloid, *colchicine* (extracted from the corm of a species of crocus, *Colchicum autumnale*) has two remarkable biological properties. The first meant a lot to those who suffered from gout, because colchicine was the first drug found that effectively relieved the excruciatingly painful inflammation of joints that occurs in this condition. However, the second effect is of more general interest, because colchicine has the remarkable effect of arresting the process of mitosis. In the presence of colchicine, the mitotic spindle is not formed, and therefore the s-chromosomes of dividing cells do not separate from one another. The chromosomes, however, continue to condense; hence, metaphase d-chromosomes seen after colchicine treatment are both shorter and thicker than normal (Fig. 2-22).

The EM helped to elucidate the mechanism by which colchicine arrests both mitosis and the progress of gouty lesions of joints. Colchicine prevents the formation of microtubules because it binds to the subunits of microtubule protein (tubulin) and prevents them from being assembled into microtubules. As a consequence, in the presence of colchicine, *microtubule formation is inhibited.*

In mitosis, colchicine inhibits the formation of both continuous and chromosomal microtubules. Hence there is nothing to push the two pairs of centrioles apart to the two poles of the cell. As a consequence, the d-chromosomes arrange themselves in a sphere around the two pairs of centrioles at the cell center and continue to shorten. In sections this arrangement of chromosomes resembles a mitotic figure and has been called a *colchicine metaphase* or a *C-metaphase* (Fig. 2-22). This effect of colchicine is reversible. When treated cells are no longer subjected to its influence, a typical spindle can form. A true metaphase follows in which the d-chromosomes become typically aligned at the equator of the spindle, followed by normal separation of the s-chromosomes from one another.

Drugs With Similar Effects on Cell Proliferation.

Certain other drugs have also been found to act in the same manner by preventing spindle formation and hence arresting cell proliferation. Two alkaloids, *vincristine* and *vinblastine*, both of which can be isolated from the periwinkle plant, have been used in treating patients with certain kinds of malignant growths in order to slow or prevent further growth and thus constitute part of the current armamenterium for treating cancer by chemotherapy. It should be appreciated, however, that drugs such as these, that inhibit the assembly of microtubules, act in a different manner from radiation in arresting cell multiplication.

Effect of Colchicine in Gout

The way colchicine alleviates the painful joint lesions of gout also deserves mention here. *Gout* is a metabolic disorder (with a familial tendency) in which *uric acid*, a

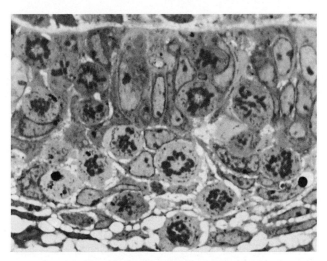

Fig. 2-22. Photomicrograph showing C-metaphases in preameloblasts and preodontoblasts of a tooth (stained with toluidine blue). This tissue was obtained from an animal 8 hours after the injection of colchicine and shows a high proportion of dividing cells trapped in a typical metaphase-like configuration. A good example is seen below *center.* (Courtesy of C. Smith)

product of purine metabolism, is not excreted rapidly enough to prevent its level rising in the blood, and under these conditions *sodium urate crystals* tend to be deposited in joint tissues. The commonest site, or at least the classic example, is in the proximal joint of the big toe. However, sodium urate crystals by themselves would not cause painful inflammation. The severe inflammation characterizing gout is due to the invasion of the affected tissues by certain white blood cells that enter the area and attempt to engulf and otherwise destroy the crystals; it is this cellular invasion that causes the acute inflammation. Colchicine prevents the formation of microtubules in these white blood cells, and without microtubules in their cytoplasm they are unable to function properly and hence cannot invade the joint tissue. This same effect on microtubules also prevents the white cells from releasing enzymes that aggravate inflammation. As a result, the administration of colchicine can alleviate or prevent the acute painful inflammation of joints, but it can also lead to undesirable diminished microtubule formation elsewhere. There are now other drugs that prevent gout by either decreasing the production of uric acid or by facilitating its excretion.

The Use of Colchicine in the Clinical Diagnosis of Chromosome Anomalies

The ability of colchicine to arrest mitosis at a stage when chromosomes are most easily identified is of great importance in another clinical area. Cells obtained, for instance, from a person's blood can be induced to proliferate in vitro, and the mitoses so obtained can be arrested with colchicine. The fact that preparations of mitotic d-chromosomes can thus be so readily obtained and studied has facilitated the development of the very important subject of medical genetics, as will be described in the next chapter.

The Use of Colchicine in Studying Cell Turnover

If a suitable dose of colchicine is injected into an animal, or added to a culture of cells in which proliferation is occurring, any cells that enter mitosis after the colchicine has taken effect cannot complete it, and as a result, mitotic figures accumulate until the drug is withdrawn. If, however, at some time before the concentration of colchicine decreases, mitotic figures are counted, the number of cells entering mitosis over the period of time allowed for the experiment can be determined. In those tissues and organs in the body in which cell proliferation is matched by cell loss or death, it is thus possible to use colchicine to estimate the turnover rate of the cell population by determining the proportion of cells that enter mitosis over a given period of time. This method, however, has now been largely superseded by the use of radioautography, an important general method that has so many applications in cell biology that it must be described in considerable detail and hence will be dealt with in the next chapter.

REFERENCES AND OTHER READING

The order of the headings follows that in which various matters are dealt with in the text (for references on the chromatin of the interphase nucleus, *see* Chap. 4).

Cell Cycle in Relation to Cell Populations and Their Turnover*

Altman, G. G., and Enesco, M.: Cell number as a measure of distribution and renewal of epithelial cells in the small intestine of growing adult rats. Am. J. Anat., *121:*319, 1967.
Beserga, R. (ed.): The Cell Cycle and Cancer. New York, Marcel Dekker, 1971.
Baserga, R.: Multiplication and Division in Mammalian Cells. The Biochemistry of Disease: A Series of Monographs, *6.* New York, Marcel Dekker, 1976.
Bertalanffy, F. D., and Lau, C.: Cell renewal. Int. Rev. Cytol., *9:*357, 1962.
Cairnie, A. B., Lala, P. K., and Osmond, D. G. (eds.): Stem Cells of Renewing Cell Populations. New York, Academic Press, 1976.

Clarkson, B., and Baserga, R. (eds.).: Control of Proliferation in Animal Cells. Cold Spring Harbor Conferences on Cell Proliferation, vol. *1.* Cold Spring Harbor Laboratory, 1974.
Fry, R. J. M., Griem, M. L., and Kirsten, W. H. (eds.): Normal and Malignant Cell Growth. New York, Springer-Verlag, 1969.
Goss, R. T.: Turnover in Cells and Tissues. *In* Prescott, D. M., Goldstein, L., and McConkey, E. (eds.): Advances in Cell Biology. vol. 1. New York, Appleton-Century-Crofts, 1970.
Leblond, C. P., Clermont, Y., and Nadler, N. J.: The pattern of stem cell renewal in three epithelia (esophagus, intestine and testis). Can. Cancer Res. Conf. (Pergamon Press), *7:*3, 1967.
Leblond, C. P., and Walker, B. E.: Renewal of cell populations. Physiol. Rev., *30:*255, 1956.
Marques-Pereira, J. P., and Leblond, C. P.: Mitosis and differentiation in the stratified squamous epithelium of the rat esophagus. Am. J. Anat., *117:*73, 1965.
Prescott, D. M.: Reproduction of Eukaryotic Cells. New York, Academic Press, 1976.
Stohlman, F., Jr.: The Kinetics of Cellular Proliferation. New York, Grune & Stratton, 1959.

Mitosis: Centrioles and Microtubules

Brinkley, B. R., and Stubblefield, E.: Ultrastructure and Interaction of the Kinetochore and Centriole in Mitosis and Meiosis. *In* Prescott, D. M., Goldstein, L., and McConkey, E. (eds.): Advances in Cell Biology, vol. 1. New York, Appleton-Century-Crofts, 1970.
Forer, A.: Actin filaments and birefringent spindle fibers during chromosome movements. *In* Goldman, R., Pollard, T. and Rosenbaum, J. (eds.): Cell Motility, Book C, Microtubules and Related Proteins. Cold Spring Harbor Conferences on Cell Proliferation, vol 3. p. 1273, 1976.
Fulton, C.: Centrioles. *In* Reinert, J., and Ursprung, H. (eds.): Origin and Continuity of Cell Organelles. vol 2, p. 170. New York, Springer-Verlag, 1971.
Margolis, R. L., Wilson, L., and Keifer, B. I.: Mitotic mechanism based on intrinsic microtubule behaviour. Nature, *272:*450, 1978.
McIntosh, J. R., Cande, W. Z., and Snyder, J. A.: Structure and physiology of the mammalian mitotic spindle. *In* Inoué, S., and Stephens, R. E. (eds.): Molecules and Cell Movement, vol. 30, p. 31. Society for General Physiologists Series, New York, Raven Press, 1975.
McIntosh, J. R., et al.: Fibrous elements of the mitotic spindle. *In* Goldman, R., Pollard, T., and Rosenbaum, J. (eds.): Cell Motility, Book C, Microtubules and Related Proteins. Cold Spring Harbor Conferences on Cell Proliferation, vol 3, p. 1261. 1976.
Niklas, R. B.: Chromosome movement: current models and experiments on living cells. *In* Inoué, S. and Stephens, R. E. (eds.): Molecules and Movement. vol. 30, p. 97. Society for General Physiologists Series. New York, Raven Press, 1975.
Porter, K. R.: Cytoplasmic microtubules and their functions. *In* Wolstenholme, G. E. W., and O'Connor, M. (eds.): Principles of Biomolecular Organization. Ciba Foundation Symposium. London, J. and Churchill, A. Ltd., 1966.
Schroeder, T. E.: Dynamics of the contractile ring. *In* Inoué, S., and Stephens, R. E. (eds.): Molecules and Movement. vol. 30, p. 305. Society for General Physiologists Series. New York, Raven Press, 1975.

---

* *See also* the references on the study of the cell cycle lineages by labeling DNA at the end of Chapter 3.

Szollosi, D.: Cortical cytoplasmic filaments of cleaving eggs: A structural element corresponding to the contractile ring. J. Cell Biol., *44:*192, 1970.

Effects of Radiation on Chromosomes and Cells

Bender, M. A., and Wolff, S.: X-ray induced chromosome aberration and reproductive death in mammalian cells. Am. Naturalist, *95:*39, 1961.

Cellular Radiation Biology. A collection of papers presented at the 18th Annual Symposium on Fundamental Cancer Research, 1964, U. of Texas, M. D. Anderson Hospital and Tumor Institute. Baltimore, Williams & Wilkins, 1965.

Elkind, M. M., and Whitmore, G. F.: The Radiobiology of Cultured Mammalian Cells. New York, Gordon and Breach, 1967.

Evans, H. J.: Chromosome aberrations induced by ionizing radiations. Int. Rev. Cytol., *13:*221, 1962.

Wolff, S.: Chromosome aberrations. *In* Hollaender, A. (ed.): Radiation Protection and Recovery. pp. 157-174, New York, Pergamon Press, 1960.

Mitotic Inhibitors

Borgers, M., and DeBrabander, M. (eds.): Microtubules and Microtubule Inhibitors. Amsterdam, North Holland, 1975.

Borisy, G. G., and Taylor, E. W.: The mechanism of action of colchicine. Binding of colchicine-H[3] to cellular protein. J. Cell Biol., *34:*525, 1967.

Brinkley, B. R., Stubblefield, E., and Hsu, T. C.: The effects of colcemid inhibition and reversal on the fine structure of the mitotic apparatus of Chinese hamster cells in vitro. J. Ultrastruct. Res., *19:*1, 1967.

Stevens Hooper, C.: Use of colchicine for measurement of mitotic rate in the intestinal epithelium. Am. J. Anat., *108:*231, 1961.

3 The Nucleus in Dividing Cells: Radioautography, Chromosome Classification, and Meiosis

In this chapter we discuss (*1*) how the DNA of chromosomes can be labeled in the S phase of the cell cycle so as to permit the turnover time of cells to be determined by radioautography and the life history of labeled cells to be traced; (*2*) the fine structure of metaphase chromosomes; (*3*) how every metaphase chromosome of the cells of man can be recognized with the LM and deviations from the normal (that is, chromosomal anomalies) can be diagnosed; and (*4*) the process of division (meiosis) in the germ cells of the female and the causes of some chromosome anomalies.

RADIOAUTOGRAPHY (AUTORADIOGRAPHY)

Radioautography is a relatively modern histological method that has enormously increased the scope of what could be learned by means of both light and electron microscopy. It is very much a modern method because it followed the developments in nuclear physics leading to the production of radioactive isotopes of various elements. In particular it required the production of isotopes of elements that were used by cells or could be attached to the substances used by cells and that could be injected safely into animals, or added to cultures, in amounts that would not interfere with the normal metabolism of cells. Since the radioactive isotope (or substance labeled with one) would enter into reactions in the same way as its nonradioactive counterpart, and at the same time emit radiation, the isotopes could be followed through the body with the various means for detecting radioactivity. One way of detecting radioactivity is based on its capacity to affect photographic film similarly to light. Radiation, however, penetrates the black wrappings used to protect film from light and affects it in the same manner as exposure to light. This explains a common practice in hospital and laboratory areas where x-ray machines or radioactive isotopes are used, for the personnel each carry a piece of photographic film shielded from light in their pockets while they work. These are regularly developed and renewed to ensure that no one on the staff is being exposed to excessive radiation.

The histological method for detecting radiation from radioactive isotopes in sectioned tissues for study with either the LM or the EM is to coat them in the darkroom with a special type of photographic emulsion and then store them in the dark for a period of time. They are then developed in the dark and fixed. As will be described in detail later, sites in the section where a radioactive isotope is present will have affected the emulsion over them and hence will appear as dark "grains" over the sites from which the radioactivity emanated. Such a preparation is called a *radioautograph* (Gr. *radio,* ray-like; *autos,* self; and *graphō,* to write). Just as a photograph (Gr. *photos,* light) refers to a record made by light, a radioautograph means a record made by rays emanating from something.

At first, only a few radioactive isotopes were available for radioautography; for example, radioactive phosphorus was an important one used in many early studies. Later, a large number became available, most notably *tritium* (*^{3}H*), a radioactive isotope of hydrogen. In due course, it became possible to incorporate ^{3}H into many different kinds of chemical compounds utilized by cells. Thus it became possible to use for radioautography not only radioactive isotopes of various elements, such as those of calcium, phosphorus, iron, and iodine (all of which enter into various cellular or tissue activities), but also innumerable other compounds concerned in cell metabolism that could also be labeled with ^{3}H.

Radioautography has thus had, and is still having, very wide application in studying what and where particular biochemical reactions occur in various parts of the body, as will be described in subsequent chapters. Here we shall concern ourselves with how one of the components of DNA can be labeled with ^{3}H and used to show where and when new DNA is synthesized in the cell cycle. We shall also explain how this method labels chromosomes for radioautographic studies so that the subsequent history of the labeled chromosomes can be followed.

Some Details About the Technic of Radioautography

Precursors and Products. The chemicals labeled with a radioactive isotope that are used to investigate biological processes are celled *precursors.* Precursors are commonly substances, similar to those available from foods, that serve as building blocks for tissue components and become incorporated into complex constituents of cells and tissues in the same way as unlabeled building blocks are incorporated. The tissue constituent into which a labeled precursor is incorporated is called a *product*, which, of course, thereafter emits radiation. Precursors are usually soluble, whereas the products commonly are not. Hence, in fixing and sectioning tissue taken from an animal given a labeled precursor, any precursor still present is washed away because it is soluble, while insoluble products remain. Any radioactivity detected in a section, therefore, is due to the presence of label in a product locked in position by fixation.

To detect sites of radioactive products in a section, advantage is taken of the fact that they serve as point sources of radiation, and the emission of electrons from them will affect photographic emulsion placed above the section. There are several methods for applying photographic emulsion to sections or spreads of whole cells. The method now most commonly used was developed by Bélanger and Leblond in Leblond's laboratory in 1946, and its development marked the birth of modern radioautography.

Tissue from animals given some kind of labeled building block (precursor) is fixed and sectioned. Indeed, the section may even be stained, but no substance capable of inhibiting the response of the emulsion, such as heavy metallic salts, should be present in the fixative or stain used. The sections are then coated in a darkroom with photographic emulsion and dried. The coated sections are left in a lightproof box for a suitable time, during which each minute amount of isotope in the section acts as a point source of radiation, bringing about ionization of the silver atoms in each crystal of silver bromide in the emulsion hit by the emitted rays. The preparation is subsequently developed and fixed like an ordinary photographic negative, and a coverslip is added (Fig. 3-1). The crystals of silver bromide that have been hit appear as little dark dots, which are commonly called *grains* (Fig. 3-1). The sites of grains in the emulsion indicate radioactivity in the sites beneath them, and indeed, by using beta emitters with short tracks, very thin sections and thin layers of emulsion, the grains seen can be related to the particular cell or tissue component directly (or almost directly) under them.

Some Factors Concerned in Obtaining Precise Localization of Radioactive Isotopes in Sections

Since a radioactive label in a tissue section serves as a point source of radiation, it gives off rays in all directions. If the label used is a high-energy emitter such as ^{32}P, an emitter of beta particles (that is, electrons) endowed with

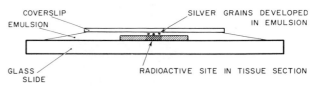

Fig. 3-1. Diagram illustrating how a radioautograph is prepared by the coating technic.

high energy, the localization in the cell spread or section is not very precise, because not only do the electrons emitted at right angles to the section affect the emulsion directly above the label, but the electrons given off by the point source at other angles also reach the emulsion even though they have to travel longer distances to reach it. Hence the emulsion for considerable distances on either side of the emitter is affected, and as a consequence the site of the label cannot be localized with precision. It is therefore desirable to use low-energy beta emitters, since they give off electrons with short tracks, which ideally are only long enough to reach emulsion directly above the label and not long enough to reach the emulsion if they extend off at various angles from the point source. This is an important reason why ^3H is so commonly used for radioautography: the electrons that it emits have a low average energy (5.7 KeV), which gives them a range in water of about 1 micrometer. It is therefore obvious that some of the emission from ^3H in the deeper part of anything except a very thin section would not reach the emulsion at all; hence, it is desirable to have the emulsion as close as possible to the tissue components in the section, and the sections of a thickness so that only the short tracks of the emitted particles passing at right angles through the section will reach the emulsion. Under optimal conditions, the emitter sites will be under the dots seen in the developed emulsion.

The Kinds of Labeled Building Blocks Used for Labeling Different Chemical Compounds of Tissues

Proteins. The usual precursor used to label newly forming protein is an amino acid, for example, leucine, into which ^3H has been incorporated. Since collagen contains proline, this particular amino acid labeled with ^3H is an excellent precursor to use to label collagen that is being synthesized.

Carbohydrates. The synthesis of glycogen can be followed by using glucose labeled with ^3H. If, after injection of labeled glucose, some radioactivity is present in control radioautographs but absent from sections that are first treated with the enzyme α-amylase, which breaks

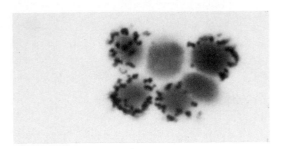

Fig. 3-2. Radioautograph of a smear of bone marrow cells obtained from an animal given radioactive iron. Since iron is a component of hemoglobin, cells synthesizing hemoglobin (precursors of red blood cells) can be identified.

down glycogen, the radioactivity observed is attributed to this polysaccharide. Radioactivity remaining in sections after α-amylase treatment is usually due to incorporation of labeled glucose into glycoproteins, proteoglycans, or glycosaminoglycans (to be described in later chapters), since glucose may be incorporated into these products as well as into glycogen.

Lipids. The synthesis of lipids may be investigated by radioautography after injection of labeled acetate or other suitable precursors. However, care must be taken to avoid dissolving out the lipids in the course of histological processing.

Inorganic Substances. The calcium phosphate deposited in cartilage or bone can be labeled with radioactive isotopes of either calcium or phosphorus (*see* Fig. 15-51). The iron that enters into the formation of the hemoglobin of developing red blood cells can be labeled with a radioactive isotope of iron (Fig. 3-2), and this is much used in the study of certain blood diseases. The hormones of the thyroid gland have iodine as one of their components, and so it is possible to follow their formation by administering a radioactive isotope of iodine, as described in Chapter 25 (p. 803).

THE STUDY OF DNA SYNTHESIS BY THE USE OF A RADIOACTIVE LABEL AND RADIOAUTOGRAPHY

Why Labeled Thymidine Is Used

The two new strands of DNA formed when a DNA molecule is duplicated (Fig. 2-6) must be synthesized out of simpler ingredients. Obviously, if one of these ingredients were to be labeled with a radioactive isotope, the synthesis of new DNA could be studied by the radioautographic method. In choosing a precursor of DNA for labeling purposes, the most important consideration is finding and using one that would not be incorporated into any other product synthesized by cells. The advantage of

using a specific precursor is that all the labeling seen in cells after incorporation of such a labeled precursor would reside in DNA. It so happens that the only product in which thymine is found in the body is DNA, and so thymine would perhaps seem to be an ideal precursor to label for study of DNA synthesis. However, pure thymine is not incorporated into newly forming DNA molecules; it is only when it is attached to sugar that it becomes incorporated. Sugar does not become attached to thymine given to an animal; it can only become attached to thymine while thymine is being synthesized in cells. However, if thymine already attached to sugar (and this is called *thymidine*) is given an animal, the thymidine will be incorporated into new DNA as it is being synthesized. So thymidine labeled with tritium is universally used to label specifically any new DNA that is being synthesized.

Since both of the original strands of a DNA molecule serve as a template against which a new strand is synthesized (Figs. 2-5 and 2-6), each one of the two doublestranded molecules of DNA resulting from DNA synthesis has one old and one new strand, as shown in Figure 2-6. If labeled thymidine is available during the period of DNA synthesis, the thymine appearing in each of the new strands is labeled; this is indicated in Figure 3-3 by an asterisk beside the T that represents the thymine carrying the label. The preexisting thymine on the old strands would of course not be labeled.

An important point to appreciate from the foregoing is that when labeled thymidine is sufficiently abundant, every new two-stranded molecule of DNA forming when it is available would incorporate some label. But the label would be present only in the *new* strand of each DNA molecule and not in the strand that was part of the previous DNA molecule. Hence, when a cell enters the process of mitosis, after doubling its DNA when the label was available, all the chromosomes of both daughter cells will carry the label, because every molecule of the DNA of which they are composed would carry some label in one of its two strands (the recently formed strand synthesized in the presence of the label). And even though labeled thymidine is incorporated only into newly forming strands of DNA, it labels DNA very satisfactorily for radioautographic studies of DNA synthesis. It is, for instance, possible to see the label over chromosomes of cells that took up labeled thymidine during the S phase and then entered mitosis. Figure 3-4 shows the way silver grains appear over and immediately beside chromosomes in a radioautograph of a spread of a mitotic cell, in which DNA synthesis took place during the preceding S phase in the presence of labeled thymidine. More commonly the label is seen over interphase cells. If the interval between giving labeled thymidine and obtaining the cells is short, label is found over cells that have not yet entered mitosis and so are still in G_2 (Figs. 3-5 and 3-6). If, however, the

Fig. 3-3. Diagram showing that if tritiated thymidine is available while the two new strands of DNA are being synthesized during the S phase (that is, the interval between the times corresponding to Figs. 2-5 and 2-6), thymine synthesized in each of the two new strands of DNA will be labeled. The label (tritium) is indicated in this figure and in Figure 3-7 by an asterisk.

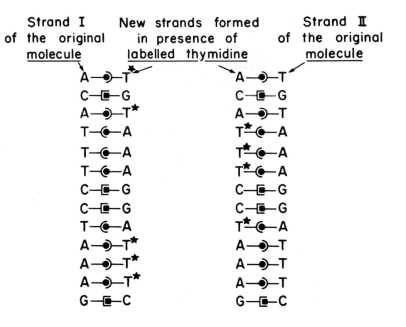

Strand I of the original molecule	New strands formed in presence of labelled thymidine	Strand II of the original molecule
A—●—T*		A—●—T
C—▣—G		C—▣—G
A—●—T*		A—●—T
T—◖—A		T*—◖—A
T—◖—A		T*—◖—A
T—◖—A		T*—◖—A
C—▣—G		C—▣—G
C—▣—G		C—▣—G
T—◖—A		T*—◖—A
A—●—T*		A—●—T
A—●—T*		A—●—T
A—●—T*		A—●—T
G—▣—C		G—▣—C

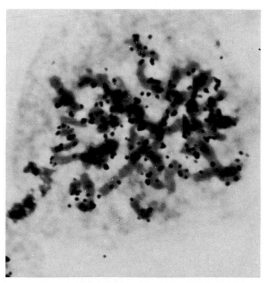

Fig. 3-4. LM radioautograph of a spread preparation of a cell from a culture given tritium-labeled thymidine. The labeled thymidine was taken up as the DNA was duplicated, and enough time elapsed for the cell to enter mitosis (metaphase). The dark grains over the chromosomes are due to the short tracks of beta particles (from the tritium) causing ionization in the overlying photographic emulsion. (Stanners, C. P., and Till, J. E.: Acta Biochim. Biophys., *37:*406, 1960)

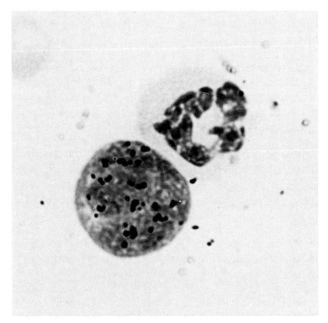

Fig. 3-5. LM radioautograph of two cells of bone marrow of a guinea pig, obtained 2 hours after the injection of tritiated thymidine. Note the black grains overlying the darker cell. Because of the track length of the beta particles emanating from the tritium, some of the grains lie outside the limits of its rounded interphase nucleus, which is located somewhat eccentrically. The light-staining cell at *upper right* (a neutrophil) is not labeled with the isotope. (Courtesy of D. Osmond and S. Miller)

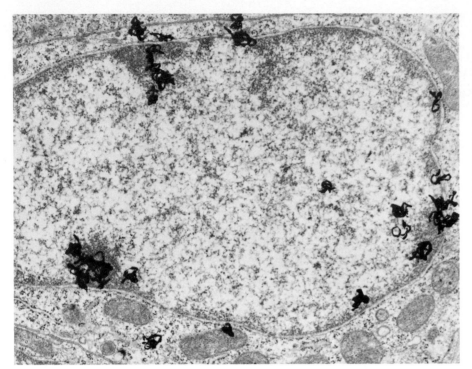

Fig. 3-6. EM radioautograph (×9,500) of an interphase epithelial cell in a crypt of small intestine, taken from a mouse soon after injection with tritium-labeled thymidine. Note the characteristic EM appearance of silver grains (black squiggles at *top, right,* and *lower* margins of the nucleus). Most of these lie over the nucleus or very close to it; they predominate over the peripheral chromatin attached to the inner aspect of the nuclear envelope. (Cheng, H., and Leblond, C. P.: Am. J. Anat., *141:*537, 1974)

cells are taken some time after giving labeled thymidine, labeled cells may have already passed through mitosis and entered G_1. Figure 3-5 is an LM radioautograph showing two interphase cells of bone marrow obtained shortly after injecting labeled thymidine into an animal. Here silver grains indicate incorporation of labeled thymidine into the DNA of one of the cells, which was in S phase at the time of labeling. Although some grains lie outside the limits of its nucleus (a result of the track length of beta particles), the label is clearly confined to one of the cells and is lacking from the other. The tritium label can be localized more precisely in cells by EM radioautography. In the EM, silver grains appear as electron-dense, characteristically squiggly areas. In Figure 3-6 they may be seen lying predominantly over the peripheral chromatin on the inner aspect of the nuclear envelope (a site occupied in the interphase by much of the nuclear DNA), again indicating that labeled thymidine was incorporated into the DNA of this interphase nucleus during the S phase when the cell was exposed to labeled thymidine.

Various Ways in Which Labeling Nuclei With Radioactive Thymidine Has Furthered Knowledge

Determination of Mitotic Activity. Before labeled thymidine became available, the extent of cell division occurring in tissues during their growth, repair, or maintenance

was commonly estimated by taking sections at different times after the injection of colchicine (described in Chap. 2) and counting the numbers of mitotic figures present. However, as noted, mitotic figures are sometimes difficult to identify, particularly when they are cut in planes other than the long axis of the cells that are dividing.

In experimental work, a more accurate estimate of the extent to which cell division is occurring in any given tissue is obtained after injecting an animal with labeled thymidine. An appropriate time is allowed for this precursor to become incorporated into replicating DNA, after which the tissue to be examined is removed and fixed and radioautographs are prepared.

Since it typically takes about 7 to 8 hours for a cell to double its DNA, it can be reasoned that, in radioautographs made from a tissue taken immediately after being subjected to labeled thymidine for, say, an hour, three general categories of cells would be labeled:

1. Cells that were in the stage of DNA duplication during the whole hour.

2. Cells that entered the stage of DNA duplication during the hour and so were exposed to the labeled thymidine for only the latter part of the hour.

3. Cells that were in the last stages of DNA duplication and finished it during the hour, so that they took up labeled thymidine for only the first part of the hour.

The period during which the cells are subjected to labeled thymidine in this type of experiment must be kept short (usually 1 hr.) so that there is not enough time for any labeled cells to have passed through mitosis, for if any labeled cells had time to divide, there would be two labeled interphase cells that could be counted instead of one. If the time is kept short, every cell labeled in the radioautograph marks a cell that is destined to undergo mitosis in the next few hours. This gives the same kind of information obtained by counting mitotic figures because it indicates the extent to which cell division is occurring in a tissue; but quantitatively, the counts would not be the same. In order to explain this, however, we shall make two assumptions: first, that it would be possible to count every mitotic figure in a section of tissue from an experimental animal and, second, that this animal was given labeled thymidine for one hour immediately before the tissue was obtained. In a radioautograph prepared from the same tissue, the labeled thymidine, as already noted, would be found only in cells that happened to be in some part of the S phase during the 1-hour exposure period. Since mitosis can take up to one and a half hours to complete, a count of mitotic figures in an ordinary section should indicate all the cells that were still in mitosis at the end of a 1.5-hour period. There would be more mitotic figures in the ordinary section than there would be labeled nuclei in the corresponding radioautograph because cells that had just begun mitosis before the hour's exposure to thymidine would not yet have finished mitosis before the section was taken, and so would still be counted, as well as all those cells that had entered mitosis during the 1-hour period when thymidine was available. Incidentally, none of the labeled cells in the radioautograph would appear as mitotic figures, since not even cells that were close to the end of the S phase at the beginning of the hour during which the thymidine was available would have had enough time after acquiring label to have begun mitosis before the hour was up; hence no labeled cells would be in mitosis when the tissue was obtained.

Establishing the Kinds of Cells That Provide New Cells in Growth, Repair, and Maintenance of Cell Populations; Tracing Cell Lineages by Radioautography. It is not as easy as might be thought to determine, in tissues where there is a mixture of cell types, which particular kind of cell is the one that responds to the need for more cells by undergoing cell division. It might be thought that the type of cell that responds could be ascertained by examining the cells seen in mitosis. But once a cell is actually in the process of mitosis, many of the usual characteristics by which it is recognized in the interphase as being of a particular type may disappear and, as a consequence, different kinds of cells, when they are in the process of mitosis, may look very much alike.

As was explained on page 42, specialized functioning cells of Category 2 do not undergo division, so when they wear out or become damaged they have to be replaced by cells formed from a pool of unspecialized cells of the same family type. The cells that multiply and serve as ancestral cells to the more specialized cells can be identified (and traced to the nondividing specialized cells) by administering labeled thymidine to several animals, all at the same time. If sufficient radioautographs are prepared from these animals at regular intervals and examined, it will be found that, say, 8 hours after the thymidine is given, the label will not be present in any specialized cells but only in unspecialized ones, which obviously must have become labeled in the S phase of a cell cycle and hence can divide. However, radioautographs taken at later times will show label in the nuclei of specialized cells, and in due course the only label seen will be in the latter type of cell. Accordingly, it is concluded that the unspecialized cells of the family are the only ones capable of dividing. Since the label only appears in the specialized cells later, when no labeled thymidine is present in the circulation for them to take up, the only way the presence of the label in them can be explained is by the development of previously labeled unspecialized cells into specialized cells.

As far as the cells of Category 1 (page 42) are concerned, no label will ever be taken up after they have fully developed. In cells of Category 3, however, if mitosis is occurring in any of them, label would be seen in some of the specialized cells soon after the tritiated thymidine was given. The extremely useful method of using tritiated thymidine to trace cell lineages does, however, suffer from the disadvantage that it eventually becomes diluted.

Why, After a Single Labeling, Label Becomes Diluted as Cells Continue to Divide

For perspective on the way DNA is propagated, it is interesting to reflect that at least one strand of some of the DNA molecules that each individual possesses at birth is still probably present and functioning in at least a few of the cells (particularly nerve cells) in adult life.

While on the whole very useful, the method of tracing cell lineages by labeling cells with thymidine suffers from one restriction, which is that if labeled cells continue to proliferate in the absence of additional label, the amount of label in the cells of further generations continues to diminish and finally reaches a point where it is no longer obvious. Why this occurs will now be explained.

When the prophase of the first mitosis after labeling begins, all the DNA molecules that have duplicated in the S phase of a cell cycle in the presence of label will carry the label in one of their two strands (Fig. 3-3). Hence, as the two s-chromosomes (chromatids) separate in the anaphase, each s-chromosome has a DNA molecule labeled in one of its two strands (one molecule of labeled DNA of Fig. 3-3 would go to one s-chromosome and the

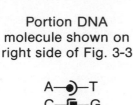

Portion DNA
molecule shown on
right side of Fig. 3-3

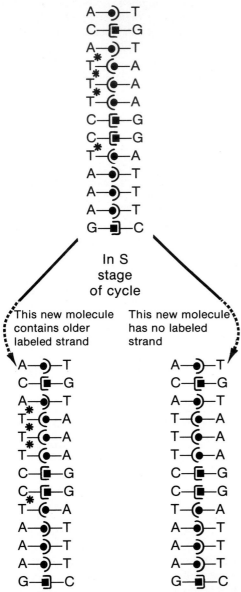

In S
stage
of cycle

This new molecule
contains older
labeled strand

This new molecule
has no labeled
strand

This molecule goes
to one s-chromosome
which will carry label

This molecule goes
to the other s-chromosome
which will carry no label

Fig. 3-7. Diagram explaining how the tritium label of tritiated thymidine, once incorporated into DNA molecules, becomes progressively diluted each time the cell containing it divides. When a DNA molecule carrying label (indicated by asterisk) in one of its strands (*top*) passes through the S phase of a cell cycle in the absence of further label, it forms one new molecule (*lower left*) that is still labeled and another (*lower right*) that carries no label. For further explanation, *see* text.

other labeled molecule to the other). So all the s-chromosomes of the two daughter cells that form will carry the label in one strand of their two-stranded DNA molecules. However, if those daughter cells now pass through another cell cycle, but this time in the absence of additional label, the label becomes diluted. When the DNA of the s-chromosomes of the daughter cells is duplicated in the S phase, but this time in the absence of additional label, the two strands of each DNA molecule that is labeled in one of its strands separate, and each acts as a template for the formation of the new strand (Fig. 3-7). The strand that was labeled thus gains an unlabeled strand beside it (*bottom left* in Fig. 3-7), so this DNA molecule is still labeled. But since the unlabeled strand also gains an unlabeled strand beside it (Fig. 3-7, *bottom right*) this DNA molecule is not labeled. So when the next prophase begins the DNA molecule of only one of each of the two s-chromosomes of the d-chromosomes will be labeled; the other s-chromosome of each d-chromosome will have no label. Since when the metaphase is reached one of the two s-chromosomes of each d-chromosome (one labeled and the other not labeled) line up in the equatorial plane, with one facing one pole of the cell and the other facing the other, it is a matter of chance which way the labeled and unlabeled s-chromosomes will face. On the average, 50 per cent will face one way and go toward one pole of the cell and the other 50 per cent will face the other way and go to the other pole. This results in only half of the chromosomes of the second-generation daughter cells possessing label, which, of course, results in less label being revealed in interphase nuclei of the daughter cells than in the nuclei of the first generation of daughter cells. Then, if one of these daughter cells passes through another cycle in the absence of further label, the chances are that the next generation of cells will only carry the label in one-quarter of their interphase s-chromosomes. So if the process of cell division continues in the absence of label, eventually only very few of the daughter cells that result from continued division will have even one labeled chromosome. This is why labeled cells can be traced only through a few divisions. If, of course, the labeled cells do not continue to divide but instead become specialized to perform some function, they will still carry their label, and this will be detectable by radioautography until the radioactivity decays.

DETERMINATION OF THE TIMES TAKEN BY CELLS IN CULTURE TO PASS THROUGH SUCCESSIVE STAGES OF THE CELL CYCLE

Unless special measures are taken to synchronize the cycles of cells being grown in cultures, these cells, even though of the same kind, will all be at different stages of the cell cycle at any given moment. It is nevertheless possible, as we shall see, to determine the durations of these stages by labeling with tritiated thymidine and preparing radioautographs. But one stage, *mitosis,* can be timed without using labeled thymidine. This is done by keeping representative cells of the culture under view with a phase contrast microscope, which permits mitosis to be observed and timed directly. Time-lapse cinemicrography is sometimes employed for this purpose since it provides a continuous film record from which numerous mitoses can be timed. As indicated in Figure 2-8B, mitosis (M) typically lasts for 1 hour but in some types of cells it takes up to 1.5 hour.

The Use of Labeled Thymidine for Estimating the Lengths of Certain Other Stages of the Cell Cycle

Determining the Duration of G_2. This is done using a technic known as *pulse labeling,* which entails adding labeled thymidine to the cell culture and then, after a brief period, changing the medium to prevent any further uptake of labeled thymidine. With this method only those cells that are in the S phase of the cell cycle during their brief exposure to labeled thymidine become labeled. The proportion of cells in S phase at this time would, of course, be small, so only a small proportion would take up the label. Moreover, the cells taking up the label would all be interphase cells ranging from those just commencing the S phase to those that had almost finished it during the exposure period. If cells were to be sampled immediately following removal of the labeled thymidine, label would be present only in interphase nuclei and these nuclei would belong to cells that were in S phase at the time of labeling; the mitotic cells in the sample would be unlabeled.

Next, if samples continued to be taken at regular intervals from the culture, with radioautographs being prepared from each successive sample, there would come a time when label would begin to appear in *mitotic d-chromosomes.* As noted, the label would be taken up by all those cells that were in S phase during labeling and they would include those just beginning S and some just finishing it at the time of labeling. Obviously the latter cells would be the first of the labeled cells to undergo mitosis and hence reveal label in their mitotic chromosomes. So the interval between (*1*) the time at which labeled thymidine was removed from the culture and (*2*) the time at which labeled mitotic chromosomes appeared would give the duration of the G_2 stage of the cell cycle.

Determining the Duration of S Phase. Since cells just ending the S phase when label was available would be the first ones to enter mitosis, it follows that those commencing S phase just before the label was removed would be the last to reveal labeled mitotic chromosomes. So if we could determine the interval between the times at which the first-labeled and the last-labeled cells entered mitosis, we would know the length of the S phase. However, although the time at which labeled mitotic chromosomes first appear is readily established, it is not feasible to determine when the last-labeled cells go into mitosis (the possibility of recognizing when the last-labeled cells enter mitosis is precluded by the very large numbers of labeled mitotic cells in the later samples). Therefore it is necessary to determine the length of the S phase in another way, as follows.

If radioautographs of consecutive samples taken at regular intervals are examined, the proportion of cells revealing label in their mitotic chromosomes will be seen to increase until virtually all the mitotic cells are labeled. But as cells consecutively complete mitosis they then go on to become labeled interphase cells. Next, the first labeled cells to finish mitosis are of course the first labeled cells that entered mitosis. Likewise, the last cells with labeled mitotic chromosomes to leave mitosis are the last labeled cells to enter mitosis. Since the time taken for mitosis is constant, it follows that if we could estimate the time that elapsed

between (*1*) the time the first-labeled mitotic cells left mitosis and (*2*) the time the last-labeled mitotic cells left mitosis, we would know the duration of the S phase, just as we would know it had we been able to determine the interval between the times of the first-labeled and last-labeled cells entering mitosis, which we cannot do. We are nevertheless able to ascertain the duration of S phase very easily by estimating the interval between (*1*) the time at which 50 per cent of the mitotic cells in the culture become labeled and (*2*) the time at which 50 per cent of the mitotic cells are last seen to be labeled. This gives the same information as would be obtained from using either of the above-mentioned procedures (had they been feasible) but it does so by using averages, so that it gives an average value for the time taken by the S phase.

Determining the Generation Time (Total Length of the Cell Cycle). If samples continue to be taken, labeled mitotic figures appear once again after falling to zero. Such mitotic cells represent the daughter cells of mother cells that took up label at the time of labeling because they were in S. The mother cells then went on to G_2, divided, and then passed through another interphase and another mitosis. The cells have thus completed one entire cycle and part of another. The time taken to complete an entire cell cycle is called the *generation time.* It represents the interval between two consecutive peaks of labeling and is commonly measured between the times in consecutive ascending curves at which 50 per cent of the mitotic figures show label.

Determining the Duration of G_1. When the durations of the other three stages have each been estimated (as outlined above), and the generation time has also been determined, the length of G_1 is readily calculated; the total time taken by G_2, S, and M is, of course, subtracted from the generation time to give G_1. The length of G_1 is reasonably constant for any given line of cells but is very variable from one cell line to another; it shows much more variation than the other three stages of the cycle. In the body, cells of Category 3 may remain for prolonged periods in an extended G_1, whereas cells of Category 2 may leave the cell cycle in G_1 in order to become specialized functioning cells.

It will be appreciated that the labeled thymidine method for estimating the lengths of the stages of the cell cycle involves sampling entire populations of cells and therefore provides average values for the cells in the population. There can be considerable variation from cell to cell within any given population, both in the relative lengths of the individual phases and in the total duration of the cell cycle.

THE FINE STRUCTURE OF METAPHASE CHROMOSOMES

The study of sections of mitotic chromosomes with the EM has not been as informative about elucidating their internal structure as the optimistic might have expected. Actually when it is realized that enormously long DNA molecules (together with associated RNA and protein covering) must somehow be very tightly crumpled, folded, or coiled to occupy the space allotted to a metaphase d-chromosome, it is not surprising that a slice cut through a chromosome would not indicate the method by which it is condensed. It might be thought, however, that if condensation were due to coiling, that this would be indicated in sections by some sort of consistent pattern in what was seen. But sectioned metaphase chromosomes

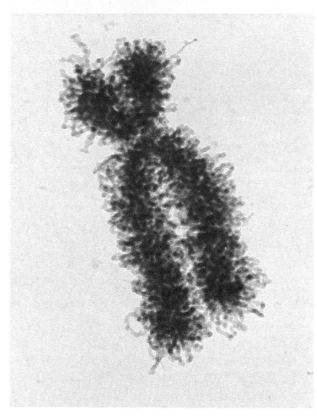

Fig. 3-8. Electron micrograph (×60,400) of a whole mount preparation of human chromosome No. 12. Each s-chromosome of the d-chromosome appears to consist of a single long fiber (20 to 50 nm. in diameter) tightly folded on itself; this accounts for the loops that can be seen around the periphery of both s-chromosomes. (DuPraw, E. J.: DNA and Chromosomes. New York, Holt, Rinehart, & Winston, 1970)

such as those seen in Figures 2-16 and 2-17 do not reveal any pattern that would be expected in a section cut through coils. They do, however, present an appearance that would be compatible with what would be seen in a slice cut through a long thread that had been crumpled together tightly into a mass. As we shall see this is not haphazard crumpling; it must be basically orderly, but not done in any easily recognized or familiar pattern. A section cut through a chromosome (as in Figs. 2-16 and 2-17) appears merely as a mass of fibrogranular material with an irregular outline. The granular appearance could be explained by the darker material being the nucleic acid of chromosomal threads and the lighter material, the protein associated with them.

Fortunately, however, there is another method for studying metaphase chromosomes with the EM. This was devised by DuPraw, who by using special technics was able to isolate and mount whole metaphase chromosomes

on grids and prepare them for examination with the EM. One of his striking micrographs of an entire human metaphase chromosome is shown in Figure 3-8. His observations indicate that each s-chromosome (chromatid) of a metaphase d-chromosome is composed of a single long thread (which he terms a *fiber*), from 20 to 50 nm. in diameter, that is tightly folded as shown in the micrograph to account for its being condensed in mitosis. This is termed the *folded fiber model* of chromosome structure. DuPraw points out from many detailed experiments that the continuous DNA molecule lying within this continuous fiber is enormously longer than the fiber itself, and hence to fit into the fiber it must be tightly coiled along its length. Since the two strands of the DNA molecule are also in a helical arrangement there are two orders of coiling within the chromatin fiber, which in turn is folded on itself (Fig. 3-8). For further details, *see* DuPraw.

HOW THE PAIRS OF CHROMOSOMES OF MAN CAN BE INDIVIDUALLY IDENTIFIED WITH THE LM AND HOW ABNORMALITIES OF NUMBER OR FORM CAN BE DETECTED

Present knowledge in this area is of particular importance, since it now constitutes an important part of cell biology, genetics, and clinical medicine.

Some Background

It is now accepted that all body cells (with a few exceptions that will be described later) of a normal person contain the same number of chromosomes, which is 46. Hence the chromosome constitution of the body can be determined by examining the metaphase chromosomes of suitable single cells. Methods to be described next make it relatively easy to obtain cells from an individual's blood and treat these in cultures so as to cause them to enter mitosis, but then stop at the metaphase stage. Spreads can be made of the metaphase chromosomes obtained from such cells. From photomicrographs of the chromosomes, a map called a *karyotype* (Gr. *karyon* + *typos,* mark or prevailing character) of the person's chromosomes can be assembled, and its examination by trained experts quickly reveals whether there is any deviation from normal in the number or form of the chromosomes. Different types of deviations are generally associated with specific kinds of abnormalities in the individuals concerned.

Chromosome abnormalities detected this way from the study of a few cells and regarded as representative of all the cells of the body must have had their origin at the level of the germ cells from which the body developed. Hence the chromosomes of the fertilized ovum from which the body developed must also have possessed the

Fig. 3-9. Photomicrograph of metaphase d-chromosomes of a normal human male. Preparation made from blood cells cultured as described in the text. (Courtesy of C. E. Ford)

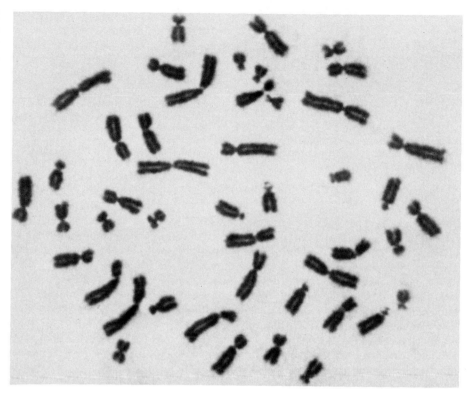

defect manifested in all the body cells. However, in individuals with a normal karyotype, chromosome abnormalities originate sometimes at the level of body cells. But for these to be detected, samples of cells must be obtained for study from the particular clone of cells derived from the body cell in which this defect developed and from which it was propagated, as will be described later. But first we shall describe the general technic employed in preparing a karyotype that permits diagnosis of chromosome defects developing at the germ cell level.

Details of the Preparation of a Karyotype

The first step is to obtain a small volume of blood from the person being investigated and then separate the white blood cells (described in Chap. 11) from it. These are then placed in a culture medium to which a plant substance called *phytohemagglutinin* is added; this has the effect of stimulating one type of white blood cell (lymphocytes) to undergo mitosis. After two or three days, colchicine is added to the culture, which, as described in the previous chapter, causes mitosis to be arrested in the C-metaphase stage. The cells are then put in a very dilute medium, which makes them swell and also causes their chromosomes to separate from one another, after which they are fixed and made to flatten and spread out on glass

by appropriate technics. The preparations can then be stained so that all the metaphase chromosomes of single cells can be examined with the LM and photographed (Fig. 3-9).

After the chromosomes of a given cell are counted, the photomicrograph can be cut up with one chromosome showing on each piece. The chromosomes can then be arranged so as to construct a *karyotype*. But first the chromosomes have to be arranged in pairs, for reasons now to be described.

The Sex Chromosomes. The fertilized ovum from which the human body develops has 46 chromosomes; hence the body of *somatic* (Gr. *soma,* body) cells that develop from it have 46 chromosomes each. The chromosomes of the fertilized ovum are derived from germ cells, half (23) from the unfertilized ovum and the other 23 from the spermatozoon that fertilized the ovum. Why germ cells have only half the number of chromosomes of somatic cells will be explained presently. Of the 23 chromosomes of a normal germ cell, one is a *sex chromosome;* the other 22 are termed *autosomes* (Gr. *autos,* self). The name of the sex chromosome of female germ cells is X. Male germ cells (spermatozoa) also each possess 22 autosomes and 1 sex chromosome but the sex chromosome may be either an X (the female sex chromosome) or a Y (the male sex chromosome). The morphology of both kinds of sex

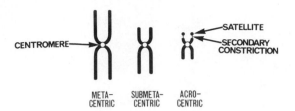

CENTROMERE

SATELLITE

SECONDARY CONSTRICTION

META-CENTRIC   SUBMETA-CENTRIC   ACRO-CENTRIC

Fig. 3-10. Diagrammatic representation of the three types of human d-chromosomes. (Adapted from Thompson, J. S., and Thompson, M. W.: Genetics in Medicine. ed. 2. Philadelphia, W. B. Saunders, 1973)

chromosomes will be described later. Maleness is dependent on the presence of a Y chromosome. Consequently, an ovum (which always has an X chromosome) when fertilized by a sperm carrying an X chromosome will have an XX combination and so will develop into a female, with each somatic cell developing from it possessing 44 autosomes and 2 X chromosomes. If, however, the sperm fertilizing the ovum has a Y chromosome, the fertilized ovum will possess 44 autosomes and an XY combination and, because of its having a Y chromosome, will develop into a male, with all the somatic cells possessing 44 autosomes, and the XY combination.

Why the Chromosomes Are Arranged in Pairs; Homologues. A chromosome spread, prepared from a body cell of a normal female, will disclose two X chromosomes, one of maternal and the other of paternal origin. Although the genetic content of the two X chromosomes is by no means identical, the metaphase chromosomes themselves have an identical appearance. Because of this each is said to be the *homologue* (Gr. *homologos,* agreeing, correspondent) of the other. Next, whereas each of the 22 autosomes of either maternal or paternal origin has at least a slightly different morphology from each of the other 21, each of the 22 autosomes of maternal origin has its counterpart (homologue) among the 22 autosomes of paternal origin, so that among the autosomes there are 22 pairs, with each member of the pair having the same appearance as its homologue. However, while homologues have the same morphology, their genetic content is not identical. So, in making a karyotype of the metaphase chromosomes of the body cells of a normal female, there are 22 pairs of autosomes and a pair of X chromosomes to place in the correct order. But in males there are only 22 pairs, because the X and the Y are not identical with one another.

Terminology Used for Classifying Chromosomes in Making Karyotypes. The first hurdle in chromosome terminology is the use of the term *arm.* This term was coined before the methods that reveal the two s-chromosomes of a metaphase d-chromosome as separate from each other

along their lengths (except at their centromeres) were available. Had such methods been available, it might have seemed more logical to describe metaphase d-chromosomes, such as the ones depicted in Figure 3-10, as having two arms and two legs, with the two arms of the chromosome extending upward from its centromere and the two legs extending downward. However, probably because only two structures were seen to extend from the centromere, one in each direction, they were called the two *arms* of the chromosomes. So the term *arm* is used to denote what we now know to be a double structure, and this can cause confusion. In making a karyotype the shorter arm (a double structure) is arranged so as to point upward and the other, longer (and likewise double) arm downward. The upper and lower arms, of course, become continuous at the centromere to which both are attached.

Next, a d-chromosome whose *centromere* (the nonstaining portion joining the two s-chromosomes, represented as a circle in each chromosome in Fig. 3-10) lies approximately halfway between its two ends, is said to be *metacentric* and its two arms are, therefore, of roughly equal length (Fig. 3-10, *left*). A d-chromosome whose centromere is closer to one of its ends is termed *submetacentric;* it, of course, has one shorter and one longer arm (Fig. 3-10, *middle*). A d-chromosome whose centromere is very near one end is referred to as *acrocentric* (Gr. *akron,* extremity); it has one very short arm and one very long arm (Fig. 3-10, *right*). No human chromosomes have centromeres right at their ends.

Satellites are small stained portions of s-chromosomes attached by a narrow nonstaining region to the ends of the short arms of certain acrocentric chromosomes (Fig. 3-10, *right*). Satellites are found on Chromosomes 13, 14, 15, 21, and 22 (but not the Y chromosome). The nonstaining regions of s-chromosomes separating the satellite portion from the remainder of the chromosome are called *secondary constrictions* (Fig. 3-10, *right*). They resemble small centromeres in the LM and enable experts to recognize the satellited chromosomes. The functional significance of secondary constrictions will be explained when we discuss how the satellited chromosomes are involved in protein synthesis (p. 100).

The cut-out photomicrographs of the 46 chromosomes of a spread, such as the ones in Figure 3-9, are first arranged in pairs and then the pairs are arranged in descending order with respect to their total lengths with their centromeres all placed along the same horizontal line (Fig. 3-11). When arm lengths are unequal, each d-chromosome is oriented with its shorter arm upward and its longer one downward (as in Fig. 3-10). The individual pairs of d-chromosomes arranged primarily in a descending order of length are then numbered serially from 1 to 22 (Fig. 3-11). Other criteria, such as those described above, permit the 22 pairs to be arranged into 7 groups.

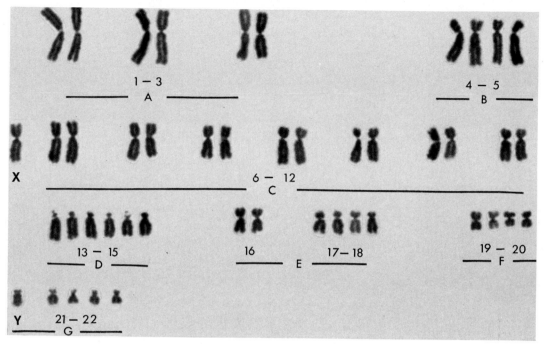

Fig. 3-11. Karyotype of chromosomes of a normal human male. (Courtesy of C. E. Ford)

These 7 groups are referred to as the 1 to 3 or *A group*, the 4 to 5 or *B group*, the 6 to 12 or *C group*, the 13 to 15 or *D group*, the 16 to 18 or *E group*, the 19 to 20 or *F group* and the 21 to 22 or *G group*. Group A, for example, consists of chromosome pairs 1 to 3, which are the longest metacentric chromsomes, and Group G includes pairs 21 and 22, which are the shortest acrocentric chromosomes. In males, group G also contains the Y chromosome (Fig. 3-11), which is an acrocentric chromosome like the others, but is usually the longest in the group, and its long arms are usually parallel to one another, rather than divergent as in the other members of the G group. The X chromosome is very similar to certain members of the 6 to 12 (C) group (Fig. 3-11).

How Each Pair of Chromosomes Can Be Individually Identified

With the methods so far described it was impossible to identify each pair of chromosomes within a group; however, more recent staining methods have now made this possible. These provide patterns of bands on chromosomes that were not seen before with older methods of staining. Such patterns have fortunately proved to be unique for each pair of chromosomes, and this enables each pair to be individually identified. Even so, banding methods do not permit any microscopic distinction to be made between the two members of a chromosome pair, since their bands are identical in appearance. For those interested in details of chromosome banding methods, the kinds currently used in cytogenetics laboratories will now be discussed.

Q-Banding. This involves the use of *quinacrine,* a derivative of the dye acridine. Under the name Atabrine, quinacrine hydrochloride had hitherto been used only as a drug for treating patients for malarial parasite or tapeworm infestations. However, quinacrine hydrochloride and quinacrine mustard, like other acridine derivatives, stain DNA and furthermore emit visible light under ultraviolet irradiation and hence are *fluorescent,* exhibiting an intense greenish-yellow fluorescence when observed under the fluorescence microscope (described in Chap. 9, p. 245).

When, in 1968, Caspersson and his coworkers first applied quinacrine mustard to fixed metaphase chromosomes, they discovered that instead of staining the chromosomes uniformly, as seen for example in Figure 3-11, it stained certain bands along the length of each chromosome. Moreover, these bands were of differing lengths and unevenly spaced in different chromosomes and hence formed a particular pattern or "fingerprint" unique to each pair of chromosomes. This, of course, permitted each chromosome pair to be identified with certainty for the first time. In addition, a particularly large and striking Q-band, as these quinacrine-stained bands are called, is evident on the distal part of the long arm of the Y chromosome. In human cells this band is visible as a brightly fluorescing spot, about 0.2 μm. in diameter,

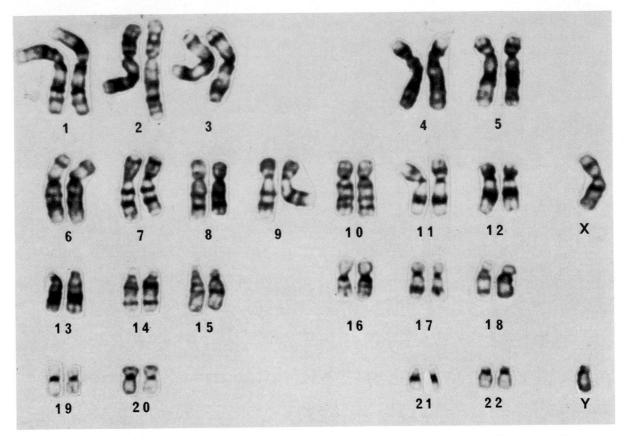

Fig. 3-12. Normal male karyotype, showing G-bands after staining by the Giemsa technic described in the text. The characteristic banding pattern permits each chromosome pair to be identified. (Courtesy of M. Seabright)

even during the interphase. This, of course, makes it possible to determine whether individual cells are from males (or, strictly speaking, from individuals with a Y chromosome), even when the cells are not dividing.

Little is known about the basis underlying staining with quinacrine mustard or quinacrine hydrochloride except that the dye has somewhat greater affinity for DNA rich in the bases adenine (A) and thymine (T) than for that rich in guanine (G) and cytosine (C). Presumably the regions of chromosomes staining as Q-bands are somewhat richer in adenine and thymine than the interband regions; Q-banding would thus reflect the gross variation in the relative content of these base pairs (A-T or G-C) along the chromosome. However, since a single DNA fiber winds back and forth upon itself in a very complex manner within a chromosome (as can be seen in Fig. 3-8), a very considerable length of the DNA thread would correspond to a Q-band.

G-Banding. The discovery of Q-banding spawned the development of alternative banding methods not requiring the special technique of fluorescence microscopy. These utilize Giemsa stain (an often-used polychromed blood stain described in Chap. 10, p. 261), but they require a special so-called denaturation treatment of the chromosome preparation before staining. This entails mild treatment of the fixed chromosomes with proteolytic enzymes, salts, heat, detergents, or urea—agents all capable of

denaturing the protein in the chromosomes. When stained with Giemsa after such treatment, a pattern of bands, called *G-bands,* may be seen on the chromosomes under an ordinary light microscope. This pattern is somewhat similar to that obtained with quinacrine staining. Figure 3-12 shows a normal male karyotype made from chromosomes stained by this procedure.

The basis of G-banding has not yet been established, but it appears to involve the local removal of proteins by denaturation, possibly in relation to the gross variation in local base pair composition of the DNA with which the proteins are associated. D. Comings has suggested that proteins remaining after the denaturation step might prevent the stain from getting into certain regions of the DNA. Hence G-bands would be parts of chromosomes where the proteins had been virtually extracted by the mild denaturation step employed, allowing free access of the stain to the DNA, and the interband regions would be placed where protein had been incompletely extracted. It is possible the DNA-associated proteins might also be involved in Q-banding. For example, less protein might be associated with A-T rich DNA, so that quinacrine could have relatively free access to the DNA in regions that stain as Q-bands. The close correspondence in position between Q- and G-bands suggests that there may be a common basis for their staining.

Another factor that may be relevant is that the regions of

chromosomes forming Q- or G-bands consist largely of heterochromatin throughout almost all the cell cycle. This is known
because they replicate their DNA slightly later than the interband regions in the S phase. The interband regions of the
chromosomes are slightly richer in G-C base pairs, and they may
be demonstrated by an alternative modification of the Giemsa
procedure that discloses them as yet another type of band,
termed the *R-bands*. Hence R-bands are complementary to
G-bands in position along the chromosome.

   C-Banding. A different sort of modification of Giemsa staining
gives a pattern altogether different from Q- and G-banding.
Here, most of the DNA is first extracted from fixed chromosomes by relatively harsh treatment with alkali, acid, salt, or heat
before staining. A short portion of each chromosome, located
close to its centromere, then stains very intensely with Giemsa
stain. The stained region, because it lies close to the centromere,
is termed a *C-band*. C-bands are evident on all but the Y
chromosome, which stains faintly and evenly. The lack of a distinct C-band on the Y chromosome, like the presence of a
brightly fluorescing spot after quinacrine staining, facilitates
identification of cells of individuals with the Y chromosome.

   Again it is heterochromatin that stains in C-bands. However,
whereas it is the heterochromatin in the arms of the chromosome
that is revealed by Q- or G-banding, it is the heterochromatin in
the centromere region that is disclosed by C-banding. It is not
understood why the Y chromosome should lack a C-band but
perhaps the centromeric heterochromatin is more diffuse in this
particular chromosome. It is known that the centromeric heterochromatin contains highly repetitive DNA that is probably
not transcribed. This heterochromatin seems to be protected in
some way from extraction by the procedure used, possibly by
nonextractable proteins. However, if this is the case, the remaining protein clearly does not prevent access of the Giemsa stain to
the DNA since it stains it as a C-band.

The Appearance of Chromosomes Stained
by Banding Methods

   Banding patterns from cytogenetics laboratories have
been combined into standardized diagrams of the major
bands to be found on each human chromosome pair. Figure 3-13 shows the principal bands on a representative
pair of chromosomes (No. 12). This figure may be compared with Figure 3-8, which shows an entire No. 12
metaphase chromosome (d-chromosome). The pair of
No. 12 chromosomes after staining for G-bands may also
be seen in the karyotype illustrated in Figure 3-12. As
will be appreciated from the karyotype illustrated in this
figure, it is frequently difficult in karyotypes prepared
from banded chromsomes to see that each of the chromosomes in a chromosome pair consists of two s-
chromosomes joined by a common centromere. A close
inspection of Chromosomes 7 and 13 in Figure 3-12 will,
however, disclose that what at first sight could be mistaken for a single banded chromosome does, in fact, consist of two s-chromosomes that have not yet begun to separate from one another.

   As well as aiding in the identification and pairing of
chromosomes in preparing karyotypes, chromosome banding made it possible to see certain abnormalities of chro-

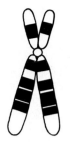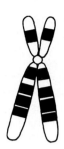

Fig. 3-13. Diagram of a pair of human d-chromosomes (No.
12), depicting their principal bands. The banding pattern was
compiled for each human chromosome from information gathered from cytogenetics laboratories, using all the banding technics available at the time. (Based on an illustration in Paris Conference [1971], Supplement [1975]: Standardization in Human
Cytogenetics. *In* Bergsma, D. (ed.): Birth Defects: Original Article Series, XI, 9, 1975. White Plains, the National Foundation)

mosome structure that had not been observed before,
such as deletions of parts of chromosomes and transloca-
tions of parts of chromosomes onto other ones. With the
development of chromosome banding it also became possible to distinguish human Chromosome No. 21 from No.
22, and this helped to further our understanding of the
chromosomal basis of certain diseases.

CHROMOSOME ANOMALIES

   The term *anomaly* (Gr. *an* + *homalos*, even) signifies a
marked deviation from a standard. The standards used for
establishing chromosome anomalies are the *numbers* and
the *morphology* of the chromosomes in cell samples.
Hence an anomaly exists in the chromosomes of a cell if it
contains more or fewer chromosomes than 46 or if any
chromosome exhibits a morphology or banding pattern
different from the normal.

   Chromosome anomalies can originate at the level of
germ cells, and hence they appear in all body cells and
can be detected in karyotypes. Anomalies, however, can
also arise at the level of somatic cells. Since chromosome
anomalies of the latter kind are *not* present in all body
cells, they remain undetected in karyotypes of cells that
are representative of all the cells of the body and are
therefore usually discovered by other means. In the following section we shall describe some anomalies that
originate at the level of germ cells and hence are disclosed
in karyotypes. Lest confusion arise, it should be emphasized that although these anomalies all originate at the
germ cell level, such anomalies are not limited to anomalies of the sex chromosomes but also include anomalies of
autosomes, for they, too, can originate at this level.

CHROMOSOME ANOMALIES THAT ORIGINATE AT THE LEVEL OF GERM CELLS

These occur in about three out of every 100 pregnancies. Some are incompatible with the continuation of pregnancy and cause spontaneous abortion or a miscarriage. In the last few decades it became possible to make karyotypes from spontaneously aborted embryos or fetuses and these karyotypes revealed many chromosome anomalies and so explained the cause of many abortions or miscarriages which before had been a mystery. However, some anomalies do not cause abortions. Probably about one out of every 200 babies born also have some kind of chromosome anomaly. The effects of various anomalies differ greatly. There are anomalies of sex chromosomes and also of autosomes; a few examples and their causes will be given later.

In order to understand anomalies that arise at the level of germ cells, it is imperative to have a reasonably extensive knowledge about the formation of germ cells and the process of *meiosis* (Gr. *meiosis*, diminution) essential to their formation.

The Difference Between Diploid and Haploid Cells

As already noted, each somatic cell of man contains 46 chromosomes constituted of 23 pairs, with one of each pair being of maternal origin (derived from the germ cell of the mother) and the other of paternal origin (derived from the germ cell of the father). Since each body cell thus has a double set of 23 homologous s-chromosomes, of the same form and banding pattern (except for the X and Y sex chromosomes in the cells of males), body (somatic) cells are said to have a *diploid* (Gr. *diplous*, twofold) number of chromosomes (46).

However, germ cells each have only one member of each of the 23 pairs of diploid cells, so they are said to have a *haploid* (Gr. *haplous*, single) number of chromosomes (23).

How Haploid Cells Develop From Diploid Cells

In both males and females the germ cells, with their haploid number of chromosomes, are derived from precursor cells that have the diploid number. In each sex this is accomplished by the precursor cell of the germ cell undergoing two consecutive divisions of a special kind called *meiosis*, which results in daughter cells with only the haploid number of chromosomes. Meiotic divisions are also referred to as *reduction divisions*, since they reduce the number of chromosomes in the daughter cells. In the male the four daughter cells resulting from meiosis are all viable *spermatozoa*, but in the female only one of the four becomes a viable egg cell; the others fail to develop and are discarded as what are termed *polar bodies*. Meiosis in the male is described in Chapter 27, page 881.

THE FORMATION OF GERM CELLS IN THE FEMALE AND THE PROCESS OF MEIOSIS

The mother cell from which haploid germ cells develop in the female is called a *primary oocyte*. How these develop is described in Chapter 26, page 838; here it is enough to state that although not formed in the ovaries, they take up residence in that site. By the time a baby girl is born, there can be as many as 2 million primary oocytes in her two ovaries. Moreover, many events of importance take place in these oocytes before the baby girl is born, as will now be described.

The first event is for each primary oocyte to pass through the S phase of a cell cycle. Since it was a diploid cell it now has enough DNA for 46 d-chromosomes as it emerges from the G_2 phase to enter the prophase of its first meiotic division. At this time, the 46 prophase d-chromosomes appear in thread-like form, and hence this first stage of the prophase of the first meiotic division is called the *leptotene* (Gr. *leptos* slender; *tainia*, ribbon) stage. Four other stages of the prophase follow.

The second event is called the *zygotene* (Gr. *zygon*, yolked) stage because in it the two members of each pair of homologous d-chromosomes (which still possess their thread-like form) seek each other out and lie beside one another along their whole lengths, as shown diagrammatically in Figure 3-14, *left*. Each pair of homologous chromosomes is thus "yolked" together in what is called a *bivalent* (L. *valentia*, strength), presumably because one of the homologues is of maternal and the other of paternal origin, so that the bivalent has the strength of two different genetic backgrounds.

The prophase of the first meiotic division then continues into what is termed its *pachytene* (Gr. *pachytes*, thickness) stage, which is characterized by each of the two thread-like chromosomes of each bivalent becoming shorter and thicker. Furthermore, in this stage it becomes apparent that each d-chromosome is actually a *double* thread, and this becomes sufficiently obvious for the next stage of the prophase to be termed the *diplotene* (Gr. *diplous*, double) stage. So at this stage each bivalent is seen to consist of two double stranded d-chromosomes, with the two strands of each lying side by side with the two strands of the other, as shown in the middle of Figure 3-14.

Crossing Over and Chiasmata

At this point it should be remembered that originally one of these double-stranded chromosomes was solely of maternal origin and the other solely of paternal origin. This is great importance because in this (diplotene) stage of the prophase of the first meiotic division, either one of the two strands of either the upper or lower arms of the double chromosomes of a bivalent may come to lie across the corresponding strand of the homologous chromosome in the bivalent, in the manner shown on the right of Figure 3-14, forming what is termed a *chiasma*, which means an X-shaped crossing. However, unlike what happens in people who may link arms in a similar fashion as they walk together, the two strands of the arms of a chromosome seem to be so fragile they commonly break at the site where they cross each other. This would result in two stumps and two detached fragments were it not for the fact that usually the damage is instantaneously repaired by the immediate uniting of each detached fragment, not with the stump from which it was detached, but with the other one. This, of course, results in portions of paternally-derived chromosomes becoming exchanged with parts of maternally-derived chromosomes and vice versa. The next stage of the first meiotic division is called *diakinesis* (Gr. *dia*, across, between or through and *kinesis*, motion). The reasons for this name, given long ago, are not clear. However, by the time this stage is reached the chromosomes of bivalents are no longer solely of paternal or maternal origin. They now have exchanged parts with one another and as a result the chromosome (each originally of either parternal or maternal origin) can confer hereditable qualities from both parents to the female germ cell that will eventually develop. Hence the phenomenon just described, and which is termed *crossing over*, is of vast importance in studying inheritance.

All of the above happens in primary oocytes before they finish the prophase of their first meiotic division. Furthermore, before a baby girl is born, these primary oocytes continue along the prophase of their first meiotic division by entering a long *rest period* in which the two chromosomes of each bivalent, which in the preceding steps had become condensed and hence visible, now become extended again so that the nucleus in this stage of the prophase may appear as if it were in interphase. Primary oocytes do not leave this resting stage until after the girl reaches approximately the age of puberty, which event is associated with the beginning of ovulation, the process by which a fully formed female germ cell is liberated from one of her ovaries about every 28 days, as will be described in Chapter 27. This means that a primary oocyte may remain in the late stage of its first meiotic division from the time of birth to at least the time of puberty, or at most for a period of 40 to 50 years. As we shall see the occurrence of a pregnancy relatively late in reproductive life, after a prolonged period during which primary oocytes have been held in a resting prophase, predisposes to the development of one type of chromosome anomaly.

The Completion of the First Meiotic Division

When at puberty the ovaries become activated by certain hormones, the process of meiosis is resumed in the primary oocytes so that a fully developed female germ cell (*ovum*) is released every 28 days or so from the surface of one of other of the ovaries. The first step is for the first meiotic division to be completed. The nuclear membrane of the primary oocyte disintegrates, a spindle forms as would occur in mitosis, and the chromosomes of the bivalents condense and then line up across the equatorial plane. The situation is similar to (but not the same as) that seen in the metaphase of mitosis. This is because instead of the d-chromosomes each separating into two s-chromosomes that would subsequently move to each end of the cell (as would occur in mitosis), the two s-chromosomes of each d-chromosome in a bivalent do not become detached from one another. Instead, it is the two *intact d-chromosomes* of each bivalent that separate from each other and move toward opposite ends of the spindle. This separation of the d-chromosomes of a bivalent from one another is illustrated in A on the left of Figure 3-15, As a result, each of the daughter cells produced at the termination of the telophase receives only 23 chromosomes (d-chromosomes) instead of the usual 46 chromosomes (s-chromosomes) and hence is haploid instead of diploid. Moreover, as is shown in Figure 3-15A, the cytoplasm becomes unevenly divided in the telophase so that only one of the two daughter cells, which is called the *secondary oocyte* (and is represented by the right half of the dividing cell in Fig. 3-15A), remains viable; the other haploid cell (the half on the left in Fig. 3-15A) becomes discarded as what is termed the *first polar body* (bottom of Fig. 3-15A).

It has already been noted that crossing over shuffles the various genes of maternal and paternal origin previously located on the chromosomes of the primary oocytes. A further mixing of these occurs in the first meiotic division, because as the bivalents line up across the equatorial plane, it is a matter of chance which way the originally

Zygotene

Diplotene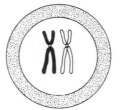

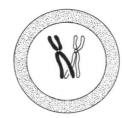

Fig. 3-14. Diagram illustrating the primary oocyte in the zygotene (*left*) and diplotene (*middle* and *right*) stages of the prophase of the first meiotic division. For clarity, only one pair of homologous chromosomes is shown. Crossing over, which may occur during the diplotene stage, is depicted on the right. The further apportionment of the s-chromosome of these homologues may be followed in Figure 3-15.

46 d-chromosomes
pair and form
23 bivalents

23 bivalents
(pairs of
d-chromosomes)

23 bivalents;
chiasmata formed
by crossing over

maternal and paternal chromosomes (which are now no longer solely maternal or paternal) face. On average, each daughter cell receives half the chromosomes originally of maternal origin and half those originally of paternal origin. In this way the genes received by an ovum from both sides of the girl's family are mixed still more.

The Second Meiotic Division

The viable daughter cell (*secondary oocyte*) resulting from the first meiotic division receives 23 d-chromosomes which would, of course, correspond to 46 s-chromosomes altogether. If it, like any somatic cell in a cell cycle, were to pass through an S phase, it would enter prophase with enough DNA to possess a total of 46 d-chromosomes or, after metaphase, 92 s-chromosomes— enough for a full complement of s-chromosomes for two daughter cells. However, the secondary oocyte does not pass through an S phase before it divides (Fig. 3-15). Instead, another division occurs without this having happened. The 23 double chromosomes line up across the equatorial plane in metaphase and the two s-chromosomes of each d-chromosome then separate from each other, as occurs in mitosis, and move toward their respective ends of the spindle. This separation of s-chromosomes from one another is illustrated in Figure 3-15B. So after the telophase there are two daughter cells each with only 23 s-chromosomes. Only one of these daughter cells (the one represented by the right half of the dividing cell in Fig. 3-15B) becomes a viable *ovum* (Fig. 3-15C); the other (the half on the left in Fig. 3-15B), as before, is not viable and is discarded as the *second polar body*.

Hence, the halving of chromosomes that has led to the characterization of meiosis as a reduction division is due to two cell divisions occurring in sequence *without there having been any S phase* (duplication of DNA) between the two (Fig. 3-15).

EXAMPLE OF AN ANOMALY OF AN AUTOSOME

It was long known that around one out of 500 babies born has a curious but characteristic facial expression, placid disposition, short hands, and certain other physical features, and that such babies would be mentally retarded. When the condition was first described, it was, unfortunately, and for no good reason, termed *mongolism* and babies so affected were called *mongoloids*. The condition is now referred to as *Down's syndrome* or *trisomy-21* syndrome. The latter and best term for this condition was adopted when it was discovered in 1959 by Lejeune and his coworkers that babies of this kind commonly have 47 chromosomes in their cells instead of the normal 46. It was established that the extra chromosome was a member of the G group and it was agreed to call it an extra No. 21 (even though Nos. 21 and 22 are very much alike). Since that time, the use of chromosome banding techniques has shown that this choice was fortuitously the right one. As there are normally two No. 21 chromosomes and the extra one made three, the condition was called *trisomy-21* which, since *soma* means body, indicates that there are three chromosome bodies of the No. 21 type present. Figure 3-16 shows these three No. 21 chromosomes (marked with arrows at the *top*, *top left*, and *top right* of the photomicrograph) in a cell from a fetus. The fetal cell was obtained during pregnancy by withdrawing through a needle some of the fluid from the amniotic cavity surrounding the fetus by a technic called *amniocentesis* (Gr. *kentesis*, puncture), which allows fetal chromosome anomalies to be detected before birth.

Trisomy-21 is most likely to occur at the stage in the first meiotic division when the two homologous chromosomes of a bivalent ordinarily separate. Probably the bivalent composed of the two homologous chromosomes No. 21 never forms; hence the two chromosomes remain as what are termed *univalents*.

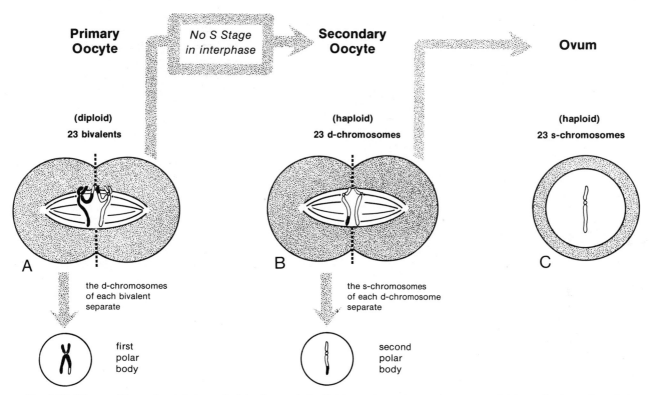

Primary Oocyte   No S Stage in interphase   **Secondary Oocyte**   **Ovum**

(diploid)
23 bivalents

(haploid)
23 d-chromosomes

(haploid)
23 s-chromosomes

A   B   C

the d-chromosomes
of each bivalent
separate

the s-chromosomes
of each d-chromosome
separate

first
polar
body

second
polar
body

Fig. 3-15. Diagram illustrating (*A*) the end of the first meiotic division and (*B*) the second meiotic division. The formation of the ovum is shown in (*C*). It is possible in this figure to follow further the apportionment of the s-chromosomes of the homologues depicted in Figure 3-14. Note that in the case illustrated, neither of the s-chromosomes that underwent exchange of arms during crossing over in diplotene (as illustrated on the *right* of Fig. 3-14) happened to end up in the ovum. There would, of course, be a 50-per-cent chance that one of them would have entered the ovum. For details, *see* text.

Univalents have an equal chance of going to either daughter cell and so both chromosomes No. 21 can end up in the same daughter cell, giving it 24 chromosomes (Fig. 3-16). The other daughter cell thus has only 22 chromosomes. The failure of two homologous chromosomes to go to two daughter cells separately is termed *nondisjunction*, and this is the usual cause of trisomy-21. Nondisjunction is, of course, an accident that can happen to any chromosome. It follows that if one of the two daughter cells that enters the second meiotic division has 24 chromosomes because of an extra chromosome No. 21 and if either of these should become an ovum and be fertilized, the baby will have cells with 47 chromosomes and suffer from the trisomy-21 syndrome. If either of the daughter cells with only 22 chromosomes should become the ovum and be fertilized it will never form a viable fetus.

Trisomy-21 is the most frequently encountered of the chromosome anomalies observed in newborn infants, although it is not a particularly common condition. How-

ever, Down's syndrome does not always require an extra complete chromosome No. 21, for the condition is sometimes caused by only an *extra piece* of chromosome No. 21 being present in the cells of the infant; this can be due to a piece of chromosome No. 21 being *translocated* to another chromosome so that the infant has not only its normal pair of chromosomes No. 21 but an *extra piece* of a chromosome No. 21 in another chromosome. The incidence of trisomy-21 increases with the age of the mother. A woman over 40 is over 50 times more likely to give birth to an affected child than a woman of 25. Her chances are, in fact, about one in 60 of doing so. The reason for this has to do with the increasingly longer time an oocyte has remained in an arrested prophase before it completes its meiotic divisions to give rise to a viable ovum. Nondisjunction can occur in the production of male germ cells but it is more unlikely. This is probably related to the fact that they are made freshly all through life and so they are not held in a suspended prophase for years as occurs in the female.

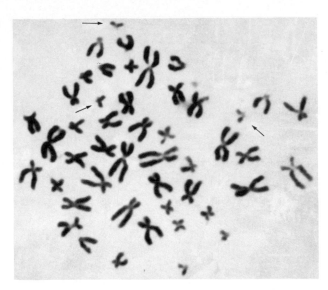

Fig. 3-16. Chromosome preparation of cell obtained by amniocentesis (for details, *see* text). The fact that there are three No. 21 chromosomes (*arrows*) shows that the fetus had the chromosome constitution of Down's syndrome, thus allowing a diagnosis to be made prenatally. (Courtesy of H. Nadler)

Some Examples of Anomalies of Sex Chromosomes

The sex chromosomes in general exert their primary effect on the development and function of the reproductive system.

One genetic function of the Y chromosome is that of directing the differentiation of the testes (the male sex glands) in embryonic life. X chromosomes, in addition to exerting genetic effects which direct development along the female type unless overpowered by a Y, have, in contrast to a Y chromosome, an extensive complement of genes which have nothing specially to do with sex, and so X chromosomes in this sense are of more general importance to a body than Y chromosomes.

The commonest anomaly of the sex chromosomes is due to an extra X being present in a male who therefore has an XXY combination in all the cells of his body. Males with this anomaly develop small testes and are infertile. For some reason not understood, having a pair of X chromosomes in their cells instead of one may affect the development of their intelligence so that in some it may be somewhat less than that of normal males. The condition is called *Klinefelter's syndrome* and, like trisomy-21, is probably to be explained by nondisjunction during one of the meiotic divisions of the oocyte which gives rise to the ovum, which leads in this instance to the pair of X chromosomes not separating but both going to the ovum which became fertilized by a spermatozoon carrying a Y chromosome. It can also arise, but less frequently, when an XY-bearing sperm (from nondisjunction at meiosis in the father) fertilizes a normal X-bearing ovum. Nondisjunction at both meiotic divisions in one of the parents can give rise to XXXY or XXXXY chromosome constituitions, conditions which clinically are indistinguishable from the regular Klinefelter's syndrome except that all of these individuals are mentally retarded.

Another condition, called *Turner's syndrome*, is seen in females that have only one X chromosome instead of a pair. This state of affairs is termed *monosomy* (only one body). Monosomies are nearly always incompatible with life but sometimes full-term babies are born with it. Two X chromosomes are required if an individual is to develop normal ovaries and hence those with an XO (O as used here means *nothing*) instead of an XX combination do not develop normal ovaries or even normal stature. Otherwise their development is essentially female though not normal in certain respects. This anomaly also can be caused by nondisjunction at the germ cell level, for if both X chromosomes of the oocyte go to one daughter cell (which is lost as a polar body), the other daughter cell has no X chromosomes left and so if it is fertilized by a spermatozoon carrying an X chromosome, the somatic cells of the individual that develops have only the one X chromosome that was derived from the male germ cell. The XO condition can probably also arise by loss of an X chromosome during spermatogenesis; if so, a spermatozoon having neither an X nor a Y would have to have fertilized a normal X-bearing ovum.

Another anomaly of interest is the male that has an XYY chromosome complement. Males with this combination tend to be tall and there is some indication that under stress the behavior of some, but not all, of such individuals may be somewhat more aggressive than that of normal males, although there is no firm evidence as yet that it is the extra chromosome that is responsible for the antisocial behavior seen in some of these individuals. Several other anomalies involving the sex chromosomes are now known. Those interested in further reading will find some references at the end of the chapter.

A Note on the Symbols Used to Denote Chromosome Anomalies

For any student pursuing this subject further it may help in reading the literature to be aware that when karyotype findings in man are being described, it is now customary to record first the total number of chromosomes. This is followed by a comma and then the sex chromosome constitution. Autosomes are mentioned only if there is an abnormality. The normal human male karyotype is thus designated as 46, XY. The karyotype of a female who has Down's syndrome with an extra chromosome No. 21 would be referred to as 47, XX, 21+ (or alternatively, 47, XX, G+) and of a male with Klinefelter's syndrome with two X chromosomes, as 47, XXY.

EXAMPLE OF AN ANOMALY INVOLVING THE FORM OF A CHROMOSOME INSTEAD OF TOTAL NUMBER

An anomaly of this type occurs as a loss (*deletion*) of part of the short arm of chromosome No. 5. It results in the infant having facial deformities of various degrees of severity, probably depending on how much of the arm of the chromosome is deleted. Another clinical feature is that the sound of the cry of the baby with this defect is unusual and resembles the mewing of a kitten, accounting for this also being called the *cri-du-chat syndrome.*

CHROMOSOME ANOMALIES THAT ARISE AT THE SOMATIC CELL LEVEL

Some Further Terminology

In addition to the terms *diploid* and *haploid* (defined on p. 76), there are some other terms to learn. One is *polyploidy*, which means many times folded or multiplied, so polyploid cells are cells that have multiples of the haploid number of chromosomes. For example, a *tetraploid* cell has four times the haploid number (double the diploid number), and so on. Still another term that is much used is *aneuploidy;* since *an-* means want or absence, *aneuploidy* means an absence of the property of being a normal multiple, so the number in a cell manifesting aneuploidy is not an exact multiple of the haploid number. Hence a human cell with say 45, 47, or any number that is not an exact multiple of 23 is an aneuploid cell. The anomalies described above, which arise at the level of the germ cells, almost all involve changes in the total number of chromosomes in the body cells and so are examples of aneuploidy, but aneuploid numbers of chromosomes can also arise at the level of somatic cells.

Polyploidy Originating in Somatic Cells

This occurs in certain somatic cell families under normal conditions; indeed there is a kind of cell to be described in a later chapter (the megakaryocyte) that is normally polyploid. Certain other types of cells, for example, liver cells, are occasionally polyploid. Seen in the interphase, a polyploid liver cell has a larger nucleus than its diploid counterpart (Fig. 3-17, *bottom* of photomicrograph). As far as is known, polyploid liver cells

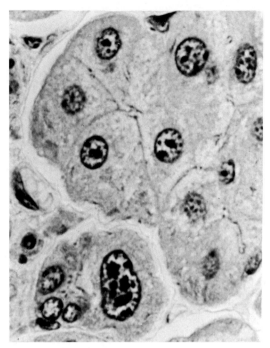

Fig. 3-17. Photomicrograph showing a liver cell (*bottom center*) that demonstrates polyploidy. The nucleus is much larger and contains more nucleoli than the nuclei of the cells above, which have the diploid number of chromosomes.

function normally. The usual cause of polyploidy is probably failure of the two s-chromosomes in each d-chromosome to separate in the metaphase of mitosis (nondisjunction), with the result that the two sets of s-chromosomes, instead of pulling to opposite ends of the cell, remain in the region of the equatorial plane until a new nuclear membrane forms and encloses them all in the same nucleus. However, there may be other ways in which polyploidy could occur. Polyploid cells are able to divide (Fig. 3-18).

Aneuploidy Originating in Somatic Cells

Aneuploidy originates at the somatic cell level under two conditions, as will now be described.

Species of higher animals, such as man, are perpetuated indefinitely because their germ cells create new individuals to carry on the species. Since bodies composed of somatic cells have a limited life span, the question arises as to whether a factor limiting their life span might not be that those cells which must multiply throughout life to maintain the structure of the body could have some inherent limitation placed on the number of times they can

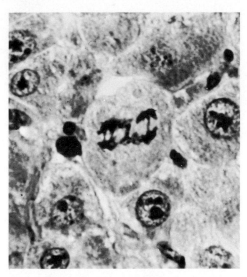

Fig. 3-18. High-power photomicrograph of regenerating rat liver, showing double the usual number of anaphase chromosomes arranged on a common spindle, which is just visible above them. This could be a tetraploid cell dividing.

reproduce themselves. It would, of course, be of great interest to know whether the kind of somatic cells that can divide, if transferred from one individual to another compatible one, would through succeeding generations demonstrate the same type of immortality as is demonstrated by germ cell lineages. One way the question of somatic cell immortality can be investigated is by cultivating somatic cells outside the body in suitable media. Studies of this kind have shown that somatic cells with proliferative capacity can indeed be propagated outside the body in nutritive media long enough to suggest that they could go on multiplying forever. But when methods for chromosomal analysis became available it also became evident that most of these lines of cells that do not die out after a few months of cultivation in vitro, but instead keep on proliferating, have acquired an aneuploid number of chromosomes and so can no longer be considered normal cells. The suspicion is thus aroused that the long-continued multiplication of somatic cells is associated with risk of some genetic change occurring in the cell that makes it less responsive to factors that would ordinarily suppress its rate of reproduction or capacity for unlimited reproduction, and which often leads to aneuploidy.

Aneuploidy and Cancer Cells

Aneuploidy occurs under conditions of the more or less continuous multiplication of cells characterizing the disease *cancer*. It is believed that cancer originates because some somatic cell undergoes a genetic change so that it multiplies under conditions in which the multiplication of normal cells would be restrained. The escape of cancer cells from growth-control mechanisms is associated more or less reciprocally with a loss of their ability to attain the kind of highly specialized structure normal cells of the same type would attain, and hence, they are usually not so proficient functionally, or if they function at all, their function is unregulated, as if they did not relate to the needs of the rest of the organism. Accordingly, cancer cells are commonly said to use energy for growth instead of function.

Since the change that turns a somatic cell into a cancer cell is a genetic change, cancer cells pass on their asocial and aggressive characteristics to their progeny and so if a cancer is not all surgically removed, or destroyed in some other fashion before it has grown for too long, its cells may be disseminated by way of blood or lymph to parts of the body distant from its origin. In these sites the cells set up new foci of invasive and destructive growth called *metastases*, and by this means cancer cells can overwhelm the body.

By losing their ability to respond to influences that control the growth of normal cells, cancer cells in a sense achieve the prerequisites for somatic cell immortality. They do not, of course, demonstrate immortality in the body in which they develop, for if they are left to multiply in that body, they will destroy it. But if they are removed, and thereafter grow in cultures, some kinds at least can be propagated indefinitely. Furthermore, if the cells of a cancer originating in an experimental animal are regularly transferred to other animals of the same strain, they will continue to multiply indefinitely, and, indeed, on continued transplantation they often experience further genetic changes by which they become even more malignant than when they originated. Some cancers have been maintained in mice by this means for decades. Cancer cells, therefore, seem to be able to reproduce themselves indefinitely.

The cells of a cancer commonly exhibit aneuploidy; indeed, the demonstration of aneuploidy in growing cells taken from the body is regarded as being a positive indication that the cells concerned are cancer cells. The absence of aneuploidy, however, does not rule out the presence of cancer, for some cancer cells may not be aneuploid—at least, not at first, but only as their multiplication continues.

From the behavior of diploid cells in cultures and cancer cells in the body, we are left with the impression that aneuploidy, originating at the somatic cell level, is probably more of less the final outcome of some genetic disorganization releasing the cells in which it occurs from the influences that ordinarily place restraints on proliferative capacity. More is said about this in Chapter 6.

An Example of a Chromosome Anomaly Originating at the Somatic Cell Level Which Involves Form Instead of Number

Patients with chronic granulocytic leukemia, a malignant disease in which there is an overproduction of certain white cells of the blood, characteristically have in the chromosome complement of their bone marrow cells a unique chromosome which, since it was discovered in Philadelphia, is referred to as the *Philadelphia* chromosome, *Ph¹*, or *Ph*. It represents a No. 22 chromosome with almost half its long arm missing; chromosome banding methods have revealed that the missing part almost always becomes translocated onto one of the No. 9 chromosomes. In all other respects the chromosomes of a patient with this type of leukemia appear normal in both number and morphology. Since the Philadelphia chromosome is present in nearly all cases of this disease and absent in other conditions, it has become valuable in the diagnosis of chronic granulocytic leukemia. It has even been found before symptoms of the disease were apparent, and it tends to persist when the patient is in remission. Somehow this chromosome anomaly, possibly being a necessary if not sufficient condition for the development of the disease, is intimately involved in the process that leads to this type of leukemia.

The Philadelphia chromosome is *not inherited* from one generation to another. It is not present in the children of patients with the disease, nor is it found (when present) in all the cells of the body. Whereas nearly all the cells of the bone marrow in these patients possess the unusual chromosome, the cells of other tissues in the same individuals have normal-looking chromosomes. This anomaly thus arises at the somatic rather than the germ cell level, probably early in the development of the disease, in a precursor of white blood cells by the translocation of part of the long arm of Chromosome 22 to another autosome (usually a No. 9 chromosome). Once this has happened, the chromosome anomaly is transmitted to all the somatic cells that thereafter develop from this altered cell. This anomaly will be mentioned again in Chapter 12.

REFERENCES AND OTHER READING

Radioautography

Kopriwa, B. M.: A semiautomatic instrument for the radioautographic coating technique. J. Histochem. Cytochem., *14:*923, 1966.

———: The influence of development on the number and appearance of silver grains in electron microscope radioautography. J. Histochem. Cytochem., *15:*501, 1967.

———: A reliable standardized method for ultrastructural electron microscopic radioautography. Histochimie, *37:*1, 1973.

Kopriwa, B. M., and Huckins, C.: A method for the use of Zenker-formol fixation and the periodic acid-Schiff technic in light microscopic radioautography. Histochimie, *32:*231, 1972.

Kopriwa, B. M., and Leblond, C. P.: Improvements in the coating technique of radioautography. J. Histochem. Cytochem., *10:*269, 1962.

Leblond, C. P., and Warren, K. B. (eds.): The Use of Radioautography in Investigating Protein Synthesis. New York, Academic Press, 1965.

Salpeter, M. M., and Szabo, M. Sensitivity in electron microscopic autoradiography. I: Effect of radiation dose. J. Histochem. Cytochem., *20:*425, 1972.

Schultze, B.: Autoradiography at the Cellular Level. Physical Technics in Biological Research, vol. 3B. New York, Academic Press, 1969.

Williams, M. A.: Autoradiography and immunocytochemistry. *In* Glauert, A. M. (ed): Practical Methods in Electron Microscopy. vol. 6, part 1. Amsterdam, North Holland, 1978.

Williams, J. R., and Van den Bosch, H.: High resolution autoradiography with stripping film. J. Histochem. Cytochem., *19:*304, 1971.

The Study of the Cell and Cell Lineages by Labeling DNA

Baserga, R.: Multiplication and Division in Mammalian Cells. The Biochemistry of Disease: A Series of Monographs, 6, New York, Marcel Dekker, 1976.

Howard, A., and Pelc, S. R.: Synthesis of deoxyribonucleic acid in normal and irradiated cells and its relation to chromosome breakage. Heredity [Supp.], *6:*261, 1953.

Mazia, M.: The cell cycle. Sci. Am., *230:*54, Jan., 1974.

Messier, B., and Leblond, C. P.: Cell proliferation and migration as revealed by radioautography after the injection of thymidine-H³ into male rats and mice. Am. J. Anat., *106:*247, 1960.

Prescott, D. M.: Comments on cell life cycle. Natl. Cancer Inst. Monogr., *14:*55, 1964.

Stanners, C. P.: and Till, J. E.: DNA synthesis in individual L-strain mouse cells. Acta Biochem. Biophys. *37:*406, 1960.

Taylor, J. H.: The time and mode of duplication of chromosomes. Am. Naturalist, *91:*209, 1957.

———: Chromosome reproduction. Int. Rev. Cytol., *13:*39, 1962.

Chromosome Structure

Comings, D., and Okada, T.: Whole mount electron microscopy of meiotic chromosomes and the synaptonemal complex. Chromosoma, *30:*269, 1970.

DuPraw, E. J.: DNA and Chromosomes. New York, Holt, Rinehart and Winston, 1970.

Paulson, J. M., and Laemmli, U. K.: The structure of histone-depleted metaphase chromosomes. Cell, *12:*817, 1977.

Prescott, D. M.: The structure and replication of eukaryotic chromosomes. Adv. Cell Biol., *1:*57, 1970.

Ris, H.: Ultrastructure of the animal chromosomes. *In* Koningsberger, V. V., and Bosch, L. (eds.): Regulation of Nucleic Acid and Protein Biosynthesis. New York, American Elsevier, 1967.

———: Chromosomal structure as seen by electron microscopy. *In* The Structure and Function of Chromosomes. Ciba Foundation Symposium 28 (New Series). New York, American Elsevier, 1975.

Wolfe, S. L.: Molecular organization of chromosomes. *In* Bittar, E. (ed.): The Biological Basis of Medicine. vol. 4. New York, Academic Press, 1967.

Chromosome Identification and Chromosome Anomalies (Including Meiosis)*

Caspersson, T., Zech, L., Johansson, C., and Modest, E.: Identification of human chromsomes by DNA-binding fluorescent agents. Chromosome, *30:*215, 1970.

Caspersson, T., and Zech, L. (eds): Chromosome Identification —Technique and Applications in Biology and Medicine. Nobel Symposium 23 in Medicine and Natural Sciences, 1973.

Comings, D. E. Chromosome organization. Postgrad. Med. J., *52* [Supp. 2]:17, 1976.

Comings, D. E., and Okada, T. A.: Architecture of meiotic cells and mechanisms of chromosome pairing. *In* DuPraw, E. J. (ed.): Advances in Cellular and Molecular Biology, vol. 2. New York, Academic Press, 1972.

Darlington, C. D., and LaCour, L. F.: The Handling of Chromosomes. ed. 6. New York, John Wiley & Sons, 1975.

Emery, A. E. H. (ed.): Antenatal Diagnosis of Genetic Disease. Edinburgh, Churchill Livingstone, 1973.

Friedmann, T.: Prenatal diagnosis of genetic disease. Sci. Am., *225:*34, Nov., 1971.

German, J.: Oncogenic implications of chromosomal instability. Hosp. Pract., *8:*93, 1973.

Golomb, H. M., and Bahr, G. F.: Analysis of an isolated metaphase plate by quantitative electron microscopy. Exp. Cell Res., *68:*65, 1971.

Kessler, S., and Moos, R. H.: Behavioral manifestations of chromosomal abnormalities. Hosp. Pract., *8:*131, 1973.

Kihlman, B. A.: Molecular mechanisms of chromosome breakage and rejoining. Adv. Cell Molec. Biol., *1:*59, 1971.

Lampert, F.: The chromosomal basis of sex determination. Int. Rev. Cytol., *23:*277, 1968.

————: Chromosome alterations in human carcinogenesis. Adv. Cell Molec. Biol. *1:*185, 1971.

McKusick, V.: The mapping of human chromosomes. Sci. Am., *224:*104, April, 1971.

McKusick, V. A., and Ruddle, F. H.: The status of the gene map of the human chromosomes. Science, *196:*390, April, 1977.

* *See* Chapter 4 for references about Barr bodies.

Mendelsohn, M., et al: Computer oriented analysis of human chromosomes, Ann. N.Y. Acad. Sci., *157:*376, 1969.

Nowell, P. C., and Hungerford, D. A.: A minute chromosome in human chronic granulocytic leukemia. Science, *132:*1197, 1960.

Paris Conference (1971), Supplement (1975): Standardization in human cytogenetics. Birth Defects: Original Article Series, XI:9, 1975.The National Foundation, New York (Also in: Cytogenet. Cell Genet. *15:*201, 1975).

Pfeiffer, R. A.: Current aspects of the banding phenomena. *In* Szabo, G., and Papp, Z. (eds.): Medical Genetics. Amsterdam, Excerpta Medica, 1977.

Ruddle, F. H., and Kuckerlapati. R. S.: Hybrid cells and human genes. Sci. Am., *231:*36, July, 1974.

Seabright, M.: The use of proteolytic enzymes for the mapping of structural rearrangments in the chromosomes of man. Chromosoma, *36:*204, 1972.

Schendl, W.: Banding patterns on chromosomes. Int. Rev. Cytol. [Supp.], *4:*237, 1974.

Sumner, A. T., Evans, H. J., and Buckland, R. A.: A new technique for distinguishing between human chromosomes. Nature [New Biol.], *323:*31, 1971.

Szabo, G., and Papp, Z. (eds.): Medical Genetics. Amsterdam, Excerpta Medica, 1977.

Thompson, J. S., and Thompson, M. W.: Genetics in Medicine. ed. 3. Philadelphia, W. B. Saunders, 1979.

Valentine, G. H.: The Chromosome Disorders. An Introduction for Clincians. ed. 3. Philadelphia, J. B. Lippincott, 1975.

Wang, H. C., and Federoff, S.: Banding in human chromosomes treated with trypsin. Nature [New Biol.], *235:*52, 1972.

Polyploidy and Aneuploidy

Beams, H. W., and King R. L.: The origin of binucleate and large mononucleate cells in the liver of the rat. Anat. Rec., *82:*281, 1942.

Herman, C. J., and Lapham, L. W.: Neuronal polyploidy and nuclear volumes in the cat central nervous system. Brain Res., *15:*35, 1969.

Thompson, R. Y., and Frazer, S. C.: The desoxyribonucleic acid content of individual rat cell nuclei. Exp. Cell Res., *7:*367, 1954.

Wilson, J. W., and Leduc. E. H.: The occurrence and formation of binucleate and multinucleate cells and polyploid nuclei in the mouse liver. Am. J. Anat., *82:*353, 1948.

4 The Interphase Nucleus

The term *interphase nucleus* is commonly used to refer to the nucleus of any cell not in the process of mitosis. It is an appropriate term for the nuclei of cells that are in cycle or that have left cycle but are capable of cycling again; both kinds of cells could be said to be between two phases of mitosis. But as already mentioned (p. 42) most of the body cells of the adult will probably never divide again, so that they are not between two phases of mitosis; hence, strictly speaking, it is not really appropriate to call them interphase cells. However, we shall use this term to denote all nonmitotic nuclei because it is often used instead of the term *nondividing cells* and also because the term *interphase*, through long use, has come to refer to the phase in which a body cell performs its specialized function.

THE DIFFERENT APPEARANCES OF INTERPHASE NUCLEI

Although interphase nuclei all contain the same basic components, they may present various appearances in different kinds of cells. Certain cell types characteristically have such small interphase nuclei that their nuclear contents become tightly packed together, so that some of their components cannot be distinguished with the LM. Some of the cells lining the sinusoids of the liver (labeled in Fig. 4-1) are of this type. The nuclei of other kinds of cells may have other unusual shapes; for example, instead of being round to ovoid (the most common shape), they may be elongated, and, in some instances, pinched along their lengths so that they resemble short strings of beads, as in the cell called a *neutrophil* (or *polymorph*) illustrated in Figure 11-2 on page 280. However, generally speaking, all nuclei are made up of the same components, and the easiest way to see these with the LM is to study cells in which the nuclei are sufficiently large to have their components spread far enough apart to allow them to be identified. Many cell types in the body have nuclei of this sort and, since we have already described interphase liver cells, we shall take them for our example and now describe the components of their nuclei in more detail. In doing so we shall compare what can be seen in the LM (Figs. 4-1 and 4-2A) with what is seen in the EM (Fig. 4-3).

THE COMPONENTS OF THE INTERPHASE NUCLEUS AS SEEN IN H AND E SECTIONS

1. With the oil-immersion objective the interphase nucleus appears to be limited by a dark blue-staining line; this is termed the *nuclear envelope* or *nuclear membrane* (labeled in Fig. 4-1).

2. Within each nucleus there are one or more rounded blue-staining bodies; these are the largest and roundest bodies within the nucleus. They are termed *nucleoli* (each one a *nucleolus*, labeled in Fig. 4-1).

3. Within each nucleus there are also numerous (often poorly defined) aggregates of blue-staining material that are of irregular shape and smaller than the nucleoli; this material is referred to as *chromatin* (labeled in Fig. 4-1) and sometimes as *chromatin granules*, although the aggregates are not sharply defined.

4. The space in the nucleus not occupied by chromatin and nucleoli was originally interpreted as containing a semifluid material and hence called *nuclear sap*. In stained sections this material is represented by very pale staining or almost clear areas (labeled in Fig. 4-1).

We shall deal first with the nuclear envelope.

THE NUCLEAR ENVELOPE (MEMBRANE)

Interpreting What Is Seen With the LM

The nuclear envelope appears in H and E sections as a substantial dark blue-purple line (Figs. 4-1 and 4-2A). Modern technics have shown that its apparent thickness and staining qualities are due to chromatin adherent to its inner surface. First, if unstained sections are treated with the enzyme DNAase (which digests DNA and hence virtually eliminates the staining of chromatin with hematoxylin) and then stained with H and E the supposed

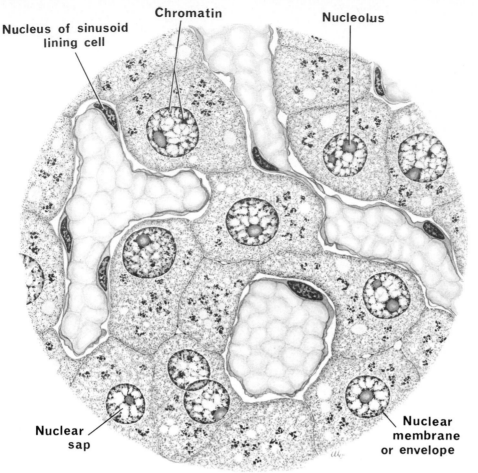

Nucleus of sinusoid lining cell

Chromatin

Nucleolus

Nuclear sap

Nuclear membrane or envelope

Fig. 4-1. Section of liver under oil immersion. The nucleus of each liver cell contains a dark-staining nucleolus (*upper right*). The remainder of the nucleus is made up of fine strands or granules of chromatin (*upper middle*), between which there are empty spaces containing nuclear sap (*lower left*). Each nucleus is surrounded by a nuclear envelope (*lower right*). Note also (*upper left*) that the nuclei of the cells lining the blood spaces are darker, smaller, and more elongated than the nuclei of liver cells; in these the chromatin is more condensed.

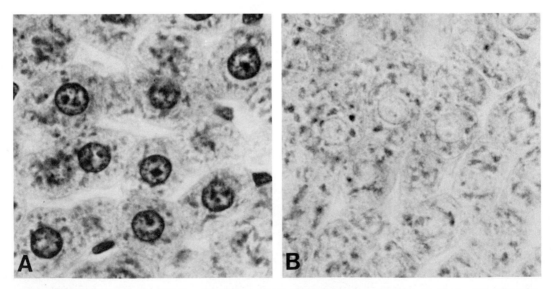

Fig. 4-2. H and E sections of rat liver (*A*) before and (*B*) after extraction with DNAase. The nuclei stain much less intensely, and the envelope appears less prominent after extraction with DNAase. (Courtesy of R. Daoust)

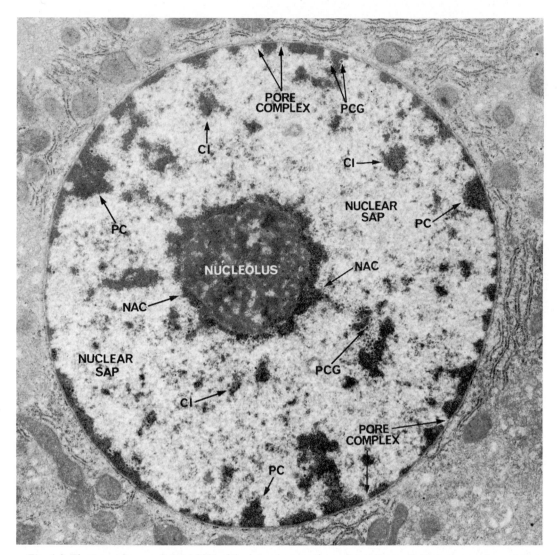

Fig. 4-3. Electron micrograph (×14,000) of the interphase nucleus of a rat liver cell. Note the condensed parts of chromosomes, forming peripheral chromatin (PC), chromatin islands (CI), and nucleolus-associated chromatin (NAC). The intranuclear channels of pore complexes can be seen as pale areas of nuclear sap between adjacent discrete masses of peripheral chromatin. Careful inspection shows perichromatin granules (PCG). (Miyai, K., and Steiner, J. W.: Exp. Molec. Pathol., *4:*525, 1965)

nuclear envelope, so obvious in Figure 4-2A, almost completely disappears, as shown in Figure 4-2B. Second, it was shown with the EM (Fig. 4-3) that a substantial amount of chromatin commonly adheres to the inner surface of the nuclear envelope and it is this that accounts for the apparent thickness and staining qualities of the membrane seen with the LM in ordinary sections.

The Appearance of the Nuclear Envelope in the EM

If the left side of the nucleus shown in Figure 4-3 is examined, it is possible to see the EM discloses that the

nuclear envelope consists of two thin membranes. This is shown to much better advantage at higher magnification in the bottom picture in Figure 4-4. Each of the membranes is about 8 nm. thick and the two are separated by a space about 25 nm. wide. The amount of substance in the membranes themselves is, of course, much too scanty to be visible in any plane of section with the LM. Indeed in places where the envelope follows a slanting course through a section, not enough electrons are scattered from an electron beam for a well-defined image to be formed in the EM. For the two membranes of the nuclear envelope to be seen clearly in an electron micrograph, the

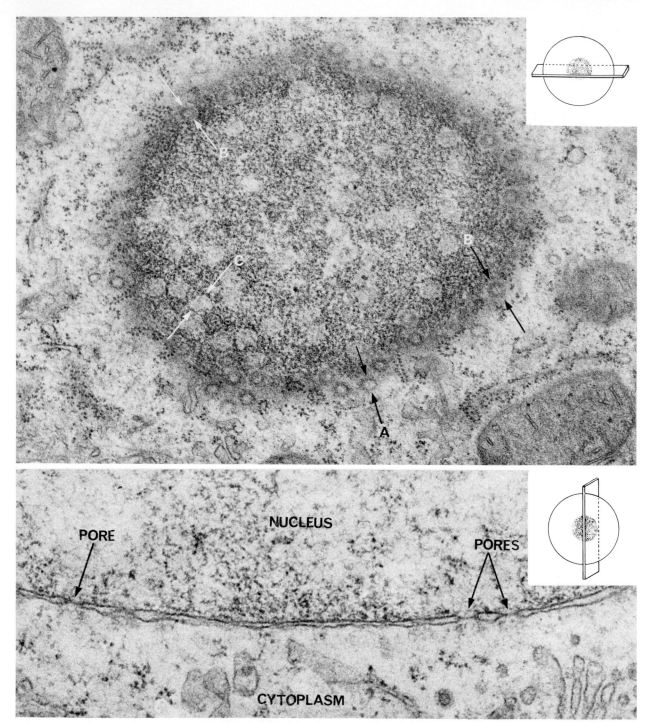

Fig. 4-4. Electron micrographs of an interphase nucleus of a liver cell (rat) showing the nuclear envelope with its nuclear pores, in different planes of section. (*Top*) Tangential section (perpendicular to the radius of the spherical nucleus, ×35,000) that shaves off a small area of the nuclear envelope as shown in the *inset* at *top right*. Note the appearance of the nuclear pore complexes where these are seen in face view. Some (A) are sectioned through their cytoplasmic aspect and hence appear to lie in the cytoplasm at a short distance from the nuclear chromatin. Others (C) are sectioned through the intranuclear channel region, so they are surrounded by peripheral chromatin. Still other pores (B) are sectioned at levels intermediate between levels A and C, and some of these would be at the level of the diaphragm closing the pore. (*Bottom*) Section cut perpendicular to the nuclear envelope (×56,000), cut as shown in the *inset*. Note the appearance of the nuclear pore complexes when cut in this plane. The diaphragm across the pores may be seen. Note also how the outer and inner membranes of the nuclear envelope are continuous with one another at the periphery of the nuclear pores. (Miyai, K., and Steiner, J.: Exp. Molec. Pathol., *4:*525, 1965)

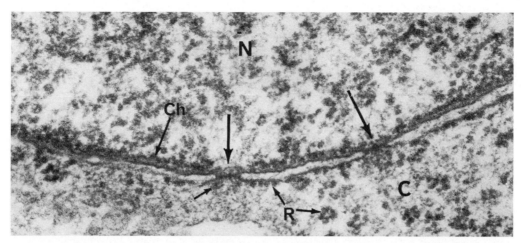

Fig. 4-5. Electron micrograph (×90,000) of a section of the nucleus cut at right angles to the nuclear envelope, showing nuclear pore complexes (*large arrows*). Note how the outer and the inner membranes of the nuclear envelope are continuous at the periphery of the nuclear pores. A thin diaphragm may be seen extending across the pore openings. A ring of dense material (*small, unlabeled arrow*) surrounds the pore and extends out into the cytoplasm (C). On the side of the nucleus (N), chromatin (Ch) is adherent to the inner aspect of the inner membrane of the nuclear envelope except at the nuclear pores. Ribosomes (R) are seen on the cytoplasmic aspect of the outer membrane and in the cytoplasm. (Courtesy of V. Kalnins)

section must be cut perpendicular to the nuclear envelope. The same problem also exists with regard to demonstrating the cell membrane by electron microscopy (refer to Fig. 5-4 on p. 110 for further explanation).

The student should now be able to reason why the two membranes of the nuclear envelope are not seen around the nucleus shown in Figure 4-4, *top*. This section shaved off a small part of a nucleus (as shown in the *inset*) and hence the nuclear envelope was cut obliquely. The electron beam, therefore, in passing through the section has only to pass through a single thickness of the membranes of the envelope and this did not scatter enough electrons from the beam for the envelope to be seen as dense lines (see also the left side of Fig. 5-4, p. 110, which illustrates this point with regard to the cell membrane).

The outer membrane of the nuclear envelope (the one next to the cytoplasm) is similar to, and connected with, a cytoplasmic membrane system called the rough-surfaced endoplasmic reticulum, which will be described in detail in Chapter 5.

Nuclear Pores

Knowledge of the biochemical interactions between the nuclear and cytoplasmic compartments of the cell indicates that there must be some means by which macromolecules of considerable size can pass between nucleus and cytoplasm. The probable pathway is through the apertures in the nuclear envelope (Fig. 4-5, *large arrows*) disclosed by the EM and termed *nuclear pores*. In face

view these appear more or less circular, but Gall showed that they are actually octagonal in outline. In most cells nuclear pores are numerous, fairly evenly distributed, and generally separated from one another by 100 to 200 nm. At the periphery of each pore, the outer and the inner membranes of the nuclear envelope are continuous with one another (Fig. 4-5). The diameter of pores in different types of cells varies from 30 to 100 nanometers. Thin tangential sections cut more or less parallel with the surface of nuclei (in which sections, as noted, the two membranes of the nuclear envelope itself cannot be seen distinctly) reveal these pores in surface view (Fig. 4-4, *top*). Detailed studies of pores show they contain rather complex structures that may be isolated from the nuclear envelope as distinct entitites. From each pore a channel projects for a short distance into the nucleus on one side and into the cytoplasm on the other. Within the nucleus condensed chromatin can be seen around the periphery of the channel (Figs. 4-4, *top*, labeled C and 4-6). On the cytoplasmic side of the nuclear pore, a channel surrounded by a ring of material of slightly increased electron density projects from the pore region (Fig. 4-4, *top*, labeled A). The whole arrangement is known as a *pore complex*.

There has been some question as to whether a nuclear pore is ever completely open, or whether there is always a very thin diaphragm extending across the pore as seen in Figures 4-4, *bottom*, and 4-5. The finding that some nuclear pores reveal no diaphragms is generally interpreted as indicating not that the nuclear pores are sometimes open, but that their diaphragms are particu-

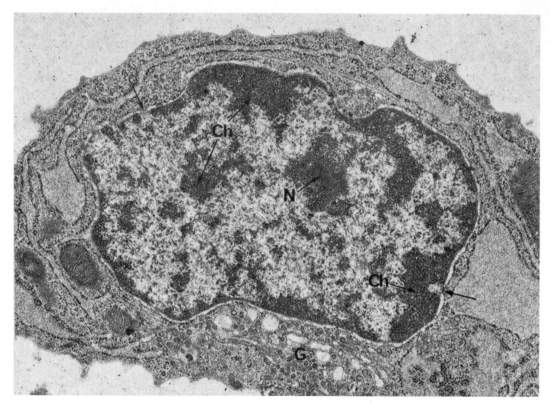

Fig. 4-6. Electron micrograph of a chondrocyte from a tracheal cartilage of a chick. The nucleus shows regions of condensed and extended chromatin. Much of the condensed chromatin is distributed along the inner surface of the nuclear membrane but some is scattered about in the nucleus in the form of chromatin islands; both types are indicated by Ch. Note that condensed chromatin is absent at the sites of nuclear pores (indicated by arrows, *lower right* and *upper left,* which point to pores). A nucleolus is labeled N. G, Golgi apparatus. (Courtesy of V. Kalnins)

larly difficult to fix and so are sometimes missing because they have not been preserved properly. Detailed information is available about the fine structure of nuclear pores of many species (*see* References and Other Reading).

The Importance of the Nuclear Envelope and Pores. It now seems obvious that in certain respects the microenvironment in the nucleus would differ from that in the cytoplasm. The nuclear envelope keeps some things out and others in. There is, however, a constant exchange of macromolecular chemical information in both directions across the nuclear envelope, and it appears likely that it is the permeability characteristics of the pore diaphragms that determine which kinds of molecules are able to pass from the nucleus to the cytoplasm and which may pass in the opposite direction.

THE CHROMATIN

The interphase nucleus of man contains 46 chromosomes which, in most specialized functioning cells of the body (such as those of the liver), are present as s-chromosomes. These exist in the interphase in a thread-like form but are variously crumpled, folded upon themselves, coiled, or otherwise formed into aggregates along their course; they correspond to the stainable chromatin granules visible in the LM. At other points along their course the chromosomes are, of course, invisible with the LM.

The Condensed Chromatin

With the EM the counterparts of the chromatin granules or the irregular masses seen with the LM are referred to as *condensed chromatin.* This is seen in three main positions with the EM. First, as noted, much condensed chromatin adheres to the inner surface of the nuclear envelope, and this is sometimes referred to as peripheral chromatin (Fig. 4-3, PC). Then, between this and the nucleolus, there are sizeable clumps of condensed chromatin scattered about in what has been termed the *nuclear sap.* Substantial dark granules represent the parts of s-chromosomes that are fully condensed. Finally, a good

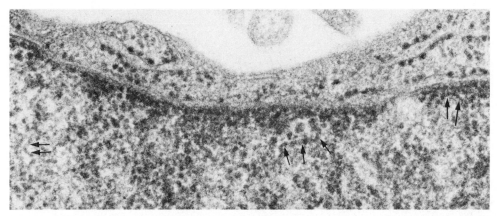

Fig. 4-7. Electron micrograph (×80,000) of part of a nucleus of a fibroblast. Extending across the middle of the micrograph is the nuclear envelope, with cytoplasm above and chromatin below it. On the lower aspect of nuclear envelope, peripheral chromatin may be seen but this is absent at the site of a nuclear pore (the pale area just to the left of the paired arrows near the right margin). Groups of arrows indicate chromatin threads cut over a short distance in longitudinal section. Note the gradual transition between the peripheral condensed chromatin and the extended chromatin lying below it. (Courtesy of V. Kalnins)

deal of condensed chromatin is clearly associated with the nucleolus, and this is appropriately termed the *nucleolus-associated chromatin* (Fig. 4-3, NAC).

The Extended Chromatin

This refers to those portions of the s-chromosomes that are extended. As already mentioned, this type of chromatin (*euchromatin*) is the important kind in the interphase cell, because the information stored in the parts of DNA molecules lying in the extended portions of interphase chromosomes is believed to be the only information transcribed during the interphase for directing protein synthesis in the cytoplasm.

However, it is difficult to study chromatin in sections of interphase nuclei with the EM, for several reasons. First, condensed and extended chromatin are not sharply demarcated from one another. Instead, as shown in Figure 4-7, gradations between densely packed chromatin and relatively open areas containing single threads are common. Next, chromatin threads curve in all directions through the nuclear sap and so it is seldom that single threads can be followed for any distance in a section; hence only short portions of these threads are seen. Third, such threads are too fine to be seen with the EM unless high magnifications are used, when it is just possible to resolve short portions of chromatin threads (indicated by grouped arrows in Fig. 4-7). The manner in which these threads relate to the folded fiber seen in each s-chromosome of condensed d-chromosomes when entire metaphase chromosomes (Fig. 3-8) are observed in the EM is a subject of current investigation. H. Ris has done

much to elucidate the structure of chromatin and his publications should be consulted for details.

The concept of only extended chromatin giving off information in the interphase to direct protein synthesis is a very important one. However, the reason for condensed portions of s-chromosomes in interphase nuclei not serving this function is not clear; the condensation of portions of the s-chromosomes is invariably associated with suppression of gene expression along these portions. Perhaps the same mechanism that suppresses gene expression also causes the chromatin thread to become condensed.

A further consideration is whether the portions of chromosomes that remain condensed and fail to direct protein synthesis might do so because they are not called upon to function. There are many indications that the genes locked up in condensed chromatin during the interphase can become functional and give information to direct new protein synthesis if they are called upon to do so. Certainly some types of body cells do express hitherto unexpressed functions. For example, at a certain stage the developing blood-forming cells of the erythrocytic series suddenly begin to synthesize hemoglobin, a protein that is not synthesized by any of their predecessors. It is possible that the expression of new functions might involve the unlocking of genes, formerly secluded in condensed chromatin, by allowing the chromatin threads bearing them to become extended. In this connection it is of considerable interest that most of the nuclear DNA is packaged into repeating globular subunits, about 12 nm. in diameter, called *nucleosomes*. In the EM these appear in suitable preparations as beads on a string. The DNA of each nucleosome is associated with histones in a complex

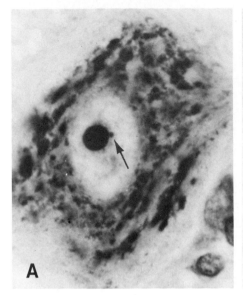
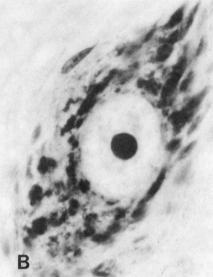

Fig. 4-8. Oil-immersion photomicrograph of nerve cells (in the anterior horn of the spinal cord) from two different cats. Note the pale appearance of the nuclei, which is due to almost all their chromatin being extended, and the prominent nucleolus in both cells. Barr and Bertram noticed that in nerve cells taken from female cats (*A*), a little round body could be found close to the nucleolus. This can be seen at the end of the arrow. The little body was not found in the nucleus of such cells taken from male animals (*B*). (Barr, M. L., Bertram, L. F., and Lindsay, H. A.: Anat. Rec., *107:*283, 1950)

arrangement, and it furthermore appears that nucleosomes may be lacking from regions of DNA that are being actively transcribed, suggesting that DNA in nucleosome-containing regions must somehow unravel in order for its genes to be expressed.

We shall go on to consider how the concept originated to the effect that condensed chromatin is genetically inactive, whereas extended chromatin is active. This concept, however, is linked with a further generalization, namely that all the chromosomes of an interphase cell must perform some important function, and it was an exception that was found to this general rule that also played a significant role in establishing the concept that only the extended chromatin is active in directing protein synthesis.

The Discovery of Barr Bodies

By the middle of this century, good light microscopes had been available for almost a hundred years, and microscopists had examined countless preparations of mammalian cells without ever observing that there was a difference in appearance between interphase nuclei of the cells of males and females that made it possible to tell the sex of the individual from which the cells were obtained. Hence, it seemed almost incredible when Barr and Bertram in 1949 described how they could establish the sex of cats by examining the nucleus in their nerve cells in ordinary sections, and furthermore pointed out that the same method was applicable to human nerve cells. They and their colleagues then examined other species and looked at different kinds of body cells. Soon Moore and Barr described a method for making smears of cells scraped from the lining of the cheek that permitted

microscopists to determine whether their nuclei contained what are now termed *Barr bodies*, which are indicative of the female sex. Research-minded students might like to know how this discovery was made.

Barr and Bertram were studying the changes in the cytoplasm of certain nerve cells of cats when the nerve fibers extending from them were stimulated. However, the pale large nucleus in these nerve cells (Fig. 4-8) helped to bring to their attention a little rounded basophilic body in the nuclei of the nerve cells of the first cats they studied. The observation that it seemed to change its position under different experimental conditions increased their interest. Commonly, however, it lay close to the nucleolus (Fig. 4-8A, indicated by arrow). As these researchers continued their experiments they continued to look for it and hence were surprised when they were unable to see it in some of the cats they later studied (as in Fig. 4-8B), while in others it was as clear as in the first ones. Puzzled by this, like the good scientists they were, they went over the careful records they had kept and discovered that the tiny body was present only in the nerve cell nuclei of female cats.

When other kinds of body cells from female cats and other female mammals were studied thoroughly, it became apparent that a similar body could be found in several other cell types. However, the common position of this little body in nerve cells (close to the nucleolus) was not typical, for in other kinds of cells it was almost always located on the inner aspect of the nuclear envelope, as shown in Figures 4-9 and 4-10; furthermore, it appears as a convex body instead of the rounded one seen in nerve cells.

Barr Bodies in Buccal Smears

To determine whether Barr bodies are present requires the examination of a considerable number of nuclei.

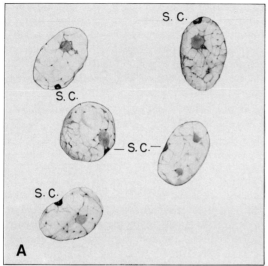 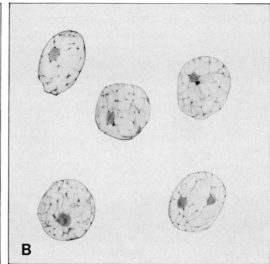

Fig. 4-9. (*A*) Oil-immersion drawing of nuclei of epithelial cells (in the stratum spinosum of the epidermis) of a female, obtained by biopsy, as they appear in a section (Harris' hematoxylin and eosin). The sex chromatin (S.C.), or Barr body, lies against the inner surface of the nuclear membrane as it does in most tissues. (*B*) A preparation in all respects similar except that the epidermis was obtained from the skin of a male. There is no sex chromatin (Barr body) visible. (Preparations by M. A. Graham and M. Barr)

Moore and Barr found that instead of having to remove bits of tissue (such as skin) from an individual and cut sections, all that was necessary in order to obtain a relatively large number of cells was to scrape cells from the inside of the cheeks, which fortunately can be done with no discomfort, using a spatula. The cells can then be smeared onto a slide, dipped into fixative (one in common use is ether-alcohol) and stained with cresyl violet. A Barr body can be recognized in such cells as a little dark mass, convex in shape and adherent to the inner aspect of the nuclear envelope (Fig. 4-9). Since its diameter is about 1 μm., it is readily visible with the oil-immersion objective in smears (Fig. 4-10) and sections (Fig. 4-9) provided the plane of section includes it. But even where present, it should not be expected that Barr bodies would be seen in every nucleus examined, for the section may not be in the right plane to include it, or inappropriate orientation of the nucleus in a smear may prevent its recognition, since the Barr body may lie on the upper or lower aspect of the flattened nucleus and not along its side, where it can be recognized most easily. Also, some nuclei of cells of normal males may show discrete masses of condensed chromatin close to the nuclear envelope that look like Barr bodies. Accordingly, since Barr bodies cannot be distinguished in every nucleus containing them, and since discrete chromatin masses resembling Barr bodies can sometimes be seen in nuclei that do not possess any, the presence or absence of Barr bodies cannot be determined with certainty by a hasty glance at single cells, but only by

Sex chromatin

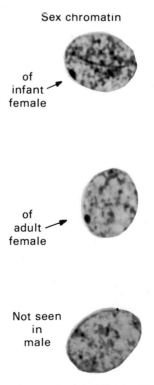

of infant female →

of adult female →

Not seen in male

Fig. 4-10. Photomicrographs (×2,000) of epithelial cells of the oral mucosa in smears stained with cresyl-echt violet. Barr bodies (*arrows*) may be seen in the upper two nuclei. (Moore, K. L., and Barr, M. L.: Lancet, *2*:57, 1955)

careful examination of about 100 nuclei, from which the percentage of cells with Barr-body-like structures may be estimated. Barr bodies, or structures resembling them, can be seen (at least with a trained eye) in up to 90 per cent of cells from chromosomally normal females, but only in about 10 per cent of cells from normal males.

The Nature of the Barr Body. The mass of chromatin now termed a *Barr body* was at first called the *sex chromatin* of the cell because of the incorrect notion that the two X chromosomes of the interphase cell would together constitute a sizeable mass of chromatin. But then as methods for studying chromosomes improved it was shown that a Barr body represented only *one* of the two X chromosomes of cells of females. The reason for its being visible in the interphase was that it remained condensed instead of becoming partly extended as did the other X chromosome and the remainder of the chromosomes in the nucleus. This finding was of great importance because by this time it was known that DNA provided the information for protein synthesis in the cytoplasm and, since female cells has two X chromosomes, one condensed and the other extended, the finding suggested that it was the extended X chromosome that gave off the information carried by an X chromosome and further that one X chromosome was all that was required to provide this information. The reason for Barr bodies not being seen in male cells thus became apparent. Since male cells have only one X chromosome, it has to be extended (in which state it is invisible as such with the LM) in order to give off the information its genes contain. (An X chromosome is concerned with much more than sex; it has over 50 genes that have nothing to do with sex and are important in both males and females.) From all this it became apparent that the term *sex chromatin* was not very appropriate for a single inactive condensed X chromosome, and so it was generally agreed to name the little body after its discoverer, so that now it is commonly called a *Barr body*.

Why one of the two X chromosomes of a female body cell should become entirely extended in the interphase while its homologue remains condensed is not understood. However, it is important for us to note here that, if one X chromosome remains condensed while the other is extended and functioning, whatever it is that suppresses gene expression in chromosomes predisposes also to condensation of the chromatin in the suppressed region. This close relation between gene inactivation and chromatin condensation is further substantiated by the finding that if genes belonging to an autosome become translocated to an X chromosome, they too become inactivated if that particular X chromosome becomes a Barr body. That a mechanism for causing chromatin to become condensed operates to cause all but one of the X chromosomes in a cell to become condensed is also apparent in certain chromosome anomalies (described in Chap. 3) in which

there are excessive numbers of X chromosomes in a cell, whether it belongs to a female or to a male. If, for example, there happen to be two X chromosomes in a male cell, one will appear as a Barr body: if there are three X chromosomes in a female cell, two will appear as Barr bodies; indeed, all but one in diploid cells will become Barr bodies.

Why Human Females Are Mosaics. Barr bodies make their initial appearance in body cells when a female embryo is about two weeks old, at which time it consists of only a few hundred cells and has become implanted in the lining of the uterus. At this time one of the two X chromosomes of its body cells can be seen to be condensed while the other is extended. Which of the two X chromosomes in a cell becomes a Barr body at this time is a matter of chance. Since the genes of the two X chromosomes may be somewhat different, because one X chromosome is derived from the father and one from the mother, the cells of an embryo in which the X chromosome from the father's side becomes active will be slightly different from those in which the X chromosome from the mother's side becomes active. After chance has determined which chromosome will be active in a body cell of the early embryo, the one that becomes active is perpetuated as the active one in all the subsequent generations of cells arising from that cell as the body develops. Hence the different clones of cells that are set up, which in due course populate the female body, are of two kinds. In one kind the paternally derived X chromosome is always active and in the other, the maternally derived X chromosome is always active. For this reason, normal human females are mosaics composed of two kinds of cells.

The Significance of Barr Body Numbers as a Sex Test. When the technics for the chromosomal analysis of mitotic cells became available and various anomalies were studied with these technics, it became apparent that Barr bodies do not always prove that an individual is female. As was described in Chapter 2, sex is not determined by whether or not individuals possess two or more X chromosomes, but by whether they possess a Y chromosome, because it is the Y chromosome that is responsible for the development of testes (the sex glands of the male). Through the use of the Barr body test, and the study of chromosome spreads, it was disclosed that there are certain chromosome anomalies in which individuals who are females do not reveal Barr bodies and some individuals who are males possess them. For example, in the anomaly known as *Turner's syndrome* (described in Chap. 3) the cells of a female have only one sex chromosome, which is an X. Since this single X chromosome would be extended and active, there would be no Barr bodies in the cells of such a female. In *Klinefelter's syndrome* (also described in Chap. 3) a male has a Y chromosome in all his cells and, in addition, he has two X chromosomes. Only one X is active and extended and the other appears as a Barr body, yet because of the Y chromosome, the individual is male. As noted, in anomalies in which there are more than two X chromosomes present in cells, only one is extended, so every additional X appears as a Barr body. Hence, strictly speaking a negative sex test, that is, establishing an absence of Barr bodies in the somatic cells of an individual, although enormously useful for detecting anomalies of the sex chromosomes, is not conclusive proof that an individual is a male. Likewise, the presence of Barr bodies in the cells of an individual, although equally useful, is not conclusive proof that the individual is a female; it is merely proof that the somatic cells of that individual contain two X chromosomes, at least. The full sex chromosome constitution of an individual can be determined only by establishing also whether or not the somatic cells also have one or more Y chromosomes; this is done by the fluorescent Y test in interphase cells (p. 73) or by studying spreads of metaphase chromosomes as outlined in Chapter 3.

The Significance of Condensed and Extended Chromatin in the Interphase Nucleus

The discovery of Barr bodies, and the development of knowledge that followed it due to the devising of technics for the chromosomal analysis of mitotic cells, not only opened up the very important aspect of modern medicine dealing with chromosome anomalies and their effects, but also lent credence to the idea that the chromatin that remains condensed in the interphase in specialized functioning cells is genetically inactive, and hence it is only extended chromatin that gives off information to direct synthesis of proteins in the interphase. Thus the condensation of chromatin would seem to be closely associated with the suppression of gene function in chromosomes.

Whereas the above evidence for its being only the extended chromatin that functions in the interphase cell was obtained by studying the sex chromosomes, substantial evidence for its being the extended chromatin of autosomes that is genetically active has come from radioautographic studies of RNA synthesis in the nuclei of specialized cells. For example, in 1964, Littau et al., using tritiated uridine to label newly forming RNA (uridine is a building block of RNA), showed that the grains appearing over the nuclei of thymus cells (lymphocytes), in which the chromatin is predominantly of the condensed type, were almost exclusively located over the small amount of chromatin that was extended. From their study they concluded that the condensed chromatin was virtually inactive as a template for the synthesis of RNA.

It seems ironic that the only chromatin visible with the LM in interphase nuclei is not the chromatin that is providing information for protein synthesis in these cells. The parts of the chromatin threads active in directing protein synthesis are probably only those that cannot be seen at all with the LM and they would lie distributed in what was originally termed the *nuclear sap*.

It is also worth noting that whereas some of the genes expressed in the extended chromatin of the nuclei of certain kinds of specialized cells may be the same as those that are active in other kinds of specialized cells, other genes may differ in expression from one kind of cell to another. Hence some of the genes that are active, and hence reside in the extended chromatin in certain kinds of cells, may be inactive and tucked away in the condensed chromatin in other types of cells. The condensed chromatin seen in different kinds of interphase nuclei therefore differs not only in amount but also in the genetic content.

HOW INFORMATION STORED IN THE DNA OF EXTENDED CHROMATIN DIRECTS PROTEIN SYNTHESIS IN THE CYTOPLASM

RIBONUCLEIC ACID (RNA)

As described on page 36, there are two kinds of nucleic acid, DNA and RNA. RNA differs from DNA not only because its sugar is D-ribose while that of DNA is 2-deoxy-D-ribose, but also because one of its four nitrogenous bases is different from one of those in DNA—instead of having thymine as one of its bases, RNA has uracil.

There are three types of RNA, which play three different roles in cells. Each type of RNA has a somewhat different molecular form, which permits it to be separated from the others.

Messenger RNA

From the four-letter alphabet, A,C,T and G, a triplet code of three-letter words is written along the strands of DNA molecules that lie in extended chromatin. The information embodied in sentences of these three-letter words prescribes which of the 20 or so amino acids available in the cytoplasm are to be strung together. Furthermore, it also specifies the order in which this is to be done, so as to form polypeptide chains in the cytoplasm that will either themselves comprise simple protein molecules or else become parts of complex protein molecules comprising many polypeptide chains. The first problem to consider is how the information on the DNA specifying which particular amino acids are to be linked together, and in what order, is conveyed to the sites of protein synthesis in the cytoplasm. This information is transcribed onto and carried out into the cytoplasm by a type of RNA, suitably called *messenger RNA (mRNA)*. The second problem is how the information conveyed to the cytoplasm by mRNA is then put into effect, by means of two other types of RNA.

Transcription by Complementary Base Pairing of DNA With mRNA. It was explained with diagrams on pages 39 and 40 that in order for a DNA molecule to be duplicated in the S phase of the cell cycle, its two strands must separate sufficiently (though not simultaneously along its whole length), as shown in Figure 2-5, so that a new strand can be synthesized along each of its two strands as shown in Figure 2-6. An important feature of this complementary base pairing is that wherever there is an A (for adenine) along a strand of DNA, a T (for thymine) is synthesized beside it as part of the new strand being formed. Similarly, wherever there is a C (for cytosine) on the original strand, a G (for guanine) forms beside it. Likewise wherever there is a T on the original, an A is formed beside it and wherever there is a G, a C forms beside it. Thus new strands are complementary to the original strands, but the new double-stranded molecules of DNA formed are identical to the mother molecules, as explained on page 40.

In the transcription of information onto a molecule of mRNA forming beside a strand of DNA, the same system of complementary base pairing applies. There are, however, two important differences between the base pairing occurring in the duplication of DNA molecules and the base pairing that takes place in the transcription of information onto forming molecules of mRNA.

First, in the duplication of DNA molecules, the whole strand of DNA must be read so that a complete new strand can be formed beside it. In other words, the duplication of DNA molecules requires the duplication of all the information stored in them. However, of the overwhelming amount of information in the DNA molecules of all the chromosomes, only a few relevant parts of the DNA molecules are transcribed onto mRNA in each type of cell. These would be the parts of the DNA molecules lying in the extended chromatin. Some of the factors possibly concerned in determining which particular parts of the DNA molecules will become transcribed in the various kinds of interphase cells (which, of course, would be essential if they were to perform different functions) are discussed in Chapter 6. Here it is enough to note that transcription onto mRNA involves relatively short regions of the DNA molecules in the chromosomes.

Second, although the same principle of transcribing information through complementary base pairing applies in both the formation of molecules of mRNA and the synthesis of new strands of DNA, as noted, RNA has one base that is different from one in DNA: it has *uracil* in place of thymine. So while a C on a DNA molecule is responsible for a G (guanine) forming in a complementary molecule of mRNA, and likewise a C is responsible for a G and a T is responsible for an A, an A (adenine) on a DNA molecule results in a U (for uracil) being incorporated into a forming molecule of RNA. So the four-letter alphabet in which three-letter words are spelled out along a mRNA molecule consists of A, C, G and U. Hence in the transcription of information from a DNA molecule to a forming molecule of mRNA, the mechanism of complementary base pairing results in a U forming on the mRNA molecule wherever there is an A on the DNA molecule. Some of the three-letter words along RNA molecules therefore contain a U and none contain a T (*see top right* of Fig. 4-11).

Messenger RNA reaches the cytoplasm, presumably by passing through the pore complexes in the nuclear envelope. It can be isolated from the cytoplasm and it appears as long thread-like strands in the EM; a portion of one is shown in Figure 5-17.

The three-letter words inscribed along DNA molecules are called *codons*, each coding for a particular amino acid. As noted, there are more possible three-letter words (codons) than there are amino acids, hence there is sometimes more than one codon for the same amino acid. Since the codons are transcribed onto mRNA by complementary base pairing, the codon on the DNA molecule for the amino acid glycine, CCT, would be transcribed by complementary base pairing onto mRNA as GGA, as shown below:

DNA molecule: CCT
mRNA molecule: GGA

The next question to consider is how the three-letter words along the molecule of mRNA bring about addition of the amino acids for which they code in the right sequence so as to form particular polypeptides or proteins. The linking together of the appropriate amino acid molecules occurs on ribosomes.

Ribosomes and Ribosomal RNA (rRNA)

Ribosomes are small electron-dense bodies of ribonucleoprotein, roughly 20 to 22 nm. in diameter, though not entirely spherical in shape (Fig. 5-17). Their nucleic acid component is a second kind of RNA, termed *ribosomal RNA, (rRNA)*. The precursor of this rRNA is synthesized in the nucleolus. Ribosomes, a type of cytoplasmic organelle, are most abundant at sites of active protein synthesis. Each ribosome is assembled from two ribonucleoprotein *subunits*, a large one and a small one (Fig. 5-24).

Ribosomes serve as essential sites where amino acids

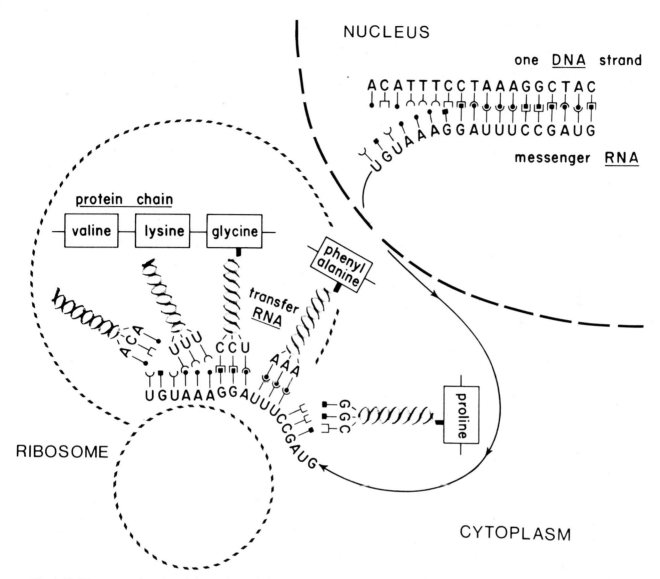

Fig. 4-11. Diagram to show how information coded on one strand of a DNA molecule in the nucleus (*upper right*) is transferred to a strand of mRNA forming beside it (*upper right*), and how the latter peels away from the DNA molecule (*upper right*) and moves out of the nucleus and into the cytoplasm toward a ribosome (*lower left*). Here the strand of mRNA is surrounded by a pool of amino acids, each of which is identified by a particular three-letter code word of tRNA; thus valine is identified by ACA, lysine by UUU, glycine by CCU, phenylalanine by AAA, and proline by GGC. The first three-letter code word inscribed along the strand of mRNA (*bottom left*) fits ACA, so valine is first selected by the mRNA. The next three-letter code word selects UUU, so that lysine is added to valine. The next word selects glycine, which is added to the protein chain. The diagram shows that phenylalanine and proline will be added next (*right side*) and that the tRNAs responsible for identifying valine and lysine (*left side*), having done their work, have become detached both from the mRNA and from the amino acids they identified.

can be linked together in the order prescribed by the codon sequence on mRNA molecules, which move along with respect to ribosomes in the cytoplasm. However, for this to occur requires the help of RNA of the third kind, which is called *transfer RNA.*

Transfer RNA (tRNA)

Messenger RNA, as described above, embodies a string of code words specifying different amino acids in a particular order so that, when these have been linked in the prescribed sequence, they will constitute a specific polypeptide or protein molecule. Ribosomes provide the machinery whereby all this can take place. But how do the amino acid molecules recognize the code words that specify them? Recognition is achieved through a go-between, which is RNA of the third kind, appropriately called *transfer RNA (tRNA)*.

Molecules of tRNA possess a characteristic shape, with two distinct arms. One of these specifically recognizes and attaches to a given amino acid. For example, in Figure 4-11, one arm of a glycine-carrying tRNA molecule (depicted as a spiral in this diagram) is attached to a glycine molecule that has just become incorporated into the polypeptide chain. The other arm of a tRNA molecule possesses a particular three-letter code word (made up from the A, C, G, and U alphabet of RNA) that by complementary base pairing will recognize and attach specifically to the complementary three-letter word (codon) at places where it occurs along the length of the molecule of RNA. Because this code word on the tRNA molecule is complementary in sequence to the codon specifying the particular amino acid, it is often called the *anticodon* part of the molecule. For example, the codon specifying glycine on a mRNA molecule is GGA (Fig. 4-11) and this pairs specifically with the CCU anticodon sequence on the molecule of glycine-carrying tRNA (Fig. 4-11). This particular kind of tRNA molecule would, of course, have a glycine molecule attached to its other arm, as depicted in Figure 4-11. Each kind of tRNA specifying a given amino acid would have its own characteristic attachment site for the amino acid and its own particular anticodon sequence for recognizing the right codon on the mRNA.

Protein Synthesis

How Polypeptide Chains Are Assembled

First, a molecule of mRNA leaves the nucleus to enter the cytoplasm, where there are ribosomes and a pool of molecules of the 20 or so amino acids. Each kind of amino acid molecule can become attached to one arm of its own kind of tRNA molecule, as described above; the other arm of the tRNA molecule bears the anticodon sequence whereby it is able to pair in complementary fashion with the mRNA three-letter codon specifying that particular amino acid. As the molecule of mRNA moves relative to the ribosome, the various amino acids specified by the code words along its course are brought together in the proper order and linked to one another to form what will become a polypeptide chain, as depicted in Figure 4-11. The molecule of tRNA carrying the amino acid molecule then becomes detached from it and, more or less simultaneously, the tRNA molecule detaches from the codon on the mRNA with which it paired. The molecule of tRNA

is then recycled, since it is now available to recombine with the same kind of amino acid and be used again.

Once a particular mRNA reaches the cytoplasm, protein synthesis occurs automatically. It is of interest that this is so even for rather inappropriate proteins induced to form by artificial means. Thus if mRNAs coding for the globin of rabbit hemoglobin or for a particular polypeptide component of bee venom are injected into cells of other species that do not ordinarily synthesize these products (frog oocytes, for example), the protein or polypeptide specified by the particular mRNA injected is thereupon synthesized (Lane). Molecules of mRNA continue to direct protein synthesis until they become degraded; different mRNAs appear to have different lifetimes, and some can persist for considerable periods as, for example, in certain cells that have lost their nuclei.

The Synthesis of RNA and Proteins in Tissues

The synthesis of RNA in cells of the body can be studied by injecting animals with tritiated uridine (a specific precursor of RNA), followed by radioautography. Likewise, the synthesis of proteins may be followed by injecting suitable tritium-labeled amino acids and preparing tissues for radioautography. Several examples of how the synthesis of particular proteins has been studied by means of radioautography are given throughout this textbook, and further details of protein synthesis are given when we consider ribosomes as cytoplasmic organelles in Chapter 5 (p. 122).

The Regulation of Protein Synthesis

The rate of protein synthesis in cells varies with changing circumstances related to varying needs of the body for growth and function. Since the synthesis of proteins in cells is directed by genes, one way of regulating the synthesis of specific proteins would be to regulate the amount of mRNA synthesized by the genes coding for them. When an increase in the synthesis of a particular protein is required, the gene directing the synthesis of that protein must do one of two things. It must either become more active than before, or it must remain active for longer periods of time. Conversely, when there is less need for the synthesis of a particular protein, the gene involved must become either less active or active for shorter periods. Accordingly it is believed that there is some sort of mechanism that turns genes "on" or "off" to relate the synthesis of specific proteins to requirements.

Next, since genes are confined to the chromatin in the nucleus, they are not in direct contact with the external environment of the cell. The demand for protein synthesis, however, often arises somewhere else in the body, not in the cells that synthesize the protein. For example, enzymes must be synthesized by secretory cells of the pancreas in amounts appropriate for the digestive process to occur efficiently in the intestine, and this has not much to do with the direct needs of the secretory cells themselves. Thus any increased demand for a given protein must somehow be signalled to the immediate environment of those cells that will respond and produce more of the protein. From the immediate environment of the cell this message must then somehow be transferred across the cytoplasm of the responding cell by chemical means to the nucleus and there reach the genes coding for the particular mRNA required for the synthesis of that protein.

The manner in which genes are turned on or off is not well understood. There are two aspects to consider. First, in specialized functioning cells the activity of each gene expressed must be regulated by mechanisms that can ensure its times and rate of functioning are appropriate to the needs of the body as a whole. A good deal is now known about how this is achieved, at least in certain instances. The second aspect is more difficult to explain. It is how and why the different genes are turned on so as to cause the various kinds of body cells to develop, and thereafter remain with the same genes turned on (or off) in their progeny, so that a spectrum of distinct cell families persists in the body. These matters are discussed in Chapter 6; here we shall go on to describe the nucleolus and the formation of ribosomal RNA from precursor molecules synthesized there.

THE NUCLEOLUS

The LM Appearance of Nucleoli

In H and E sections nucleoli are readily seen in nuclei that are reasonably large and have well-dispersed chromatin (Figs. 4-1 and 4-2A). However, they are commonly obscured in smaller nuclei that have much condensed chromatin, since within the thickness of an ordinary section this may lie above and below, as well as to each side of the nucleoli. Nevertheless, even though nucleoli cannot be seen with the LM in H and E sections of certain cells, ultrathin sections examined with the EM show them to be present.

When apparent in H and E sections, nucleoli appear very basophilic. Since the RNA of ribosomes is synthesized in nucleoli, it might be thought that the basophilia of nucleoli would be due to rRNA. But if sections are treated with DNAase and then stained, most of the basophilia of nucleoli disappears (Fig. 4-12B). Furthermore, after treatment with RNAase, most of the basophilia remains (Fig. 4-12A). Hence most of the basophilia that otherwise might be attributed to the nucleoli them-

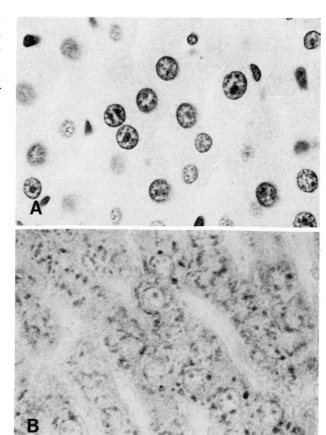

Fig. 4-12. Oil-immersion photomicrographs of two sections of liver, stained with H and E. The upper section (*A*) was treated with RNAase before staining and the lower one (*B*) with DNAase. Note that nucleoli can still be seen in the nuclei in (*A*) even though the RNA has been removed from them. That the appearance of nucleoli in (*A*) is due to DNA is indicated by the fact that they stain only faintly when the nucleolus-associated chromatin is removed from them with DNAase, as shown in (*B*). (Courtesy of R. Daoust)

selves is due to nuclear chromatin condensed around them and hence termed *nucleolus-associated chromatin* (Fig. 4-3, NAC).

Size

It is of interest that the total amount of nucleolar substance was found, in Purkinje cells of the nervous system, to be always similar whether there was one, or more than one, nucleolus in the nucleus (Shea). Hence, the greater the number of nucleoli present, the smaller they are. However, whereas the total amount of nucleolar substance of cells of the same kind and in approximately the same state of function is probably similar, there is much evidence indicating that nucleoli tend to be larger than normal in cells actively engaged in protein synthesis. The cells of rapidly growing cancers, in which protein synthesis for growth is very active, often reveal very large nucleoli (*see* Fig. 4-16, *upper left corner*).

Nucleolar Organizers and the Function of the Nucleolus

The nucleolus is the site where the RNA of ribosomes is synthesized. As explained earlier, messenger RNA (mRNA) is synthesized along molecules of DNA of the extended chromatin. Ribosomal RNA (rRNA) is also synthesized along DNA molecules of extended chromatin, but only beside the parts of certain chromosomes that lie within the substance of the nucleolus. The regions of the chromosomes that perform this function are called *nucleolar organizers,* probably because when new nucleoli are formed in cells following mitosis, nucleoli are formed in association with them. The chromosomes that can serve this function are Nos. 13, 14, 15, 21, and 22. These chromosomes, as was noted in Chapter 3, page 72, are the ones with satellites.

The fact that there are several chromosomes possessing nucleolar organizers accounts for there sometimes being several nucleoli in the same nucleus. However the nucleoli tend to fuse to become a single body. A single large nucleolus is the result of the several nucleolar organizers of the satellited chromosomes being close together when they transcribe for rRNA, so that the rRNA formed in association with different chromosomes becomes confluent.

The Synthesis of rRNA in the Nucleolus

What is seen with the EM in the different parts of the nucleolus will be easier to interpret if we first describe the synthesis of rRNA in that organelle.

The Nucleolar Genes. In discussing the triplet code, we described a gene (actually, only one type of gene, called a *structural gene*) as being a portion of a DNA molecule coding for the amino acid sequence of a particular polypeptide or protein.

Earlier in this chapter we described how the code of such a gene is transcribed onto mRNA and how when this moves to the cytoplasm it directs the linking, in the correct order, of the amino acids specified by the code. Since various assortments of proteins are synthesized in different cells, differing assortments of mRNA are also produced in these cells. However, the rRNA of ribosomes is believed to be of exactly the same composition in all kinds of body cells, regardless of the proteins they are synthesizing. Its role in protein synthesis, unlike that of mRNA, is nonspecific. Accordingly, there must be segments of DNA molecules in every body cell, carrying ex-

actly the same code, that are responsible for rRNA being transcribed beside them. These segments are not concerned with transcribing the mRNA that directs the synthesis of particular polypeptides and hence do not conform to the usual concept of a structural gene; nevertheless, since they do transcribe RNA, they represent a type of structural gene and are termed *nucleolar genes.* They are distributed repetitively along the DNA of the extended chromatin of those portions of chromosomes corresponding to the *secondary constrictions* of metaphase satellited chromosomes.

In the nucleolus the molecules of rRNA synthesized along the nucleolar genes undergo certain changes that are necessary for later incorporation of the rRNA into ribosomes. These changes involve the first-formed units (molecules) of rRNA being cleaved into various classes of subunits, as will be described presently. The rRNA units and their subunits are designated in terms of their sedimentation coefficients, as determined by centrifugation, in Svedberg units (S). (This coefficient is related to molecular weight.) The rRNA that is first formed along the course of the nucleolar organizers has a sedimentation coefficient of 45S and, being the largest detectable class of rRNA molecule in the nucleolus, it is regarded as the precursor from which all the rRNA subunits are formed, as will be explained later. But first we shall describe how formation of 45S precursor rRNA molecules along nucleolar genes was demonstrated with the EM.

EM Studies on the Formation of rRNA. The oocytes of amphibians possess certain distinctive features that make them particularly suitable for EM studies of rRNA synthesis, the principal one being that they contain multiple extrachromosomal nucleoli (not attached to chromosomes) that contain large numbers of copies of nucleolar genes. From such isolated nucleoli Miller and Beattie were successful in obtaining remarkable electron micrographs of strands of DNA containing the genes coding for rRNA (Fig. 4-13). These disclose 45S precursor rRNA molecules forming alongside the "sentences" coding for rRNA repeated along these particular regions of the DNA. Each sentence coding for rRNA appears to be separated from the next one by an inactive segment of DNA. The micrograph (Fig. 4-13) depicts many molecules of rRNA in 45S precursor form being synthesized simultaneously on each of the many sentences coding for rRNA written along the DNA strand. The synthesis of rRNA molecules, as seen in the electron micrograph, has almost gone to completion at one end of each sentence and is just beginning at the other, which accounts for each sentence on the DNA, together with the rRNA made from it, having an appearance similar to that of a Christmas tree (Fig. 4-13). Several sentences along a strand of DNA, each coding for many molecules of precursor rRNA, look like a whole series of Christmas

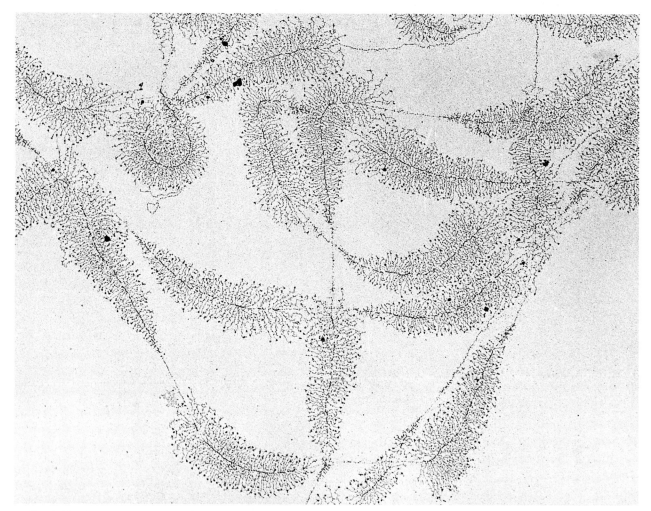

Fig. 4-13. Electron micrograph (×25,000) of nucleolar genes isolated from an oocyte of the spotted newt, *Triturus viridescens. See* text for description and explanation. (Courtesy of O. Miller, Jr., and B. Beatty)

trees arranged end to end, with the branch-free bottom of the trunk of each (which represents DNA that is not transcribed) touching the tip of the next (Fig. 4-13). The branching portion of the trunk of each tree would contain the portion of a DNA strand coding for rRNA and the branches of each tree would consist of increasing lengths of the rRNA being synthesized.

The Incorporation of rRNA Subunits Into Ribosomes. Ribosomes can each be readily separated into two *ribosomal subunits.* One is referred to as the *60S,* or *large, subunit* (corresponding to a molecular weight of almost 3 million) and the other as the *40S,* or *small, subunit* (which corresponds to a molecular weight of just over 1 million). Each of these subunits contains protein as well as rRNA. As far as the rRNA itself is concerned, the large (60S) subunit probably contains as many as three different classes of rRNA (with sedimentation coefficients of 28S, 7S, and 5S re-

spectively), while the smaller (40S) subunit contains 18S rRNA. The 45S precursor rRNA molecules of both types of subunits are produced in the nucleolus but their cleavage products are incorporated into ribosomal subunits in the cytoplasm.

The steps involved from the initial synthesis of the 45S rRNA until rRNA is finally incorporated into ribosomal subunits are complex. From the precursor (45S) rRNA synthesized along the nucleolar genes, segments are cleaved in a stepwise fashion and it is these shortened rRNA molecules that become incorporated, together with proteins, into the subunits of ribosomes in the cytoplasm. First, a small (5S) segment is split off from the 45S precursor rRNA molecule. Then the 41S portion remaining is split further into a 32S and a 20S segment. The 32S segment represents the precursor molecule of the 28S rRNA component of the large subunit of the ribosome, while the 20S portion corresponds to the precursor of the 18S rRNA of the small subunit. The 5S and 7S segments of rRNA also formed by cleavage of rRNA are probably incorporated along with the 28S rRNA into the large subunit of ribosomes.

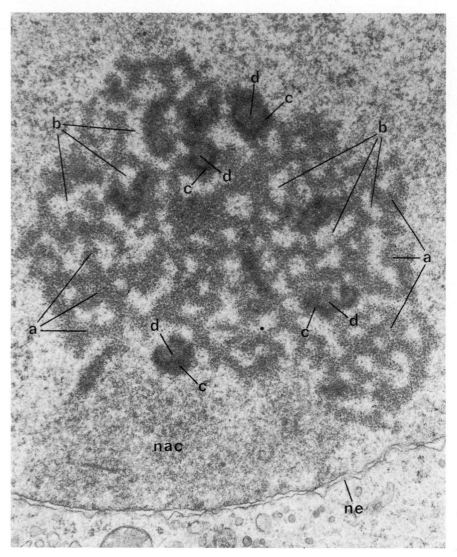

Fig. 4-14. Electron micrograph (×26,000) of part of the nucleus of a mouse oocyte (in the prophase of meiosis). Note the sponge-like appearance of the nucleolus in ultrathin section. It consists of dark material (a) and its interstices are filled with light material (b). For an explanation of the rings of dark material (c) and the cores of less dense material (d), *see* text. The nuclear envelope (ne) and nucleolus-associated chromatin (nac) are also shown. (Courtesy of L. Chouinard)

Proteins become associated with the 45S rRNA shortly after its synthesis. The 45S rRNA then undergoes cleavage and the cleavage products together with these proteins accumulate in the nucleus. Ribonucleoprotein particles containing 32S rRNA and protein tend to accumulate in the nucleolus before moving out into the cytoplasm. There is controversy about how nucleoproteins reach the cytoplasm, but it is widely believed that it must be via the nuclear pores.

The Fine Structure of the Nucleolus

With the EM the nucleoli of different kinds of cells present a variety of appearances, so that many cell types need to be studied in order to gain an understanding of the basic structure of this organelle. We shall begin by describing the typical structure of the nucleolus as seen in an ultrathin section of a mouse oocyte, as illustrated in Figure 4-14.

The first feature to note is that the rounded, homogeneous body seen with the LM (Fig. 4-1) appears not as a solid mass but as a network of electron-dense material (Fig. 4-14, a), lying free (that is, with no surrounding membrane) in the substance of the nucleus. In the interstices of this network there is a light material (Fig. 4-14, b) corresponding to nuclear sap, and this appears as little irregular islands surrounded by dark material.

The Form of the Dark Material and Its Two Components. Not all LM studies indicated that the nucleolus was solid; from the use of special technics it seemed that it might

Fig. 4-15. Electron micrograph (×22,000) of an interphase nucleus of *Allium cepa* (onion), which shows fibrillar centers to advantage. Four are indicated by arrows. The fibrillar centers contain several electron-dense bodies that appear to be sections of the chromatin thread of the nucleolus-organizing portion of a chromosome. The electron density of these is similar to that of the chromatin appearing as dark material scattered around the nucleolus. The organization of the fibrillar and granular material in this type of nucleolus is different from that of the nucleolus shown in Figure 4-14, for the granular material (gr) is located around the periphery and toward the center of the nucleolus, with some in between. The fibrillar component (fr) is disposed in patches associated with the fibrillar centers. (Courtesy of L. Chouinard)

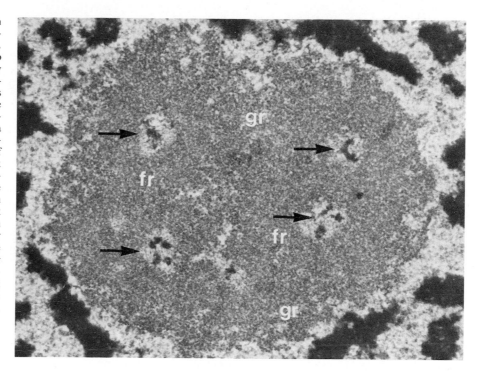

contain something with the shape of a crumpled cord, so this was called a *nucleonema* (Gr. *nema*, thread). When the EM disclosed a network of dark material in the nucleolus, it was assumed that this material corresponded to the crumpled thread. However, if the dark material were in the form of a crumpled cord, sections of it would be expected to be surrounded by light material, but the reverse is true for, as noted, it is the light material (Fig. 4-14, b) that appears as islands within the dark material (Fig. 4-14, a). Hence it seems that the dark material forms a spongework with light material occupying the spaces. Accordingly, if there is any such thing as a nucleonema, it is represented not by the network of dark material seen in EM sections but by something less dense winding about within the dark material.

The Pars Granulosa. As is apparent from Figure 4-14, much of the material in the dark network (the part labeled a) has a granular appearance; this is therefore referred to as the *pars granulosa.* Its granularity is due to accumulated ribonucleoprotein particles, containing the 32S rRNA that goes on to become the 28S rRNA of the large subunits of ribosomes. The ribonucleoprotein particles probably leave the nucleolus from the periphery of the granular material, where it borders on the nuclear sap (Fig. 4-14, b) surrounding and permeating the nucleolus.

The Pars Fibrosa. The second component of the dark material consists of extremely fine, electron-dense fila-

ments (containing much rRNA), packed tightly together. Chouinard has shown that these dense, closely packed filaments (Fig. 4-14, c) are arranged in aggregates around cores of less dense material (Fig. 4-14, d), termed *fibrillar centers.* The dense filamentous material, seen in sections as rings (Fig. 4-14, c) surrounding these centers, is considered to represent (at least in part) the 45S rRNA just synthesized along nucleolar genes. The granular material at the periphery of the rings is probably a result of proteins becoming associated with the rRNA and changing its configuration, forming particles resembling the granules of the pars granulosa. Hence the border between the pars fibrosa and the pars granulosa is not sharply defined; it is a zone of transition where the fibrillar material is changing into granular material.

Fibrillar Centers. These are the less dense regions (Fig. 4-14, d) surrounded by thick rings of dense fibrillar material (Fig. 4-14, c). Rounded fibrillar centers represent cross (or slightly oblique) sections through cords of material of moderate electron density (indicated by arrows in Fig. 4-15). These contain electron-dense threads of chromatin, as can be seen in Figure 4-15, where the chromatin in the cores of the cords has about the same electron density as chromatin outside the nucleolus. Moreover, after treatment with DNAase, neither the fibrillar centers nor the nuclear chromatin are as electron dense. This substantiates the concept of the DNA of the nucleolar

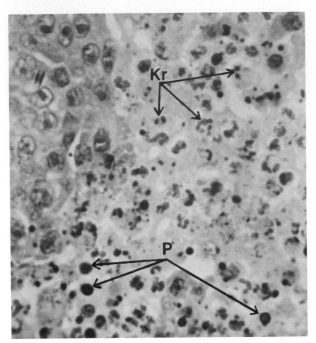

Fig. 4-16. High-power photomicrograph of part of a malignant tumor. The cells at *top left* were still alive and growing (note their large nucleoli) when the specimen was taken, but those on the right side had died previously, and, as a consequence, their nuclei had undergone changes indicative of cell death. Some nuclei have shrunken into rounded dark-staining bodies (P); this is termed *pyknosis*. Other nuclei have become broken up into fragments (Kr) and this is termed *karyorrhexis*. Areas of tissue in which the cells die during life are described as being necrotic. *See also karyolysis* (Fig. 4-17).

organizer, from which rRNA is transcribed, winding its way (perhaps associated with other components) through the fibrillar centers of the nucleolus, coding along its course for 45S rRNA, which is formed as a sheath of electron-dense fibrillar material around it. In other words, it appears likely that the chromatin strands in the fibrillar centers are the counterparts of the trunks of the "Christmas trees" shown in Figure 4-13 and that the branches of these trees become the dark fibrillar material (Fig. 4-14, c) surrounding the centers.

The Light Component of the Nucleolus. The light areas in the nucleolus appear mostly as islands but around the periphery of the nucleolus they are commonly continuous with the nuclear sap (Fig. 4-14). Hence it is debatable whether the light component should be regarded as part of the nucleolus at all, or merely as regions of nuclear sap (to be described presently) incorporated as a result of local fusion of various regions of the dark component as the sponge-like nucleolus develops. The manner in which a nucleolus forms may be studied by following it through mitosis.

The Behavior of the Structural Components of the Nucleolus During Mitosis

Some clues to the functional significance of the various structural components of the nucleolus have been obtained through studies of their behavior during mitosis. As is well known the nucleolus, as an organized entity, usually disappears at late prophase and is formed anew in the daughter nuclei at late telophase. This occurs in intimate association with a specific region, the *nucleolar-organizing region,* on the satellited chromosomes. In late prophase the intranucleolar chromatin begins to condense and the fibrillar and granular material of the nucleolus disperses into the surrounding nuclear sap. From early prophase to midtelophase the nucleolus comprises no more than the chromatin of the nucleolar organizers, but then this chromatin gradually extends and dense fibrillar material (*pars fibrosa*) again becomes deposited around it. The subsequent growth of the nucleolus through late telophase is due to the increasing quantity of fibrillar material and also to the addition more peripherally of granular material (*pars granulosa*). The nucleolus exhibits all the features of the mature interphase nucleolus by the end of telophase. Hence the chromatin containing the DNA that codes for rRNA in the nucleolar organizers is the only component of the nucleolus showing any continuity from one cell generation to the next.

THE NUCLEAR SAP

So far, we have considered three of the main components of the nucleus: (*1*) the nuclear envelope, (*2*) chromatin and chromosomes, and (*3*) the nucleolus. We shall now briefly mention the fourth component, the *nuclear sap* (labeled in Fig. 4-1). This term originated from light microscopy to denote the content of the seemingly empty spaces in nuclei, long before it became known that extended chromatin lies suspended in these spaces during the interphase, giving off its genetic information.

The nuclear sap is a colloidal protein solution that stains poorly for the EM and scarcely at all with H and E. It provides a medium for rapid diffusion of metabolites and the movement of ribosomal ribonucleoprotein, mRNA, and tRNA toward the nuclear pores.

NUCLEAR CHANGES INDICATIVE OF CELL DEATH

Needless to say, all the cells in a section cut from fixed materials are dead. However, when the histologist or pathologist refers to *dead* cells in a section, he is talking not about fixed cells but cells that had died while the body was still alive.

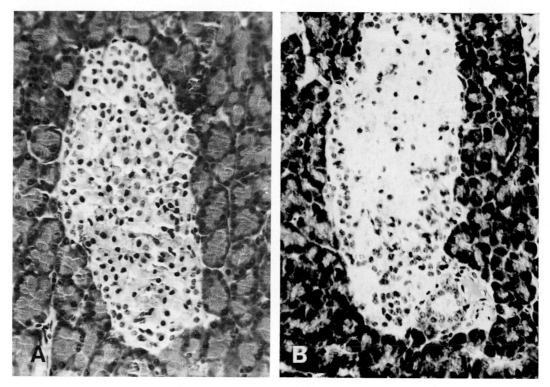

Fig. 4-17. Medium-power photomicrographs of section of pancreas obtained from rats some hours after they had been given alloxan, an agent that destroys many of the cells of the islets of Langerhans. (*A*) The nuclei of the cells in the islet may be seen; there are some examples of *pyknosis*. (*B*) The nuclei have mostly dissolved away; this illustrates *karyolysis*.

Dead cells may be encountered in the living body for two main reasons. First, in some tissues it is normal for cells to die and be replaced by others; this occurs, for example, in the outer layer of the skin. Likewise, certain of the white cells of the blood have only a short life span and die within the body. Accordingly, in tissue removed from a healthy body, it is normal to see nuclear changes indicative of cell death in sites where it is normal for cells to die. Second, dead cells may be present as a result of disease. For example, an artery supplying a particular part of a tissue can become plugged as a result of disease, whereupon the cells in the region supplied by the artery may die from lack of oxygen and nutrients. In such regions the nuclei of the cells demonstrate characteristic changes indicative of cell death. Rapidly growing cancers, for example, commonly have central zones of dead tissue (*necrotic* zones, from the Gr. *nekros*, corpse), due to the blood supply to the middle of the large mass of cells becoming inadequate. Dead cells in such a region may be seen in Figure 4-16.

Although there are also cytoplasmic changes in dead cells, the most positive indication that cells are dead is given by the appearance of their nuclei. The nuclear changes indicating cell death are of three general kinds. The commonest is called *pyknosis* (Gr. for condensation) and entails shrinkage of the nuclear material into a homogeneous and darkly staining (*hyperchromatic*) mass (Fig. 4-16, P). It is important that the student learn how not to confuse a nucleus showing pyknosis with a nucleus containing much condensed chromatin or with a poorly fixed mitotic figure. When difficulty is encountered in this respect, it is advisable to examine the cytoplasm also of the cell in question, for, if the cell is dead, the cytoplasm too will commonly present an abnormal appearance, as may be seen in Figure 4-16. Often it will lack detail and present a generally "muddy" appearance; moreover, it may be harder to distinguish cells as separate entities, as is the case in the middle of Figure 4-16.

In other instances, cell death is indicated by the nucleus breaking up into fragments, a type of nuclear change called *karyorrhexis* (Gr. *karyon + rhexis*, breaking). Thus instead of shrinking, nuclei may completely disintegrate (Fig. 4-16, Kr), with the ultimate formation of such tiny fragments of nuclear material that these are sometimes referred to as nuclear "dust."

The third appearance presented by nuclei in dead or dying cells is that of dissolving away. This type of nuclear change, which is illustrated in Figure 4-17B, is termed *karyolysis* (Gr. *lysis*, dissolution).

REFERENCES AND OTHER READING

The Nuclear Envelope

Feldherr, C.: Structure and Function of the Nuclear Envelope. DuPraw, E. J. (ed.): Adv. Cell Molecular Biology. vol. 2. New York, Academic Press, 1972.

Franke, W. W.: Structure, biochemistry and functions of the nuclear envelope. Int. Rev. Cytol. [Suppl.], *4:*72, 1974.

Gall, J. G.: Octagonal nuclear pores. J. Cell Biol., *32:*391, 1967.

Kessel, R. G.: Structure and Function of the Nuclear Envelope and Related Cytomembranes. *In* Progress in Surface and Membrane Science. vol. 6, p. 243. 1973.

Maul, G. G.: Ultrastructure of pore complexes of annulate lamellae. J. Cell Biol., *46:*604, 1970.

Stevens, B., and André, J.: The nuclear envelope. *In* Handbook of Molecular Cytology. Lima-de-Faria, A. (ed.): Frontiers of Biology. vol. 15. Amsterdam, North Holland, 1969.

Wischnitzer, S.: The annulate lamellae. Int. Rev. Cytol., *27:*65, 1970.

The Interphase Nucleus

Brown, S. W.: Heterochromatin. Science, *151:*417, 1966.

Dalton, A. J., and Haguenau, F. (eds.): Ultrastructure in Biological Systems. vol. 3. The Nucleus. New York, Academic Press, 1968.

DuPraw, E. J.: DNA and Chromosomes. New York, Holt, Rinehart and Winston, 1970.

Gurdon, J. B.: Transplanted nuclei and cell differentiation. Sci. Am., *219:*24, 1968.

Gurdon, J. B., and Brown, D. D.: Toward an in vitro analysis of gene control and function. *In* T'so, P. (ed): Symposium on Molecular Biology of the Genetic Apparatus. vol. 2. Amsterdam, North Holland, 1976.

Harris, H.: The reactivation of the red cell nucleus. J. Cell Sci., *2:*23, 1967.

Milner, G. R.: Nuclear morphology and ultrastructural localization of deoxyribonucleic acid synthesis during interphase. J. Cell Sci., *4:*569, 1969.

Ris, H.: Chromosomal structure as seen by electron microscopy. *In* The Structure and Function of Chromosomes. Ciba Foundation Symposium 28 (New Series). New York, American Elsevier, 1975.

Respective Significance of Condensed and Extended Chromatin (Including Barr Bodies) in the Interphase Nucleus

Barr, M. L.: The significance of the sex chromatin. Int. Rev. Cytol., *19:*35, 1966.

Barr, M. L. and Bertram, E. G.: A morphological distinction between neurons of the male and female, and the behaviour of the nucleolar satellite during accelerated nucleoprotein synthesis. Nature, *163:*676, 1949.

Lewis, K. R., and John, B.: The chromosomal basis of sex determination. Int. Rev. Cytol., *23:*277, 1968.

Littau, V. C., Allfrey, V. G., Frenster, J. H., and Mirsky, A. E.: Active and inactive regions of nuclear chromatin as revealed by electron microscope autoradiography. Proc. Nat. Acad. Sci., *52:*93, 1964.

Mittwoch, U.: The Sex Chromosomes. New York, Academic Press, 1967.

Moore, K. L. (ed): The Sex Chromatin, Philadelphia, W. B. Saunders, 1966.

DNA, RNA, and Protein Synthesis

Bostock, C.: Repetitious DNA. Advances in Cell Biology, vol. 2, p. 153. New York, Appleton-Century-Crofts, 1971.

Brown, D. D.: The isolation of genes. Sci. Am., *229:*20, 1973.

DeRobertis, E. D. P., Nowinski, W. W., and Saez, F. A.: Cell Biology. ed. 5. Philadelphia, W. B. Saunders, 1970.

Dowben, R. M.: Cell Biology. New York, Harper & Row, 1971.

DuPraw, E. J.: The Biosciences: Cell and Molecular Biology. Cell and Molecular Biology Council, Stanford, Calif., 1972.

Franke, W. W., and Scheer, U.: Morphology of transcriptional units at different states of activity. Philos. Trans. R. Soc. Lond. [Biol. Sci.], *283:*333, 1978.

Gurdon, J. B., Wyllie, A. H., and DeRobertis, E. M. The transcription and translation of DNA injected into oocytes. Philos. Trans. R. Soc. Lond. [Biol. Sci.], *283:*375, 1978.

Lane, C.: Rabbit hemoglobin from frog eggs. Sci. Am., *235:*60, Aug., 1976.

Loewy, A. G., and Siekevitz, P.: Cell Structure and Function. ed. 2. New York, Holt, Rinehart and Winston, 1970.

Novikoff, A. B., and Holtzman, E.: Cells and Organelles. New York, Holt, Rinehart and Winston, 1970.

Oudet, P., et al.: Nucleosome structure. Philos. Trans. R. Soc. Lond. [Biol. Sci.], *283:*241, 1978.

Pardue, M. L., Bonner, J. J., Lengyel, J. A., and Spradling, A. C.: Drosophila salivary gland polytene chromosomes studied by in situ hybridization. *In* Brinkley, B. R. and Porter, K. R. (eds.): International Cell Biology 1976–1977. New York, Rockefeller University Press, 1977.

Rae, P. M. M.: The distribution of repetitive DNA sequences in chromosomes. DuPraw, E. J. (ed.): Advances in Cell and Molecular Biology. vol. 2. p. 109. New York, Academic Press, 1972.

Rich, A., and Kim, S. H.: The three-dimensional structure of transfer RNA. Sci. Am., *238:*52, Jan., 1978.

Rosenberg, E.: Cell and Molecular Biology, An Appreciation. New York, Holt, Rinehart and Winston, 1971.

Stein, G. S., Stein, J. S., and Kleinsmith, L. J. Chromosomal proteins and gene regulation. Sci. Am., *232:*46, Feb., 1975.

Watson, J. D.: Molecular Biology of the Gene. ed. 2. New York, W. A. Benjamin, 1970.

The Nucleolus

Busch, H., and Smetana, K.: The Nucleolus. New York, Academic Press, 1970.

Chouinard, L. A.: Localization of intranucleolar DNA in root meristematic cells of *Allium cepa*. J. Cell Sci., *6:*73, 1970.

———: A light- and electron-microscope study of the nucleolus during growth of the oocyte in the prepubertal mouse. J. Cell Sci., *9:*637, 1971.

———: Behaviour of the Structural Components of the Nucleolus During Mitosis in *Allium cepa*. *In* Advances in Cytopharmacology. vol. 1. New York, Raven Press, 1971.

Ghosh, S.: The nucleolar structure. Int. Rev. Cytol., *44:*1, 1976.

Miller, O. L., Jr.: The visualization of genes in action. Sci. Am., *228:*34, March, 1973.

Miller, O. L., Jr., Beatty, B. R., Hamkalo, B. A., and Thomas, C. A., Jr.: Electron microscopic visualization of transcription. Cold Spring Harbor Symp. Quant. Biol., *35:*505, 1970.

5 Cytoplasm and Its Organelles

Although the nucleus, by synthesizing specific mRNA molecules, directs the kind of work a cell will do, the various specialized functions of interphase cells are performed by their cytoplasm. The performance of work requires energy, which ultimately is obtained through the oxidation of foodstuffs in the cytoplasm. For this to occur, both nutrients and oxygen must be absorbed by the cytoplasm of a cell from its environment. The nutrients reach the bloodstream from the intestine, where the food eaten is broken down into its chemical building blocks, and these are then absorbed into the blood. Oxygen is absorbed into the blood from the air in the lungs, which is repeatedly changed through respiratory movements. Most body cells, however, do not lie directly beside blood capillaries, but are separated from them by intercellular substances permeated with tissue fluid through which nutrients and oxygen diffuse to reach the cells (Fig. 5-1). Waste products, of course, diffuse in the reverse direction. By this arrangement the border of the cytoplasm of each cell has constant access to the nutrients that either serve as fuel for oxidation or as building blocks for the synthesis of new cell substance or some secretory product of the cytoplasm. We shall now deal with the various components of the cytoplasm, the most important of which are called *organelles*.

THE ORGANELLES OF THE CYTOPLASM

A particular part of the body carrying out some special function is called an *organ*. The lungs, liver, kidneys, for example, each have a specialized structure that enables them to play a specific role in the body. Likewise there are specific structures in the cytoplasm whose particular structure allows them to carry out some specific function necessary for the metabolism of the cell, and so these are called *organelles* (meaning little organs). As will be explained presently, most of the cytoplasmic organelles are membranous structures.

The nature, function, and distribution of the cytoplasmic organelles had to await the development of the tools of modern cell biology for their elucidation. The technics of most assistance in this regard were (*1*) electron microscopy, (*2*) cell fractionation, by means of which biochemists could obtain relatively pure fractions containing particular organelles from disrupted cells and hence could study the particular metabolic reactions with which they

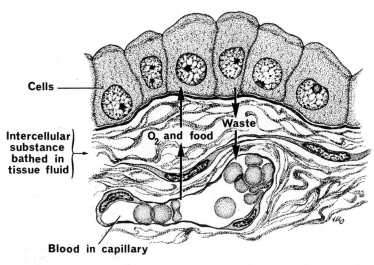

Fig. 5-1. Diagram of the routes by which food and oxygen in blood capillaries reach cells not adjacent to capillaries, and how waste products from the metabolism of cells travel in the opposite direction. Both routes depend on substances diffusing through the tissue fluid permeating the intercellular substances between capillaries and cells.

107

were concerned, and (*3*) radioautography, which enabled the particular metabolic reactions occurring in these organelles to be studied directly. Two of these methods have already been described, and cell fractionation is mentioned again in this chapter; other technics are described in later chapters, where appropriate to the topic being discussed.

The major membranous cytoplasmic organelles are:
1. The cell (or plasma) membrane
2. Mitochondria
3. The rough-surfaced endoplasmic reticulum (rER)
4. The Golgi apparatus
5. Lysosomes
6. Coated vesicles
7. The smooth-surfaced endoplasmic reticulum (sER)

The major nonmembranous organelles are:
1. Free ribosomes and polyribosomes
2. Microtubules
3. Centrioles, cilia, and flagella (structures assembled from microtubules)
4. Filaments (including microfilaments and intermediate and other types of filaments)

THE OTHER COMPONENTS OF THE CYTOPLASM

Inclusions

In addition to organelles, there are, in some kinds of cells, certain materials in the cytoplasm not regarded as part of the metabolic machinery or the physical structure of the cytoplasm; these are termed *inclusions*. Stored glycogen or fat, pigments of various sorts, and so on are all included in this category and are described at the end of this chapter.

The Cytosol

The organelles and cytoplasmic inclusions are all suspended in a solution of proteins and other substances that includes the building blocks from which larger molecules are made. For example, the proteins from which the organelles are assembled, the soluble enzymes concerned in the intermediary metabolism of the cell, and the substrates and products of enzymatic activity are all present in this component. Other smaller molecules and ions, many of which are important for cell function and the maintenance of the intra- and intercellular environments of the cell, are also present. This nonorganelle component of cytoplasm is generally termed the *cytosol*. It varies in overall viscosity, and this increases with the number of microfilaments it may contain. The terms *cytoplasmic matrix* or *ground substance* are sometimes also used for this part of the cytoplasm.

Before describing the membranous organelles it should be explained that some of the nonmembranous organelles may be associated with membranes. Thus cilia and flagella are partly enclosed by the cell membrane, and at least some types of other filaments may be attached to cell membranes.

Since so many of the organelles are membranous structures, we shall first discuss the general significance of membranes.

THE IMPORTANCE OF MEMBRANES

If all the enzymes and substances within a cell were allowed to mix freely, the metabolic reactions on which the viability and functions of cells depend could not occur, at least not very efficiently. Life is only possible in cells if its various enzymes and substances are arranged in an orderly way and kept from mixing freely with one another. This is done by means of membranes. The membranes that serve this purpose within the cell are the delicate walls of the membranous organelles; they allow the contents of the membranous organelle to remain chemically different from the cytosol in which it lies. The walls of organelles are such that they selectively restrain the passage of certain molecules or ions through them, while permitting free passage of others. Many enzymes are firmly bound to membranes and are thus disposed in orderly arrays within or along membranes, an arrangement that permits the efficient processing of substances. This arrangement also ensures that the products of the reactions that these enzymes catalyze are segregated on the appropriate side of the membrane, commonly the side away from the cytosol.

The fact that so many fluids of different composition are thus separated from one another within the cytoplasm has led to a terminology whereby the different components separated are said to be in different *compartments*. However, this term does not necessarily mean an enclosed space in a structural sense.

We shall begin our study of the cytoplasmic organelles by describing the membrane that surrounds the cell and abuts on the tissue fluid.

THE CELL MEMBRANE (PLASMA MEMBRANE, PLASMALEMMA)

Can the Cell Membrane Be Seen With the LM?

In the usual diagram of a cell it is customary to indicate its periphery with a line and label it the "cell membrane." Furthermore, in drawings of groups of cells the borders between the adjacent cells are also usually indicated by lines. Such illustrations tend to give the impression that the cell membrane can be seen readily with the LM and hence is much more substantial than it really is. Actually, the cell membrane is only 9 to 10 nm. thick and is thus much too thin for a cross section of it to be resolved with the LM. Indeed, as the reader may already have noticed, the borders between the cells of liver are often not seen at all. We are, therefore, led to ask what is responsible for the lines that can sometimes be seen between adjacent cells.

Although it complicates the discussion somewhat, it should first be explained that the cell membranes of adjacent cells are not in continuous direct contact with one another. The space between them, which is somewhat wider than each of the membranes bordering it, is generally filled with a carbohydrate-rich material, the nature of which is described under *cell coat*. In cells that are close together, this material is analogous to the filling of a sandwich, with the slices of bread corresponding to the cell membranes of adjacent cells. However, this sandwich of cell membranes, even with its filling, would still be too thin for a cross section of it to be resolved with the LM (Fig. 5-2A). Why is it then sometimes seen in a stained section? The reason is that it absorbs stain and, where the stained sandwich slants through the substance of the section, its slanting sides may provide large enough expanses for some color to be seen (as shown in Fig. 5-2B). It should be remembered that a paraffin section is roughly half as thick as the cells through which it is cut. There is then, relatively speaking, a considerable distance over which the sandwich can be seen if it slants obliquely from the top of the section to its bottom.

How the Cell Membrane Appears in the EM

The EM readily allows a single cell membrane (9 to 10 nm. in thickness) to be identified as a distinct entity when cut at an angle approaching a cross section. In low-magnification electron micrographs, a cell membrane cut at right angles (or even at an angle approaching a right angle)

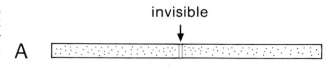

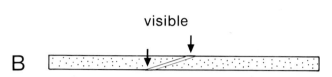

Fig. 5-2. Diagram (not to scale) illustrating how cell membranes too thin for their cross-sectional dimension to be resolved, and hence *invisible* in (*A*), may be *visible* with the LM in sections cut as in (*B*), where the membranes cross the section obliquely and can therefore be seen over a much larger area.

appears in a micrograph as a single dark line. At higher resolution, a cell membrane that passes from top to bottom of the section, exactly or nearly at a right angle to the plane of section, shows in a micrograph as two dark lines with a light line between them, as shown in Figure 5-3. Since its appearance is that of a three-layered structure it came to be spoken of as a *trilaminar* (or *trilamellar*) membrane. As we shall see, this appearance is due to artifact.

The Unit Membrane

The trilamellar type of membrane seen in the electron microscope became known as a *unit membrane*. The same trilamellar type of structure can be found in the membranes of all the membranous cytoplasmic organ-

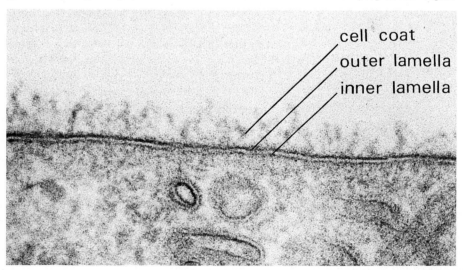

Fig. 5-3. High resolution electron micrograph (×200,000) of the cell membrane and cell coat. The trilaminar unit membrane structure consisting of a dense inner lamella, a dense outer lamella, and a light-staining lamella between the two is clearly visible. Cell coat covers the cell membrane on the outside. (Courtesy of M. Weinstock)

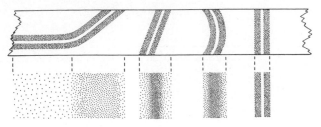

Fig. 5-4. Diagram illustrating why cell membranes seen in electron micrographs may not always show the trilaminar unit membrane structure. The upper part of the diagram shows cell membranes passing through a section at various angles and the lower part shows the corresponding images seen in the electron microscope. Note that a typical unit membrane appearance is seen only when the membrane passes through the section at right angles to the plane of the section, as shown at far right. (*See* text for more detailed explanation.)

elles. However, their membranes, being about 7 nm. thick, are somewhat thinner than the cell membrane, which as noted is about 9 to 10 nm. thick. Each is also slightly different in chemical composition and has different enzymes associated with it, depending on the organelle from which it comes. The enzymes membranes contain are characteristic for the organelles concerned and thus helpful in isolating, assaying, and identifying the various membranous organelles obtained by cell fractionation procedures.

The appearance of a unit membrane in an electron micrograph varies with the angle at which it passes through the section. Depending on this angle, a membrane may (*1*) be almost invisible, or appear as (*2*) a fuzzy dark line, or (*3*) a fairly distinct dark line, or (*4*) a trilamellar structure, as in Figure 5-4.

In considering why this should be so, it must be remembered that everything in a section examined in the EM is in focus at the same time, and that contrast is seen in the EM only because some components encountered in a section as the electron beam passes through it are more electron-dense and so scatter more electrons than other components beside them. With this in mind we shall now refer to the examples shown in Figure 5-4, in which an electron beam from above passes through trilamellar membranes disposed at various angles to the plane of section. What is seen in a micrograph is shown immediately below each example.

First, at the *left*, the membrane lies parallel with the section so that the electron beam would pass through only a single thickness of the membrane. The membrane is so very thin that this would not scatter many electrons. The site of the membrane would, therefore, not appear greatly different from sites where a membrane was not present, as is shown beneath the section.

Next (moving to the *right*), the membrane is shown

slanting through the section. Here electrons would have to pass through more membrane substance than where the membrane was flat. As is shown by moving still further to the *right* in Figure 5-4, more and more electrons are scattered as the angle of the membrane approaches a right angle. A membrane that passes through the section at close to a right angle could scatter enough electrons to appear as a single dark line. A membrane that passed from the top of the section to the bottom at approximately a right angle, but pursued a slightly curving course would also appear as a dark line with fuzzy edges (*second to right* in Fig. 5-4). Finally only a straight membrane that passes through the section at a right angle would reveal its trilamellar structure, because in such a preparation the middle layer of the membrane would not scatter as many electrons as the more electron-dense layers on each of its sides (Fig. 5-4, *right*).

Relation of the Appearance of Membranes in the EM to Present Concepts of Membrane Structure

Development of Knowledge. Early physiological experiments showed that cells immersed in solutions of various osmotic pressures would swell or shrink, indicating that they must be surrounded by a membrane with special permeability properties. It was also noted that the cell membrane was in general permeable to materials that were soluble in lipid. Experimental data of many kinds, as well as theoretical considerations, led to the concept of the membrane being composed for the most part of lipid, more specifically by two rows of *phospholipid* molecules arranged more or less perpendicular to the surface of the membrane so that their nonpolar, or *hydrophobic*, ends meet and their polar (*hydrophilic*) ends face aqueous solutions on either side of the membrane. The lipid in the membranes was believed to be associated with protein, but the structural relation between these two components was unknown.

This classic concept of the membrane was well established before cell membranes were seen in the EM. When the EM became available, cell membranes were first seen as single black lines. Since osmium was used to blacken fats for LM studies, and since osmium tetroxide was the common fixative used for electron microscopy, it was assumed that the single black line seen with the EM was due to the lipid layer being rendered electron-dense by the osmium.

Consequently, as the EM resolution improved and the membrane was revealed as a trilamellar structure (Fig. 5-3), it was disturbing to find that after osmium fixation, the outer layers were electron-dense and not the middle layer, as had been assumed. The reason for the electron density of the layers of the unit membrane being more or less opposite to what would be expected after osmium fixation is not clear. However, after very brief exposure to osmium tetroxide, the membrane stains as a single dense line even at high resolution (Robertson). So it has been suggested that whereas the osmium would interact first with the hydrophobic region of the lipid bilayer, more prolonged contact might lead to osmium leaving this part of the bilayer by diffusion to become associated with the hydrophilic portions of the lipid molecules (and probably also the hydrophilic parts of the protein molecules of the membrane) so as to produce two parallel dense lines, one on each aspect of the bilayer.

Some Physical Properties of the Cell Membrane

The cell membrane is not permeable to macromolecules; hence, the proteins in the cytoplasm cannot escape into the tissue fluid. But the proteins in the cell exert osmotic pressure and this would continuously draw water into the cell if the tissue fluid did not contain other substances in solution to counterbalance the osmotic pressure generated within the cell. The counterbalancing factor is the osmotic pressure exerted by the greater concentration of inorganic ions outside the cell than inside it, and for this to be maintained requires that some mechanism exist to maintain different concentrations of ions on the two sides of the membrane. This difference in concentration results in yet another feature, namely, that since ions bear electrical charges, there is a difference in electrical potential between the two sides of the membrane (in nerve and muscle cells this is as much as 85 millivolts), with the tissue fluid side being more positive than the cytoplasmic side. For a difference of electrical potential to be sustained, a cell membrane would have to possess dielectric properties. This property, as well as another, namely, its relative permeability to substances that dissolve in lipids, fitted with the concept of the membrane having a substantial content of lipid, because lipid has good dielectric properties.

The Sodium-Potassium Pump. Whereas the concentrations of some dissolved substances present on either side of the cell membrane may be accounted for by diffusion from sites of higher to lower concentration, the relative concentrations of certain water-soluble substances, in particular inorganic ions, cannot be explained this way. For example, not only is there a higher concentration of sodium ions in the tissue fluid outside the membrane, but there is also a higher concentration of potassium ions in the cytoplasm than in the tissue fluid. This difference in concentration of sodium and potassium ions is maintained by what is called the *sodium* (or *sodium-potassium*) *pump.* The transfer of ions is brought about by a special enzyme that uses energy supplied by the cell. It pumps sodium ions out through the cell membrane and hence keeps their concentration lower on the inner than on the

outer side of the membrane. Concomitantly, this enzyme picks up potassium ions on the outside and releases them on the inner side of the membrane, but it does not necessarily carry as many potassium ions inward as sodium ions outward.

It is also accepted that glucose, amino acids, and fatty acids, as well as certain other ions, also require special enzymes in the cell membrane to transport them from the tissue fluid into the cytoplasm, and that these mechanisms consume energy. Such energy-requiring, enzyme-mediated systems are called *active transport mechanisms.*

The Molecular Structure of the Cell Membrane as Revealed by Special Histological Techniques

If the middle layer of the cell membrane were a continuous layer of lipid molecules it would, of course, be difficult to understand how substances not soluble in lipid could be transported through it. The passage of such substances would be more easily explained if there were some protein molecules in the lipid bilayer, for then substances not soluble in lipid would not have to pass through the lipid to gain access to the cell. In this connection, a model of the cell membrane has been proposed, and generally accepted, in which some *protein* molecules are present in the lipid bilayer and extend all the way from one side of the membrane to the other (Fig. 5-5). These protein molecules can be demonstrated by the freeze-etch technic,* and the presence of protein agrees with

---

The Freeze-Etch Technic. It is possible to obtain a view of various surfaces of cellular membranes by means of what is termed the *freeze-etch* or *freeze-fracture* replica technic. Although the technic is elaborate, the essentials are that a small piece of tissue is frozen rapidly in liquid nitrogen and transferred to an apparatus in which a vacuum can be produced and in which the tissue can be fractured by a knife. In this manner a tissue surface resulting from having a portion of frozen tissue split away from it is exposed. The fractures usually occur along membranes in such a way that the membranes are split in half so that their interior is exposed. The vacuum is then usually allowed to act on the surface of the frozen and fractured tissue for a brief period, during which it becomes etched because of the vacuum evaporating ice from it. This etching can expose the outside surface features of a membrane as well as surfaces split in the fracturing step (Fig. 5-6).

All the surfaces thus exposed are then covered with a thin deposit obtained by evaporating a metal over them; this can be so done that the mist evaporating from the metal is applied at an angle to the fractured and etched surface and, as a result, more is deposited on one side of structures projecting from the surface than on the other (which is said to be in the shadow). After a shadowed metal replica of the fractured and etched surface is thus obtained, the tissue is digested away and the metal replica is washed and mounted on a grid, and examined in the EM. No fixation or sectioning is required for this method and large areas of membrane can be examined.

outside

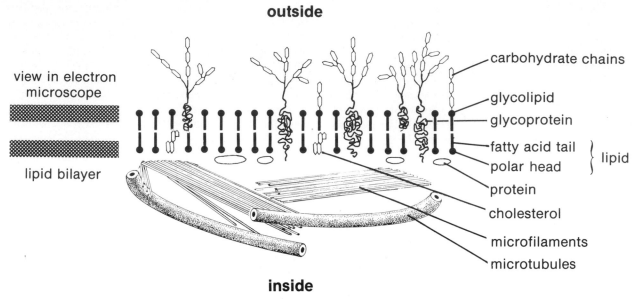

view in electron microscope

lipid bilayer

carbohydrate chains

glycolipid

glycoprotein

fatty acid tail ⎫ lipid

polar head ⎭

protein

cholesterol

microfilaments

microtubules

inside

Fig. 5-5. Diagram illustrating the molecular structure of the cell membrane.

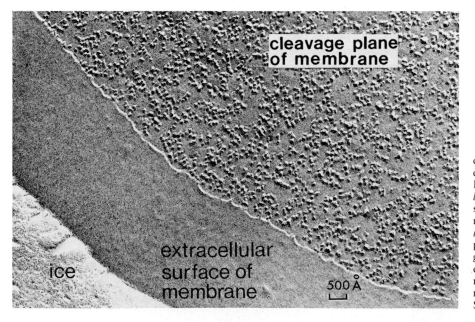

cleavage plane of membrane

ice

extracellular surface of membrane

500 Å

Fig. 5-6. Electron micrograph of the cell membrane of an erythrocyte after freeze-etching. Residual ice remains at the *lower left.* To the *right* of this, the smooth outer surface of the cell membrane may be seen. The *upper right* shows the cleavage plane of the membrane, in which globules of protein, 9 nm. in diameter, lie exposed. The smooth regions between these globules represent lipid. (Courtesy of P. Seeman)

biochemical analyses of membrane composition and organization. The EM freeze-etch technic reveals small globular bodies, embedded in the middle (lipid) layer of the membrane (Fig. 5-6), that can be digested with trypsin, an enzyme that digests protein. Some of these protein globular bodies constitute channels of protein continuity between the outside and the inside of the cell. Furthermore, biochemical studies indicate that some of the same

glycoproteins (also present in the cell membrane) become labeled whether it is the outer or the inner surface of the membrane that is exposed to the label. This indicates that these glycoprotein molecules extend right through the membrane and that different parts of these molecules are exposed at either surface. Such molecules are illustrated in Figure 5-5. Some of the cell membrane proteins (or groups of these proteins) could be enzymes that participate in active transport mechanisms operating across the membrane. It appears that the surrounding lipid is necessary in order for some of these enzymes to function. Other protein molecules are only partly embedded in the lipid bilayer and do not extend all the way through it. Thus, in addition to these proteins totally embedded in the lipid bilayer, which are called *integral* or *intrinsic membrane proteins,* and which require detergents to remove them, there are others more loosely bound to the cytoplasmic side of the lipid bilayer; these are called *peripheral* or *extrinsic membrane proteins* and can be separated easily from the membrane. Some of the integral membrane protein molecules passing through the lipid bilayer may be anchored, directly or indirectly, to filamentous structures in the cytoplasm such as microfilaments and microtubules (Fig. 5-5).

The Asymmetry of the Cell Membrane. Yet another feature of the cell membrane that has recently come to light is that there are certain differences between its inner and outer halves. In other words, the cell membrane is not the symmetrical structure first suggested by its appearance in electron micrographs. For example, all the carbohydrate-containing portions of the glycoprotein and glycolipid molecules project from the *outer surface* of the membrane (Fig. 5-5) and these contribute to what is known as the *cell coat*. The outer half of the membrane also contains the various molecules called *receptors* that interact with specific molecules in the environment of the cell. It is through the interaction of receptors and these specific molecules that the cell may be either triggered into action or shut down if it is already active. Furthermore, it has been found that, besides proteins and lipids, membranes commonly contain a significant amount of *cholesterol* and most of this seems to be disposed in the *inner half* of the membrane (Fig. 5-5). More recent evidence indicates that the proteins in the outer and inner halves of the membrane are not identical (*see* Fox) and the relative amounts of the various kinds of phospholipids are different in the outer and inner halves of the lipid bilayer. Occasionally, it can even be seen directly by electron microscopy that the membrane is asymmetrical. For example, the cell membrane of the cells lining the urinary bladder does not stain evenly, for the outer half of the membrane (that abuts on the lumen of the bladder) stains much more densely than the inner half that faces the cytoplasm of these cells.

Surface Flow. It is possible experimentally to bring about fusion between two different kinds of cells and also between cells of two different species (even human cells with cells of another species). When this is done, certain characteristic molecules on the surface on one type cell mix quickly with those on the other (the surface molecules of each kind can be identified by immunological means). Within less than an hour, at body temperature, the molecules intermix to such an extent that it is impossi-

ble to tell which part of the resulting combined cell surface has come from which cell. Experiments of this sort indicate that the lipid bilayer behaves like a *fluid* and that, at least under some conditions, the protein molecules embedded in it can flow from one region of the cell membrane to another.

THE CELL COAT

Development of Knowledge

Plant cells, it will be recalled, live in compartments, and carbohydrate is an important or chief component of the compartment walls. The cell membranes of bacteria are coated with carbohydrate of physiological importance; for example, if their cell coats are removed, the bacteria are affected by osmotic pressures that would not affect them if their coats were intact. With the advent of the PAS technic and other methods for demonstrating glycoproteins, several observers found that many of the cells lining the surfaces inside the body had on their free surface a thin layer of glycoprotein material. Such findings, however, did not necessarily prove the existence of a cell coat in these sites, since it is common for secreted mucus to adhere closely to epithelial cells. With the advent of the EM, more convincing evidence appeared and many cell types were demonstrated to possess a *cell coat* (Fig. 5-3). The microvilli of the intestine (microvilli are tiny finger-like processes covered with cell membrane, that project from the free surfaces of lining absorptive cells and thus increase the absorptive area of the free surface) are covered with a particularly thick and easily demonstrable cell coat, which appears as a "fuzz" and is composed of filamentous material of low electron density (Fig. 5-7), very closely associated with the cell membrane.

It was one matter to accept the existence of a cell coat on wet epithelial surfaces, but another to accept the idea of a carbohydrate-containing cell coat being a heritage that virtually all body cells would demonstrate to some degree. Nevertheless, observations suggesting this began to accumulate, and, when Rambourg and Leblond examined over 50 different types of body cells in rats, they found that all had demonstrable cell coats, thus establishing the universality of this surface component. Cell coats appeared as thin films along all cell surfaces, whether these surfaces abutted on the surfaces of other cells (as shown in Fig. 5-8) or were free. One exception only was found: the cell coat was not seen at sites between adjacent cells where they form special types of junctions (described in Chap. 7). It should be emphasized here that in most cases special technics are required to demonstrate the cell coat; hence, it is not seen in routine electron micrographs of most cells.

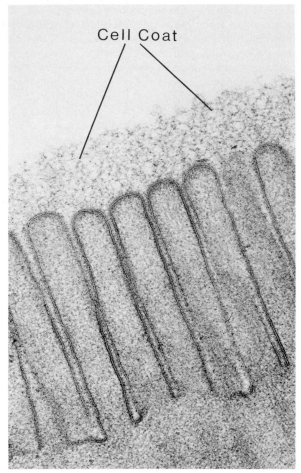

Cell Coat

Fig. 5-7. Electron micrograph (×75,000) of part of an epithelial lining cell of small intestine (cat). The cell membrane adjacent to the lumen of the intestine is thrown into finger-like projections that are parallel and close to one another; these are microvilli. Between adjacent microvilli, and covering their tips, there is a surface layer called the cell coat. (Courtesy of S. Ito)

The Nature of the Cell Coat

The cell coat has been studied by histochemical technics with both the LM and the EM and also by biochemical analysis of material obtained from cell surfaces after treatment with various enzymes. The use of the PAS technic with the LM and the PA-silver technic with the EM indicates that the coat contains carbohydrate. Chemical studies have led to the identification of sialic acid as one of the major components, and the cell coat is made up predominantly of sialic-acid-containing glycoproteins. Most of these are anchored in the lipid bilayer of the cell membrane, as shown in Figure 5-5, so that their carbohydrate chains, together with the part of the protein molecule to which they are anchored, project out into the cell

coat. The carbohydrate chains of glycolipids also seem to project into the cell coat. There thus appears to be a very intimate relationship between the cell coat and the cell membrane just below it.

The Functions of the Cell Coat

It is generally accepted that the cell coat on the cell surface probably acts as an adhesive, helping to hold cells together, often in very specific manner. It is interesting that when most of the cell coat is enzymatically removed from cells, they still remain viable and can regenerate their lost coat in a relatively short period of time. If, on the other hand, even the tiniest holes are made in the cell membrane, the cell dies. The cell coat probably also plays an important role in allowing cells to recognize other cells of their own kind so that they can form aggregates with them. As Moscona has shown, if cells of different kinds but from the same animal are dissociated and then mixed together in culture, the cells of any given kind, such as cartilage cells, seek each other out and adhere to one another. Indeed, cells of the same specialized type, but from different species, recognize each other much better than do cells of the same species but of different specialized types. Thus cartilage cells from different species associate better with one another than they do with any other kind of specialized cells from the same animals. It is also by their cell surfaces or coats that

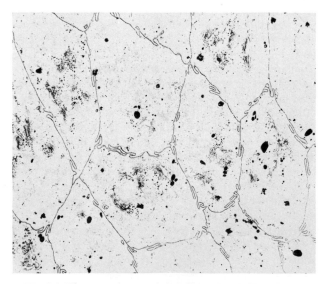

Fig. 5-8. Electron micrograph (×2,600) of epithelial cells of intestine, stained by the PA-silver methenamine technic for glycoprotein. The black lines between adjacent cells represent the glycoprotein of the cell coats. Note also how these epithelial cells interdigitate with one another. The nuclei of cells are not visible in this type of preparation. (Courtesy of C. P. Leblond and A. Rambourg)

foreign cells (for example, in organ transplants from other individuals) are recognized in the body so that immunological mechanisms are set into operation leading to their rejection. The surface by which the foreign cell is recognized depends on integral membrane glycoproteins whose carbohydrate-containing ends are exposed at the cell surface.

The Formation and Maintenance of the Cell Coat

This is discussed later, in connection with the Golgi apparatus.

A NOTE ON THE ORDER IN WHICH THE REMAINDER OF THE CYTOPLASMIC ORGANELLES WILL BE PRESENTED

We shall deal in turn with the members of a group of organelles that includes mitochondria, ribosomes, rough-surfaced endoplasmic reticulum, the Golgi apparatus, lysosomes, coated vesicles, and the smooth-surfaced endoplasmic reticulum. These organelles are being considered in this order because, at least in some instances, knowledge of the function of one organelle aids in understanding the function of subsequent ones. After considering the above-mentioned group of organelles, we shall go on to deal with the remainder.

As already noted, the elucidation of the structure, and sometimes even the very existence, of most of the organelles had to await the introduction of the EM into the study of histology. Next, the development of radioautography, particularly at the level of electron microscopy, allowed many of the chemical building blocks of tissues to be traced to the organelles specifically concerned with their metabolism. But thorough biochemical investigation of the roles played by the various organelles depended on the development of methods whereby each type of organelle could be separated from broken-up cells, not only in good condition and in sufficient quantities, but also in a pure enough state for biochemical analyses and functional studies to be done. The method by which organelles are isolated from cells is termed *cell fractionation*. This procedure will be described before dealing with the organelles because much information about the cytoplasmic organelles was obtained from cell fractionation studies.

CELL FRACTIONATION

The steps in cell fractionation are illustrated in Figure 5-9. As noted, this method has become a potent technic enabling biochemists to isolate different cell organelles in a relatively pure form. Moreover it allows them to deter-

mine their chemical composition and enzyme content, and from these data draw conclusions about their function in the cell. As a first step, the cells are disrupted by homogenization in a suitable medium that preserves the organelles and prevents them from aggregating. Very often this is a sucrose solution. Although mitochondria and many other cell organelles remain intact, interconnected networks of membranes such as endoplasmic reticulum, as well as the cell membrane, get broken into fragments. These fragments of membrane, however, each tend to seal up so as to form a rounded vesicle of variable size.

As a next step, the cell homogenate is subjected to a series of centrifugations of increasing speed and duration, a process called *differential centrifugation*. Depending on their size, density, and shape, different organelles sediment at the bottom of the centrifuge tube at different speeds. A sediment that forms at a given speed is called a *pellet* and can be obtained for examination. The structures that are large and dense, such as nuclei, sediment most rapidly, whereas smaller, less dense structures, such as vesicles of endoplasmic reticulum, require higher speeds and longer times to sediment. Therefore, at the lower speeds nuclei will sediment while the other cell organelles remain in suspension. At higher speeds the mitochondria and lysosomes will be sedimented and at very high speeds and long periods of centrifugation, even particles as small as ribosomes will form a pellet. These pellets can be examined by electron microscopy to determine the degree of purity of the fractions obtained. All the fractions are contaminated by other organelles to some extent. If sufficient purity has nevertheless been achieved, the fractions can then be subjected to biochemical analysis to determine the chemical composition and enzymatic activity of the isolated type of organelle.

More recently, a technic of cell fractionation called *density gradient centrifugation* has been introduced in which the centrifugation is done through layers of sucrose of increasing concentrations and therefore increasing densities. During centrifugation, the organelles of the homogenate position themselves at those levels in the centrifuge tubes where their density matches the density of the sucrose solution. This technic has enabled biochemists to separate organelles of similar size but different densities.

The Term Microsome. This term unfortunately has become a cause of confusion. From its derivation, a *microsome* means a small body. This word was introduced in the early days of centrifuging broken-up cells, before the characteristic structure of the organelles had been established by electron microscopy, to denote small bodies that could be centrifuged down from cell homogenates and studied biochemically. This unfortunately led to the concept that there were organelles called microsomes in cells. It is now known that what were

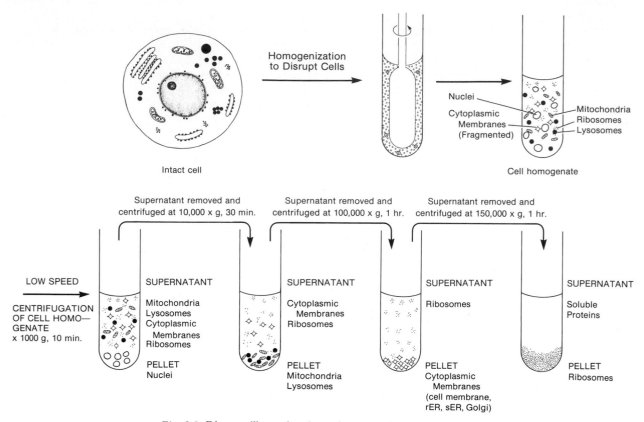

Fig. 5-9. Diagram illustrating the various steps in cell fractionation.

called microsomes were mixtures of broken-up organelles that now have their own names; hence there are no specific organelles in cells that should be called microsomes, as is sometimes assumed by those still unfamiliar with the fine structure of cytoplasm. Later on in this chapter we shall comment further on the organelles from which these so-called microsomes are obtained.

MITOCHONDRIA

At the beginning of this chapter it was noted that the energy required to sustain the viability and functions of cells is almost entirely derived from the oxidation of nutrients which, together with oxygen, pass from the tissue fluid through the membranes of cells to enter the cytoplasm (Fig. 5-1). The oxidation of nutrients takes place in membranous organelles long ago termed *mitochondria* because of their thread-like (Gr. *mitos,* thread) appearance in the LM.

Mitochondria house the chains of enzymes responsible for what is termed cell respiration. These enzymes cata-

lyze reactions that provide the cell with an important energy-rich compound known as *adenosine triphosphate (ATP)*. This compound accomplishes its energy-providing function by transferring one of its energetic terminal phosphate groups to another molecule. The ATP is thereby changed to adenosine diphosphate (ADP). Within mitochondria ADP is recharged by the addition of another phosphate group to become ATP again and so regains its energy-providing function.

Since mitochondria through their production of ATP are responsible for providing most of the energy required for the cell, they are often referred to as the powerhouses of the cell. Further details of their function in relation to their structure will be given later. Here, however, we shall describe their structure.

Early Studies With the LM

Although even with the stains commonly used today mitochondria are not evident in cells, Altmann, near the end of the last century, managed to stain them selectively by using acid fuchsin. Altmann, who is now regarded as a

Fig. 5-10. Photomicrograph (×2,440) showing changes in the shape of mitochondria in living fibroblasts, as seen under phase contrast. The same cell was photographed at 4-minute intervals. Note the remarkable changes in the shape of the mitochondria, especially in the regions below and to the left of the nucleus. (Chèvremont, M.: Cytologie et Histologie. ed. 2, p. 142. Liège, Desoer, 1966)

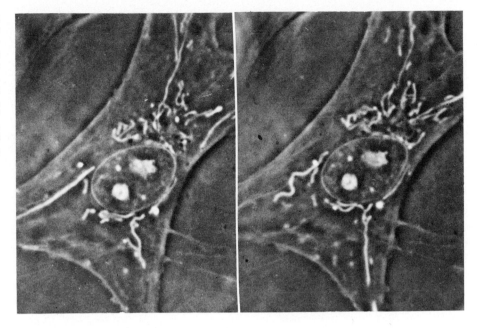

biological prophet, was able to demonstrate these organelles in a great variety of cells, terming them *bioblasts* and suggesting that they were elementary forms of life that were present in all kinds of cells and that, like bacteria (which they resemble), they were probably capable of independent existence. His contemporaries, however, were mostly antagonistic to his views and as a result he became so withdrawn that he avoided them to the point where he was referred to as "the ghost" in the laboratory. His career ended sadly. Curiously enough new evidence, obtainable only with modern knowledge and methods, is providing support for some of his prophetic views.

Studies With Supravital Stains

In this century it was found that mitochondria could be demonstrated in fresh, unfixed tissue by *supravital stains.* For these to act, a cell must be alive, because a supravital stain combines selectively with a cell component only because of a particular vital process in the cell component with which it becomes involved. The supravital stain most commonly used is Janus green, which imparts a transient blue-green color to mitochondria until the cell dies. (It should be noted that *supravital stains* differ from *vital stains* which will be described on p. 253.)

Studies With the Phase Contrast Microscope

Mitochondria can be studied profitably in living cells under phase contrast (described on p. 18). By the time phase microscopes became available, many laboratories had tissue culture facilities that provided single layers of flattened-out living cells suitable for examination with this instrument, which enhances contrast between cell components that are roughly similar in optical densities. Mitochondria can be seen readily in such cells. In living cells they constantly move and change shape; this feature is strikingly illustrated in the photomicrographs of living cells shown in Figure 5-10.

Fine Structure

The EM showed that mitochondria were membranous structures bounded by two membranes, an outer and an inner one, as shown in Figures 5-11 and 5-12, and in diagrammatic form in Figure 5-13. The membranes are each of the unit type and are about 7 nm. thick and hence slightly thinner than the cell membrane (Fig. 5-12). The outer membrane is thought to play a role in controlling the movement of substance into and out of the mitochondrion, the uptake of substrates, and the release of ATP.

The inner membrane is thrown into folds that project like shelves into the inside of the mitochondrion (Figs. 5-11 and 5-12); these projections, shown in three-dimensions in Figure 5-13, are termed *cristae.* Obviously in thin sections a mitochondrion will be cut only infrequently in longitudinal section throughout its whole length, as is the one shown in Figure 5-11. Most will be cut in cross or oblique section (Figs. 5-12 and 5-14); hence, deciding their size, shape, and structure from thin sections would require making reconstructions of them from serial sections, or at least a rather thoughtful exercise in three-

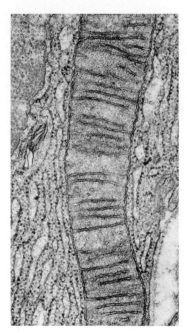

Fig. 5-11. Electron micrograph of part of a mitochondrion from an acinar cell of the pancreas. (Courtesy of H. Warshawsky)

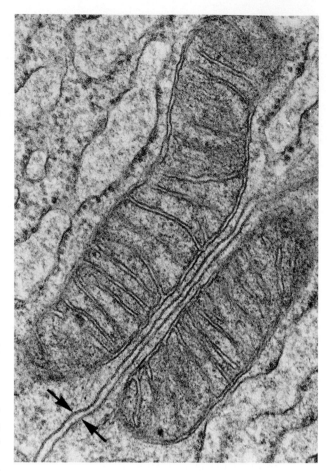

Fig. 5-12. Electron micrograph (×86,000) of mitochondria from the tracheal epithelium of a newborn rat, showing their cristae and matrix. The cell membranes (*arrows*) of two adjacent cells can also be seen, with a narrow intercellular space between them. (Courtesy of M. Weinstock)

dimensional visualization. Mitochondria usually vary considerably in size in any one cell type, but most are from 0.4 to 1 μm. in diameter. In different cell types the size, shape and number of the cristae vary considerably. In liver cells, for example, the cristae are short and extend only about halfway across mitochondria (Fig. 22-21); in other cells, such as muscle cells, the cristae may extend completely across mitochondria (Fig. 18-12). Some cell types have mitochondria with large numbers of cristae and others have mitochondria in which the cristae are tubular in form instead of being shelf-like.

The interior of each mitochondrion is filled with a fluid that in electron micrographs appears slightly denser than the surrounding cytoplasm; this is termed the *mitochondrial matrix*. Occasional spherical or ovoid electron-dense *granules* are seen lying in it (Fig. 5-14). These granules are accumulations of such cations as calcium and magnesium and their presence testifies to the ability of mitochondria to concentrate cations. Some of these ions are required for the functioning of mitochondrial enzymes.

Numbers, Distribution and Renewal of Mitochondria

Mitochondria are usually very numerous in cells. However, their numbers differ in relation to the energy requirements of different kinds of cells; thus some, for ex-

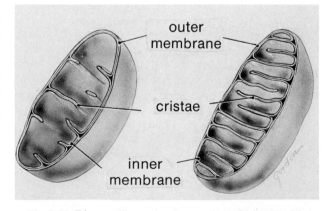

Fig. 5-13. Diagram illustrating the structure of mitochondria in three dimensions.

ample, lymphocytes, have only a few, whereas a liver cell possesses several hundred. The number of cristae in the mitochondria also reflect the energy requirements of cells. Cells with mitochondria having numerous cristae (such as muscle cells) have higher energy requirements than cells whose mitochondria have fewer cristae. Moreover, although mitochondria in general are found throughout the cytoplasm in many kinds of cells, they are aggregated particularly in those parts of the cell that have the highest requirement for ATP.

There is continual renewal of mitochondria throughout the cell cycle. In rat liver cells they are replaced in about 10 days. It is believed that mitochondria divide by fission, similar to that involved in the division of bacteria; that is, a partition develops across the middle of a mitochondrion and the two halves separate along this partition.

Mitochondrial Structure in Relation to the Enzymes Concerned in Cell Respiration

From early research it was found that there were two pathways by which sugar could be metabolized to yield energy in mammalian cells: (*1*) an anaerobic (without air) pathway, now generally termed *glycolysis*, which enabled sugar to be metabolized in the absence of oxygen, and (*2*) an (aerobic) pathway in which oxygen was utilized, now called *oxidative phosphorylation*, that yielded much more energy (ATP) than the anaerobic one. As more was learned it became established that although there were two pathways in the cell they were not side-by-side alternatives as at first believed; instead, the two pathways are arranged in tandem, with the anaerobic pathway preceding the aerobic. It is now accepted that sugar absorbed by cells is, without the help of oxygen, degraded by a series of steps catalyzed by enzymes to pyruvic acid (pyruvate) and that the reactions involved occur in the cytoplasmic matrix and result in the formation of a small amount of ATP and a low energy yield as compared with that from the aerobic pathway which normally follows. It is the reactions of the second (aerobic) pathway that accomplish what is known as *cell respiration*, and this takes place in mitochondria. Glycolysis and cell respiration are, of course, dealt with in detail in biochemistry courses, and the brief comment given here is only to relate certain of the processes involved to mitochondrial structure.

Sites of Enzymes. The end products of glycolysis (after being somewhat altered) are taken through the mitochondrial membranes into the mitochondrial matrix, where the enzymes of the Krebs cycle are located. These enzymes catalyze a host of different reactions concerned with the breakdown of the end-products of glycolysis and of amino and fatty acid metabolism. Within mitochondria, the end-products of glycolysis are gradually broken down to CO_2 by the enzymes of the Krebs cycle. During this process

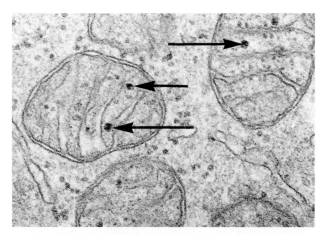

Fig. 5-14. Electron micrograph (×80,000) of mitochondria of an epithelial cell (chick trachea), showing cristae and spherical dense granules (indicated by arrows) lying in the matrix between them. (Courtesy of V. Kalnins)

there is a release of several hydrogen ions, which are captured by the coenzyme nicotinamide adenine dinucleotide (NAD). The electrons of the hydrogen are then passed along a series of respiratory enzymes called flavoproteins and cytochromes and ultimately combine with protons and oxygen to form water. The energy obtained from this passage of electrons is utilized at several sites along the series to permit the phosphorylation that regenerates ATP from ADP and inorganic phosphate. For this reason the reactions involved in electron transport are closely coupled with those of phosphorylation, and as a result ATP is produced in a very efficient manner. It is not surprising therefore to find that the enzymes concerned in electron transport and oxidative phosphorylation are arranged in integrated complexes on the inner mitochondrial membrane and its cristae. This arrangement is believed to be one that would permit special step-by-step enzymatic processes to occur. The energy-rich ATP finally produced is made available to the cytoplasm outside the mitochondria.

Negative Staining of Mitochondria

In an attempt to obtain information about the location of various enzymes concerned in cell respiration, mitochondrial cristae have been examined in the EM by means of *negative staining*—a technic that has also given much new information about the structure of other cell organelles, macromolecular complexes, and viruses. The negative staining procedure involves surrounding a particle with electron-dense material. In a micrograph the object itself is thereby delineated with electron-dense material so that it appears light against a dark background.

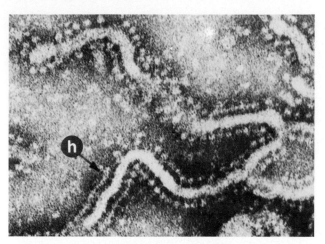

Fig. 5-15. Electron micrograph (×192,000) of a *negatively stained* preparation of mitochondrial cristae, showing a number of white-appearing cristae covered on both surfaces by toadstool-like structures, the heads of which are visible as small round white objects (h) lined up at a specific distance from the cristae. The heads are attached to the membrane by thin stalks. (Parsons, D. F.: Science, *140:*985, May, 1963)

When the inner membranes of mitochondria are studied in this way they appear as shown in Figure 5-15. Both sides of the cristae are seen to be covered with toadstool-like projections of the inner mitochondrial membrane; they have heads 9 nm. in diameter and stems 3 to 4 nm. wide. It is thought that these projections contain an enzyme concerned in the phosphorylation of ADP to ATP.

Mitochondria as Symbionts; Nucleic Acids in Mitochondria

As already noted, Altmann in the last century was scorned for his beliefs about the nature of mitochondria. However, subsequent findings have done much to vindicate him, for mitochondria have now been shown to contain not only DNA and RNA but also ribosomes slightly different from those found elsewhere in the cytoplasm. Hence mitochondria possess the means for a considerable degree of independent existence. Their DNA, RNA, and ribosomes are in forms similar to those found in bacteria. It is now accepted that mitochondrial DNA provides the information for the synthesis of many, but not all, of the proteins of a mitochondrion (the information for the rest being supplied by the nucleus); thus they are at least semiautonomous organelles. Hence the concept that long ago they originated from bacteria that invaded animal cells, where they became symbionts and added much to the total metabolic capacity of animal cells, looks quite attractive at the present time.

FREE RIBOSOMES AND POLYRIBOSOMES

Ribosomes lying free in the cytoplasm, either singly or in small groups known as polyribosomes (now commonly abbreviated to polysomes), together constitute a class of cytoplasmic organelles. But before dealing with these we should, in order to avoid possible confusion, mention that ribosomes (but not free ribosomes) also enter into the structure of another class of cytoplasmic organelle called the rough-surfaced endoplasmic reticulum, where they are attached to a membrane. We shall go on to deal with that organelle after we have described free ribosomes and polyribosomes.

The Relation of Free Ribosomes and Polyribosomes to Diffuse Cytoplasmic Basophilia Observed With the LM

Long before the EM became available, histologists and histopathologists observed that the cytoplasm of certain kinds of cells exhibited more basophilia than that of others; furthermore, they noticed that the basophilia could be either diffuse or localized. With the advent of the EM, it was found that the diffuse basophilia was due to the presence of free ribosomes and polyribosomes in the cytoplasm, whereas localized basophilia was due to rough-surfaced endoplasmic reticulum, in which organelle the ribosomes, as noted above, are attached to a membrane. We shall now deal with free ribosomes and their function and the situations in which they are numerous enough to cause diffuse basophilia.

The Function of Free Ribosomes

This is to participate in the synthesis of the proteins of the cytoplasmic matrix (cytosol) and the protein subunits of certain organelles, including those from which microfilaments and microtubules are made. Since all of these proteins are always being catabolized, they must be constantly renewed. In addition, free ribosomes are essential for the extra amounts of protein that are required when growth occurs. Proteins synthesized by free ribosomes include many special cytoplasmic proteins found only in specific cell types as, for example, the hemoglobin in red blood cells.

Situations in Which There Are Enough Free Ribosomes in the Cytoplasm to Render It Diffusely Basophilic

Although free ribosomes are present in every kind of living cell (except mature red blood cells), and although free ribosomes are basophilic because of their content of rRNA, there are not enough of them in most kinds of cells to impart noticeable basophilia to the cytoplasm. There are, however, special situations in which there are enough

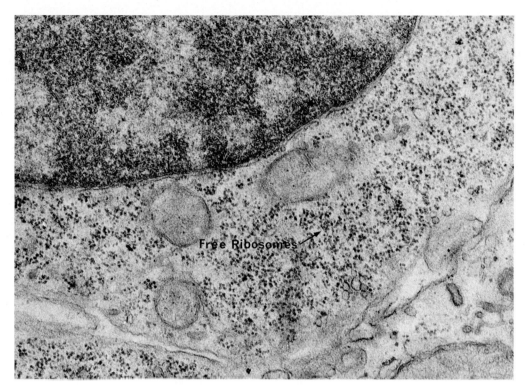

Fig. 5-16. Electron micrograph (×40,000) showing part of an erythroblast (rat). The cytoplasm has many free ribosomes arranged into groups forming polyribosomes for the synthesis of hemoglobin. (Courtesy of A. Jézéquel)

free ribosomes in the cytoplasm to make the cytoplasm appear basophilic in H and E sections.

In Rapidly Growing Cells. It was observed long ago with the LM that the cytoplasm of rapidly growing cancer cells was often diffusely basophilic. In 1955, Howatson and Ham made an early EM study of two types of rapidly growing cancer cells and showed that their cytoplasm revealed a relative abundance of particles of the type that later became termed free ribosomes. As might be expected, diffuse basophilia of the cytoplasm is frequently also seen in rapidly growing normal cells of developing embryos and, in postnatal life, in the cytoplasm of cells that are proliferating rapidly to bring about the repair of an injury.

In Connection With the Synthesis of Hemoglobin. Fully formed red blood cells have lost their nuclei and almost all the cytoplasmic components they had at earlier stages of development. Indeed, mature red blood cells are not much more than biconcave bags of cell membrane, filled with the protein hemoglobin which, as has already been mentioned, serves as an oxygen carrier. The cell that gives rise to red blood cells is called an *erythroblast* (Fig. 5-16). At this stage of development the cell still possesses

a nucleus, the DNA of which gives off information via mRNA to the cytoplasm, and its cytoplasm is intensely basophilic because, as the EM shows, it contains many free ribosomes (Fig. 5-16). An erythroblast is primarily concerned with the synthesis of hemoglobin, which in due course will be the only major component left in the cytoplasm. So almost all the abundant free ribosomes dispersed throughout its cytoplasm represent sites of hemoglobin synthesis. Hemoglobin is of course a special protein and not one of those required for normal cell maintenance and growth.

Free Polyribosomes

It was in connection with the synthesis of hemoglobin that the arrangement of ribosomes into functional units called *polyribosomes (polysomes)* was first observed; this was done by Warner and his coworkers, who devised special ways of extracting intact clusters of ribosomes from developing red blood cells. They found that the free ribosomes concerned in hemoglobin synthesis tended to be arranged in clusters, the average number of which (in the instance of hemoglobin synthesis) seemed to be five.

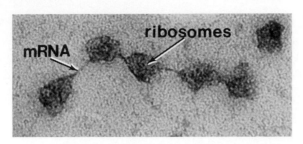

Fig. 5-17. Electron micrograph (×400,000) of a polyribosome isolated from red blood cell precursors (stained with uranyl acetate). Note the thread of mRNA connecting the five ribosomes. (Courtesy of H. Slater and A. Rich)

Furthermore, as shown in Figure 5-17, the free ribosomes in a polyribosome are connected by a fine thread, which is a molecule of mRNA coding for hemoglobin. Electron micrographs of sections of erythroblasts also show that the ribosomes are arranged in little groups or clusters, as is shown in Figure 5-16.

In order for a particular polypeptide molecule to be synthesized, the correct amino acids have to be linked together one at a time and in a certain order. One amino acid can be joined to another only at the site of a ribosome. Hence the long molecule of mRNA, which carries the code specifying which amino acids are to be joined together and the order in which they are to be joined, has to move along in relation to a ribosome, so that the successive amino acids called for in its code can be joined to the forming end of the polypeptide chain already assembled. If only a single ribosome were attached to each molecule of mRNA, only a single polypeptide molecule would result at the end of protein synthesis. If, however, there were, say, five ribosomes located at different points along the same mRNA molecule, five molecules of the polypeptide could be assembled simultaneously as these ribosomes moved along and, as a result, five complete molecules could be synthesized in roughly the same time that it would take to make one protein molecule if only one ribosome were available.

The ribosomes of polyribosomes are commonly arranged in whorls or spirals. Compared to other protein macromolecules, the hemoglobin molecule is relatively small and requires only a short molecule of mRNA to code for it. Strictly speaking, it is only the globin chains of hemoglobin that are synthesized on ribosomes. Therefore, only relatively small numbers of ribosomes become attached to the mRNA molecule along which the globin moiety is synthesized. As might be expected, the polyribosomes concerned in the synthesis of larger protein molecules have a larger number of ribosomes, because their molecules of mRNA are longer and hence there is room for more ribosomes. Indeed the number of ribosomes

seen in a polyribosome provides information about the size of the protein macromolecule being synthesized. Ribosomes, polysomes of various sizes, and the large and small subunits of ribosomes can now all be isolated in relatively pure form by cell fractionation procedures previously described (Fig. 5-9) and hence can be studied independently of other cell components.

THE ROUGH-SURFACED ENDOPLASMIC RETICULUM (rER)

The term *rough-surfaced endoplasmic reticulum* was not coined until cytoplasm could be studied in sections with the EM. However, long before this happened something had been seen in its place in cytoplasm with the LM. Since it is of the greatest importance for a microscopist to be able to translate mentally what is seen with the LM into what is seen with the EM, we shall first outline how our knowledge about the rough-surfaced endoplasmic reticulum developed. This of course, started long before its name was coined and its intricate structure elucidated with the EM.

Development of Knowledge From LM Studies

Early microscopists noticed that the cytoplasm of many different kinds of cells often revealed localized deposits of some component with as much affinity for basic stains as the nuclear chromatin. This component was given several names, only two of which need now be mentioned. It was referred to as the *basophilic component* of cytoplasm or as *ergastoplasm* (Gr. *ergon*, work), because it was thought it performed some special work for the cell.

When the Feulgen reaction became available for specifically identifying DNA, it was found that the basophilic material in cytoplasm was Feulgen-negative and hence not DNA. However, it was shown to absorb ultraviolet light of a wavelength that indicated it contained nucleic acid. Then, when the enzymes DNAase and RNAase became available, it was found to be digested by RNAase but not DNAase, so it became obvious that it was RNA. The way this component appears in the LM in a liver cell is shown in color at the upper left corner of Plate 1-1 (where it is labeled *cytoplasmic RNA*) and in black and white in Figure 5-18A (where it is not labeled but appears as irregular darkly staining areas in the cytoplasm). These areas disappear after extraction with RNAase (Fig. 5-18B)

One of the places where this material is easily seen is in certain secretory cells of the pancreas, and this is where we shall describe its appearance in detail. However, until the student has studied and become familiar with the structure of the pancreas as an organ, it may not be very

Fig. 5-18. Photomicrographs of liver cells stained with toluidine blue (*A*) before and (*B*) after extraction with RNAase. This enzyme, which is specific for RNA, removes the irregular patches of basophilic material in the cytoplasm, indicating that their basophilia is due to the presence of RNA. The staining of nuclei, however, is very little affected by this treatment, since most of their staining is due to DNA rather than to RNA. (Courtesy of R. Daoust)

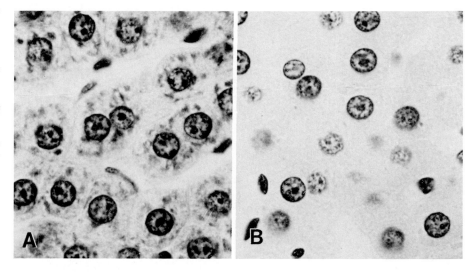

easy to locate these cells. We shall therefore first describe enough about the microscopic structure of the pancreas to enable the student to find the right kind of cells to study. For those who wish further information about the pancreas, it is described in detail as an organ in Chapter 22.

Some Guidance for Finding Pancreatic Cells That Reveal Basophilic Cytoplasmic Material

Most of the cells of the pancreas are of a type that produces and secretes the precursors of enzymes, which are proteins. These enzymes are delivered via the pan-

creatic duct into the intestine, where they act to digest certain foods. The cells synthesizing the enzymes are arranged in small rounded groups resembling bunches of grapes and hence called *acini* (L. *acinus,* grape). Each acinus has a central lumen that connects to a duct extending from it much as a stem extends from a grape; this duct carries the secretion away to the pancreatic duct. The acini and their ducts are oriented in random fashion so that a given section slices through acini and ducts at all angles. It takes some hunting with the low-power objective to find an acinus cut more or less in cross section like the one in the rectangle in Figure 5-19A. A high-power photomicrograph of a cross section of a similar acinus is

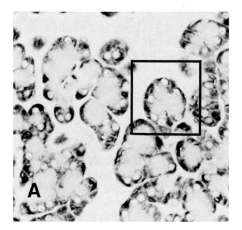
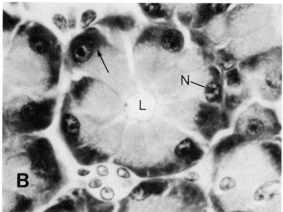

Fig. 5-19. (*A*) Medium-power photomicrograph of pancreas (stained with toluidine blue). A cross section of a single acinus is seen in the rectangle. (*B*) A high-power photomicrograph of a single pancreatic acinus (stained with H and E). Note the central lumen (L) of the acinus; the unstained secretory granules to be discharged into it fill those parts of the cells near the lumen. The nucleus (N) near the base of each cell and the basophilic region (*arrow*) between the nucleus and the base of the cell are clearly visible.

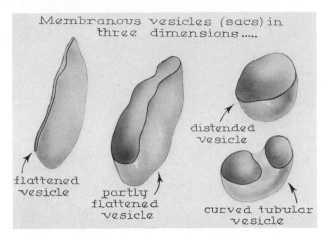

Membranous vesicles (sacs) in three dimensions.....

distended vesicle

flattened vesicle

partly flattened vesicle

curved tubular vesicle

Fig. 5-20. Diagram illustrating in three dimensions the various shapes of cytoplasmic membranous vesicles. The cut surface of each vesicle shows what it would appear like in a section. The large flattened vesicles (as at *left*) are termed cisternae.

shown in Figure 5-19B. Here it will be seen that a cross section of an acinus resembles a pie that has been cut into pieces but not yet served. Each piece of pie represents a secretory cell. The secretion is produced in several steps, soon to be described, and the product passes through the tip of each cell into the central lumen of the acinus (L in Fig. 5-19B), which connects with the duct that drains the secretion away. The nucleus of each secretory cell is located near its broad base, and the basophilic component of the cytoplasm is disposed between the nucleus and the sides and base of the cell. In these sites it appears as a purple-blue material in H and E sections (Fig. 5-19B, *arrow*).

Development of Knowledge and Terminology From EM Studies

Before it became feasible to cut sections thin enough for the EM, Porter and his coworkers grew cells in culture in which the cytoplasm at the cell margins was spread so thinly that they were able to examine it with the EM (after it was fixed). In it they observed a lace-like network of what appeared to be strands and vesicles, which they named the *endoplasmic reticulum (ER)*. The term *reticulum* indicates that the strands and vesicles are arranged in a network (L. *rete*, net) and *endoplasmic* is used to denote its location within (Gr. *endon*, within) the cytoplasm.

When it became possible to study the ER in sections with the EM, the network was shown to consist of hollow membranous structures: either *tubules* or bladder-like structures termed *vesicles* (L. *vesicula*, a small bladder).

Figure 5-20 illustrates some of the latter in three dimensions. Large flattened vesicles of the ER are commonly termed *cisternae*. Although there are different amounts of ER in different kinds of cells, virtually all kinds of cells contain at least a little of it. Furthermore, when studied in sections with the EM, it soon became apparent that there were two kinds of ER, the *rough* and the *smooth*. Here we shall deal only with the rough type *(rER)* because it possesses ribosomes that appear basophilic in LM preparations and are responsible for the protein synthesis that takes place in the rER. The cytoplasmic basophilia seen in stained sections with the LM, for example in the basal parts of the acinar cells of the pancreas (Fig. 5-19B), is accounted for by large numbers of ribosomes, most of which are attached to rER in such areas.

The Appearance of Rough-Surfaced ER in Micrographs

As shown in Figures 5-21 (diagram) and 5-22 (electron micrograph), the rER is seen with the EM to be in the form of membranous cisternae, the outer walls of which are studded with ribosomes. These ribosome-studded cisternae are packed fairly closely together and generally lie parallel to one another (Figs. 5-21 and 5-22). Secretion can be seen within the lumina of the cisternae (Fig. 5-22); it appears a little more electron-dense then the cytoplasmic matrix between cisternae. Although most of the ribosomes in this area are attached to the outer surface of the flattened vesicles of the rER, there are also some free ribosomes between adjacent cisternae.

The Function of the Rough-Surfaced ER

The synthesis of protein occurs on the ribosomes attached to the outer aspect of the membranous walls of the cisternae of the rER. Here, amino acids, tRNA, and mRNA are all present together with the ribosomes to participate in the reactions by which amino acids are linked together according to the instructions coded along the mRNA. The reason for the close association of ribosomes and membranous vesicles (cisternae) of the rER is, of course, that if special proteins are to be synthesized and exported from the cell, they must be segregated from the cytosol in membranous vesicles as they are synthesized. Furthermore, if these special proteins are to be released from the cell they must be kept segregated from the cytosol in membranous vesicles until they are emptied through the cell membrane. Thus the special proteins synthesized within the cell to serve purposes outside it have a different status from the proteins synthesized in connection with free ribosomes or polysomes. The latter proteins are, of course, produced within the cytosol and not segregated from it.

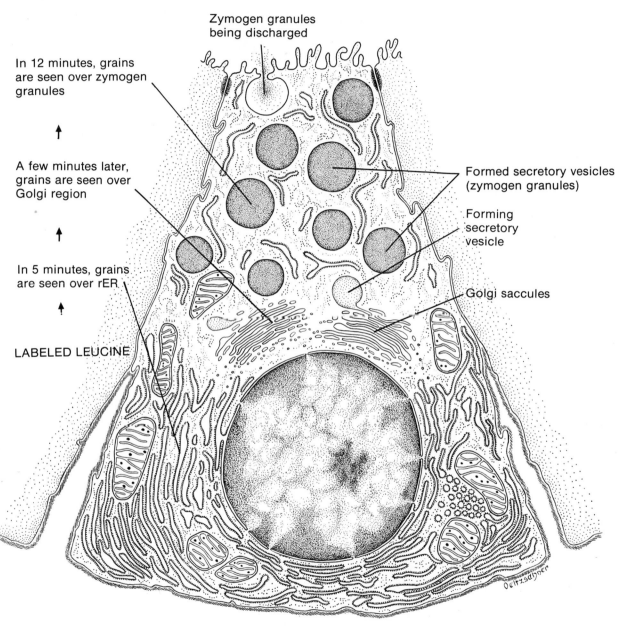

Lumen of acinus

Zymogen granules
being discharged

In 12 minutes, grains
are seen over zymogen
granules

↑

A few minutes later,
grains are seen over
Golgi region

↑

In 5 minutes, grains
are seen over rER

↑

LABELED LEUCINE

Formed secretory vesicles
(zymogen granules)

Forming
secretory
vesicle

Golgi saccules

Base of acinar cell of pancreas

Fig. 5-21. Diagram of an acinar cell of the pancreas, showing the sites where grains are seen in radioautographs prepared from samples of tissue taken at different times after injecting an animal with tritiated leucine. (Courtesy of C. P. Leblond)

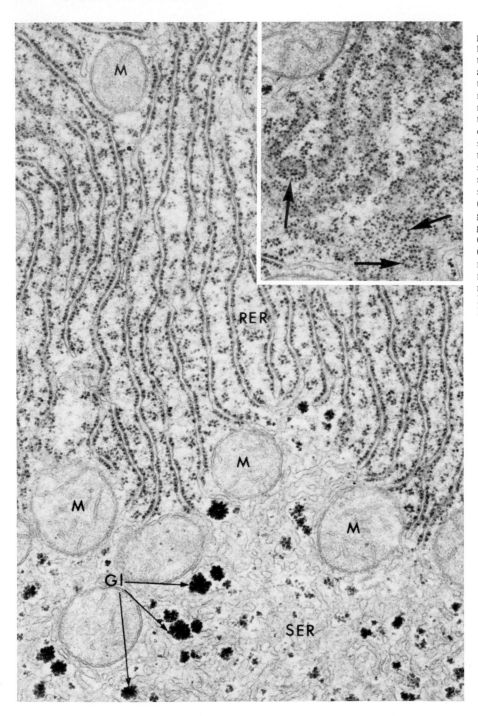

Fig. 5-22. Electron micrographs showing the rough-surfaced endoplasmic reticulum in the cytoplasm of a liver cell (from a rat treated with cortisone). In the large micrograph (×38,000), note the parallel cisternae of rough-surfaced endoplasmic reticulum (RER), the outer surface of which is studded with ribosomes. The lumen of each cisterna contains recently synthesized protein, eventually to be secreted. Note also the smooth-surfaced endoplasmic reticulum (SER) in the bottom of the micrograph. Mitochrondria (M) and glycogen (Gl) may also be seen. (Inset) A grazing section (×37,000) through the cisternae of rER shows a face view of the ribosomes studding the rER. Arrows indicate polysomes (*see also* Fig. 5-23). (Cardell, R.: Anat. Rec., *180:*309, 1974)

The Polysomes of the Rough-Surfaced ER

The ribosomes of the rER, as in most free polysomes, are arranged in clusters and often whorls (Figs. 5-22, *inset,* 5-23), in association with mRNA molecules. The larger subunit of each ribosome is attached to the membrane of the rER itself; the smaller one projects out into the cytoplasmic matrix (Fig. 5-24). Since polysomes are on the outer surfaces of the cisternae, it seems reasonable to assume that as the amino acids are linked to form polypeptide chains, the protein being synthesized is delivered through the membranous walls into the lumen of these cisternae (Fig. 5-24). Possibly there would be something like a pore in the membrane through which the end of a newly forming polypeptide molecule could enter the cisterna as rapidly as it was being lengthened by the ribosomes on the exterior of the membrane. By cell fractionation (Fig. 5-9), rER can be isolated in a relatively pure form, although it does break up into little membrane-bound vesicles with ribosomes on the outside upon preparation of cell homogenates. Moreover, by using detergents it is possible to remove the ribosomes of the rER so that they too can be separately analyzed by biochemical technics.

The Signal Hypothesis

The question arises as to why, depending on the type of protein synthesized, some polysomes are bound to membrane while others exist free in the cytoplasm. There is some evidence that all polysomes initially lie free in the cytoplasmic matrix, but those synthesizing membrane-segregated proteins attach to membranes of the rER soon after the synthesis of the protein begins. They appear to be able to do this because the *initial* segments of all kinds of membrane-segregated protein molecules synthesized have a specific "signal" (as illustrated at the top of Fig. 5-24), probably a particular amino acid sequence, that permits these protein molecules to bind to certain sites on the rER membrane. The same "signal" (amino acid sequence) also allows this type of protein to pass through the membrane of rER. Once the protein gets through the rER membrane, this initial segment may be cleaved and hence removed from the protein molecules by a special enzyme within the cisternae. Integral proteins and glycoproteins (*see* p. 113) that become parts of the rER membrane may be formed in much the same way, only here, instead of passing right through the membrane, they would stop when only part way through.

After synthesis on the ribosomes and passage into the cisternae of rER, other modifications occur in the protein molecule. As already mentioned, the initial signal portion may be removed and the molecule also folds up through the formation of S-S bonds. These steps prevent it from leaving the membrane-bound compartment again, thus making the step unidirectional. Then sugars, such as glucosamine and mannose, may be added at appropriate places on the polypeptide chain.

The Distribution of Rough ER in Different Types of Cells

Some rER is present in every kind of nucleated cell, because the outer membrane of the nuclear envelope is

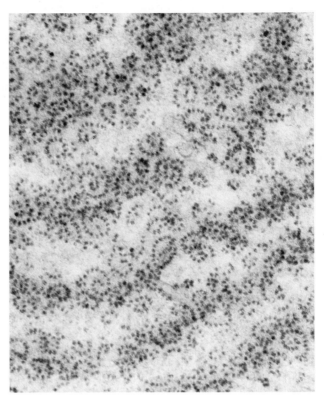

Fig. 5-23. Electron micrograph of part of a cell from the cortex of an adrenal gland of a human fetus, showing polyribosomes attached to the outer surface of cisternae of rER, which have been cut in grazing section. The individual ribosomes are arranged to form spiral polyribosomes. The membranes of the rER are not seen here in cross section due to the plane of section. (Courtesy of E. Yamada)

identical with the membrane of the rER, having ribosomes attached to it, as shown in Figure 4-5 (on p. 89). The greatest amounts of rER are found in such secretory cells as the acinar cells of the pancreas (Fig. 5-21) and liver cells (Fig. 5-22). However, many other kinds of cells not always thought of as secretory cells also synthesize and secrete protein into their environment; for example, *fibroblasts* of connective tissue which secrete proteins and the other substances that constitute the intercellular substances occupying the spaces between the cells of connective tissue, *osteoblasts* of bone which elaborate proteins that become part of the organic intercellular substance of bone, and *plasma cells* which make and secrete circulating antibodies. Some of the hormones (those that are proteins) also are made by cells with a well-developed rER. In all kinds of cells rER is required for the synthesis of the enzymes contained within little membrane-bound vesicles called *lysosomes*, which we shall soon consider. Accordingly, although the rER is most highly developed

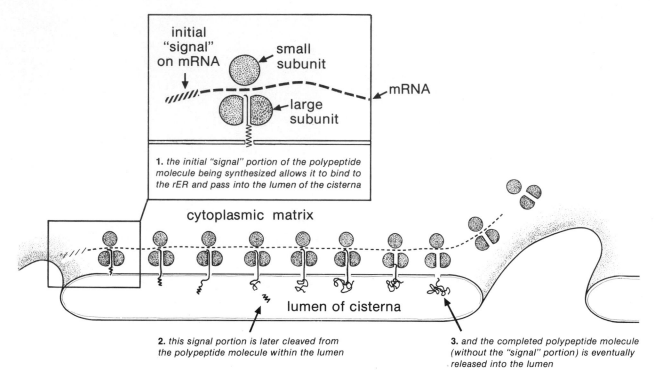

Fig. 5-24. Diagram illustrating protein synthesis by ribosomes on the outer aspect of a cisterna of rER, according to the signal hypothesis (*see* text). Note how the product becomes segregated within the lumen of the cisterna.

in cells that are obviously secretory, it is an essential component of all nucleated cells, for it is required for synthesis and segregation of proteins required within the cell as well as for products that will be secreted into the environment.

The Fate of the Membrane-Segregated Protein Synthesized in the rER

As will be described in the next section on the Golgi apparatus, the protein synthesized in the cisternae of the rER is delivered to, and emptied into, another membranous organelle termed the *Golgi apparatus*. This process is accomplished by small vesicles, termed *transfer vesicles* and containing the protein, budding off from the rER and moving to, fusing with, and emptying their contents into the membranous structures of which the Golgi apparatus is composed (Figs. 5-25 and 5-26). It is not certain whether a few of these transfer vesicles that bud off from the rER may bypass the Golgi and go directly to the cell membrane, fuse with it, and empty their contents outside the cell. Within the Golgi region the product formed in the rER is both chemically modified and physically packaged into small membranous vesicles

(Fig. 5-21, *secretory vesicles*), in which form it is delivered to sites where the final product will serve its function.

THE GOLGI APPARATUS

The elucidation of the structure and functions of the Golgi apparatus required not only the advent of the EM but also the development of the technic of radioautography and some understanding of the enzymes involved in adding carbohydrate to proteins. Accordingly, most of the definitive information is of recent origin and much still remains to be learned. It is now known that the Golgi apparatus is a very important membranous organelle that is not part of the endoplasmic reticulum. Although present in all cells, its size varies greatly in different kinds of cells.

Development of Knowledge

In 1898, Camillo Golgi, an Italian neurologist, working with a microscope and not much more equipment than might be found in a kitchen, made a discovery that started

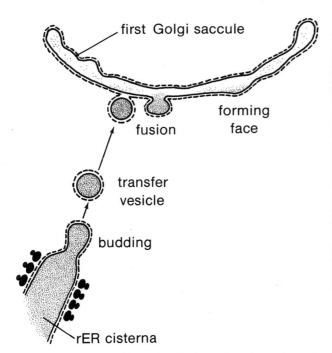

Fig. 5-25. Diagram illustrating the formation of transfer vesicles from the rER and their subsequent fusion with the forming face of the Golgi, by which means they carry newly synthesized protein from the rER to the first Golgi saccule.

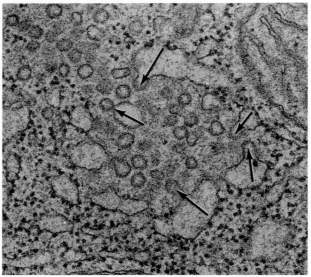

Fig. 5-26. Electron micrograph (×70,000) showing the region in a secretory cell where cisternae of rER abut on the periphery of the Golgi apparatus. In several sites (*arrows*), smooth-surfaced transfer vesicles are budding from rER. They transport protein from the rER to the Golgi apparatus. (Palade, G. F.: Proc. Natl. Acad. Sci. U.S.A., *52*:613, 1964)

him on the path to sharing a Nobel prize many years later. He had fixed some pieces of brain tissue in a bichromate solution and had followed this by impregnating them with a silver salt. When he examined this tissue with his microscope he found some dark material in the cytoplasm that seemed to be arranged in a network, so he referred to this as the reticular apparatus of the cell. Subsequent studies on other kinds of cells confirmed the existence of this organelle, but not that it always formed a network, and so it became known as the *Golgi apparatus* or *Golgi complex*. Most people now refer to it simply as the *Golgi*. Later this organelle was demonstrated in cells immersed in osmium tetroxide. Many studies indicated that its position and form were different in different kinds of specialized cells. In secretory cells, such as the acinar cells of the pancreas, it was located between the nucleus and the apex of the cell through which the secretion is delivered (Fig. 5-27). In other kinds of cells without such polarized secretory activities, parts of the apparatus were sometimes distributed about in the cytoplasm, but generally lay fairly close to the nucleus. In the following years an enormous number of papers were published about the Golgi, without much further information being disclosed. However, in the light of what is now known from the EM and radioautography, the prophetic views of Bowen and

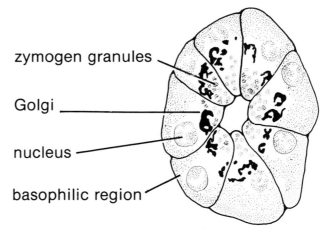

Fig. 5-27. Drawing of a pancreatic acinus specifically stained to demonstrate the Golgi apparatus in the acinar cells. Note that the Golgi apparatus lies between the nuclei and the zymogen granules toward the apical borders of these cells. (Based on a preparation by C. P. Leblond and H. Warshawsky)

Hirsch (in the 1920s and 1930s respectively) should be mentioned, for both surmised that the Golgi apparatus must function as the site of aggregation and condensation for secretory products made elsewhere in the cell.

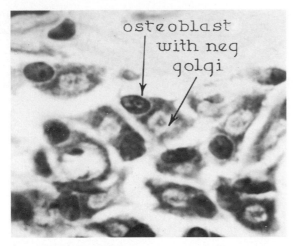

osteoblast
with neg
golgi

Fig. 5-28. Medium-power photomicrograph of osteoblasts in a section of bone (stained with azure-eosin-hematoxylin). This shows osteoblasts beginning to lay down bone near the site of a fracture. The osteoblasts show pale areas (negative Golgi regions) in their basophilic cytoplasm.

Negative Golgi Images

In laboratory work a student may have the opportunity to examine with the LM a section prepared by a technic that demonstrates the Golgi apparatus. However, in any event, although routine methods such as H and E do not stain the apparatus itself, they do often reveal the existence of a somewhat lighter staining region next to the nucleus that marks the site where it exists. These lighter staining regions, which are termed *negative Golgi images,* are seen to best advantage in cells elaborating secretions (Fig. 5-28). The paleness is due to the Golgi apparatus not containing any ribosomes. But in secretory cells the cytoplasm adjacent to the apparatus generally has a heavy content of rER, which makes it basophilic, so the Golgi-containing area appears lighter in contrast.

The Fine Structure of the Golgi Apparatus

The general features of the fine structure of the Golgi will be described here; special features will be considered later.

Just as the unit of structure of the rER is a flattened membranous vesicle studded on its outer surface with ribosomes and termed a *cisterna,* the unit of structure of the Golgi is likewise a flattened membranous vesicle, but since it has no ribosomes attached to its outer surface, it is distinguished from a cisterna by being called a *saccule.* The difference in appearance between cisternae of rER and saccules of the Golgi apparatus in electron micrographs of ultrathin sections is illustrated in Figure 5-21.

Next, a Golgi saccule is commonly visualized as having the form of a saucer. Just as saucers may be stacked one upon another in a kitchen, the saucer-like saccules of the Golgi are commonly present in the cytoplasm in stacks (Fig. 5-21). But unlike a stack of real saucers, the saucers (saccules) of a Golgi stack generally look as if they were stacked upside down and are slightly separated from one another. Furthermore, the bottom two saucers and the top two saucers of the stack are somewhat different from the ones in between them, as will be described later.

Seen in three dimensions, a stack of Golgi saccules would appear as shown in Figure 5-29. (The rounded secretory vesicles at the top of this illustration will be described later.) However, if a section is cut through a stack of Golgi saccules, each saccule will appear only as two lines which, of course, represent its membranous walls, one on one side of the saccule and one on the other (Fig. 5-21). The substance within the lumen of the saccule does not show. So in a section of a stack there is a thin space between each saccule as well as a thin space between the opposing walls of each saccule. There may be from three to ten saccules in a stack.

Continuity Between Golgi Stacks. The Golgi apparatus rarely consists of only one stack of saccules; commonly it consists of several. It has been generally assumed, until relatively recently, that the Golgi stacks in a cell were isolated from one another, because connections between stacks were not apparent in the ultrathin sections used for the EM. However, if it were possible to employ thicker sections, connections between what appear to be isolated structures in ultrathin sections might be seen beneath or above the level at which a single ultrathin section may have been cut. The examination of somewhat thicker sections has now become possible with the development of the million volt electron microscope. Because of its great penetrating power, this type of EM permits much thicker sections to be studied than was previously possible with conventional EMs. Such studies have shown some lateral connections between adjacent stacks.

As already mentioned, osmium tetroxide will impregnate the Golgi apparatus of cells. Friend showed, however, that only part of the apparatus is stained with it, namely, the first saccule at the bottom of a stack. Rambourg and Clermont took advantage of this property to examine this saccule in 2-μm.-thick sections in the million volt electron microscope. They found, in eight different cell types, that the first saccule in each of the stacks showed continuity with the first saccule in the nearby stacks and hence the Golgi apparatus constituted an irregular network within the cell. In nerve cells, the picture they obtained was that of a reticulated apparatus around the nucleus, very much like the one originally described by Golgi. In other cells only a single irregular network on

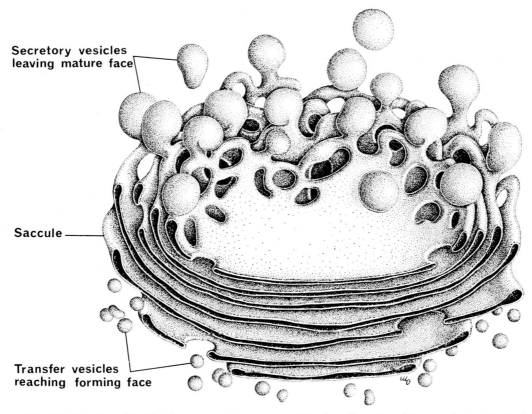

Fig. 5-29. Drawing of the Golgi apparatus of a secretory cell in three dimensions. The transfer vesicles bud off from the rER, which would be below. The secretory vesicles that bud off from saccules on the mature face become, in the instance of acinar cells, the so-called zymogen granules. (Drawn from a model by J. Kephart; illustration courtesy of C. P. Leblond)

one side of the nucleus was seen. At high magnifications, the first (bottom) saccule appears fenestrated, as was already known; the fenestrae are commonly so wide that Rambourg and Clermont describe this saccule as being composed of a tubular network.

While the first saccule of a stack shows continuity with the first saccule of some of the other Golgi stacks in the cell, the situation with regard to the other saccules of the different stacks is more complex; they may be connected with either the corresponding or a different saccule in another stack. Hence the Golgi stacks are not isolated from one another but instead connected in a network to form the Golgi apparatus.

The Position of the Golgi Stacks in Different Kinds of Cells. In specialized secretory cells, such as the acinar cells of the pancreas (Figs. 5-21 and 5-27), the Golgi apparatus is located above the nucleus and occupies a position between the rER (which is close to the base of the cell) and the apex of the cell through which the secretion, produced

in the rER and modified in the Golgi, is delivered. In cells where secretory activity is not so definitely polarized, Golgi stacks do not have such a specific location, but although they may be scattered about in a few kinds of cells, in most types they lie close to the centrioles. The number of stacks in a cell varies, large nerve cells having the most. But all kinds of cells need to have a Golgi apparatus because, as we shall soon see, this is essential for the maintenance of their cell membranes and cell coats.

The Two Faces of Golgi Stacks. A stack of saccules is said to have two *faces:* one is called the *forming, immature,* or *cis* (L., on this side of, near) *face,* which is usually (but not always) convex and the other is termed the *mature,* or *trans* (L., beyond) *face,* which is generally concave. In Figure 5-29, the forming face seen at the base of the drawing is associated with small rounded vesicles, whereas the mature face at the top is associated with larger rounded vesicles. In Figure 5-21, the forming face is oriented toward the base of the cell (toward the nucleus) and is close to the rER. The mature face, on the other hand, faces the apex of the cell, the direction in which secretion is delivered (Fig. 5-21).

The Formation and Maintenance of Golgi Stacks. For perspective about the Golgi it is important to realize that it is devoid of ribosomes and hence does not synthesize the membranous saccules of which it is composed. Its formation, maintenance, and capacity for function all depend on the rER. The membrane of which Golgi saccules are composed is synthesized in the rER and reaches the forming face of a Golgi stack by means of little vesicles called *transfer* (or intermediate) *vesicles*. These bud off from the rER (Figs. 5-25 and 5-26) at sites where it has lost its ribosomes. They then move toward the forming face of a Golgi stack where their membranous walls fuse with those of the bottom saccule, which explains why this face is called the *forming face* of a Golgi stack.

Since it has become established that the two sides of any given membrane are not the same as each other, it has become important to understand how membranes can fuse to permit their proper "sidedness" to be preserved in the new membranous structure to which they both contribute their membrane. As shown in Figure 5-25, the outer side of the membrane of both the transfer vesicle and the first Golgi saccule first meet and fuse, after which the fused outer halves open at the site of fusion to allow the inner halves of the two membranes to meet and fuse. At the fused site, the inner halves of the two membranes than open up so that the contents of the transfer vesicle can now be emptied into the first Golgi saccule. Furthermore, the membranous wall of the vesicle opens up completely to become part of the membranous wall of the first Golgi saccule, by which process the membranous wall of the saccule is expanded with the appropriate aspects of the membrane facing inside and outside, respectively.

The Turnover of the Saccules in a Stack; Why Golgi Stacks Must Be Continuously Renewed. Vesicles filled with secretion that may serve various purposes bud off more or less constantly from the mature face of a Golgi stack. As a consequence, the membrane of the top saccule of a stack is constantly being lost. Since the Golgi cannot itself synthesize more membrane, the membrane lost at the mature face can only be compensated for by new membrane being added to the first saccule at the forming face. This means that there is a turnover of saccules. As the membrane of the saccule at the top of the mature face is "used up" by forming membranous vesicles that bud off from it, membrane from the next saccule beneath must in due course become the membrane of the saccule at the mature face. Likewise, membrane from the bottom saccule, as more and more membrane is added to it by transfer vesicles, becomes the membrane of the saccule just above it. Hence there is a turnover of the membrane of the saccules of a Golgi stack with new membrane being added at

the forming face and membrane from the top saccules being lost at the mature face as it gives rise to secretory vesicles (also called secretory granules).

The Source of the Contents of the Golgi Saccules. The protein content of the fluid in the Golgi saccules is all derived from the rER by way of transfer vesicles but it may be modified between the time it enters the saccule on the forming face and the time it leaves in a secretory vesicle from the mature face. Some of the carbohydrate component of the contents of the Golgi saccules is also derived from the rER, but most is added in the Golgi saccules, where certain enzymes, called *glycosyl transferases*, in the membranous walls of the saccules add carbohydrate groups to the protein molecules. In cells that secrete sulfated glycosaminoglycans, the sulfate is also added in the Golgi saccules. Hence the Golgi plays a key role in the synthesis of cell secretions containing glycoproteins or glycosaminoglycans. The fluid vehicle for such macromolecular components is, of course, derived from the fluid entering the rER from the cytosol. Its relative amount and hence the concentration of the components in it appear to be determined by the movement of fluid between the interior of the Golgi saccules and the cytosol.

How Membrane-Segregated Protein Moves From the Forming Face to the Mature Face. The protein content of the fluid released into the bottom saccule by transfer vesicles conceivably could reach the saccule on the mature face in either of two ways: first, if there were no connections between adjacent saccules, it could make this journey only by the particular saccule in which it was contained moving from the bottom to the top of the stack. Second, if the saccules within a stack were somehow interconnected, it would be possible for proteins to move through the connecting portions from one saccule to another. However, if proteins do move in this fashion, it would appear that, instead of moving from one saccule to the next within the same stack, they might be more likely to pass laterally from any given saccule in one stack to other saccules at the next level in nearby stacks. This more indirect route would be more compatible with the recent finding of Clermont and Rambourg that although direct connections between adjacent saccules seem to be lacking within stacks, tubules that connect Golgi saccules laterally with their counterparts in other stacks (and not shown in Fig. 5-21) appear to anastomose in such a way that they could allow the passage of secretory materials from saccules of a given stack to saccules at other levels in nearby stacks.

It will be appreciated that during the process of delivering their content of protein to the bottom saccule at the forming face, transfer vesicles contribute membrane to the bottom saccule by fusing with it. So it might be expected that protein would be delivered to the bottom sac-

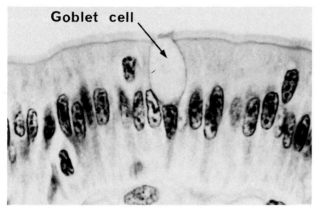

Goblet cell

Fig. 5-30. Photomicrograph (×800) of the epithelium lining the small intestine (dog), stained with H and E, showing a goblet cell. The nucleus of the goblet cell lies below the bowl part of the goblet.

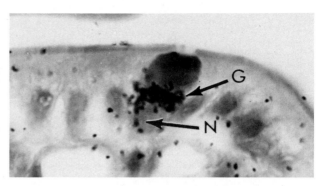

G

N

Fig. 5-31. Radioautograph of the epithelium lining the small intestine (rat), 5 minutes after intravenous injection of ^{3}H-glucose, showing grains in a goblet cell over the Golgi region (G), which lies just above the nucleus (N) of the cell. (Courtesy of G. C. Bennet)

cule at the same rate as membrane was lost from the mature face, because membrane is required for the formation of secretory vesicles. It could also be reasoned that, whether there were any interconnections between the saccules or not, protein would not enter the saccule at the forming face any faster than protein could be emptied into this saccule from transfer vesicles; hence it might be thought that the turnover time of the protein in the saccule would match the turnover time of the membrane of the saccule. There is, however, some evidence indicating that the turnover rate of the saccule membrane is in fact somewhat slower than that of the protein content of the saccules.

How It Was Established by Radioautography that the Carbohydrate in Cell Secretions Was Mostly Synthesized by Golgi Saccules

In order to discuss this, we must first describe a type of secretory cell called a *goblet cell* that is highly specialized to elaborate a glycoprotein secretion.

Goblet Cells. The small intestine is lined by a single layer of epithelial cells taller than they are wide and arranged side by side (Plate 1-1, *middle*). These cells are of two types, (*1*) pale-staining cells specialized to absorb the products of digestion and (*2*) goblet cells, which are specialized to secrete mucus and lie scattered among cells of the first type. As explained in Chapter 1, mucus is a thick, slippery material made from glycoprotein and which stains magenta with the PAS technic, as shown in Plate 1-1, *middle.* The mucus secreted by goblet cells flows over the lining of the intestine to cover and protect the free surface of the absorptive cells. The characteristic

shape of a goblet cell is due to its basal part, which contains the nucleus, being narrow and hence appearing as the stem of a goblet, while the part of the cell between the stem and the free surface (the bowl of the goblet) is so distended by bubble-like, membrane-enclosed globules of mucus that it bulges sideways, pressing into the sides of the absorptive cells beside it (Fig. 5-30).

The Role of the Golgi in Goblet Cells. Clues indicating that the Golgi apparatus might have some function in adding carbohydrate to cell secretions came from several sources. For example, the PAS technic often revealed the presence of carbohydrate in the Golgi region of various types of cells. Finally, Neutra and Leblond showed that when radioactive glucose was administered to animals, radioautographs of tissues containing goblet cells revealed grains over the Golgi regions of the goblet cells, and this occurred in tissues taken from animals and fixed less than 5 minutes after the radioactive glucose was given (Fig. 5-31). These results indicate that when labeled glucose is made available to goblet cells, it almost immediately becomes incorporated into carbohydrate macromolecules in the Golgi region, which, in goblet cells, is located just above the nucleus. When the fate of this macromolecular material was followed by radioautography, it was found that it subsequently enters the bowl portion of the goblet cell and later still is liberated through the free surface of the cell in its mucus secretion.

Further evidence has indicated that most of the carbohydrate component of the glycoprotein secretion is being continually added to the protein material in all the Golgi saccules, the protein, of course, being derived from the rER. However, it was found that the addition of some of the sugar residues in the carbohydrate side-chains of glycoproteins begins in the rER soon after protein chains

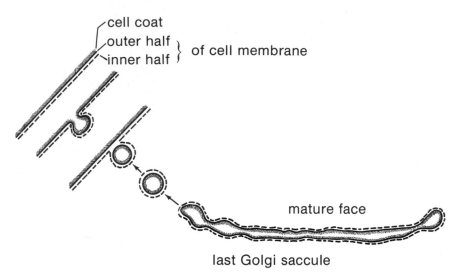

Fig. 5-32. Diagram illustrating how vesicles budding from the Golgi saccules can contribute cell membrane and cell coat to the cell surface by fusing with it. Note that the outer half of the vesicle membrane becomes the inner half of the cell membrane.

synthesized on ribosomes are released into the cisternae of the rER. Usually, N-acetylglucosamine first and then mannose are added in the rER; later in the Golgi apparatus, galactose, fucose, and sialic acid are all added to complete the carbohydrate side-chains of the glycoproteins. This is done by glycosyl transferases and, as might be expected, the Golgi membrane is a particularly rich source of these enzymes. It should be pointed out that, unlike the polypeptide chains of proteins synthesized by single ribosomes in one location, the carbohydrate side-chains of glycoproteins are built up successively at different sites by the various transferases adding sugars one at a time, in a stepwise manner, during the time the protein travels through the cisternae of the rER and from there through the Golgi apparatus.

Since much of the carbohydrate is added to the content of the Golgi saccules as it moves through a stack, those saccules nearer the mature face should contain more carbohydrate than the saccules near the forming face. Rambourg, Hernandez, and Leblond showed that the contents of the first two or three saccules on the forming face of a stack give only a weak reaction for carbohydrate by the periodic acid-silver technic (this technic for electron microscopy corresponds to the PAS technic commonly employed to demonstrate carbohydrate for light microscopy). The reaction of the contents of the saccules increased in intensity as the mature face was approached and the most intense reactions were found in the last (the most mature) saccule of the stack.

How Special Vesicles Could Add Both Membrane and Cell Coat to the Cell Surface. During the growth of tissues by means of cell proliferation there is a need for the synthesis of new cell membrane because, following cell division, the daughter cells quickly enlarge. There is also a need for

more cell coat to cover the surfaces of the increased number of cells. The manner in which this is accomplished has been investigated by Bennett and Leblond by radioautography, using ^{3}H-fucose as a precursor to trace the formation of glycoprotein. The columnar (absorptive) cells lining the intestine were studied, for these enlarge rapidly after dividing and also have a prominent cell coat (Fig. 5-7). Two minutes after a ^{3}H-fucose injection into an animal, radioactivity could be detected in the Golgi apparatus of these cells, where this sugar is taken up during glycoprotein synthesis. Presumably fucose is the last sugar to be picked up by the glycoprotein molecules since it is located at the end of the carbohydrate side chains. Within 20 minutes most of the radioactivity had appeared on all the cell surfaces, indicating that the glycoprotein had migrated from the Golgi apparatus to the cell coat. The carrier involved seems to be a type of secretory vesicle whose membrane would provide additional cell membrane and whose glycoprotein content would provide additional cell coat, as illustrated in Figure 5-32. It is to be noted in studying this illustration that the contents of the vesicle (future cell coat) are surrounded by the side of the Golgi membrane that is the counterpart of the outer side of the cell membrane. So when the vesicle meets the cell membrane, the outer side of the vesicle (the counterpart of the inner half of the cell membrane) fuses with the latter. The fused site then breaks open and allows the inner side of the vesicle membrane to fuse with the outer side of the cell membrane, and when this fused site opens up the contents of the vesicle (cell coat material) are emptied onto the outer side of the cell membrane where it belongs. (The inner side of the membrane of a secretory vesicle is, of course, the counterpart of the outer side of the cell membrane).

The liberation of the contents of a vesicle onto the surface of a cell by this sort of mechanism is often referred to as *exocytosis*. Observations on nongrowing liver cells suggest that there may be a renewal of cell membrane and cell coat even in nongrowing cells by this same mechanism. It is also interesting that the membranes of the saccules on the mature face of the Golgi, the face from which new membrane is added to the cell membrane, resemble the cell membrane in thickness, whereas those of the saccules on the immature face are considerably thinner and hence more like those of the rER. This suggests that another function of the Golgi may be to modify the membrane formed in the rER so that it becomes similar to, and capable of fusion with, the cell membrane. Phospholipids, sterols, and proteins in the membrane of the Golgi saccules are present in amounts intermediate between those of the rER and those of the cell membrane.

Histochemical Studies of the Golgi Region at the EM Level

The identification and characterization of various phosphatases in what has been considered to constitute the Golgi have been very informative. A brief summary of the histochemical method commonly used may help in understanding the structure and function of the Golgi.

Thick slices (50 to 75 μm.) cut on an instrument called a "chopper" are incubated with a substrate of the enzyme under study, as well as with some lead nitrate. (For example, thiamine pyrophosphate is used as a substrate for the detection of thiamine pyrophosphatase; nucleosides, usually uridine diphosphate, may be used for nucleoside diphosphatase, and glycerophosphate serves as a substrate for acid phosphatase). These various enzymes, where present, split off phosphate ions from their respective substrates and the phosphate ions combine with the free lead ions to form a precipitate of lead phosphate. The washed tissue is sectioned for examination in the EM. Since the lead present in the precipitate is a heavy metal, it appears electron-dense in the EM and this permits the intracellular localization of the enzyme concerned.

More details can now be added to the general description of the fine structure of the Golgi stacks, in particular with regard to the location of certain enzymes. First, as shown in Figures 5-33 and 5-34, what have been regarded as the two last saccules at the mature face of a Golgi stack are different from the others in at least some types of cells. In these, the next-to-last saccule is parallel to the rest of the stack, but what would be regarded as the last saccule is irregularly shaped and commonly extends some distance from the stack. The next-to-last saccule, while being oriented parallel to the other saccules, is more highly fenestrated and, by histochemical methods, can be shown to contain two enzymes lacking in the rest of the Golgi apparatus, namely thiamine pyrophosphatase and nucleoside diphosphatase. The last irregular saccule,

where present, was named by Novikoff the *GERL*, for reasons to be explained presently. It is characterized by the presence of an enzyme that can act on many more phosphate-containing substances than the two just named, but only under slightly acidic conditions; this is the enzyme acid phosphatase.

Why these particular enzymes are present in some Golgi saccules and not others is not entirely clear, but this presumably is related to the role these enzymes play in either helping to synthesize or modify the contents of the Golgi saccules before their contents leave the mature face of the Golgi in *secretory vesicles*, or in rounding out the enzyme complement of the saccule contents so that the secretory vesicles arising from it will be able to perform their respective functions.

Before describing how secretory vesicles are formed and released from the Golgi, however, some further comment on terminology is required.

Definition of Secretions and Terminology Used in Connection With Their Production. Although secretion was listed on page 4 as one of the basic physiological properties of all cells, it should now be explained that in those multicellular organisms in which there is a division of labor, with cells being specialized so that their particular structure is adapted to the performance of certain functions, the function of what is now understood as secretion is limited to only certain cells specialized to perform this function. As a result only certain cells of the body are classified as secretory cells.

From its derivation (L. *secretio* from *secernere*, to separate), the term *secrete* means to separate something from something else. There are, of course, many substances that are separated from cells, but these are not necessarily termed secretions. A long established view has been that for anything to be termed a secretion it must serve a useful purpose somewhere in the body; this concept helps to distinguish between cell secretions and cell excretions, because the latter are regarded as waste products of metabolism that must eventually be disposed of within the body or eliminated from it. The waste products of metabolism, moreover, escape the confines of the cell by passing through the plasmalemma from the cytosol to the tissue fluid outside the cell. Secretions, however, as useful products synthesized within a cell for use elsewhere, have their origin in the rER (as described in the preceding text) and from then on are always contained in membranous vesicles of one sort or another. First, membranous vesicles (transfer vesicles) containing secretion bud off from the rER; these then fuse with Golgi saccules and empty their contents into them. Then, after passage through the Golgi, other vesicles bud off from the uppermost Golgi saccule and move to the plasmalemma where their membranous walls fuse with the plasmalemma and their contents are thereby emptied to the exterior of the cell. Thus

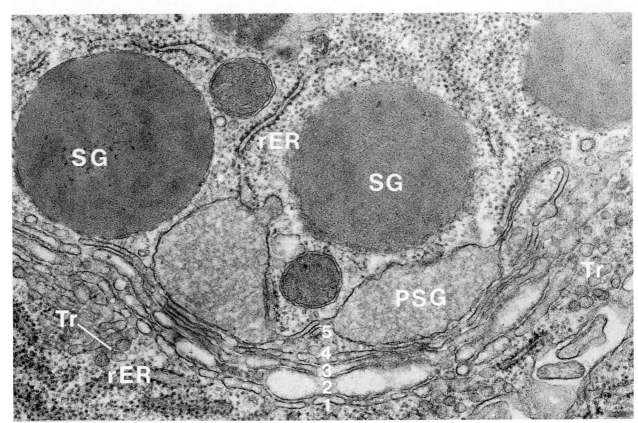

Fig. 5-33. Electronmicrograph (×37,500) of part of a secretory cell of a rat parotid gland, showing a Golgi stack and adjacent organelles. For explanation of the features seen, refer to the caption for Figure 5-34 (*opposite*). (Courtesy of A. R. Hand; from Leblond, C. P., and Bennet, G.: *In* Brinkley, B. R., and Porter, K. R. (eds.): International Cell Biology 1976–1977. p. 326. New York, Rockefeller Press, 1977)

secretions are always segregated from the cytosol, whereas waste products of metabolism are not. The process by which secretions are extruded from cells is sometimes called *exocytosis* probably because the term *phagocytosis* (Gr. *phagein,* to eat, *cyte,* cell, and *osis,* process) refers to the process by which a cell engulfs an extracellular particle with its plasmalemma and then draws the enveloped particle into its cytoplasm. So the term *exocytosis* was coined to denote the process by which a substance enclosed by membrane within the cell is extruded in the reverse fashion from the cell cytoplasm to the exterior of the cell.

What Are Secretion Granules? Secretion was first studied with the LM and EM in sections of fixed tissue. In such preparations the contents of secretory vesicles (because they contain protein) are coagulated by the fixative employed and so would appear in sections as granules. Accordingly, it became common to speak of what we now know to be secretory vesicles as *secretion granules.* In life, of course, they are not granules but little membranous sacs of fluid that can now be isolated from cells

as such by appropriate methods. Nevertheless, the secretory vesicles leaving the Golgi are generally termed *secretory granules* and portions of Golgi saccules that are swollen and about to bud off from them are commonly termed *prosecretory granules.* However, the vesicles that bud off from the rER to fuse with the bottom saccule of a Golgi stack are referred to not as granules but as *vesicles* because when they were discovered it was already appreciated that they were membranous bags of fluid. But this was not the case when the more obvious secretory vesicles were first seen and named secretion granules. These various structures, of course, are *all* secretory vesicles of one kind or another, and we think they all should be referred to as such, but for the time being we must make some concessions to the older terminology.

Finally, in order to understand lysosomes, which we shall soon consider, it should be understood that it is possible for an organelle to synthesize a secretion and bud off vesicles containing it without these vesicles ever leaving the cell. Some of the secretory vesicles budding off from the Golgi, and which are termed *lysosomes,* are destined

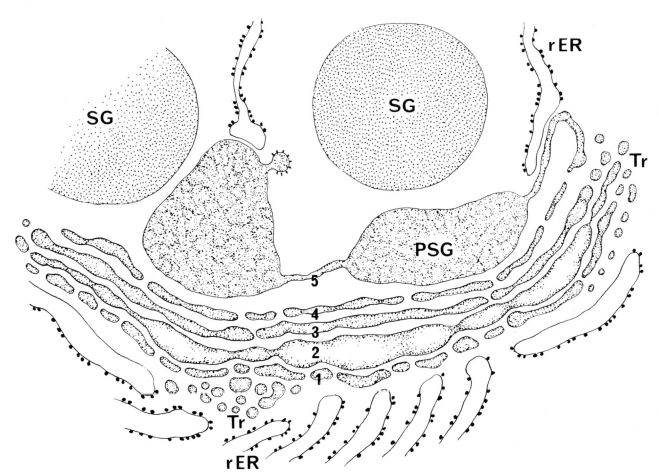

Fig. 5-34. Diagram of the Golgi apparatus in a secretory cell of a parotid gland of a rat (shown in Fig. 5-33). Near the lower margin, the ends of the associated cisternae of rER along the forming face of the stack may be seen; these ends lack ribosomes. Transfer vesicles (Tr) may be seen between the cisternae of rER and the forming face of the Golgi. The first Golgi saccule (1) is heavily fenestrated; the second is distended. The third and fourth are flattened, and the fourth (the next-to-last) is more fenestrated than either the second or the third. The fifth saccule (the last one on top of the stack) is known as the GERL saccule. It extends along the mature face in a less regular manner than the other saccules. Note that it is irregularly distended so as to form prosecretory granules (PSG), which are also called condensing vacuoles. These eventually become released as secretory granules (SG). The regions of the cisternae of rER that come into intimate contact with the GERL saccule are also free of ribosomes. (Courtesy of C. P. Leblond)

to do their work inside the cell. Hence in thinking of secretion it must be realized that not all vesicles budding off from the Golgi are destined to liberate their contained secretions extracellularly. So we now have to realize that secretion can occur at the level of organelles as well as the cellular level, so that all cell secretions are organelle secretions but not all organelle secretions end up as cell secretions.

Next, the first step in the formation of a secretory vesicle from a Golgi saccule is that a portion of the saccule becomes distended with secretion and this, or a part of the distended portion, buds off as a secretory vesicle. However, before it buds off it is commonly referred to,

not as a *prosecretory vesicle*, but as a *prosecretory granule* for reasons just described (Figs. 5-33 and 5-34). In life it is not, of course, a solid structure. When these structures bud off from the Golgi they sometimes become smaller, probably because of absorption of fluid from them into the cytosol. At this stage, or just preceding it, the prosecretory granules are sometimes referred to as *condensing vacuoles*, which is a very confusing term because a vacuole (L. *vacuus,* empty) is a small *space* or *cavity*, whereas a secretory vesicle is a membranous *structure* containing fluid and not just a hole in the cytoplasm. Having explained the awkward terminology, we can now discuss the GERL concept.

The GERL Concept

As noted previously, the last saccule on the mature face of Golgi stacks, in at least a substantial number of kinds of cells, is somewhat different in form from the other saccules of the stack and, moreover, it has a different complement of phosphatases. Elucidation of the differences between this particular saccule and the others has, to a great extent, been due to the many studies of Novikoff, who named it *GERL*. The G in GERL indicates that its location and morphology relate it very closely to the Golgi apparatus. Indeed, it is from the membranous wall of the GERL saccule that prosecretory vesicles (granules) first appear as bulbous distensions.

The ER in GERL indicates that this saccule also has a close relation with the rER, as has been clearly demonstrated by Novikoff and his coworkers. It is evident that ribosome-free regions of cisternae of rER lie very closely apposed to the GERL saccule and some are even insinuated into the fenestrations of the saccule. Because of this close association, the possibility of such or other cisternae of rER actually opening into the GERL saccule has been raised and recent investigations have been directed toward obtaining more information as to whether such connections exist. In any event, Clermont and Rambourg have recently succeeded in demonstrating tubular connections linking the next-to-last saccule at the mature face of the Golgi stack with the GERL saccule of the stack, and so it seems likely that such tubules would be able to carry secretory products to the GERL saccule from the Golgi saccules beneath it.

Finally, the L in GERL stands for *lysosomes*. Since the GERL saccule contains the enzyme acid phosphatase and since lysosomes (vesicles containing hydrolytic enzymes and which are budded off from the Golgi to function in the cytoplasm, as described in the next section) are commonly identified by their content of acid phosphatase (Fig. 5-35), it seems logical to assume that lysosomes, too, are formed from the GERL.

The GERL concept has raised some interesting questions. It seems logical to think that a very close association between ribosome-free rER and the membranous walls of what is considered to be the last saccule of the mature face of a Golgi stack must be of particular significance. If it were proven beyond all doubt that there were at these points direct connections between the rER and the GERL, the possibility would be raised of there being a more direct route for enzymes produced in the rER to reach the site from which they would be delivered in secretory vesicles into the cytosol, where they might either remain within the cell as lysosomes or reach the plasmalemma as secretory vesicles (granules). Since the present evidence indicates that the contents of the saccules of a Golgi stack are delivered into the GERL (where a GERL is present) before they leave the Golgi in secretory vesicles, the further possibility is raised that the GERL might act as a sort of mixing bowl for enzymes from two sources. Furthermore, if the existence of connections between the rER and the GERL is ever firmly established, the possibility

of the GERL as the last saccule of a Golgi stack having a dual origin would also be raised. These and other questions about the Golgi will probably be settled during the life span of this edition of this textbook.

LYSOSOMES

Some General Features

Lysosomes are membranous organelles present in almost all kinds of cells. Their numbers, however, vary greatly from one cell to another, depending on its type and function. They were given their name because they are little bodies (Gr. *soma*, body)—actually they are membranous vesicles containing various enzymes that are hydrolytic (Gr. *lysis*, dissolution) and hence called hydrolases; these act to catalyze reactions in which H_2O is used to break down large molecules into smaller components (for example, proteins into amino acids).

Since the hydrolytic enzymes of lysosomes are capable of lysing the various components of the cytoplasm, it is fortunate that their content of enzymes is separated from the rest of the cytoplasm by their membranous walls.

In healthy cells lysosomes serve an important digestive function; they are concerned with degrading certain substances which may originate either from within or from without the cell. This function, as will be explained later, is the reason why they have a variety of appearances. Moreover, intracellular digestion is accomplished without their enzymes escaping into the cytoplasmic matrix. But when a cell, because of oxygen lack or for some other reason, approaches death or dies, the lysosomes quickly liberate their enzymes into the surrounding cytoplasm and bring about the digestion of the cell and even some of the materials in the environment of the cell. Thus the enzymes of lysosomes are believed to be largely responsible for the profound changes initiated in cells and tissues after death and account for what is termed *autolysis* or the *portmortem degeneration* of tissues.

As more is learned about lysosomes, it will become increasingly evident that they not only carry out essential roles in regard to maintaining the health of normal cells but are also of great importance in the defense of the body against certain bacterial invaders. Furthermore, they are important because they can also contribute to causing certain *inflammatory lesions*.

Development of Knowledge About Lysosomes

In contrast to the organelles already described, the LM provided no direct evidence at all for the existence of lysosomes. That there were such organelles in cytoplasm was first postulated by Christian de Duve in 1955 from biochemical data. Shortly before this time, de Duve and his associates were examining by biochemical methods the enzyme content of various fractions separated from homogenates of rat liver cells by differential centrifugation, described earlier in this chapter (Fig. 5-9). They were interested particularly in investigating the enzymes of the fractions that contained mitochondria. By refinements of the centrifugation procedures, they managed to obtain a fraction which, although similar to mitochondria in sedimentation characteristics, contained enzymes different from those of mitochondria. In this fraction they unexpectely found a number of hydrolytic enzymes, including acid phosphatase. They then performed biochemical experiments which led them to postulate that the hydrolytic enzymes would be contained in vesicles about 0.4 μm. in diameter, and that each of these vesicles would be limited by a membrane that prevented the enzymes reacting with substrates in the cytoplasm. Realizing that the little bodies in this fraction were not mitochondria but, instead, a new type of cytoplasmic organelle, they proposed the name *lysosome* for this organelle.

Identification of Lysosomes With the EM

Subsequently, the fractions containing acid phosphatase were examined in the EM. As was anticipated, lysosomes proved to be membranous organelles about 0.5 μm. in diameter. Since that time, Novikoff and others have studies lysosomes in a great variety of cells by combining the histochemical test for acid phosphatase with electron microscopy. Although lysosomes contain several other hydrolytic enzymes—namely proteases, nucleases, glycosidases, lipases, phospholipases, certain sulfatases and phosphatases—acid phosphatase is the most easily tested for by a histochemical technic (Fig. 5-35) and its demonstration in a more or less spherical membranous organelle is usually taken to indicate that the organelle is a lysosome. The presence of acid phosphatase can be determined by a procedure that indicates the location of the enzyme by the deposition of an electron-dense precipitate (Fig. 5-35). The appearance of lysosomes in routine EM sections not specially stained for acid phosphatase is shown in Figure 5-36.

Formation of Lysosomes

Lysosomes are similar to secretory vesicles (zymogen granules) of acinar cells of the pancreas in that they are membranous vesicles filled with digestive enzymes. It is therefore not surprising that they are formed in the same way. The enzymes of lysosomes, being proteins, are synthesized in the rER and from there are moved via transfer vesicles to the forming face of the Golgi. As already outlined, the enzymes later come to be contained in bulbous distensions of the edge of the saccule on the mature

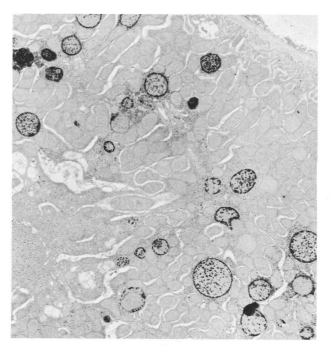

Fig. 5-35. Electron micrograph ($\times 7,600$) of part of a kidney cell (rat), illustrating how lysosomes can be shown to contain acid phosphatase by the Gomori technic. This histochemical procedure leads to the deposition of lead where acid phosphatase was present. Lead salts are very electron-dense, so the sites of their deposition appear black in this type of preparation. (Novikoff, A. B.: Ciba Symposium on Lysosomes. p. 36. Boston, Little, Brown & Co., 1963)

face of the Golgi and then bud off to constitute membranous vesicles (lysosomes) filled with enzymes, as was illustrated in Figures 5-21 and 5-29. Lysosomes are also rich in glycoprotein, most of the carbohydrate component of which is acquired during passage of the protein through the Golgi.

Terminology Used to Designate Lysosomes of Different Appearances and Stages of Function

A lysosome that buds off from the mature face (or GERL saccule) of a stack of Golgi saccules is termed a *primary lysosome* (Fig. 5-37A and center of Fig. 5-38). A primary lysosome may interact with material brought into the cell from outside, or with broken-down organelles or unwanted substances arising within the cell, as described below. When the primary lysosome fuses with another vesicle containing material from either source, the resulting vesicle (which contains both the material to be digested and the lysosomal enzymes) is generally referred to as a *secondary lysosome.*

There is some controversy about the morphological

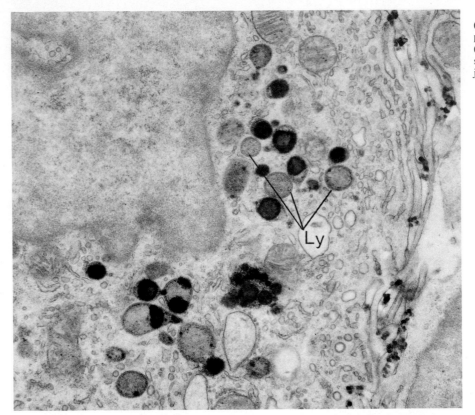

Fig. 5-36. Electron micrograph (×18,000) of a portion of a macrophage (rat), showing lysosomes (Ly) as seen with routine EM staining. (Courtesy of C. Nopajaroonsri and G. Simon)

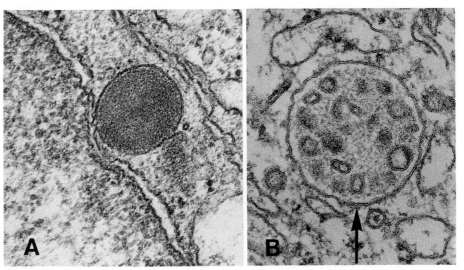

Fig. 5-37. (*A*) Electron micrograph showing a primary lysosome in a thyroid cell (courtesy of C. P. Leblond). (*B*) Electron micrograph (×90,000) showing a multivesicular body (*arrow*) (Friend, D. S., and Farquhar, M. G.: J. Cell Biol., *35*:357, 1967).

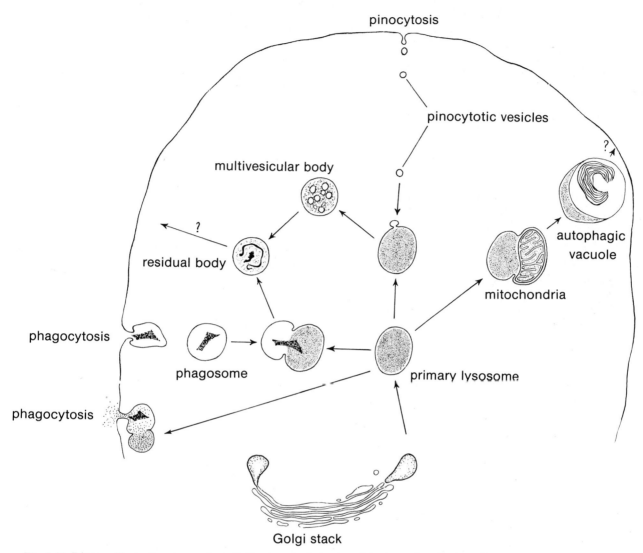

Fig. 5-38. Diagram illustrating phagocytosis (*left*), pinocytosis (*top*), and the formation of primary lysosomes from the Golgi apparatus (*bottom*). Various fates of ingested materials contained in vesicles that meet and fuse with primary lysosomes are depicted. Likewise, the various possible fates of secondary lysosomes are depicted. During phagocytosis, lysosomal enzymes sometimes escape into the environment of the cell if lysosomes fuse with phagocytic vacuoles before they pinch off completely (*lower left*).

features of primary lysosomes, since structurally heterogeneous vesicles may contain enzymes characteristic of lysosomes. A primary lysosome is illustrated in Figure 5-37A.

Particulate or nonparticulate matter of macromolecular dimensions is brought into the cell from outside by a process called *phagocytosis*.

Phagocytosis. As already noted, this term refers to the process by which a cell takes up a particle or macromolecular aggregate from its exterior into its substance. The various steps involved are illustrated in Figure 5-39 and

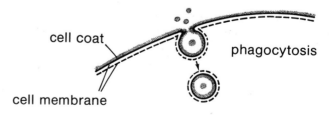

Fig. 5-39. Diagram illustrating phagocytosis. Pinocytosis (uptake of fluid) occurs by a similar process.

on the left of Figure 5-38. When a particle comes into contact with the cell membrane, it is engulfed and surrounded on all sides by cell membrane, so that it comes to be contained in a little membranous bag called a *phagocytic vesicle*. This vesicle, with the particle in it, becomes detached from the cell membrane and sinks deeper into the cytoplasmic matrix, whereupon the vesicle and its contents become known as a *phagosome* (an eaten body) (Fig. 5-38).

In Phagocytosis, the Inner Half of the Cell Membrane Becomes the Outer Half of the Vesicular Membrane. The process of phagocytosis illustrates an important fact about the "sidedness" of any membranous structure that develops from the cell membrane as an invagination. Figure 5-39 shows the outer half of the cell membrane as a solid line and the inner half as a dotted line. It is readily apparent from this diagram that it is the inner half of the cell membrane that becomes the outer half of the vesicular membrane. It should be noted that in the instance of both the cell membrane and the vesicular membrane the aspect of the membrane facing the cytoplasm is the same (the inner half of the cell membrane).

The Fate of Phagosomes; Secondary Lysosomes

When a phagosome, containing for example a bacterium, meets a lysosome the exposed cytoplasmic halves of the membranes of the two vesicles meet, and the complete membranes fuse at their site of contact so that the lysosome discharges its contents through an opening at the site of fusion into the phagosome. Thus the two vesicles become one. The membranous vesicle formed this way is termed a *secondary lysosome*. Additional primary lysosomes may meet with and fuse with this secondary lysosome and several secondary lysosomes also may coalesce. The enzymes contributed by primary lysosomes act to digest the material carried into the cell by phagosomes. Whatever is left over after digestion in the secondary lysosome becomes known as a *residual body* (Fig. 5-38). Residual bodies may finally be extruded from the cell by *exocytosis*.

If the foreign material entering the cell is contained in pinocytotic vesicles (Gr. *pinein*, to drink; *osis*, process: meaning the way in which fluid is engulfed in vesicles, as in phagocytosis), the course of events is not as clear. One hypothesis is that somehow the pinocytotic vesicles get inside the lysosomes. These small, seemingly intact vesicles which appear within the lysosomes are surrounded by the hydrolytic enzymes characteristic of lysosomes. This body thereupon becomes known as a *multivesicular body* (Figs. 5-37B and 5-38) and is, of course, another type of secondary lysosome. Presumably, its contents are eventually digested.

Next, as a result of wear and tear, mitochondria and pieces of rER and other organelles may become functionless and segregated from the rest of the cytoplasm by a membrane. These organelle-containing, membrane-bound portions of cytoplasm, like phagosomes, coalesce with lysosomes and undergo digestion (Fig. 5-38, *right*). The resulting structures may take on an endless variety of appearances because they can contain various kinds of cell organelles, in different degrees of digestion (Fig. 5-40). Usually, parts of membranes can be recognized because they persist longer than the other components of the organelles (*see* Fig. 5-40). These bodies are referred to as *autophagic vacuoles* or *cytolysosomes*. Figure 5-40 shows one with a mitochondrion within it; Figure 5-41 shows one at a later stage, when only relatively resistant whorls of lipid-containing membrane known as *myelin figures* can be demonstrated in it. Later the contents of these autophagic vacuoles may be ejected from the cell by exocytosis. If they persist in cells for long periods of time, they may accumulate, in addition to lipid products, a pigment called *lipofuscin*, particularly in the cells of heart muscle, nervous tissue, and liver (this pigment is described in more detail later in this chapter). Lysosomes and their activities thus provide a type of intracellular demolition system that normally works to do away with cytoplasmic structures as they wear out and begin to disintegrate. Normally, of course, the cytoplasmic structures thus disposed of have their places taken by new ones being formed at the same time.

Lysosomal Storage Diseases

One of the more impressive findings indicating that lysosomes play a significant role in the metabolism of at least several kinds of body cells is the discovery that several diseases result from their not performing their normal function in this respect. As a consequence, certain substances (notably certain lipids and glycogen) normally produced in cells are not properly catabolized (degraded) by lysosomes; hence these substances accumulate in the cytoplasm to the point where the function of the cell is seriously impaired. It has been shown that accumulation of these substances in cells is not due to their overproduction; the fault lies in the lysosomes not possessing some enzyme normally present in them. Furthermore, the absence of a particular enzyme is to be explained as a result of a genetic defect in those who develop such a disease and this defect can be inheritable. Accordingly, genetic counselling has become important with regard to the prevention of certain of these diseases. *Tay-Sach's disease* is one of the most important of this group. It is caused by the lack of one particular enzyme in lysosomes, the enzyme normally concerned with the degradation of a

Fig. 5-40. Electron micrograph (×57,000) of part of the cytoplasm of a hepatocyte of a rat 3 days after partial hepatectomy. In the center are two autophagic vacuoles, each surrounded by a membrane. The autophagic vacuole on the left contains a clearly recognizable but markedly altered mitochondrion and some glycogen. The content of the one on the right is no longer recognizable. Autophagic vacuoles are secondary lysosomes in which obsolete cytoplasmic components are undergoing degradation. (Courtesy of A. Jézéquel)

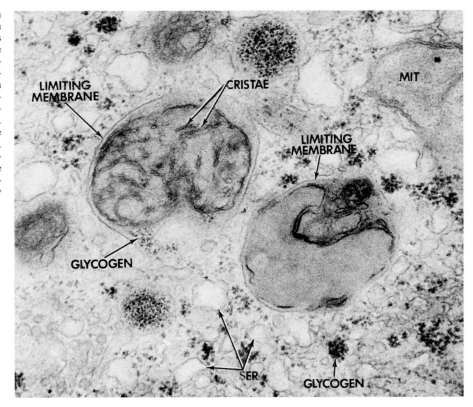

galactoside in cells such as the nerve cells of the brain. Because this enzyme is lacking, secondary lysosomes of nerve cells become filled with concentric dense laminae representing the substance the nerve cells cannot digest. Their cytoplasm becomes so filled with residual bodies stuffed with this undigested material (Fig. 5-42) that their function becomes increasingly impaired.

COATED VESICLES

Discovery and Definition

Certain rounded, free membranous vesicles in the cytoplasm have what appears to be a bristly or fuzzy coating applied to their outer (cytoplasmic) side. Such vesicles have been termed *coated vesicles.*

Sites of Formation

Coated vesicles arise from several different membranous surfaces: the cell membrane, Golgi saccules, condensing vacuoles, or rER.

The Cell Membrane. The cell membrane covering the free surface of the cells that line the vas deferens (Fig.

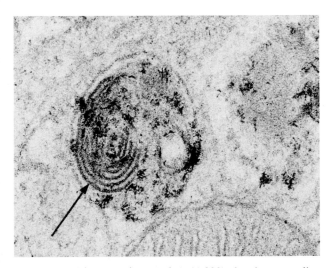

Fig. 5-41. Electron micrograph (×41,000) showing a myelin-like figure (*arrow*) in a secondary lysosome that has been identified by its histochemical reaction for acid phosphatase. (Goldfischer, S., Essner, E., and Novikoff, A.: J. Histochem. Cytochem., *12:*72, 1964)

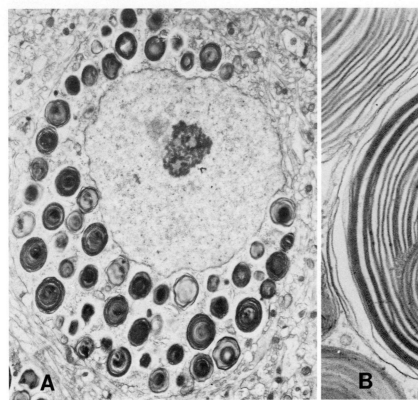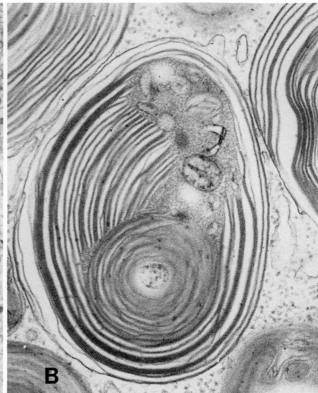

Fig. 5-42. Membranous cytoplasmic inclusion bodies in nerve cells of a patient with Tay-Sach's disease. (*A*) Micrograph (×8,000) of neuron from the cerebral cortex packed with numerous membranous cytoplasmic bodies composed of concentric, electron-dense lamellae. (*B*) Micrograph (×70,000) of a typical membranous cytoplasmic body from a brain cell of this patient. These laminated dense bodies are a distinctive feature of the brain cells of patients with Tay-Sach's disease. (Terry, R. D., and Weiss, M.: J. Neuropath. Exp. Neurol., *22:*18, 1963)

27-18) is thrown into many little folds and declivities, as shown at the upper margin of Figure 5-43. Friend and Farquhar used a protein that could be recognized in electron micrographs to show that protein solution in the deepest parts of the folds became engulfed by the cell membrane by pinocytosis in the same way as particles are engulfed during phagocytosis (Fig. 5-39). By this means a vesicle was formed that enclosed the protein. The vesicle then became detached from the cell membrane and made its way into the cytoplasmic matrix (Fig. 5-43). What is particularly interesting here, however, is that the inner (cytoplasmic) aspect of the cell membrane at these sites has associated with it a material that appears bristly in sections, with the bristles projecting into the cytoplasmic matrix (Fig. 5-43). Since these vesicles form at the cell membrane the bristly material on the inner (cytoplasmic) side of the cell membrane remains on the cytoplasmic side (the outside) of the resulting vesicle, so that the bristles project outward from the vesicle into the cytoplasmic matrix (*see* Fig. 5-43, *arrow*).

The Golgi Apparatus. Coated vesicles of small to moderate size are sometimes seen close to the edges or upper surface of the flattened saccules at the mature face of the Golgi apparatus. These seem to form in much the same manner as noncoated vesicles, by budding.

Secretory Vesicles. As was described in connection with the Golgi apparatus, secretory vesicles bud from the uppermost saccule on the mature face and move into the cytoplasm. Weinstock and Leblond found in ameloblasts that, as the secretory vesicles (condensing vacuoles) become smaller because of their contents becoming condensed, small portions of their membranous wall developed a bristly appearance. They believe that these bristly portions of membrane bud off as small coated vesicles from the secretory vesicles as they become smaller and require less membrane to surround their contents.

Rough-Surfaced Endoplasmic Reticulum. Transfer vesicles, as noted, bud off from the ends of cisternae of rER close to the Golgi apparatus (Fig. 5-26). The outer surface of the transfer vesicles forming in this fashion is free of ribosomes but some transfer vesicles develop a fuzzy coating.

Since fuzz-coated vesicles can arise from the Golgi, and certain transfer vesicles are also fuzz-coated and able to fuse with the lowermost saccule of the Golgi, there is sometimes difficulty in deciding whether a coated vesicle is budding off from, or fusing with, a Golgi saccule. This can often be settled by observing whether any are connected to the saccule by a stalk; if so, it is probably a site where coated vesicles are being formed. Moreover, vesicle formation occurs primarily from saccules at the mature face, whereas fusion with saccules occurs at the forming face.

The Nature of the Coat on the Vesicle

In sections the coat may seem to be bristly on some vesicles and fuzzy on others. Sections cut obliquely through an object, or in a plane close to and parallel with its surface, can often help in determining its three-dimensional structure, as can such technics as negative staining. From studies made using these methods, it appears that the bristly outer surface of a coated vesicle is not due to bristles projecting from its outer surface (like the quills of an emotionally disturbed porcupine), but to a honeycomb or basket-like arrangement of the material on the cytoplasmic surface of the vesicle.

The coat of a coated vesicle should not be confused with the cell coat. The cell coat is found on the outside of the cell membrane (Figs. 5-3 and 5-7), whereas the coat of a vesicle forms on the inner side, that is, the cytoplasmic side of the cell membrane, and remains on the cytoplasmic side in the fully formed coated vesicle (Fig. 5-43). It is the content of a type of secretory vesicle that adds to the cell coat as vesicles from the Golgi apparatus fuse with, and open their contents onto, the surface of a cell (Fig. 5-32). The coat of a coated vesicle, however, is derived from something residing in the cytoplasmic matrix, as is illustrated by the formation of coated vesicles from the cell membrane of the cells lining the walls of the vas deferens (Fig. 5-43).

The Function, Fate, and Significance of Coated Vesicles

There is much evidence to indicate that the coated vesicles forming from the cell membrane (Fig. 5-43) allow many different cell types to take up protein from their environment. This formation of coated vesicles also prevents cell membrane from accumulating at sites of extensive exocytosis. An extreme example of this is to be found at synapses (connections between nerve cells), where countless synaptic vesicles, a type of secretory vesicle, keep fusing with the cell membrane and would undoubtedly keep increasing the size of the region unless

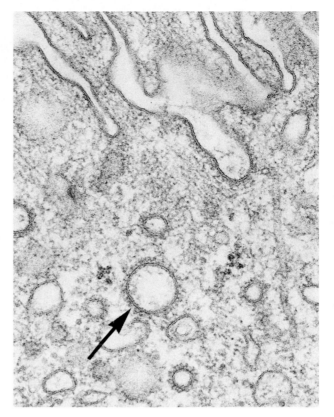

Fig. 5-43. Portion of an epithelial lining cell of the vas deferens, close to its free surface. A large coated vesicle (*arrow*) is seen close to the center. Note its "bristle" coat, and also that the closest large pit above it (*upper right*) shows a similar bristle coat on the cytoplasmic side of the cell membrane. This is therefore a site where coated vesicles are forming. (Friend, D. S., and Farquhar, M. G.: J. Cell Biol., *35:*357, 1967)

accumulation were matched by removal of cell membrane by coated vesicles. Why coated vesicles should also be formed from membranous organelles of the cytoplasm is not clear, unless it is again to reduce the amount of membrane in them or to permit recycling of membrane.

THE SMOOTH-SURFACED ENDOPLASMIC RETICULUM (sER)

The amount of sER in cells varies in relation to their type and only in certain cell types is it prominent. It differs from the rER structurally in two ways: first, the outer surfaces of its membranes are not studded with ribosomes. Second, instead of consisting mostly of fairly large vesicles, flattened or otherwise, the sER consists almost entirely of tubules arranged in an anastomosing network and pursuing tortuous courses in the cytoplasm (Figs.

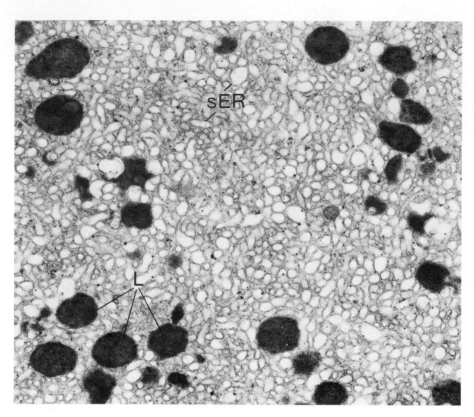

Fig. 5-44. Electron micrograph (×15,400) of part of a steroid-producing cell from the zona reticularis of human adrenal cortex. Note the interconnected tubules of smooth endoplasmic reticulum (sER), which pursue a tortuous course through the cytoplasm. The electron-dense, membrane-bound bodies (L) are lipofuscin granules. Lead citrate stain. (Courtesy of M. J. Phillips)

5-44 and 5-45). The tubules of the sER are often continuous with vesicles and cisternae of the rER.

Functions

The sER carries out a wide variety of functions, which suggests that there are many different types of sER, each specialized for a particular function. Since it possesses no ribosomes, the sER is not concerned with the synthesis of protein; instead it has a role in the metabolism and/or segregation of other kinds of chemical entities, as follows.

The Synthesis of Lipids. The sER is concerned with the synthesis of lipids and compounds of the cholesterol family. Accordingly, sER is abundant in cells that synthesize and secrete lipids, lipoproteins, and steroid hormones (Fig. 5-44). As explained in Chapter 25, the steroid hormones are related chemically to cholesterol.

Liver cells probably produce most, if not all, the lipoprotein found in blood. The sER of liver cells is believed to be concerned in the formation of its lipid component.

Another example of the sER having function in relation to fat metabolism is provided by the cells absorbing fat from the intestine. As mentioned at the beginning of this chapter, fat is digested in the intestine, which results in its being broken down to simpler components that can be ab-

sorbed by the absorptive cells lining the small intestine. Within the cytoplasm of these cells, however, the simpler components are synthesized back into fats again and this occurs in the sER. The tiny droplets of fat thus formed are later secreted by the cells into the tissue fluid, where they are known as *chylomicrons*. From the tissue fluid they make their way into lymphatics and via this route eventually reach the bloodstream.

Drug Detoxification. That the liver is concerned with the detoxification of certain drugs has been accepted for a long time, and studies with the EM indicate that the sER plays a significant role in the process involved. For example, barbiturates such as phenobarbital, on being given to experimental animals, have been shown to greatly increase the amount of sER. A larger and more extensive sER can detoxify this drug faster. It is believed that the sER functions in detoxifying many other drugs in similar fashion. The resistance or sensitivity of a person to a given dose of a drug depends in part on the time it takes for the drug to be broken down and made inactive. This in turn depends on the amount of sER present in the liver cells of the individual when the drug is given.

Glycogen Formation. Glycogen, when present, lies as deposits in the cytoplasmic matrix; commonly these are found in close association with the sER (Fig. 5-45). Al-

Fig. 5-45. Electron micrograph (×27,000) of a region of the cytoplasm of a liver cell, illustrating the close association of glycogen (g) with the smooth-surfaced endoplasmic reticulum (sER), but not with the rough-surfaced endoplasmic reticulum (rER). (Cardell, R.: Internat. Rev. Cytol., 48:221, 1977)

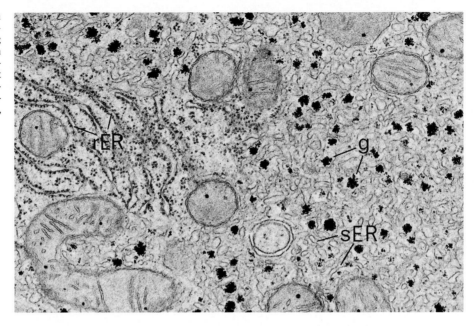

though the cytoplasm of liver cells contains patches of both rER and sER (Fig. 5-45), glycogen is found associated only with the latter. As can be seen in Figure 5-45, the tubules of the sER extend throughout the regions where glycogen is present. There is evidence that enzymes required for the synthesis of glycogen in the liver are present in the membrane of the sER.

Calcium Storage. As described in detail in Chapter 18, contraction in striated and cardiac muscle cells is regulated by the concentration of calcium ions available to the contractile elements. The sER in these muscle cells surrounds the contractile elements and releases the calcium ions to bring about contraction, and then it sequesters them again to bring about relaxation. Enzymes that pump calcium into the sER are present in its membrane and other proteins within the sER have a high capacity for binding calcium. In other cells, however, most of the calcium is stored in the mitochondria.

Other Functions. In certain cells of the stomach, which will be considered later, the sER seems to be involved in the mechanism by which chloride ions are concentrated in connection with the production of free hydrochloric acid.

Formation

Since the sER is continuous with the rER in certain sites, and since there are no arrangements for protein synthesis along the smooth kind, it would seem reasonable to assume that rER membrane is formed first and then transforms, by losing its ribosomes, into endoplasmic reticulum of the smooth type. The fact that in many places the membrane of the sER remains continuous with that of the rER also supports this concept.

MICROTUBULES, CILIA, FLAGELLA, AND CENTRIOLES

Development of Knowledge

Cilia, flagella, and centrioles were all given their respective names when they were discovered long ago with the LM. However, it was not until it became possible to study these structures with the EM that it was found that they were all organized from what appeared to be tiny tubules, which were thereupon named *microtubules.* For a few years it was not known that microtubules are also present as individual entities, dispersed throughout the cytoplasm, because these were more difficult to fix than those organized into cilia, flagella, and centrioles. These dispersed microtubules are referred to as *cytoplasmic microtubules.*

CYTOPLASMIC MICROTUBULES

Morphology

Microtubules, which are present in all kinds of cells except bacteria and certain algae, are slender filamentous structures about 24 nm. in diameter and of variable length (Fig. 5-46). They tend to be straight, probably have a certain amount of rigidity, and are sufficiently elastic to bend

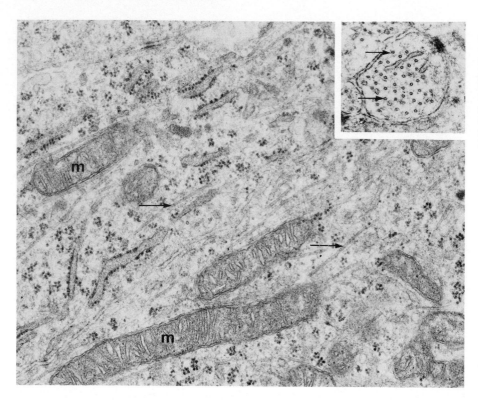

Fig. 5-46. Electron micrograph of part of an ependymal cell (rat) showing numerous microtubules (*arrows*) in longitudinal section. Mitochrondria (m), rER, and polysomes are also evident in the cytoplasm. (*Inset*) Nerve cell process (×40,000) showing numerous microtubules in cross section (*arrows*). (Courtesy of V. Kalnins)

without breaking. When they are seen in cross section they appear as tiny circles because their walls are denser than their central parts (*see* Fig. 5-46, *inset*). Furthermore, with special staining procedures, each microtubule is seen to consist of 13 rod-shaped components termed *protofilaments* arranged parallel to the long axis of the microtubule. This subunit structure of microtubules may be seen very clearly in the section of a centriole (a structure composed of microtubules) in Figure 2-12 (p. 48).

The distribution of cytoplasmic microtubules can be readily investigated by making an antibody to the protein *tubulin* from which microtubules are assembled and using this antibody, after labeling it with a fluorescent dye, to localize the microtubules. (A full description of what antibodies are and how they are made and labeled is given on p. 246). Using this technic, the distribution of microtubules in whole cells, particularly flat ones grown in cultures, can be demonstrated (Fig. 5-47).

Functions

Cytoplasmic microtubules act to some extent as a skeleton for the cell. Cells may be of many different shapes, some even star-shaped, and the maintenance of characteristic shape in different kinds of cells is due substantially to the way the cytoplasmic microtubules are distributed within them. As an aid to their serving a skeletal function, most of these microtubules are anchored in a

region near the centrioles (Fig. 5-47, C). Cytoplasmic microtubules, however, are not the only organelle to serve a supportive role within the cell, for the *terminal web* (described later) also functions to some extent in this respect.

A second function of microtubules may be to facilitate transport of various particles and perhaps even large macromolecules throughout the cytoplasm. In many cells the pathways along which such components move seem to be related to the manner in which the microtubules are disposed. It is therefore thought that microtubules form some sort of arrangement whereby the movement of particles is restricted to specific courses, much as the movement of trains is restricted to tracks.

One type of cell that has extensive cytoplasmic processes extending from its main body of cytoplasm is the nerve cell; here a fine process (a nerve fiber) may be several feet in length. As shown in the *inset* of Figure 5-46, which is a cross section of a nerve fiber, these processes too have microtubules within them to provide support and perhaps provide direction to the flow of material synthesized close to the nucleus and constantly moving toward the extremity of the process, as described in Chapter 17 (p. 496).

Microtubules are also concerned with the development of cell shape. When a cell elongates, the microtubules become longer because of the addition of new microtubule subunits to one of their ends; this also occurs dur-

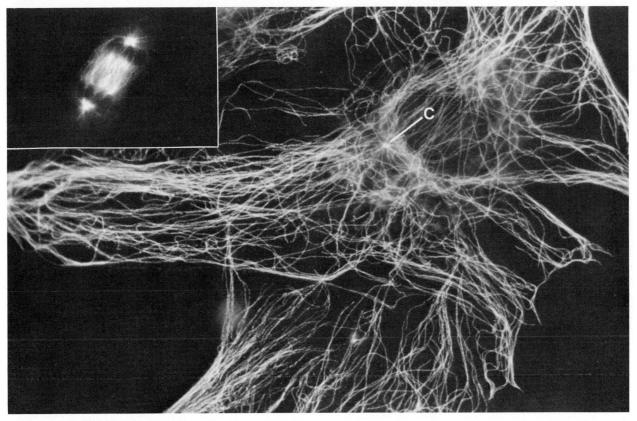

Fig. 5-47. Immunofluorescence photomicrograph (×3,000) of mouse embryo fibroblasts in tissue culture. Antibody to microtubule protein (tubulin) was employed to demonstrate the distributions of (*1*) cytoplasmic microtubules during interphase (*large photomicrograph*) and (*2*) spindle microtubules during anaphase (*inset*). The nucleus of the interphase cell lies toward the top right corner of the large photomicrograph; the centrioles (labeled C) appear as a brightly fluorescent spot to the lower left of the nucleus. Both mitotic spindle and centrioles are evident in the anaphase cell (*inset*); the two sets of daughter chromosomes appear dark against the fluorescing microtubules of the spindle. Note that during mitosis the cytoplasmic microtubules seen during the interphase are absent. (From the work of J. A. Connolly)

ing spindle formation in mitosis, when microtubules grow in length and push the two pairs of centrioles apart to increase the length of the spindle. Forces generated between adjacent microtubules can also cause them to slide past each other, as occurs when they bend in ciliary movement.

The Formation of Microtubules

As described in connection with the formation of the spindle in mitosis, microtubules are assembled from a specific protein called *tubulin* that is present in relatively high concentrations in a soluble form in the cytoplasm of all cells. This protein has a molecular weight of around 55,000. In order for molecules of tubulin to form microtubules, they first unite in pairs called *dimers;* these dimers, in turn, become assembled into the walls of the microtubules. In the cytoplasm, tubulin in the form of

dimers is present in solution in equilibrium with the microtubules, as follows:

$$\text{tubulin dimers} \rightleftharpoons \text{microtubules}$$

Hence microtubules, except those of cilia, centrioles and basal bodies (which are fairly stable), are always breaking down into tubulin, and tubulin is always being assembled back again into microtubules. This is of great interest in connection with the action of two drugs, *colchicine* and *vinblastine*, that affect mitosis and other processes which depend on the presence of microtubules; indeed, vinblastine is so effective that it is used in the treatment of certain malignancies to arrest the division of cells.

It has been found that one of these drugs, colchicine, acts by binding fairly specifically to the tubulin dimers in solution in the cell and which, of course, form the pool of tubulin from which new microtubules would ordinarily be

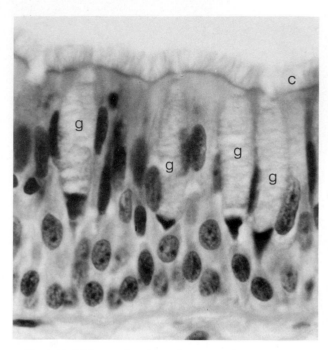

Fig. 5-48. Oil-immersion photomicrograph of the epithelial lining of the human trachea, pseudostratified ciliated columnar epithelium with goblet cells (g). Note the numerous cilia (c) on this type of epithelium. (Courtesy of B. Smith)

These centers are particularly common near the centrioles. When cytoplasmic microtubules are made to disappear by colchicine, and the colchicine is then washed out, the reassembly of these microtubules can be followed. From such experiments it was found that their assembly begins in the centriolar region and continues by the addition of more tubulin to one of their ends. The cytoplasmic microtubules disappear when a cell goes into mitosis and instead microtubules of the spindle become assembled (Fig. 5-47). When mitosis is over, the cytoplasmic microtubules reappear by growing out from the centriolar region. Thus assembly and depolymerization must be under very strict control to ensure that the right arrangements pertain at the right time and in the right places. The availability of other proteins (microtubule-associated proteins) associated with tubulin in the wall of the microtubules may regulate microtubule assembly and determine how much tubulin becomes assembled into microtubules at any one time.

CILIA AND FLAGELLA

Cilia is the plural form of the Latin for eyelid, which is *cilium.* Since eyelashes extend from the free border of the eyelid, it is not surprising that, when microscopes became available and it was noticed that certain unicellular organisms and cells in the body had hair-like processes extending from their free surfaces, these processes would be termed *cilia.*

General Distribution and Function of Ciliated Cells

Ciliated cells are one of the kinds of cells present in cellular membranes lining wet surfaces in the body. In the upper part of the respiratory tract the lining membrane contains goblet cells that secrete mucus (a slippery fluid) and ciliated cells (Fig. 5-48) that move the mucus along the surface. This arrangement permits the free surface of the upper respiratory tract, for example, to be always covered with a film of mucus, in which the cilia of the ciliated cells are immersed. The cilia beat rhythmically in such a way as to move the film of mucus in one direction, with the result that particles inhaled in the air are caught in the mucus and moved along the tubes or cavities so that they can be disposed of without damaging the delicate structure of the lungs.

Structure of Ciliated Cells As Seen With the LM

Ciliated cells are commonly longer than they are wide (Fig. 5-48) and their sides are apposed to the sides of the cells that surround them. Cilia are found only on the free surface of each, the surface that abuts on a lumen or cav-

assembled. However, if small amounts of this drug become bound to soluble tubulin, the latter can no longer aggregate into microtubules. Since microtubules are constantly breaking down into tubulin, and since, in the presence of this drug, tubulin becomes incapable of being assembled into microtubules (which is why this drug inhibits spindle formation), the action of the drug in interphase cells quickly leads to the disappearance of the microtubules from the cytoplasm; only the microtubules organized into the more permanent structures such as centrioles and cilia persist. However, the process is reversible, for, if the drug is washed away from cells or metabolized, the assembling of new microtubules from the pool of soluble tubulin in the cells begins anew. Vinblastine, which causes the tubulin to aggregate into crystal-like structures in the cytoplasm and hence makes it unavailable for polymerization, also has the same effect, that is, it prevents the microtubule subunits from polymerizing into microtubules.

Initiation Sites

It is thought that the formation of microtubules is initiated at special sites distributed throughout the cytoplasm, called *microtubule organizing centers (MTOC).*

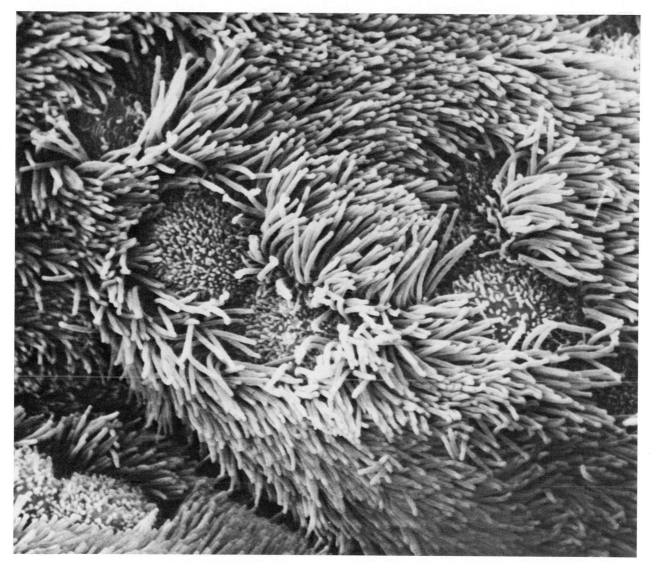

Fig. 5-49. Scanning electron micrograph (×7,000) of ciliated cells of the oviduct (mouse), showing the three-dimensional appearance of ciliated cells. A few nonciliated cells can also be seen; these have microvilli on their surface. (Courtesy of Dirksen, E. R.: *In* Hafez, E. S. E. (ed.): Scanning Electron Microscopic Atlas of Mammalian Reproduction. Tokyo, Igaku Shoin, 1975)

ity (Fig. 5-48). There may be several hundred cilia on a single cell, as becomes strikingly evident when ciliated cells are observed in the scanning EM (Fig. 5-49). Commonly cilia are from 5 to 15 μm. long and around 0.2 μm. in diameter. Accordingly, individual cilia can be discerned but their internal structure cannot be resolved with the LM (Fig. 5-48). However, the LM, used in conjunction with special staining, revealed that there was a little body in the cytoplasm beneath each cilium, to which it appeared to be connected, and this was called its *basal body*. It is these bodies arranged in a row which give the

dense appearance to the cytoplasm just below the cell surface (Fig. 5-48).

The Development and Fine Structure of Cilia

The EM revealed that the cilia develop from centrioles and indeed that the basal body of a cilium is a centriole.

It will be recalled that centrioles (described in Chap. 2 on p. 48 in connection with mitosis) are short cylindrical structures (Figs. 2-12 and 2-13). The wall of each is composed of nine longitudinally disposed and parallel

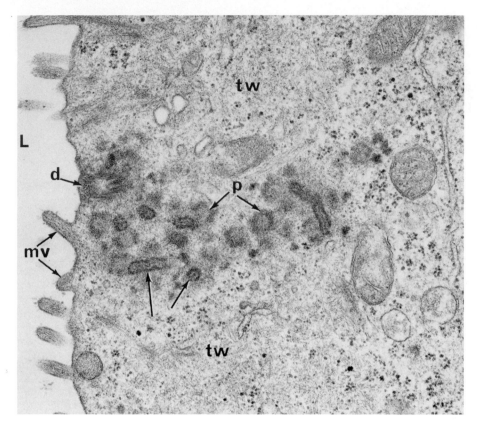

Fig. 5-50. Electron micrograph (×40,000) of the luminal surface of a cell from chick trachea, showing assembly of centrioles in preparation for ciliation; mv, microvilli; tw, terminal web; L, lumen of trachea. Clusters of immature centrioles called procentrioles (p) may be seen in the apical portion of the cell. The procentrioles assemble around cylindrical structures called centriolar organizers (*arrows*), near the two original centrioles (d). Microtubules have not yet formed in the procentrioles. (Courtesy of J. Marshall and V. Kalnins)

bundles of microtubules, each bundle containing three microtubules (Fig. 2-12). A bundle of three closely grouped microtubules is termed a *triplet*. The nine triplets of a centriole are held in position by fibrillar material so that together they form the wall of a cylinder. As noted previously, centrioles are commonly present in interphase cells in pairs, which are located either close to the nucleus and the Golgi apparatus or near the cell surface.

The Basal Body

To develop a ciliated surface, a cell must first assemble enough centrioles to have one for each of the several hundred cilia that will form. A cell in which such an assembly of multiple centrioles is taking place is shown in Fig. 5-50. After the baby centrioles develop to full size, they migrate toward the free surface of the cell and become aligned just below it. Next, microtubules of the ciliary shaft (which is often called an *axoneme*) grow out from the distal end of each centriole (which is now called a *basal body*) and become the core of a cilium that will project, enclosed by the cell membrane, from the free sur-

face of a ciliated cell (Fig. 5-51). At about this time, structures that anchor the basal body, and hence the cilium, develop under the basal body. These structures are called *rootlets* because of their position in relation to the cilium, and they present a variety of appearances in different species, one of which may be seen in Figure 5-51. In addition, a striated structure called a *basal foot* is attached laterally to the basal body (Fig. 5-51). Cytoplasmic microtubules are often attached to the free end of the basal foot.

The Growth of the Shaft

The ciliary shaft (axoneme) grows toward the surface as a result of the two innermost tubules of each triplet of the basal body increasing in length as new tubulin is added to their distal ends. A pair of microtubules such as this is called a *doublet*. Since the third microtubule of each triplet of the basal body does not increase in length, there is a difference in the cross section appearance of the basal body and the axoneme of the cilium, for a cross section of the former shows a ring of nine triplets (Fig. 5-52) whereas a cross section of the shaft reveals a ring of nine doublets (Fig. 5-53). There is another difference also: two

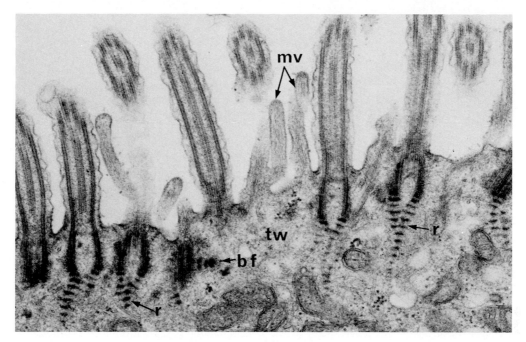

Fig. 5-51. Electron micrograph on the luminal surface of a ciliated cell of duck trachea, showing cilia in longitudinal and oblique sections. The basal bodies of the cilia lie embedded in the apical cytoplasm of the cell. Rootlets (r) are attached to their basal ends, and a basal foot (bf) projects from their sides. Microtubules may be seen inside the ciliary shafts (axonemes). Microvilli (mv) with cores composed of microfilaments (to be described later) are present between the cilia. (Courtesy of J. Marshall and V. Kalnins)

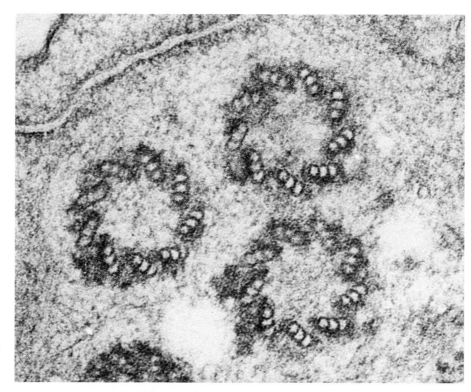

Fig. 5-52. Electron micrograph (×74,000) of part of a ciliated cell of rat trachea, sectioned just below and parallel to its surface, showing three basal bodies cut in cross section. The nine triplets of microtubules in their walls are clearly visible. Note that their appearance is identical with that of centrioles (Fig. 2-12). (Courtesy of V. Kalnins)

153

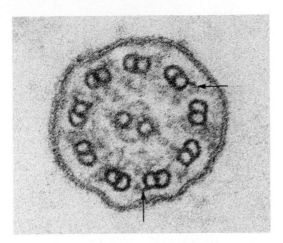

Fig. 5-53. Electron micrograph (×220,000) of a cilium from a ciliated cell of rat trachea, cut in cross section, showing the nine peripheral doublets and the two central singlet microtubules of the axoneme. On the doublets short arms (*arrows*) with ATPase activity can be seen. The unit membrane structure of the cell membrane surrounding the cilium is also evident. (Courtesy of V. Kalnins)

single microtubules develop in the central region of the shaft. These are termed *singlets* and they also grow toward the surface. They can be seen in a cross section of the shaft (Fig. 5-53) but not in a cross section of the basal body (Fig. 5-52). The doublets and singlets are held together so as to form a bundle by fibrous connections between them.

The Movement of Cilia

Rows of cilia commonly beat in sequence so that they propel a sheet of mucus in one direction across the cell surface. Measurements made in the nose show that a particle caught in the mucus may be moved by as much as 6 mm. or more per minute. A cilium, while fairly rigid, beats in one direction; then it relaxes and is pulled back in the other direction to its starting position to complete a cycle in about $\frac{1}{25}$ of a second. It then becomes rigid and beats forward again. The downbeat is called the *effective stroke* (the stroke that propels the mucus), whereas the return stroke is called the *recovery stroke*. The question arises, however, how this back-and-forth motion of cilia moves mucus in only one direction. This is because on its effective stroke the cilium remains stiff and pushes mucus ahead of it. But on its return stroke it relaxes and bends and so it is, as it were, crouched down so that it slides easily back into position without disturbing the overlying mucus, whereupon it straightens and stiffens for its next forward stroke. The effective stroke is in a direction per-

pendicular to an imaginary line joining the two singlet microtubules.

The mechanism of ciliary action is now becoming clear. There are short arms (marked with arrows in Fig. 5-53) on each of the doublets and it is possible to remove and study these by biochemical methods. Such methods have revealed that they contain the enzyme ATPase and are therefore involved in releasing energy from ATP, so that work can be done in their immediate neighborhood. Since microtubules themselves are not contractile, the work resulting in ciliary movement involves the doublets of microtubules in the cilium (Fig. 5-53) sliding in relation to one another. In living cells the ATPase-containing arms of one doublet touch the adjacent doublet and provide the force for this sliding mechanism between adjacent doublets. When this covering cell membrane is removed from isolated cilia, the doublets can be induced to slide past each other by adding ATP. In the intact cilium, however, this sliding is restrained by interconnections between the doublets and hence attempts of adjacent doublets to slide past each other result in the bending of the whole cilium.

Cells that Develop a Single Cilium

In contrast to cells that develop hundreds of cilia, there are many kinds in the body that develop only one cilium; it is usually rudimentary or incomplete and probably nonmotile. For its formation, the pair of centrioles of a cell migrate to the cell surface, where only one of them gives rise to a ciliary shaft and hence becomes a basal body (Fig. 5-54). The purpose of this single cilium is not clear. However, in certain instances the single cilium may undergo extensive modification, as occurs in the receptor cells of the organs of special sense. These modified cilia become very important parts of the arrangement by which nerve impulses are initiated as a result of exposure to certain forms of energy. For example, the rods and cones of the eye, which represent modified cilia, are receptive to light energy, as described in Chapter 28.

Flagella

Another example of a single cilium becoming highly developed is manifested in what are termed *flagella*. Like cilia, flagella are found on many kinds of unicellular organisms where they too serve as a means of propulsion for the organism. Cilia and flagella are much alike; they differ chiefly in that the flagella (L. *flagellum*, whip) are somewhat longer than cilia. Also, whereas a cell may have very large numbers of cilia, it commonly has only one or two flagella. In mammals the only cells with flagella are spermatozoa, each having only one flagellum.

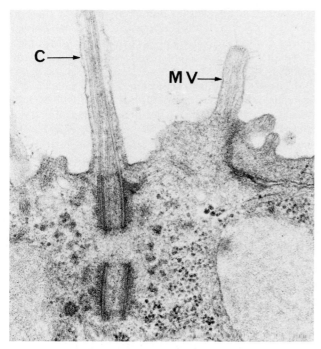

Fig. 5-54. Electron micrograph (×40,000) showing the apical part of a mucus-secreting cell from rat trachea with a single cilium (C) extending from one of the two centrioles (which are cut in longitudinal section). Microvilli (MV) also project into the lumen of the trachea. The pale-staining area at *lower right* is a mucus granule. (Courtesy of J. Marshall and V. Kalnins)

tures different from microtubules. Though often associated with one another, filaments and microtubules differ in their functions. An analogy sometimes employed to indicate their functional relation to each other is that microtubules act as the "bones" of the cell, whereas certain types of filaments are like "muscles," since they provide for movement. The two however are not directly attached to each other, so the analogy should not be taken too literally.

There are three main categories of filaments. Those of the first category are termed *microfilaments*. These are 5 to 6 nm. in diameter and composed of a protein called *actin*. Actin filaments were first demonstrated in muscle cells, but more recently they have been shown to be present in a wide variety of cells. Two other proteins, *tropomyosin* and *troponin,* have been found in small amounts in association with actin filaments (Fig. 5-55). They are probably essential for the function of microfilaments, which is to participate with the second kind of filament in contractile mechanisms in cells.

The second kind of filament is referred to as the *myosin filament* because myosin is the protein of which they are composed. Myosin filaments are found in close association with actin filaments in muscle, where they are thicker than the actin filaments, being 10 nm. in diameter. However, in other kinds of cells they vary a good deal in width. Myosin and actin filaments are involved in the contractile movements of cells.

FILAMENTS

Definitions and General Features

The words *fiber*, *fibril* and *filament*, from their derivation, all mean elongated, thread-like structures. In practice these terms are used in microscopy to refer, in the order given above, to thread-like structures of decreasing diameters. The words, however, do not have precise meanings with regard to size; for example, a thread-like structure readily seen with the naked eye or with the low power of the LM is generally termed a *fiber*. Those resolved only by the high power of the LM are in general termed *fibrils*. The larger of those resolved only with the EM are usually also termed *fibrils*, while those of the smallest diameters are termed *filaments*. Filaments of more than one kind exist in cells, but not in equal numbers in all kinds of cells. In some, filaments are arranged in networks or bundles large enough to be seen with the higher powers of the LM in suitably stained preparations.

To avoid possible confusion, it should be emphasized that filaments constitute a category of threadlike struc-

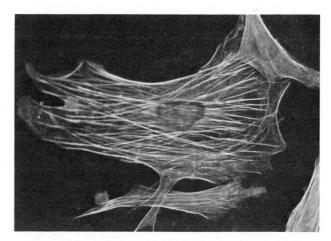

Fig. 5-55. Immunofluorescence photomicrograph (×3,000) of a mouse embryo fibroblast in tissue culture. Antibody to tropomyosin was employed to demonstrate the distribution of bundles of tropomyosin-containing actin microfilaments in the cytoplasm. These bundles lie just below the cell membrane and are more common on the underside of the cell, where it is attached to the substrate. (From the work of L. Subrahmanyan and A. Jorgensen)

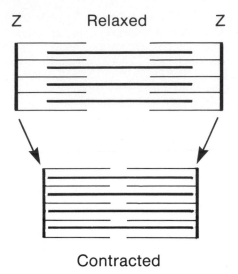

Fig. 5-56. Diagram of a sarcomere of striated muscle, showing the change in arrangement of the thick and thin filaments during contraction. For details, *see* text.

Filaments of the third category are called *intermediate filaments*. They range from 7 to 10 nm. in diameter. As we shall see when we describe the cells of the different tissues, intermediate filaments are found in many different kinds of cells. Often they are bundled together to form what have been termed *fibrils* that can be seen with the EM. They are not directly involved in contractile mechanisms. In many instances they seem to "come and go" because of being formed and disassembled. They can contribute to the form of a cell by constituting networks through various parts of the cytosol, thereby supporting the organelles and maintaining cell shapes, and in smooth muscle cells they probably also transmit pull to the cell membrane.

Microfilaments and Myosin Filaments and Their Relation to Contraction

Development of Knowledge. It has long been known that muscle cells are long and narrow and that on stimulation they shorten and thus perform work. For the first half of this century it was generally believed that contraction depended on longitudinally oriented components that would shorten when the cell was stimulated and hence pull the two ends of a muscle cell closer together. However, early in the second half of the century studies of striated muscle cells with the EM revealed that whereas they did contain longitudinally oriented filaments, contraction was not the result of shortening of these filaments. Instead, it was found to depend on there being two kinds of filaments, one (the *microfilaments)* composed

primarily of actin and the other of myosin. Both kinds are arranged so as to interdigitate and interact with one another. The fine structure and mechanism of contraction of striated muscle is of course, dealt with in much more detail in Chapter 18.

In the cytoplasm of striated muscle cells there are longitudinal fibrils called *myofibrils* housing both kinds of filaments. Each myofibril is a longitudinal series of tiny segments—contractile units called *sarcomeres* (Gr. *sarcos*, flesh; *meros*, part)—the ends of which are marked by structures called *Z lines* that extend across the myofibril. As can be seen in the upper part of Figure 5-56, half the thin, actin-containing filaments in each sarcomere are attached to each Z line and extend toward the middle of the sarcomere without reaching it, so that a gap is evident between their free ends in the middle third of the sarcomere during relaxation. The thicker myosin filaments, however, occupy the middle two-thirds of the sarcomere. Both their ends are free and these extend (both ways) between the free ends of the actin filaments for a short distance, as may be seen in Figure 5-56, *top*. During contraction (Fig. 5-56, *bottom*), the actin-containing filaments slide farther in between the myosin filaments until their free ends almost meet in the middle of the sarcomere. This sliding pulls the two Z lines at the limits of each sarcomere closer together, thereby shortening the myofibrils and hence the muscle fiber.

Stimulation of the muscle fiber liberates calcium ions from the sER into the myofibril and it is these calcium ions that cause the actin filaments to become interactive with the myosin filaments and utilize energy from ATP to bring about contraction.

Contractile Phemenomena in Other Types of Cells

When it was shown that the contractile mechanism in muscle, where it is studied to best advantage, depended on filaments sliding past each other, the question was raised whether contractile phemenona in other kinds of cells similarly depended on filaments sliding along one another. In cells other than those specialized to contract this constituted a problem that was much more difficult to study. Since it was obvious from studies on muscle that contraction depended on the interaction of actin filaments with myosin filaments, it was of interest that filaments with a diameter of 6 nm. were found in many other kinds of cells. Furthermore, it was shown experimentally that these filaments would bind parts of myosin molecules, indicating they contained actin. Myosin filaments, and also other proteins concerned in regulating contraction in muscle cells (for example, tropomyosin and troponin), have also been demonstrated in a variety of nonmuscle cells (Fig. 5-55). The myosin filaments, however, are harder to fix and therefore to demonstrate than the actin-containing filaments. These two types of filaments appear to be closely associated in many kinds of cells and are believed to interact in a manner similar to that occurring during the contraction of muscle cells.

Actin is found in relatively high concentrations in many kinds of nonmuscle cells, but it is not clear at present how much of this protein is in the form of microfilaments and how much exists in its soluble form. It is believed that regions of the cytoplasm with a high content of microfilaments are more rigid that parts with only a few microfilaments, and attempts are now being made to explain such activities as ameboid movement on the basis of local polymerization of actin into microfilaments, accompanied by depolymerization of these filaments in other parts of the cytoplasm. The outermost zone of the cytoplasm just below the cell membrane (the so-called *ectoplasm* or *cortex* described by early microscopists) is relatively rigid and gel-like and has been shown to be particularly rich in these microfilaments. Moreover, it is thought that some integral proteins of the cell membrane may be attached, either directly or indirectly, to actin filaments just beneath the cell membrane (Fig. 5-5), since when integral membrane proteins are induced to aggregate by experimental means, the actin and myosin present in this region aggregate below the aggregating membrane protein. Contractile activities involving actin-like filaments are now considered to be responsible for changes in shape and certain types of movement, including ameboid movement, observed in many kinds of living cells in the body and in cell cultures.

Role of Microfilaments in Cell Division

In describing the telophase of mitosis in Chapter 2, it was noted that the separation of a dividing cell into two daughter cells depends on a *contraction furrow* developing in the midsection of the mother cell and deepening until the cell becomes pinched in two. At this stage a bundle of microfilaments, called a *contractile ring*, appears; it encircles the cell like a ring at the bottom of the furrow, just below the cell membrane (Fig. 2-11E). This suggested that the microfilaments of the ring might be responsible for causing the furrow to deepen, eventually pinching the mother cell into two daughter cells.

In 1969, Schroeder added some cytochalasin (a drug isolated from certain fungi) to dividing marine eggs in which a furrow was developing and observed that the ring of microfilaments became disorganized and the furrow failed to form properly. As a result, the eggs did not pinch into two and each ended up with two nuclei. This, of course, suggested that the cytochalasin had prevented division into two daughter cells by causing disorganization of the actin-containing filaments in the contractile ring.

Another well-known process, the retraction of blood clots, which is important for stopping bleeding, also appears to involve actin and myosin filaments in little bodies called *platelets*, as will be described in Chapter 10.

Contractile Mechanism in Nonmuscle Cells

The nature of the contractile process in muscle makes it seem likely that such movements as those described above would depend on actin-containing microfilaments remaining unchanged in length but moving in relation to some other component. In this connection it is of interest that only the thin, actin-containing filaments in the contractile units of striated muscle (Fig. 5-56) are anchored in the Z lines. The myosin filaments of the contractile unit merely cause the actin filaments to slide along them. It is therefore conceivable that a less well organized arrangement might exist in other kinds of cells, whereby myosin molecules or filaments could cause adjacent actin filaments to slide along them. If the actin filaments had one end anchored somewhere, for example, in the cell membrane as is the case in microvilli (*see* below), movement within the cytoplasm could occur. Whatever the contractile mechanism in cells other than muscle cells, evidence is accumulating that, as in muscle cells, it requires ATP and calcium ions for its operation.

The Microfilaments of Microvilli

The free surface of certain body cells, in particular absorptive cells that constitute much of the lining of the intestine, was long ago observed with the LM to be less smooth in appearance than the free border of the other cells. Since these cells seemed to be covered with a layer of something possessing fine striations disposed at right angles to the free surface, they were said to have *striated borders*.

With the EM the striated border proved to consist of innumerable little finger-like processes of cytoplasm, each covered with a cell membrane, projecting from the cell surface into the lumen of the intestine (Fig. 5-7). These were termed *microvilli* (L. *villus*, tuft of hair). (The reason for the *micro-* in this term is that there are also certain much larger structures called *villi* in the lining of the small intestine). By visualizing microvilli in three dimensions, the student should be able to appreciate how it would be possible, in looking at EM sections such as Figure 5-51 where microvilli are cut almost longitudinally, to tell that they are finger-like processes and not folds; oblique sections of these structures would not be encountered and glancing sections as seen in this micrograph would seldom be observed if the structures cut were folds.

Microvilli enormously increase the surface through which the absorption of nutrients can take place in the

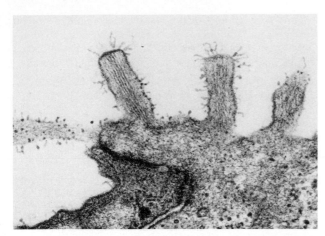

Fig. 5-57. Electron micrograph (×60,000) of the apical surface of an epithelial cell of the trachea of a chick, showing microvilli. Actin-containing microfilaments can be seen in the microvillus on the *left*. Note how they are attached to the cell membrane at the tip of the microvillus. (Courtesy of V. Kalnins)

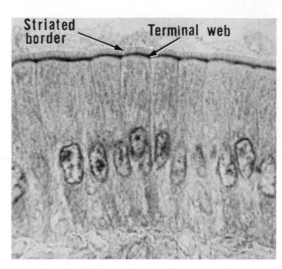

Fig. 5-59. Photomicrograph of absorptive cells lining the rat intestine, stained with tannic and phosphomolybdic acids and amido black to show the terminal web of the cells. The striated border can also be seen immediately above the terminal web.

small intestine. Moreover, some microvilli are found on almost all cells in the body (Figs. 5-50, mv, and 5-51, mv), although they are rarely as large or uniformly arranged as in the absorptive cells of small intestine, as shown in Figure 5-7. Only when they constitute a striated border are they noticeable with the LM.

The Fine Structure of Microvilli. Microvilli are 0.1 μm. in diameter and of variable length. As can be seen in Figure 5-57, they have a core composed of actin-containing filaments, 6 nm. in diameter, anchored to the cell membrane at the tips of microvilli in much the same way as actin filaments are anchored to the Z lines at the ends of sarcomeres of muscle cells (described on p. 546). Myosin filaments have also been discovered in the cytoplasm just below microvilli, and it is believed that interaction of

the actin filaments (microfilaments) in the microvilli with myosin filaments just below the surface could cause the microvilli to bend or shorten.

It is not uncommon for the beginner to mistake the fine structure of microvilli for that of cilia. A glance at Figure 5-51 however will illustrate how these two different kinds of structures may be distinguished from one another. Microvilli are shorter than cilia and, furthermore, they lack the basal bodies (centrioles) and internal microtubules of cilia. Instead of microtubules, a less well organized bundle of microfilaments is seen in microvilli cut so as to reveal these in their cores (Fig. 5-57).

INTERMEDIATE (10 NM.) FILAMENTS

In addition to microtubules, actin-containing microfilaments, and myosin filaments, many cell types contain filaments 7 to 10 nm. in diameter. Much less is known about these *intermediate* filaments than about the others. They are particularly common in nerve cells and their supporting (glial) cells, but they occur to some extent in all cells (Fig. 5-58). Those in nerve cells contain a protein of molecular weight 68,000 whereas those present in other cell types may have a protein with a molecular weight of 54,000 as their major component. It is interesting that colchicine, which causes the disappearance of microtubules, also induces large aggregates of 10-nm. filaments to form in many cell types. There are indications that this class may be a heterogeneous group of different filaments varying considerably in chemical composition and function (*see* review by Gilbert).

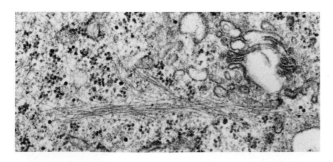

Fig. 5-58. Electron micrograph (×60,000) of part of the cytoplasm of an epithelial cell (trachea of chick), showing a bundle of intermediate filaments (10 nm. filaments). (Courtesy of V. Kalnins)

Fig. 5-60. Electron micrograph (×38,500) of part of the cytoplasm of a liver cell of a rat that had eaten a meal a few hours previously. Note the multiparticulate rosette appearance of the α-particles of glycogen (g) deposited in this region, which contains abundant sER. (Cardell, R.: Internat. Rev. Cytol., *48*:221, 1977)

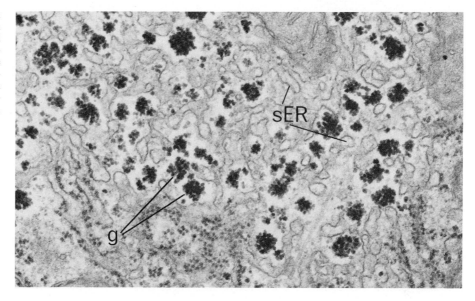

Terminal Web

Certain regions of the cytoplasm, in particular that just below the cell membrane in columnar epithelial cells, are very rigid and contain an especially high concentration of microfilaments, intermediate (10 nm.) filaments, and myosin filaments. Some of the intermediate filaments, called *tonofilaments,* are connected to desmosomes, which are localized specializations of the cell membrane attaching cells to one another in certain tissues of the body, described in Chapter 7. The microfilaments forming the cores of microvilli extend down into the terminal web.

The concentration of the various types of filaments constituting the terminal web is so dense that the other organelles, especially the larger membranous ones, are excluded from this region. Because of this, the region was given a special name, the *terminal web*. It is possible to stain this region in absorptive cells so that it can be seen just below the striated border with the LM (Fig. 5-59). Although the filaments are more concentrated under the apical end of the cell, they also occur to a lesser extent under all parts of the cell membrane and some extend deep into the cytoplasm.

CYTOPLASMIC INCLUSIONS

STORED FOODS

Of the three basic foodstuffs—carbohydrate, protein and fat—only carbohydrate and fat are stored in cells as inclusions.

Carbohydrate is stored chiefly in liver cells and to a lesser extent in muscle and other cells. In all instances it is stored in the form of *glycogen* that exists as deposits in the cytoplasmic matrix, as described in connection with liver cells in Chapter 1 and illustrated in Plate 1-1 and Figure 1-19. The storage of glycogen in liver cells will be considered in more detail when we describe the liver as an organ. When stained, glycogen appears in electron micrographs in either of two forms. In the first, which is referred to as *α-particles*, it consists of rosettes of electron-dense particles (Fig. 5-60, g). The other kind, known as *β-particles*, and which is found for example in muscle cells (Fig. 5-61, g), exists as single electron-dense granules a little larger than ribosomes.

Fat is stored primarily in cells known as *adipose* or *fat cells*. These are the cells of a special tissue known as *fat or adipose tissue* that will be considered in detail when we study connective tissue. Fat sometimes accumulates in liver cells and other types of cells also (Fig. 1-20).

PIGMENTS

The value to the medical student of becoming interested in normal and abnormal color of various parts of the body, and the basis for the color, is very great. A most important factor, and sometimes the chief one in the clinical diagnosis of some diseases, is the changed color of some part of the body. Color is of even greater importance to the pathologist that to the clinician. A good part of the description of the gross appearance of diseased organs at operation or at autopsy relates to their changed color.

Color in any tissue is due chiefly to the kind and amount of pigment it contains. Pigments in cells have gen-

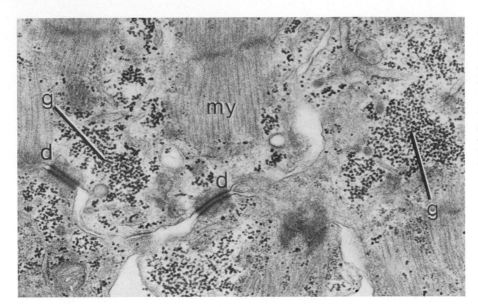

Fig. 5-61. Electron micrograph (×25,500) of rat heart muscle storing glycogen. Note the single particles (β-particles) of glycogen (g) characteristic of muscle cells lying in the cytoplasm between the contractile elements (myofibrils, labeled my) of the muscle. The dark structures (d) are desmosomes, junctions that hold cardiac muscle cells together (these will be described in Chap. 7). (Courtesy of I. Taylor)

erally been classed as inclusions, but in the instance of some pigments this is debatable. In disease conditions certain pigments derived from cells may be found in extracellular spaces as well as in the cells in which they were formed.

It is important to realize what constitutes a pigment. There are many ingredients of cells that, while colorless in life, take on brilliant colors after they are treated with stains. These are not pigments. To qualify as a pigment, a material must possess color in its natural state; hence, a pigment, to be seen, does not need to be treated with stains. However, pigments are sometimes colored further or differently by stains.

Fortunately, there are only a few broad groups of pigments with which the student should become familiar.

CLASSIFICATION

Pigments are usually classified into two groups, *exogenous* and *endogenous*. *Exogenous* (Gr. *ex*, out; *genein*, to produce) pigments are those that have been generated outside the body and subsequently taken into it by one route or another. *Endogenous* (Gr. *endon*, within) pigments are generated inside the body from nonpigmented ingredients.

Exogenous Pigments

Exogenous Lipochromes. These are pigments that are lipid-soluble, and hence they color fats (Gr. *lipos* + *chroma*, color). The best known example is *carotene*, the pigment that gives carrots their attractive orange color.

Carotene. This pigment is formed in several kinds of vegetables. There are several types of carotene, and different vegetables form somewhat different kinds. The kind in carrots is yellow in color, but in tomatoes, carotene is more red. The carotenes are soluble in fat and so are taken up from foods, whereupon they color certain body components that contain fat. For example, the color of egg yolks is due to the carotene absorbed by chickens from the vegetable food that they eat. Likewise the (natural) yellow color of butter is due to the carotene eaten by cows, which is dissolved into the fat of the cream they produce. The body fat of man often has a yellow tinge because of its content of carotene.

Several forms of carotene are provitamins and may be converted into vitamin A in the body, which is one good reason for eating fresh vegetables or drinking vegetable juices. Occasionally, however, individuals do not practice moderation in this respect. It is possible to eat so many carrots or tomatoes, or to drink so much vegetable juice, that the skin of the body takes on a yellow (or even reddish) color due to its great content of carotene. The condition caused by excessive consumption of carotene is called *carotenemia* (meaning carotene in the blood) and individuals with this condition may at first glance be thought to have jaundice. It is an unusual condition in adults*, but is sometimes seen in babies given too much vegetable juice.

---

* Regarding carotenemia, interested students will find "The Orange Man," an article which appeared in The New Yorker magazine (vol. 43, May 27, 1967), intriguing as a good mystery story and very much more informative.

Dusts. A second important group of exogenous pigments is provided by the various kinds of dusts that gain entrance to the respiratory tract. Pigmentation of parts of the respiratory system by this means is of course pathological. We shall comment briefly on this matter in Chapter 23.

Minerals. Certain minerals taken by mouth or absorbed through the surface of the body may also lead to pigmentation. For example, too much silver applied to body surfaces in the treatment of certain diseases may lead to an accumulation of silver and hence a gray pigmentation of the body. Lead can be absorbed and impart a blue line to the gums.

Tattoo Marks. These consist of inorganic pigments driven deep into the skin with needles, where they become fixed in position in phagocytic cells called *macrophages.*

Endogenous Pigments

The most important of these is *hemoglobin*, the iron-containing pigment in red blood cells. This serves as the oxygen carrier of the body and is discussed in detail in Chapter 10. Here is is enough to note that pink cheeks and red lips are due to this pigment, which is in the red blood cells that are circulating in capillaries just below the surface of these parts of the body. Certain altered forms of hemoglobin of a different color from the normal are also discussed in Chapter 10.

Pigments From the Destruction of Hemoglobin. Under normal conditions, red blood cells do not survive for more than four months in the circulatory system. As they wear out, they are phagocytosed by macrophages in the spleen, liver, and bone marrow. In the cytoplasm of these large cells, the iron-containing hemoglobin is broken down into an iron-containing pigment called *hemosiderin* and a noniron-containing one called *bilirubin* (further details are given on p. 717).

Hemosiderin. This is golden brown and occurs in the cytoplasm of macrophages in the form of granules or small irregular masses. By histochemical tests for iron, hemosiderin can be shown to contain this element; this permits it to be distinguished from the other golden and brown pigments of the body.

Whereas hemosiderin is normally present to some extent in the macrophages of the spleen, liver, and bone marrow, it becomes greatly increased in these sites in diseases in which red blood corpuscles are broken down much more rapidly than usual. It may even appear in large quantities in other kinds of cells under certain pathologic conditions.

Bilirubin. Bile is a yellow-to-brown fluid secreted by the liver and stored and concentrated in the gallbladder; eventually, it passes into the intestine, where it plays an important role in absorption and digestion. Its coloring matter is *bilirubin*, a yellow-to-brown pigment which becomes oxidized to biliverdin, a green pigment. In some birds a considerable amount of biliverdin is present in the bile, enhancing the tendency of the bile to be green, but in man only a little biliverdin is normally present, so that human bile is yellow to brown.

It was once believed that bilirubin was manufactured by the liver cells that secrete it, but with further studies it became apparent that bilirubin, like hemosiderin, is a breakdown product of hemoglobin and hence formed in the sites where old, worn-out red blood corpuscles are destroyed. Unlike hemosiderin, however, bilirubin contains no iron and is more soluble; hence it does not tend to remain in the cytoplasm of macrophages that destroy red blood cells but instead dissolves into the blood, from which it is continuously removed by the cells of the liver to be transferred to bile.

The first tangible lead indicating that bilirubin was derived from hemoglobin was given by Virchow, the great pathologist, over 100 years ago. He observed that crystals of a yellow pigment tended to form in tissues of the body that were the sites of previous hemorrhages. He named the pigment that crystallized out among the old, breaking-down red blood corpuscles *hematoidin* and concluded that it was derived from hemoglobin. Not content with microscopic examinations alone, he subjected this pigment to chemical tests and made the remarkable discovery that hematoidin, as far as these tests could demonstrate, was the same thing as the pigment that colors bile (*bilirubin*). Yet for many years afterward, hemoglobin was not accepted as the origin of bile pigment, and many decades passed before his view gained general acceptance.

Melanin. This is usually a brown-to-black pigment found chiefly in the skin and its appendages and in the eye. It is also present in the *substantia nigra*, a part of the brain. In white races it appears in skin in appreciable amounts after exposure to sunlight (suntan). Melanin accounts for the dark color of the Negro; here, too, the degree of pigmentation is increased by sunlight. The color of brown eyes is due to melanin and deep in the eye melanin is used as a light-proofing material much in the same way as photographers use black paper and black paint.

Melanin is a nitrogenous substance that in pure form contains no sulfur or iron. The formation of melanin will be considered in detail in Chapter 20 (p. 626). Cells that make melanin are termed *melanocytes.* They contain an enzyme capable of acting on a colorless precursor brought to the cell by way of the blood and tissue fluid, converting it into melanin.

Lipofuscin. This is a pigment that contains lipid, permitting it to be stained with certain fat stains. It is itself

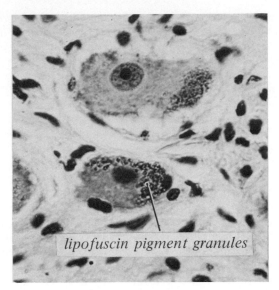

Fig. 5-62. High-power photomicrograph of two nerve cell bodies in a ganglion. The cytoplasm contains accumulated granules of lipofuscin pigment.

golden brown in color (L. *fuscus*, brown) and appears in the form of aggregates, sometimes called *granules* (Fig. 5-62). This pigment is relatively common in heart muscle, nerve and liver cells, and its amount increases with age, which has led to the concept that it represents a "wear-and-tear" product that is not readily degraded in the cytoplasm or excreted. Deposits of lipofuscin commonly have hydrolase activity, and the pigment is contained in residual bodies. Although lipofuscin is commonly classified as an *endogenous lipochrome* pigment, it is usually referred to simply as *lipochrome pigment*.

REFERENCES AND OTHER READING

Fine Structure of Cells and Tissues

Fujita, T., Tokunaga, J., and Inoué, H.: Atlas of Scanning Electron Microscopy in Medicine. Amsterdam, Elsevier, 1971.
Lentz, T. L.: Cell Fine Structure. Philadelphia, W. B. Saunders, 1971.
Porter, K. R., and Bonneville, M. A.: An Introduction to the Fine Structure of Cells and Tissues. ed. 4. Philadelphia, Lea & Febiger, 1973.
Rhodin, J. A. G.: Histology, A Text and Atlas. New York, Oxford University Press, 1974.

Cell Membrane, Cell Surface and Cell Coat

Burger, M.: Surface properties of neoplastic cells. Hosp. Prac., July, 1973.

————: Surface changes in transformed cells detected by lectins. Fed. Proc., *32:*91, 1973.
Chapman, D.: Lipid dynamics in cell membranes. Hosp. Prac., February, 1973.
De Pierce, J. W., and Karnovsky, M. L.: Plasma membranes of mammalian cells. A review of methods for their characterization and isolation. J. Cell Biol., *56:*275, 1973.
Fox, C. F.: The structure of cell membranes. Sci. Am., *226:*30, 1972.
Frye, C. D., and Edidin, M.: The rigid intermixing of cell surface antigens after formation of mouse-human heterokaryons. J. Cell Sci., *7:*319, 1970.
Hughes, R. C.: Glycoproteins as components of cellular membranes. Prog. Biophys. Molec. Biol., *26:*189, 1973.
Lucy, J. A.: The fusion of cell membranes. Hosp. Prac., Sept., 1973.
Marchesi, V. T., Jackson, R. L., Segrest, J. P., and Kahane, I.: Molecular features of the major glycoprotein of the human erythrocyte membrane. Fed. Proc., *32:*1833, 1973.
Martinez-Palomo, A.: The surface coats of animal cells. Int. Rev. Cytol., *29:*29, 1970.
Nicolson, G. L.: The interactions of lectins with animal cell surfaces. Int. Rev. Cytol. *39:*90, 1974.
Nicolson, G. L., Giotta, G., Lotan, R., Neri, A. and Poste, G.: The membrane glycoproteins of normal and malignant cells. *In* Brinkley, B. R. and Porter, K. R. (eds.): International Cell Biology 1976–1977. New York, Rockefeller University Press, 1977.
Nicolson, G. L. and Poste, G.: The cancer cell: dynamic aspects and modifications in cell surface organization. Parts I and II. N. Engl. J. Med., *295:*197, 1976; *295:*253, 1976.
Pinto da Silva, P., and Branton, D.: Membrane splitting in freeze-etching. J. Cell Biol., *45:*598, 1970.
Porter, K. R., Prescott, D., and Frye, J.: Changes in surface morphology of Chinese hamster ovary cells during the cell cycle. J. Cell Biol., *57:*815, 1973.
Rambourg, A., and Leblond, C. P.: Electron microscope observations on the carbohydrate rich cell coat present at the surface of cells in the rat. J. Cell Biol., *32:*27, 1967.
Revel, J. P., Henning, U. and Fox, C. F. (eds.): Cell Shape and Surface Architecture. Progress in Clinical and Biological Research, vol. 17. New York, Alan R. Liss, 1977.
Singer, S. J.: Proteins and membrane topography. Hosp. Prac., May, 1973.
Singer, S. J., and Nicolson, G. L.: The fluid mosaic model of the structure of cell membranes. Science, *175:*720, 1972.
Taylor, R. B., Duffus, P. H., Raff, M. C., and de Petris, S.: Redistribution and pinocytosis of lymphocyte surface immunoglobulin molecules induced by anti-immunoglobulin antibody. Nature (New Biol.), *233:*225, 1971.

Mitochondria

Bandlow, W., Schweyen, R. J., Thomas, D. Y., Wolf, K., and Kaudewitz, F. (eds.): Genetics, Biogenesis and Bioenergetics of Mitochondria. Berlin, Gruyter, 1976.
Goodenough, U., and Levine, R.: The genetic activity of mitochondria and chloroplasts. Sci. Am. *223:*22, Nov., 1970.
Margulis, L.: Symbiosis and evolution. Sci. Am., *225:*48, August, 1971.
Racker, E.: The membrane of the mitochondrion. Sci. Am., *218:*32, Feb. 1968.
Tedeschi, H.: Mitochondria: Structure, Biogenesis and Transducing Functions. Cell Biology Monographs, Vol. 4. Wein, Springer-Verlag, 1976.

Wainio, W.: The Mammalian Mitochondrial Respiratory Chain. New York, Academic Press, 1970.

Williams, C., and Vail, W.: Ultrastructural transitions in energized and de-energized mitochondria. Adv. Cell Molec. Biol., *2*:385, 1972.

Ribosomes, Rough-Surfaced Endoplasmic Reticulum, Protein Synthesis, and Protein Secretion

Blobel, G.: Synthesis and segregation of secretory proteins: the signal hypothesis. *In* Brinkley, B. R. and Porter, K. R. (eds.): International Cell Biology 1976–1977. New York, Rockefeller University Press, 1977.

Jamieson, J. D., and Palade, G. E.: Production of secretory proteins in animal cells. *In* Brinkley, B. R. and Porter, K. R. (eds.): International Cell Biology 1976–1977. New York, Rockefeller University Press, 1977.

Leblond, C. P., and Warren, K. B.: The use of radioautography in investigation protein synthesis. New York, Academic Press, 1965.

Nonomura, Y., Blobel, G., and Sabatini, D.: Structure of liver ribosomes studied by negative staining. J. Molec. Biol., *60*:303, 1971.

Novikoff, A. B.: The endoplasmic reticulum: a cytochemist's view (a review) Proc. Natl. Acad. Sci. U.S.A., *73*:2781, 1976.

Palade, G. E.: Intracellular aspects of the process of protein secretion. Science, *189*:347, 1975.

Warner, J. R., Knoff, P., and Rich, A.: A multiple ribosomal structure in protein synthesis. Proc. Natl. Acad. Sci. U.S.A., *49*:122, 1963.

Weinstock, M. and Leblond, C. P.: Synthesis, migration and release of precursor collagen by odontoblasts as visualized by radioautography after [^{3}H] proline administration. J. Cell Biol., *60*:92, 1974.

The Golgi Apparatus

Bentfeld, M. E., and Bainton, D. F.: Cytochemical localization of lysomal enzymes in rat megakaryocytes and platelets. J. Clin. Invest., *56*:1635, 1975.

Bergeron, J. J. M., Ehrenreich, J. H., Siekevitz, P. and Palade, G. E.: Golgi fractions prepared from rat liver homogenates. II. Biochemical characterization. J. Cell Biol. *59*:73, 1973.

Decker, R. S.: Lysomal packaging in differentiating and degenerating anuran lateral motor column neurons. J. Cell Biol., *61*:599, 1974.

Gonatas, N. K., Kim, S. U., Stieber, A., and Avrameas, S. Internalization of lectins in neuronal GERL. J. Cell Biol., *73*:1, 1977.

Hand, A. R.: Morphology and cytochemistry of the Golgi apparatus of rat salivary gland acinar cells. Am. J. Anat., *130*:141, 1971.

Hand, A. R., and Oliver, C.: Cytochemical studies of GERL and its role in secretory granule formation in exocrine cells. Histochem. J., *9*:375, 1977.

Leblond, C. P. and Bennett, G.: Role of the Golgi apparatus in terminal glycosylation. *In* Brinkley, B. R. and Porter, K. R. (eds.): International Cell Biology 1976–1977. New York, Rockefeller University Press, 1977.

Morré, D. J.: Membrane differentiation and the control of secretion: a comparison of plant and animal Golgi apparatus. *In* Brinkley, B. R. and Porter, K. R. (eds.): International Cell Biology 1976–1977. New York, Rockefeller University Press, 1977.

Neutra, M., and Leblond, C. P.: Synthesis of the carbohydrate of mucus in the Golgi complex, as shown by electron microscope radioautography of goblet cells from rats injected with ^{3}H-glucose. J. Cell Biol., *30*:119, 1966.

——: The Golgi apparatus. Sci. Am., *220*:100, February 1969.

Northcote, D. H.: The Golgi apparatus. Endeavour, *30*:26, 1971.

——: The Golgi complex. *In* Bittar, E. E. (ed.): Cell biology in Medicine. New York, John Wiley & Sons, 1973.

Novikoff, A. B., Mori, M., Quinatana, N. and Yam, A.: Studies of the secretory process in the mammalian exocrine pancreas. I. The condensing vacuoles. J. Cell Biol., *75*:148, 1977.

Novikoff, A. B., and Novikoff, P. M.: Cytochemical contributions to differentiating GERL from the Golgi apparatus. Histochem. J., *9*:525, 1977.

Novikoff, P. M., and Yam, A. Sites of lipoprotein particles in normal rat hepatocytes. J. Cell Biol., *76*:1, 1978.

Rambourg, A., Clermont, Y., and Marraud, A.: Three-dimensional structure of the osmium-impregnated Golgi-apparatus as seen in the high voltage electron microscope. Am. J. Anat., *140*:27, 1974.

Schacter, H.: The subcellular sites of glycosylation. Biochem. Soc. Symp., *40*:57, 1974.

Schenkein, I., and Uhr, J. W.: Immunoglobulin synthesis and secretion. I. Biosynthesis studies of the addition of the carbohydrate moieties. J. Cell Biol., *46*:42, 52, 1970.

Whaley, W. G., Dauwalder, M., and Kephart, J. E.: Golgi apparatus: influence on cell surfaces. Science, *175*:596, 1972.

Lysosomes

Allison, A.: Lysosomes and disease. Sci. Am., *217*:62, 1967.

Arstila , A., Jauregui, H., Chang, J., and Trump, B.: Studies on cellular autophagocytosis. Lab Invest., *27*:162, 1972.

Bainton, D.: Sequential degranulation of the two types of polymorphonuclear granules during phagocytosis of microorganisms. J. Cell Biol., *58*:249, 1973.

Bainton, D. F., Nichols, B. A., and Farquhar, M. G.: Primary lysosomes of blood leukocytes. *In* Dingle, J. T. and Dean, R. T. (eds.). Lysosomes in Biology and Pathology. vol. 5. Amsterdam, North Holland, 1976.

Brady, R. O.: Hereditary fat metabolism diseases. Sci. Am., August 1973.

DeDuve, C.: Lysosomes in pathology and therapeutics. Abstracts, International Symposium on Lysosomes, Hakone, Japan, p. 4, 1972.

——: Biochemical studies on the occurrence, biogenesis and life history of mammalian peroxisomes. J. Histochem. Cytochem., *21*.941, 1973.

Dingle, J. T., Fell, H. B., and Dean, R. T. (eds.): Lysosomes in Biology and Pathology, vols. 1 to 5. Amsterdam, North Holland, 1975–1976.

Hirsch, J. G.: Lysosomes and mental retardation. Quart. Rev. Biol., *47*:303, 1972.

Holtzman, E.: Lysosomes: A Survey. Cell Biology Monographs vol. 3. Wein, Springer-Verlag, 1976.

Novikoff, A. B.: Lysosomes: a personal account. *In* Hers, G., and Van Hoof, F. (eds.): Lysosomes and Storage Diseases. p. 1. New York, Academic Press, 1973.

Novikoff, A. B., and Holtzman, E.: Cells and Organelles. New York, Holt, 1970.

Rajan, K. T.: Lysosomes and gout. Nature, *210*:959, 1966.

Phagocytosis, Pinocytosis, and Coated Vesicles

Bowers, B., and Olszewski, T. E.: Pinocytosis in *Acanthamoeba castellanii*. Kinetics and morphology. J. Cell Biol., *53:*68, 1972.

Cornell, R., Walker, W. A., and Isselbacher, K. J.: Small intestine absorption of horse radish peroxidase. Lab. Invest., *25:*42, 1971.

Friend, D. S., and Farquhar, M. G.: Functions of coated vesicles during protein absorption in the rat vas deferens. J. Cell Biol., *35:*337, 1967.

Goldstein, J. L., Brown, M. S., and Anderson, R. G. W.: The low-density lipoprotein pathway in human fibroblasts. Biochemical and Ultrastructural Correlations. *In* Brinkley, B. R. and Porter, K. R. (eds.): International Cell Biology 1976–1977. New York, Rockefeller University Press, 1977.

LaBella, F. S.: Pinocytosis — Addresses, Essays, Lectures, New York, MSS Information Corp., 1973.

Lagunoff, D.: Macrophage pinocytosis. The removal and resynthesis of a cell surface factor. Proc. Soc. Exp. Biol. Med., *138:*118, 1971.

Rodewald, R.: Intestinal transport of antibodies in the newborn rat. J. Cell Biol., *58:*189, 1973.

Simionescu, N., Simionescu, M., and Palade, G. E.: Permeability of muscle capillaries to exogenous myoglobin. *57:*424, 1973.

Werb, Z., and Cohn, Z. A.: Plasma membrane synthesis in the macrophage following phagocytosis of polystyrene latex particles. J. Biol. Chem., *247:*2439, 1972.

Williams, R. C., Jr., and Fudenberg, H. H. (eds.): Phagocytic Mechanisms in Health and Disease. New York, Intercontinental Medical Book, 1972.

Smooth Endoplasmic Reticulum

Black, W. H.: The development of smooth surfaced endoplasmic reticulum in adrenal cortical cells of fetal guinea pig. Am. J. Anat., *135:*381, 1972.

Cardell, R. R.: Smooth endoplasmic reticulum in rat hepatocytes during glycogen deposition and depletion. Int. Rev. Cytol., *48:*221, 1977.

Cardell, R. R., Jr., Badenhausen, S., and Porter, K. R.: Intestinal triglyceride absorption in the rat. An electron microscopical study. J. Cell Biol., *34:*123, 1967.

Christensen, A. K.: Fine structure of testicular interstitial cells in humans. *In* Rosenberg E., and Paulsen, C. (eds.): The Human Testis. p. 75. New York, Plenum Press, 1970.

Higgins, J. A., and Barrnett, R. J : Studies on the biogenesis of smooth endoplasmic reticulum membranes in livers of phenobarbital treated rats. J. Cell Biol., *55:*282, 1972.

Kappas, A., and Alvares, A. P.: How the liver metabolizes foreign substances. Sci. Am., *232:*22, June, 1975.

Kelly, A. M.: Sarcoplasmic reticulum and T-tubules in differentiating rat skeletal muscle. J. Cell Biol., *49:*335, 1971.

McNutt, N. S., and Jones, A. L.: Observations on the ultrastructure of cytodifferentiation in the human fetal adrenal cortex. Lab Invest., *22:*513, 1970.

Microtubules

Borgers, M., and DeBrabander, M. (eds.): Microtubules and Microtubule Inhibitors. Amsterdam, North Holland, 1975.

Borisy, G. G., and Taylor, E. W.: The mechanism of action of colchicine. Binding of colchicine -H³ to cellular protein. J. Cell Biol., *34:*525, 1967.

Brinkley, B. R., Stubblefield, E., and Hsu, T. C.: The effects of colcemid inhibition and reversal on the fine structure of the mitotic apparatus of Chinese hamster cells in vitro. J. Ultrastruct. Res., *19:*1, 1967.

Dustin, P.: Microtubules. Berlin, Springer-Verlag, 1978.

Fujiwara, K., and Tilney, L. G.: Substructural analysis of the microtubule and its polymorphic forms. Ann. N.Y. Acad. Sci., *253:*27, 1975.

Goldman, R., Pollard, T., and Rosenbaum, J. (eds.): Cell Motility. Book C Microtubules and Related Proteins. Cold Spring Harbor Conferences on Cell Proliferation, vol. 3. Cold Spring Harbor Laboratory, 1976.

Olmsted, J. B., and Borisy, G. G.: Microtubules. Ann. Rev. Biochem., p. 507, 1973.

Porter, K. R.: Cytoplasmic microtubules and their functions. *In* Wolstenholme, G. E. W., and O'Connor, M. (eds.): Principles of Biomolecular Organization. Ciba Foundation Symposium. London, Churchill, 1966.

Soifer, D. (ed.): The biology of cytoplasmic microtubules. Ann. N.Y. Acad. Sci., *253:*1, 1975.

Tilney, L. G., Bryan, J., Busch, D. J., Fujiwara, K., Moosekar, M. S., Murphy, D. B., and Snyder, D. H.: Microtubules: evidence for 13 protofilaments. J. Cell Biol., *59:*267, 1973.

Yamada, K. M., Spooner, B. S., and Wessels, N. K.: Axon growth: roles of microfilaments and microtubules. Proc. Natl. Acad. Sci. U.S.A., *66:*1206, 1970.

Centrioles, Cilia, and Flagella

Baba, S., and Hiramoto, Y.: A quantitative analysis of ciliary movement by high speed microcinematography. J. Exp. Biol., *52:*675, 1970.

Fulton, C.: Centrioles. *In* Reinert, J., and Ursprung, H. (eds.): Origin and Continuity of Cell Organelles. Vol. 2, p. 170. New York, Springer-Verlag, 1971.

Gibbons, I. R.: Structure and function of flagellar microtubules. *In* Brinkley, B. R. and Porter, K. R. (eds.): International Cell Biology 1976–1977. New York, Rockefeller University Press, 1977.

Kalnins, V. I., and Porter, K. R.: Centriole replication during ciliogenesis in the chick tracheal epithelium. Z. Zellforsch., *100:*1, 1969.

Olmsted, J. B.: Microtubules and Flagella. *In* Brinkley, B. R., and Porter, K. R. (eds.): International Cell Biology 1976–1977. New York, Rockefeller University Press, 1977.

Pickett-Heaps, J.: The autonomy of centriole: fact or fallacy. Cytobios, *3:*205, 1971.

Sleigh, M. A. (ed.): Cilia and Flagella. London, Academic Press, 1974.

Sorokin, S. P.: Reconstructions of centriole formation and ciliogenesis in mammalian lungs. J. Cell Sci., *3:*207, 1968.

Summers, K. E., and Gibbons, I. R.: Adenosine triphosphate-induced sliding of tubules in trypsin treated flagella of sea urchin sperm. Proc. Natl. Acad. Sci. U.S.A., *68:*3092, 1971.

Warner, F. D.: Macromolecular organization of eukaryotic cilia and flagella. Adv. Cell Molec. Biol., *2:*193, 1972.

Wolfe, J.: Basal body fine structure and chemistry. Adv. Cell Molec. Biol., *2:*151, 1972.

Filaments

Beams, H. W., and Kessel, R. G.: Cytokinesis: a comparative study of cytoplasmic division in animal cells. Am. Sci., *63:*279, 1976.

Bhenke, O., Forer, A., and Emmerson, J.: Actin in sperm tails and mciotic spindle. Nature, *234:*408, 1971.

Bonneville, M. A., and Weinstock, M.: Brush border development in the intestinal absorptive cells of *Xenopus* during metamorphosis. J. Cell Biol., *44:*151, 1970.

Fine, R. E., and Bray, D.: Actin in growing nerve cells. Nature, New Biol., *234:*115, 1971.

Gilbert, D.: 10 nm. Filaments. Nature, *272:*577, 1978.

Goldman, R., Pollard, T., and Rosenbaum, J. (eds.): Cell Motility. Book A Motility, Muscle and Non-muscle Cells and Book B Actin, Myosin and Associated Proteins. Cold Spring Harbor Conferences on Cell Proliferation, vol. 3. Cold Spring Harbor Laboratory, 1976.

Holtzer, H., and Sanger, I. W.: Cytochalasin B. Problems in interpreting its effect on cells. Develop. Biol., *27:*443, 1972.

Huxley, H. E.: The relevance of studies on muscle to problems of cell motility. *In* Cell Motility Book A Motility, Muscle and Non-muscle Cells. Cold Spring Harbor Conferences on Cell Proliferation, vol. 3. Cold Spring Harbor Laboratory, 1976.

Inoué, S. and Stephens, R. E. (eds.): Molecules and Cell Movement. Society of General Physiologists Series, vol. 30. New York, Raven Press, 1975.

Perdue, J. F.: The distribution, ulstrastructure and chemistry of microfilaments in cultured chick embryo fibroblasts. J. Cell Biol., *58:*265, 1973.

Pollard, T. D.: Cytoplasmic contractile proteins. *In* Brinkley, B. R. and Porter, K. R. (eds.): International Cell Biology 1976–1977. New York, Rockefeller University Press, 1977.

Spooner, B. S., Yamada, K. M., and Wessels, N. K.: Microfilaments and cell locomotion. J. Cell Biol., *49:*595, 1971.

Taylor, D. L.: Dynamics of cytoplasmic structure and contractility *In* Brinkley, B. R. and Porter, K. R. (eds.): International Cell Biology 1976–1977. New York, Rockefeller University Press, 1977.

Tilney, L. G.: Actin: its association with membranes and the regulation of its polymerization. *In* Brinkley, B. R. and Porter, K. R. (eds.): International Cell Biology 1976–1977. New York, Rockefeller University Press, 1977.

Wessels, N. K.: How living cells change their shape. Sci. Am., *225:*76, 1971.

Zucker-Franklin D., and Grusky, G. G.: The actin and myosin filaments of human and bovine blood platelets. J. Clin. Invest., *51:*419, 1972.

Glycogen, Lipid, Pigments, and Inclusions

Biava, C.: Identification and structural forms of human particulate glycogen. Lab. Invest., *12:*1179, 1963.

Bissell, D. M., Hammaker, L., and Schmid, R.: Hemoglobin and erythrocyte catabolism in rat liver: the separate roles of parenchymal and sinusoidal cells. Blood J. Hematol., *40:*812, 1972.

———: Liver sinusoidal cells. Identification of a subpopulation for erythrocyte catabolism. J. Cell Biol., *54:*107, 1972.

Bjorkerud, S.: Isolation of lipofuscin granules from bovine cardiac muscle. J. Ultrastruct. Res. (Suppl.), *5:*5, 1963.

Cardell, R. R.: Smooth endoplasmic reticulum in rat hepatocytes during glycogen deposition and depletion. Int. Rev. Cytol., *48:*221, 1977.

Frank, A. L., and Christensen, A. K.: Localization of acid phosphatase in lipofuscin granules and possible autophagic vacuoles in interstitial cells of the guinea pig testis. J. Cell Biol., *36:*1, 1968.

Harrison, P.: Ferritin and haemosiderin. *In* Iron Metabolism. p. 148. Ciba International Symposium, Berlin, Springer-Verlag, 1964.

Malkoff, D., and Strehler, B.: The ultrastructure of isolated and in situ human cardiac age pigment. J. Cell Biol., *16:*611, 1963.

Palay, S. L., and Revel, J. P.: The morphology of fat absorption. *In* Meng, H. C. (ed.): Lipid Transport. pp. 33-43. Springfield, Ill., Charles C Thomas, 1964.

Revel, J. P.: Electron microscopy of glycogen. J. Histochem. Cytochem., *12:*104, 1964.

Seiji, M., Birbeck, M. S. C., and Fitzpatrick, T. B.: Subcellular localization of melanin biosynthesis. Ann. N.Y. Acad. Sci., *100:*497, 1963.

Senior, J. R.: Intestinal absorption of fats. J. Lipid Res., *5:*495, 1964.

Silagi, S.: Control of pigment production in mouse melanoma cells *in vitro*. J. Cell Biol., *43:*263, 1969.

Wood, E. N.: An ordered complex of filaments surrounding the lipid droplets in developing adipose cells. Anat. Rec., *157:*437, 1967.

6

Cell Differentiation and Its Relation to Gene Expression, the Control of Cell Populations, and the Development of the Four Basic Tissues of the Body

The first part of this chapter introduces some interrelated areas of cell biology that are now attracting a vast amount of research. Attempting to deal briefly with these in a simple way and at an elementary level is a hazardous procedure, particularly if a few of one's own ideas are included. Nevertheless, these are areas of biology that students of today are bound to encounter in their various studies, and indeed they should know something about them to understand the subject matter of the next portion of this book, which deals with the tissues.

CELL DIFFERENTIATION AND ITS RELATION TO GENE EXPRESSION

The ancestry of the millions of somatic cells in a human body can all be traced back to a single cell: the fertilized ovum. Among these millions of cells, about 100 different kinds can be recognized by microscopy. Two processes must therefore occur in the development of the body. First, an enormous amount of cell proliferation must take place, which would require millions of mitoses. Second, as the cells increase in number they must become different from one another. Furthermore, for the body to become composed of parts arranged in a standard pattern with such structures as muscles, tendons, and bones, and such organs as the brain, liver, heart, kidney, and lungs, all developing in the right places, the cells derived from the fertilized ovum must become different from one another in different sites, in a very orderly way. Before discussing how the pattern develops and the possible factors involved, we must first comment on the terminology used in this area.

Potentiality and Differentiation

The word *potentiality* in ordinary use refers to capabilities not yet realized. With regard to a cell it is used specifically to denote the extent to which it can serve as the ancestral cell for different kinds (not numbers) of cells. Since the fertilized ovum serves as the ancestral cell for all the kinds of cells that develop in the body, it is said

to be a *totipotential* cell. How long does totipotentiality last in its descendants?

Commonly the two daughter cells resulting from its first mitotic division adhere to one another and both contribute to the subsequent development of an embryo. But occasionally after this division the two daughter cells separate and each develops into an embryo; this, of course, results in the development of identical twins and shows that after one division, both daughter cells retain totipotentiality. Furthermore, the first four cells all may occasionally separate, resulting in the birth of identical quadruplets. Very, very rarely, five identical quintuplets are born—all of which shows that through the first three mitotic divisions the cellular descendants of the fertilized ovum can retain totipotentiality. But if daughter cells remain together and cell division continues, the formation of a clump of cells called a *morula* (L. *morus,* mulberry) (Fig. 6-1B) is soon formed. The cells of the clump destined to become body cells become different from one another, generally more or less imperceptibly, and in doing so cease being totipotential cells. Cells that become different from, and have lost some of the potentiality of, the cell from which they were derived are said to have undergone some degree of *differentiation*. So cells, as a result of differentiation, gain some new properties but lose some of their former potentiality.

The Terms *Differentiation* and *Modulation*

There are examples in the animal kingdom of apparently differentiated cells, under extraordinary circumstances, seeming to revert to an earlier stage of differentiation in which they multiply and regenerate, for example, a lost appendage. It has therefore been suggested that it is possible for differentiated cells to "dedifferentiate," in which process they regain potentiality. However, for them to demonstrate any potentiality they possessed previously only indicates they have never lost it: they merely assumed a different form from that in which they existed before they seemingly differentiated. If a cell merely becomes different in its physical form without losing any of its potentiality, it is generally said to have undergone *modulation* (L. *modulatus*, regulated or arranged). This term was probably coined to denote what happens when the physical form of a cell becomes altered in order for it to fit into its environment. Modulation can occur without the cell losing any potentiality.

Differentiation in the developing embryo commonly occurs in steps and along different cell lineages. Because of cells differentiating in steps, cells can exist in different states of differentiation and hence possess different potentialities. The end cells that form as a final result of the last step of differentiation, such as those of Category 1 (p. 42) and those of Category 2 (p. 42), retain no potentiality. The stem or progenitor cells of Category 2 type cells retain not totipotentiality but a restricted potentiality which limits them to forming cells only of their respective family types. Cells of Category 3 retain no potentiality; they merely reproduce themselves as such.

There is, however, one exception to the rule that the cells derived from the fertilized ovum undergo differentiation and hence lose some of their potentiality; this exception involves the cells which are not destined to be body (*somatic*) cells but *germ* cells. These retain totipotentiality. Hence among the cells of the little clump of cells that forms early in the development of a female embryo, some do not undergo any differentiation. These cells, as the embryo develops, multiply and migrate in large numbers into the developing ovaries where after puberty they begin to develop further into mature female germ cells. That these cells in the ovaries retain full potentiality is demonstrated not only by their being shed after puberty as haploid *germ cells* (p. 76), which if fertilized develop into embryos, but also by the fact that very occasionally one (as a diploid cell) may give rise to a tumor while it is still in the ovary without its ever having been fertilized. Such a tumor often becomes large enough to require removal by surgery. A cut through one may reveal a hodgepodge of the kinds of tissue found in the normal body. Bits of skin, hair follicles and hair, ill-formed teeth, bits of bone and cartilage may all be present, along with some nerve tissue, parts of eyes, and so on. Obviously the cell from which the tumor developed was a totipotential cell, but the cells derived from it did not develop in the orderly manner that characterizes the development of the normal embryo. It is of interest that the cells of such tumors that develop in ovaries all contain Barr bodies.

DEVELOPMENT OF KNOWLEDGE ABOUT POSSIBLE MECHANISMS OF DIFFERENTIATION

After the concept of genes was established, it became evident that a genetic mutation could occur in a cell without its being lethal. Such a cell often could continue to divide but it would of course, propagate its genetic defect to its descendants. So, one of the first concepts of how body cells became different from one another during development was that an orderly sequence of mutations, involving gene deletions, occurred to account for the formation of different cell families. Thus the cells of each family would contain fewer genes than the cells from which they developed. It was assumed also that different genes would be lost by different cells so the cells of different cell families that developed this way would express different physical and functional features. One of the attractive features of this hypothesis was that it would explain how different families of cells were able to perpetuate their own kind, because the members of each family would only be able to transmit their own particular genes to subsequent members of that family and so give rise only to cells of the family to which they belonged. This concept, of course, required a belief that the genes and the chromosomes of each family of cells in the body were different from those of other cell families.

After the relation of genes to DNA become established and modern methods of chromosome analysis became available, it became apparent that there was no supportive evidence for the mutation theory of differentiation. First, it was shown that the DNA content of all body cells was the same and second, body cells of different kinds were found to have the same assortment of chromosomes as all the other body cells. Probably these and other factors aroused the suspicion that the genetic and chromosomal content of all body cells might be identical, even though the structure and functions of cells were different. This suggested that the body cells of any cell family were different from those of other families because different genes were *expressed* (the remainder being *suppressed*) in different kinds of cells. This, of course, also raised the problem of how to explain why once a certain set of genes was expressed in a given cell family, only those same genes would be expressed in subsequent generations of that cell family. There are now some answers to the questions that arose.

The first question explored was that of trying to ascertain if the chromosomes of a specialized body cell still retained and, under suitable circumstances, could be made to express, the totipotentiality of a fertilized ovum. An impressive way of doing this would be to show that the chromosomes of a cell, sufficiently differentiated to have become a particular type of body cell could, under the right circumstances, direct the formation of an entire body. The simplest way to do this would be to remove the nucleus from a fertilized ovum and by means of transplantation technics substitute for it the nucleus of a cell that had undergone some degree of differentiation; then it could be ascertained whether an entire body could develop from it. This, of course, would be a formidable research project. However, methods for performing microsurgery were developed by which the equivalent of reduction gears made it possible to transmit relatively coarse movements of the fingers into much finer movements of instruments required for such a delicate type of operation which, of course, is performed under the field of a microscope. Micropipettes are used to advantage in this type of work; with the development of these micromanipulation technics, investigators began transplanting nuclei from one type of cell to another. Frogs are commonly used because their eggs are large and easy to obtain, as are the embryos, and furthermore, an adult frog develops in less than a year, so that conclusions can be drawn from experiments relatively quickly. Briggs and King (1952) are considered to have been the first to successfully transplant a nucleus in animal cells. In 1962, Gurdon transplanted single nuclei from the intestinal lining cells of tadpoles into enucleated frog eggs and was able to demonstrate that a normal frog would develop from such an egg. He also showed that nuclei removed from cells that were grown in tissue culture from the skin of adult frogs when transplanted to enucleated eggs gave the same result. For details, *see* Gurdon.

As a result of the findings outlined above and other kinds of evidence that have since been obtained, it is now generally conceded that, as far as the problem of differentiation is concerned, it is evident that all body cells in the developing embryo and in postnatal life have exactly the same complement of genes, This finding requires some clarification of the meaning of the term *potentiality*. In common usage, this term does not refer to genetic potentiality but to *cell potentiality*. The reason for cells losing totipotentiality as they differentiate is not due to cells losing genes but because the function of certain genes (probably most genes) in the various kinds of cells that develop in a body remain suppressed. For any as yet undifferentiated cell to differentiate into one particular kind of specialized cell, it is essential that the genes it possesses that would direct it into becoming a different kind of cell remain suppressed. For example, if the genes that would direct a cell into developing into, and functioning as, a brain cell, were also "turned on" in a cell in which the genes that would cause it to become a liver cell were already turned on, the results would be chaotic, Hence, for cells that have complete gene potentiality to become body cells with restricted potentialities requires that only certain genes be turned on and that the great bulk of other genes (that would make it become some other kind of cell) be turned off and for all practical purposes turned off permanently. This probably explains why there is so much condensed chromatin in nuclei; it probably houses the vast number of genes that are for the most part permanently turned off in that particular cell.

The above suggests that the turning on of genes that would cause one particular kind of cell to develop some-

how acts to ensure that the genes that would cause it to develop into any other kind of cell be turned off permanently. This in turn suggests that, as cells differentiate along a specific pathway, there is some kind of negative feedback resulting from the turning on of its genes that direct it along this pathway of differentiation to keep other genes turned off, even though the cell was later exposed to conditions that might otherwise have turned them on. The above-described phenomenon of the turning on of genes that will result in a cell's becoming a certain kind is described in the language of embryology by saying that such a cell is *committed*, which means that it will develop into only a certain kind of cell and not be susceptible to influence by any factors that might otherwise have turned on other genes and made it some other kind of cell. However, before discussing this further, we shall comment on what causes different genes to be turned on (or off) in different cells as a body develops.

THE ROLE OF CYTOPLASM IN THE EXPRESSION AND SUPPRESSION OF GENES

Unlike what happens with regard to the chromosomes when cells of an early embryo undergo mitosis — in which process each daughter cell receives exactly the same complement of genes — the cytoplasm of a cell is not always divided equally either qualitatively or quantitatively. It has been known for a long time that unequal amounts of cytoplasm may be present in the daughter cells that result from cell divisions that occur in the earliest stages of embryonic development. It also became obvious, first in the study of invertebrates, that the different distribution of different specific regions of the cytoplasm of a fertilized ovum to daughter cells was associated with their differentiation into different kinds of cells. It was shown that this was also true in vertebrates in early embryonic development. For interested graduate students, Gurdon gives substantial information on this topic, which is of the greatest interest.

Next, it is generally assumed that, later on in embryonic development or in postnatal life, when any cell divides, the two daughter cells that form are identical with each other and with the mother cell that divided. It is furthermore generally assumed that if daughter cells become different from one another subsequently it is due to their being exposed to different microenvironments. It is obvious that any different environment which could affect the differentiation of a cell would have to do so by adding something to the cytoplasm or by creating some change in some other manner in the cytoplasm that would then set in motion some mechanism that acted in the nucleus to cause the expression of genes not formerly expressed, at least to any substantial degree. However, there are some exceptions to the rule that the daughter cells resulting from a division are identical. There was a concept in the past to the effect that there could sometimes be what was termed a *differentiation division* which resulted in the two daughter cells being different from one another. This was generally visualized as being caused by an unequal division of genetic material so that one daughter cell was different from the other because it possessed a different genetic content. But, as matters turned out, this was not the answer. Gurdon gives a fascinating account of an example of what we think would be considered as a differentiation division, but it is not due to an unequal distribution of genetic material but rather to an unequal distribution of cytoplasm. He notes that in the grasshopper, when cells called neuroblasts (because they serve as the progenitor cells of certain kinds of nerve cells) divide, one daughter cell always differentiates into a fully mature nerve cell while the other always remains as a neuroblast. Gurdon then describes how Carlson in 1953 had been able, by using a fine needle, to rotate the metaphase spindle that developed in the grasshopper neuroblast so that the s-chromosomes (chromatids) that would ordinarily have gone to one pole of the dividing cell would go to the other and vice versa. When mitosis was completed after this operation, it was found that the daughter cell that formed at the pole of the cell that would ordinarily (without the spindle having been turned around) have remained as a neuroblast still did so, while the daughter cell at the other pole of the cell developed into a nerve cell, as it would have done without this intervention. Hence what might have otherwise been conceived of as being a differentiation division, involving an unequal distribution of genetic material, was shown to be due to *the cytoplasm at the two ends of the cell being different,* with that at one end always involving the activation of genes that caused the differentiation of the cell into a nerve cell and that at the other pole not exerting this effect.

The above-described experiment not only provides information to the effect that the cytoplasm can affect gene expression, it also provides information regarding the phase of the cell cycle in which this effect would be exerted. In this instance the cytoplasmic effects must have been exerted after the spindle had been rotated, otherwise the results would have been opposite to those obtained. Since neither of the sets of metaphase chromosomes facing the two ends of the cell were affected until after the spindle was rotated, it would seem unlikely that the cytoplasmic effect was exerted on metaphase chromosomes; instead, the most likely time would seem to be when segments of the condensed chromatin of anaphase chromosomes began to become extended in the telephase in order to transcribe for protein synthesis. The probability would therefore seem to be that the two daughter cells that resulted from mitosis would have somewhat different

segments of their s-chromosomes in an extended state.

The finding described, while most impressive with regard to demonstrating the ability of cytoplasm to affect gene expression, should be regarded as only an illustration of how cytoplasm affects gene expression so as to cause differentiation in early embryonic life. In later embryonic life, and in postnatal life, the microenvironment of the cytoplasm seems to become the important factor in turning genes on or off in the nucleus. However, for the microenvironment of a cell to affect genes, the cell microenvironment must somehow affect the cytoplasm. This could be achieved several ways. For example, something new in the microenvironment can be absorbed by the cytoplasm. Or, its concentration in the microenvironment could change so as to alter the metabolism of the cell. There would be many possibilities, as will be mentioned later. But for an environmental influence to be effective in causing gene expression or suppression, a cell has to be competent. So before proceeding further, another term must be defined and explained.

Competence and Commitment

A cell that can respond to an environmental influence by becoming a cell of a different kind is said to possess *competence* with regard to responding to that particular influence. A cell that does not respond to any environmental influence by becoming different from the type it was before is said to be *committed* or *determined.* We shall give some examples.

The cells of the outer part of the skin are committed. This sometimes creates an awkward situation for the plastic surgeon, for if he transplants whole skin from one part of the body to another, the transplanted skin in its new site will continue to produce the features (for example, hair) that is produced in its original site. However, the tissue that would develop into a particular kind of skin when left in its normal site in early embryonic life, if transplanted to some other site in the embryo, will produce the kind of skin that would normally develop at the site to which it is transplanted. Such a tisssue, for example, embryonic skin, is said to be *competent* because it is receptive to being affected by its environment, and hence its genetic expression becomes different from what it would have been had the tissue been left in its normal site.

Another seemingly very simple example of microenvironment affecting differentiation and hence gene expression in competent cells is illustrated in the development and repair of bones, to be described in detail in Chapter 15. The surfaces of a bone are all covered or lined with the stem cells of bone which are committed to forming either bone or cartilage, but competent to respond to an environmental influence which directs their differentiation into one tissue or the other. When a bone is broken, those near the break multiply rapidly. In the cellular mass that forms to repair the break, those near capillaries differentiate into bone-forming cells while those farther away differentiate into cartilage-forming cells. In-vitro experiments have shown that oxygen concentration is probably the factor that determines which way the stem cells differentiate in this instance.

The above example is given to illustrate that environmental influences that invoke differentiation in competent cells need not be unknown specific agents that defy detection—although some may be—but rather include the supply of known substances that become more available as development proceeds. However, in all instances, agents in the microenvironment that affect gene expression or suppression must somehow act through the agency of the cytoplasm.

Finally, as already described, in each step in differentiation there is a loss in potentiality in the cell that differentiates. As a result there is an increase in the degree to which differentiating cells become determined. Hence determination, along with differentiation, occurs in steps so that although all *end cells* (p. 42), are determined, not all determined cells are necessarily end cells. For example, stem cells in postnatal life, even pluripotential types, are determined with regard to the kinds of cells that can develop from them.

HOW THE CYTOPLASM OF DETERMINED CELLS CAUSES THEM TO PRODUCE DAUGHTER CELLS THAT ARE SIMILARLY DETERMINED

It is easy to visualize that a cell that has become determined will produce daughter cells that are determined in the same way, that "like produce like." But it is not so easy to explain why daughter cells should be determined the same way as their mother cell. If, as was believed in the past, the differentiation of the mother cell into a special type of cell had depended on the occurrence of a genetic mutation, the subsequent determination of its daughter cells could be explained readily. But now that we have accepted that the genetic complement of all cells is the same, we have to explain why genes that are selectively turned on or off in a determined cell are also turned on or off in its daughter cells. It would be easy to assume that genes that have been turned off or on in a mother cell would be duplicated as genes that were turned on or off. However, this possibility seems most unlikely because in the S phase of the cell cycle *all* of the DNA of cells must be duplicated, and in this process each strand of each DNA molecule must transcribe *all* of their genes on the newly forming strands of DNA, including those genes normally quiescent in the condensed chromatin. For genes to transcribe they must be unblocked. What therefore seems more likely than the genes being reproduced in a "turned-on" or "turned-off" form in the S phase is that the intracytoplasmic environment in both of the daughter cells that result from a mitosis is the same as that of the mother cell; hence, after the S phase it turns on or off the same genes that were turned on or off in the mother cell. Determination in different cell lineages would therefore seem to be dependent on the *constancy of the cytoplasm through successive generations.* If cytoplasmic factors did not control gene expression, how could a differentiated nucleus give rise to a complete frog when it is transplanted into an enucleated egg?

GENE EXPRESSION AND DIFFERENTIATION

The function of structural genes in interphase cells is to code for amino acids in sequences that will be transcribed onto mRNA. The code words in turn are translated in the cytoplasm so as to direct the synthesis of particular polypeptides and proteins. Some proteins synthesized in cells serve nonenzymatic functions, but most of them serve as enzymes.

In order for different kinds of cells to develop in a given body as a result of differentiation, the proteins synthesized in some cells must be different from those produced in others. However, not all of them are different because all the cells in the body must synthesize the enzymes required for the fundamental metabolic processes on which the life of its cells depends. But also for the different cells of a body to perform their various specialized functions, they must synthesize the different particular proteins, including enzymes, required for these different functions. Since the synthesis of proteins is dictated by gene expression, it would, therefore, seem that there are two categories of genes. The first kind, which function in all the cells of the body to direct their basic metabolism, would seem to be relatively unaffected directly by factors that evoke differentiation. But the category of genes directing the synthesis of the proteins that account for cells being different from one another would have to be capable of being variously affected during development so that differentiation could occur. Furthermore, when a set of such genes is turned on in a given competent cell it results in the cell's becoming committed, which would seem to indicate that the genes concerned continue thereafter to be selectively expressed or repressed in it and its progeny (if any).

It should be mentioned here that there is a vast number of genes for the differentiation process to draw on. The chromosomes in the various cells of man possess an enormous pool of genes that for the most part are *repressed and reside in the condensed chromatin* of interphase cells. However, it would seem that the genes that are in condensed chromatin in one kind of cell are not necessarily always the same ones that are repressed in other kinds of cells. It would seem moreover that, as cells pass through different stages of differentiation, genes previously in the form of condensed chromatin would appear in the form of extended chromatin, while some previously in the extended form would now become a part of the condensed chromatin.

Finally, a phenomenon termed *induction* appears to be a very important factor in turning on the genes that are responsible for synthesis of the special proteins that cause the cells of the body to become different from one another. So we shall now discuss induction.

The Term *Induction*

As used in science this word generally denotes the phenomenon by which an effect is produced in something by an outside influence. So if cells are caused to differentiate to some degree because of some factor in their immediate environment, the differentiation is said to be the result of *induction*. Hence differentiation, except in the very early stages of embryonic development, is generally believed to occur as a result of induction, that is by the external microenvironment of cells exerting effects which, mediated through or by the cytoplasm, result in different gene expression in cells that are competent to respond to these inductive factors. As mentioned above, it would seem that inductive influences would, therefore, act by turning on the class of genes that directs the synthesis of the particular special proteins produced in specialized lines of cells that thereafter characterize them.

The Basis for Induction

In looking for the kinds of agents that would cause differentiation, we have to look for environmental factors that could modify the expression of genes within the cell in such a way as to cause it to synthesize new proteins. An illuminating example has been found from experimental studies on prokaryotes, specifically bacteria. However, since bacteria do not undergo differentiation as occurs in eukaryotes, the example we are about to describe is not an example of an outside influence inducing differentiation. But it is an example of how an outside environmental influence can change the expression of genes and hence the synthesis of proteins within a cell. This is the kind of phenomenon that has to be understood if the cause or causes of differentiation of eukaryotic cells is ever to be satisfactorily established. The example to which we refer is termed *the induction of an enzyme* and the work we shall briefly describe stems in great part from the brilliant research of Jacob and Monod. The following account is provided for those interested in this aspect of cell biology.

Some Aspects of the Control of Gene Expression in Bacteria

Bacteria synthesize two kind of enzymes, (*1*) constitutive and (*2*) inducible. The constitutive enzymes are those concerned with catalyzing the chemical reactions on which the basic metabolic life of bacteria depend. The genes that code for the production of these enzymes do not require any special environmental factors except proper nutrients to ensure their expression. However, the inducible enzymes are normally produced in only minute or trace amounts. Nevertheless, the fact that these proteins are present in any amount indicates that genes that code for their synthesis must be present in the DNA of the bacteria concerned. The bacteria commonly used for studies in this area are of a kind called *E. coli*. Normally the wild type of *E. coli* utilize glucose for their metabolism. If, however, glucose is not available to them they can utilize lactose but only after it has been converted to glucose, which requires the availability of an enzyme, β-galactosidase, that is ordinarily present in them in minute amounts. However, if only lactose is available this enzyme is produced in large amounts. As this phenomenon was investigated, it became evident that the way the substrate of an enzyme induces the activity of the gene that codes for the amino acid sequence of the enzyme β-galactosidase (an inducible enzyme) is not as simple or direct as might have been expected.

It was found for example that certain galactosides that were not hydrolyzed by β-galactosidase would nevertheless turn on the gene responsible for directing its synthesis. It thus became evident that it was not any participant in the reactions instituted by β-galactosidase that turned on the gene but the galactoside itself. But as matters turned out, the galactoside does not act directly on the gene that codes for the synthesis of β-galactosidase, as was shown by subsequent studies on various mutants of *E. coli*. For example, mutants were discovered that formed large amounts of β-galactosidase even though no galactoside was available to induce the enzyme. This was in turn found to be due to the absence in these mutants of a protein called a *repressor* which was coded for by another gene called an *inhibitory* (or *repressor*) gene and which was located close to the gene that coded for β-galactosidase. (The latter type of gene that codes for the synthesis of the enzyme is termed a *structural gene*.) These findings showed that the reason β-galactosidase was produced in *E. coli* in only small amounts under normal conditions of glucose availability was that the structural gene that codes for it is normally inhibited, not directly, but indirectly, as will soon be explained, by the repressor protein that was coded for by the repressor (inhibitory) gene.

Further work revealed that the matter was even more complicated, for it was found that the genetic defect in the mutants that kept on producing β-galactosidase in the absence of an inducer was not in the repressor gene as had at first been suspected. Instead it was found to be in still another gene, called the *operator* gene, whose normal function is to activate the structural gene that codes for β-galactosidase. The reason certain mutants kept on producing galactosidase in the absence of an inducer was found to be that in them the operator gene did not bind the repressor protein. Hence the operator gene was not inhibited by the repressor protein, and as a result it kept the structural gene continuously transcribing for β-galactosidase synthesis.

It was also found that the repressor protein has, as it were, two binding sites. It can bind either to the operator gene or to the inducer. When bound to the latter, it forms a repressor-inducer complex, and in this form it cannot bind to the operator gene and block its activity. So under conditions of lactose availability and glucose non-availability, the inducer is present and ties up the repressor protein. The operator gene is thus unblocked and hence activates the structural gene that transcribes for β-galactosidase, which is thereupon produced. When the substrate is used up or when there is not enough of it to bind and block the action of the repressor protein, the latter then blocks the operator gene, and hence the structural gene that codes for β-galactosidase is turned off.

It was also established that two other enzymes were induced by lactose beside β-galactosidase, both of which contributed to facilitating the hydrolysis of lactose — one by facilitating entry into the bacterial cell and another whose mode of action is not entirely clear. The genes that code for them are believed to be in sequence with the structural gene that codes for β-galactosidase along the DNA molecule. The whole arrangement constitutes what is termed the *lac operon model*.

Possible Implications With Regard to Differentiation of Eukaryotic Cells

Since the topic under discussion here is differentiation and since differentiation does not occur in bacteria, it might be thought that studies on prokaryotic cells would provide no clue as to how differentiation occurs in eukaryotic cells such as those of man. Furthermore, whereas many highly differentiated eukaryotic cells lose their ability to proliferate, bacteria continue to multiply as long as they are fed. So it might be asked why the study mentioned above could provide any clue as to how differentiation could diminish or stop the proliferation of cells in which it occurs, and hence serve as an intrinsic mechanism for controlling cell populations, a hypothesis we shall soon present. We think, however, that the findings described above are helpful in obtaining some insight into both of these matters. Hence before mentioning that the regulation of gene expression in eukaryotic cells dif-

fers in many respects from that disclosed in bacteria, we shall comment on how we think the bacterial model helps to visualize what could happen in differentiation in eukaryotes.

It seems to us to be very helpful to assume that in eukaryotic cells there would, as in bacteria, be two general categories of genes: one of constitutive, and the other of inducible, genes. It seems helpful, moreover, to assume that the constitutive group would be concerned with directing such protein synthesis as is required for providing the physical structure and metabolic processes required for the basic life processes of a cell and for cell multiplication. Next, the vast number of different genes of the inducible group could be visualized as being concerned with directing the synthesis of the various special proteins that are required for differentiated cells to perform various specialized functions. Thus, the constitutive genes could account for undifferentiated cells living and multiplying. But then when cells encounter microenvironmental influences that exert inductive effects, which in the instance of eukaryotic cells could be enormously complicated but would include the induction of enzymes, the inductive influence would account for groups of inducible genes being turned on to bring about the synthesis of the special proteins required for specialized function.

For those interested in pursuing the topic of the control of gene expression in both prokaryotic and eukaryotic cells, and in a description of a model of gene expression in cells of the latter type, a most interesting, informative and accessible account of this topic is to be found in Lehninger's *Biochemistry* (*see* References and Other Reading).

The Relation of Differentiation to Cell Multiplication

It is an old generalization about differentiation that it is associated with some restriction or even a complete cessation of multiplication in the cell in which it occurs. This association is so prevalent that it suggests a cause-and-effect relationship. For example, when inducible genes (which direct the synthesis of special proteins required in differentiated cells for specialized function) are turned on, it may somehow institute a *negative feedback* on the constitutive genes which beforehand would have been directing protein synthesis for *continued* cell multiplication. The fact that products synthesized under the direction of inducible genes in bacteria can exert a negative feedback effect in blocking genes in the bacterial genome, together with the fact that gene interaction can be so complicated to achieve an effect, would seem to raise the possibility that a negative feedback from products synthesized under the direction of inducible genes could turn off constitutive genes and hence slow or stop further cell growth.

In man, perhaps the most dramatic example of the occurrence of differentiation that involves the synthesis of a special protein responsible for a cell's specialized function, and seeming inhibition of any further cell division, is observed in the formation of erythrocytes (red blood cells). This will now be described briefly. The most undifferentiated cell of the series of cells concerned in erythrocyte formation that can be recognized at the level of the LM is called a *proerythroblast*. Examples of this cell dividing are numerous. Its cytoplasm reveals ribosomes, a finding which is consistent with the translation equipment essential for the function of constitutive genes. Next, proerythroblasts begin to differentiate into what are termed *erythroblasts*. The cytoplasm of these reveals not only an abundance of free ribosomes but also an increasing number of polyribosomes along which specialized proteins can be synthesized. In this instance the polyribosomes are associated with the beginning of the synthesis of hemoglobin, which is the special protein produced by this cell and which serves to perform its particular specialized function as a carrier of oxygen. As the amount of hemoglobin produced in the cytoplasm increases, the proliferative ability of the cell diminishes and indeed, when the production of the specialized protein in the cell has been completed, the constitutive genes no longer support even the life of the cell and its dead nucleus is eventually extruded from it. Thereafter the erythrocyte survives as a non-nucleated cell serving its specialized function without a nucleus for about four months before it is worn out and phagocytosed. Hence, in the instance of the formation of the erythrocyte, it would seem that the turning on of the inducible genes directing the synthesis of the special protein that allows the cell to perform its specialized function, together with the subsequent accumulation of this protein in the cytoplasm, must somehow bring about a negative feedback effect on the constitutive genes which leads not merely to a suppression of cell multiplication but in this instance also to death of the nucleus.

Finally, no matter what mechanism is involved, there must be some mechanism whereby differentiation inhibits the activity of the constitutive genes that direct synthesis for growth. If this were not so, differentiated cells would continue to proliferate as rapidly as undifferentiated cells, and as a result the body would grow to such enormous proportions as to be incompatible with its life processes. It therefore seems reasonable to assume that the turning on of inducible genes, which direct the synthesis of special proteins required for the specialized function that a differentiated cell is to perform, must result in a negative feedback to the constitutive genes, which suppress their activity in directing synthesis for further cell multiplication. This, in our opinion, would constitute an *intrinsic mechanism* for the control of the population of differentiated cells. We shall now pursue this topic further.

WHAT HAPPENS IF THE INTRINSIC CONTROL MECHANISM DOES NOT DEVELOP OR FUNCTION

We have already noted that if there were no intrinsic mechanisms to control cell growth, the body would grow to a size incompatible with life. We shall next deal with what can happen if there is even a single cell in the body that is affected so that thereafter its growth is not controlled by an intrinsic mechanism. Such a cell could continue to grow and proliferate, propagating its own kind, and, unless it and its progeny are effectively treated and eliminated, its progeny eventually overwhelm and destroy the body. This is what happens in what is commonly called *cancer* which, of course, is one of the most important causes of death. As we shall describe, a cancer cell in most instances does not become differentiated to the same extent as its normal counterpart, and indeed an important basis for determining the relative malignancies of different cancers by microscopic examination depends on assessing the extent to which the cells of the cancer are differentiated. Estimates of this can be made at the level of either light or electron microscopy, and several criteria can be used for this purpose, but attempting to describe these would be beyond the scope of this book. However, since we have described the fine structure of cells in some detail, it may be worthwhile to note that the activity of what we have termed the constitutive genes in causing cell growth is mediated through the agency of free ribosomes. These may be relatively abundant in cancer cells. But the amount of rER in the cytoplasm of cancer cells would be less, because the development of this organelle reflects the extent of synthesis of special proteins, which may be enzymes or, in some instances, the precursors of intercellular substances. So it could be hypothesized that the extent of development of rER, in cells of a type in which it is normally prominent, would be a reflection of the activity of what we would term inducible genes in directing specialized cell functions, and hence cancer cells in general could not be expected to contain as great a complement of this organelle as their normal counterparts.

Some Terminology

The cellular growth called a *cancer* is more properly termed a *neoplasm* (Gr. *neos*, new; *plassein*, to form), because this word denotes a growth of *new (abnormal)* cells in the body. Since the neoplasm may form a lump, neoplasms are commonly called *tumors* (L. *tumere*, to swell) even though swellings can be the result of many causes, for example, a bump on the head into which tissue fluid is exuded. Hence most swellings are not neoplasms. We should also note here that there are two main classes of neoplasm, benign and malignant. Here we shall deal only with the malignant variety.

The cells of a malignant neoplasm have long been commonly described as exhibiting *anaplasia* (Gr. *ana,* up, backward + *plassein*), which indicates that their cells are not differentiated to the same degree as their normal counterparts. Indeed a common synonym for anaplasia is *undifferentiation.* Hence neither the internal organization nor the functional capacities of anaplastic cells are well developed, as already noted. More recently a further relevant feature has been established. If normal cells are grown in vitro they respect each other's presence; hence, if one cell abuts on another it acts as if it had good manners and does not push it aside or try to climb over it. This property of normal cells is termed *contact inhibition.* Anaplastic cells, however, do not exhibit this property; when grown in cultures with normal cells they push them aside and climb over them.

The Changed Genome in Neoplastic Cells

It is now generally conceded that cells manifest anaplasia because they have an altered genome. Neoplasia is not due merely to a change in the gene expression of a normal genome, it is due to a changed genome. This fact has been established by chromosome analysis and measurements of the DNA content of cancer cells, most of which (but not all) show variations from the normal in these respects. Another indication of an altered genome is that neoplastic cells transmit their anaplastic nature to their progeny. Why should such genetic changes develop in the body? Since it has been shown that normal cells, cultivated in vitro, will proliferate through only a given number of divisions before they die out — unless a mutant cell appears among them, which will then continue to proliferate — there is some thought to the effect that the reason for neoplasia as an increasingly common cause of death as people become older is that mutations are more prone to occur in cells after they have divided many times. However, it also became known that similar cell mutations could be induced at younger ages by extrinsic agents which gained entrance to the body, beginning with the observation, made long ago, that those whose occupation it was to sweep clean the chimneys of coal-burning fireplaces developed a high incidence of skin cancer, and next the observation that extracts of coal tar painted on the ears of rabbits would induce skin cancer. A vast amount of research has been performed which shows that there are carcinogenic hydrocarbons and many other agents that can cause mutant cells to arise if the body is suitably exposed to them. The discovery of radium and the early use of x-ray examination, moreover, led to the subjection of individuals to what we now know to be harmful amounts of radiation that would cause enough damage to the DNA in their chromosomes for mutant neoplastic cells to originate in their tissues. It was also noticed that even undue exposure to ultraviolet light by whites who exposed their skin to too much sunlight in tropical and subtropical countries caused an increase in the incidence of skin cancer. It is now known that carcinogenic substances can even be produced within the body. The present crusade against industrial pollution and inhaling cigarette smoke is witness to the realization that chemical or physical factors can act somewhere in the cell, often over long periods of time, to produce effects that become progressively obvious when the affected cells are called upon to proliferate, and that these affected cells often increasingly manifest an anaplastic nature because of their DNA having been altered.

The feature of gene expression by the altered genome of neoplastic cells that is of particular interest to the present discussion is that the synthesis of those kinds of proteins that account for cells becoming more differentiated and specialized in their functioning is *diminished,* whereas there is a corresponding relative *increase* in the expression of genes that account for the synthesis of the proteins required for growth. Hence if there is a normal intrinsic mechanism operating that involves a negative feedback of some kind (by means of which the expression of the inducible genes directing the synthesis of enzymes for specialized cell functions normally suppresses the expression of the constitutive genes that direct the synthesis of proteins for growth), a question is posed as to which set of genes is primarily affected in the genetic change that causes neoplasia. It would seem, at least superficially, that because neoplastic cells are characterized by their abundant growth, the constitutive genes that direct growth have not been damaged, by say, a carcinogen. What would seem likely is that the inducible genes, which direct the synthesis of the special proteins characterizing specialized cells, would be the ones gradually damaged by carcinogens, and as a result there would not be proper negative feedback from these to control the expression of the constitutive genes. So what to us would seem worth serious consideration (in view of the hypothesis outlined here) is the likelihood that it would be some change in the inducible genes that would be the genetic change responsible for neoplasia.

There is, however, another mechanism by which neoplasia can be induced, at least in certain experimental animals: this is by viruses, which we shall now consider briefly.

Viruses

Unlike bacteria, viruses are not independently living agents, for they cannot propagate in nutritive, nonliving media. In order to be propagated, they must gain entrance to living cells, generally of specific types and in particular species. A virus is a particle of genetic material, which may be either DNA or RNA, surrounded by a protective coat of protein with or without lipid or carbohydrate. The nucleic acid of a virus particle provides the code for the duplication of the particle, but for this to lead to the production of more virus particles the code requires the translation equipment of a living cell, which, when parasitized by a suitable virus particle, may obligingly and preferentially lend its equipment for the synthesis of more virus particles. Viruses are responsible for many communicable diseases in man. They produce disease by gaining entrance to certain specific types of cells in which virus particles are produced in such numbers that the cells are destroyed. This is called a *necrotizing* (Gr. *nekrosis*, death) type of lesion. Fortunately, however, because virus is thus liberated from the killed cells into the fluids of the body, it is generally brought into contact with the cells concerned with producing antibodies (as described in detail in Chap. 13), and so before long antibodies that react specifically with the virus are produced in quantity and combine with any free virus to render it noninfective. As a consequence, recovery from the virus disease generally ensues, and commonly individuals that suffered from a viral disease are left with enough specific antibody to be immune from further infections, as in the case of measles or chicken pox.

Oncogenic Viruses

Since viruses commonly cause disease by producing necrotizing lesions and kill the cells they infect, it seemed strange that some viruses could cause neoplasia in certain animals. Such viruses are referred to as *oncogenic* (Gr. *onco*, mass or bulk; *genesis*, production of) viruses. It was at first thought that tumor-producing (*oncogenic*) viruses must be of a special kind that failed to multiply rapidly in the cells that they infected. Hence, instead of destroying the cells, it was thought they might irritate the cells sufficiently to stimulate their continuous multiplication. But this was not the answer. After several decades of research it was shown that there were viruses that either in cell cultures or newborn animals could elicit two different responses. In the instance of certain DNA viruses it was shown they could either produce necrotizing lesions and so destroy the cells they infected (a typical virus lesion) or their DNA (or some part of it) could become incorporated into the genome of the cell they infected and thus change the genome so that the cell thereafter was neoplastic. When polyoma virus, so-called because it causes several different kinds of malignant tumors when injected into newborn mice, was injected into newborn hamsters, it was found to cause both necrotizing lesions and malignant transformations of what seemed the same kinds of cells in the kidneys. Further-

more, whereas abundant virus particles could be seen with the EM in the necrotizing lesions, virus particles were not observed in the cells of the neoplasm that it initiated. Hence its DNA was no longer being reproduced in virus particles but only as part of the genome of the cell.

It was subsequently shown that certain RNA viruses could also cause neoplasia in a somewhat similar manner, in that a viral enzyme termed *reverse transcriptase* forms a DNA copy of the viral RNA, and this DNA copy can thereafter become an integral part of the genome of the infected cells and so cause them to exhibit neoplastic behavior.

The finding in experimental animals that virus-derived nucleic acid could become part of the genome of the cell, and thereafter be propagated as part of the genome of the neoplastic cells to which it gave rise, raised great hopes that many or all human tumors would be shown to be due to this cause. If so, they might be susceptible to prevention through the means by which so many virus diseases are now prevented. But, alas, this hope has not been realized. Indeed, as yet no human neoplasia has been conclusively proven to be due to a virus. However, it could be said that since the virus in the form of recognizable virus particles can disappear from the tumors that it causes by integrating its nucleic acid into the genome of a cell, there are difficulties in establishing whether a human tumor might have been caused by a virus.

What we are concerned with here, however, is whether the genetic change responsible for neoplasia is some primary alteration in the constitutive or in the inducible genes. It might be hoped that the study of virus-induced tumors would give some clue about this. In considering the matter superficially, it might seem that since DNA viruses proliferate at a prodigious rate in necrotizing lesions, the DNA of a tumor virus that became incorporated into the genome of a cell might combine with the constitutive genes and have the effect of promoting their growth-directing functions. However, there is evidence to the effect that DNA tumor viruses induce neoplasia by acting in cells that have not yet differentiated, which suggests they may act on inducible genes, and in such a way as to prevent the differentiation that would ordinarily have the effect of restraining growth. Some examples follow.

The Organs in Which Virus-Induced Neoplasms Appear in Experimental Animals

For many of the viruses studied in experimental animals, certain requirements have to be met if they are to induce neoplasia. Commonly, the virus has to be injected into newborn animals (which also must be born of mothers that were free of virus so that the offspring will have no antibodies to the virus). In the instance of polyoma virus, huge neoplasms may develop in the kidneys as little as ten days after a newborn is injected. In mice, neoplasms appear much later. Common ones appear in the salivary glands and later still in the mammary glands. It may be of significance that none of these three organs has completed its development at birth. In all three differentiation, which in other sites occurs in fetal life, continues after birth.

The salivary glands do not develop their specialized secretory units until shortly after birth. The mammary glands do not develop their functional differentiated forms until they are stimulated to do so by sex hormones at the time of puberty, and this is the time when tumors develop in mice given polyoma virus at birth. It is of particular interest that the kidneys, in which polyoma virus injected into newborn hamsters causes relatively enormous malignant tumors to develop very rapidly, have not at the time of birth finished their development, and so this still continues on for a brief period into postnatal life. The same virus injected into older animals does not cause kidney tumors. So, in these instances the virus incites neoplasia in organs where the differentiation that occurs in most organs only in prenatal life is still taking place. Since the neoplastic cells in these particular cases do not differentiate, it is difficult to escape the conclusions that (*1*) the virus-derived genes in the genome somehow interfere with the proper turning on of the inducible genes directing the synthesis of special proteins for differentiation, and (*2*) the intrinsic mechanism that would ordinarily control growth does not develop properly in the virus-infected undifferentiated cells.

Summary

In normal cells differentiation is in general associated with some degree of restriction, or even cessation, of further proliferation. This leads us to hypothesize that there may be some sort of feedback instituted after the inducible genes that direct the synthesis of special proteins required for differentiation become expressed. Such a feedback would diminish or stop the expression of the constitutive genes directing the synthesis of the proteins required for further growth. If so, this would constitute an *intrinsic mechanism* for the control of cell multiplication. In malignant neoplasia, although there are differences in the extent to which differentiation occurs (which is more or less related to the cell line in which the neoplasia develops), it can be safely generalized that differentiation is greatly impaired while the capacity of the cells for proliferation seems relatively unrestricted. Neoplastic cells thus have altered gene expression compared with their normal counterparts. Gene expression in them seems to be directed more toward the synthesis of proteins for continued growth and cell renewal and less for the proteins required for the normal pattern of differentiation and the performance of specialized functions. Hence in neoplastic cells an intrinsic mechanism by which differentiation would control cell multiplication does not appear to function effectively. In any event, it is important to realize that the behavior of neoplastic cells is not typically due to failure of their external environment to control their growth; they behave as they do because their growth does not seem to be restrained by the development of the intrinsic mechanism that ordinarily operates in cells that differentiate.

Next, there are also *extrinsic mechanisms* that can regulate normal cell multiplication and hence control the size of cell populations, so we shall next deal briefly with these.

EXTRINSIC MECHANISMS CONTROLLING THE PROLIFERATION OF CELLS

The term *homeostasis* (Gr. *homeo*, unchanging; *stasis*, standing) refers to the way the internal environment of the body is maintained in a stable condition. For example, the numbers of red and white cells in the blood are maintained at more or less constant levels even though these cells die and require continuous replacement. Hence the production of new cells must be regulated to match their death rate. The blood sugar level stays relatively constant even though sugar is being constantly metabolized and only supplied to the body by the eating of meals, usually supplemented by snacks at irregular intervals. Other mechanisms maintain a constant pH in all the body fluids. Furthermore, the relative sizes of the various organs in the healthy body remain fairly constant throughout life. The maintenance of homeostasis therefore requires that the number of various specialized cells in the body, and the functions demanded of them, be under various control mechanisms that maintain stable conditions.

How are the numbers and activities of different groups of specialized cells controlled? In many instances a signal is given to them to increase their functional activity, for which an increase in cell numbers may be required. In some instances the signal may be perceived by the cells that perform the function but in others, it may be perceived by monitors elsewhere and be delivered by a very circuitous route to the cells that are to be stimulated.

Hormonal Mechanisms

A relatively simple example is provided by the cells of the parathyroid glands. These cells secrete a hormone into the bloodstream that has the effect of raising the level of calcium in the blood. If the blood calcium level falls, this drop is sensed by the cells of the parathyroid glands, which thereupon secrete more hormone. If, however, an animal is on an inadequate diet of calcium, the secretion of more hormone may not be able to raise the blood calcium to a normal level. It seems that the cells of the gland then try even harder, because they then undergo division and increase their numbers for still greater function. Hence the monitoring of decreased function can lead to both increased functional activity and an increase in the population of cells that perform special tasks.

A more complicated situation exists with regard to the maintenance of a normal number of red blood cells in the circulation. When people who live at low altitudes move to mountainous areas, their red blood cells (which transport oxygen to the body cells) become increased in number. This, of course, serves a useful purpose because there is not as much oxygen in the air at high altitudes, so having more red blood cells enables more oxygen to be taken up by the blood as it passes through the lungs. But how does the body of a person moving to a high altitude detect the fact that insufficient oxygen is being delivered to the various parts of the body and how is corrective action instituted? The cells sensing low oxygen (*hypoxia*) in the blood are located in the kidneys. They react by secreting more of a hormone termed *erythropoietin,* which acts on blood-forming cells so as to increase the rate of formation of red blood cells (the mechanism is explained in Chap. 12). When enough extra ones are formed, the oxygen tension becomes raised to normal and the sensor cells then return to making their usual low levels of erythropoietin.

The Responses of the Various Categories of Cell Populations to Increased Demand for Function

In considering this matter further it is helpful to think of how increased demand for function affects the cell populations of the three categories of cells described on page 42. Nerve and striated muscle cells do not divide in adults, so increased demand for function in this instance cannot lead to their proliferation. However, as everyone knows, exercise increases the size of muscles. This is because the cells of muscles become larger instead of more numerous. It would be of interest to know whether nerve cells, of the brain in particular, respond in some way to increased function. Whereas they cannot divide, it is not impossible, as will be discussed in Chapter 17, that they may respond to increased use by developing more processes, which could provide for more connections between them and so, let us hope, help a person think more effectively so as to solve problems of increasing complexity.

The fully differentiated functioning cells of Category 2 are unable to divide. Hence, if there is a need for more of them or the function they perform, there must be some mechanism whereby the particular stem cells responsible

for their origin are caused to proliferate more rapidly than usual, so that more are available to differentiate into end cells and so increase the function or numbers of end cells.

The Control of Stem Cell Populations

At first thought it might seem that an increase in any stem cell population would be due to their reception of a message that would directly stimulate their proliferation. However, from our foregoing discussion on the possibility of an intrinsic mechanism, whereby the turning on of genes for directing the synthesis of the special enzymes required for differentiated function could exert a negative feedback on the genes directing growth, the possibility of another type of control is suggested. First, stem cells, though committed, are not themselves highly differentiated. It might, therefore, be expected that they would not have developed specialized functional activities and hence do not utilize the set of genes that directs the synthesis of the special proteins found in the functional end cells into which they differentiate. Hence stem cells might be expected to lack, at least to some extent, the negative feedback that would repress their constitutive genes directing growth. Why then should they not continually proliferate, instead of merely replenishing their numbers as required? In view of the foregoing, the possibility comes to mind that in the instance of stem cells, proliferation may be controlled at least to some degree by some externalization of the negative feedback that functions in their differentiated progeny. For this to happen, the feedback would have to reach and affect the particular kind of stem cells involved and so keep their proliferation in check. According to this view, if it could be assumed that when the population of end cells becomes unduly reduced and their functional activities thus impaired, there would be a temporary lack of feedback, with the result that their stem cells would proliferate and differentiate into functioning end cells. The feedback from these would then in turn suppress the proliferation of their stem cells. It is of interest that Lord et al. have described an inhibitor of stem cell proliferation.

With regard to the cells of Category 3, in which category the functioning cells of most hormone-producing (endocrine) glands are to be found, we shall find that the functions of most of these are monitored elsewhere and that their functional activity and to some extent the size of their cell populations are controlled by chemical messengers that reach them by circuitous routes, as described in Chapter 25.

The Control of Organ Size

Another possibility that might be considered with regard to the control of cell populations is whether or not the cell populations of different tissues and organs might not be controlled by some mechanism dependent on the total mass of each population being maintained in more or less constant relation to that of the others. It is to be noted that in normal adults the various organs do indeed in general maintain the same general size in relation to each other. It has also been noted that if this is changed artificially, a normal size ratio tends to be restored. For example, it is well known that if two-thirds of the liver of an experimental animal is removed, the liver becomes restored to its normal size, and not beyond its normal size, within relatively few days as a result of extensive proliferation of liver cells. Likewise, it has been observed that if one kidney of an experimenal animal is removed, the remaining kidney nearly doubles in size in a relatively short period of time. One concept that has been proposed to explain this phenomenon is that cell proliferation is controlled by what are termed *chalones* (Gr. *chalan*, to relax).

Chalones

These were originally visualized as antimitotic agents that are cell or tissue specific but not species specific. Specialized cells were postulated to produce their specific chalones. This chalone, when retained by a cell, inhibits its division. However, chalone was believed to be able to leave the cell and diffuse to other adjacent cells or even enter the circulation. If large numbers of specialized cells are lost from the body, as, for example, happens when a large part of the liver is removed, the total amount of chalone produced by the liver cells would be much less than normal. Since the chalone within liver cells was conceived of as being in equilibrium with that in the blood plasma in which liver cells are bathed, the concentration in both the blood and liver cells would thus fall to a low level. Since not enough would stay in the remaining liver cells to suppress their proliferation, they would proliferate until there were enough of them to produce a normal concentration of liver chalone in the blood plasma in which they are bathed, whereupon they would cease proliferating. The growth of one kidney following removal of the other can be explained in terms of the same general concept.

Substances considered to be chalones are obtained for experimental studies by making extracts of the various tissues and organs. However, chalones have not as yet been obtained in pure form. Such information as is available has been interpreted to suggest that they are proteins or glycoproteins with a molecular weight around 30,000 to 50,000, but some may be polypeptides with a much smaller molecular weight. As noted, chalones are believed to be specific with regard to different cell types, tissues, or organs. Hence a chalone that would control the

population of cells of the liver would have no effect on the cells of the kidney, and vice versa. Chalones, however, are not believed to be species specific, and hence a chalone prepared from one species would in all likelihood function in another, which facilitates experimental work with them.

The Epidermal Chalone

Much of the evidence for the existence and function of chalones has come from studies on epidermis, which is the multilayered membrane of epithelial cells that forms the outer part of the skin. In the epidermis the outer cells are always being worn away and lost, so the cellular content of the epidermis must be kept intact by proliferation of cells of the deep layer, at least some of which may be regarded as the stem cells of epidermis. Evidence for an epidermal chalone was obtained by Bullough and Lawrence in 1960. The epidermal chalone is believed to diffuse directly from one cell to another and perhaps locally through the amorphous intercellular substance of the underlying connective tissue. Many experiments seem to show that a loss of epidermal cells, which would reduce the local concentration of chalone in the epidermal area (because it diffuses out of cells) causes proliferation to occur in those that remain. In one experiment the epidermis was removed from one side of the wing of an African fruit bat, whereupon the rate of cell division was greatly increased in the epidermis on the other side of the wing (because chalone presumably diffused through the wing from the untouched side to the other so that its concentration would be reduced on the untouched side). The action of the epidermal chalone, however, is somewhat more complicated than that of others, for it seems to require the help of a hormone (which is probably epinephrine) to form a complex that is stable enough to inhibit cell division. This may explain why it is difficult to obtain a section of epidermis that demonstrates mitotic figures if the tissue is taken during the day (cell division in the epidermis generally occurs at night, a phenomenon termed diurnal mitotic rhythm). The suggested reason for this is that daytime, for most of us, is associated with activity and stress, which accounts for secretion of more epinephrine than during the night, when sleep is the rule. Hence, during the day there is enough epinephrine in the blood to form a complex with epidermal chalone, and this complex is stable enough to block cell division in the epidermis.

The Possible Role of Chalones in Repair

Why, at the site of an injury there should be a local and often rapid proliferation of cells, that in due course restores the original continuity of the tissue involved, has puzzled investigators for decades. But the evidence for the local release of substances that stimulate local growth in repair phenomena is probably no more substantial than the concept that the local cells are released from some mechanism which ordinarily holds their proliferation in check. The chalone concept suggests that repair could be instituted by release of tissues from the effect of their specific chalones that, of course, had diffused away from uninjured cells close to the wound. Indeed it has been claimed that applying epidermal chalone to an epidermal injury slows its repair.

Summary

Since the chalone hypothesis deals with the control of various cell populations in cell states in which there is an extensive division of labor, it, like the same kind of problem that occurs in human societies in which there is a division of labor and expanding population, should likewise arouse our interest and attention. With regard to cell populations, we may be so conditioned by our knowledge of hormones that we visualize them as circulating agents that act only by stimulating the function and growth of the cells they specifically affect, that we disregard the possibility of agents having the opposite effect. However, the concept of chalones stimulates us to think that there may be another side to the coin and that there may be agents that circulate and suppress growth activities in certain sites so as to keep different cell populations in balance. There are, however, criticisms of the chalone hypothesis. For example, chalones have not been obtained in pure form. But the effects of many hormones were established before they were obtained in pure form. It is, however, unfortunate (but understandable) that when chalones were first described they were termed antimitotic agents. Now that the existence of clear-cut antimitotic agents (such as colchicine and other drugs that block the assembly of microtubules upon which the process of mitosis is dependent) is established, and in the absence of any information which would suggest the chalones act on the mitotic process itself, this definition of chalones should be abandoned. If chalones exist, it would seem most probable that they must act directly or indirectly at the level of genes, and at some stage of the cell cycle other than mitosis. However, it may be that the term *chalone* has acquired meanings and associations over past years that render it unsuitable for designating agents produced in the body that presumably must suppress gene expression related to cell multiplication; hence it might be prudent to use a more general term for such agents, for example, *inhibitors*. However, the important thing is to appreciate that there must be mechanisms by which the sizes of cell populations are controlled and that there is a great need

for more information on this subject. Those who originated the chalone concept had vision.

AN INTRODUCTION TO THE FOUR BASIC TISSUES AND THEIR EMBRYONIC ORIGIN

The final section of this chapter deals with prenatal development, in particular with the origin and development of the four basic tissues of which the postnatal body is composed and with which the subject matter of the next 12 chapters is concerned.

Except for the very early development of the embryo, in which the cytoplasm of the fertilized egg is unequally divided (both quantitatively and qualitatively) in forming the cells to which it gives rise, the story of the development of the four basic tissues and the subtypes which form within them is the story of induction bringing about commitment, and various steps in the differentiation, of cells along different pathways of development.

It is to be appreciated that differentiation in the embryo (and also in postnatal life) is associated with a great variety of developing cells changing from being competent to being more committed and less competent. Furthermore, in embryonic life there is a time element involved. Cells that are competent to respond to a given influence at one stage of their development are not competent to respond to that influence before reaching a certain stage of differentiation. In other words, many environmental influences have to exert their effects at specific times for them to be effective. This is important because sometimes the differentiation of cells into a particular type must occur at a given time because cells of this type are in turn essential to act as an environmental influence that will bring about the differentiation of yet other cells that appear in their neighborhood at this particular time.

The inductive phenomena occurring in embryonic development are so complex and often so imperfectly understood that we shall not attempt to describe them in relation to the events that follow one another as an embryo develops.

It should, however, be emphasized that while the induction of enzymes may be one way induction is accomplished, a host of other inductive factors are also involved. Some could be of a general nature, such as the availability of nutrients or oxygen, particular salt concentrations and pH levels, and hormones, as well as possible chemical messengers not yet defined, and so on. Of particular importance is the way mesenchyme somehow influences the development of other forming tissues to which it lies adjacent. However, as noted, induction in embryonic development is such a complex problem that, while accepting that it is the important factor involved in bringing about the changes we shall describe, we shall not

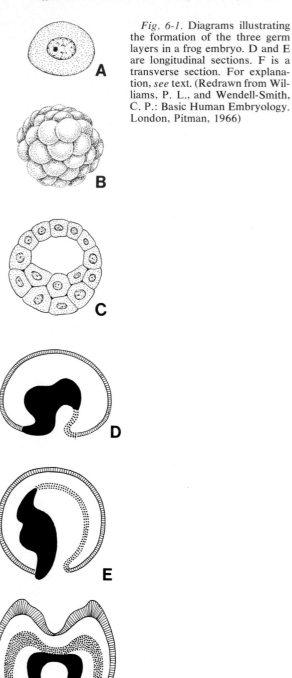

Fig. 6-1. Diagrams illustrating the formation of the three germ layers in a frog embryo. D and E are longitudinal sections. F is a transverse section. For explanation, *see* text. (Redrawn from Williams, P. L., and Wendell-Smith, C. P.: Basic Human Embryology. London, Pitman, 1966)

(*3*) nervous tissue, and (*4*) muscle tissue. These develop in embryonic life from what are termed the three *germ layers* of the developing embryo. It is necessary in histology to know something about the way the four basic tissues develop in prenatal life from the three germ layers. It is also important for those who have not studied embryology to know something about the way the three germ layers develop from the fertilized ovum. This, however, can be described much more simply in amphibians than in man, and for discussing the development of the tissues from the three germ layers the amphibian embryo suits our purposes well.

The Formation of the Three Germ Layers

A fertilized amphibian ovum (Fig. 6-1A) undergoes a series of divisions (*cleavages*) to develop into a *morula* (Fig, 6-1B), so-called because it resembles a mulberry (L. *morus*). The cells of the morula are not all of the same size because as already mentioned, the large store of yolk in the cytoplasm of the fertilized ovum is apportioned unequally as it divides to form the cells of the morula (Fig. 6-1B). Those in its lower half obtain much yolk, which makes the cells there larger than those in the upper half. The morula at this time is described as having two poles, with the smaller cells surrounding the *animal pole* and the larger yolky cells aggregated toward the *vegetative pole*.

As a result of the continuing mitosis, the morula enlarges in such a way as to develop a central cavity that makes it into a hollow sphere (Fig. 6-1C). It was long ago termed a *blastula* (Gr. *blastos,* germ) when it was found it would develop (germinate) into an embryo. The cavity within it is termed a *blastocoele* (Gr. *koilos,* hollow). At this time the cells of the wall nearer the animal pole became smaller and smaller because they continue to divide more rapidly than those nearer the vegetative pole, and hence this part of the blastula (top of Fig. 6-1D) becomes greatly thinned. In Figure 6-1 the site of these cells is indicated by the two parallel lines joined by cross lines at right angles to them. The site thus indicated marks the origin of *ectoderm* (Gr. *ektos,* outer; *derma,* skin), one of the three germ layers. However, the wall of the blastula near its vegetative pole consists of several layers of yolk-containing cells. The sites occupied by these is shown in solid black in Figure 6-1D. As is seen in Figure 6-1D, E, and F, the wall of the blastula at the site (solid black in these figures) becomes invaginated into the developing embryo. This process continues (Fig. 6-1E) so that the invaginated portion of what was part of the wall of the blastula becomes an inner lining of a tube that will become the intestine (Fig. 6-1F). Thus the cells represented by solid black become the *endoderm* (Gr. *entos,* inside), the second of the three germ layers. Since the invagination encroaches into the blastocoele, what was the origi-

attempt to explain how and why it does so in each instance.

As mentioned in Chapter 1, the body is composed of four basic tissues: (*1*) epithelium, (*2*) connective tissue,

nal blastocoele cavity becomes smaller and smaller and in due course becomes obliterated. The new cavity within the invagination (Fig. 6-1E) is termed the *archenteron* (Gr. *arch,* first; *enteron,* intestine) because its wall of yolky cells forms the lining of what will become the gut.

Next, some smaller cells of the animal pole type give rise to the third germ layer, the *mesoderm* (Gr. *mesos,* middle). The site of these cells is shown in stipple in Fig. 6-1D, E, and F. They move inward at the lip of the opening into the archenteron and proliferate to constitute (at first) a part of the wall of the archenteron (Fig. 6-1E). But some then migrate out of this wall and proliferate in such a way as to form a cellular filling (stippled in Fig. 6-1F) that separates the outer wall of the blastula from the wall of the archenteron, which, as noted, goes on to form a tube (black in Fig. 6-1F). Hence the structure that at the blastula stage (Fig. 6-1D) had only one layer for its wall now has three layers in its wall, as shown in Figure 6-1F. To summarize: there are (*1*) an outer layer (cross-hatched in Fig. 6-1F) which is constituted of cells of the animal pole and is called *ectoderm;* (*2*) an innermost layer of cells that constitutes the wall of the archenteron and, in due course, forms a tube (black in Fig. 6-1F); this layer of cells is termed the *endoderm* (or *entoderm*); and (*3*) a middle layer between the ectoderm and the endoderm. This layer, stippled in Figure 6-1F, is at first termed the *chorda-mesoderm* because as the developing embryo enlongates its cells form (among other things) a long structure lying axially along the developing embryo, called the *notochord,* around which the vertebrae subsequently form. Other cells of this middle layer, which in due course comes to be called *mesoderm,* form most of the muscle of the embryo and also its skeleton and other connective tissue structures. It is obvious that the possibilities for inductive phenomena between the cells of the different germ layers and the various lines of cells that develop from them from here on can have an enormous influence in determining the further steps in development.

Before long, the embryo attains a more or less oval outline in cross section and is covered with a layer of ectoderm (Fig. 6-1F). Within this lies the developing gastrointestinal tube, lined with *endoderm.* The outer part of the wall of the gastrointestinal tube (black in Fig. 6-1) is derived from tissue that is in turn derived from mesoderm. Between the endoderm and the ectoderm, the mesodermal cells are more compact dorsally than ventrally, which is where the body cavity, the *coelom,* will form. The denser mesoderm forms the vertebrae and a little farther away it gives rise to most of the muscles of the body. The remainder of the mesoderm gives rise to the connective tissue of the body. In forming this, as well as some muscle, the mesoderm first gives rise to a soft tissue called *mesenchyme* (Gr. *mesos,* middle; *enchyma,* infusion), which consists of undifferentiated mesenchymal

cells separated from one another by a gelatinous intercellular substance that they form. Mesenchyme will be discussed in detail in Chapters 8 and 9.

THE DEVELOPMENT OF THE FOUR BASIC TISSUES FROM THE THREE GERM LAYERS

The four basic tissues are (*1*) epithelium, (*2*) connective tissue, (*3*) nervous tissue, and (*4*) muscle tissue. Before describing their origins from germ layers, we shall comment briefly on the way the tissues were classified.

The Basis on Which the Tissues Were Classified

The thinking student will soon find the classification of the four basic tissues of the body unsatisfactory in certain respects, but the point to make here is that the four tissues were not classified on the basis of their embryological origin from the three germ layers, but chiefly on their microscopic structure and the functions they perform. However, it so happens that most epithelial tissue develops from ectoderm and endoderm, but not all of it, because some is derived from mesoderm. Connective tissue is derived from mesoderm. Muscle tissue is almost entirely derived from mesoderm, but a little is derived from ectoderm. Nerve tissue is derived from ectoderm. But, as we shall see, what is termed muscle tissue is not pure muscle because of its being composed of a mixture of pure muscle fibers and connective tissue. Likewise, some of what is termed nerve tissue has mesoderm-derived connective tissue mixed with structures that developed from ectoderm. Nevertheless the classification of the tissues, though imperfect, is enormously useful.

EPITHELIAL TISSUE (EPITHELIUM)

From its derivation the term *epithelium* (Gr. *epi,* upon; *thele,* nipple) refers to something that covers (is upon) nipples (the nipples here referred to when the term was coined were the little capillary-containing connective tissue papillae that project into the transluscent epithelium covering the lips; the blood in these capillaries just beneath the surface gives the lips their color). From this beginning the term *epithelium* came to be used for all covering and lining membranes in the body that are composed of contiguous cells. The epithelial part of the skin (which is its outer part) develops from ectoderm. The continuous layer of cells that lines the intestinal tract is derived from endoderm while that lining the peritoneal (body) cavity is derived from mesoderm. However, while the latter is true epithelium because it is a cellular lining membrane, it is generally termed

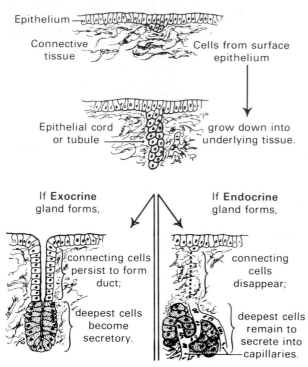

Fig. 6-2. Diagrams illustrating how exocrine and endocrine glands develop.

mesothelium because of its origin from mesoderm. Likewise, the epithelium that lines the blood vessels and the heart and is also derived from mesoderm is not generally called epithelium but *endothelium*. These distinctions were believed to be useful, not because the normal appearances of these types are different from similar ectoderm or endoderm-derived epithelium but because they behave differently from ectoderm or endoderm-derived epithelium under certain pathological conditions.

All covering and lining epithelial membranes are composed of cells joined together by cell junctions, the types of which will be described in the next chapter. Epithelial membranes are all supported by connective tissue, the capillaries of which are responsible for nourishing the epithelial cells of the membrane (Fig. 7-1), while the intercellular substances of connective tissue support both the capillaries and the epithelium. External epithelial membranes, however, except for those of the lips and a few other sites, are not translucent, so blood in capillaries cannot be seen through the epithelium of the skin except in special circumstances when the capillary bed of the underlying connective tissue becomes expanded as, for example, in blushing or sunburn.

GLANDS

Some or all of the epithelial cells of many membranes elaborate a secretion onto the free surface of the membrane. An example is the epithelial membrane that lines the intestine, which must always be kept wet. However, in many body sites the need for secretion is too great to be satisfied by the limited number of secretory cells that can be accommodated in a covering or lining membrane, and furthermore they are not suited to the function of some membranes. To provide for extra secretion, the cells of the epithelial membrane at these body sites, during the development of the embryo, grow into the underlying developing connective tissue (as illustrated in Fig. 6-2) to form structures that were called *glands* (L. *glans,* acorn) because some of the first that were studied were shaped like acorns.

Exocrine and Endocrine Glands

The most common type of gland is the *exocrine* (Gr. *ex,* out or away from; *krinein,* to separate). As this name suggests, an exocrine gland delivers its secretion onto the surface from which the gland originated and hence *outside* the substance of the body. To do this exocrine glands possess tubes called *ducts* that convey the secretion produced in the more deeply located secretory cells to the surface (Fig. 6-2, *lower left*).

The other type of gland is of the *endocrine* (Gr. *endo-* + *krinein,* to separate) type. These develop in the same way as exocrine glands except that the cellular connection with the surface (which they do at first have and which in an exocrine gland would become a duct) is lost; hence endocrine glands have no ducts (Fig. 6-2, *lower right*). Endocrine glands therefore are constitued of islands of epithelial secretory cells surrounded by connective tissue and hence can only deliver their secretions into the substance of the body. Most of their secretory cells have a close association with the blood capillaries of connective tissue (Fig. 6-2, *lower right*) into which their secretions gain entry and are thus carried all over the body. Endocrine secretions are chemical substances generally called *hormones* (Gr. *hormaein,* to arouse to activity or spur on), which in very small amounts exert important physiological effects in the various parts of the body to which they are carried by the blood in both prenatal and postnatal life, as described in Chapter 25.

MESODERM AND CONNECTIVE TISSUE

Connective tissue develops from *mesenchyme,* a derivative of mesoderm. Since it is derived from the middle germ cell layer, it is in a good position to nourish and support epithelial membranes and glands that develop from ectoderm and endoderm. Blood cells, the heart, and the blood vessels of various sizes, through which blood is pumped all through the body, are also formed from cells that develop in the mesenchyme and hence throughout life *blood circulates in vessels that are confined to connective tissue.* As might be expected in the development of any epithelial glandular structure, epithelial cells and connective tissue develop in close association with one another (Fig. 6-2); hence the epithelial cells are provided with nutrients.

As already mentioned, connective tissue is unique because many varities of it consist chiefly of nonliving materials called *intercellular substance* (p. 9) produced by certain kinds of connective tissue cells. Details are given in Chapters 8 and 9. The cartilage and bone of the skeleton, as well as ligaments, fasciae and tendons, all develop from mesenchyme and represent types of connective tissue that consist chiefly of intercellular substance. In these the chief role of the connective tissue cells is to produce and maintain the intercellular substances. But there are other kinds of connective tissue that are essentially cellular, and in these there are other particular kinds of connective tissue cells that are concerned, not with producing intercellular substances, but with other functions, in particular with the various reactions that defend the body against foreign agents of many kinds. Among these are the white cells of the blood. All blood cells as well as all blood vessels are of mesenchymal origin.

ECTODERM AND NERVOUS TISSUE

At a very early stage of development the mid-dorsal ectoderm of the embryo becomes depressed axially along the midline of the embryo (Figs. 6-1F and 6-3) to form the *neural plate.* This plate of ectodermal cells sinks more deeply to form the *neural groove* (Fig. 6-3). The edges of the groove then come together and fuse so that the groove becomes a tube lying just below the ectodermal surface (Fig. 6-3). This tube extends all the way from the head to the tail of the developing embryo. In the head region the walls of the tube thicken to develop into the brain (a gross cross-section of which is illustrated in Fig. 6-3). Along the remainder of its course toward the tail region, the wall of the tube thickens to become the *spinal cord* (labeled in Fig. 6-3). As described in more detail in Chapter 17, the ectodermal cells of the walls of the tube give rise in both sites to nerve cells (called *neurons*) and cells that support them (called *neuroglia* cells from the Gr. *glia*, glue). Small masses of nerve tissue become detached along the tube where the edges of the groove become fused, and

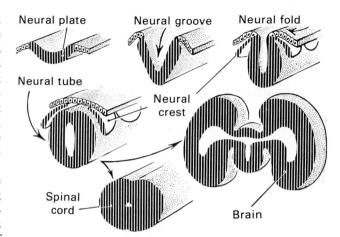

Fig. 6-3. Diagrams illustrating how ectoderm forms a neural plate (*top left*), which then goes on to develop a neural groove (*top middle*) and later becomes the neural tube (*middle left*). In the head region the neural tube develops into the brain (*lower right*) and in the remainder of the body it forms the spinal cord (*bottom middle*).

these remain scattered along the tube on each side of its posterior aspect to become what are known as the *cerebrospinal ganglia* (Gr. *ganglion,* a knot-like mass). They too are composed of nerve cells and supporting cells.

Cytoplasmic fibers grow out from the bodies of the nerve cells that develop in the ectodermally derived tube of nerve tissue that becomes the brain and spinal cord, and other nerve fibers grow out from the bodies of the nerve cells of the ganglia. There is also some migration of nerve cells to certain body parts. The nerve fibers that grow out from the tube and ganglia enter the mesoderm that is becoming connective tissue. Here each nerve fiber becomes surrounded by a sheath of delicate connective tissue. Nerve fibers commonly become grouped together to become the nerves (in which the nerve fibers are individually and collectively ensheathed with connective tissue). These are the nerves seen in dissections of the various parts of the body.

MESODERM AND MUSCLE TISSUE

Muscles are composed of muscle cells, which are called *muscle fibers* because they are elongated. The muscle fibers in a muscle are individually surrounded by a delicate connective tissue that brings a blood supply close to them. Bundles of fibers and whole muscles are also wrapped in connective tissue. The various wrappings of muscle fibers fuse at the ends of muscles to provide attachments to tendons composed of strong connective tissue, or connective tissue structures of other types that attach the muscles to the structures on which they pull. Both the muscle fibers and the connective tissue wrappings are regarded as part of muscle tissue and both arise from the middle germ layer.

REFERENCES AND OTHER READING

Gene Expression

Gurdon, J. B.: The Control of Gene Expression in Animal Development. Cambridge. Harvard University Press, 1974.
Jacob, F., and Monod, J.: Regulatory mechanisms in the synthesis of proteins. J. Mol. Biol., *3:*318, 1961.
Lehninger, A. L.: Biochemistry, ed. 2. New York, Worth Publishers, 1975.

Carcinogenesis (General)

Farber, E.: Carcinogenesis—cellular evolution as a unifying thread. Cancer Res., *33:*2537, 1973.

Viral Carcinogenesis In Vivo and Its Relation to Differentiation

Axelrad, A. A., et al.: Induction of tumors in Syrian hamsters by a cytopathogenic virus derived from a C3H mammary tumor. J. Natl. Cancer Inst., *24:*1095, 1960.
Ham, A. W., et al.: The histopathological sequence in viral carcinogenesis in the hamster kidney. J. Natl. Cancer Inst., *24:*1113, 1960.
Howatson, A. F., et al.: Studies *in vitro, in vivo,* and by electron microscopy of a virus recovered from a C3H mouse mammary tumor. Relationship to polyoma virus. J. Natl. Cancer Inst., *24:*1131, 1960.
McCulloch, E. A., et al.: Carcinogenesis in vivo by polyoma virus. Can. Cancer Conf., *4:*253, 1961.

Cell Differentiation and Its Relation to Neoplasia

Saunders, G. F. (ed): Cell Differentiation and Neoplasia. New York, Raven Press, 1977. (A very complete and up-to-date reference on this topic is to be found in this publication of the papers presented at a relatively recent symposium held on this subject, which is now the object of so much research.)

Chalones and Inhibitors

Bullough, W. S.: Chalone control systems. *In* Lobue, J., and Gordin, A. S. (eds.): Humoral Control of Growth and Differentiation. New York, Academic Press, 1973.
Houck, J. C. (ed): Chalones. Amsterdam, North-Holland, 1976.
Lord, B. I., Mori, K. J., Wright E. G., and Lajtha, L. G.: An inhibitor of stem cell proliferation in normal bone marrow. Br. J. Haematol., *34:*441, 1976.
Mauer, H. R.: Chalones: Specific regulators of eukaryote tissue growth. *In* Talwar, G. P. (ed.): Regulation of Differentiated Function in Eukaryote Cells. New York, Raven Press, 1975.

PART THREE

THE TISSUES OF THE BODY

In this section of the book we describe the microscopic structure and the general functions of the four basic tissues and their various subdivisions.

7 Epithelial Tissue

What the Student Should Learn from this Chapter. Pehaps the first thing to be learned is the appearance of the main types of epithelial membranes and glands in sections taken from representative parts of the body, so that they will be easily recognized in the laboratory. Of equal importance is appreciation of how the microscopic structure of the different membranes and glands is related to their general functions.

What the Student Should Not Attempt to Learn from this Chapter. It should be explained that in order to demonstrate the main types of epithelial membranes and glands, it is necessary to use sections of organs or specialized structures assembled from the tissues of the body. But students on seeing illustrations of these may assume they are supposed at this time to learn the microscopic structure of the entire organ or specialized structure illustrated and not merely that of the epithelium they illustrate. This task will come later after learning the nature and microscopic structure of all four tissues. Hence in the following, in order to demonstrate different kinds of epithelial membranes, we shall use illustrations of skin, intestine, kidney, cervix of uterus, trachea, and urinary bladder. Learning the microscopic structure in relation to function of all these organs should not however be attempted here; it will be considered in Part Four of this book, after we have dealt with all the tissues. Nevertheless, this is not meant to imply that one should not learn anything about these things while studying the tissues, but to reassure the student that they will be dealt with again in detail in Part Four, when all the facts are in so that the task will be much easier. For example, skin is composed of three major components, namely an epithelial membrane of a special type, epithelial glands, and connective tissue. But it also contains some muscle and nerve tissue. So although one cannot avoid learning something about skin here, no attempt will be made to describe it in detail until Chapter 20.

EPITHELIAL COVERING AND LINING MEMBRANES

The origin and general nature of epithelial tissues are described on page 181. As noted, it is helpful to classify epithelium into two divisions: (*1*) covering and lining membranes and (*2*) glands.

We shall deal here with membranes and begin by explaining the difference between a covering and a lining.

A Lining Is Always a Covering but a Covering Is Not Always a Lining. These terms are easily misused with regard to epithelial and other membranes in other tissues. The term *lining* can only be used with reference to hollow structures that have two surfaces, an outer and an inner, for it refers only to a membrane that covers the inner surface of a hollow structure. Hence the term *covering* can only be used with reference to an inner surface if it is made clear that one is speaking of a surface and not the structure itself. If some substructure projects into the cavity of a main structure lined by membrane, the substructure must be said to be covered, not lined, by the membrane lining the main structure, because it is its outer surface that projects into the cavity.

General Features of Epithelial Membranes in Relation to Their Functions

Composition. Epithelial membranes are composed entirely of cells. For epithelial cells to constitute a continuous membrane their edges are connected together by what are termed *cell junctions,* as will be described presently. Such membranes are of different thicknesses. As a glance at Figure 7-3 will show, some are only one cell thick, and the cells of such membranes may be either very thin (Fig. 7-3a) or else tall (Fig. 7-3c). Other types of membranes, however, may be several cells in thickness (Fig. 7-3f and 7-1).

How Epithelial Membranes Are Supported and Nourished. As shown in Figure 7-1, which illustrates a thick membrane, there are *no capillaries* among the epithelial cells of a membrane. Hence for oxygen and nutrients to reach its cells they must diffuse through the intercellular substance of the underlying connective tissue from its capillaries (Fig. 7-1). The intercellular substances of the underlying connective tissue also provide support for the membrane. Attachment is provided to the connective tissue by a component termed a *basement membrane,* a thin and somewhat complex layer of intercellular material lying

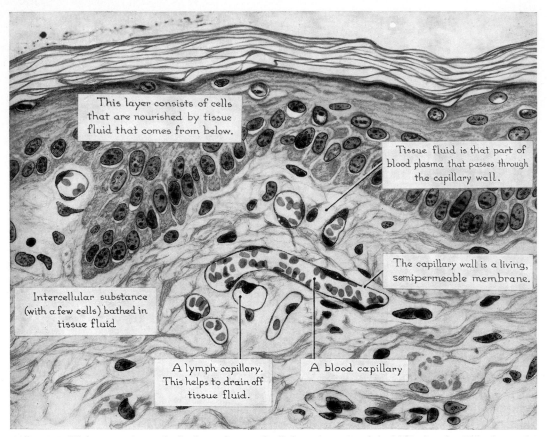

This layer consists of cells that are nourished by tissue fluid that comes from below.

Tissue fluid is that part of blood plasma that passes through the capillary wall.

Intercellular substance (with a few cells) bathed in tissue fluid.

The capillary wall is a living, semipermeable membrane.

A lymph capillary. This helps to drain off tissue fluid.

A blood capillary

Fig. 7-1. High-power (retouched) photomicrograph of the outer part of the skin of a pig. This shows the epidermis above and the capillaries surrounded by intercellular substance below, and explains how tissue fluid must migrate from capillaries to nourish the epithelial cells (epidermis).

between the epithelium and the connective tissue. This does not stain very well with H and E but is sometimes seen as a pale, seemingly structureless band (labeled in Fig. 7-9). It is, however, stained to advantage by the PAS technic, as shown in Figure 7-2, B.M., where it lies beneath a single layer of epithelial cells. The nature of the basement membrane and the way it is formed is described in the next chapter on connective tissue (page 222).

The outermost layer of the kind of epithelium illustrated in Figure 7-1 is composed of a protein called *keratin* and because it gradually wears away it must be constantly replaced. This requires that the deepest cells in the membrane divide so that new cells move from the deepest layer to the more superficial layers. As cells approach the layer of keratin they die and become converted into keratin as described in more detail in the chapter on skin (Chap. 20).

Functions. A basic function of epithelial membranes is protecting the connective tissue they cover. However, in some instances, certain cells of a membrane also serve a

secretory or absorptive function. For instance, occasional secretory cells may be interspersed among other supporting cells of a membrane as shown in Figure 7-3d. Here the secretory cells provide a viscous fluid that flows over the surface of the other cells of the membrane to keep it wet and slippery.

While providing protection, some epithelial membranes also serve a second and very important function of selective absorption. For example, absorptive cells of the epithelial membrane lining the small intestine absorb only certain components of the contents of the intestinal tube. The epithelial cells then pass the materials they absorb into the body substance, where it is taken up either by blood or lymphatic capillaries. Likewise, in the kidney we find examples of the epithelial walls of the tubules selectively resorbing certain components from a filtrate of blood plasma so that these are conserved and not lost in the urine.

Moreover, very thin epithelial membranes in some sites (Fig. 7-3a) may permit passage of fluid through them and so serve more or less as dialyzing membranes that permit

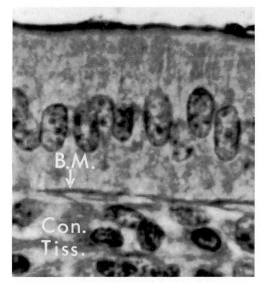

Fig. 7-2. Photomicrograph of mouse intestinal epithelium, stained by the PAS technic. Mucus on the free surface of the cells is stained, as is the basement membrane (B.M.) between the epithelial cells and the connective tissue (Con. Tiss.) beneath.

water and ions to pass through them but hold back macromolecules. Examples are given in later chapters.

Since the main purpose of epithelial membranes is to provide protection, it may help to note that this is of two main kinds. First, some membranes must withstand much wear and tear. For example, the esophagus, the tube through which chewed food has to pass to reach the stomach, has a protective lining several cells in thickness, of the type shown in Figure 7-3f; this is particularly necessary in animals that swallow chewed-up bones. However, a second kind of protection is needed on surfaces exposed to air, such as skin, to prevent the cells beneath the membrane from becoming dried out. This is provided by the multilayered epithelial membrane having an outer layer of cells that have become converted into relatively impervious *keratin* (Fig. 7-1, *top*). This outer layer not only protects the underlying cells from becoming dehydrated but also keeps the body from soaking up water when one has a bath. The epithelial membrane of the skin is also thick; this and its outer layer of keratin make it protective against wear and tear. Calluses are mostly keratin and they are formed where there is much wear.

Protection against body cells drying out because of contact with air is also essential in the respiratory tract. However, it is done differently here. The epithelium lining the nasal passageways through which air is drawn and expelled is richly provided with secretory cells that produce mucus to keep the surface wet. Furthermore, there are many little glands beneath the surface whose ducts open onto it to provide extra fluid to keep it always wet.

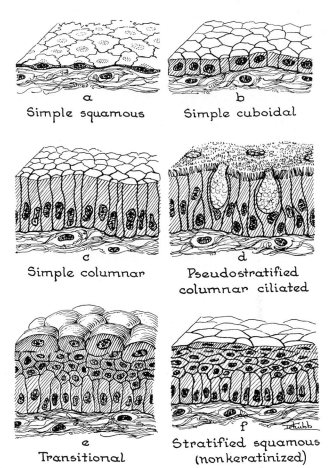

Fig. 7-3. Three-dimensional illustrations of the various types of epithelial membranes found on wet surfaces.

The tubes leading to the lungs also have a similar lining of epithelium and also many glands to keep their inner surface wet. In the respiratory portion of the lungs, where there is interchange of oxygen and carbon dioxide between blood in capillaries and air in air sacs, the lining of these sacs must be very thin because gasses must diffuse back and forth between blood and air. In this instance, dialyzed fluid exudes from the capillaries and through the thin epithelium lining the air sacs and thus always keep their inner surface wet. From the foregoing it is obvious that the kinds of epithelium found in differing covering or lining membranes are adapted to performing the particular functions required. Specific examples are given in later chapters.

We now name and describe the different types of epithelial membranes found in the body.

The Terms Simple, Stratified, and Pseudostratified Epithelium. If an epithelial membrane consists of only a single layer of cells it is said to be a *simple epithelium* (Fig.

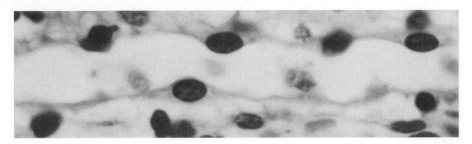

Fig. 7-4. Photomicrograph of part of a kidney tubule (thin-walled portion of loop of Henle) of rabbit kidney, showing simple squamous epithelium. Note that the cytoplasm is very thin and the nuclei bulge out into the lumen.

7-3a, b, and c). If, however, it is two or more layers of cells in thickness, as shown in (*e*) and (*f*) of Figure 7-3, it is said to be *stratified epithelium*. If some cells of a membrane reach from its bottom to its surface but others extend from the bottom only part way to the surface, the membrane is said to be *pseudostratified;* an example is shown in (*d*) of Figure 7-3. The reason for this name is that in a section an observer can see two rows of nuclei, due to the nuclei of the shorter cells forming a row closer to the bottom of the membrane than the row of nuclei belonging to the taller cells; the two rows of nuclei give the false impression of there being two layers of cells.

Epithelial membranes are classified not only as to whether they are simple, stratified, or pseudostratified but also according to the kinds of cells they contain. We shall first describe the classes of epithelium found on wet surfaces.

SIMPLE EPITHELIAL MEMBRANES

Simple Squamous Epithelium

An epithelial membrane composed of a single layer of very thin cells, as illustrated in Figure 7-3a, is termed a *simple squamous epithelium* (squamous means scale-like). This type of epithelium generally does not appear to advantage in sections cut through it at right angles (Fig. 7-4). The nuclei of squamous cells are thicker than the cytoplasm and create bulges on the membrane (Fig. 7-4). In this plane of section (cut at right angles to the membrane), the cytoplasm of simple squamous cells is so thin that it sometimes cannot be seen at all with the LM and hence only the somewhat flattened nuclei, distributed along the surface, may be visible.

Because simple squamous epithelium usually does not show to advantage in sections, the endothelium lining blood vessels or the mesothelium lining the great body cavities (pleural, pericardial and peritoneal) is often studied instead. The organs in the body cavities are covered by a similar layer of mesothelium and in between the layer of squamous epithelium (mesothelium) lining the

cavity and that covering the organs there is a thin film of fluid that allows movement of the organs within the cavity. Mesothelium can be prepared and studied in flat mounts, which allows the surface of the membrane to be examined directly. In this type of preparation it has the appearance of the flat surface seen from above in Figure 7-3a, after suitable staining (for example, after staining with silver nitrate, which blackens the borders between adjacent cells).

The medulla of the kidney is a good site for studying sections of simple squamous epithelium, but it may be difficult for the inexperienced student to find good examples (like the one in Fig. 7-4) until the kidney has been studied as an organ.

Simple Cuboidal Epithelium

The cells of simple cuboidal epithelium do not actually have the shape of cubes. Cuboidal epithelium was given its name because of the way it appeared in sections cut through it at right angles. As shown in Figure 7-3b, the cut surfaces of the cells in such a section are indeed roughly square. But in the surface view provided by Figure 7-3b, the cells have an irregular hexagonal appearance and hence are not true cubes.

Simple cuboidal epithelium is not found in very many sites in the body other than the ovary, where it forms a covering for that organ, and the epithelium lining small collecting tubules in the medulla of the kidney (Fig. 7-5).

Simple Columnar Epithelium and the Various Ways Its Structure Is Modified for Special Functions

There are several subtypes of simple columnar epithelium. In all these the basic structure is similar in that the cells are more tall than wide and are joined together side by side by means of cell junctions. As shown in Figure 7-3c, a surface view shows that the cells of simple columnar epithelium also tend to be hexagonal, which permits them to be fitted together efficiently.

Unmodified Simple Columnar Epithelium. Examples are not very numerous and are found only in sites where the

Fig. 7-5. Photomicrograph of part of the wall of a collecting tubule of rabbit kidney, showing simple cuboidal epithelium.

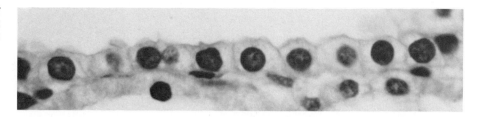

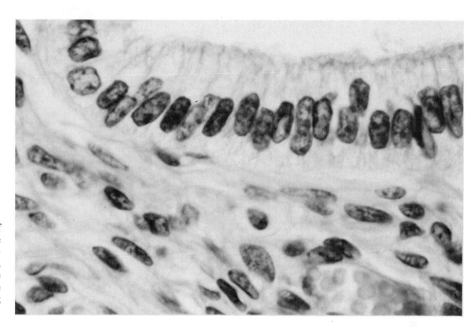

Fig. 7-6. Photomicrograph of the lining of the canal of the uterine cervix, showing simple columnar secretory epithelial cells, all of which are alike. Note the proximity to the epithelium of the blood vessel in the underlying connective tissue (*bottom right*).

chief function of the epithelium is to provide protection along some wet surface and not to engage to any great extent in secretory or absorptive activities. Here the cells all resemble one another. Their cytoplasm stains lightly in H and E sections. One place to find epithelium of this type is in some ducts of glands (Fig. 7-27, *center*). Here, however, the simple columnar cells may be secretory to some extent, elaborating watery secretions.

Most simple columnar epithelium, however, is modified to perform, in addition to a protective function, either specialized secretory or absorptive functions. We shall now consider some examples.

Secretory Simple Columnar Epithelium. In this subtype all the cells are specialized to secrete mucus. Since they cannot all individually bulge sideways when full of mucus they all remain columnar in shape. Two sites where this type of epithelium is found are (*1*) the lining of the stomach and (*2*) the lining of the cervical canal of the uterus (Fig. 7-6). In H and E sections the cytoplasm of all the cells in an epithelial membrane of this type have much the same light and somewhat frothy appearance, caused by the cytoplasm being packed with membrane-bounded

vesicles of mucus destined for secretion from the free end of the cell; since mucus does not stain with H and E, the cytoplasm superficial to the nucleus in cells of simple columnar epithelium of this type appears pale and vacuolated (Fig. 7-6). With the PAS technic the cytoplasm stains similarly to that of goblet cells (described below).

Simple Columnar Epithelium Composed of Both Secretory and Absorptive Cells. This is ideal for lining for the small intestine, because, if effective absorption is to occur, the membrane can be only one cell thick. Also, since it is subjected to a good deal of wear and tear, it helps to have its surface coated with mucus, a protective slippery fluid. Since absorptive cells (specialized for absorption) are interspersed with mucus-secreting goblet cells, there are enough goblet cells to provide a protective coating of mucus over the whole inner surface of the membrane as is shown in the PAS stained preparation in Figure 7-7.

Goblet Cells. As already described in Chapter 5 and illustrated in Figures 5-30 and 5-31, where mucus-secreting cells are interspersed with some other kind of cell—in this instance, absorptive cells—a mucus-secreting cell can assume the form of a goblet because the portion

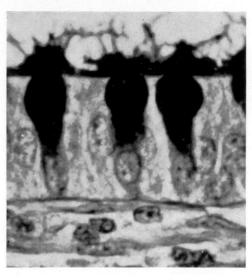

Fig. 7-7. Photomicrograph of intestinal epithelium (mouse) stained by the PAS technic. Three goblet cells are evident, with their secretion flowing over the free surfaces of the adjacent absorptive cells. The basement membrane extends along the lower aspect of the epithelium where it abuts on the connective tissue beneath.

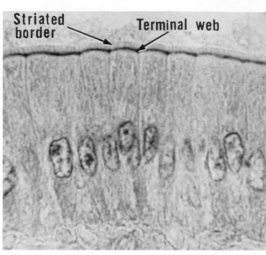

Fig. 7-8. Photomicrograph of simple columnar absorptive epithelial cells (rat intestine) stained with tannic and phosphomolybdic acids and amido black to show the terminal web in the cells. Note also the striated border immediately above the terminal web.

packed with membranous vesicles of mucus can expand to assume a bowl-like shape by indenting the cytoplasm of the absorptive cells beside it. The nuclei of goblet cells, as is shown in Figure 7-7, lie in the narrow stem-like portions of the cells, close to their bases.

Absorptive Cells, Striated Borders, and Microvilli. The absorptive cells of intestinal epithelium may be seen with the LM to be covered with a thin layer with a refractive index different from the underlying cytoplasm (Fig. 7-8). In good preparations it was possible with the LM to see fine striations (lines or stripes) in this layer, perpendicular to its free surface (Fig. 7-8), so it was termed a *striated border*. With the advent of the EM, the striations on the free surface of the cells were found to be due to minute finger-like projections termed *microvilli* (Fig. 5-7), described on page 157. (The beginning student should be careful to distinguish the term *striated*, as in striated border, from the term *stratified*, which means more than one layer in thickness).

Simple Columnar Ciliated Epithelium. Another combination of cells found in simple columnar epithelial membranes is that of goblet cells intermixed with ciliated cells. The fine structure of the latter is described on page 151 and illustrated in Figures 5-50 to 5-54 inclusive (pp. 152–155). The cilia beat in such a way as to move mucus along the membrane. This type of epithelium is found in some parts of the upper respiratory tract, but it is not as common here as another type which is called pseudostratified columnar ciliated epithelium.

PSEUDOSTRATIFIED EPITHELIUM

Pseudostratified Columnar Ciliated Epithelium With Goblet Cells

As already described, in pseudostratified epithelium some of the cells in contact with the basement membrane do not reach the surface (Fig. 7-3d), but many do reach the surface, and this gives a false impression of being stratified because sections cut at right angles to its surface show nuclei at two levels. Pseudostratified columnar epithelium with goblet cells forms the lining for most of the upper respiratory tract and is seen to advantage in a section of trachea (Fig. 7-9). As can be seen in this illustration, the cells reaching the surface are either ciliated or goblet cells. The mucus secreted by the latter forms a film on the inner surface of the respiratory passages and serves as a dust-catcher to prevent dusts being inhaled into the lungs; it also moistens the dry air inspired. The cilia serve a very useful function by beating so as to move the mucus containing the dust particles upward to a point at which it can be swallowed or otherwise eliminated. The cells that do not reach the surface probably serve as stem cells for the taller kind of cells when these are lost from the membrane.

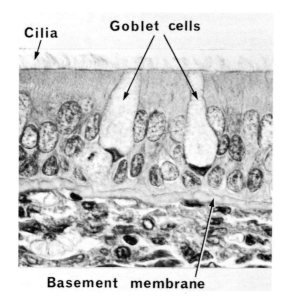

Cilia **Goblet cells**

Basement membrane

Fig. 7-9. Photomicrograph of pseudostratified columnar ciliated epithelium (dog trachea). Note that not all the cells in this type of epithelium are tall enough to reach the surface.

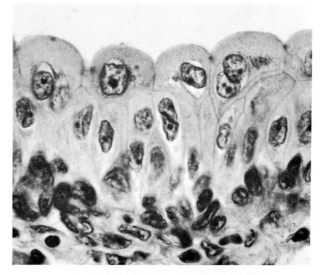

Fig. 7-10. Photomicrograph of transitional epithelium of the urinary bladder (dog). Note how the rounded surface cells of this type of epithelium bulge into the lumen when the epithelium is not stretched.

STRATIFIED EPITHELIAL MEMBRANES

Stratified epithelial membranes (membranes two or more cells in thickness) withstand more wear and tear than membranes of the simple type. But because they are stratified, they cannot serve efficiently as absorptive membranes; furthermore, their stratified structure makes them ill adapted to perform secretory functions. Hence such secretion as is found on stratified membranes is provided by glands situated below the membrane and opening through the membrane by way of ducts. Therefore, stratified membranes serve chiefly to protect, and they differ from one another because they provide different kinds and degrees of protection in different places.

Stratified Squamous Nonkeratinizing Epithelium

This type of membrane (Fig. 7-3f) is found on wet surfaces subject to considerable wear and tear, where absorptive function is not needed. The fluid required to keep the surface wet is provided by glands in the connective tissue under the epithelium. The inside of the mouth and esophagus are both lined with this type of epithelium, as are the crypts of the palatine tonsil where the epithelium is kept wet by saliva, which provides protection from coarse foods. Part of the epiglottis is covered, and the vagina lined, with this type of epithelium.

Stratified squamous nonkeratinizing epithelium is not, as its name implies, composed of successive layers of squamous cells. As shown in Figure 7-3f, the deepest cells (constituting the basal layer that abuts on the basement membrane) are *columnar*. Just above this layer the cells are *polyhedral* (many sided), and it is only toward the surface that the cells assume a *squamous* shape; so only the more superficial cells in stratified squamous nonkeratinizing epithelium are actually squamous.

Stratified Columnar Epithelium

This is found on very few wet surfaces in the body, where presumably more protection is required than would be afforded by simple columnar epithelium and where some slight absorption of fluid from the surface is required so that stratified squamous nonkeratinizing epithelium could not be used. For example, whereas ducts of moderate size are usually lined with simple columnar epithelium, the larger ducts of glands are commonly lined by stratified columnar epithelium. In a few sites stratified columnar epithelium is ciliated.

Transitional Epithelium

This is somewhat similar to stratified squamous nonkeratinizing epithelium when stretched but when not stretched the more superficial cells become rounded instead of squamous in shape (Figs. 7-3e and 7-10). Such a membrane can be stretched without the superficial cells pulling apart from one another; they merely become drawn out into broader, thinner cells. Hence transitional

Keratin

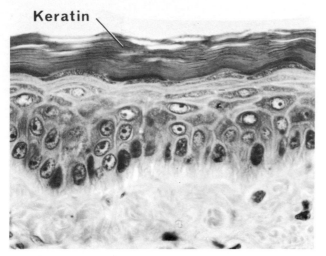

Fig. 7-11. Photomicrograph of thin skin (ear of monkey), showing stratified squamous keratinizing epithelium.

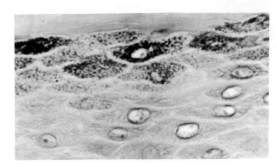

Fig. 7-12. Photomicrograph of thick skin (human), showing the granular layer (stratum granulosum) at a magnification high enough for its keratohyalin granules to be discerned.

epithelium is well adapted to lining tubes and hollow structures subject to being expanded from within, such as the urinary bladder, in which it is best studied (Fig. 7-10). The surface cells of the transitional epithelium in the urinary bladder are commonly polyploid or multinucleated (Leuchtenberger et al.; Walker) but it is not clear why this should be so.

Stratified Squamous Keratinizing Epithelium (The Usual Covering of Dry Surfaces)

This epithelium (Figs. 7-1 and 7-11) resembles stratified squamous nonkeratinizing epithelium except the more superficial cells undergo metamorphosis into a tough nonliving layer of *keratin* tightly attached to the underlying living cells. The epithelial part of the skin (the *epidermis*) provides a good example of stratified squamous keratinizing epithelium (Fig. 7-1). In skin, keratin serves several purposes. As noted, it is virtually waterproof and hence prevents evaporation from the cells beneath it; likewise, it keeps the body from imbibing water in the bathtub. Since it is tough and resilient, it protects the underlying living epithelial cells from wear and tear and being impervious to bacteria it constitutes a first line of defense against infection. Over the soles of the feet and the palms of the hands the stratified squamous epithelium of the skin is thicker and the keratin in particular is very thick; this helps the epithelium withstand the great wear to which these particular surfaces are exposed.

In all but the thinnest membranes of stratified squamous keratinizing epithelium there is a particular layer of cells, called the *granular layer*, slightly below the layer of keratin. Its cells are more or less diamond-shaped with

their long axes parallel to the surface. This layer received its name because in H and E sections its cells reveal blue-staining granules (Fig. 7-12), called *keratohyalin granules*, involved in the transformation of cells into keratin. This type of epithelium is discussed further in Chapter 20.

HOW (1) THE CELLS OF EPITHELIAL MEMBRANES AND GLANDS AND (2) THE CONTIGUOUS CELLS OF CERTAIN OTHER TISSUES ARE HELD TOGETHER

The way contiguous cells are held together, as for example in epithelial membranes, was not elucidated until the matter could be investigated with the EM; in the 1960s and 1970s this instrument disclosed that this function is performed by special structures termed *cell junctions*. Three main kinds of junctions, all serving special purposes, were described as follows.

1. *Occludens junctions* (commonly called *tight junctions*). In these the outer aspects of the cell membranes of adjacent epithelial cells are fused along ridges that extend along them in a characteristic pattern so as to provide a perfect or near-perfect seal between the cells.

2. *Adherens junctions* (which include what are termed *desmosomes,* soon to be described). In these the cell membranes of adjacent cells are not fused together but adhere to each other very firmly, through the medium of some intercellular component that holds them together.

3. The last type of junction to be discovered was termed a *nexus* (L. bond), but is now more commonly referred to as a *gap junction* because there is a very narrow gap between the adjacent cell membranes at these sites. However little tubular structures penetrate both cell membranes so as to provide tiny interconnecting passageways between the adjacent cells through which ions and small molecules can pass directly from one cell to the

next without entering the intercellular space. This arrangement allows electrical and chemical signals to be transmitted through whole series of cells united by junctions of this type. We shall now describe the three types of junctions in more detail.

Occludens (Tight) Junctions; Structure in Relation to Function

The Zonula Occludens. The single layer of columnar epithelial cells lining the intestine (Fig. 7-8) constitues a continuous barrier between the contents of the intestine and the internal environment of the body. It is of the greatest importance that only certain substances present in the lumen be absorbed into the body; other substances that could be toxic must be prevented from passing through this membrane. The ability to select what is being absorbed is a property of the lining absorptive cells. Hence it is imperative that no separations be allowed to occur between the individual lining cells concerned with absorption, since this would allow unwanted substances to bypass the absorptive cells. So there has to be some sort of effective seal between such cells. To understand the nature of the seal, it may be helpful to glance at Figure 7-3c. This three-dimensional diagram shows that simple columnar epithelial cells are more or less hexagonal in shape, at least sufficiently so for them to be packed side by side without having any spaces between them. Before the EM was available, it was thought that little crevices would be present between the cell membranes of the contiguous cells where the lateral borders of these cells extended up the sides of the cells to turn a right angle and continue on as the free surface. Indeed, it was at one time postulated that crevices did exist there, and that these were filled with an intercellular cement substance that prevented any leakage from the intestine through the potential route between the lining cells. However, the EM revealed that this was not the case; instead, leakage was prevented at these sites by fusion of the cell membranes of the contiguous cells to form what were called *zonulae occludentes.* The reason for the word *zonula* being adopted for this purpose will be obvious if the reader glances at Figure 7-3c, which shows how the regions of fusion between the lateral borders of contiguous cells would completely encircle every cell close to the luminal surface like a girdle or belt. Where this type of junction does not completely encircle a cell, however, it is referred to simply as an *occluding* or *tight junction* (without any reference to its being a zonula).

The special role of the zonula occludens in constituting a seal was confirmed experimentally when it was shown that such junctions prevented electron-dense marker substances from entering the lumen of the intestine from the intercellular space and vice versa.

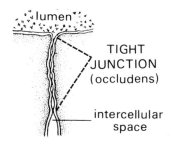

Fig. 7-13. Diagram of a tight junction (zonula occludens), showing the ridges within the junction along which the cell membranes of the adjacent epithelial cells are fused.

More recently it has been found by means of the EM-freeze-etch technic (described on p. 111) that at tight junctions adjacent cell membranes are fused only where networks of matching ridges project from adjacent cell membranes and meet each other, as illustrated in Figures 7-13, 7-14, and 7-15. The most likely interpretation at the molecular level is that certain integral membrane protein particles in the adjacent cell membranes are arranged side by side to constitute special sealing strands that interlock and adhere to one another tightly across the gap, something like teeth in a zipper, with the result that the intercellular space in this particular region is obliterated all along the strands (Staehelin and Hull). Moreover, it has been found that not all junctions of this type are equally tight and the greater the number of fused ridges in a junction, the better the seal the junction makes. Hence in the very impermeable kind of tight junction found, for instance, in the intestine (Fig. 7-14) or urinary bladder, there are up to a dozen or so anastomosing ridges, while in the more leaky kind, such as may be found between endothelial cells of capillaries in a few regions of the body (Fig. 7-15) or between epithelial cells of kidney tubules, only one to three ridges are seen.

The Fascia Occludens. From its origin (L.), *fascia* means a band. Thus the term *fascia occludens* is used to denote discontinuous (patchy) bands of fusions between cell membranes of adjacent cells. Examples are to be found between the endothelial cells comprising the lining of blood capillaries in most parts of the body (other than a few exceptional regions as noted above). Fascia occludens junctions do not, of course, constitute an uninterrupted seal between the contiguous lining cells of such capillaries, because the cell membranes are not fused between the junctions. As explained in later chapters, in between these junctions there are potential slits through which tissue fluid can exude and white blood cells sometimes migrate from the blood into the connective tissue in which the capillaries lie.

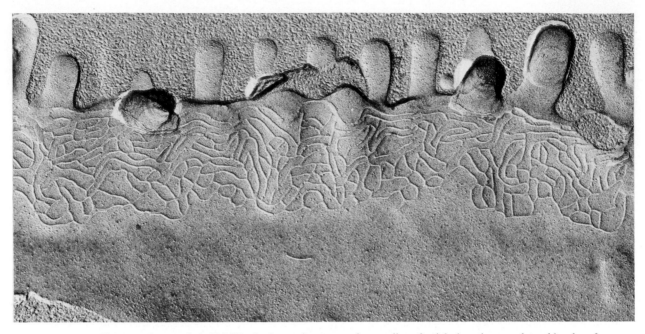

Fig. 7-14. Electron micrograph (×50,000) of a freeze-fracture surface replica of a tight junction on a lateral border of an epithelial cell lining the large intestine of a *Xenopus* tadpole. Note the multiple interconnecting strands (ridges) in this nonleaky kind of tight junction. (Hull, B. E., and Staehelin, L. A.: J. Cell Biol., *68*:688, 1976)

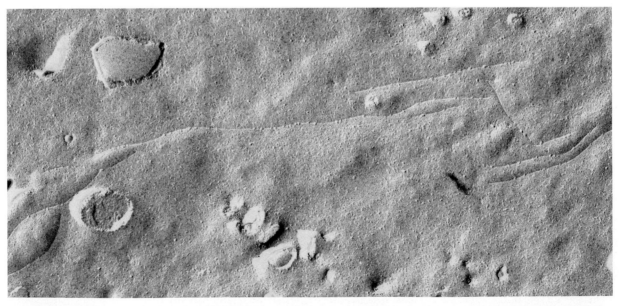

Fig. 7-15. Electron micrograph (×50,000) of a freeze-fracture surface replica of a tight junction on a lateral border of a capillary endothelial cell in the gut region of a *Xenopus* tadpole. Note that there is only a single interconnecting strand in most of the junctional network so that this is a relatively leaky kind of tight junction. (Courtesy of B. Hull)

Junctions of the Adherens Type

In this kind of junction there is no direct contact between the apposed cell membranes of the contiguous cells, but they are joined by intercellular bonding material that serves to hold the membranes of the two cells firmly together. Indeed it is the adherens type of junction that is the last to part company under conditions that cause cells to separate from one another. There are two different kinds of adherens junctions:

The Zonula Adherens (Belt Desmosome). In shape this resembles the zonula occludens, being disposed as a girdle right around epithelial cells. In the junctional complex between absorptive cells of the intestine the zonula adherens (Fig. 7-16, Z.A.), now often referred to as a *belt desmosome,* lies fairly close to the luminal surface just deep to the zonula occludens. The space of about 20 nm. between the apposed cell membranes in this type of junction is filled with intercellular material of low electron density and as yet undetermined composition, by means of which the two cell membranes adhere to one another (Fig. 7-16). Electron-dense material coats the cytoplasmic surface of the cell membranes and 7-nm. actin-containing cytoplasmic microfilaments appear to be closely associated with this kind of junction.

The Macula Adherens (Desmosome). This was termed a *macula* because it takes the form of a spot (L. *macula,* spot), and not a girdle or band, on the cell membranes of contiguous cells. However, it is now customary to refer to such junctions simply as *desmosomes* (Gr. *desmos,* band or ligament; *soma,* body). The term *spot desmosome* is sometimes employed when it is necessary to make a distinction between a spot-shaped adherens junction and a belt desmosome (zonula adherens). In the spot-shaped desmosome, the kind of junction implied when the word desmosome is used alone, bundles of intermediate (10-nm.) filaments, termed *tonofilaments,* are anchored in disk-shaped *plaques* on the cytoplasmic side of the cell membranes and probably play an important role in transmitting and distributing tensile forces. Desmosomes are, of course, particularly common in tissues, such as lining membranes, subject to much wear and tear and moreover are important in holding muscle cells together in the heart. In the absorptive cells lining the intestine desmosomes (Fig. 7-16, M.A.) are present scattered along the cell membrane deep to the zonula adherens.

Epithelial Appearances Attributable to Desmosomes. The most striking appearance is to be found in sections of thick, stratified, squamous keratinizing epithelium, as shown in Figure 20-4, page 618. Here, desmosomes are responsible for the cells in the layer just above the basal layer having a prickly appearance in the LM that led to their being described as *prickle cells.* This unusual ap-

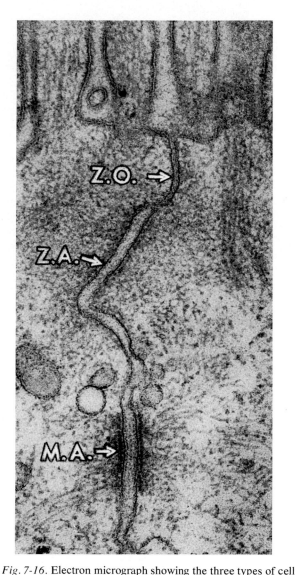

Fig. 7-16. Electron micrograph showing the three types of cell junctions on the lateral borders of intestinal epithelial cells close to the lumen. These junctions would all lie near the tip of the arrow in Figure 7-8 indicating the terminal web. Below the microvilli at *top* (which project into the lumen) a *tight junction* (zonula occludens, Z.O.) completely encircles each cell; here, fused ridges along the adjacent lateral cell membranes (*see* Fig. 7-14) seal the lumen of the intestine from intercellular space. Deep to the tight junction and in the region of the terminal web a *belt desmosome* (zonula aherens, Z.A.) also entirely encircles each cell. At *bottom,* a spot-shaped desmosome (macula adherens, M.A.) is seen. The two kinds of adherens junctions illustrated here both serve to bond the cells together securely. The three different types of junctions (Z.O., Z.A., and M.A.) are sometimes collectively referred to as a *junctional complex.* (Farquhar, M. G., and Palade, G. E.: J. Cell Biol., *17:*375, 1963)

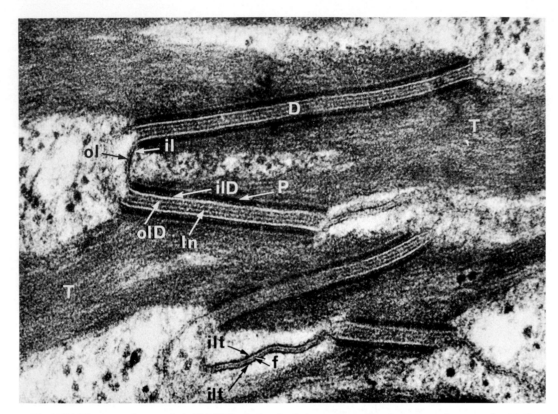

Fig. 7-17. Electron micrograph (×114,000) of a border between two cells of stratum spinosum of epithelium from human palate, showing desmosomes and tight junctions between the cell at *left* and the one at *right,* which interdigitate along a zigzag line. Four large, well-developed desmosomes (D) are seen. Between the top desmosome (D) and the next, the outer half (ol) and inner half (il) of the cell membrane of the right-hand cell may be discerned. This membrane makes a hairpin turn and the outer layer continues into one of the lines seen within the desmosome (olD). Similarly, the inner layer is continuous with another line (ilD), which is immediately adjacent to a thick band of cytoplasmic material, the attachment plaque (P). Bundles of tonofilaments forming tonofibrils (T) insert into the attachment plaque on either side of the desmosome. In the middle of the desmosome an electron-dense intermediate line (In) is seen lying centrally in the intercellular space. For further interpretation of the lines seen in a desmosome, *see* text. At *bottom center* the adjacent cell membranes form a tight junction. This is characterized by two outer parallel thicker lines, representing the inner halves (ilt) of the membranes, and a central thinner line (f), representing the site of the network of fusion ridges of the adjacent cell membranes. (Wilgram, G. F., and Weinstock, A.: Arch. Dermatol., *94:*456, 1966)

pearance is attributable to two factors. First, over most of their surface, these cells become slightly separated from one another as a result of shrinkage on fixation; this is probably to be explained by the fact that during life there would be a film of tissue fluid between the cells of this layer. Second, the spaces between these cells are crossed by many narrow processes containing fibrillar material, the purpose of which is seemingly to hold the contiguous cells together at these sites (Fig. 20-4). Before this appearance was investigated with the EM, it was assumed that the bundles of fibrillar material, which were termed *tonofibrils,* would extend right through the cell membrane to attach contiguous cells to one another. However, the EM revealed that the cell membrane was not interrupted

by such bundles; furthermore the appearance seen in the LM was due to the fact that whereas there were indeed bundles of filaments (*tonofilaments*) in each cell, such bundles terminated in plaques on the cytoplasmic aspect of the cell membrane without penetrating the membrane itself. Moreover, the bundles of filaments ending in these plaques were aligned with similar bundles in adjacent cells, and the cell membranes of contiguous cells were bonded with one another at the sites of the plaques so as to constitute spot-shaped desmosomes. Since such sites are the only ones where the contiguous cells are firmly bonded together, they are the only places where the cells do not separate on fixation; hence desmosomes confer the prickly appearance on these cells when they are seen in

Fig. 7-18. Diagrams illustrating the structure of a desmosome (*left*) and a hemidesmosome (*right*), and showing how tonofilaments are anchored in the electron-dense plaques of these structures.

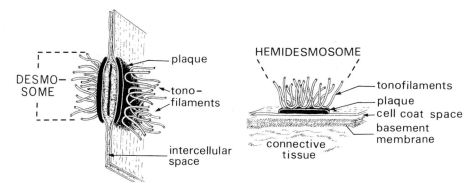

the LM. We shall now go on to describe the details of the fine structure of this type of junction.

Fine Structure. Patterns consisting of parallel electron-dense lines are seen in section of desmosomes of certain types of epithelium. First, a dark line may extend along the midline of the intercellular gap, which is about 30 nm. wide in desmosomes. This line is prominent only in desmosomes of certain kinds of epithelium, such as those shown in Figures 7-16, M.A. and 7-17, where it is labeled In. It was once regarded as an interface where the outer borders of the cell coats of the two cell membranes are condensed or otherwise modified to secure effective mutual attachment, but there is now some indication that it may represent a central layer containing yet another kind of filament attached to the plaques on either side and linking them together across the intercellular gap (Staehelin and Hull). The lighter line seen in Figure 7-17 on each side of the central dark one (In) would correspond to cell coat material. External to each light line is a cell membrane which, being cut in cross section, has the appearance of two dark lines (labeled ilD and olD in Fig. 7-17), with a central light line. The cytoplasmic aspect of each cell membrane is greatly thickened with the electron-dense material of the plaque (Fig. 7-17P). As depicted in Figure 7-18, intermediate (10 nm.) filaments (the so-called *tonofilaments*) are inserted into this dense plaque material and then loop back out again into the cytoplasm. The positions of desmosomes on the cell surface are well demonstrated by the technic of shadow-casting,* which

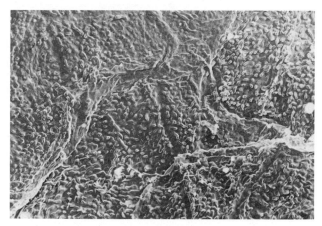

Fig. 7-19. Electron micrograph showing desmosomes on cells deep in the epithelium (epidermis) of skin, as seen by the shadow cast replica technic. Every site of attachment by a desmosome to a contiguous cell is seen as a small projection of the cell surface. By this technic it has been estimated that there is a desmosome on every square μm. or so of cell surface on this type of cell. (Courtesy of R. Buck)

shows how abundant these junctions are on certain kinds of cells (Fig. 7-19).

The Hemidesmosome. Certain regions of the cell surface of epithelial cells have the structure of half-desmosomes (Fig. 7-18, *right*) and are therefore termed *hemidesmosomes* (Gr. *hemi*, half). These are found in sites where a cell, instead of being attached by a complete desmosome to a neighboring cell, is attached to extracellular material, commonly a basement membrane, and so has only been able to make half a desmosome. It therefore seems that a complete desmosome is made jointly by contiguous cells.

---

* *Shadow Casting of Surface Replicas.* The cell surface is first coated with a carbon film, which conforms readily to its surface contours, and the cellular material is digested away so as to leave only a replica of the surface. A heavy metal such as gold is then applied at an angle so that fronts of elevated regions are more thickly coated than regions behind the high points, which are said to be in the shadow. In the EM the thinly coated parts of the replica (the regions in the shadow) scatter fewer electrons than the thickly coated fronts of the high points. However, photographic reversal in the printing of the electron micrograph makes the

thinly coated shadows appear darker than the other regions and hence gives a positive image of the surface contours of the surface being studied.

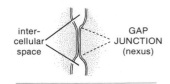

Same after filling
extracellular spaces
with lanthanum hydroxide

enlarged interpretation
showing cylindrical structures
of junction

Fig. 7-20. Diagrams illustrating
the structure of a gap junction as
it appears in a routine EM section
(*top*) and after filling the intercellular spaces with lanthanum
(*bottom*). Complementary integral membrane proteins in apposing cell membranes interlock so as
to form the walls of characteristic
cylindrical structures containing
central pores, as shown at *bottom*.

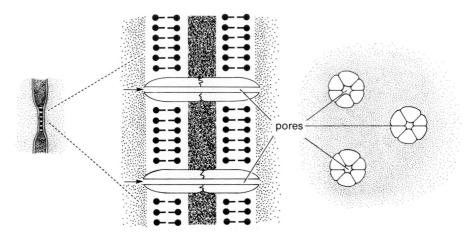

longitudinal section   surface view

Gap Junctions (Nexuses) — Structure in Relation to Function

As noted, the word *nexus* means a bond, but since all types of junctions in a sense act as bonds, the term *gap junction* is preferable. This term was probably coined to distinguish this type of junction from the tight junction, because in many instances junctions originally thought to be tight junctions on further study turned out to be gap junctions, and indeed the difference between these two kinds of junctions in routine EM sections is not easy to see. However, with high resolution electron microscopy it can be seen that at gap junctions the cell membranes are not fused together as they are in tight junctions, but separated by a narrow gap of about 2 nm. — hence the name *gap junction.*

Much of the information gained about the gap region of these junctions was obtained by two special EM methods. First, an electron-dense marker substance (lanthanum hydroxide) was injected into the intercellular space bordering on a gap junction. By infiltrating between the two cell membranes, it negatively stained and hence outlined

little structures arranged side by side, but separated somewhat from one another, in the midline (the gap region) of the junction. The ends of each of these strucutres moreover were found to project through the cell membranes of the two cells that met in the junction (Fig. 7-20). A second way the gap region was investigated was by the EM freeze-fracture-etch technic (described on p. 111). Fractures through the gap region revealed the same structures as projections on the surface of the cell membrane. Furthermore, injecting dyes into the cells that met in gap junctions indicated that there were interconnecting passageways between the two cells linked by the junction. Accordingly it is believed that the structures outlined by lanthanum are cylindrical in shape, with open channels extending through their middles. It is likely that they are complex structures composed of complementary integral membrane proteins of the apposed cell membranes that interlock across the intercellular gap to form the walls of little tubular channels (Fig. 7-20) directly linking the cytoplasm of the adjacent cells. The communicating channels through the centers of the numerous connecting structures in a gap junction permit the direct passage of ions from the cytoplasm of one cell to that of the next and hence conduct electrical impulses without delay. Furthermore, substances of low molecular weight (such as fluorescein) are able to pass directly via gap junctions from one cell to another without having to go through the intercellular space. Like desmosomes, gap junctions are spot-like in outline; they do not form zonulae.

As we shall see there are gap junctions between the muscle cells of the heart and these are instrumental in permitting the wave of depolarization sweeping over the heart to activate contraction of its different parts in proper sequence. Gap junctions also serve a similar function in conducting waves of contraction along the muscle cells in the wall of the intestine. They also serve a role in nervous tissue, and have been observed in certain epithelial structures and between the processes of adjacent bone cells. Their importance in the body requires no further proof than to say that without them our hearts would not work. We should add here that the other types of cell junctions are equally important, because if it were not for the occludens type we would absorb toxic substances from our intestines and without the adherens type our skin and many other structures would fall apart.

THE MAINTENANCE OF CELL POPULATION IN EPITHELIAL MEMBRANES

The site of formation of new cells for the maintenance or repair of an epithelial membrane varies in different types of membranes.

Simple Squamous or Cuboidal Epithelia

The degree of specialization attained by cells of these membranes is not very great and does not seem to result in diminution of their capacity to divide. The cells of membranes of these types are representative of our Category 3 type of cell. Perhaps the best example of cell growth in a simple epithelial membrane is manifested when there is an injury to tissue containing capillaries, because in these instances new tubes of endothelium grow out from pre-existing endothelium to form new capillaries, a phenomenon that can be observed with the LM in living preparations.

Simple Columnar Epithelia Composed of Only Secretory Cells (as in the Lining of the Stomach) or of a Combination of Secretory Cells and Absorptive Cells (as in the Lining of the Small Intestine)

In these instances the cells of the membrane have all undergone a degree of specialization that seems to have caused a loss of their ability to divide; hence, their replacement in maintenance and repair is due to stem cells

multiplying and differentiating to take the place of those specialized cells that die or are lost from the surface.

The stem cells in such membranes are all located in little crypts or glands that extend down from the membrane into the connective tissue on which the membrane rests. Proliferation of cells in the crypts or glands leads to cells being pushed up so as to become surface cells. Details are given in connection with the organs in which these types of epithelia are found.

Pseudostratified Epithelia

It is believed that the stem cells responsible for dividing and being able to differentiate into goblet or ciliated cells to take the place of those that wear out are the short cells (Fig. 7-3d) lying in amongst the bases of the goblet and ciliated cells.

Stratified Epithelia

Cells are continuously lost from the free surface of such membranes. In thick stratified membranes at least certain cells of the deepest layers are sufficiently unspecialized to be able to divide and serve as stem cells. The proliferation of these cells permits their progeny to move toward the free surface of the membrane, becoming more specialized to provide protection but losing their ability to divide as they approach the surface. A most interesting study (Marques-Pereira and Leblond) revealed that in the rat esophagus, which is lined by stratified squamous epithelium, the only cells of the membrane that divided were those of the basal layer. Moreover, when a cell of the basal layer divided there was no set rule as to what happened to the two daughter cells. Both could move toward the surface and differentiate into cells of the outer layers. Or both could remain in the basal layer to provide for more stem cells. Or one could move up and differentiate and leave the other to serve as a stem cell. This indicates that it is a matter of chance whether daughter cells of stem cells differentiate or remain as stem cells; they all have the capacity to do either.

The Repair of Epithelial Membranes

Although the cells of epithelial membranes are firmly attached to the surfaces they cover, they manifest a surprising degree of plasticity and behave as if they had a mission to cover immediately any site normally covered with epithelium, should it ever become uncovered. Although ultimately the proper covering of any bare connective tissue surface depends on mitosis occurring in epithelial cells to provide new cells to take the place of those lost, the epithelial cells adjacent to a site where membrane has been lost do not wait for mitosis to occur but almost immediately begin to migrate toward and over the bare area. They remain attached to each other as a layer but become thinner so that in the form of a wedge they can spread over as much of the bare area as possible. This is the first step in epithelial migration; the second is that mitosis occurs behind the advancing edge of migrating epithelium, providing more cells to help push the advancing edge along and cover the entire surface where membrane is required. Details will be given when we study the repair of skin wounds and burns.

A Second Source of Stem Cells for Stratified Epithelial Membranes. It might be thought that if a scrape or burn removed or destroyed a large patch of epithelium from the skin, for it to be re-covered the basal cells of the surrounding epithelium would have to proliferate to supply new cells that would, in turn, continue to proliferate so as to spread over the denuded area and cover it again with epithelium. If the area to be re-covered is very small, this method of repair suffices. But if it were the only method for repair, it would take a very long time for a sizeable scrape or a burn to be re-covered, and while this was taking place the uncovered connective tissue would not only remain a site for potential infection but also would form a nasty scar.

Fortunately, there is a second source of stem cells providing new epithelium for sizeable areas that are denuded. As we shall see when we study the skin, the cells of the numerous hair follicles and sweat glands (both of which extend deep into the connective tissue below the epidermis and hence their deeper parts commonly escape injury) undergo division, and cells from this source multiply and migrate onto the surface and serve as stem cells to form a new stratified epithelium, as shown on page 636. As a result a localized scrape or burn that destroys the surface epithelium over a given area heals from multiple foci and infiinitely faster than it would if epithelium had to grow in from the edges of the injury for the entire denuded area to be re-covered. Furthermore this occurs with formation of far less scar tissue than would otherwise be the case.

GLANDS

As already noted, there are two main divisions of epithelial tissue: (*1*) covering and lining membranes, which were dealt with in the preceding section, and (*2*) glands, with which we deal here.

Development. The way in which glands develop from epithelial membranes is described and illustrated (Fig. 6-2) in Chapter 6.

Classification of Glands. Although glands can be classified in several different ways, there are two main types: (*1*) *exocrine* glands, which are provided with ducts that convey their secretions to the epithelial surface from which they originated and hence out of the substance of the body and (*2*) *endocrine* glands, which have no ducts and so have to secrete into the body substance (generally capillaries) and are therefore also called *ductless glands* (refer to Fig. 6-2). Exocrine glands are classified further as follows.

EXOCRINE GLANDS

Exocrine glands consist of two main epithelial components, (*1*) groups of specialized cells called *secretory units* that synthesize the particular secretion made by the gland and (*2*) tubular ducts that conduct the secretion produced by the secretory units to some surface on to which the secretion is emptied (refer back to Fig. 6-2, *lower left*). Actually the cells of the epithelial walls of the ducts may alter the concentration of the secretion, but the important components of a secretion are usually proteins or glycoproteins synthesized by the cells of the secretory units.

Exocrine glands are classified several ways. We shall give some examples.

Simple and Compound Glands

If a gland has only one *unbranched* duct it is said to be a *simple gland* (Fig. 7-21, *lower left*). If, however, it has a *branched* duct system so as to be able to convey secretion from a large number of secretory units it is called a *compound gland* (Fig. 7-21, *lower right*). Compound glands are of course much larger than simple glands. One of the few examples of a simple gland that has a distinguishable secretory unit and an easily recognized duct is a sweat gland. The unbranched but coiled secretory unit lies deep in the skin, where it empties into a tube of about the same size (its duct), which takes a more or less coiled course to the surface of the skin. The coiled secretory unit and a coiled portion of the duct of a sweat gland are shown on page 622, where sweat glands are described in detail.

Many compound glands are large enough to be termed *organs.* Both the liver and the pancreas are large compound glands with extensive branching duct systems. The duct system of a large compound gland can be likened to a tree. The main duct is like the trunk of a tree. Smaller ducts extend from the trunk like branches and in turn give rise to smaller and smaller branches. These eventually terminate at secretory units the products of which they drain away to the site where the main duct (corresponding to the trunk) opens on some surface. For example, the main ducts of the pancreas and liver both empty their contents into the small intestine.

Tubular, Acinous, and Alveolar Glands

If the clusters of cells that constitute the secretory unit or units of a gland are tubular in shape (Fig. 7-21), the gland is said to be a *tubular gland*. But if the secretory units are more rounded in shape, the gland is said to be an *acinous* (L. *acinus*, grape or berry) or an *alveolar* (L. *alveolus*, little hollow sac) *gland*. Although in the past some distinction was made between acini and alveoli, it is now usual to call them all *alveoli* except those in the pancreas which are still, because of custom, termed *acini*. If glands contain both tubular and alveolar secretory units, or units that have some characteristics of each, they are called *tubuloalveolar glands* (Fig. 7-21).

Mucous, Serous, and Mixed Glands

It was noticed long ago that the secretion of some glands was somewhat viscous and slippery and so glands making this kind of secretion were called *mucous glands*. It was also noticed that the secretion of another kind of gland was relatively clear and watery, which must have reminded someone of whey (the thin fluid left after the cream and curd are removed from milk), and so glands of this type were given the name *serous* (L. *serum*, whey) *glands*. Serous glands commonly secrete various enzymes in their whey-like secretions. Both mucous and serous secretions emerge from the ducts of certain glands, and because such glands possess both kinds of secretory units (mucous and serous) they are termed *mixed glands*.

It is important in histology to learn how to distinguish between serous and mucous secretory units in sections and also to learn the appearance in sections of a curious combination of mucous and serous secretory cells in the same secretory unit, so these will now be described in turn.

Serous Secretory Units. Instruction on how to locate a secretory unit in an H and E section of the pancreas, a gland in which the secretory units are all of the serous type, is given on page 123 in connection with Figure 5-19.

When a serous secretory unit cut in cross section is seen with the oil-immersion objective (as already noted in Chap. 5), it resembles a pie cut into pieces but not yet served (Fig. 5-19). Each piece of pie corresponds to a single secretory cell with a roughly triangular outline. A lumen is present in the center of each acinus where the apices of the secretory cells meet. However, in fixed tissue this is so small it is difficult and often impossible to see with the LM.

The cytoplasm at the base of each cell is basophilic because of its content of free ribosomes and rER. The nucleus is rounded and lies close to the base of the cell but not directly against it (Fig. 5-19). In properly fixed preparations the cytoplasm toward the apex of each cell can be seen to contain eosinophilic *zymogen granules* (Z in Fig. 7-22). As described in Chapter 5, these are membrane-bounded vesicles containing a semifluid material

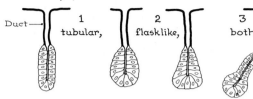

If secretory portion is:

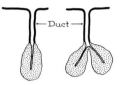

it is a tubular exocrine gland.

it is an alveolar or acinous gland.

it is a tubulo-alveolar gland.

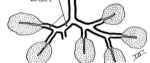

If duct doesn't branch:

it is a simple gland.

If duct branches:

it is a compound gland.

Fig. 7-21. Diagrams showing the different kinds of secretory units of exocrine glands and the difference between simple and compound glands.

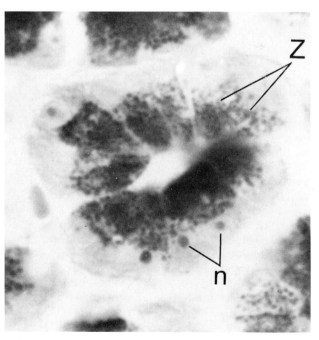

Fig. 7-22. High-power photomicrograph of a serous secretory unit of rabbit pancreas, stained with eosin-azure to demonstrate zymogen granules (Z). Nucleoli (n) of secretory cells have also stained. (Courtesy of B. Smith)

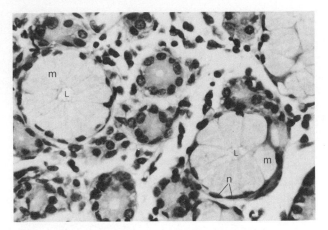

Fig. 7-23. Medium-power photomicrograph of human submaxillary gland, showing two mucous secretory units (m) cut in cross section. The lumina (L) of the units and flat basal nuclei (n) are also indicated.

that on fixation is coagulated. The fine structure and mechanism of secretion in these cells are described in detail in Chapter 5, page 128.

Mucous Secretory Unit. The cross sectional appearance of a mucous secretory unit differs from that of a serous secretory unit. Whereas the nuclei of serous cells are rounded, those in mucous secretory units are flattened, almost to the point of appearing disk-like; furthermore, they are squeezed up against the bases of the cells that contain them (Fig. 7-23n). The cytoplasm of mucous cells also looks different from that of serous cells. Thus the cytoplasm at the base of the cells is much less basophilic than in serous cells and that between the nucleus and the apex of a mucous cell contains membrane-bounded vesicles of mucus as in goblet cells.

The glycoprotein in the secretory vesicles of mucous cells does not stain well with H and E, and hence mucous cells appears pale and vacuolated (Fig. 7-23). The contents of the vesicles do, however, stain with the PAS technic, so useful for demonstrating glycoproteins.

Radioactive sulfur injected into animals can be demonstrated by radioautography in the secretory cells of mucous glands; indeed, in low-power radioautographs, some mucous glands stand out like a sprinkling of black ink drops on a white page. This uptake of radioactive sulfur is due to some glycoproteins synthesized by mucous cells containing sulfur. Other radioautographic studies of glycoprotein secretion by goblet cells, using glucose labeled with tritium, are described in Chapter 5 (page 133).

Mixed Glands. Some exocrine glands deliver serous and mucous secretions through their ducts. This is due to these glands possessing both serous and mucous secretory units and/or secretory units assembled from both mucous- and serous-secreting cells (Fig. 7-24). The latter type of secretory unit usually consists of mucous units capped by crescent-shaped aggregations of serous cells (sd in Fig. 7-24), so these units are called *serous demilunes* (L. *demidius*, half; *luna*, moon). Obviously for the secretory product of these serous cells to gain entrance to the lumen there must be passageways between the mucous cells separating them from the lumen of the mucous unit. These passageways are probably tiny intercellular canals between adjacent mucous secretory cells or between adjacent serous and mucous cells. However, they are not usually seen in ordinary preparations.

Myoepithelial (Basket) Cells. Secretory units of either mucous or serous types can be shown by special technics to be cradled in a loose basket made up of the cytoplasmic processes of special cells lying between the bases of the secretory cells and the basement membrane in between the secretory unit and the surrounding connective tissue. These cells have a central region containing the nucleus and many long cytoplasmic processes that extend to encircle the secretory unit (Fig. 7-25). Although these cells are of epithelial origin, it seems very probable that their cytoplasmic processes are contractile, not only because of their shape and position, but also because filaments have been seen in them with the EM. Therefore it is assumed that the function of these cells is to promote expression of secretion from secretory units into ducts. The cytoplasmic processes comprising the basket cannot be seen well in ordinary sections but are demonstrated to advantage by alkaline phosphatase (Fig. 7-25), an enzyme they contain.

The Terms *Parenchyma* and *Stroma* Used With Reference to Glands and Organs

The epithelial component of a gland is termed its *parenchyma* (Gr. something poured in) and the connective tissue component in which the secretory units and ducts are embedded is called its *stroma* (Gr. *stroma*, anything laid out for something to lie on). The stroma thus provides support by virtue of its intercellular substances and carries blood vessels and nerve fibers into the gland or organ.

Support for a gland as a whole is provided by (*1*) a capsule of surrounding connective tissue and (*2*) partitions of connective tissue extending in from the capsule and dividing the gland substance into segments "fenced off" in three dimensions by connective tissue. The capsule and partitions contain enough intercellular substance to make them strong. In some glands large sectors are fairly widely separated from one another and termed *lobes,* but if the fenced-off areas lie closer to one another they are called *lobules* (little lobes).

Fig. 7-24. Medium-power photomicrograph of a mixed gland (human submaxillary gland), showing mucous secretory units (m) with serous demilunes (sd). The lumen (L) of a mucous secretory unit is also indicated.

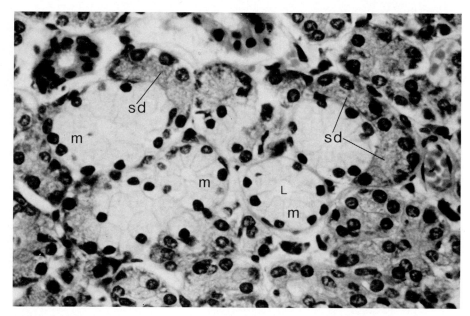

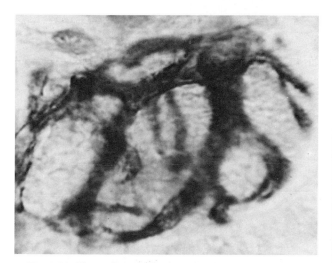

Fig. 7-25. Photomicrograph (×2,250) of a myoepithelial (basket) cell in submaxillary gland of rat, stained by the Gomori method for alkaline phosphatase. The cytoplasmic arms of the cell appear black. (Leeson, C. R.: Nature, *178*:858, 1956)

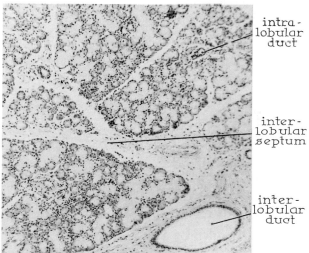

Fig. 7-26. Low-power photomicrograph of a salivary gland of mixed type, showing interlobular septa, lobules containing secretory units, and intra- and interlobular ducts.

A connective tissue partition of the sort described above is termed a *septum*. Hence connective tissue partitions between lobes are termed *interlobar septa,* and those between lobules, *interlobular septa* (Fig. 7-26).

Interlobular and Intralobular Ducts. The septa in some glands converge toward the place where the main duct leaves the gland. Hence, septa support the main branches of the duct as they pass from the interior to the exterior of the gland. The branches of the duct system conveyed in interlobular septa (lying between lobules) are termed *interlobular ducts;* they are easily recognized because they are large, have a thick epithelial lining and a large lumen and are surrounded by the connective tissue of the partition conveying them (Fig. 7-26). Smaller branches of the duct system lying within lobules are termed *intralobular ducts;* these drain into the interlobular ducts of the septa. Intralobular ducts (Fig. 7-27) are smaller than interlobular ducts (Fig. 7-26). Furthermore, they are not

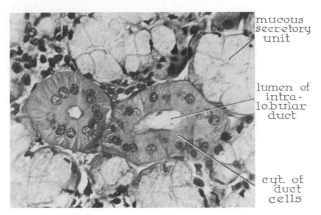

Fig. 7-27. High-power photomicrograph of a mucous gland, showing two intralobular ducts cut more or less in cross section.

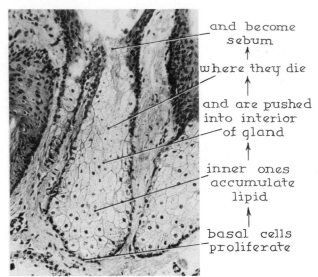

Fig. 7-28. Medium-power photomicrograph of a sebaceous gland in skin. This is a holocrine gland in which whole cells become the secretion sebum. Sebaceous glands open into hair follicles.

surrounded by as much connective tissue as the interlobular ducts because they do not run in partitions (Fig. 7-27). However, a small amount of connective tissue is present and it connects the intralobular ducts with the septa into which they pass, thus providing support for the ducts lying within the substance of lobules.

Blood Vessels in the Stroma. The larger blood vessels supplying a gland usually enter and leave by way of the connective tissue septa; they can easily be distinguished from ducts because they are lined by squamous cells, whereas ducts are lined by columnar cells. The blood vessels within lobules supply capillary networks in the delicate connective tissue surrounding the epithelial secretory units and these capillaries provide the secretory cells with oxygen and nutrients. In fixed tissue, however, the capillaries are commonly collapsed and difficult to see.

Merocrine, Holocrine, and Apocrine Glands

Another classification of glands is based on the manner in which they were first thought to produce their secretion. Since giving the derivation of the terms *merocrine* and *apocrine* might be more confusing than helpful, we shall merely comment on the meanings of these terms.

Merocrine Glands. These have secretory cells of the type discussed in Chapter 5: for example, the acinar cells of the pancreas and goblet cells. Here the secretion is a product of the cell and is delivered through the cell membrane in membranous vesicles in such a way as to keep the cell membrane intact (Fig. 5-21), so that clearly there is no loss of cytoplasm in the secretory process.

Holocrine Glands. Holocrine (Gr. *holos,* all) is fortunately a very specific term. It means that in order for a holocrine gland to secrete, whole cells must become detached and die and become the secretion of the gland. This of course is a very drastic process and holocrine glands are far from common; indeed, the sebaceous

glands of the skin are the only common example in the whole body. Each sebaceous gland is a little sac (Fig. 7-28) with a lining of epithelial cells that proliferate; by this process more and more cells are forced into the interior of the sac while at the same time their cytoplasm becomes filled with a pale fatty material (Fig. 7-28), termed *sebum,* which the cells manufacture as they move from the wall toward the interior of the sac. Here they die and break down (Fig. 7-28), thereby constituting the secretion of the gland, which is squeezed out via the hair follicles to lubricate the skin (details are given in Chap. 20).

Apocrine Glands. When only the LM was available it was thought that in certain glands the delivery of a secretion into the lumen of a secretory unit required some loss of the superficial cytoplasm of the secretory cell so that it too became part of the secretion. However the EM has shown that the concept of cells losing some of their cytoplasm in the secretory process was exaggerated, and indeed it is probable that most glands in the past termed apocrine are really merocrine. The so-called apocrine sweat glands in certain regions of the skin (p. 621) are a case in point. Here, as might be expected, cytoplasm is not lost during release of the secretory product.

The Control of the Secretory Activity of Exocrine Glands

There are two kinds of control mechanisms, one mediated by the nervous system and the other by hormones. Some exocrine glands are primarily under the first kind of control and others under the second.

Fig. 7-29. Diagrams showing how the different types of endocrine glands store secretion and how a clump of cells can become a follicle.

How a clump of cells can become a follicle

Capillaries

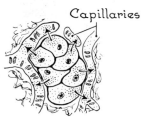 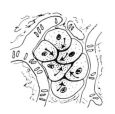 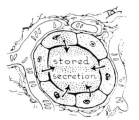

Endocrine cells commonly secrete into capillaries,

but, to store secretion, cells may secrete in opposite direction.

Then they expand the clump into a follicle.

The secretory activity of glands, unlike the activity of one's muscles, is not under voluntary nervous control. People by taking thought can neither stop themselves from sweating nor prevent their mouths from becoming dry if they become nervous while making a speech. The nervous control of the secretory activity of exocrine glands is mediated by what is termed the involuntary or *autonomic* division of the nervous system, which functions more or less automatically, except that it is affected by emotional states, as described in Chapter 17.

The hormonal control of the secretory activity of exocrine glands is seen, for example, in the gastrointestinal tract. The presence of certain foods in the stomach causes an appropriate hormone to be secreted into the bloodstream; this then instructs certain glands farther down the tract to secrete digestive juices so that when the contents of the intestinal tract arrive there they will be further digested.

ENDOCRINE GLANDS

The development of endocrine glands is described on page 182 and illustrated in Figure 6-2. The structure of endocrine glands is considerably simpler than that of exocrine glands because they possess no ducts. Since their secretory cells all discharge their secretion into capillaries, the secretory cells must all be so arranged as to abut on capillaries. This is accomplished by the disposition of secretory cells either in straight or irregular cords separated from one another by capillaries, or in little clumps surrounded by capillaries (Fig. 6-2, *bottom right*).

Intracellular Storage

All endocrine glands store their secretion to some extent. This is accomplished in most of them by intracellular

storage. Secretion granules are found in the cells of many endocrine glands where they are temporarily stored in the cytoplasm before they are secreted. For example, β cells of the islets of Langerhans of the pancreas—the cells that produce the hormone insulin, which regulates the level of the sugar in the blood—store enough of their secretion (insulin) to kill a person if it were all released into the blood at the same time; it would have this effect because it would cause the level of sugar in the blood to fall suddenly to a critically low level incompatible with life.

Extracellular Storage

Another way a secretory product or its precursor can be stored is exemplified in the thyroid gland. Here the cells of what would otherwise be a clump form an extracellular pool of secretory product in the middle of the clump. Hence this secretion comes to be stored extracellularly in what is termed a *follicle* (L. small bag), as shown in Figure 7-29, *right*.

Capsules, Trabeculae, and Blood Supply

Endocrine glands too are enclosed by *capsules* of connective tissue, and usually projections of the capsule extend into the substance of the gland as *trabeculae* (L. little beams) to provide it with internal support and carry blood vessels into it. Trabeculae account for the lobulated appearance of some endocrine glands in sections. Capillaries are abundant in the delicate connective tissue between the cords or clumps of secretory cells (Fig 7-29).

Functions of Endocrine Glands

Although most endocrine glands make hormones, a gland can properly be termed endocrine even if it does not make a hormone, provided it secretes a useful product into the substance of the body. The liver, for example, secretes sugar into the bloodstream and so can also be included in the list of endocrine glands.

GLANDS THAT ARE BOTH EXOCRINE AND ENDOCRINE

The liver, as just mentioned, secretes a useful substance (sugar) into the bloodstream; in addition it possesses a duct system into which its cells secrete bile. So it is both an endocrine and an exocrine gland. The pancreas provides an even better example. It arises from an epithelial outgrowth of the epithelial lining of the intestine. This epithelial outgrowth branches repeatedly to become a duct system, but it also gives rise to two kinds of secretory units: serous ones, in which the secretory portions remain exocrine and connected with the end branches of the duct system, and little groups of cells, the islets of Langerhans, that do not develop a lumen but become arranged into irregular cords and clumps richly provided with capillaries. These islands of cells secrete their hormones directly into the many capillaries with which they are provided; they thus constitute the endocrine portion of the pancreas.

THE CONTROL OF THE SECRETORY ACTIVITY OF ENDOCRINE GLANDS

When we study the endocrine system in detail in Chapter 25 and discuss each gland and the hormone or hormones it makes in some detail, we shall discuss how the secretion of each and every hormone is controlled within narrow limits. For those who are curious about this matter, however, we next describe the principal mechanism by which the secretion of most hormones is regulated. This is termed *feedback inhibition.*

Feedback Inhibition

The term *feedback* originated to designate an arrangement whereby some of the output of a circuit—for example, in a radio receiver—is fed back into the input of the circuit. When the term *inhibition* was combined with *feedback,* a term evolved that seemed useful to describe many of the regulatory mechanisms operating in the body, in which the final product of some reaction is fed back, not into the input but, instead, to *depress the output* of the reaction. (This kind of reaction has already been mentioned in connection with the turning off of genes in Chapter 6.) In other words, feedback inhibition mechanisms can operate in such a way that when the product from some reaction begins to increase over normal levels,

the increased product automatically inhibits the reaction that produces the product. Then, as the product continues to be utilized, its amount will begin to fall below normal levels, at which point there is not enough product to inhibit the reaction, which then automatically increases production of the product. Such mechanisms can be very sensitive and regulate within narrow limits the concentration in the bloodstream of various products, including hormones and the products whose levels hormones control. The concept of feedback inhibition helps a good deal in understanding the control of secretion of most endocrine glands (and other regulatory mechanisms in the body). But the matter is complicated with regard to endocrine glands, because in some instances, as will be described in Chapter 25, two or more endocrine glands and their hormones are sometimes involved in a chain-like way in the feedback mechanism controlling the secretion of some hormones.

Finally, nerve cells have been added to the list of cells that can produce hormones, as described in later chapters.

REFERENCES AND OTHER READING

The general purpose of this chapter is to describe the various arrangements in which epithelial cells are disposed in various types of covering or lining membranes and various types of glands. The information presented has mostly been of a general nature and scarcely justifies listing references and other reading not previously given. Other relevant sources will be listed after we study the various systems of the body, in which we deal with epithelial arrangements in relation to their functions in different systems. However, since cell junctions are described in some detail in this chapter, some references to further reading on them follow.

Cell Junctions

Bullivant, S.: The structure of tight junctions. Electron Microscopy 1978. vol. 3, p. 659. Papers presented at Ninth International Congress on Electron Microscopy. Toronto, Microscopical Society of Canada, 1978.

Claude, P., and Goodenough, D. A.: Fracture faces of zonulae occludentes from tight and leaky epithelia. J. Cell Biol., *58:*391, 1973.

Douglas, W. H. J., Ripley, R. C., and Ellis, R. A.: Enzymatic digestion of desmosomes and hemidesmosome plaques performed on ultrathin sections. J. Cell Biol., *44:*211, 1970.

Farquhar, M. G., and Palade, G. E.: Junctional complexes in various epithelia. J. Cell Biol., *17:*375, 1963.

Gilula, N. B.: Gap junctions and cell communication. *In* Brinkley B. R. and Porter, K. R. (eds.): International Cell Biology 1976–1977. New York, Rockefeller University Press, 1977.

Hull, B. E., and Staehelin, L. A.: Functional significance of the variations in the geometrical organization of tight junction networks. J. Cell Biol., *68:*688, 1976.

Keeter, J. S., and Pappas, G. D.: Gap junctions in embryonic skeletal muscle. Anat. Rec., *175*(2):355, 1973.

Lentz, T., and Trinkaus, J. P.: Differentiation of the junctional complex of surface cells. J. Cell Biol. *48:*455, 1971.

Loewenstein, W. R.: Permeability of the junctional membrane channel. *In* Brinkley, B. R. and Porter, K. R. (eds.); International Cell Biology 1976–1977. New York, Rockefeller University Press, 1977.

McNutt, N. S., Hershberg, R. A., and Weinstein, R. S.: Ultrastructure of intercellular junctions in adult and developing cardiac muscle. Am. J. Cardiol., *25:*169, 1970.

————: Further observations on the occurrence of nexuses in benign and malignant human cervical epithelium. J. Cell Biol., *51:*805, 1971.

McNutt, N. S., and Weinstein, R. S.: The ultrastructure of the nexus, A correlated thin-section and freeze-cleave study. J. Cell Biol., *47:*666, 1970.

————: Membrane ultrastructure at mammalian intercellular junctions. Progr. Biophys. Molec. Biol., *26:*47, 1973.

Overton, J.: Experimental manipulation of desmosome formation. J. Cell Biol., *56:*636, 1973.

Pappas, G. D.: Junctions between cells. Hosp, Prac., August 1973.

Revel, J. P.: Morphological and chemical organization of gap junctions. Electron Microscopy 1978. vol. 3, p. 651. Papers presented at Ninth International Congress on Electron Microscopy. Toronto, Microscopical Society of Canada, 1978.

Staehelin, L. A.: Structure and function of intercellular junctions. Int. Rev. Cytol., *39:*191, 1974.

Staehelin, L. A. and Hull, B. E.: Junctions between living cells. Sci. Am., *238:*140, May, 1978.

Suzuki, F., and Nagano, T.: Development of tight junctions in the caput epididymal epithelium of the mouse. Dev. Biol., *63:*321, 1978.

Weinstein, R. S., and McNutt, N. S.: Cell junctions. N. Engl. J. Med., *286:*521, 1972.

8 Loose Connective Tissue

With this chapter we begin the study of a group of related tissues requiring several chapters to describe and all classed under the general heading of Connective Tissues. However, before describing the loose kind of connective tissue we shall first comment on the nature of connective tissues in general.

Some General Features of Connective Tissues. It was mentioned in Chapter 1 that connective tissue was given its name because it connects other tissues together. Moreover, it was explained that the reason for its being able to connect other tissues together, and also to bear weight, was that certain of its cells produced nonliving intercellular substances, some of which are very strong, and that this intercellular substance was responsible for holding the body together and giving it form.

The next point to make is that a great many other functions are performed by the subtypes of tissue in the connective tissue category and that some of these subtypes do little or no connecting. Even some of the connecting types of connective tissue contain cells that perform other functions. To discuss this briefly we shall first list the main groups of tissue classed as connective tissues. These are: (*1*) ordinary connective tissue, (*2*) adipose (fat) tissue, (*3*) blood cells and the blood cell-forming tissues, (*4*) cartilage, and (*5*) bone.

Ordinary connective tissue, as we shall see, is very important for connecting things together in the body. Adipose tissue, however, while serving a role in filling certain crevices in the connective tissue and acting in many sites as a cushion, does not do much connecting; its main function is to store fat for the body. Since neither blood cells (Chaps. 10 and 11) nor the blood cell-forming tissues (Chaps. 12 and 13) serve any connecting functions, it is questionable whether they should be included in the connective tissue group or regarded as a special (fifth) category of tissues. The probable reason for their being considered subtypes of connective tissue is their embryonic origin. Mesenchyme, described in Chapter 6, could be regarded as the connective tissue of the early embryo and, since blood cell-forming tissues (and hence blood cells) develop from mesenchymal cells, both kinds of tissues are developmentally linked with the connective tissue group. Cartilage, bone, and joints (Chaps. 14, 15, and 16) all very obviously play connective tissue and supporting roles dependent on intercellular substances and so can be classified without reservation as connective tissues.

To explain the purpose of this chapter, it should be mentioned that there are two kinds of *ordinary* connective tissue, (*1*) *loose* and (*2*) *dense*. The dense kind consists almost entirely of intercellular substance, in which the cells that produced it lie embedded. The dense kind is very strong and constitutes tendons, aponeuroses, ligaments, and the deep connective tissue layer of the skin. These will all be dealt with in later chapters. The loose kind of ordinary connective tissue, however, is not so specialized, and indeed provides representation not only of all the important kinds of intercellular substances and cells that produce them, but also of a great many other kinds of cells that have other functions. In fact, it will take the whole next chapter to describe these cells and explain their various origins and functions. So in this chapter we shall confine ourselves to describing the several kinds of *intercellular substances* formed in loose connective tissue, which can be regarded as prototypes for those found in the other types of connective tissue. We shall discuss in detail a second and very important function performed by intercellular substance, that of serving as a means for diffusion of nutrients and waste substances between the blood in capillaries and the cells of tissues. We shall, moreover, describe the source of the fluid (called *tissue fluid*) held by the intercellular substance that permits diffusion of nutrients and waste products to occur. We shall also deal with factors regulating the formation and resorption of this essential fluid, and explain how certain conditions can cause excess amounts of it to accumulate. Finally, we shall describe the basement membranes that lie between epithelial or other structures on the one hand and loose connective tissue, with its tissue fluid, on the other.

Sites Where Loose Connective Tissue Are Found. Loose connective tissue is the histological term for what is called *areolar* (L. for small space) *tissue* by gross anatomists. It is found almost everywhere as a thin filling between apposed body parts that can move slightly with respect to one another. For example, it forms an external wrapping for blood vessels, nerves, muscles, and fasciae. Indeed, it is present between so many parts that an anatomist once noted that dissecting the body so that its various parts can be examined consists chiefly of cutting areolar tissue. It seems this tissue was given the name *areolar* because when structures joined by it are gently pulled apart along their lengths, air bubbles are drawn into it as it is stretched, creating an impression that small spaces (areolae) must have existed that filled with air when the tissue was stretched.

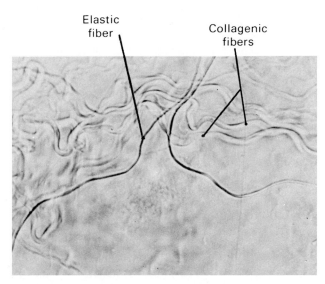

Fig. 8-1. Collagenic and elastic fibers in a fresh, unstained, teased preparation of loose connective tissue. The elastic fibers are more refractile than the collagenic fibers.

THE STUDY OF LOOSE CONNECTIVE TISSUE IN SPREADS AND SECTIONS

Unstained Spreads

Tissue for making spreads can be readily obtained from a recently killed laboratory animal (such as a mouse) by reflecting the skin and subcutaneous tissue from a thigh; loose connective tissue can then be obtained from the site where these tissues were separated from the muscle. Once removed, the tissue can be mounted on a slide in isotonic saline, teased apart, and a coverslip added. With the ordinary LM not much contrast is obtained, but more is seen if the condenser diaphragm is stopped down more than usual. Two kinds of fibers can usually be discerned in such a preparation, as illustrated in Figure 8-1. Fibers of the wider, wavy kind are composed of the protein *collagen* and hence are termed *collagenic fibers*. They vary in width, the largest being around 10 μm., and are composed of *collagenic fibrils* arranged side by side. The latter can sometimes be seen—for example, if a fiber is cut and its end is frayed—but, under normal conditions, ends of collagenic fibers are not seen in a spread. The second kind of fiber seen in unstained spreads is narrower than collagenic fibers, the largest being about 1 μm. in diameter. Such fibers are termed *elastic fibers* because they can be stretched by tensile force and on being released they snap back, like stretched rubber bands, to their original lengths. Because of their higher refractive index they appear darker than the collagenic fibers in unstained spreads (Fig. 8-1).

Unfixed collagenic fibers are white in the gross and therefore are sometimes called *white fibers;* unfixed elastic fibers, however, are slightly yellow and hence are termed *yellow fibers.*

Characteristics of Collagen. Since collagen is such a tough protein, a considerable content of it in meat makes meat tough. If collagen is boiled in water, however, it becomes hydrated and converts into gelatin, which is soft; this is the reason why tough (collagen-rich) meats are more tender when cooked in stews for a long time. Collagen can also be made into leather by digesting the epithelium from the hides of animals and then treating the remaining dense connective tissue with tanning agents that render collagen even more resistant to chemical change. Before World War II, skin burns were often treated by painting them with tannic acid, which literally tanned the collagen of the burned area to constitute a relatively impervious dressing. However, this treatment was abandoned when it became apparent that patients sometimes absorbed enough tannic acid from the painted area to damage their livers. Furthermore, histological studies showed that the tannic acid could penetrate the burned region of the skin so deeply that it could actually increase the damage inflicted by the burn.

The Flexibility of Loose Connective Tissue. It is sometimes too readily assumed that the flexibility of loose connective tissue, such as that underlying the skin, is due primarily to its elastic fibers. Most of the flexibility of loose connective tissue, however, is due to its collagenic fibers not being straight as fibers are in tendons; instead they pursue rather wavy courses, so that the tissue can be stretched somewhat without trying to stretch any collagenic fibers. Hence collagenic fibers limit the extent to which loose connective tissue can be stretched. Elastic fibers, however, which are generally straight, are stretched by most movements and hence important in returning stretched loose connective tissue to its former position once the stretching force is removed.

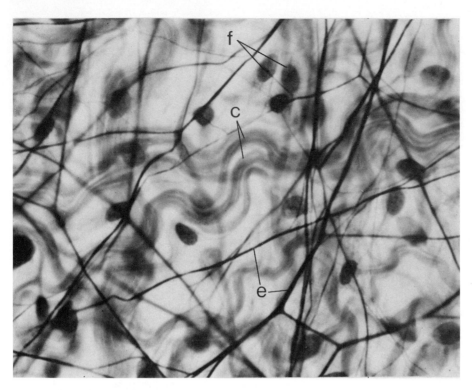

Fig. 8-2. Photomicrograph of an areolar tissue spread, stained with resorcin-fuchsin, Weigert's hematoxylin, and eosin. Note the wavy collagenic fibers (c), branched elastic fibers (e), and nuclei of fibroblasts (f).

THE STAINING OF COLLAGENIC, ELASTIC, AND RETICULAR FIBERS IN SECTIONS

Stained Spreads

Unless phase microscopy is used, cells and other features of loose connective tissue cannot be seen to advantage in unstained material. However, spreads can be fixed and stained. Figure 8-2 shows part of one spread stained so as to demonstrate elastic fibers to advantage, and it shows that unlike collagen fibers these fibers branch. The use of stain, moreover, discloses the nuclei of numerous cells scattered throughout the intercellular substance of the tissue. These belong mostly to *fibroblasts,* the cells that produce the elastic and collagenic fibers of loose connective tissue; these cells, as well as the fine structure of the fibers they produce, will be described in detail in the next chapter.

Collagenic fibers stain pink in H and E sections. When it is important to distinguish collagenic fibers from other components (such as muscle fibers) also staining pink with eosin, other staining methods are sometimes used (those commonly employed include Mallory, Van Gieson, and Masson stains). It is possible to distinguish collagenic fibers from reticular fibers (see below) by PAS staining because collagenic fibers, unlike reticular fibers, fail to stain with the PAS reaction.

Elastic fibers take up very little eosin and cannot be distinguished from the other kinds of intercellular fibers in H

and E sections. Their poor staining is due to elastin having a relatively low content of polar amino acids. In the walls of certain types of blood vessels, however, elastin exists as fairly large fibers and layers *(laminae)* that are commonly thick enough to be refractile and stain pink in H and E sections. In order to demonstrate elastic fibers in ordinary connective tissue it is necessary to employ selective stains such as orcein or resorcin-fuchsin (Fig. 8-2). The appearance of collagenic and elastic fibers in electron micrographs will be described when we consider the composition and formation of these fibers in the next chapter.

Reticular Fibers. These are very fine branched fibers that are characteristically arranged in delicate networks, which accounts for their name (L. *rete,* net). The interstices of the network are commonly of a size that will hold individual cells in place (Fig. 8-3). But reticular fibers are not a very consistent component of loose connective tissue. They nevertheless do assume some importance (*1*) where loose connective tissue is associated with capillaries, nerves, or muscle fibers, (*2*) in the blood cell-forming tissues, where reticular fibers support individual free cells, and (*3*) in certain epithelial glands such as the liver where there is a requirement for delicate support of secretory cells. Furthermore, reticular fibers commonly are present in substantial numbers in association with basement membranes (described at the end of this chapter) in between epithelia and their supporting loose connective tissue. So we shall next briefly describe the chemical composition and special staining characteristics of these fibers.

Reticular fibers are not recognizable in H and E sections. They are most readily demonstrated by silver impregnation technics, whereby they can be distinguished from collagenic fibers because they stain black, whereas collagenic fibers stain yellow to pale brown. The silver impregnation technic involves treating a tissue first with a solution of a reducible silver salt and then with a reducing agent. The latter acts similarly to the developer used for photographic negatives, converting the silver salt into metallic silver, with the result that components (such as reticular fibers) that take up the silver salt appear black.

Because reticular fibers stain differently from collagenic fibers with silver technics it was once assumed that they were of different composition from collagenic fibers. But when they were studied with the EM it was found that they exhibited the same periodicity (a term meaning a repeating pattern, explained in the next chapter) as collagenic fibers, and this finding indicated a molecular structure identical with that of collagen. However, it was also noted with the LM that reticular fibers, if present in sufficient quantities, would stain positively with the PAS technic, and this suggested that they contained or were associated with glycoprotein. It was found, moreover, from chemical studies that reticular fibers had a relatively large carbohydrate content (4%), which is about 10 times that of collagenic fibers. However, it appears this polysaccharide is present as a coating on the re-

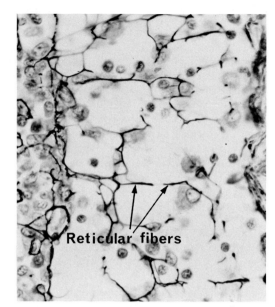

Fig. 8-3. Reticular fibers of a lymph node, stained by the PA-silver technic. (Courtesy of Y. Clermont)

ticular fibers, and this explains why they stain with silver impregnation technics. Reticular fibers of the spleen, stained by a silver technic and examined in the EM, showed in both grazing and cross section (Fig. 8-4) that silver was deposited at the periphery of the fibers, which

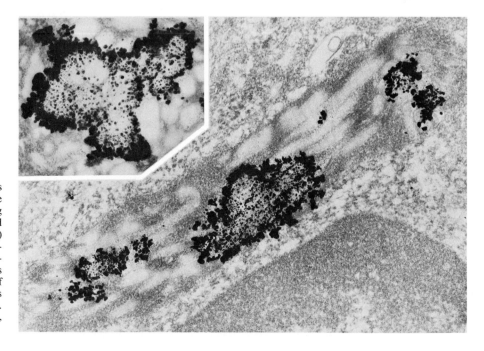

Fig. 8-4. Electron micrographs showing reticular fibers from the spleen of a mouse in grazing (tangential) section (×65,000) and cross section (×105,000, *inset*) following impregnation of the tissue with silver. Note that the electron-dense silver precipitate lies predominantly in the coating of the fiber. The pale unstained areas in the fiber are collagen fibrils. (Snodgrass, M. J.: Anat. Rec., *187:*191, 1977)

indicates that it is due to their coating that reticular fibers stain differently from collagenic fibers.

Before all these observations were made it was thought that reticular fibers were composed of a protein (reticulin) that was different from collagen. Now it is believed that the substance of a reticular fiber is in fact collagen; however, reticular fibers differ in being of fine caliber and in possessing a coating of glycoprotein and proteoglycan.

Whereas fibroblasts probably form reticular fibers in loose connective tissue, there is evidence that in the blood cell-forming tissues these fibers may be formed by what have been called *reticular cells*, described in Chapters 12 and 13.

THE AMORPHOUS COMPONENT OF THE INTERCELLULAR SUBSTANCE OF LOOSE CONNECTIVE TISSUE

From the study of loose connective tissue by any method, it was obvious that its cells and fibers must exist in an aqueous medium, for otherwise the cells would die. So it was postulated that they were bathed in a fluid, called *tissue* (or *extracellular*) *fluid*, that was derived from the blood circulating through nearby capillaries. It was also established that the amount of this fluid present in the tissue was determined by the balance between the hydrostatic pressure of the blood along the length of the capillaries and the osmotic pressure of the blood plasma within the capillaries, as will be explained in detail presently. However, it was not known, and still is not always appreciated, that this tissue (extracellular) fluid is for the most part held in position in loose connective tissue by something of the nature of a soft gel. It took a long time for the presence of this particular component to be established and even longer for its chemical nature to be determined. Indeed, the composition of this material has been the subject of a great deal of modern research, and much of what is now known will be described not only in this chapter but also in subsequent ones on connective tissue.

Development of Knowledge. This began in 1934, when S. Bensley reported an experiment in which she injected a small volume of fluid containing some living paramecia into some loose connective tissue, whereupon it formed a little bleb. She removed the tissue containing this and observed that the paramecia moved about vigorously in the bleb but nevertheless remained confined to it. Whenever they approached its edge they bumped into something invisible. Furthermore the bleb of fluid remained for some time as an entity, which indicated that it was obviously surrounded by something. As a result of these and other findings it was concluded that there must be some substance, structureless though it seemed, between the fibers in loose connective tissue and so it was called the *ground*

substance of loose connective tissue. Later it became usual to refer to this as the *amorphous component* of intercellular substance (in contrast to the fibrous components) and as we shall see it is of profound importance to the functions of the tissue. However, in order to explain why it is so important, we must first describe the structure of loose connective tissue as disclosed by its study in sections.

THE STUDY OF THE INTERCELLULAR SUBSTANCES OF LOOSE CONNECTIVE TISSUE IN SECTIONS

This is more difficult than might be imagined, for two reasons. First, areolar tissue is so commonly disposed in the body in thin layers between other structures that a haphazard slice through body tissue cuts and discloses it where it is more or less squeezed between the structures it separates. For example, in adipose tissue there are little partitions of loose connective tissue separating the fat tissue into lobules (one such partition is labeled a *connective tissue septum* in Fig. 9-14). These septa are almost always cut so that they appear as thin layers that do not reveal much substance for microscopic study. Second, for tissues to be sectioned they must first be fixed and dehydrated. Since the amorphous component of the intercellular substance contains mostly fluid held in place by relatively little substance, the spaces holding the fluid during life tend to collapse when the fluid is removed from them during dehydration. So what is seen in sections of most thin layers of loose connective tissue is a very shrunken and distorted misrepresentation of what was there during life. However, in some body sites there are depots of loose connective tissue that are supported strongly enough to avoid undue shrinkage when fixed and dehydrated, even though the fluid in the amorphous intercellular substance is removed. In such sites, the spaces occupied by the amorphous component remain, but appear empty. In our experience, the loose connective tissue directly below the epithelial covering of the skin is a good place to find loose connective tissue that has not undergone excessive shrinkage, as shown in Figure 7-1, which should be consulted again at this time. Furthermore, because this loose connective tissue is situated immediately below the covering layer of stratified squamous keratinizing epithelium, sites where it appears to advantage are easy to locate.

As shown in Figure 7-1, a feature of loose ordinary tissue here is that it contains blood and lymph capillaries. All around these, wavy collagenic fibers are seen, between which there are seemingly empty spaces. In life these spaces are filled with the amorphous component of loose connective tissue and the chief component of this is

Fig. 8-5. Demonstration of the effect of spreading factor (hyaluronidase) of testicular extract on the extent of spread of injected dye through loose connective tissue (superficial fascia). This rat was injected subcutaneously in two sites: (*1*) with saline containing India ink as a marker (dorsolateral site) and (*2*) with aqueous extract of rat testis containing India ink (dorsal site). Note that the marker has spread more widely from the dorsal site, due to the spreading factor in the testicular extract. (Courtesy of W. Harris)

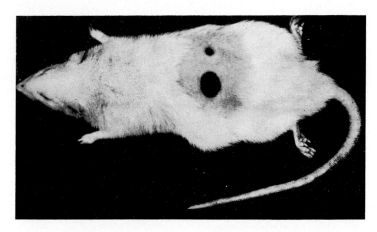

tissue fluid, which exudes from blood capillaries. In ordinary H and E sections there is no sign of the carbohydrate-containing amorphous substance that in life retains the tissue fluid in the spaces between the intercellular fibers.

THE FURTHER DEVELOPMENT OF KNOWLEDGE ABOUT THE AMORPHOUS COMPONENT OF INTERCELLULAR SUBSTANCE

Around the time when Bensley reported her experiments with paramecia (see above), another discovery was made that also proved to have an important bearing on this matter. In 1928 Duran-Reynals noted that when he injected a rabbit's skin with an extract made from a testis of an animal infected with a certain disease, the disease spread very rapidly in the connective tissue of the injected skin. Later studies showed the rapid spread was not necessarily due to the disease agent, for it was found that an extract of normal testis tissue would cause dye injected together with it into the connective tissue of the skin to spread rapidly (Fig. 8-5). From these experiments Duran-Reynals postulated the existence of a *spreading factor* that could be extracted from testicular tissue. For many years its chemical nature remained a mystery. In the meantime, Meyer was investigating the chemistry of the intercellular substances, including the amorphorus ground substance of loose connective tissue. He identified the chief component of ground substance as being essentially polysaccharides that were at first called *acid mucopolysaccharides*. In due course one of these was shown to be a substance termed *hyaluronic acid*, which will be described in detail presently.

Hyaluronidase. As research on the mucopolysaccharides continued, the mystery of the spreading factor was solved. Meyer found that certain kinds of bacteria produced an enzyme capable of depolymerizing hyaluronic acid and named the enzyme *hyaluronidase*. Subsequently it was shown this enzyme was responsible for the spreading effect of testicular extracts. By depolymerizing hyaluronic acid in the ground substance, it removed the chief obstacle to the spread of particulate or dissolved matter through the intercellular substances of loose connective tissue. As a consequence of this finding, the enzyme was for a while used clinically to facilitate the spread and absorption of certain injected drugs, particularly local anesthetics. However, this practice was largely discontinued because it can cause local anesthetics to spread too widely and affect the body unfavorably.

PRESENT CONCEPTS OF THE AMORPHOUS COMPONENT OF THE INTERCELLULAR SUBSTANCE OF LOOSE CONNECTIVE TISSUE

The ground substance in which the fibers and cells of loose connective tissue are embedded is now conceived of as being a semifluid viscous gel. This gel consists of macromolecules, predominantly *polysaccharides*, and a relatively large amount of tissue fluid associated with these macromolecules and representing the aqueous phase of the gel.

As already mentioned, after the essentially polysaccharide nature of ground substance was established, the general term *acid mucopolysaccharides* was used for the substances concerned. The prefix *muco-* was adopted because it was in common use with reference to slippery viscous solutions physically resembling mucus. The polysaccharides of ground substance were termed *acid* mucopolysaccharides because they were made up of carbohydrate groups that were mostly acidic in nature. The term *mucopolysaccharide* is still used to some extent, particularly because certain diseases were found to be characterized by the disordered production of mucopolysaccharides by the cells responsible for their synthesis, and so this group of disorders involving the disordered metabolism of mucopolysaccharides was termed the *mucopolysaccharidoses* (Gr. *-osis,* a process, often a disease process). However, as the chemistry of the acid mucopolysaccharides became further clarified, more accurate biochemical terms for these substances were coined and adopted (see below).

Two kinds of acid mucopolysaccharides were discovered, with an important distinction between them being that one kind was not sulfated while the other was. It was established that the nonsulfated variety in loose connective tissue was hyaluronic acid. The repeating disaccharide unit of this particular polysaccharide is N-acetylglucosamine linked to glucuronic acid. The unbranched polysaccharide chain of the hyaluronic acid molecule (one end of which is attached to a small peptide) is extremely long, and in aqueous solutions it is irregularly coiled or kinked upon itself so as to occupy a relatively huge molecular domain 400 nm. in diameter. Furthermore, it is believed that the macromolecules of hyaluronic acid intermingle with sister macromolecules so as to form a molecular network, the interstices of which are filled with tissue fluid, which serves as the aqueous phase of the gel. As described later, there is an upper limit to the volume of tissue fluid that can serve as a component of the gel, so that excess tissue fluid has to be accomodated as pools of free fluid in the midst of the gel.

The Newer Terminology

Glycosaminoglycans. Hyaluronic acid is now classified as a glycosaminoglycan (*-glycan* is a term meaning polysaccharide). The *glycosamino-* part of the term reflects the fact that the polysaccharide molecule is made up of *repeating disaccharides,* each of which consists of a hexuronic acid linked with an amino sugar (hexosamine).

Sulfated Glycosaminoglycans. It has already been mentioned that what were termed acid mucopolysaccharides were classified into two groups, the nonsulfated kind (hyaluronic acid) and the sulfated kind. Since it is has become usual to call acid mucopolysaccharides *glycosaminoglycans,* the latter kind are now called *sulfated glycosaminoglycans.*

There are four kinds of sulfated glycosaminoglycans. These exist in different relative amounts in the amorphous components of the various connective tissues, including the dense varieties of ordinary connective tissue and also cartilage and bone. As well as containing tissue fluid and so providing a means for diffusion, sulfated glycosaminoglycans may serve an additional function with regard to support because some of them constitute very firm gels. They will be dealt with again later when we describe the tissues in which they play a prominent role (particularly cartilage) and will merely be listed here because they exist in relatively minor amounts in the

amorphous component of loose connective tissue. They are: *(1) heparan sulfate,* which is chemically similar to heparin (described in the next chapter), but less highly sulfated, and is also somewhat similar to hyaluronic acid in composition, but some of its glucosamine is sulfated instead of being acetylated; *(2) chondroitin-4-sulfate* and *(3) chondroitin-6-sulfate,* both of which are characterized by a disaccharide unit consisting of N-acetylgalactosamine and glucuronic acid; and *(4) dermatan sulfate,* which has a repeating disaccharide unit containing sulfated N-acetylgalactosamine and iduronic acid. Hence, with the exception of hyaluronic acid, all the glycosaminoglycans of the ground substance are sulfated.

Proteoglycans. Under normal conditions, the glycosaminoglycans other than hyaluronic acid (that is, the sulfated glycosaminoglycans) are almost all bound to proteins so as to form complexes known as *proteoglycans.* These differ from glycoproteins (which in small quantities are also present in the ground substance) in always containing regularly repeating disaccharide units, whereas the polysaccharide moieties of glycoproteins are made up of several different monosaccharides not arranged in the form of repeating disaccharide groups. The structure of proteoglycans is complex and is discussed in more detail when we describe the matrix of cartilage (pp. 467–468). The point to be made here is that any reference to a *proteoglycan* implies a macromolecular complex, a large part of which consists of sulfated glycosaminoglycans. Although the polysaccharide chain of hyaluronic acid is attached to a peptide, hyaluronic acid is not classed as a proteoglycan.

The Staining of Glycosaminoglycans

Sulfated glycosaminoglycans are sufficiently acidic (anionic) to take up some hematoxylin in H and E sections, as will be seen when we study cartilage. However, the concentration of sulfated glycosaminoglycans is too low in the ground substance of loose connective tissue for any effective staining with hematoxylin. Other methods have to be used to demonstrate its nonsulfated glycosaminoglycan, namely hyaluronic acid. Even with these there is still difficulty in staining hyaluronic acid because its mass is so small in relation to the huge space its molecules encompass; thus it is greatly diluted in ordinary sections. Special methods are often employed to fix sufficient amounts of it for staining and three staining methods are commonly employed for its demonstration.

The first utilizes basic (cationic) stains with a particularly high affinity for acidic (anionic) sites, an example being the copper phthalocyanin dye, alcian blue. Alternatively, metachromatic (Gr. *meta,* after; *chroma,* color) cationic dyes can be used; these stain glycosaminoglycans a color different from that of the dye itself. Toluidine blue, for instance, imparts to glycosaminoglycans a purple color (this is thought to be due to the close packing of dye molecules as they become adsorbed onto closely spaced anionic sites). A third method for detecting glycosaminoglycans, Hale's colloidal iron method, is a two-stage procedure based first on specific binding of colloidal ferric iron to the anionic groups of glycosaminoglycans at low pH, followed by a routine staining method for iron.

Unlike glycoproteins, neither glycosaminoglycans nor proteoglycans are PAS positive. This is because the 1,2-glycol groups of hexuronic acids require much longer for oxidation into aldehyde by periodic acid than is generally allowed in the PAS procedure. It is thus possible to distinguish histochemically the glycoproteins from the glycosaminoglycans in the amorphous intercellular component of connective tissue. Since glycoproteins lack a preponderance of acidic (anionic) groups, they fail to show the cationic staining and metachromasia exhibited by glycosaminoglycans. However, they can just about be detected in the ground substance by the PAS technic, which stains them a very faint magenta color.

THE IMPORTANCE OF THE AMORPHOUS COMPONENT OF INTERCELLULAR SUBSTANCES

First, the capacity of the amorphous component for retaining relatively large quantities of tissue fluid ensures a supply of suitable medium by means of which nutrients and oxygen can diffuse from capillaries to cells not located directly beside capillaries. Furthermore, it provides a means whereby waste products of cellular metabolism can diffuse in the reverse direction and be carried toward blood and lymph capillaries, to be disposed of elsewhere in the body. Second, the relative amounts of particular amorphous intercellular substances present, whether hyaluronic acid and/or proteoglycans, determine to an important degree the histological character of the different kinds of connective tissue in the body. Hence the cells of the various kinds of connective tissue, including cartilage and bone, differ from one another in particular with regard to the amounts and kinds of glycosaminoglycans they synthesize and secrete. Third, the relative amount of amorphous component in the connective tissues seems to be related to aging. In the fetus and the newborn this is relatively abundant in relation to collagen and elastin. But its relative proportion diminishes throughout life, as can be noted particularly in the skin, the connective tissue portion of which gradually becomes thinner and wrinkled with age. Hence a physician in asking a patient's age wisely glances at the skin of their hands for confirmation.

The Relation of Tissue Fluid to the Glycosaminoglycans of Loose Connective Tissue. The fluid within a cell is termed *intracellular fluid* and that between cells and capillaries is termed *tissue fluid*, or *intercellular* (or *extracellular*) *fluid*. As noted, tissue fluid bathes the intercellular substances of connective tissue and is retained in its amorphous com-

ponent by the molecular chains of glycosaminoglycans, which are entangled with those of neighboring molecules so as to constitute a more or less continuously interconnected network with a considerable capacity for holding tissue fluid in its interstices. However, between the extensive domains occupied by glycosaminoglycan molecules, there are tortuous channels through which tissue fluid with its dissolved substances can permeate. These channels permit limited circulation of tissue fluid through the macromolecular maze, and as it circulates there is probably some interchange of fluid between that sequestered in the maze and the relatively free fluid circulating slowly through the channels.

The Difference Between the Circulation of Tissue Fluid and Diffusion Through Tissue Fluid. Tissue fluid circulates through the channels. However, substances of high molecular weight, if present, find few such channels wide enough to move along and so must take long and indirect routes. Furthermore, they may experience frictional effects where they approach the walls of the channels, and the charge distribution and general shape of their molecules may also impede their progress. As a consequence of having to negotiate this molecular labyrinth, particles such as infecting bacteria and viruses and many substances of high molecular weight do not readily circulate (unaided) through the ground substance.

Substances of low molecular weight, ions and gases in solution in the tissue fluid, however, can circulate readily through the channels; moreover, they readily diffuse through the tissue fluid contained in the glycosaminoglycan molecular mesh. Likewise, such substances diffuse through the cytoplasm of capillary walls. Tissue fluid itself, however, passes from the blood in capillaries almost entirely by way of fine slits between the endothelial cells of capillary walls.

Edema. As we shall see, under several kinds of altered physiological conditions the rate of production of tissue fluid exceeds its rate of resorption, whereupon excess tissue fluid accumulates in loose connective tissue and causes it to swell. Any substantial excess causes there to be more tissue fluid in the amorphous material than can be accommodated by the glycosaminoglycan molecular network. This results in excess free tissue fluid in the intercellular substance, which is termed *edema* (Gr. *oidema*, a swelling). Clinically, edema is detected by gently but firmly poking the fingers into the skin at a site where an excess is suspected. Where there is a normal content of tissue fluid in the underlying connective tissue, removal of the fingers is followed by the depressed site quickly returning to its normal position. However, with an excess of tissue fluid in the tissue, the site remains as a depressed pit (hence the term *pitting edema*) for a considerable time. This is because the pressure of the fingers has forced free tissue fluid out of the region into the adjacent tissue. If there had not been any excess of tissue fluid,

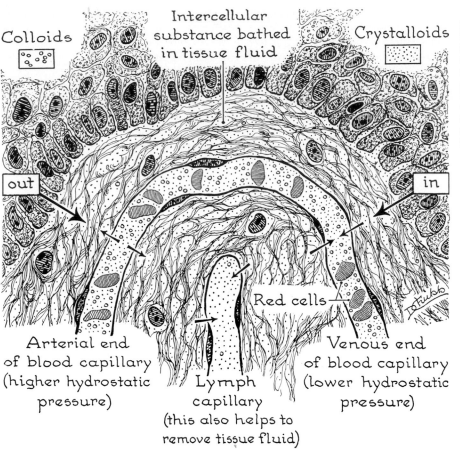

Colloids

Intercellular substance bathed in tissue fluid

Crystalloids

out

in

Arterial end of blood capillary (higher hydrostatic pressure)

Lymph capillary (this also helps to remove tissue fluid)

Red cells

Venous end of blood capillary (lower hydrostatic pressure)

Fig. 8-6. Diagram illustrating how tissue fluid is formed by capillaries and absorbed by capillaries and lymphatics. The proteins of the blood are represented as small circles and the crystalloids of blood and tissue fluid as dots. Under normal conditions only very little colloid escapes from capillaries, and such colloid as escapes is returned to the circulation by way of the lymphatics.

there would have been too little free tissue fluid displaced for this to happen, for if one presses on tissue in which the tissue fluid is to all intents and purposes contained within the glycosaminoglycan network, the fluid is not noticeably displaced by this amount of pressure.

The volume of tissue fluid accumulating in connective tissues varies in relation to the subtype of tissue. Some, for example loose connective or adipose tissue, offer little resistance to being spread apart from within while others, such as dense connective tissue (as in a tendon), resist expansion. In most sites edema tends to be self-limiting because the more a tissue becomes swollen, the more resistance it offers to becoming stretched further.

We shall go on to describe the main causes of edema, but first it is necessary to explain the normal production and absorption of tissue fluid.

THE FORMATION AND ABSORPTION OF TISSUE FLUID

As explained in detail in Chapter 19, blood from the heart is forced under considerable pressure along arteries, tubes with strong walls that branch to supply blood to all parts of the body. The arteries become smaller and smaller as they branch and finally terminate in tiny tubes called *arterioles* with narrow lumina and relatively thick walls. The arterioles reduce pressure like the nozzle of a hose which, if tightened down, permits only a gentle stream to pass through it under low pressure. Arterioles empty into capillary beds and hence the blood in capillaries is under very low pressure compared with that in arteries. Capillary beds are composed of anastomosing, thin-walled tubes that drain into venules, which in turn empty into veins draining blood back to the heart.

The fine structure of capillaries and other blood vessels will of course be considered in detail in Chapter 19. Here it is enough to visualize a single capillary pursuing a curving course through loose connective tissue, like the main one in Figure 7-1 and the one in Figure 8-6. The wall of a capillary is essentially made up of a layer of squamous epithelial cells (like those shown in Fig. 7-4), which develop from mesenchyme and are called *endothelial* cells. The cytoplasm of each endothelial cell is very thin, so that the nucleus bulges in much the same way as the yolk bulges in a fried egg (Fig. 7-4). The edges of the endothelial cells, while always in close apposition, are joined to each other here and there by junctions of the occludens type (fascia occludens). Except in a few parts of the body (such as the brain) these tight junctions do not completely encircle each endothelial cell but are discontinuous, leaving fine potential slits between the edges of adjacent cells where the tight junctions are not present. These slits, however, are so narrow they only permit the passage of water and crystalloids and gases in solution. Under normal conditions, they are not wide enough to permit the exit of the large macromolecules present in blood plasma, so that very little protein escapes.

We now have to explain why a contest between two different kinds of pressure would cause tissue fluid to exude through these tiny slits at one end of the capillary and be drawn back through these slits at the other. The two pressures concerned are *(1) hydrostatic* and *(2) osmotic*.

As already noted, blood is emptied into capillaries from arterioles under relatively low hydrostatic pressure, for otherwise it would burst their delicate walls. Nevertheless, it is under slight pressure. Next, blood is a somewhat viscous fluid, not only because it contains cells but also because blood plasma contains macromolecules of protein and hence is a colloidal solution. As a result of its viscosity, blood experiences some resistance to its flow along narrow capillaries and, as a result, the hydrostatic pressure it is under falls steadily as it moves from the arterial end of a capillary to the venous end. So the hydrostatic pressure tending to force water out through the minute slits between adjacent endothelial cells of the capillary wall becomes less and less along the length of the capillary.

Next, the protein macromolecules in blood plasma exert osmotic pressure. It is well known, for example, that if the wide end of an inverted funnel is covered with a semipermeable membrane (which permits the passage of water and substances of small molecular weight, but not protein macromolecules), egg albumin (a colloidal protein solution) placed in the funnel, by virtue of its osmotic pressure, will draw water through the semipermeable membrane against the force of gravity. The plasma of blood acts like this egg albumin in exerting osmotic pressure and hence is always drawing tissue fluid back into capillaries against the force of hydrostatic pressure. However, as shown on the left in Figure 8-6, at the arterial ends of capillaries the hydrostatic pressure is greater than the osmotic pressure of the blood plasma and hence water (tissue fluid) is forced out through the slits between endothelial cells to become tissue fluid. But at the venous end of the capillary the hydrostatic pressure has dropped to somewhat less than the osmotic pressure exerted by the colloids of blood so that water (tissue fluid) here is drawn back into the capillary (right of Fig. 8-6). This, of course, leads to circulation of tissue fluid through the

channels of the glycosaminoglycan network of the surrounding ground substance.

Some Basic Causes of Edema

Obstruction to the Return of Blood Via Veins. As shown in Figure 8-7A, if venous drainage from capillaries is obstructed, the hydrostatic pressure rises all along the length of the capillaries involved so that more tissue fluid is produced and at the same time less (or none) is absorbed at their venous ends because the greater osmotic pressure within the capillary at its venous end is no longer sufficient to overcome the increased hydrostatic pressure present within the capillary (Fig. 8-7A). This condition can arise in a more or less localized area because of the veins draining that part of the body becoming obstructed, or it can be generalized when a diseased heart becomes unable to pump blood into the arterial system as rapidly as it is being returned to the heart via the veins.

Lymphatic Obstruction. As is shown in Figure 8-7B, obstructed lymphatics can cause edema for two reasons. First, they do not return their usual quota of tissue fluid to the venous system; second, obstructed lymphatics cannot drain away such blood protein as normally escapes from blood capillaries; hence the tissue fluid comes to contain more and more protein, which raises its osmotic pressure so that the differential between the osmotic pressure in the tissue fluid and the venous ends of capillaries become less and less, which results in less and less tissue fluid being returned to the blood at the venous ends of capillaries. This type of edema is most dramatically illustrated in a tropical disease called elephantiasis, in which parasites may invade and obstruct the lymphatics of parts of the body which thereupon become enormously swollen.

Insufficient Protein in the Blood Plasma. As illustrated in Figure 8-8A, if there is too little protein in the blood plasma, its osmotic pressure in the venous ends of capillaries is too little to draw tissue fluid produced at their arterial ends back into them. This condition can arise from plasma protein being lost from the body more rapidly than it is formed because of some disease condition, for example, a large weeping wound or kidney disease that permits protein to leak into the urine. It can also be due to insufficient production of blood protein as a result of starvation or lack of protein in the diet.

Increased Permeability of Capillaries. This can occur at or close to sites damaged by an extensive burn or crushed in an accident. In and around such sites damaged capillaries leak plasma and this can so reduce the blood volume that the amount returned to the heart becomes insufficient for it to pump efficiently. This in turn leads to further complications, as the student will find when he later comes to consider the clinical problem of shock. One

(Text continues on p. 222.)

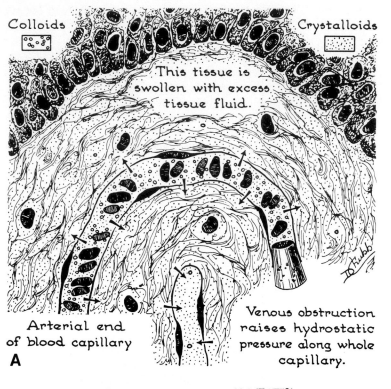

Colloids

Crystalloids

This tissue is
swollen with excess
tissue fluid.

Arterial end
of blood capillary

Venous obstruction
raises hydrostatic
pressure along whole
capillary.

A

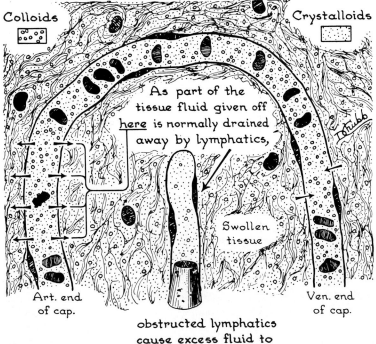

Colloids

Crystalloids

As part of the
tissue fluid given off
here is normally drained
away by lymphatics,

Swollen
tissue

Art. end
of cap.

Ven. end
of cap.

obstructed lymphatics
cause excess fluid to
accumulate in tissue.

B

Fig. 8-7. (A) Diagram showing how an obstruction to the outflow of blood from capillaries (back pressure on veins) can cause an increased amount of tissue fluid to form from the capillaries and also interfere with its absorption. (B) Diagram showing how the obstruction of lymphatics may cause an increased amount of tissue fluid to be present in the tissues they normally drain. The amount of colloid in the tissue fluid becomes increased when lymphatics are obstructed because such colloid as normally escapes from capillaries is ordinarily drained away by the lymphatics.

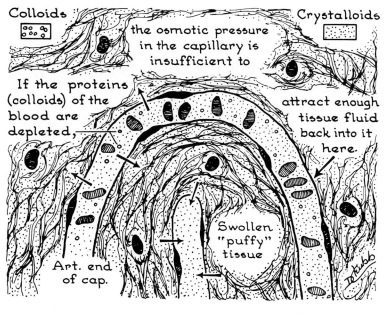

Colloids | Crystalloids

the osmotic pressure in the capillary is insufficient to

If the proteins (colloids) of the blood are depleted,

attract enough tissue fluid back into it here.

Swollen "puffy" tissue

Art. end of cap.

A

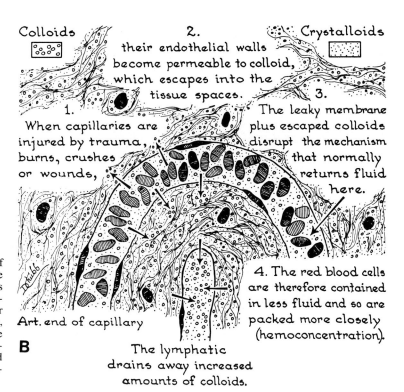

Colloids | 2. | Crystalloids

their endothelial walls become permeable to colloid, which escapes into the tissue spaces.

1. When capillaries are injured by trauma, burns, crushes or wounds,

3. The leaky membrane plus escaped colloids disrupt the mechanism that normally returns fluid here.

4. The red blood cells are therefore contained in less fluid and so are packed more closely (hemoconcentration).

Art. end of capillary

B

The lymphatic drains away increased amounts of colloids.

Fig. 8-8. (*A*) Diagram showing how a lack of colloid in the blood increases the amount of tissue fluid. (*B*) Diagram showing how plasma escapes when the endothelial walls of capillaries are damaged by burns, crushes, nearby wounds, or other means. As plasma leaks away from the capillary, the proportion of red blood cells to plasma in the blood becomes increased. This is called hemoconcentration. Under conditions of this sort, increased amounts of colloid are drained away by the lymphatic capillaries.

consequence of such plasma loss is shown in Figure 8-8B. Because blood cells are not lost along with the plasma, they become relatively concentrated in the plasma remaining. This is called *hemoconcentration* and it can be corrected by the intravenous administration of blood plasma.

THE FORMATION OF LYMPH

More tissue fluid is usually produced at the arterial ends of capillaries than is absorbed at their venous ends. However, loose connective tissue does not normally become swollen with tissue fluid because the extra amount produced (over and above what is absorbed) is drained away by a second set of capillaries termed *lymphatic capillaries,* so called because the tissue fluid that seeps into them is known as *lymph* (L. *lympha*, clear water).

Lymphatic capillaries (Fig. 8-6) form networks of great complexity and drain into larger lymphatic vessels. These eventually open into two lymphatic ducts returning the lymph collected from the whole body to large veins at the root of the neck. Hence that part of the tissue fluid absorbed by the lymphatic capillaries is eventually returned to the confines of the blood circulatory system again, but by a somewhat circuitous route.

Lymphatic capillaries are involved in regulating the quality of the tissue fluid as well as its quantity. It is generally agreed that the blood capillaries do in one way or another allow a little protein to escape from the plasma into the amorphous intercellular substance. Indeed, were it not for the lymphatic drainage of tissue fluid, this escaped blood protein would accumulate in tissue fluid and by virtue of its osmotic pressure would tend to increase the water content of the tissue. Thus by continually draining away protein, lymphatic capillaries keep blood proteins from accumulating in the intercellular compartment.

It might be thought that the increased hydrostatic pressure of the tissue fluid in swollen (edematous) tissue might lead to a collapse of its lymphatic capillaries and so interfere with lymphatic drainage. However, this is prevented because the endothelial cells lining the lymphatic capillaries are attached to collagenic *anchoring fibers* extending through the surrounding tissue. Thus as the tissue becomes spread apart by edema fluid, these fibers pull on the walls of lymphatics in all directions so as to hold them open.

BASEMENT MEMBRANES

In routine sections a seemingly structureless special layer (labeled basement membrane in Fig. 7-9) was often noticed between an epithelial membrane and the connec-

tive tissue immediately beneath it. Since it was positioned immediately below the bases of the epithelial cells, this layer was termed a *basement membrane* (BM). This "classic" example of a BM was at first thought to consist of a homogeneous condensed layer of intercellular substance produced by the fibroblasts of the underlying connective tissue. When the PAS method became available it was observed that such basement membranes were PAS positive and this tended to support the concept of the membrane being composed of a single layer. However, the EM showed that the deeper part of what was then considered a basement membrane was actually composed of a matted network of reticular fibers. It also disclosed a single homogeneous, electron-dense layer 50 to 100 nm. thick, positioned immediately above the reticular fibers (as depicted in Fig. 8-10). This was called the *basal lamina* (L. *lamina*, flat layer), so as to distinguish it from a basement membrane, which term was then used to include the underlying layer of reticular fibers as well as the basal lamina. The basal lamina was found to always follow the contours of the basal surface of the epithelium, as can be seen in Figure 8-9, and was separated from it by a space about 40 nm. wide corresponding to the thickness of the cell coat of the epithelial cells.

Next, by means of the immunofluorescence technic for locating specific proteins (p. 245) it was found that certain constituents of the basement membrane could be detected in the epithelial cells above it and this, of course, suggested that the basal lamina was synthesized by the epithelial cells and not by the underlying connective tissue cells, as had previously been believed. It was therefore intriguing when chemical investigations showed that the basal lamina contained collagen—which, however, was of a different form from that in the connective tissue below. (As explained in the next chapter, p. 231, a unique form of collagen termed *Type IV collagen* is characteristic of basal laminae). Furthermore, the basal lamina was found also to contain two different glycoproteins, one of a high and one of a low molecular weight. The presence of these glycoproteins could account for the basal lamina being PAS positive, and because the reticular fibers beneath the basal lamina would also be PAS positive, it could be expected that an entire BM might appear as a single PAS positive "membrane."

As research continued, the EM disclosed that basal laminae in some parts of the body lacked evident mats of reticular fibers beneath them. Indeed basal laminae could even be found between two layers of epithelial cells of different origins; for example, as we shall see, the endothelium of capillaries of kidney glomeruli is covered with a layer of visceral epithelium, and sandwiched in between these two layers is a basal lamina through which the fluid that will eventually become urine is filtered. At first it was customary to refer to such basal laminae,

Fig. 8-9. Electron micrograph (×16,400) of part of the wall of a bile duct (rat liver), showing the basal lamina (bl) of the epithelial cells of the duct. Part of a liver cell (hepatocyte) is seen at *top left;* the large nucleus at *center* belongs to an epithelial lining cell of the duct (lumen at *bottom right*). Note how the duct is encircled by the continuous basal lamina, which follows closely the contours of the basal surface of the lining epithelium. Lead citrate stain. (Courtesy of M. J. Phillips)

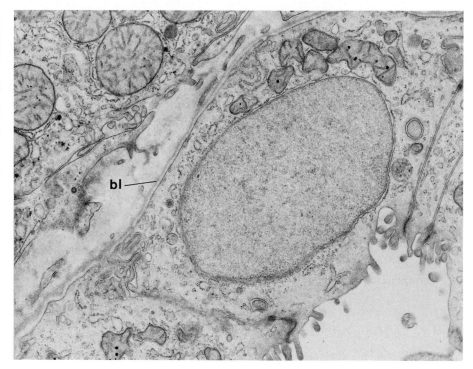

which are not supported by mats of reticular fibers, as basement membranes. But since a classic basement membrane has two layers with two different origins, the tendency now is to term these single layers *basal laminae* and reserve the term *basement membrane* for those types that have the two-layered structure.

A prominent basement membrane is found beneath the epithelium covering the cornea of the eye (Fig. 28-5, 1). It was at first believed that this basement membrane would be formed by the underlying connective tissue cells of the cornea. But Dodson and Hay showed that epithelial cells

of the cornea when cultivated in vitro are themselves capable of synthesizing the material of this basement membrane.

Finally, we shall also find that basal laminae are associated with nerve and muscle fibers and not only epithelial cells.

Summary of Basement Membrane Structure. A diagram depicting what would be seen at the EM level in a "classic" (two-component) basement membrane lying beneath parts of two epithelial cells is shown in Figure 8-10. This shows the following structures, from top to bottom.

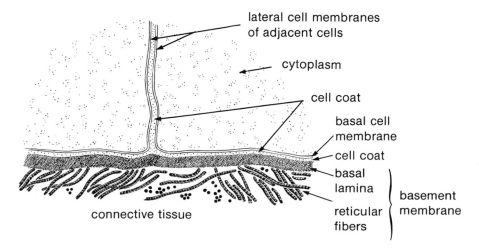

Fig. 8-10. Diagram showing the components of the basement membrane along the basal surface of an epithelial membrane. These components would all be demonstrable in the EM with appropriate staining procedures.

First, there is the *cell membrane* (a double line labeled in Fig. 8-10) of the basal cells. Second, beneath this there is the *cell coat* that covers the cell membrane. Third, there is the *basal lamina* and fourth, the mat of associated *reticular fibers*. The two latter layers (the basal lamina and the reticular fibers) constitute the two layers of the classic *basement membrane*. However, as noted, in some body sites the basement membrane seems to be represented only by a basal lamina.

Functions of Basement Membranes. Basement membranes (and/or basal laminae) have two principal roles: *(1)* to provide elastic support and *(2)* to act as filtration or diffusion barriers. A particularly good example of a basement membrane serving the first function is the capsule surrounding the lens of the eye. This lens capsule (which corresponds to a well-developed basement membrane) not only supports the lens but must also possess considerable elasticity, since it has to be able to expand when the lens accommodates for distant vision and then return to its original shape afterward. Under the basal layer of the skin epithelium (epidermis) there is again a well-developed flexible basement membrane that doubtless serves to bond the epithelium strongly to the collagen in the dermal connective tissue beneath. Next, since basement membranes in a sense separate the cells of other tissues from the connective tissue that nourishes them, it is obvious that they must permit the passage of tissue fluid and the diffusion of substances of low molecular weight. Moreover, it will become evident when we consider the role of the basement membrane in the glomeruli of the kidneys that basement membranes selectively filter out macromolecular substances on the basis of their molecular weight and if they fail to perform this function properly, it may have very serious consequences for the body.

For references and other reading *see* lists at end of Chapter 9.

9 The Origins, Morphologies, and Functions (Including Immunological Functions) of the Cells of Loose Connective Tissue

Loose connective tissue permeates almost everywhere in the body and provides intimate support for blood vessels and nerves of all sizes. Moreover, loose connective tissue is the usual arena in which the process of inflammation occurs when any body part is invaded by bacteria or other pathogenic microorganisms. Therefore, its cells must not only provide for the formation of its intercellular substances, which enable it to perform its supportive and nutritive functions, but they must also perform defensive roles. Thus, there is a division of labor among the cells of loose connective tissue. We shall in this chapter deal first with the cells involved in its formation and maintenance, and then with those of its cells that are concerned primarily in immunological and inflammatory reactions. The other cells involved in immune responses will be considered in detail in subsequent chapters.

If enough samples of loose connective tissue (from reasonably mature animals) are studied in stained spreads or sections, at least eight kinds of cells may be recognized with the LM by their morphology (aided sometimes by observing the positions they occupy). For convenient reference they are all illustrated and labeled in Figure 9-1. It should be understood, however, that this illustration is a composite drawing showing one of each sort of cell that might only be found by studying a great many spreads or sections; hence they would not all be seen in a single field as depicted in the illustration. The cells are thus best studied in the laboratory by finding a good example of each one somewhere in a spread or section. We shall describe the appearance of each kind in detail and explain the relation of its structure to its function, but first we must discuss the origins of connective tissue cells.

Origins. Some of these cells are formed directly from the mesenchyme that occupied the same site in prenatal life. Certain others, however, though their ancestral cells were mesenchymal cells, developed elsewhere in the body and then entered the bloodstream, from which they migrated into loose connective tissue later, either as it developed or at some time in postnatal life. So what we term the cells of loose connective tissue represent a mixed cell population of natives and immigrants. Since all of these cells are nevertheless derived either directly or indirectly from mesenchyme, we shall first briefly discuss mesenchyme.

Mesenchyme. This embryonic tissue was given its name (Gr. *mesos*, middle; *enchyma*, infusion) because it was thought to develop exclusively from mesoderm, the middle germ layer. While almost all of it does, some was later shown to develop from ectoderm, particularly in the head region. Characteristically, mesenchyme is depicted as a loose network of more or less star-shaped cells with very pale staining cytoplasm. The processes (labeled in Fig. 9-2) of many of these cells connect with those of adjacent cells. The cells are usually fairly widely separated from one another by a jelly-like amorphous intercellular substance (Fig. 9-2, ics) which, as development proceeds, is seen to contain some delicate fibers. In some sites, as we shall see when we study the development of cartilage, mesenchyme may become condensed with its cells lying closer together, and mesenchyme being an embryonic tissue, the cells undergo frequent mitoses (labeled in Fig. 9-2). Mesenchymal cells are either directly or indirectly ancestral to all the cells of loose connective tissue, which include (*1*) endothelial cells, (*2*) pericytes, (*3*) fibroblasts, (*4*) smooth muscle cells, (*5*) fat cells, (*6*) plasma cells, (*7*) mast cells, and (*8*) macrophages.

ENDOTHELIAL CELLS AND HOW THEY DEVELOP FROM MESENCHYMAL CELLS

The first endothelial cells to appear in the embryo are commonly associated with the formation of the precursors of blood cells. The most common place for this to occur in most species is in the yolk sac of the early embryo. One way this happens is for certain of the mesenchymal cells to form a clump of free cells (the progenitor cells of blood cells); the nature of these is described in Chapter 12. The mesenchymal cells surrounding such a clump become flattened, and these encircling cells become joined to one another by cell junctions to form a large capillary-like tube. The free cells in the lumen of the vessel and the flattened mesenchymal (now endothelial) cells that surround them together con-

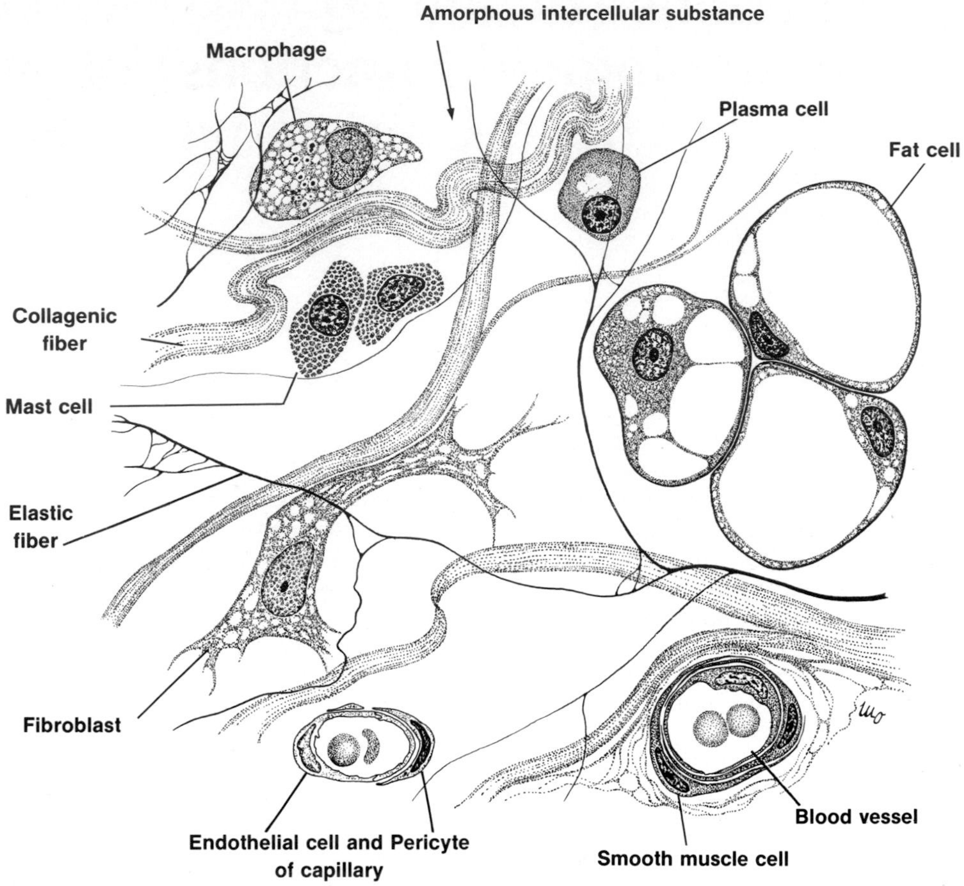

Macrophage

Amorphous intercellular substance

Plasma cell

Fat cell

Collagenic fiber

Mast cell

Elastic fiber

Fibroblast

Endothelial cell and Pericyte of capillary

Smooth muscle cell

Blood vessel

Fig. 9-1. Diagrammatic representation of cells that may be seen in loose connective tissue. These cells are embedded in an amorphous intercellular component bathed in tissue fluid that originates from capillaries.

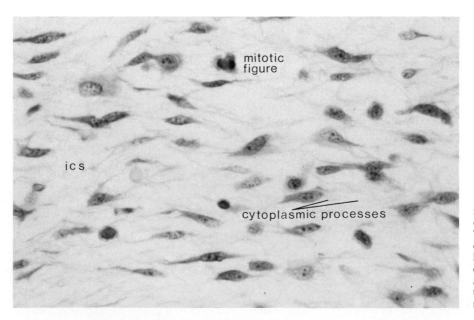

mitotic figure

i c s

cytoplasmic processes

Fig. 9-2. Photomicrograph of mesenchyme (developing loose connective tissue) of an embryo. This tissue is very soft because its cells are embedded in a relatively large volume of amorphous intercellular substances (ics). A cell at *top* is undergoing mitosis. Note the thin cytoplasmic processes of mesenchymal cells.

stitute what has long been termed a *blood island*. However, since it is our purpose at this point to describe the formation not of blood cells but of endothelium, it should here be explained that primitive capillaries consisting of endothelium do not form exclusively around primitive blood cells, because in some sites mesenchymal cells also gather around tiny pools of fluid to form capillaries, as shown in Figure 9-3.

The formation of wide capillary-like tubes, with walls consisting of endothelial cells differentiated from mesenchymal cells, marks the beginning of the formation of the blood-circulatory system. As more and more endothelial tubes form from mesenchyme, they connect with one another. Then other mesoderm-derived cells begin to condense around them and differentiate into muscle cells, and by this means the heart, arteries, and veins are formed. The arteries are connected to veins by capillaries and the endothelial cells of these proliferate to form capillary networks throughout the developing tissues. Hence while endothelial cells develop at first by the differentiation of mesenchymal cells into endothelial cells, the great development of the capillaries, arteries, and veins, which comes later, is not directly from mesenchyme but from the subsequent proliferation of endothelium and its surrounding cells; these grow all through ordinary connective tissue as it continues to develop. Endothelial cells thus retain a great capacity for proliferation.

A single endothelial cell may be large enough to completely encircle a capillary (Fig. 9-4, *right*) but commonly is not; hence a capillary wall examined in cross section may show two separate sites where cell junctions are

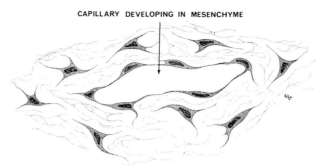

CAPILLARY DEVELOPING IN MESENCHYME

Fig. 9-3. Diagram illustrating the way flattened mesenchymal cells lining a space in mesenchyme differentiate into the endothelial cells of a capillary.

present, as does the one on the left side of Figure 9-4. In most parts of the body the interdigitating edges of contiguous cells are joined together tightly (but not continuously) by occludens junctions of the fascia type. As already mentioned, at the sites between these junctions there are very fine slits just wide enough to permit the passage of substances in simple solution, but narrow enough to hold back most of the protein macromolecules of the blood plasma, so that tissue fluid, as already mentioned, contains only a low concentration of protein. In some body sites the capillaries provide a second way for tissue fluid to cross their walls, since the cytoplasm of their endothelial cells is riddled with openings about 60 to 80 nm. in diameter. Capillaries of this type are said to be

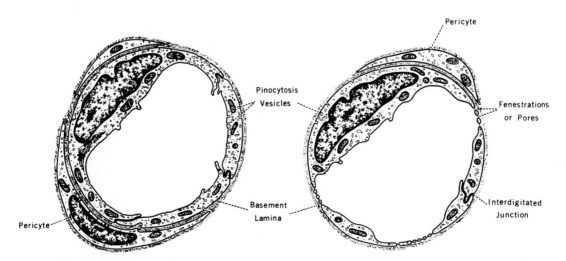

Fig. 9-4. Diagrams illustrating the structure of a muscle capillary of the continuous type (*left*), and a visceral capillary of the fenestrated type (*right*). (Fawcett, D. W.: Comparative observations on the fine structure of blood capillaries. *In* Orbison, J. L., and Smith, D. (eds.): Peripheral Blood Vessels, p. 17. Baltimore, Williams & Wilkins, 1963)

fenestrated (L. *fenestra,* window) to distinguish them from the *continuous* type (compare the right diagram with the left one in Fig. 9-4). It is believed, however, that each fenestra is not open as it seems, but closed over with a thin *diaphragm* that is seldom visible in a micrograph. However, the fenestrated capillaries in the kidney glomeruli appear to be an exception to this general rule, since there the fenestrae do lack diaphragms.

The fine structure of the endothelium of capillaries, the larger blood vessels, and the heart will be described in more detail when we consider the circulatory system (Chap. 19).

Finally, endothelial cells are generally viewed as fully determined cells having no potentiality to form other kinds of connective tissue cells. However, they retain a great ability to divide and so are able to maintain a continuous lining for the whole circulatory system and form new capillaries when required.

PERICYTES (PERIVASCULAR CELLS)

A question that arises from all kinds of connective tissue cells developing directly or indirectly from mesenchyme, and hence all being related to one another, is whether any of them in postnatal life retains enough mesenchymal potentiality to be able to differentiate into any other kind of cell of connective tissue. Different views have been held. For example, it was argued in past decades that macrophages could undergo a transformation (differentiation) into fibroblasts. This view is no longer held. Still other kinds of cell transformations have been postulated but are no longer accepted. The fact remains, however, that some curious things happen in ordinary connective tissue that prove that some cells retaining considerable mesenchymal potentiality must be present in it even in adult life. The type of loose connective tissue cell that in our opinion is best qualified to fit this category is the one we are about to describe, the *pericyte.*

Development of Knowledge

Around the turn of the century, the distinguished histologist Felix Marchand described the cells now termed *pericytes* as *adventitial cells* (L. *adventicius,* coming from abroad) because they were located along the sides of capillaries (Fig. 9-1, pericyte) but did not seem to be derived from them. Furthermore, he considered that they were not end cells but retained a certain amount of mesenchymal potentiality and could hence serve as a source of certain other types of connective tissue cells. Somewhat later, the equally distinguished histologist Alexander Maximow also conceived of there being rela-

tively undifferentiated mesenchymal cells persisting as such in the connective tissues in postnatal life; these he termed *undifferentiated mesenchymal cells.* Like Marchand, Maximow believed these cells were closely associated with capillaries.

Some mention must be made here of the kinds of events occurring in ordinary connective tissue that seem to require the presence of relatively undifferentiated mesenchymal cells for their explanation. For example, a fragment of bone tissue occasionally develops in ordinary connective tissue, usually in association with an old operation scar or beside some calcified deposit in an artery wall. For bone to form requires the presence of special cells called *osteoblasts,* bone-forming cells normally present only in bone tissue. It has been shown, as described in detail on page 394, that it is possible to induce bone formation in connective tissue by implanting decalcified bone in it. Sequential histological studies indicate that the osteoblasts responsibe for forming bone in these sites develop from cells that grow into the area along with capillaries (*see* references for Ectopic Bone in Chap. 15). Next, when connective tissue is damaged, its repair may require the formation of new blood vessels. As already noted, capillary endothelium is prolific and grows rapidly into wound areas to form new capillary beds. As time goes on, however, some of these capillaries become larger blood vessels, such as arterioles or venules, which possess smooth muscle cells in their walls (Fig. 9-1, blood vessel). It has now been shown that the *pericyte* is the most likely candidate for forming the smooth muscle cells that appear under these conditions. Finally, in the repair of wounds there is sometimes a great deal of growth of what appear to be fibroblasts (which we shall soon describe) for they are the cells that synthesize and secrete the intercellular substances of loose connective tissue. It is often assumed that fibroblasts mature enough to have formed intercellular substances still retain the ability to divide. However, it is questionable whether mature functioning fibroblasts account for all the new fibroblasts that appear in repair processes. It now seems very probable that capillary-associated pericytes, proliferating along with endothelial cells in the repair process, serve as the chief progenitor cells for the fibroblasts (Ross et al.).

The Microscopic Appearance of Pericytes

With the LM, the nuclei of pericytes appear several times longer than wide and show no particular distinctive features (Figs. 9-1 and 9-4), and their cytoplasm is pale in H and E sections. With the EM the cytoplasm is seen to extend from the main cell body in the form of processes wrapped around the capillaries with which they are associated (Fig. 19-22), as described in more detail on page 605, where the fine structure of small blood vessels is described. The cytoplasm of pericytes, as shown in Figs. 9-4 and 19-22, is disposed so as to envelop the capillary wall. It was once thought that these cells were contractile like smooth muscle cells, but it is now generally believed that the usual cell in this position is not itself contractile but that as a pericyte it can develop into a contractile smooth muscle cell if the capillary develops into an arteriole or large venule.

FIBROBLASTS AND THE SYNTHESIS OF THE INTERCELLULAR SUBSTANCES OF ORDINARY CONNECTIVE TISSUE

The word *fibroblast* (L. *fibra,* fiber, and Gr. *blastos,* germ) was coined to denote the cell type that formed fibers of ordinary connective tissue. Later, when the amorphous component of the intercellular substance of ordinary connective tissue was also recognized, it was conceded that this too was produced by fibroblasts.

Lest confusion arise later, it should be emphasized here that whereas fibroblasts produce the intercellular substances of ordinary connective tissue they are not the *only* kinds of cells able to form collagenic and elastic fibers and amorphous intercellular substance. For example, the collagen, glycosaminoglycans, and proteoglycans of cartilage and bone are produced by relatives of fibroblasts, called chondroblasts and osteoblasts respectively. Furthermore, in the blood cell-forming tissues reticular fibers are believed to be produced by special cells called reticular cells. In addition, it is now known that smooth muscle cells can form elastin, the protein in elastic fibers. Hence it is only in the ordinary connective tissues that fibroblasts are allotted the important task of producing intercellular substances, and even here the smooth muscle cells of small blood vessels also produce some elastin.

The Degree to Which Fibroblasts Have Differentiated and Become Committed

The position taken here is that a fibroblast is a committed cell that can produce only intercellular substances of ordinary connective tissue. If, for example, bone happens to develop somewhere in ordinary connective tissue, we do not believe (as is so often assumed by others) that it is formed by a fibroblast undergoing a transformation into an osteoblast. Instead, we take the position that this is to be explained by the persistence of relatively undifferentiated cells in ordinary connective tissue, which the evidence now indicates are the pericytes.

The next question is whether fibroblasts can serve their function of producing intercellular substances and still remain able to divide. There are many indications

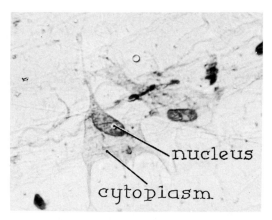

Fig. 9-5. Photomicrograph of a teased preparation of areolar tissue, lightly stained with methylene blue, showing two fibroblasts.

suggesting that eventually after a fibroblast has surrounded itself with the intercellular substance it has produced it loses its ability to divide. For example, it has been found that during the repair of a tendon, in which there are old fibroblasts lying between the bundles of collagenic fibers they previously made, repair is effected by ingrowth of young fibroblasts (probably derived from pericytes). These grow into the damaged site along with the capillaries that invade the site of injury (p. 368). Accordingly, there is a tendency to refer to old fibroblasts that have almost completed their task of producing intercellular substances as *fibrocytes.* Furthermore, as already mentioned, there are indications that many of the new cells seen undergoing mitosis where ordinary connective tissue is being repaired develop from pericytes. It therefore seems that when the genes directing the synthesis of intercellular substances are turned on in a fibroblast, those directing its growth and proliferation become repressed as outlined in Chapter 6.

THE MICROSCOPIC FEATURES OF FIBROBLASTS

Appearance in Stained Spreads

If teased spreads of freshly obtained loose connective tissue (prepared as for the study of fibers) are stained lightly with a basic dye such as methylene blue, fibroblasts similar to the ones illustrated in Figures 9-1 and 9-5 are readily seen, since fibroblasts are the commonest cells in loose connective tissue. The pale-staining cytoplasm of fibroblasts often extends irregularly from around the nucleus in the form of processes; however, the latter are probably accentuated in Figure 9-5 by teasing so that the

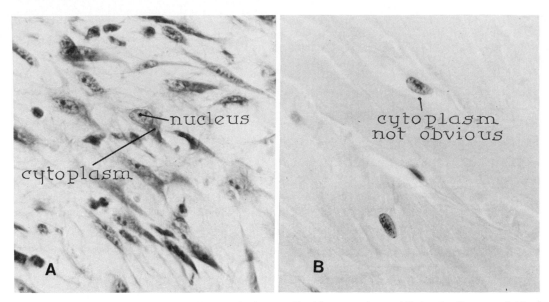

Fig. 9-6. (*A*) Medium-power photomicrograph of young fibroblasts growing rapidly in a healing wound. Note that the cytoplasm of young, actively growing fibroblasts is visible in H and E sections. (*B*) Photomicrograph of mature connective tissue in the deeper part of the skin. Most of this tissue consists of collagenic fibers. Only the nuclei of fibrocytes (old fibroblasts) can be seen to advantage in such tissue.

processes of the cells are more prominent here than they would be in life. Some fibroblasts have a fusiform shape. The nuclei of fibroblasts in this type of preparation are generally ovoid and pale; their chromatin is finely granular and nucleoli can generally be seen.

Appearance in H and E Sections

Old fibroblasts (*fibrocytes*) are surrounded by collagenic fibers, mostly made some time previously (Fig. 9-6B). Little or no cytoplasm can be seen in these old cells whose presence is revealed only by their pale nuclei (Fig. 9-6B). Their nuclei are more or less flattened ovoids; therefore, if cut in some planes, they appear much thinner than they do in others, and if they are cut in cross section, they appear smaller than if cut longitudinally.

A young fibroblast differs from a fibrocyte in an H and E section in having abundant basophilic cytoplasm surrounding its nucleus, as shown in Figure 9-6A. From the main cell body less basophilic processes extend for considerable distances (Fig. 9-6A). Furthermore, the nucleus of a young active fibroblast generally has a prominent nucleolus (Fig. 9-6A). Thus the appearance of a young fibroblast (abundant basophilic cytoplasm and a large nucleolus) is that of a cell actively synthesizing protein. This could be protein for further growth (for the formation of more fibroblasts, because *young* fibroblasts can divide) or protein destined for secretion (for the production of intercellular substances). After a fibroblast has produced its

quota of intercellular substance, its cytoplasm becomes pale, as already noted (Fig. 9-6B), and it is then commonly called a *fibrocyte*. Fibrocytes, however, have been shown to take up labeled proline, an amino acid required for the synthesis of collagen, which would indicate that fibrocytes, although they do not divide, may still be able to secrete some intercellular substance.

THE ORIGIN OF FIBROBLASTS

In embryonic development, fibroblasts are believed to arise directly from the mesenchymal cells originally present in the sites at which these fibroblasts are later found. However, studies on the repair of connective tissue in postnatal life indicate that mitoses resulting in formation of new fibroblasts also occur in the less differentiated pericytes closely associated with small blood vessels. Furthermore, there has been controversy over the years as to whether certain blood cells (monocytes) enter damaged regions of connective tissue and there differentiate into fibroblasts that assist in the repair process. Ross et al., using parabiotic rats (rats joined together so as to share a common bloodstream), have shown in an ingenious experiment that neither monocytes nor any other blood cells labeled with thymidine become fibroblasts in the repair of a wound. They believe that the fibroblasts repairing a wound are of local origin and that they arise mostly from pericytes, which are less differentiated than fibroblasts but can serve as their precursors.

THE SYNTHESIS AND SECRETION OF PRECURSORS OF FIBROUS INTERCELLULAR SUBSTANCES

It is possible that from reading the chapter on cytoplasm, in which the mechanism of secretion was described in connection with epithelial cells, the student may assume that secretion is characteristic only of epithelial cells. However, several kinds of connective tissue cells are also secretory and later we shall find that certain kinds of muscle cells and also nerve cells perform secretory functions. So in beginning to study the fine structure of the fibroblast, it is most important to realize that it is a *secretory* cell and that what has been said previously about secretion in Chapters 5 and 7 is relevant here too. The essential difference between a fibroblast and an epithelial secretory cell is that the fibroblast does not secrete its products onto a free surface through a particular region of its cell surface, but through sites all over its surface. Fibroblasts can secrete three main products, procollagen, glycosaminoglycans, and proelastin. They can also secrete a microfibrillar protein that becomes incorporated into elastic fibers.

Some Basic Biochemistry of Collagen

Collagen molecules are relatively long (about 280 nm.) and narrow (about 1.5 nm.) and consist of three polypeptide chains wound together in the form of a triple helix. The chains are termed alpha chains and each consists of sequences of three amino acids repeated along its course. The first amino acid of each sequence may be any of a variety of amino acids other then the next two to be mentioned. The second amino acid is either proline or lysine, and the third is always glycine.

Four types of collagen are recognized,* each differing slightly in the composition of its alpha chains. In *Type I* collagen, which is characteristic of ordinary connective tissue and bone, there is a minor difference in amino acid composition and sequence between one alpha chain and the other two which are identical to one another. In basement membrane collagen (*Type IV*), the amino acid composition and sequence are somewhat different again, while in *Type II* collagen (found in cartilage) and *Type III*

---

* The four types of collagen have the following distribution in the body:

Type	Location
I	Ordinary connective tissue (both loose and dense kinds) and bone
II	Hyaline cartilage
III	Fetal dermis, also arteries and certain other sites
IV	Basement membranes

collagen (found for example in arteries), there are further minor differences in alpha chain composition. In all but Type I collagen, however, the three alpha chains of the collagen molecules are identical with one another. The Type IV collagen of basement membranes has a much higher content of carbohydrate side chains than that found elsewhere. It also has a higher content of hydroxylysine and hydroxyproline.

Collagen is unusual because it contains such a high proportion of proline and glycine and it is unique because a considerable amount of the proline and lysine is hydroxylated. The function of the hydroxyproline in collagen is not known but advantage can be taken of the fact that it is present (to any great extent) only in collagen. First, whether cells are capable of producing collagen can be investigated by determining whether they contain the enzymes required for hydroxylating proline. Second, and of clinical significance, is the fact that it can also be determined whether collagen is being broken down in the body at an excessive rate, for hydroxyproline then appears in quantity in the urine. Since bone contains a good deal of collagen, conditions in which excessive amounts of bone are being resorbed can be detected by this means.

The function of the hydroxylysine is better known. First, the hydroxylysine of one collagen molecule can attach to the hydroxylysine of other collagen molecules and this accounts for the cross linking of collagen molecules that gives collagenic fibers their strength. Second, the hydroxylysine molecules provide for the attachment of short carbohydrate chains of galactose and glucose.

THE STEPS IN THE SYNTHESIS AND SECRETION OF PROCOLLAGEN IN THE CYTOPLASM OF CELLS

Collagen is synthesized in the form of a precursor known as *procollagen*. The synthesis of the alpha chains of procollagen occurs in association with polyribosomes of the rER. When first synthesized, these chains are somewhat longer than later because a tailpiece of about 13 nm. is added to each as it is produced. A number of proline and lysine residues in the chains become hydroxylated within 3 minutes of being incorporated into the chain being synthesized, and it takes only about 5 to 6 minutes for a complete chain to be synthesized. These facts have been established by biochemical investigations. Further information was derived from radioautographic studies using ^{3}H-proline as a marker in both fibroblasts and odontoblasts. The latter are the cells that produce the dentin in teeth. There are certain advantages for studying the synthesis of collagen in odontoblasts because they are long, narrow cells that synthesize procollagen the same way as fibroblasts but secrete the finished product only through one of their ends. Hence in odontoblasts there is, as it were, a production line along

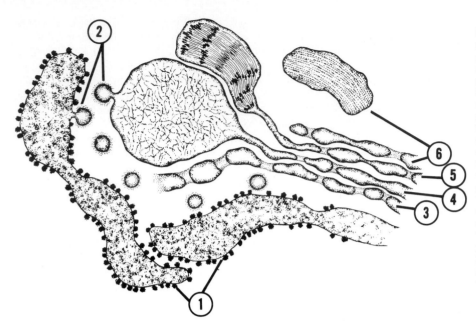

Fig. 9-7. Diagrammatic drawing of part of the Golgi region of a collagen-secreting cell. From *bottom* to *top,* note: (1) cisternae of rER studded with ribosomes; (2) transfer vesicles, one of which is budding from a cisterna, another fusing with a distended portion of a Golgi saccule; (3) the first saccule of a stack of Golgi saccules at *upper right;* (4) the second saccule with a distended portion filled with entangled threads; (5) the third saccule with a distended portion filled with parallel threads; and (6) the fourth saccule, and above it a structure with discrete striations, which is a distended portion that has separated from it; here the parallel threads have aggregated. This structure is a secretory vesicle, and its contents will be released at the cell surface. (Courtesy of M. Weinstock and C. P. Leblond)

which the stages of procollagen synthesis and its secretion can be followed by radioautography. The process illustrated in Figure 9-7 was based on studies on odontoblasts and shows the various steps occuring in the cytoplasm, culminating in the secretion of procollagen. The information presented here, however, is just as applicable to fibroblasts, which will be illustrated a little later.

Weinstock and Leblond found labeled proline (one of the amino acids essential for collagen synthesis) in the rER of odontoblasts 2 to 5 minutes after its injection into animals. This time would be in accord with the concept of the alpha chains being synthesized in the rER (*left* and *bottom* in Fig. 9-7, labeled 1). After 10 minutes, they found label in small transfer vesicles at the periphery of Golgi saccules (labeled 2 in Fig. 9-7). The saccules themselves (particularly the one large one at the left end of layer 4 in Fig. 9-7) contained thin entangled threads but in no organized arrangements. Somewhat later the threads became arranged so that they were parallel (the large saccule at the left end of layer 5 in Fig. 9-7), and after 20 minutes label was found over saccules that contained rigid parallel threads (as in the large one associated with layer 6 in Fig. 9-7). It should be mentioned here that physical chemical work has disclosed that alpha chains have a variable shape, whereas the triple helix is a rigid structure. Accordingly, the interpretation of Weinstock and Leblond is that alpha chains have a variable shape when they enter saccules at the forming face of the stack, so they appear as entangled threads (Fig. 9-7, large dilation near center of illustration), but within the Golgi saccules they become combined into the triple helices of procol-

lagen and then appear as rigid parallel threads (vesicle at left of layer 5 in Fig. 9-7). These threads aggregate into relatively thick rods. By 35 minutes the rods are within free vesicles presumably derived from Golgi saccules and in which the label is located (labeled 6 in Fig. 9-7, *farthest upper right*). These secretory vesicles (also sometimes called secretory granules) contain aggregates of procollagen and in due course deliver it to the cell surface. It is suggested that at the cell surface the tailpiece formerly attached to each alpha chain is split off by enzymatic action (by a peptidase) and thus the procollagen molecules are converted to *tropocollagen* molecules, which soon become arranged into what are termed *collagenic fibrils.*

THE FINE STRUCTURE OF FIBROBLASTS

Having followed the process of procollagen synthesis in the diagram made from the study on odontoblasts (Fig. 9-7) should make it easier to interpret what is seen in fibroblasts. A micrograph of part of one is shown in Figure 9-8. A portion of the nucleus (N) may be seen at the lower left of the micrograph. Along the top and right borders of the micrograph large flattened vesicles of rER are present; these are the sites where the alpha chains of procollagen are being synthesized. The Golgi region can be seen slightly left of center. Transfer vesicles bring the alpha chains of procollagen to deeper Golgi saccules and as the Golgi saccules move outward, portions of them become distended spherical vesicles (S) containing entangled threads. The threads later become straight and parallel, and the vesicle containing them (C) becomes cylindri-

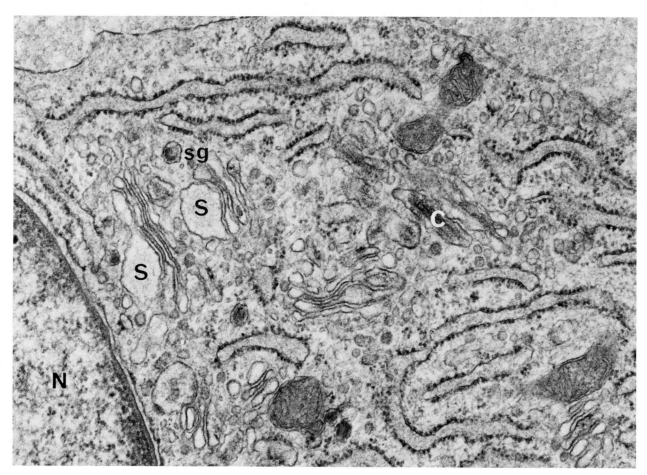

Fig. 9-8. Electron micrograph (×42,000) of a portion of an active fibroblast (from rat periodontal ligament). The nucleus (N) is seen at *lower left*. The Golgi region occupies the middle of the micrograph. As well as the stacks of Golgi saccules, it is possible to see spherical distentions (S) containing entangled threads, and cylindrical distentions (C) containing parallel threads, which probably consist of procollagen molecules. The contents of the cylindrical vesicles will condense and be seen later in secretory granules (sg). (Courtesy of M. Weinstock)

cal. As their contents condense further, these vesicles appear as secretory granules (sg in Fig. 9-8). Thus procollagen is secreted onto the surface of the fibroblast, where procollagen molecules will be trimmed down to size, becoming tropocollagen molecules that in turn will be assembled into collagenic fibrils.

THE FINE STRUCTURE, FORMATION, AND GROWTH OF COLLAGENIC FIBRILS

As was noted in Chapter 8, collagenic fibers, as seen with the LM, are often seen at their frayed ends to be composed of smaller thread-like structures called *fibrils*. However, the EM discloses that still finer fibrils, beyond the limits of resolution obtained with the LM, are present in collagen. The very smallest fibrils seen with the EM are only about 7nm. in diameter, which could be accounted for by less than a dozen tropocollagen molecules being grouped together in a side-by-side, overlapping array within a bundle. However, the EM reveals many collagenic fibrils much thicker than the small ones, but these do not seem to be made up of bundles of smaller fibers arranged side by side. Instead, small fibrils *grow* into larger ones by accretion of further molecules of tropocollagen along their sides in a special arrangement, to be described presently.

Next, the EM discloses that the collagenic fibrils exhibit what is termed *axial periodicity*, which means they reveal cross-banding units repeating every 64 nm. along their lengths. The most obvious feature of the cross banding is that along the length of a collagenic fibril a dark cross band is followed by a lighter cross band (followed in

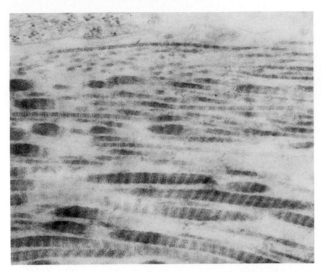

Fig. 9-9. Electron micrograph (×76,000) of newly polymerized collagenic fibrils beside a fibroblast, the edge of whose cytoplasm is seen at *top left.* Note that the fibrils closest to the cytoplasm are narrower than those farther away; hence they increase in diameter after they are first polymerized outside fibroblasts. (Fernando, N. V. P., and Movat, H. Z.: Lab. Invest., *12:*214, 1963)

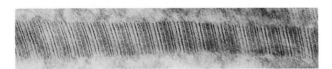

Fig. 9-10. Electron micrograph (similar magnification to Fig. 9-11) showing a collagenic fibril in thin section after conventional (positive) EM staining. Although traversed by finer cross banding, the gap and overlap regions illustrated in Figure 9-11 can be identified, but the dark segments here are overlap regions and the light segments, gap regions. For an explanation of the finer cross banding, *see* Hodge and Petruska. (Courtesy of H. Warshawsky)

turn by another dark one and another light one, and so on), as shown in Figure 9-9. With more sophisticated technics, still finer banding can be demonstrated within these dark and light bands (Fig. 9-10). The explanation for cross banding follows.

Cross banding in collagenic fibrils was first seen with the EM, not in sections, but in shadow cast mounts of collagenic fibers treated so as to break them up into fibrils. Once this periodicity of collagenic fibrils was discovered, a search was begun to find an explanation for it. First, it was found that collagen could be dissociated into its component molecules, and next, that these molecules could be reassembled again by appropriate biochemical procedures into fibrils exhibiting the same axial periodicity as natural collagen. The molecules into which collagen could be dissociated were termed *tropocollagen* mole-

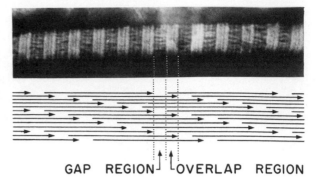

GAP REGION ⌐OVERLAP REGION

Fig. 9-11. (*Top*) Electron micrograph (×175,000) of an isolated, negatively stained collagenic fibril showing alternating light and dark regions. These are the reverse of those seen in Figure 9-10. Here, the dark segments are gap regions and the light ones are overlap regions. One dark and one light segment together correspond to one 64-nm. period. (*Bottom*) Diagram illustrating the arrangement of tropocollagen molecules as suggested by Hodge and Petruska to account for the 64-nm. periodicity (*see* explanation in text). (Courtesy of A. Howatson and J. Almeida)

cules; they are what come to lie just outside fibroblasts. An interesting question then arose, namely, how molecules of tropocollagen, which were found to be 280 nm. long, could be assembled side by side so as to account for the 64-nm. periodicity of collagenic fibrils.

A periodicity of 64 nm. could theoretically be attained in fibrils constituted of molecules 280 nm. in length if these were arranged side by side in a paralled but staggered fashion, with each molecule overlapping the neighboring one by one quarter of its length but without meeting the ends of the molecules ahead of or behind it—the kind of arrangement depicted in the lower part of Figure 9-11. Moreover, this hypothesis, proposed by Hodge and Petruska, would explain how molecules 280 nm. in length could be fitted together in a staggered fashion so as to give rise to cross bands along the course of a fibril. These cross bands are seen most clearly in negatively stained preparations of collagenic fibrils, as shown in the upper part of Figure 9-11. Here basic repeating light and dark segments are seen; one dark plus one light segment constitute one *unit* (*period*), and each light segment accounts for slightly less than half a unit. It should be recalled that in negative staining (described on p. 119) the stain enters and demonstrates regions that are least dense in content or may even represent actual spaces. Accordingly, the electron-dense stain enters the places where the collagen fibrils are least dense in content; the dark (negatively stained) segments, as shown in the diagram at the bottom of Figure 9-11, are not as dense in content as the light segments. Thus, as can be seen from the diagram, each light segment has five tropocollagen molecules passing through it for every four that pass through a dark segment. By this arrangement every tropocollagen molecule extends over approximately four and a half units, that is, across five light segments but only four dark ones (Fig. 9-11, *bottom*).

The gap regions (negatively stained in Fig. 9-11, *top*) between the ends of the tropocollagen molecules are referred to as holes. However, in life they must be filled with something, and the usual assumption is that they contain amorphous intercellular substance.

The pattern in collagenic fibrils seen after the usual sort of EM staining is, of course, just the reverse of what is seen by negative staining. As may be seen from Figure 9-10, conventional (positive) staining gives a complex pattern of cross bands with an underlying basic dark-light periodicity of 64 nm. in the opposite position to that obtained by negative staining. In other words, with the usual (positive) staining, the light segments correspond to the gap regions and the dark segments appear dark because they are more dense in content, lacking gap regions. However, besides this basic light-dark periodicity, as is evident in Figure 9-10, an additional rather complex pattern of finely spaced electron-dense cross bands is superimposed on the basic pattern of light and dark segments. It is known that certain sequences of polar amino acids are repeated several times along the length of the tropocollagen molecules; where such sequences are in register with one another they give rise to these fine darkly stained bands superimposed on the basic 64-nm. axial periodicity.

Growth in Width of Collagenic Fibrils

At a site where a fibroblast is forming collagen, the fibrils closest to the fibroblast are the narrowest, while those farther away are considerably thicker (Fig. 9-9). It might be thought that the larger fibrils could form by fusion of smaller ones forming immediately beside the fibroblast. However, the cross banding would not then necessarily be in register all the way across them. The fact that the bands are invariably in register, even in large fibrils, suggests that each fibril grows by apposition, with further tropocollagen molecules joining those already assembled in the same staggered fashion. The longitudinal striations seen in the negatively stained fibril illustrated in Figure 9-11 probably indicate the width of individual tropocollagen molecules.

THE FORMATION OF ELASTIC FIBERS

The Fine Structure of Elastic Fibers

As can be seen from Figure 9-12, elastic fibers (labeled E at *upper* and *lower right*) appear very different from collagenic fibers (two fibrils of which are labeled C at *top left* of micrograph). Unlike collagenic fibers, which in the EM can be seen to consist of numerous fibrils, each with a characteristic axial periodicity, elastic fibers are single structures lacking any periodicity. The central region of the fiber is occupied by the amorphous protein *elastin,* which appears pale because it has very little affinity for the heavy metal salts employed for routine EM staining. However, surrounding the fiber and embedded in it are numerous thread-like, more electron-dense components termed *microfibrils* (labeled M in Fig. 9-12). As can be seen right of *center* in Figure 9-12, where an elastic fiber is sectioned obliquely, the microfibrils are tubular in shape and have a diameter of about 11 nm.; as noted, they lack the axial periodicity characteristic of collagenic fibrils.

Thus elastic fibers contain two protein components. The principal protein, *elastin,* constitutes the amorphous component of the fiber. Its amino acid composition is in some respects similar to that of collagen. However, its content of polar amino acids is much lower and, although rich in proline and glycine, it possesses little hydroxyproline and no hydroxylysine. Moreover, it is characterized by having two unique amino acid derivatives called *desmosine* and *isodesmosine,* which, as we shall see, form the cross links in elastin.

The second component of elastic fibers is the *microfibrillar protein.* This differs from elastin and collagen and is relatively rich in polar amino acids; hence it stains better than the elastin in electron micrographs. However, it lacks the hydroxylysine and hydroxyproline found in collagen. It has a high content of carbohydrate (about 5%), indicating it is probably a glycoprotein.

How Elastin Becomes Molded Into Fibers

Most of the elastin in the body is formed in the walls of blood vessels, particularly the larger arteries, where it represents much of the vessel wall. In blood vessel walls, elastin is formed primarily by muscle cells. In ordinary connective tissue, however, elastin, like the other intercellular substances, is formed by fibroblasts. A precursor of elastin, called *proelastin,* is synthesized in much the same way as procollagen. But before elastic fibers can be formed from this, fibroblasts must first lay down bundles of microfibrils, since these act as scaffolds that mold the shape of the newly secreted amorphous material (elastin) into fibers. Without microfibrils, elastin would probably never form into anything other than irregularly shaped blobs and could not become more or less cylindrical fibers. The scaffold of microfibrils is assembled in close proximity to the fibroblast, sometimes along a groove in its surface. Once the scaffold is laid down, the amorphous material (elastin) starts to form into a fiber and some

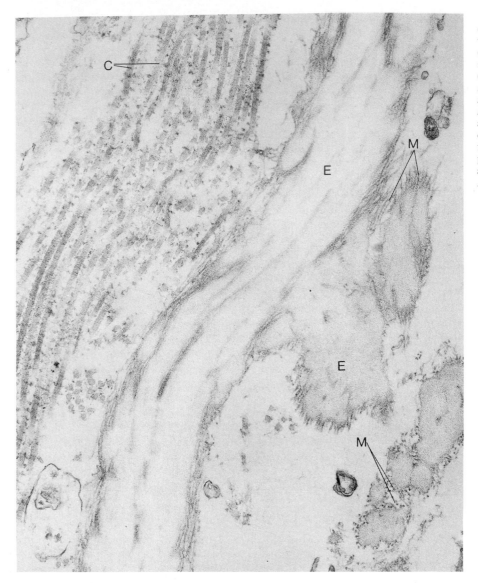

Fig. 9-12. Electron micrograph (×60,000) of elastic fibers in the wall of a developing artery (guinea pig). Elastic fibers (E) are seen here in longitudinal section (stretching from *top right* to *bottom left*), oblique section (*center right*), and cross section (*bottom right*). Microfibrils (M) surround and penetrate the amorphous elastin, molding it as it forms into fibers. Collagen fibrils (C) are also present at *upper left*. (Ross, R., and Bornstein, P.: Sci. Am., *224*:44, June, 1971)

bundles of microfibrils become buried in it while others remain as a sheath around the fiber (Fig. 9-12).

The proelastin secreted by fibroblasts appears to be converted into *tropoelastin* much as procollagen is converted into tropocollagen, that is, by enzymatic removal of a tailpiece of the molecule. Another enzyme in the intercellular space, called lysyl oxidase, then links the lysine groups of four tropoelastin molecules together, leading to the formation of the desmosine (and isodesmosine) that cross link tropoelastin molecules to form elastin. As in collagen, cross linking in elastin increases with age and this eventually may have serious consequences because it reduces the elasticity of the walls of arteries.

THE SYNTHESIS AND SECRETION OF GLYCOSAMINOGLYCANS AND PROTEOGLYCANS

These components of the ground substance of connective tissue are also synthesized by fibroblasts. Their protein portions are synthesized in the rER, and carbohydrate chains are mostly added in the Golgi, from which the completed products are delivered to the cell surface by secretory vesicles. It is not clear whether there is any chemical association between amorphous intercellular substances and tropocollagen before or during assembly of tropocollagen into fibrils. However, there is a physical association between them, since the amorphous inter-nucleus

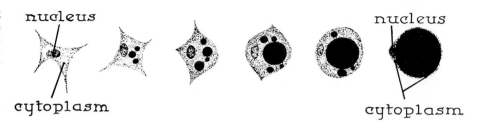

Fig. 9-13. Diagram illustrating how a cell of white fat changes in appearance as it synthesizes and stores fat. Note that it finally acquires a signet-ring appearance, shown at *farthest right.*

cellular substance is present in the gaps (the so-called holes) between the ends of tropocollagen molecules and also, of course, between fibrils.

SMOOTH MUSCLE CELLS

Since smooth muscle cells will be dealt with at length in Chapter 18, we shall not describe them here. All that need be noted at this time is that they have a fusiform shape, with a centrally located elongated nucleus and dark pink cytoplasm in H and E sections. In loose connective tissue they are present both as components of arterioles that empty into capillary beds and also in the walls of large venules that drain these capillary beds. In both they are arranged so as to encircle the lumen of the vessel just outside its endothelial lining. Attempts to identify them are best left until we have described muscle (Chap. 18) and blood vessels (Chap. 19).

FAT CELLS AND ADIPOSE TISSUE

Fat cells are also known as *adipocytes.* Although single or small groups of fat cells are normal constituents of loose connective tissue, when a tissue consists almost entirely of fat cells organized into lobules, the tissue is termed *adipose tissue.*

Fat Cells as Representatives of a Special Cell Lineage

Since fat cells may seem to lie more or less haphazardly in loose connective tissue, it was often assumed they could develop from fibroblasts. However, there is evidence that they represent a special line of connective tissue cells. If fat is transplanted from a part of the body where fat normally accumulates to a site where it does not ordinarily do so, the transplanted cells do not revert to fibroblasts in their new location but instead continue to function as fat cells. Accordingly, it seems that the reason for fat accumulating in certain sites, for example, over the belly or buttocks, is that, instead of developing into fibroblasts, the mesenchymal cells in the developing connective tissue of these parts of the body differentiate along a

different line; hence fat cells represent a special type of cell. Obese individuals possess a larger number of fat cells than thin people. Fat cells are long lived; since mitosis of the cells destined to become fat cells is virtually complete by about 2 to 3 weeks after birth, mature fat cells do not divide in the adult. However, tissue culture studies indicate that cells with a capacity for forming new fat cells are present in adipose tissue in adult life; these may well be the pericytes described earlier in this chapter.

THE MICROSCOPIC FEATURES OF FAT CELLS

The first indication of a mesenchyme-derived cell taking on the function of a fat cell is the appearance of droplets of fat in its cytoplasm. In H and E sections these are seen as little holes. But in frozen sections the fat is retained and may be stained with special fat stains as described in Chapter 1 and illustrated in Plate 1-1, *bottom right.* In Figure 9-13, the droplets are indicated in black. As this illustration shows, in the common type of fat cell the droplets fuse with one another as they increase in number and, eventually, a single relatively huge droplet of fat so expands the cell that the cytoplasm is reduced to a thin film, and even the nucleus becomes somewhat stretched. The diameter of a fat cell thus filled with stored fat may be as much as 120 μm. The appearance of such a cell in cross section (if the section passes through the region of the nucleus) is of a signet ring worn on a finger; the nucleus accounts for the signet and the ring is represented by the greatly thinned cytoplasm that surrounds the fat (Fig. 9-13, *right*). Even though the cytoplasm is thinned its total amount is believed not to be reduced.

Morphology of Adipose Tissue

This variety of connective tissue consists of fat cells that are organized into groups called *lobules.* The lobules of fat cells are separated from each other and supported by partitions of loose connective tissue, called *septa,* which extend between them and support them (Fig. 9-14). This connective tissue stroma also conducts blood vessels and nerves into the adipose tissue. Within a lobule

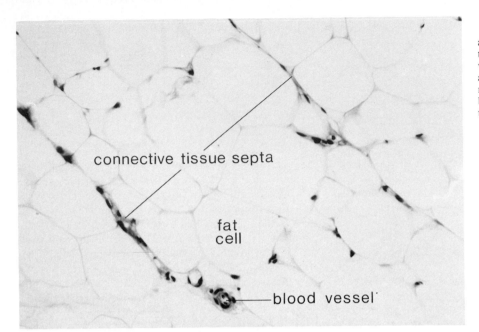

connective tissue septa

fat
cell

blood vessel

Fig. 9-14. Photomicrograph of a section of adipose tissue (omentum), showing lobules packed with fat cells. The lobules are separated from one another by connective tissue septa carrying blood vessels (and also nerves) to the tissue.

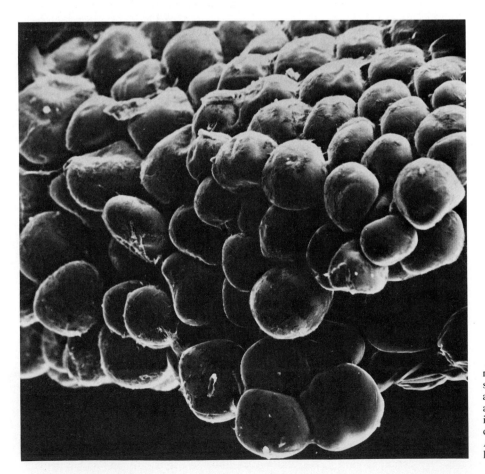

Fig. 9-15. Scanning electron micrograph (×400) showing the surface of part of a lobule of white adipose tissue (rat). The fat cells are large in diameter and spherical in shape, due to their single large droplet of stored fat. (Courtesy of A. Angel, R. Mills, and M. Hollenburg)

the individual fat cells are supported by a stroma that consists of nets of delicate reticular and collagenic fibers containing abundant capillaries in their meshes, and by this means capillaries and nerve fibers are brought into intimate contact with fat cells. Mast cells are also commonly present in the connective tissue stroma. About 50 per cent of the cells of adipose tissue are not fat cells but cells of the stroma. In H and E sections the fat cells have of course lost their content of fat through processing and the capillaries between them may have had their blood squeezed out because of the procedures involved in preparing the section.

The way fat cells are packed together in lobules is illustrated in a striking manner by means of scanning electron microscopy, which shows that the rounded fat cells, each containing a large fat droplet, are packed together in lobules much as grapes are packed together in bunches for shipment (Fig. 9-15).

The Fine Structure of Fat Cells

The layer of cytoplasm of a fat cell storing its full complement of fat is so thin that its organelles are to some extent displaced by the principal fat droplet in the middle of the cell to the region closer to the nucleus, where there is more cytoplasm. As can be seen in Figure 9-16, which is a micrograph of a fat cell storing only a small amount of fat, organelles can be seen particularly in the cytoplasm adjacent to the nucleus. Free ribosomes, both kinds of endoplasmic reticulum, a Golgi apparatus, and mitochondria can all be found in fat cells. Mitochondria are the most prominent organelles; in Figure 9-16 they appear as rods because of the low magnification. They serve an important function in fat cells, as will soon be described.

TYPES OF FAT AND THEIR GENERAL FUNCTIONS

There are two main types of adipose tissue, *white* and *brown*. *White* is the common type in mammals and accounts for almost all that of man. It sometimes may be off-white or even yellow because it contains carotene. *Brown* adipose tissue is very scanty in man but is relatively abundant in some mammals. It is brown in life because it has a very rich capillary blood supply and because its cells contain many mitochondria and are therefore rich in cytochromes (mitochondrial enzymes that, like hemoglobin, contain a colored component). Brown adipose tissue is mainly concerned with regulating body temperature in the newborn and serving as a source of heat production in certain animal species during arousal from hibernation. It will be described in further detail in due course when we discuss the effects of the hormone epinephrine on fat metabolism.

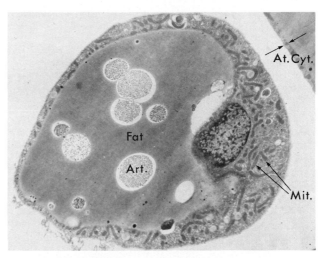

Fig. 9-16. Electron micrograph (×3,000) of a fat cell from a free cell preparation of white fat cells. This cell contains less lipid than would be found in most fat cells; were it otherwise, the cytoplasm would be so attenuated it would by very difficult to see its organelles (as is evident at *upper right*, where part of the cytoplasm of another fat cell with larger lipid content is seen; note that here the cytoplasm, labeled At. Cyt., is very attenuated). The clear (granular) areas in the lipid are artifacts (Art.) Note that mitochondria (Mit.) are numerous in fat cells. (Angel, A., and Sheldon, H.: Ann. N.Y. Acad. Sci., *131:*157, 1965)

White adipose tissue comprises 15 to 20 per cent of the body weight of adult males and 5 per cent more in females. In a sense it can be spoken of as a large organ that is metabolically very active, being primarily engaged in the uptake, synthesis, storage, and mobilization (mobilization means to make mobile so its calories become available as fuel in other parts of the body) of neutral lipid (fat). In fat cells at body temperature the fat is in the form of oil. It consists of triglycerides, which comprise three molecules of fatty acid esterified to glycerol. Triglycerides have the highest calorie content of all food, hence the fat in fat cells constitutes a store of high-calorie fuel that is relatively light in weight. Moreover, for those who live in cold countries, fat helps to insulate those parts of the body lying beneath it. In addition, fat serves as an excellent filler of various crevices in the body and provides cushions on which certain parts of the body can rest comfortably.

HOW FAT IS SYNTHESIZED BY FAT CELLS

The fat stored in a fat cell is synthesized by that particular cell from building blocks brought to it in the bloodstream. The fat in the diet, as well as carbohydrates and proteins, can provide these building blocks.

The Fate of Fat in the Diet. Neutral fats (triglycerides) consumed in the diet are digested chiefly by the enzyme *lipase*, secreted by the pancreas into the duodenum. Its actions is facilitated by bile, which is secreted by the liver into the same site. Bile components help to emulsify the fat so that the action of the lipase is more effective. As a result of digestion, some fat is broken down to fatty acids and glycerol, while the remainder is broken down only as far as monoglycerides. The fatty acids are absorbed through the apical cell membrane of the absorptive epithelial cells lining the intestine. Within these cells, glycerol-phosphate is synthesized and combined in the sER with fatty acids, forming new triglycerides. Monoglycerides, too, are absorbed and recombined with fatty acids in the sER to form triglycerides.

Details about fat absorption are given in Chapter 21 (p. 688), but here we should mention that newly reconstituted triglyceride (neutral fat) is transported to the lateral cell membranes of the intestinal epithelial cells in vesicles that bud off from the sER in which it is formed. Thus the fat droplets within intestinal epithelial cells are enclosed by membrane derived from the sER. When they reach the cell membrane, however, these membrane-bound droplets fuse with it and discharge their contents as naked droplets into the intercellular space between each epithelial cell and the next. In this manner the fat droplets soon gain entrance to the tissue fluid beneath the epithelium and travel with it as it drains into the lymphatic capillaries in the underlying connective tissue. After a fatty meal the droplets of newly synthesized fat may be numerous enough to make the lymph milky in appearance; indeed, if a great deal of fat has been consumed, even the plasma of the blood may become milky when the lymph reaches the bloodstream. Because this milky appearance of the "juice" (lymph) from the lymphatics was found to be due to the presence of tiny fat droplets, about 1 μm. in diameter, the droplets in it were termed *chylomicrons* (Gr. *chylos*, juice; *micros*, small). In addition to triglycerides, chylomicrons contain phospholipids, cholesterol ester, and some protein, which is complexed with the lipid as lipoprotein.

As the blood containing chylomicrons passes through capillaries, the chylomicrons become exposed to *lipoprotein lipase*, an enzyme associated with the endothelial lining cells of these vessels; this breaks down their triglycerides into fatty acids and glycerol again. When this happens in a capillary in fat tissue, the fatty acids may be absorbed by a fat cell and be combined with glycerol-phosphate synthesized by the fat cell.

After chylomicrons have been cleared from the blood there is still lipid in the blood in the form of *lipoproteins* (lipid complexed with protein) produced chiefly by the liver and synthesized in part from lipid obtained from chylomicrons absorbed by that organ. The lipoproteins serve as a source of fatty acids for the body cells; they are obtained locally by cells because of the local action of lipoprotein lipase on the lipoproteins brought to cells via the capillaries.

The Formation of Fat From the Fatty Acids of the Chylomicrons and Lipoproteins of the Blood. Most of the lipid in fat cells is derived from this source, as follows. Under the action of lipoprotein lipase, free fatty acids are released from the chylomicrons or lipoproteins of blood and pass into the cells of adipose tissue. Within fat cells, fatty acids are rapidly reconverted into triglycerides by means of a coupling reaction involving glycerolphosphate; this substance is available only from the glucose metabolism occurring in the fat cell. The glycerol released from the breakdown of the triglycerides coming to the cell cannot be recombined with the fatty acids because adipose tissue lacks the enzyme (glycerol kinase) essential for this to happen; hence, the glycerol-phosphate required for producing triglycerides within fat cells is dependent on carbohydrate being metabolized in the same cell.

Unlike the situation in the absorptive epithelial cells of the intestine, the lipid droplets in fat cells are not enclosed by a unit membrane. However, in fat cells the fat droplets are sometimes seen to be covered by a special type of investing layer that appears to consist of an orderly array of fine filaments. New fat first appears in the cytoplasm in the form of very fine droplets that can be isolated from homogenates of fat cells, constituting what biochemists call *liposomes*. Their diameter varies from being half to twice that of chylomicrons, which they somewhat resemble when seen in the EM.

The Fates of Carbohydrate and Protein in the Diet. In the intestine carbohydrates are broken down by enzymes to monosaccharides, while proteins are degraded to amino acids. These products are absorbed through the epithelial cells of the intestine and reach the blood circulation; they too (particularly glucose) can serve as building blocks for fat. Both glucose and amino acids pass through the cell membranes of fat cells by means of specific transport mechanisms.

The Formation of Fat From Glucose or Amino Acids. As mentioned in Chapter 5 in connection with mitochondria, glucose is broken down in the cytoplasmic matrix by a series of reactions termed *glycolysis*, and the products of this are oxidized by enzymes within the mitochondria to provide most of the energy required by the cell. However, certain of the products of the breakdown of both glucose and amino acids in the cytoplasmic matrix can be converted to long chain fatty acids which, as already explained, are combined with newly synthesized glycerolphosphate to become triglycerides.

How Fat Is Broken Down Again in Fat Cells, With the Release of Fatty Acids That Other Body Cells Can Use for Fuel. When calorie intake is restricted for any reason the energy requirements of the cells of the body are met by drawing on the food reserve stored in fat cells. Furthermore, under the influence of a lack or an excess of certain hormones (to be described shortly) fatty acids are released from fat cells and used for fuel. The mechanism by which fat is broken down is dependent on the action of another enzyme system called *tissue lipase*, distinct from the lipoprotein lipase system. The tissue lipase system consists of a hormone-sensitive triglyceride lipase and a monoglyceride lipase.

Under ordinary conditions the triglyceride lipase remains dormant and must be activated before it is able to break down triglyceride molecules. This activation occurs following the interaction of a lipolytic hormone—e.g., epinephrine or norepinephrine—with its specific receptor on the cell surface. As a result of this interaction, the levels of intracellular cyclic AMP (a substance that acts as a chemical messenger to tell the cell it has been stimulated by a hormone) rise and this is thought to be responsible for the activation of tissue lipase. The functioning of this system breaks down the triglyceride of the fat globule at its surface, and the fatty acids thus released either are metabolized or pass through the membrane of the fat cell to enter the circulation. Here they bind to albumin, which acts as a carrier, and are thus transported to other cells to supply them with fuel.

EFFECTS OF HORMONES ON ADIPOSE TISSUE

Several hormones have effects on adipose tissue. For example, the different distribution of fat in males and females suggests that sex hormones affect the site at which fat cells will develop. It is also known that hormones from the adrenal cortex can affect fat distribution. In fact many hormones either indirectly or, perhaps, directly affect adipose tissue one way or another. The two most important are *insulin* and the hormone from the adrenal medulla called *epinephrine*. The effect of the latter is mimicked by stimulation of the sympathetic fibers of the autonomic nervous system which terminate around fat cells and release the substance norepinephrine locally, as will be described later. But first we shall consider the effects of insulin.

Effects of Insulin. As will be described in detail later, the hormone insulin is produced by cells in the islets of Langerhans of the pancreas and the amount secreted is regulated by the amount of glucose that is present in blood. Hence when a person eats a lot of carbohydrate it leads to more insulin being secreted into the bloodstream, whereas under conditions of fasting or a reducing diet, insulin secretion by the pancreas is greatly reduced. Insulin, in addition to other effects, greatly influences fat cells. The latter have what are termed *insulin receptors* on their cell membranes and when the insulin in blood becomes sufficient it combines with enough receptors on fat cells to cause several different reactions to be triggered so as to make them synthesize and store fat. The reactions triggered include an increase in uptake of glucose and synthesis of fat from it and increased activity of the enzyme lipoprotein lipase and hence increased delivery into the fat cells of fatty acid from chylomicrons and lipoprotein lipid. At the same time insulin slows the mobilization of fat from fat cells by depressing the action of the enzymes concerned in breaking down the fat stored in the cell.

It is of interest that the capacity of the cells that produce insulin to respond to the increased amounts of glucose in the blood varies in people, and, if these cells are overstrained by demands for increased function, which can occur in people who have limited capacities in this regard, the cells that produce insulin may undergo degeneration. Thus people with limited capacities for producing insulin are prone to develop diabetes and should live on regulated diets if they are to avoid diminishing their limited capacity to produce insulin. It is easily understood why people with diabetes become thin, because insulin is so important in facilitating both the synthesis and storage of fat in fat cells as well as blocking its breakdown. Under conditions of a limited carbohydrate intake, less insulin is produced in the body and so it is easy to understand why limiting their carbohydrate intake keeps normal people from becoming fat and why those who have cells competent to produce lots of insulin and who cannot resist consuming too many sweets and starches become fat.

EFFECT OF NERVE STIMULATION ON ADIPOSE TISSUE

Information about the effects of epinephrine and stimulating the sympathetic division of the autonomic nervous system (described in Chap. 17) on adipose tissue was fa-

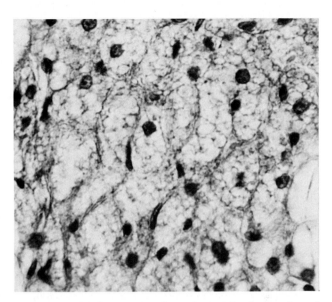

Fig. 9-17. Medium-power photomicrograph of a section of brown fat (rat). In this type of fat the nuclei of the cells (seen here as black rounded structures) tend to be located more centrally, and the globules of fat do not all fuse together. The cytoplasm therefore has a vacuolated appearance.

cilitated by studying brown fat, formerly termed the *hibernating gland* because of its superficial resemblance to glandular tissue.

Brown Fat. This type of fat is characterized histologically by its fat being in multiple droplets in the cytoplasm (Fig. 9-17). Since the many droplets do not coalesce into one large one, this arrangement is termed *multilocular* (L. *locus*, place or site) in contrast to that seen in white fat cells, in which the lipid forms only a single droplet and hence the arrangement is referred to as *unilocular*. Brown fat cells reach only about one-tenth the diameter of white fat cells and differ from them also in having more and larger mitochondria. The greater content of mitochondria in brown fat is important for its role as a heat-producing tissue. A little brown fat is commonly found in the mediastinum, along the aorta, and under the skin between the scapulae. The cells in brown fat have a very rich supply of nerve fibers from the sympathetic division of the autonomic nervous system.

The hormone *epinephrine* (produced by the adrenal gland, particularly during emotional states) and a similar substance, *norepinephrine* (liberated at the periphery of fat cells when the sympathetic nerve fibers supplying them are stimulated), both affect the metabolism of fat cells profoundly. Their first effect is to cause the formation of more cyclic AMP, a derivative of ATP that mediates the effects of many hormones, as discussed in Chapter 25 (p. 783). The cyclic AMP in turn augments the activity of tissue lipase, which releases fatty acids from stored triglycerides.

Epinephrine and norepinephrine appear to be involved in the arousal of animals from hibernation, in which state their metabolic rate is very sluggish. In this instance, fatty acids accumulating in the fat cell act so as to uncouple the oxidation process from the production of ATP, with the result that a large proportion of the energy generated appears as heat. This carefully controlled inefficiency is a very important part of the mechanism of *heat production* and is a property unique to brown adipose tissue; it is vital in survival of the newborn human infant and the warming-up process of hibernating animals.

PLASMA CELLS

The plasma cell was long ago classed as a cell of loose connective tissue. It was easily recognized in H and E sections, being a relatively large, rounded cell with an eccentrically placed nucleus and a large amount of basophilic cytoplasm (Fig. 9-18), and was commonly present in the loose connective tissue of certain parts of the body. However, even though considered a cell of loose connective tissue, it was noted that plasma cells were present in even larger numbers in the kind of blood cell forming tissues known as lymphatic tissue (which includes tonsils, lymph nodules, lymph nodes, and the spleen, as described in subsequent chapters). So plasma cells came to be regarded as components of lymphatic tissue as well as loose connective tissue.

Development of Knowledge About the Origin and Function of Plasma Cells

In the first half of this century, plasma cells were regularly described in textbooks of histology and pathology, but until 1947 their function was not known. Furthermore, it was still later before their origin was known with any certainty. Establishment of their function and origin has had a great deal to do with the development of modern immunology. Indeed it is now almost meaningless to describe the plasma cells of loose connective tissue without becoming involved in discussing them as part of the cellular basis for modern immunology — which is an aspect of histology of great importance, interest, and value as a background for the later formal study of immunology. Therefore, to relate histology as effectively as possible to immunology, the subsequent portion of this chapter and the following several chapters are arranged so as to provide such information as the student might wish to obtain on this particular aspect of histology. We shall begin with appropriate comment on the general nature of immunology and then go on to describe the morphology of plasma cells.

The Term Immunology. The word *immunity* from its derivation (L. *immunis*) means *safe* or *exempt* from infection. The study of immunity (immunology) began long ago when it was discovered that individuals who had recovered from communicable diseases were in most instances safe from getting the same disease under similarly infectious conditions. This, of course, raised the question of why having one bout of the disease protected the individuals from having other bouts of the same disease.

In due course it was established that the individual developing immunity had certain proteins, termed *antibodies*, in his blood plasma that reacted specifically with the kind of organism responsible for the disease and in such a way as to render these organisms inocuous should they again enter his body.

Much was learned about antibodies before their cellular origin was determined; for example, it was learned that they were a type of globulin, a particular kind of protein in the blood plasma. Accordingly, antibodies are now usually referred to as *immunoglobulins*. Moreover, it was discovered they were specific for the infecting organism, and tests were devised for their detection. In some cases antibodies would be formed when killed disease organisms, or organisms otherwise treated to stop them propagating, were injected as *vaccines,* and so it became possible to *immunize* individuals against certain communicable diseases. Nevertheless, all this time the cellular source of antibodies was unknown, even though pathologists and histologists were already by then very familiar with the appearance of plasma cells and knew they were seen at sites exposed to infection, namely loose connective tissue under the wet epithelia lining the intestine and respiratory tract, including the tonsils, and in lymph nodes and the spleen (as described in following chapters). However, by the second half of this century evidence was eventually obtained that plasma cells were responsible for producing antibodies, and so their true significance became established.

THE MICROSCOPIC FEATURES OF PLASMA CELLS

Appearance of Plasma Cells in H and E Sections. Plasma cells are easily recognized. If lying free in tissue they are rounded (Fig. 9-18), but where pressed upon by other cells their outlines may be more angular (Fig. 9-19). A plasma cell has much cytoplasm relative to the size of its nucleus, which is commonly round and eccentrically placed in the cell (Fig. 9-18,N). Sometimes, however, it may appear to lie in the center of the cell because the section sliced an eccentric nucleus in the upper or lower part of the cell. Much of the chromatin in the nucleus is condensed, and the peripheral chromatin (c in Fig. 9-18) is often arranged like the numerals on a dial, giving the nucleus a characteristic "clockface" appearance (Fig. 9-18). A prominent nucleolus (n in Fig. 9-18) may also be

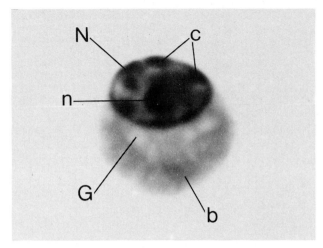

Fig. 9-18. Oil-immersion photomicrograph of a plasma cell from human large intestine. Note the characteristic features of a plasma cell: the clockface appearance of the nucleus (N) due to peripheral chromatin granules (c); a prominent nucleolus (n); basophilic cytoplasm (b); and a negative Golgi image (G). This cell is rounded in outline because it was not pressed upon by other cells.

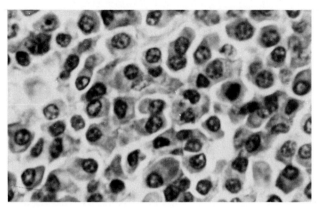

Fig. 9-19. Photomicrograph showing numerous plasma cells that have accumulated in loose connective tissue below the epithelium of a tonsil. Their angular outlines are due to the close packing of the cells.

seen. The cytoplasm is intensely basophilic (b in Fig. 9-18) and often reveals a negative Golgi image (Fig. 9 18 G). The intense basophilia of the cytoplasm is due to its abundant rRNA. In mature plasma cells acidophilic droplets or bodies, termed *Russell bodies,* are sometimes seen.

Fine Structure. Antibodies (immunoglobulins) are synthesized and secreted by plasma cells. Hence, as might be expected, the cytoplasm of plasma cells shows great specialization for the synthesis of a protein secretion, being replete with cisternae of rER (Fig. 9-20) which may be flattened or somewhat dilated. In sections cut at appropriate angles the ribosomes can be seen to be arranged in the form of spirals (polyribosomes).

The Golgi region of plasma cells is customarily large (Fig. 9-20). Centrioles are seen in this region, close to the nucleus (Fig. 9-20). Immunoglobulins contain some carbohydrate; some of this is added to protein in the rER and the remainder is added in the Golgi. The secretory vesicles originate in the same manner as they do in the acinar cells of the pancreas; namely, secretion accumulates at the edge of a flattened Golgi saccule where a vesicular structure buds off to become a free secretory vesicle. The secretory vesicles (Fig. 9-20) then deliver their contents at the cell surface. Russell bodies seen with the LM may represent abnormally large accumulations of secretion within the rER; one opinion is that they signify the plasma cell is beginning to degenerate.

The other features of plasma cells, as seen with the

EM, are not unusual except that the cell membrane often extends from the cell in finger-like processes.

The immunoglobulins secreted by the plasma cells of loose connective tissue and lymph nodes would have to reach the bloodstream by way of lymph. Plasma cells in the spleen, as we shall learn in Chapter 13, have more direct access to blood.

THE DEVELOPMENT OF PLASMA CELLS AS A RESPONSE TO ANTIGENS ENTERING BODY TISSUES

What Is an Antigen? From its derivation (Gr. *anti,* against and *gennan,* to produce) the word *antigen* refers to a substance against which something is produced (in this case, a specific antibody) if that substance enters the tissues of the body and comes into contact with body fluids and cells. However, for a given substance to incite antibody formation and hence serve as an antigen it must possess certain features. First, it must be in the form of macromolecules. Antigens are commonly proteins of relatively high molecular weight, with all but a few antigens having a molecular weight over 5,000. Some antigens are proteins complexed with polysaccharides. Second, for any kind of macromolecular substance to incite antibody formation in a given individual, it must be foreign to his body in the sense that its molecules must differ from any of the macromolecules that developed normally in that particular body and were exposed to the body fluids during embryonic and fetal life. It must be understood that as the body develops, countless different macromolecules are synthesized in it. These do not act as antigens in that body. When the task of producing the body (and all the great variety of macromolecules that are in it) is finished — and this is generally close to the time of birth — the body develops the ability to recognize further (different) macromolecules that get into it and is able to react to them by developing plasma cells.

These foreign macromolecules are antigens and plasma cells developing in response to the presence of each new kind produce

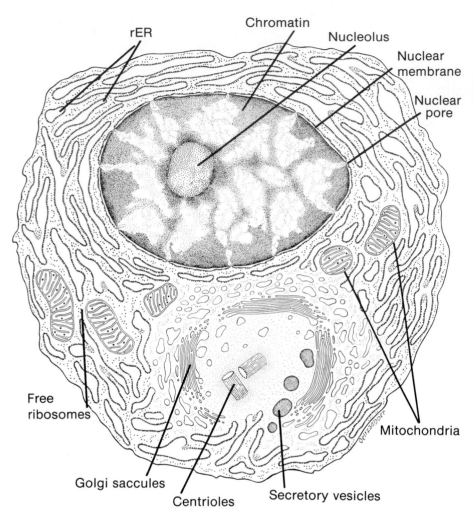

rER

Chromatin

Nucleolus

Nuclear membrane

Nuclear pore

Free ribosomes

Mitochondria

Golgi saccules

Centrioles

Secretory vesicles

Fig. 9-20. Diagram of a plasma cell illustrating its fine structure. The abundant rough-surfaced endoplasmic reticulum (rER) indicates the degree of synthesis of antibody destined for secretion. The extremely well developed Golgi region indicates that the secretion is delivered via this organelle. (Courtesy of C. P. Leblond)

specific antibody that combines specifically with them. With very few exceptions, disease organisms do not gain entrance to the body until after birth, and since their macromolecules are different from those with which the body is familiar, disease organisms are regarded as antigens by the body. In addition to the antigens of viruses, bacteria, protozoa, and other types of disease organisms, foreign macromolecules of certain inert materials gaining entrance to the body—for example, dusts and pollens that somehow get through epithelial covering and lining membranes to enter the connective tissues—may also act as antigens. Furthermore, certain chemical substances—for example, certain drugs—absorbed in a normal way by the body may as haptens become combined with body proteins to constitute macromolecules having configurations different from those normally present in the body, and so these too become antigens and incite the formation of antibodies.

Plasma cells are responsible for producing the antibodies circulating in the blood; these antibodies are termed *humoral* antibodies (L. *humor,* liquid). There is, however, another kind of cellular mechanism concerned in immunity that does not depend on humoral antibodies. This other kind (described in Chap. 13) is seen, for example, in the rejection of transplants of tissue from one person to another and is mediated not by plasma cells but by cells of another type that go directly to transplants of foreign tissue (which are antigenic), where they destroy the foreign cells of the graft.

HOW IT WAS ESTABLISHED THAT PLASMA CELLS PRODUCE ANTIBODIES

In describing the approach used to establish this, we should first explain that the method used was an example of what is now referred to as an *immunofluorescence technic.* Such methods are relatively new and have enabled many formerly undetectable substances (including the antibody made by plasma cells) to be localized within cells or tissues in a specific manner. Some of the background that led to their development will now be given.

Development of Knowledge. The limiting factor restricting the resolving power of the LM is, as noted in Chapter 1, the wavelength of light. It is curious that it was due to attempts to improve the resolution of the LM by utilizing light of shorter wavelength (in the ultraviolet range) that immunofluorescence technics evolved. Some progress had already been made toward obtaining better resolution by employing ultraviolet light when it was realized that an electron beam, because of its extremely short wavelength, if used instead, could provide far greater resolution than light of even the shortest wavelengths. The use of light of short wavelength nevertheless did lead to the development of a new kind of histological technic, but for another reason, as we go on to explain.

It is a physical characteristic of some chemicals that they absorb light energy of short wavelength and emit it as visible light, a property called *fluorescence.* Extensive use is made of this in fluorescence microscopy, as will be discussed below.

The Fluorescence Microscope. Although basically similar to an ordinary LM, the fluorescence microscope is equipped with a mercury vapor lamp emitting very intense light, including some in the ultraviolet range. This is filtered through a special filter that cuts out all wavelengths except those needed to elicit fluorescence. The wavelengths used are long enough to pass through glass lenses. Since light of the longer wavelengths in the ultraviolet range is employed, some of it, after passing through the nonfluorescing parts of the section, continues on through the glass lenses of the objectives and eyepieces. Accordingly, to prevent injury to the eyes from this invisible light, the appropriate barrier filters that exclude ultraviolet rays but permit passage of light in the visible range must be inserted below the eyepieces used for inspecting sections. Moreover, a similar filter must also be used for photographing fluorescence in sections; otherwise, enough ultraviolet light could enter the camera to fog the film.

Fluorescent-Labeled Proteins. What made the fluorescence microscope so useful to histologists was the finding that certain dyes, notably fluorescein (which emits a brilliant green fluorescence) or lissamine rhodamine (which emits red light), could be attached chemically to protein molecules. After being applied to cells or tissues, or being injected into animals, a fluorescent-tagged protein could, for example, be sought and localized in cells or tissues using a fluorescence microscope. The technic became extremely useful when it was discovered that the fluorescent dye could just as readily be attached to a specific antibody (a protein) and that the antibody retained its specificity after labeling. Thus, it became possible to prepare fluorescent-labeled reagents that would react *immunologically,* and therefore specifically, with the particular component being studied. The specificity of the technic is due to antibody molecules being able to recognize and stick to molecules of the antigen against which they were made, which is like a lock and key arrangement, in which one region of the antibody molecule "fits" the antigen molecule in a precise manner. Methods based on this principle are referred to as *immunofluorescence technics.*

It also became possible to use immunofluorescence to

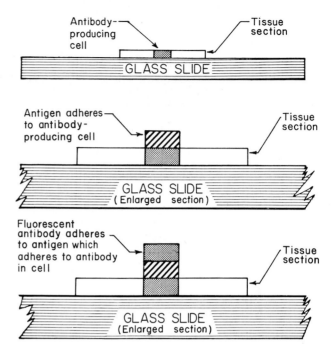

Fig. 9-21. Diagram illustrating the three steps in the immunofluorescent sandwich technic. The relative sizes of the components illustrated are not drawn to scale.

detect sites of localization of antibodies as well as antigens in body tissues. By means of an immunofluorescence technic, Coons and his associates, in 1955, were able to show that the antibody formed in response to an injected antigen was produced by plasma cells. The ingenious method they devised for this purpose was named the immunofluorescent sandwich technic for reasons that will soon be obvious.

The details of the method are as follows. An animal is injected with the antigen to be studied and sections are prepared from tissue samples removed and fixed in a special manner. Either frozen or routine paraffin sections may be used (Sainte-Marie). When sections containing antibody-forming cells (as shown in Fig. 9-21, *top*) are flooded with a solution of the same antigen that was injected, the antigen adheres to the cells making the antibody (Fig. 9-21, *middle* diagram). The sections are washed to remove any antigen that has *not* combined with antibody and then are flooded with fluorescent-labeled antibody to this particular antigen. This, of course, sticks to the antigen adhering to the specific antibody in the cells (as shown in Fig. 9-21, *bottom*), so that these cells can be identified under a fluorescence microscope (*see* below). The appearance of such cells may be seen in Fig. 13-17. This indirect method is referred to as the *immunofluorescent sandwich technic* because it involves building up a sandwich, with a layer of antigen in between two layers of antibody.

Immunofluorescence Technics. Two other important immunofluorescent technics are widely used for studying macromolecular components and products of cells and tissues. They have had so many useful applications in histological studies that a brief description of them is warranted here.

If the chemical component being studied is of high molecular weight it will usually be antigenic when injected into an animal of another species. This being the case, it is relatively easy to isolate the antibody (immunoglobulin) fraction from the blood serum of the injected (immunized) animal, and this antibody can be labeled with a fluorescent dye without destroying its antigenic specificity. The labeled antibody can then be used as a specific reagent for locating the antigen against which it was made, a method called the *direct fluorescent antibody technic*. To raise a specific antibody, the component being studied must first be freed of all contaminants, for otherwise the impurities would lead to the formation of unwanted antibodies that would detract from the specificity of the method. The purified antigen is repeatedly injected at appropriate intervals into an experimental animal, commonly a rabbit or mouse, which responds by producing increasing amounts of specific antibody.

A more versatile and sensitive immunofluorescence technic widely used in investigative work is the *indirect fluorescent-labeled antibody technic*. To understand the basis of this method, it should be appreciated that the immunoglobulins of one species, like any other protein, are recognized as foreign when injected into animals of a different species; accordingly, a further antibody is made against the injected immunoglobulin. Moreover, it is possible to raise an antibody that will react with *all* the immunoglobulins produced by a given species, regardless of their specificities, if it is directed against the constant region of the foreign antibody molecule. (The structure of antibody molecules is considered in Chap. 13, pp. 327–328). Thus, a single fluorescent-labeled antibody preparation can be prepared that will react with immunoglobulins of *all specificities* of a given species.

In the indirect method, the particular antigen being studied is treated first with an unlabeled specific antibody raised in a certain species and then with a fluorescent-labeled immunoglobulin directed against all antibodies of that species. This method is very sensitive due to the number of antibody molecules bound at each step in the procedure and is economical because it requires only one fluorescent-labeled antibody reagent for investigating all kinds of antigens.

The Origin of Plasma Cells

Plasma cells of loose connective tissue do not develop from the original mesenchyme of the part of the body where they subsequently appear. They are immigrants because they develop from a type of blood cell termed *B-lymphocytes* that enter the part of the body where the plasma cells are subsequently seen.

The factors and processes involved in causing B-lymphocytes to develop into plasma cells and produce specific antibodies are described in Chapter 13.

MAST CELLS—RELATION TO HEPARIN, HISTAMINE, ANAPHYLAXIS, AND ALLERGIES

From its derivation *mast* relates to feeding and was applied by Ehrlich in 1877 to certain cells of connective tissue he thought looked so stuffed with granules, he imagined they might have been overeating. The granules, however, are not prominent in H and E sections, so the number of mast cells in routine sections of connective tissue is often underestimated. Mast cells with their granules are readily demonstrated by injecting methylene blue into the connective or adipose tissue of a suitable animal (such as a rat) and making a whole mount of the teased tissue. Many mast cells will then be seen lying along small blood vessels and elsewhere, as shown in Figure 9-22A. Under high power these cells are indeed seen to be stuffed with granules, which stain blue-purple with methylene blue. The mast cells commonly rupture in making the preparation so the granules may be strewn about (Fig. 9-22B). Even fixation can cause degranulation. The nucleus of the mast cell may be difficult to see in whole preparations because it is obscured by the granules; however, it is readily seen in sections.

Mast cells are so common and large in the rat that there is a tendency to think that the mast cells of all species, including man, would be similar and as numerous. However, this is not the case and mast cells show considerable variation from species to species. In human skin, for instance, they are rounded or fusiform and their granules are relatively small.

Mast cell granules contain several important substances, including at least two of major physiological and pharmacological significance. Their characteristic staining properties are due to their content of *heparin*, which represents as much as 30 per cent of their total content. *Histamine*, whose extremely important role in the body will be explained later, accounts for a further 10 per cent of their content. Mast cells of some species (rat and mouse) contain a third substance, *serotonin*, but in humans this third potent pharmacological agent is present in blood platelets but not mast cells. Before describing the fine structure of mast cells we shall comment on heparin.

Development of Knowledge About Heparin

About 60 years ago it was discovered that a substance that could be isolated from liver would prevent blood from clotting, so this was called heparin (Gr. *hepar*, liver). Since a prevalent cause of death is *thrombosis* (clotting of the blood as a result of blood platelets aggregating, which blocks blood vessels), this discovery of heparin aroused hopes that it might serve to prevent thrombosis—and indeed the hope was realized, for it was found that not only did heparin prevent clotting but it also helped to stop platelet aggregation. Hence administration of heparin to individuals threatened with fatal thrombosis has saved many lives. This also introduced the era of blood vessel surgery, for operations on blood vessels involve great risk of a thrombus forming. Besides heparin, other anticoagulants are also now available.

Heparin Found to Be a Sulfated Glycosaminoglycan. As was mentioned in the previous chapter, glycosaminoglycans stain metachromatically. In the late 1930s heparin was found to be metachromatic. Since the cytoplasmic granules of mast cells

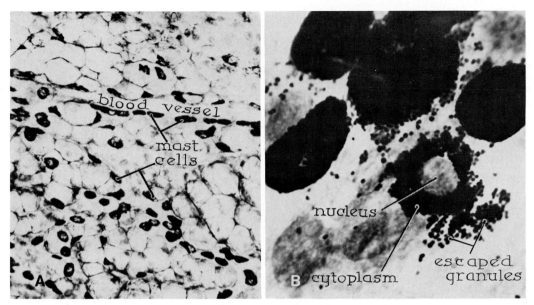

Fig. 9-22. (A) Low-power photomicrograph of a fat tissue spread (rat) containing a blood vessel, stained with methylene blue to demonstrate mast cells. Note that many mast cells are distributed along the vessel. *(B)* Oil-immersion photomicrograph of an areolar tissue spread (rat), stained with methylene blue. Several dark-stained mast cells are seen. Granules are commonly so densely packed in mast cells that no details can be seen. However, the lowermost mast cell has ruptured, so some of its granules have escaped, revealing its nucleus.

were by this time also known to be metachromatic, they were soon suspected of being the source of the heparin extractable from tissues. It was then shown that the amount of heparin obtainable from a tissue was directly related to the number of mast cells it contained and so, as matters turned out, heparin extracted from liver was found not to be a product of the liver cells but of mast cells in the loose connective tissue component of the liver.

Next, there was suspicion that mast cells did not synthesize sulfated glycosaminoglycan but merely phagocytosed it from the intercellular substance of the loose connective tissue in which they resided. However, two solid pieces of evidence soon indicated that mast cells actually synthesize the heparin they contain. The first came from the study of mast cell tumors (mastocytomas), which are not uncommon in dogs. Mast cell tumors have been grown in tissue culture and transferred from one culture to another many times, and all the while the cells of the tumors continued to produce heparin. The second line of evidence came from radioautographic studies in which radioactive sulfur given to animals was taken up quickly by mast cells, an indication that the mast cell itself is the site where sulfur becomes incorporated into sulfated glycosaminoglycans.

Possible Normal Function of the Heparin in the Granules of Mast Cells. It is surprising that, from the evidence available, there is no indication that heparin normally plays a role in keeping blood from clotting in the vascular system. It has not been possible to demonstrate enough heparin in the blood to suggest that it serves any normal function in this respect. It is therefore somewhat of a problem to know what purpose mast cells serve in producing heparin. Two possibilities might be considered.

First, it might be thought that mast cells would secrete their sulfated glycosaminoglycan into the ground substance. How-

ever, the sulfated glycosaminoglycans of the ground substance all differ to some extent from heparin, so there is no evidence that mast cells have anything to do with forming intercellular substance.

Second, it was found that injecting heparin dissipates chylomicrons (which, as noted, make plasma milky) so that the plasma quickly clears; that is, heparin has a *clearing action* on plasma. Subsequent work showed that an enzyme, lipoprotein lipase (earlier described under Adipose Tissue on p. 240), produced by endothelial cells of capillaries, is responsible for degrading chylomicrons in plasma and furthermore that heparin increases the activity of this enzyme, probably by acting as a cofactor with it. Since heparin seems to be required for adequate activity of this enzyme along capillaries, it would appear that heparin released from mast cells serves to promote the clearing of chylomicrons by lipoprotein lipase.

THE FINE STRUCTURE OF MAST CELLS

The rounded nucleus of a mast cell lies more or less centrally and is not unusual in any respect (Fig. 9-23). The mast cell itself is irregular in outline, with cytoplasmic processes extending from it (right border of cell in Fig. 9-24), and it lacks a surrounding basal lamina. The cytoplasm contains numerous mitochondria (Fig. 9-24) and a little sER; some rER and a well-developed Golgi are also present (Fig. 9-25). The main feature of the cytoplasm, however, is its great content of large, character-

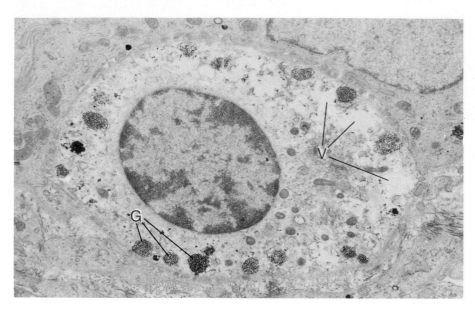

Fig. 9-23. Low-power electron micrograph of a partially degranulated mast cell situated in loose connective tissue just under the epithelial lining of the human stomach. Its rounded nucleus lies near the center of the cell. The cytoplasm shows characteristic granules (G) and also vacuoles (V) left where some of its granules have been released. (Steer, H. W.: J. Anat., *121*:385, 1976)

istic granules, about 0.2 to 0.8 μm. in diameter, each enclosed by a membrane (Fig. 9-25). The heterogeneous granules (labeled G in Figs. 9-23 and 9-24) contain either particles or lamellar structures. Some empty vacuoles (V in Figs. 9-23 and 9-24), representing discharged granules, and a few disintegrating granules (Fig. 9-24, DG) are also seen. Degranulation does not appear to be an essential finding in histamine release but vacuolation is a reliable indication that such release has occurred. The Golgi plays an important role in the synthesis and sulfation of the sulfated glycosaminoglycan heparin stored in the granules; secretory vesicles containing electron-dense material similar to that seen in the granules are found budding off from the Golgi saccules (Fig. 9-25).

THE RELATION OF MAST CELLS TO HISTAMINE, ANAPHYLAXIS, AND ALLERGIES

Development of Knowledge

To protect individuals from certain infectious diseases vaccines can be prepared from the causative organisms, modified so as not to transmit disease but still remain antigenic, then be injected before exposure to the disease. This immunizes such individuals against getting the disease when exposed to it. As we know, this widely used approach to the prevention of disease, which is accordingly said to be a *prophylactic* (Gr. *prophylasso*, to be on guard) measure, has on the whole been remarkably successful in controlling many potentially lethal or crippling diseases.

Late in the last century, however, it was found that a second injection of such an antigen sometimes had a deleterious effect, and indeed could be fatal. Richet in 1893 gave this effect a name; he unfortunately termed it *anaphylaxis*, because he conceived it to be the opposite of prophylaxis.

Anaphylaxis is easily demonstrated in guinea pigs. If a guinea pig is injected with a particular antigen and then after 10 to 14 days injected again with the same antigen, it goes into what is called *anaphylactic shock*. This is manifested by difficulty in breathing and a rapid pulse rate; moreover, the animal may soon die from an inability to breathe. The reason for respiratory failure is that the muscle cells encircling the smaller tubes (bronchioles), through which air is drawn into the lungs, become so contracted that their lumens become too narrow to permit an adequate volume of air to enter, and in particular to leave, the lungs.

Another effect observed in anaphylaxis is that thin-walled vessels, such as venules and blood capillaries, become dilated and leaky, so that plasma escapes from them. As a result (in man), blebs of plasma may form from these vessels in the loose connective tissue directly under the epithelium of the skin, resulting in a condition called *urticaria*.

Attempts to determine why muscle cells in bronchioles should contract and why thin-walled vessels should leak after a second injection of an antigen were greatly facilitated by the discovery, around 1914, that most of the events characterizing anaphylaxis could be duplicated in guinea pigs by injecting them with a substance just discovered called *histamine*.

HISTAMINE AND ITS RELEASE FROM MAST CELLS

The Effects of Histamine. Histamine, an amine derived from the amino acid histidine, has a profound effect on visceral (smooth) muscle, causing it to contract. It also causes the endothelial cells lining venules and capillaries to part company slightly where their edges are not joined by tight junctions. As a result, these thin-walled vessels dilate and leak plasma. Histamine also has certain other deleterious effects in the body.

How It Was Established that Histamine Is Synthesized by Mast Cells. In 1955, West and Riley introduced the concept of mast cells containing histamine as well as heparin.

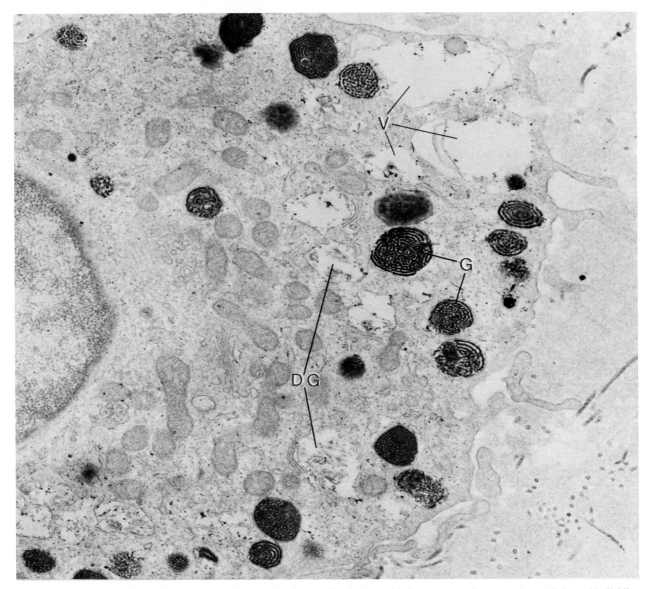

Fig. 9-24. Electron micrograph of a portion of a partially degranulated mast cell in loose connective tissue beneath the epithelial lining of the stomach (human). Numerous cytoplasmic processes project from the border of the cell. Note the large typical granules (G), the disintegrating granules (DG), and the empty vacuoles (V) left in the cytoplasm where some of its granules have been discharged. (Steer, H. W.: J. Anat., *121*:395, 1976)

Experiments similar to those done with heparin showed that mast cells were the chief repositories of histamine in tissues. For example, a correlation was found in various tissues between histamine and mast cell content and fractions containing mast cell granules were shown to contain histamine. Moreover, it was shown that agents inducing histamine release would also cause mast cells to liberate their granules. Finally, it was found that mast cells contained the enzymes necessary for producing histamine from its precursor and, furthermore, that the content of histamine in mast cell tumors, after many transfers, became increased and not decreased, as would happen if mast cells did not synthesize the histamine they contain.

The Relation of Histamine Release to Antigens and Antibodies. From the knowledge available, it therefore seemed probable that injecting a guinea pig with a second

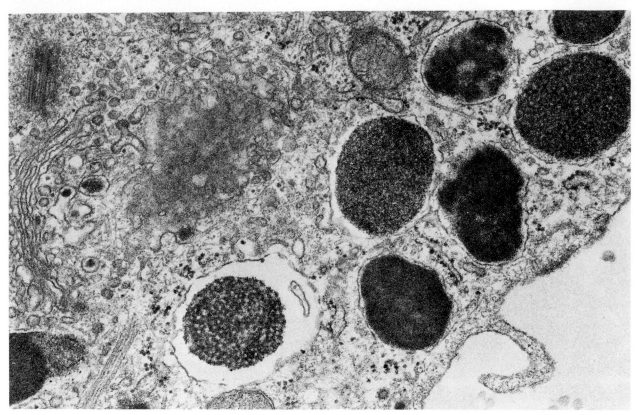

Fig. 9-25. Electron micrograph of a portion of an undegranulated mast cell. At *left* there is a stack of Golgi saccules. Just to the right of the Golgi small granules, each enclosed by a membrane, can be seen. Farther to the right there are typical large membrane-bound granules. (Courtesy of C. P. Leblond)

dose of an antigen about two weeks after the first dose caused its mast cells to release histamine (Fig. 9-26) and this in turn caused symptoms and signs of anaphylaxis. This may be explained as follows. The first dose of antigen induced the formation of specific antibody to that antigen. Next, some of these antibody molecules became attached to mast cells in such a way that the antigen binding sites on these molecules remained exposed and therefore able to interact with the antigen. This is achieved by the mast cell having surface receptor sites for what is known as the *constant region* of the antibody molecule (explained on p. 328), so that when antibody molecules become attached, they do so with their variable region, the one with antigenic specificity, sticking out. Then, when more of the antigen was injected, it quickly combined with the specific antibody on the mast cells to form an *antigen-antibody complex*. Antigen-antibody complexes formed this way on mast cells cause them to release their granules (Fig. 9-26), and, since the granules contain histamine, signs of anaphylaxis are thereby produced.

It should be noted here that there are some species differences and also that mast cells release other important substances in addition to histamine. Mast cells of rats and mice, for instance, produce and release another amine, *serotonin* (5-hydroxy-tryptamine), which is derived from tryptophan. Like histamine, this is also *vasoactive* (meaning it has an effect on the diameter of blood vessels). Furthermore, it should be appreciated that mast cells are not the only cells containing histamine. As we shall see in Chapter 11, certain blood cells called *basophils* also have granules that not only appear similar to those of mast cells but also contain both histamine and heparin.

Anaphylaxis sometimes occurs in man and may be lethal. It has occurred chiefly in individuals sensitized prior to receiving a second injection of a substance, two doses of which would not normally present any problem. Sometimes the individual does not know, or cannot remember, that he has been injected or had some other effective contact with that particular substance before; hence the physician should carefully watch any patient given an injection of, for example, penicillin or tetanus antitoxin to see if he has been previously sensitized to it. If he begins to go into anaphylactic shock, very prompt treatment is essential.

ALLERGIES

We all absorb some kinds of macromolecules that may serve as antigens, through little discontinuities in the epithelial linings of our respiratory tracts and intestines. Pollens, dusts, and so on, absorbed anywhere along the respiratory tract, can incite the formation of specific antibodies, with the result that subsequent reexposure to the same antigens may set off antigen-antibody reactions.

Those who react to antigens absorbed into the body by manifesting reactions are said to be *sensitive* or *allergic* to those antigens, and in general such people are said to be hypersensitive. *Hay fever* is a common manifestation of an allergy; people who suffer from hay fever are commonly sensitive to pollen from ragweed, which is prevalent in the air at the time of year when hay is cut. There are literally hundreds of possible allergy-causing antigens to which people may be exposed in everyday life.

Allergic disease, which affects one out of every five persons, is now known to be mediated by a class of immunoglobulin called *IgE* (there are several other classes, as will be described in Chap. 13). IgE is produced in response to certain antigens called *allergens* entering the body. Plasma cells synthesizing IgE are found mainly beneath the wet epithelial linings of the respiratory and gastrointestinal tracts, where the antigens may gain entrance to the underlying loose connective tissue through breaks in the epithelium.

While much remains to be learned about the mechanism of allergic disease, it is known that mast cells (and the basophils of blood, which are described in a later chapter) have a *high affinity for IgE antibodies.* This type of antibody becomes attached to the surface of mast cells in the way already mentioned so as to leave the antigen-combining sites of the antibody molecules exposed. So if the antigen in question re-enters the body, it can readily react with these sites. The combination of the antigen with the IgE antibody bound to the cells triggers the release of histamine and other chemical mediators (described later), producing the familiar symptoms of allergic disease. The severity of the symptoms (which depend upon the part of the body involved) can usually be controlled by administering antihistaminic drugs (*antihistamines*) that act as follows.

Antihistamines. These do not act by preventing histamine from being liberated from mast cells, but instead by occupying the receptor sites for histamine on cells that would otherwise ordinarily respond to it. Thus the histamine liberated from mast (or

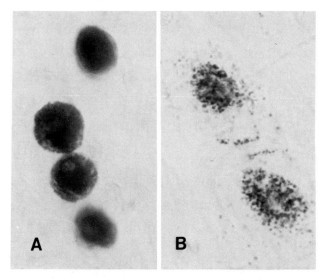

Fig. 9-26. Photomicrographs of mast cells from a rat (*A*) before and (*B*) after undergoing an antigen-antibody reaction at their surface. Toluidine blue stain. In (*B*), the mast cell granules have been scattered. This event is accompanied by histamine release. (Humphrey, J. H., and White, R. G.: Immunology for Medical Students. ed 2. Oxford, Blackwell Scientific Publications, 1964)

other) cells is prevented from having as great an effect on cells that respond to it.

Desensitization. The treatment of allergies by lengthy desensitization procedures is based, at least partly, on the rationale that injections of minute but gradually increasing doses of the antigens to which a patient is allergic will eventually produce more of another class of antibody called *IgG* (also described in Chap. 13). IgG antibody is the type most commonly produced during any sustained immunization procedure and it does not show the same tendency to stick to the surface of mast cells or basophils, and therefore does not cause release of histamine. However, it can compete with IgE for the allergen and thus it blocks reaction of IgE with the allergen. Thus when hypersensitive individuals are producing enough blocking antibody (IgG), this combines with the minute quantities of antigen they absorb from the outside world so that it never reaches and reacts with the IgE on their mast cells and basophils. The release of histamine and consequent allergic symptoms may in this way be avoided.

Allergic Individuals. The question arises as to why some people are hypersensitive to antigens that cause no problem in others. There is probably a genetic basis for this, but its mechanism is not clear. It may be that certain individuals inherit a greater tendency to make more IgE antibody than others (and indeed the level of circulating IgE is higher in hypersensitive than normal individuals), or that they inherit the tendency to respond to certain antigens that happen to be allergenic. Perhaps allergic individuals have both tendencies.

Histamine and Serotonin. As already noted, certain other cells besides mast cells contain histamine; thus *basophils* of blood and *blood platelets* of certain species contain appreciable amounts of it. In some species, (but not in man), mast cells also contain *serotonin*; this acts like histamine in some respects but differently in others. Serotonin, however, is more commonly present in blood platelets and some is found in human platelets. Its release from platelets can be triggered by antigen reacting with antibody on the surface of the platelets.

OTHER CHEMICAL MEDIATORS RELEASED FROM MAST CELLS

Mast cells liberate several different substances acting as mediators not only in allergies but also in inflammation. Besides histamine, two other mediators are particularly important.

The first of these has effects similar to those of histamine. However, unlike histamine, which has rapid but short-lasting effects on both smooth muscle and vascular permeability, this particular mediator has a much more long-lasting effect and hence is called the *slow-reacting substance of anaphylaxis (SRS-A)*. Chemically, it is an acidic, sulfur-containing lipopeptide. Instead of being stored in mast cells, SRS-A is formed anew in response to an antigen-antibody interaction at the surface of these cells.

The other important mediator selectively attracts *eosinophils* (a type of blood cell) toward it when released from mast cells and hence is said to be *chemotactic* (Gr. *taksis*, orderly arrangement) with respect to eosinophils. Accordingly, this substance (an acidic peptide that, like histamine and heparin, is stored in mast cells) is called the *eosinophil chemotactic factor of anaphylaxis (ECF-A)*.

Mast cells are very much involved in the process of inflammation, a subject with which we deal in Chapter 11. In that chapter we shall explain how mast cells contribute to the signs and symptoms of an acute inflammatory reaction.

For those requiring further information about the part mast cells play in hypersensitivity reactions of the type that we have been considering above, we shall go on to explain briefly how mast cells defend the body against infection.

THE ROLE OF MAST CELLS IN BODY DEFENSES

Mast cells, as noted, lie along small blood vessels in connective tissue, particularly alongside venules and capillaries, which are the vessels from which tissue fluid escapes into the ground substance. The tissue fluid, on leaving these vessels, would of course take with it at least small quantities of any foreign antigen gaining access to the body and subsequently entering the general circulation. It is significant also that many mast cells are found in the loose connective tissue under the wet epithelial linings of the respiratory tract and intestine, where foreign antigens may enter through local breaks in the epithelial membrane. Hence mast cells are strategically placed for guarding the possible entry points for antigens from the bloodstream (via tissue fluid) or through local discontinuities in epithelial membranes.

Mast cells in these locations will have been sensitized with IgE to particular foreign antigens that have already entered the body (and moreover elicited the production of IgE specific for these antigens). Thus they serve as sentinels on the lookout, as it were, for the reappearance of the same antigens. When these again enter the body they cause mast cells primed with IgE specific for these antigens to liberate their content of chemical mediators and thereby invoke the many facets of the inflammatory reaction (described in Chap. 11). In general this reaction serves to render the foreign antigen harmless to the body and eliminate the source of antigen if it is within the body. Hence mast cells are to be regarded as an important component of the body's defense mechanism for ridding itself of infecting organisms. Furthermore, it seems that it is only when the body overreacts to foreign antigens, as for example in the overproduction of IgE in response to the entry of a particular antigen, that signs of immediate hypersensitivity are manifested.

In due course it will be apparent why such hypersensitivity reactions are self-limiting. In this connection it should be mentioned here that one of the mechanisms that restrains inflammation in hypersensitivity reactions depends on the release of the eosinophil chemotactic factor ECF-A from mast cells, which as noted serves to attract eosinophils into the affected region. As explained in more detail in Chapter 11, eosinophils possess several enzymes that degrade mediators liberated by mast cells and so they rapidly dampen the inflammatory effects of these mediators when they too arrive on the scene.

THE ORIGIN AND MAINTENANCE OF THE MAST CELL POPULATION

Mast cells are generally regarded as being derived from cells that retain considerable mesenchymal potentiality, cells for which we think the likely candidate would be the pericyte. Mast cells do not seem to be related to the basophils of blood, which they resemble insofar as the content and mechanism of release of their granules are concerned. Moreover, their origin is different since they do not arise from the pluripotential stem cell from which basophils are derived. It is not known whether any stem cell is involved in maintaining their numbers; however, here again the pericyte has come under suspicion, if for no other reason but that pericytes, like mast cells, are located alongside capillaries. There is in-vitro evidence to indicate that cells of the thymus gland (or their products) may play some role in mast cell differentiation (Ginsberg and Sachs).

The population of mast cells undergoes very slow turnover, because mast cells are relatively long-lived. Mitotic figures are seldom seen in these cells; however, since mast cells are able to go through DNA synthesis (Walker), it may be that mitosis is not so rare but only obscured by the heavy content of granules in the cytoplasm of these cells.

MACROPHAGES

The concept of *phagocytosis* (Gr. *phagein*, to eat; *osis*, process) was first elaborated by Metchnikoff, a Russian zoologist and anatomist. In 1882 he pushed some rose thorns into starfish larvae and followed the course of events with his microscope. He found that on the second day certain mobile cells had gathered around the foreign material. Subsequently it was found that a special kind of cell in loose connective tissue could perform this phagocytic function, and several different names were given to it, including *clasmatocyte, histiocyte,* and *macrophage.* The latter, which means "big eater," is now the most widely used. Macrophages are not the only kind of phagocyte; in the next chapter we shall also describe the "little eaters" (*microphage* was the early name given to the blood cell now known as a *polymorph* or *neutrophil*).

THE MICROSCOPIC FEATURES OF MACROPHAGES

Macrophages that are relatively young, free, and active tend to assume an oval shape, like those illustrated in Figure 9-27. When they are older and compressed by other tissue elements, they may become elongated and have angular contours (which is probably the reason why macrophages were given so many different names). In oval macrophages the nucleus commonly lies toward one end and it generally has the form of an indented oval (Fig. 9-27). Its chromatin is more condensed than that of a fibroblast but less than that of a plasma cell; its size is smaller than that of a fibroblast but larger than that of a plasma cell.

The Vital Staining of Macrophages

The identification of macrophages under experimental conditions was greatly facilitated by the development of *vital staining* which, as its name implies, means a method in which living cells become stained because of some vital activity (in this instance, phagocytosis). The dye trypan blue is widely used; this may be injected either directly into connective tissue or may be administered intravenously or injected into the peritoneal cavity. When this is done, the dye is phagocytosed by macrophages and can be seen as blue material in their cytoplasm. Such vital stains are colloidal dyes and it is because they are in the

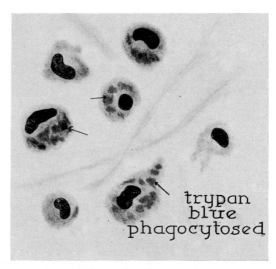

Fig. 9-27. Illustration of the oil-immersion appearance of a group of macrophages after phagocytosing trypan blue, following injection of trypan blue and some bacteria into loose connective tissue. The nuclei of macrophages are commonly indented, small, and deeply stained.

form of macromolecular aggregates that they are phagocytosed. Particles in colloidal suspension are phagocytosed just as effectively, so colloidal silver or diluted India ink are also frequently employed for vital staining of macrophages.

THE DISTRIBUTION OF MACROPHAGES IN THE BODY

By describing macrophages as one of the important cells of loose connective tissue, we may inadvertently give the impression that they are not present or important in other tissues. This would be unfortunate because macrophages are widely distributed, being essential components of many other tissues, in particular the blood cell forming tissues. Indeed when vital stains are administered intravenously, vitally stained macrophages are found in so many organs and sites they have been sometimes regarded as comprising what has been termed *the macrophage system.* Hence we shall necessarily comment more on macrophages in later chapters when dealing with tissues or organs in which they are present and serve some function.

THE FUNCTIONS OF MACROPHAGES

As all the foregoing suggests, a very important function of macrophages is to phagocytose waste or foreign macromolecular or particulate matter, for example, worn-out

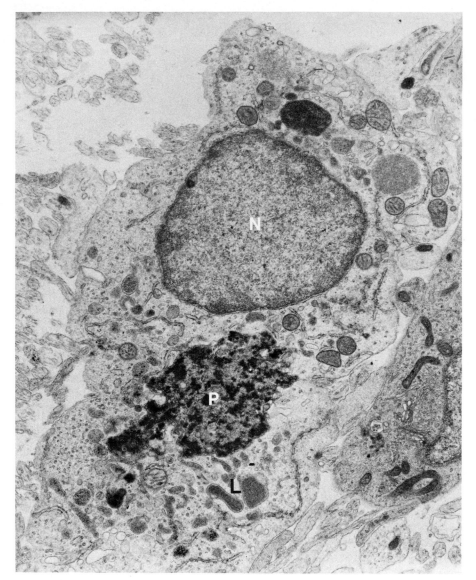

Fig. 9-28. Electron micrograph of a macrophage (rat). Note its irregular outline and the eccentric position of its nucleus (N). Directly beneath the nucleus a prominent dark phagosome (P) can be seen. Its content appears to be a remnant of the nucleus of a phagocytosed cell. Farther below are various types of dense bodies and at *bottom center* a group of lysosomes (L) can be seen. Some of these lysosomes (the ones just above the letter L) seem to be elongating toward the phagosome. The rER is not prominent in macrophages (Imamoto, K., and Leblond, C. P.: J. Comp. Neurol., *180:*139, 1978)

red blood cells or carbon particles in the lungs of heavy smokers. Macrophages are also able to engulf and destroy infecting bacteria; hence they participate in inflammatory reactions (pp. 285–286). Moreover, antibody molecules made against such bacteria can become bound to surface receptor sites on macrophages in such a way that the antigen-binding sites of the antibody molecules remain exposed (that is, the same way they are bound to mast cells). This, of course, constitutes a way in which macrophages can specifically "recognize" other bacteria of the same kind, and it facilitates elimination of these bacteria if they reinfect the body.

The process of phagocytosis is illustrated in Figures 5-38 and 5-39. As shown, phagocytosis is accomplished by extensions of the cell membrane engulfing a particle with which the cell makes contact. The little vacuole formed by these extensions meeting one another so as to enclose the particle is termed a *phagosome*. This buds off (internally) from the cell membrane so as to become contained within the cytoplasm. As described in connection with lysosomes (Fig. 5-38, p. 141), phagosomes can become fused with primary lysosomes, which leads to digestion of the phagocytosed material if it succumbs to the hydrolytic enzymes of the lysosome.

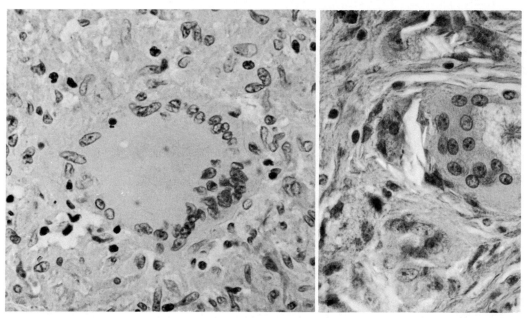

Fig. 9-29. Photomicrographs of giant cells. The one at *left* is typical of the kind forming in sites infected with the tubercle bacillus. The one at *right,* of which only a portion is shown, is seen in what is termed a nonspecific granuloma. (Courtesy of T. Brown)

The role of macrophages in immune responses will be dealt with further in Chapter 13 (p. 351).

THE FINE STRUCTURE OF MACROPHAGES

Macrophages present a variety of appearances. The boundaries of some free macrophages of loose connective tissue are seen with the EM to be very irregular because of numerous pseudopodia, surface folds, and finger-like processes projecting from them in various directions. Furthermore, invaginations of the cell membrane may extend deeply into the cytoplasm and, if cut in oblique or cross section, may appear as empty vesicles. It has been shown that most, but not all, of these invaginations retain continuity with the cell surface.

As may be seen from Figure 9-28, the rER is not very well developed in macrophages. The Golgi stacks, however, are at least of moderate size. Some macrophages have numerous free ribosomes, others have few. Mitochondria, of course, are also present. However, just as spotting vital staining helps in the recognition of macrophages in the LM, finding *phagosomes* helps in recognizing macrophages in the EM. For example the macrophage in Figure 9-28 shows a large phagosome (labeled P) below the nucleus. Furthermore, macrophages contain a relative abundance of lysosomes of the several types described in connection with lysosomes in Chapter 5; for

example, there is a group of lysosomes (labeled L) just below, and in association with, the phagosome in Figure 9-28.

THE ORIGIN OF MACROPHAGES

For a long time it was generally assumed that macrophages of loose connective tissue were derived from mesenchymal cells that preexisted in the sites where loose connective tissue developed, and hence that macrophages were natives as far as the cell population of loose connective tissue was concerned. However, modern methods such as radioautography have cast new light on their origin and disclosed that macrophages develop in loose connective tissue, and other sites as well, from blood cells of a type called *monocytes* (described in Chap. 11) entering loose connective tissue and other sites from the bloodstream. Hence, like plasma cells, macrophages are now believed to develop in loose connective tissue from an immigrant type of cell.

FOREIGN BODY GIANT CELLS

Particles or masses of foreign material in loose connective tissue too large to be phagocytosed by individual macrophages may incite the formation of *foreign body giant cells.* These are very large and contain from two to a

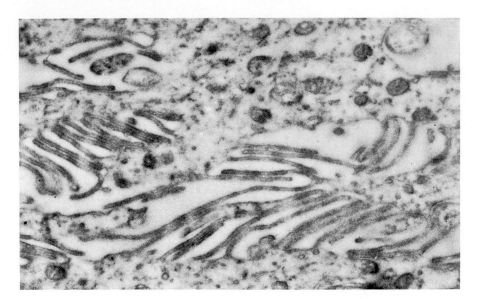

Fig. 9-30. Electron micrograph (×24,000) of parts of macrophages adjacent to a site where agar-agar was injected into subcutaneous tissue (rabbit). The cell borders of the macrophages are in all probability fusing to form a giant cell. Note how thin plate-like processes extending from the surfaces of the macrophages interdigitate with one another. (Courtesy of A. Howatson)

great many nuclei (Fig. 9-29). They originate from the fusion of monocytes or macrophages, as has been observed directly in tissue cultures. Their purpose seems to be to provide a cell large enough to enclose, wall off, or otherwise deal with large amounts of foreign material or debris too big to be incorporated into a single macrophage.

Giant cells of this type are common in the lesions of *tuberculosis* (Fig. 9-29, *left*). These cells are probably incited to form because of tubercle bacilli being phagocytosed by groups of macrophages which, on being injured by the bacilli, may fuse to form giant cells. The central region then undergoes necrosis, leaving a ring of macrophage nuclei around the periphery (Fig. 9-29). Giant cells of various appearances form from macrophages in several other low-grade inflammatory conditions, for instance in nodular lesions called *granulomas* (Fig. 9-29). They also form in connection with walling off foreign bodies. It is easy to produce foreign body giant cells experimentally by injecting foreign material, such as agar, into loose connective tissue; they soon form around the larger masses of injected material and completely surround the smaller masses. If this is done in animals given vital stains such as trypan blue before the material is injected, the stain can be found later in some of the foreign body giant cells. Sometimes this leads to the assumption that foreign body giant cells themselves are phagocytic. However, if vital stains have been given, the cells fusing to form giant cells could have accumulated vital stain before they fused. In our experience foreign body giant cells, once formed, do not seem very active so far as further phagocytosis of vital stain is concerned. They could, of course, perform

functions dependent on the action of the hydrolytic enzymes of their lysosomes.

Giant Cells Formed From Macrophages as Normal Functioning Body Cells

As will be described in Chapter 15, the remodeling of bones that occurs throughout life, though mostly during the growing period, involves both the resorption of preexisting bone and formation of new bone. It was formerly thought that bone was resorbed by multinucleated cells developing from the same cells as those that became bone cells. It has now been shown, however, that these huge cells called *osteoclasts* are formed as a result of the fusion of macrophages. So multinucleated giant cells resulting from the fusion of macrophages are not necessarily the result of foreign bodies (or materials) gaining entrance to the body; instead they can be normal functioning cells serving a physiological function.

Mechanism of Fusion

One way (though not necessarily the only way) macrophages fuse is by extending regular, thin cytoplasmic folds; such folded membranes were first observed in macrophages by Palade in 1955. While studying the formation of giant cells around injected foreign material, Howatson and Ham (unreported experiments) noted that folds of some adjacent macrophages interdigitated with one another (Fig. 9-30), suggesting that this was the way they fused with one another in the vicinity of foreign bodies.

REFERENCES AND OTHER READING FOR CHAPTERS 8 AND 9

Fibroblasts, Collagenic Fibers, and Reticular Fibers

Fernando, N. V. P., and Movat, H. Z.: Fibrillogenesis in regenerating tendon. Lab. Invest., *12:*214, 1963.

Fullmer, H. M.: The histochemistry of the connective tissues. Internat. Rev. Connective Tissue Res., *3:*1, 1965.

Gillman, T.: The Dermis. *In* Champion, R. H., Gillman, T., Rook, A. J., and Sims, R. T. (eds).: An Introduction to the Biology of the Skin. Oxford, Blackwell Scientific Publications, 1970.

Hodge, A. J., and Petruska, J. A.: Recent studies with the electron microscope on ordered aggregates of the tropocollagen macromolecules. *In* Aspects of Protein Structure. p. 289. New York, Academic Press, 1964.

Hodge, A. J., and Schmitt, F. O.: The tropocollagen macromolecule and its properties of ordered interaction. *In* Edds, M. V., Jr. (ed.): Macromolecular Complexes. pp. 19–51. New York, Ronald Press, 1961.

Jackson, S. F.: Connective tissue cells. *In* Brachet, J., and Mirsky, A. E. (eds.): The Cell. vol. 6, p. 387. New York, Academic Press, 1964.

Movat, H. Z., and Fernando, N. V. P.: The fine structure of connective tissue. I. The fibroblast. Exp. Mol. Pathol., *1:*509, 1962.

Peacock, E. E., Jr., and Van Winkle, W., Jr.: Surgery and Biology of Wound Repair. Philadelphia, W. B. Saunders, 1970.

Ramachandran, G. N., and Reddi, A. H. (eds.): The Biochemistry of Collagen. New York, Plenum, 1976.

Ross, R.: Collagen formation in healing wounds. *In* Montagna, W., and Billingham, R. E. (eds.): Advances in Biology of Skin: Wound Healing. p. 144. London, Pergamon Press, 1964.

———: Connective tissue cells, cell proliferation and synthesis of extracellular matrix – A review. Philos. Trans. R. Soc. Lond. [Biol. Sci.], *271:*247, 1975.

Ross, R., Everett, N. B., and Tyler, R.: Wound healing and collagen formation. V. The origin of the wound fibroblast studied in parabiosis. J. Cell Biol., *44:*645, 1970.

Snodgrass, M. J.: Ultrastructural distinction between reticular and collagenous fibers with an ammoniacal silver strain. Anat. Rec., *187:*191, 1977.

Weinstock, M., and Leblond, C. P.: Synthesis, migration and release of precursor collagen by odontoblasts as visualized by radioautography after ³H-proline administration. J. Cell Biol., *60:*92, 1974.

Elastic Fibers

(*See also* references on Elastin in Chapter 19)

Fahrenbach, W. H., Sandberg, L. B., and Eleary, E. G.: Ultrastructural studies on early elastogenesis. Anat. Rec., *155:*563, 1966.

Greenlee, T. K., Ross, R., and Hartman, J. L.: The fine structure of elastic fibers. J. Cell Biol., *30:*59, 1966.

Hashimoto, K., and DiBella, R. J.: Electron microscopic studies of normal and abnormal elastic fibers of the skin. J. Invest. Dermatol., *48:*405, 1967.

Kewley, M. A., Steven, F. S., and Williams, G.: The presence of fine elastin fibrils within the elastic fiber observed by scanning electron microscopy. J. Anat., *123:*129, 1977.

Kirkaldy-Willis, W. H., Murakami, H., Emery, M. A., Mungai,
J., and Shnitka, T. K.: Elastogenesis in the cranial patagium of the wing of the chick. Can. J. Surg., *10:*348, 1967.

Low, F. W.: Microfibrils, fine filamentous components of the tissue space. Anat. Rec., *142:*131, 1962.

Ross, R., and Bornstein, P.: Elastic fibers in the body. Sci. Am., *224:*44 (June), 1971.

Taylor, J. J., and Yeager, V. L.: The fine structure of elastin fibers in the fibrous periosteum of the rat femur. Anat. Rec., *156:*129, 1966.

Aging of Connective Tissue

Engel, A., and Larsson, T. (eds.): Aging of Connective and Skeletal Tissue. Thule International Symposia. Stockholm, Nordiska Bokhandelns Forlag, 1969.

Hall, D. A.: The Aging of Connective Tissue. New York, Academic Press, 1976.

Sobel, H.: Ageing of the ground substance in connective tissue. Advances Geront. Res., *2:*205, 1967.

Amorphous Intercellular Substance

Bensley, S. H.: On the presence, properties and distribution of the intercellular ground substance of loose connective tissue. Anat. Rec., *60:*93, 1934.

Bergeron, J. A., and Singer, M.: Metachromasy: an experimental and theoretical re-evaluation. J. Biophys. Biochem. Cytol., *4:*433, 1958.

Chain, E., and Duthie, E. S.: Identity of hyaluronidase and the spreading factor. Br. J. Exp. Pathol., *21:*324, 1940.

Curran, R. C.: The histochemistry of mucopolysaccharides. Int. Rev. Cytol., *17:*149, 1964.

Duran-Reynals, F.: Some remarks on the spreading reaction. *In* Asboe-Hansen, G. (ed.): Connective Tissue in Health and Disease, p. 103. Copenhagen, Munksgaard, 1954.

Mancini, R. E.: Connective tissue and serum proteins. Int. Rev. Cytol., *14:*193, 1963.

Meyer, K.: The biological significance of hyaluronic acid and hyaluronidase. Physiol. Rev., *27:*335, 1947.

———: The chemistry of the ground substances of connective tissue. *In* Asboe-Hansen, G. (ed.): Connective Tissue in Health and Disease. p. 54. Copenhagen, Munksgaard, 1954.

———: The chemistry of the mesodermal ground substance. Harvey Lect., Ser. 51, p. 88, 1955.

Tissue Fluid, Lymph, and Lymphatic Capillaries

(*See also* References for Chap. 19 and textbooks of physiology)

Drinker, C. K., and Field, M. E.: Lymphatics, Lymph and Tissue Fluid. Baltimore, Williams & Wilkins, 1933.

Leak, L. V.: Electron microscopic observations on lymphatic capillaries and the structural components of the connective tissue-lymph interface. Microvascular Res., *2:*391, 1970.

Pullinger, B. D., and Florey, H. W.: Some observations on the structure and function of lymphatics. Br. J. Exp. Pathol., *16:*49, 1935.

———: Proliferation of lymphatics in inflammation. J. Pathol. Bact., *45:*157, 1937.

Rouviere, H.: Anatomy of the Human Lymphatic System. Translated by M. J. Tobias. Ann Arbor, Edwards Bros., 1938.

Blood Capillaries

See References for Chapter 19.

Edema

For references *see* textbooks of physiology, pathology and medicine.

Basement Membranes

Davies, P., Allison, A. C., and Cardella, C. J.: The relation between connective tissue cells and intercellular substances, including basement membranes. Philos. Trans. R. Soc. Lond. [Biol. Sci.], *271:*363, 1975.

Kefalides, N. A.: Chemical properties of basement membranes. Intern. Rev. Exp. Pathol., *10:*1, 1971.

Rambourg, A., and Leblond, C. P.: Staining of basement membranes and associated structures by the periodic acid-Schiff and periodic acid-silver methenamine techniques. J. Ultrastruc. Res., *20:*306, 1967.

Adipose Tissue

Angel, A., and Sheldon, H.: Adipose tissue organelles: isolation morphology and possible relation to intracellular lipid transport. Ann. N.Y. Acad. Sci., *131:*157, 1965.

Fawcett, D. W.: A comparison of the histological organization and histochemical reactions of brown fat and ordinary adipose tissue. J. Morphol., *90:*363, 1952.

Hayward, J. S., Lyman, C. P., and Taylor, C. R.: The possible role of brown fat as a source of heat during arousal from hibernation. Ann. N.Y. Acad. Sci., *131:*441, 1965.

Menschik, Z.: Histochemical comparison of brown and white adipose tissue in guinea pigs. Anat Rec., *116:*439, 1953.

Napolitano, L.: The differentiation of white adipose cells. J. Cell Biol., *18:*663, 1963.

Napolitano, L., and Fawcett, D.: The fine structure of brown adipose tissue in the newborn mouse and rat. J. Biophys. Biochem. Cytol., *4:*685, 1958.

Palay, S. L., and Revel, J. P.: The morphology of fat absorption. *In* Meng, H. C. (ed.): Lipid Transport. pp. 33–43. Springfield, Charles C Thomas, 1964.

Senior, J. R.: Intestinal absorption of fats. J. Lipid Res., *5:*495, 1964.

Sheldon, H.: The fine structure of adipose tissue. *In* Rodahl, K., and Issekutz, B. (eds.): Fat as a Tissue. p. 41. New York, McGraw-Hill, 1964.

Sheldon, H., and Angel, A.: Some considerations on the morphology of adipose tissue. *In* Meng, H. C. (ed.): Proc. Internat. Symp. on Lipid Transport. p. 155. Springfield, Charles C Thomas, 1964.

Sheldon, H., Hollenberg, C. H., and Winegrad, A. I.: Observations on the morphology of adipose tissue. Diabetes, *11:*378, 1962.

Sidman, R. L., and Fawcett, D. W.: The effect of peripheral nerve section on some metabolic responses of brown adipose tissue in mice. Anat. Rec., *118:*487, 1964.

Sidman, R. L., Perkins, M., and Weiner, N.: Noradrenaline and adrenaline content of adipose tissue. Nature, *193:*36, 1962.

Smith, R. E., and Hock, R. J.: Brown fat: thermogenic effector of arousal in hibernation. Science, *140:*199, 1963.

Thompson, J. F., Habeck, D. A., Nance, S. L., and Beetham, K. L.: Ultrastructural and biochemical changes in brown fat in cold exposed rats. J. Cell Biol., *41:*312, 1969.

Wood, E. N.: An ordered complex of filaments surrounding the lipid droplets in developing adipose cells. Anat. Rec., *157:*437, 1967.

Plasma Cells

(*See also* References for Chap. 13)

Coons, A. H., Leduc, E. H., and Connolly, J. M.: Studies on antibody production: I. A. method for the histochemical demonstration of specific antibody and its application to a study of the hyperimmune rabbit. J. Exp. Med., *102:*49, 1955.

dePetris, S., Karlsbad, G., and Pernis, B.: Localization of antibodies in plasma cells by electron microscopy. J. Exp. Med., *117:*849, 1963.

Fagraeus, A.: Antibody production in relation to development of plasma cells; in vivo and in vitro experiments. Acta Med. Scand., *130:*3, 1948.

Movat, H. Z., and Fernando, N. V. P.: The fine structure of connective tissue. II. The plasma cells. Exp. Mol. Pathol., *1:*535, 1962.

Rifkind, R. A., Osserman, E. F., Hsu, K. C., and Morgan, C.: The intracellular distribution of gamma globulin in a mouse plasma cell tumor as revealed by fluorescence and electron microscopy. J. Exp. Med., *116:*423, 1962.

Sainte-Marie, G.: Study on plasmocytopoiesis. I. Description of plasmocytes and of their mitoses in the mediastinal lymph nodes of ten-week-old rats. Am. J. Anat., *114:*207, 1964.

Immunofluorescence Technics

Hijmans, W., and Schaeffer, M. (eds.): Fifth International Conference on Immunofluorescence and Related Staining Techniques. Ann. N.Y. Acad. Sci., *254:*1, 1975.

Kawamura, A., Jr. (ed.): Fluorescent Antibody Techniques and Their Application. ed. 2. Baltimore. University Park Press, 1977.

Nairn, R. C. (ed.): Fluorescent Protein Tracing. ed. 3. Edinburgh, Livingstone, 1969.

Sainte-Marie, G.: A paraffin embedding technic for studies employing immunofluorescence. J. Histochem. Cytochem., *10:*250, 1962.

Sternberger, L. A.: Immunocytochemistry. Foundations of Immunology Series. Englewood Cliffs, Prentice-Hall, 1974.

Mast Cells

Austen, K. F., and Orange, R. P.: Bronchial asthma: the possible role of the chemical mediators of immediate hypersensitivity in the pathogenesis of subacute chronic disease. Am. Rev. Respir. Dis., *112:*423, 1975.

Beaven, M. A.: Histamine. Part I. N. Engl. J. Med., *294:*30, 1976; Part II *Ibid.*, *294:*320, 1976.

Combs, J. W.: Maturation of rat mast cells. An electron microscope study. J. Cell Biol., *31:*563, 1966.

Fawcett, D. W.: An experimental study of mast cell degranulation and regeneration. Anat. Rec., *121:*29, 1955.

Fernando, N. V. P., and Movat, H. Z.: The fine structure of connective tissue. III. The mast cell. Exp. Mol. Pathol., *2:*450, 1963.

Ginsberg, H., and Sachs, L.: Formation of pure suspensions of mast cells in tissue culture by differentiation of lymphoid cells from the mouse thymus J. Natl. Cancer Inst., *31:*1, 1963.

Ishizaka, T., Okudaira, H., Mauser, L. E., and Ishizaka, K.: Development of rat mast cells in vitro I. Differentiation of mast cells from thymus cells. J. Immunol., *116:*747, 1976.

Mota, I.: The behaviour of mast cells in anaphylaxis. Int. Rev. Cytol., *15:*363, 1963.

Selye, H.: The Mast Cells. Washington, Butterworth, 1965.

Smith, D. E.: The tissue mast cell. Int. Rev. Cytol., *14:*327, 1963.

Steer, H. W.: Mast cells of the human stomach. J. Anat., *121:*385, 1976.

Weinstock, A., and Albright, J. T.: The fine structure of mast cells in normal human gingiva. J. Ultrastruc. Res., *17:*245, 1967.

Zweifach, B. Z., Grant, L., and McCluskey, R. T. (eds.): The Inflammatory Process. ed. 2. vols. 1 to 3. New York, Academic Press, 1974.

Macrophages and Foreign Body Giant Cells

(*See also* References and Other Reading for Chapter 5 under "Phagocytosis, Pinocytosis and Coated Vesicles" and under "Lysosomes.")

Carr, I.: The Macrophage. A Review of Ultrastructure and Function. New York, Academic Press, 1973.

Cline, M. J.: The White Cell. Cambridge, Harvard University Press, 1975.

Haythorn, S. R.: Multinucleated giant cells with particular reference to the foreign body giant cell. Arch. Pathol. Lab. Med., *7:*651, 1929.

Osmond, D. G.: The origin of peritoneal macrophages from the bone marrow. Anat Rec., *154:*397, 1966.

Page, R. C.: The macrophage as a secretory cell. Int. Rev. Cytol., *52:*119, 1978.

Palade, G. E.: Relations between the endoplasmic reticulum and the plasma membrane in macrophages. Anat. Rec., *121:*445, 1955.

Pearsall, N. N., and Weiser, R. S.: The Macrophage. Philadelphia, Lea & Febiger, 1970.

Sampaio, M. M.: The use of Thorotrast for the electron microscopic study of phagocytosis. Anat. Rec., *124:*501, 1956.

Volkman, A., and Gowans, J. H.: The origin of macrophages from bone marrow in the rat. Br. J. Exp. Pathol., *46:*62, 1965.

10 Blood Cells: Erythrocytes and Platelets

Blood cells represent a category of *free* connective tissue cells because they are not normally attached to each other or to any other kinds of cells. Moreover, they are not held in position by intercellular substance as are most kinds of connective tissue cells. Blood cells are formed in the hematopoietic tissues (as described in following chapters) and when they enter the bloodstream they are suspended in, and carried along by, the *blood plasma*, which is the fluid portion of the blood. They are classified into two main categories, the *red* and *white* blood cells. Tiny bodies—*blood platelets*—are also suspended in plasma; they will be described after red blood cells. Although fresh isolated red cells seen under the microscope are straw colored, the large numbers present in blood make it appear red. They are commonly called erythro-cytes (Gr. *erythros,* red). White cells are called leuko-cytes (GR. *leukos,* white) even though fresh ones are colorless; when they are packed together they appear white.

Mature erythrocytes have no nucleus; the nucleus they possessed during development is extruded as they mature, before entering the circulation. Leukocytes, however, possess nuclei whose characteristics help in distinguishing one kind from another.

Platelets, unlike erythrocytes and leukocytes, are not whole cells. They are membrane-covered fragments of cytoplasm liberated from certain very large cells that in man are housed in the red bone marrow. Although platelets are only fragments of cells, they perform, as we shall see, several very important functions.

Erythrocytes and platelets perform their role in the blood whereas most leukocytes perform their various functions only when they leave the blood to enter the connective tissues. Thus leukocytes are blood cells chiefly in the sense that they use the blood as a means of transport, from the time they enter the bloodstream until they leave it to perform their work. We shall consider leukocytes in detail in the next chapter.

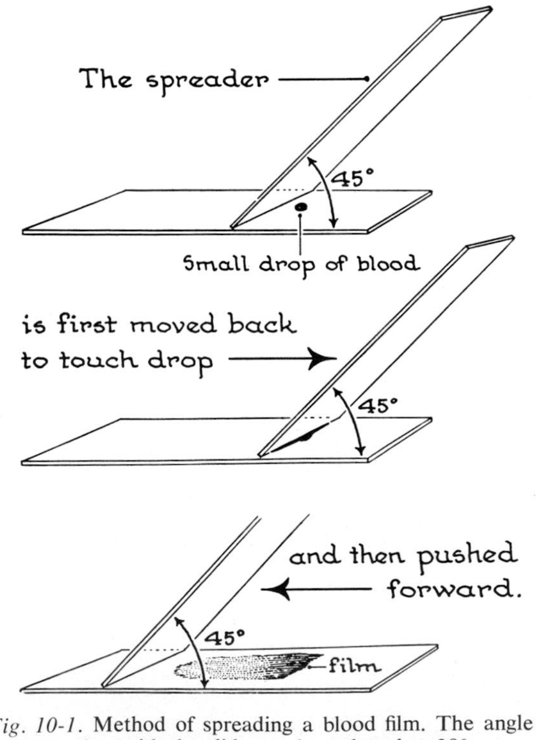

THE USE OF BLOOD FILMS FOR THE IDENTIFICATION AND STUDY OF ERYTHROCYTES, PLATELETS, AND LEUKOCYTES

Although blood cells can be identified in sections, they can be studied to much better advantage by spreading some blood very thinly on a clean glass slide, drying it, and then staining the cells spread out and flattened on it. Preparations made this way are called stained *blood films* (*smears*).

To obtain blood for making a blood film the cleaned finger (or earlobe) is punctured lightly, and the first drop or two of blood that well up are wiped away with sterile gauze. Then, a tiny drop (the first drops are too large) wells up from the puncture. Blood films (smears) are made differently in different laboratories. One way is to touch the tiny drop with one surface of a very clean slide (held by its edges and avoiding contact of the slide with the skin) so that most of the drop adheres to the slide midway between its sides and a short distance from one end (Fig. 10-1, *top*).

Fig. 10-1. Method of spreading a blood film. The angle the spreader makes with the slide can be reduced to 30°.

Fig. 10-2. Diagram illustrating the shape of a red blood cell (cut in half).

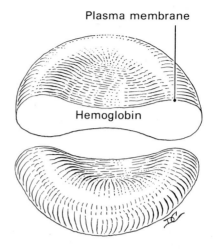

Plasma membrane

Hemoglobin

A second clean slide, called the spreader, is now put in the position indicated in Figure 10-1 (many consider that a spreader should be at an angle of 30° to the slide). The edge of the spreader should be pressed against the other slide rather lightly. The spreader is now drawn back until the edge in contact with the first slide touches the drop of blood, which thereupon spreads quickly along the line of contact between the slides. The spreader is then pushed steadily forward, still with only light pressure on it, and by this means the drop of blood is drawn out into a thin film.

The angle at which the spreader is held in relation to the first slide determines to some extent the thickness of the film. The greater the angle, the thicker the film. Furthermore, a film is thicker if the spreading is done rapidly. A film is usually thicker toward the end of the slide from which the film is spread (Fig. 10-4).

After a film has dried in air, it is generally stained with what is often called a "blood stain." Glance at Plate 11-1 to see that the erythrocytes are pink to red in color, circular in form, and nonnucleated. The leukocytes are nucleated and much less numerous. Although there are different varieties of blood stains, each commonly exists as a single solution. Enough blood stain is added to a slide to cover the film, and then after a short time twice as much distilled water, adjusted to pH 6.4 to 6.6 with a phosphate buffer, is added to dilute the stain. After the diluted solution has been allowed to act for a few minutes, the slide is rinsed and dried. Then it can be studied with the high-power objective either with or without a coverslip.

Development of Blood Stains. In 1891, Romanovsky tried the effect of mixing an acid stain (eosin) with a basic stain (methylene blue). Curiously enough, the mixture acted as a better stain for blood than if the ingredients were applied separately. With it he was able to stain malarial parasites inside red blood cells (a great help in diagnosing malaria); indeed, one part of the parasite was colored a violet shade, which could not be attributed directly to eosin or methylene blue. Another dye seemed to have been produced. Then Unna found if he treated methylene blue with alkali and heat, it would impart a violet color to tissues. Methylene blue treated to produce this new dye (or dyes) was said to be *polychromed* as described on page 3. Next, polychromed methylene blue was mixed with eosin and this was better still. But such mixtures soon precipitate. So, for convenience, they are allowed to do so, and the precipitate is then dissolved in methyl alcohol; this is roughly what is in the bottle of blood stain in the laboratory. However, in alcoholic solution it is not an effective stain. But when water is added to it on the slide, the compound previously in solution in methyl alcohol partly passes into aqueous solution, and some dissociation occurs into anions and cations, and both carry color. So for a brief period the stain acts as if the ingredients had just been freshly mixed. Later on, of course, it tends to form a precipitate again, but by this time staining has been completed, and the slide should have been washed.

ERYTHROCYTES

Erythrocytes (red blood cells) are the commonest type of blood cell, being from 500 to 1,000 times more numerous than leukocytes. In absolute numbers there are about 5 million erythrocytes per cubic millimeter of blood.

Shape

The human erythrocyte has the shape of a *biconcave disk* (Fig. 10-2), but other shapes are found in other species. In certain diseases erythrocytes with altered shapes make their appearance (Fig. 10-3B), hence determining the shapes of erythrocytes is of diagnostic importance.

Size and Volume

The diameter of erythrocytes is usually measured in blood films (Fig. 10-1). Since they have the shape of biconcave disks they lie flat on the slide, so drying does not greatly affect their size. In normal blood the diameter of erythrocytes has a mean value of 7.2 μm. and does not vary by much more than 0.5 μm. from this mean value (Fig. 10-4). Thus a glance at the size distribution of erythrocytes (which is called a Price-Jones curve) reveals any abnormalities of size that might occur.

An erythrocyte smaller than 6 μm. in diameter is termed a *microcyte* (Gr. *mikros*, small), as illustrated in

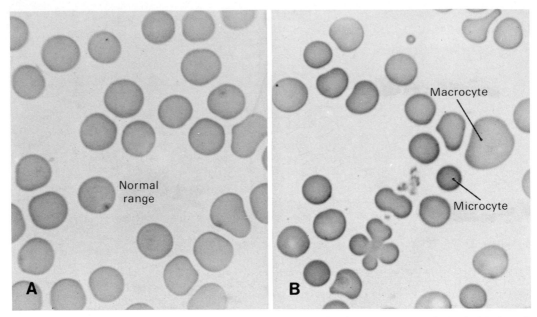

Fig. 10-3. Oil-immersion photomicrographs of stained films of rabbit blood. (*A*) Normal blood with the cells varying in size only slightly and, except where pressed upon by other cells in the film, having a normal shape. (*B*) Blood obtained from an animal after TNT poisoning. It shows a great range in size of red blood cells, with both microcytes and macrocytes present. It also shows red cells of abnormal shapes (poikilocytes).

Figure 10-3B, whereas an erythrocyte larger than normal (from 9 to 12 μm, in diameter) is termed a *macrocyte* (Gr. *makros,* large), also illustrated in Figure 10-3B. Thus a shift in size range toward smaller erythrocytes is called a *microcytic* condition, and toward bigger ones a *macrocytic* condition (Fig. 10-5). In some conditions both microcytes and macrocytes may be present concurrently (Fig. 10-3B).

With the introduction of electronic counting instruments in hematology laboratories it is now common practice to measure the red cell volume instead of size, since the volume of the red cell has diagnostic significance; accordingly, the terms *microcyte* and *macrocyte* have come to mean also erythrocytes of smaller and larger volume, respectively.

Structure and Composition

The factors determining and maintaining the shape of an erythrocyte are the particular molecular constituents of its cell membrane and the constitution of the colloidal complex with which it is filled. Moreover, these confer pliability and elasticity so that the red cell can undergo deformation when necessary in negotiating passage through networks of vessels with small lumina.

More than half (66%) of the content of the erythrocyte is water and about 33 per cent is the protein *hemoglobin.* This protein contains a protein moiety, *globin,* joined to

the pigment *heme.* Although only 4 per cent of hemoglobin actually consists of heme, its combination with globin results in the combined entity (hemoglobin) being colored; hence hemoglobin too is spoken of as a pigment. A little other protein, several enzymes, and some lipid also exist in the cell along with hemoglobin.

It may seem curious that erythrocytes containing only a soft jelly would maintain their biconcave shape, and that the molecular constitution of the jelly could be such as to be an important factor in making the cell assume this shape. However, the fact is that a change in the chemical constitution of hemoglobin can be responsible for the cells taking on a different shape. For example, there is a disease (called *sickle cell anemia*) in which the erythrocytes may assume the form of sickles. In this form they are destroyed easily, and so individuals with this disease do not have enough erythrocytes and suffer from *anemia* (a subject dealt with in more detail later). In 1949 Pauling and his colleagues discovered that hemoglobin in sickle cells was slightly different from normal and the difference was sufficient to make the cells assume a shape different from a biconcave disk when the hemoglobin is deoxygenated. Hereditary factors are responsible for the condition; hence this disease provides an example of how an altered sequence in a DNA molecule, resulting in one amino acid (valine) being substituted for the usual one (glutamic acid) in the hemoglobin molecule, can cause a disease.

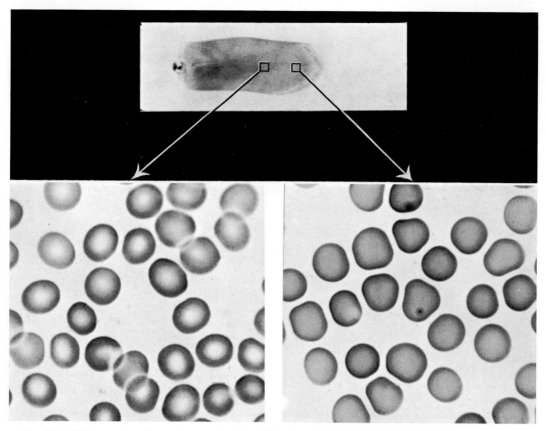

Fig. 10-4. Oil-immersion photomicrographs of red blood cells at different sites in a blood film. (*Lower left*) These show the pale areas characteristic of normal red cells. Such pale areas show only where the film is thick enough for occasional red cells to be superimposed on one another. (*Lower right*) Appearance of red cells at a place where they are spread very thinly. No cells are superimposed here and the central pale areas cannot be seen.

Each erythrocyte, of course, is surrounded by a plasmalemma which prevents the escape of the colloidal protein material of the cell into the plasma. It also exhibits great selectivity with regard to the passage of ions. Features of the red cell membrane are illustrated in Figure 5-6 (p. 112).

Rouleau Formation

If fresh blood is placed on a slide and covered with a coverslip, the broad surfaces of erythrocytes often adhere to one another, with the result that numbers of erythrocytes may become arranged together like coins in a pile. These arrangements of adherent erythrocytes are termed *rouleaux* and they are probably manifestations of surface tension forces. They are seen primarily under conditions in which certain plasma proteins (globulins) are increased. However, if circulating blood is examined under the microscope, rouleaux are also sometimes normally seen where the circulation is not rapid. They are not permanent, and the erythrocytes in them can become separated again with no harm having been done to them.

Behavior in Solutions of Different Osmotic Pressures

The osmotic pressure of plasma equals that of erythrocytes, and so plasma is said to be *isotonic* (Gr. *iso*, equal; *tonos*, tension) with regard to them. In plasma, then, there is no tendency for the erythrocytes to absorb water from the plasma or vice versa. It is possible to prepare salt solutions that are *isotonic* with erythrocytes. If a salt concentration of a solution is below that of erythrocytes, it is said to be *hypotonic* (Gr. *hypo*, under), if above it, *hypertonic* (Gr. *hyper*, above, over), in relation to them.

Hemolysis

Erythrocytes are fairly resistant to slight changes in osmotic pressure, but in a solution that is sufficiently hypo-

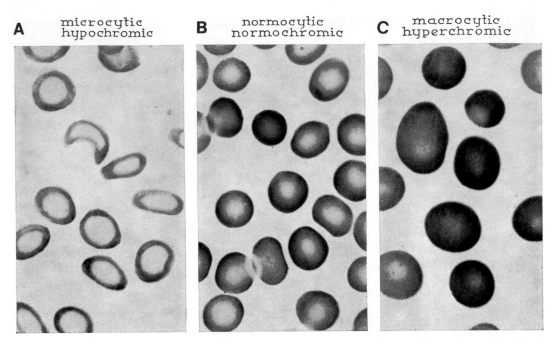

Fig. 10-5. Oil-immersion photomicrographs (same magnification) of three different films of human blood. (*A*) Blood from a patient with microcytic hypochromic anemia due to iron deficiency; the red blood cells are small and their central pale area greatly enlarged. (*B*) Normal blood. (*C*) Blood obtained from a patient with pernicious anemia. The red blood cells, though fewer than normal, tend to be larger and so *appear* to be overfilled with hemoglobin.

tonic, they swell and assume a spherical shape. Another phenomenon then occurs: their membranes become incapable of retaining hemoglobin, and this escapes into the surrounding fluid, coloring it. This is known as *hemolysis* (Gr. *lysis*, solution). The cell membrane remains to constitute what is termed the *ghost* of the cell.

Hemolysis can be induced by means other than hypotonic solutions. Certain chemicals, particularly lipid solvents, exert a hemolytic effect. Snake venom, a potent source of lipolytic enzymes, is a hemolytic agent. The plasma of some species hemolyzes the erythrocytes of others. Antibodies made by injecting the erythrocytes of one animal into a genetically dissimilar one will hemolyze the erythrocytes of the first; this phenomenon involves the fixing of complement as described in Chapter 11 (p. 285).

It should also be mentioned, however, that some hemoglobin release is normal in such sites as the spleen, where worn-out red cells are always being phagocytosed by macrophages.

Fragility

The erythrocytes in any given sample of blood are not equally susceptible to hemolysis. For instance, a solution of saline may be prepared in a concentration that will hemolyze only some cells; for all to be hemolyzed, the strength of the solution must be reduced further. Hence erythrocytes are said to vary in their *fragility* (their susceptibility to hemolysis). The fragility of erythrocytes becomes altered in certain diseases; hence fragility tests are of use in diagnosis.

Crenation

If erythrocytes are immersed in a hypertonic solution, water is drawn from them into the solution. This results in shrinkage and because they shrink irregularly, so that their outlines contain notches and indentations, they are said to be *crenated* (L. *crena*, a notch).

THE ROLE OF ERYTHROCYTES IN TRANSPORTING OXYGEN

Oxygen (at atmospheric pressure) does not dissolve to any great extent in plasma. Hence, if the circulatory system contained nothing more than plasma, only a small fraction of the amount of oxygen needed by the cells of the body would dissolve into it as it was pumped through the capillaries of the lungs, which are exposed to freshly inspired air. Blood is enabled to pick up large amounts of oxygen in the lungs by the hemoglobin in its erythrocytes. Hemoglobin is able to combine rapidly with oxygen to form the compound *oxyhemoglobin*. So because of the hemoglobin in erythrocytes blood can absorb relatively large amounts of oxygen as it passes through the lungs and constantly supply oxygen to all the cells of the body.

Hemoglobin, fortunately, does not bind oxygen very firmly. So when oxyhemoglobin reaches the various tissues of the body, where the cells are constantly using oxygen, the hemoglobin releases a good part of its oxygen. When oxygen is thus divorced from oxyhemoglobin, the hemoglobin remaining is called *deoxyhemoglobin;* this, on reaching the lungs as it continues on its route through the circulatory system, is again in contact with a high concentration of oxygen, and is prepared to reunite with it and become oxyhemoglobin again.

Why Hemoglobin Must Be Confined in Cells

One of the main reasons for this is that erythrocytes contain, in addition to their content of hemoglobin, many enzymes responsible for keeping the hemoglobin in the reduced form in which it is able to carry oxygen. These enzymes must be kept in intimate association with the hemoglobin in order to maintain it in its reduced form. Moreover, hemoglobin macromolecules are relatively small and, if free in plasma, would leak through the endothelial membranes of the blood vascular system. Hence, if hemoglobin becomes free in plasma, it escapes into the tissues and then into the urine. This gave the name "red-water fever" to a disease of cattle in which a minute parasite invades the erythrocytes and so damages them that their hemoglobin escapes first into the plasma and then into the urine, which becomes colored. In certain human diseases—for example, in "black-water fever," which is a virulent type of malaria—enough erythrocytes may be damaged to produce a similar condition. There are further advantages in having hemoglobin enclosed by the cell membrane of erythrocytes. For example, erythrocytes are involved in the transport of carbon dioxide from the tissues to the lungs, where it escapes into the air. Their use in this respect is dependent on their not losing their content of the enzyme carbonic anhydrase.

How the Structure of Erythrocytes Is Adapted to Their Function

Erythrocytes must absorb and release oxygen and carbon dioxide very quickly from the surface of the cell membrane. Therefore it is important that the interface between each erythrocyte and plasma be as extensive as possible, which is realized by the biconcave form of the erythrocyte. This gives a surface area 20 to 30 per cent greater than that of a sphere containing the same amount of hemoglobin. Furthermore, if erythrocytes were spheres, the distance over which a gas would have to diffuse to reach the surface would be greatly increased. The non-nucleated state of the erythrocyte is also advantageous in that it allows the whole cell to contain hemoglobin and so be more efficient per unit volume.

The rounded edges of the erythrocyte protect it from injury, and its resilient elastic structure allows it to bend rather then break as it strikes bifurcations in capillary networks (this may be watched under the microscope in the web of a living frog's foot, suitably mounted).

Pink Cheeks and Red Lips

It is the oxyhemoglobin in the erythrocytes in capillaries below the surface that imparts pinkness to cheeks and varying degrees of redness of lips and mucous membranes. The degree of color so imparted depends on many factors: the number of capillaries open in the capillary bed, their closeness to the surface, the transparency of the overlying tissue, and, finally, the proportion of oxyhemoglobin in the blood.

Blue Lips

Deoxygenated hemoglobin, however, has a bluish tinge. Normally, as blood passes through capillaries, not enough deoxygenated hemoglobin is formed for the blue color to show. However, in a normal person exposed to severe cold, the local circulation in the lips may be closed down sufficiently for the amount of deoxyhemoglobin to be increased in the superficial capillaries, so the blue shows. In certain diseases the oxygenation of blood in the lungs is seriously impaired so that blood containing a considerable amount of deoxyhemoglobin is delivered to capillaries all over the body. A sufficient absolute amount of deoxyhemoglobin may under certain disease conditions impart a blue color to all surfaces of the body that are ordinarily pink or red. This is termed *cyanosis* (Gr. *kyanos*, blue).

Carbon Monoxide Poisoning

Hemoglobin has a great affinity for certain other gases besides oxygen, notably carbon monoxide. This dangerous gas forms a firm union with hemoglobin and so oxygen cannot be transported to the tissues. Hence a person breathing air containing even low levels of carbon monoxide gradually comes to have more and more of his hemoglobin bound to it and therefore unavailable for the transport of oxygen. (This happens all too often on cold nights in parked cars in which the motor is kept running to keep the heater on.) Carbon monoxide-hemoglobin is a bright red color, and the cherry-red lips of the carbon monoxide victim, whose tissues are in reality starved for oxygen, provide a sad paradox.

HOW THE OXYGEN-CARRYING CAPACITY OF THE BLOOD OF A PERSON IS DETERMINED

In the practice of medicine it is frequently necessary to determine whether or not a patient is suffering from inability of the blood to transport oxygen properly. Aside from relatively rare instances in which hemoglobin is chemically altered, it is obvious that the oxygen-carrying capacity of the blood could be diminished by there not being (*1*) enough erythrocytes in the blood, or (*2*) enough hemoglobin in the red cells, or (*3*) both. The usual tests made are (*1*) estimating the number of erythrocytes present per cubic millimeter of blood and (*2*) estimating the amount of hemoglobin per 100 ml. of blood.

Erythrocyte Counts

These are made using a suitably calibrated blood pipet, with an expanded mixing bulb in the middle, to draw up a measured volume of blood for dilution. Then a large volume of counting fluid is drawn into the pipet to dilute the blood for counting. After careful mixing in the bulb the first few drops of unmixed diluent (in the stem of the pipet) are discarded and a sample of the diluted blood is run into a counting chamber, called a *hemocytometer* because blood cells are counted in it. This is a special type of ruled slide divided up into squares of given sizes for counting different kinds of blood cells. Since the thickness of the sample is determined by the height at which the coverslip is supported, the volume of diluted fluid above the ruled squares is known and hence by counting the numbers of erythrocytes in such squares the number of erythrocytes per cubic millimeter of blood may be readily calculated. This method is, of course, time consuming, and for large numbers of routine blood cell counts in hospital hematology laboratories electronic counting instruments capable of doing a count in a fraction of the time it takes with a hemocytometer are employed. A count of 4 to 5 million erythrocytes per cubic millimeter of blood is considered normal for women and from 4.5 to 5.5 million is normal for men.

Hematocrit Estimation

A rapid method of determining whether an individual has a normal complement of red blood cells is to centrifuge a small volume of blood so as to estimate the packed red cell volume. This is termed determining his *hematocrit* (Gr. *haima*, blood; *krino*, to separate) since it involves separating the blood cells (erythrocytes account for almost all the packed blood cell volume) from the plasma; the hematocrit is the percentage of the blood sample volume occupied by erythrocytes. Average hematocrit values for

normal women are about 41 per cent and for normal men about 47 per cent.

Hemoglobin Estimation

Several methods are available that permit the amount of hemoglobin per unit volume of blood to be determined from a single drop; from this the total amount of hemoglobin per 100 ml. of blood is calculated. Women normally have about 13.5 g. and men normally have about 15 g. hemoglobin per 100 ml. blood.

ANEMIA

If the amount of hemoglobin in circulating blood is significantly reduced, the condition is said to constitute *anemia* (Gr., without blood). A lack of hemoglobin can be due primarily to a lack of erythrocytes or to a lack of hemoglobin itself.

In order to consider the problem further, certain facts must be taken into consideration.

The Life Span of Erythrocytes

Erythrocytes have a limited life span; in man this is 120 days. After their lifetime in the circulatory system, they must be removed from it to prevent their disintegrating bodies from cluttering up the circulatory system. Worn-out erythrocytes are removed from the bloodstream by macrophages in the spleen, bone marrow, and liver.

Since erythrocytes are constantly removed from the circulation as they wear out, their numbers in the blood would steadily fall if new ones were not delivered into the blood at the same rate. Hence anemia could occur primarily as a result of an uncompensated increase in the rate of removal of erythrocytes from blood or a decrease in the rate at which they are formed and liberated into blood. In other words, some anemias are due primarily to an increased rate of erythrocyte destruction or loss from the body that is not compensated for by just as great an increase in the rate of their production, while other anemias could be due primarily to a deficient rate of production.

In order to ascertain whether it is the rate of erythrocyte production or the rate of erythrocyte destruction that is at fault, much useful information can be obtained by making what is termed a *reticulocyte count*.

The Reticulocyte Count

In a normal blood film, stained with an ordinary blood stain, almost all erythrocytes are clear pink in color. But from 1 to 2 per cent of the erythrocytes will demonstrate a blue tinge. Such an erythrocyte is said to be a *polychromatophilic erythrocyte* (a red cell that loves many colors; Plate 11-1). We shall now explain what causes the blue tinge in a red cell.

The nucleated precursor cells giving rise to erythrocytes are larger cells called *erythroblasts* that synthesize the hemoglobin later found in their progeny, the erythrocytes. For synthesizing hemoglobin they have abundant polyribosomes (Fig. 5-16), which render their cytoplasm intensely basophilic in the LM. However, they divide several times in forming erythrocytes and in so doing the polyribosomes become divided up so that there are only enough in immature erythrocytes to impart a trace of basophilia to the cytoplasm.

Polychromatophilic erythrocytes are difficult to identify in films stained with ordinary blood stains. A much better way to identify the cells is to employ supravital staining with brilliant cresyl blue. This stain may be mixed with a fresh drop of blood and a blood film made that may be subsequently stained with an ordinary blood stain. Brilliant cresyl blue reacts in a curious manner with such rRNA as persists so as to produce a thread-like blue structure that sometimes looks like a wreath (Fig. 10-6), but if the rRNA is scanty it may constitute no more than a few scattered dots (Plate 11-1, *bottom right*). Due to the notion that this appearance might be due to a preexisting reticular network in this type of cell, such cells were termed *reticulocytes* and the name has remained ever since even though we now know that the network is really an artifact due to the staining procedure. The *reticulocyte* is, of course, the same cell as a polychromatophilic erythrocyte seen after staining with an ordinary blood stain (Plate 11-1). The use of radioautography following administration of labeled amino acid has shown that reticulocytes are still capable of a significant level of protein synthesis, so they would also contain some mRNA and tRNA in addition to rRNA.

The rRNA present in reticulocytes liberated from the bone marrow into the circulation soon fades away; it remains only for about two days in immature erythrocytes.

Precise data about the numbers of reticulocytes released from the bone marrow into the circulation under normal conditions are not easily ascertained. However, when erythrocyte production is increased, since the storage space in the marrow is not correspondingly increased, more reticulocytes are liberated into the blood. Thus the reticulocyte count goes up when more erythrocytes are produced, and reticulocyte counts can be used to monitor the rate of red cell production.

Under otherwise normal circumstances, any condition that causes an increased rate of erythrocyte destruction (or loss by hemorrhage) is compensated for by an increase in the rate of erythrocyte production. So if, for example, the reticulocyte count remains high day after day,

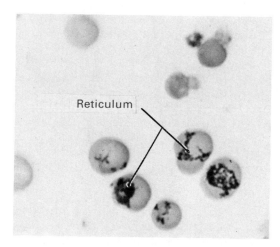

Fig. 10-6. Oil-immersion photomicrograph of a blood film stained with brilliant cresyl blue to show reticulocytes. The blood used was obtained from an experimental animal regenerating large numbers of new erythrocytes.

it can be assumed that the rate of destruction of erythrocytes is increased, or that erythrocytes are being lost from the circulation in some other fashion. In other words, the reticulocyte count can be used not only to provide information about the rate of erythrocyte production but also, in conjunction with daily erythrocyte counts, about the rate of erythrocyte destruction or loss. For example, reticulocyte counts can be used to monitor whether products such as the explosive TNT, toxic to cells of the erythrocytic series, are being absorbed by those who handle them.

How Anemias Are Classified

Sooner or later, the medical student must learn to examine a blood film and say whether it indicates a *hypochromic microcytic anemia* or a *macrocytic anemia* or some other kind of blood disorder designated by this type of terminology. What do these terms mean?

Macrocytes and microcytes have already been defined. If in any anemia the erythrocytes tend to be substantially larger than normal, the anemia is said to be macrocytic; if smaller than normal, microcytic; and if of normal size, normocytic. The terms *hyperchromic, normochromic,* and *hypochromic* refer to the total amount of hemoglobin in the red cells, which of course is what accounts for their depth of color in films. We shall elaborate.

Since an erythrocyte has the shape of a biconcave disk, it is thinner in the middle than at the edge and so its central region stains lighter than its periphery (Fig. 10-4, *left*). However, this appearance is seen only in the proper part of a well-made film that is just thick enough for occasional cells to partly overlap one another (Fig. 10-4, *left*); the lighter-staining central area cannot be seen properly where the cells are spread too thinly (Fig. 10-4, *right*).

If the central pale area represents roughly a third of the diameter of the erythrocyte and the peripheral region shows fairly intense staining, the erythrocytes are said to be *normochromic* (normal in color) (Fig. 10-5B). Some anemias are characterized by a reduction in the number of erythrocytes, but such cells as are present are normochromic; hence they are said to be *normochromic anemias*. However, in a much more common type of anemia, the erythrocytes exhibit enlarged central pale areas and poorly stained peripheral zones (Fig. 10-5A). The cells so altered are said to be *hypochromic* (undercolored); hence the anemias with which they are associated are called *hypochromic anemias*. In still other anemias there are fewer cells than normal but these are well filled with hemoglobin. It is doubtful if red cells can be overfilled, and so the reason these anemias are called *hyperchromic* is that the cells are generally larger and, since they are well filled, they take on a deeper color (Fig. 10-5C).

Films of normal blood usually exhibit an occasional erythrocyte of abnormal shape. The general term for such a cell is a *poikilocyte* (Gr. *poikilis*, manifold). In the anemias, poikilocytes are common; hence, anemic blood is often said to exhibit *poikilocytosis* (Fig. 10-3B). In some anemias the abnormal shape is named more specifically— for example, the type in which erythrocytes tend to be shaped like sickles, which has already been mentioned.

The Different Effects of a Deficiency of Iron and of Vitamin B_{12}

In any given anemia, knowing whether the hemoglobin content is reduced more or less than the erythrocyte count is helpful in indicating the possible cause of the anemia. For example, iron is an essential ingredient of hemoglobin, and so when iron is deficient, the production of hemoglobin is reduced. However, iron is not as necessary for the production of erythrocytes as it is for the formation of hemoglobin, so in iron-deficiency anemias the hemoglobin content of blood is reduced more than the number of erythrocytes; hence the cells are poorly filled with hemoglobin, and the anemia is said to be of the *hypochromic* type (Fig. 10-5A). On the other hand, certain dietary factors (vitamin B_{12} and folic acid) seem to be more necessary to the production of erythrocytes than for the production of hemoglobin, so that, when either one of these substances is lacking, there is more difficulty in producing red blood cells than in producing hemoglobin; hence those cells that are produced under these conditions are filled to capacity with hemoglobin, and the anemia is of the *hyperchromic macrocytic* type (Fig. 10-5C). The anemias in this category are all caused by a defi-

ciency of vitamin B_{12} or folic acid in the body. An interesting example is pernicious anemia, which is caused by a failure to secrete a specific factor needed to absorb vitamin B_{12} and consequent failure to absorb this vitamin in the intestine. However, if the vitamin is injected into patients with pernicious anemia, they recover, and the condition recurs only if injections are discontinued. There is no point in feeding the vitamin by mouth because those afflicted cannot absorb it. (Vitamin B_{12} is present in liver extracts.)

The Control of Erythrocyte Production by Erythropoietin

A glycoprotein hormone known as *erythropoietin* affects the production of cells of the erythrocyte series. It is discussed in Chapter 12.

PLATELETS

PLATELETS, FIBRIN, AND THE HEMOSTATIC MECHANISM

Platelets Are Fragments of Cells

Platelets are little fragments of cytoplasm that, as described in Chapter 12, become detached from the cytoplasm of very large cells called *megakaryocytes* in the bone marrow in such a way that each platelet is completely covered with cell membrane. They have no nuclear components. In this respect the blood of mammals differs from that of birds, for in the latter there are very small nucleated cells, called *thrombocytes* (Gr. *thrombos*, clot) that serve the same function as the platelets of man. Platelets, however, are also sometimes called *thrombocytes* even though they are not whole cells. Their numbers in circulating blood are estimated at 250,000 to 350,000 per cubic millimeter. Two are shown in Figure 10-7, but before describing their structure we should first comment on their functions.

THE ROLE OF PLATELETS IN ARRESTING BLEEDING

When a person cuts himself, blood flows from vessels severed at the site of the injury. But unless the vessels are relatively large the flow of blood soon ceases. Although other factors also operate to achieve this end—for example, the circular muscle of the vessel wall becomes constricted so as to narrow the lumen of the vessel—the primary reason for the cessation of bleeding is that platelets settle out and adhere to the inner surface of the vessel in the region of the cut. This, of course, narrows the opening through which blood can escape and, as blood continues to flow through the narrowed opening, more and more platelets adhere to those already attached to the lining so that the lumen soon becomes completely occluded by what is termed a *platelet plug*. This process is called *platelet aggregation*.

The Terms Aggregation and Coagulation

As noted, the clumping of platelets occurring when platelets pile up and adhere to one another is termed *aggregation*. But this process is almost always associated with the formation of threads of the fibrous protein *fibrin* derived from a precursor in the plasma by a mechanism termed *coagulation*. Accordingly, platelets not only aggregate, they are also concerned in initiating coagulation.

A blood vessel, however, does not have to be severed in order for platelets to adhere to its lining. The arteries of many people as they become older undergo a degenerative change (the condition referred to as *arteriosclerosis*), which often affects the lining of arteries in such a way that it no longer presents a smooth uninterrupted endothelial surface to the blood flowing along it; as a consequence, platelets on coming into contact with certain components of the artery wall may begin to adhere to its lining. If platelets continue to accumulate at such a site, they, together with fibrin forming in association with them as a result of coagulation, may eventually entirely occlude the lumen of the vessel. If the vessel in which this occurs is a coronary artery of the heart, part of the heart muscle becomes deprived of a supply of oxygen and the person involved experiences what is commonly termed an *acute coronary attack*. If the same process occurs in an artery supplying the brain, the individual is said to have suffered a *stroke*.

Before describing the microscopic structure of platelets and the relation of their fine structure to their function, we should comment very briefly on blood coagulation for those readers who have not yet studied physiology, in which subject it is dealt with at length.

Coagulation

In contrast to *aggregation*, which occurs in flowing blood, *coagulation* is commonly associated with stagnant blood. Coagulation is responsible for the clot that forms when blood is drawn from the body and left in a test tube. Coagulation also occurs in blood that escapes from vessels and becomes pooled in a tissue space in the body. For example, when a bone is broken, blood vessels are torn and some blood leaks into the tissues in and around the fracture. In blood escaping from the vascular system, just as in blood in a test tube, an extensive mesh of fine

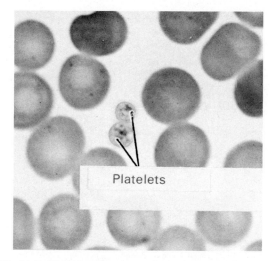

Fig. 10-7. Oil-immersion photomicrograph of a stained film of human blood. Two platelets are seen adhering to one another.

fibers of *fibrin* (Fig. 10-8) appears. The erythrocytes present in this blood become trapped in the network of fibrin and can be seen there for a short time (Fig. 10-8A), after which they disintegrate. Blood in which fibrin forms as above is said to have *clotted*.

Why blood should stay fluid when it is in the blood vessels but clot when it is removed has always been a fascinating problem and it is now known that a host of factors are involved, a thorough discussion of which is more the subject matter of physiology, clinical hematology, and biochemistry than histology. However, we must give at least a very abbreviated account of the process of coagulation, because platelets are involved in it.

The Clotting Mechanism

One of the proteins of blood plasma is *fibrinogen*. Under normal conditions fibrinogen exists in solution. Also, there is in plasma a globulin called *prothrombin*, which under ordinary conditions is inactive. However, at sites of injury a component commonly called tissue *thromboplastin* is liberated, and (although many factors are involved) the net result is that the release of tissue thromboplastin triggers the conversion of prothrombin to thrombin, which acts to cause soluble fibrinogen to become polymerized into insoluble threads of fibrin. These threads, seen with the EM, show axial periodicity (Fig. 10-9); the periods, however, are shorter then those seen in collagen, being about 25 nm. in length. Since tissue thromboplastin comes from the damaged tissue, it is said to be an *extrinsic* factor; that is, a factor not originating in blood.

The coagulation mechanism, however, can be triggered

Fibrin threads

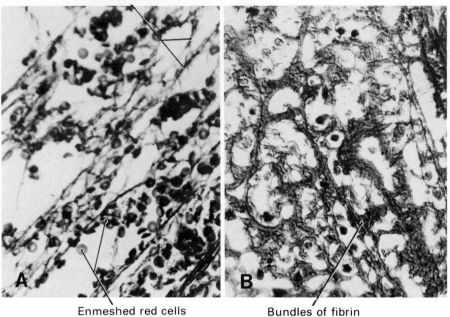

A

B

Enmeshed red cells

Bundles of fibrin
threads

Fig. 10-8. High-power photomicrographs of a region into
which bleeding occurred. (*A*)
Fine threads of fibrin form a mesh
entangling many red blood cells.
(*B*) Fibrin threads in coarser bundles.

by an *intrinsic* factor originating in blood. Platelets can play a part in leading to the formation of this substance. It is an intrinsic factor that triggers coagulation when blood comes into contact with a foreign substance, as it does if it is put in a glass test tube.

It should now be clear that, as a platelet plug begins to form on the inner surface of a diseased artery or at the edge of a cut vessel, both extrinsic and intrinsic factors could operate to trigger coagulation so that the formation of fibrin (coagulation) commonly occurs at sites of plate-let aggregation.

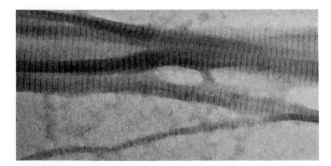

Fig. 10-9. Electron micrograph (×69,000) of bovine fibrin, clotted in vitro by the addition of thrombin to fibrinogen solution, and stained with phosphotungstic acid. Note the 25-nm. axial periodicity of fibrin threads. (Courtesy of C. Hall)

Thrombosis—White and Red Thrombi

An aggregated mass of platelets adhering to the inner surface of a blood vessel is known as a *white thrombus* because masses of platelets, in their fresh state, are white in color. A white thrombus can form only in flowing blood; it grows by abstracting fresh supplies of platelets from the blood that passes over it. Furthermore, it is different in nature from the *red thrombus* that forms when still blood coagulates. Aggregation, then, tends to form a white clot, which consists primarily of fused platelets; coagulation, a red clot that consists primarily of strands of fibrin that enmesh innumerable erythrocytes. Since platelets, when they aggregate, liberate a substance which triggers the formation of thromboplastin, it is easy to see why red thrombi are often associated with white thrombi.

Having dealt briefly with coagulation we can now describe the morphology of platelets and the relation of their fine structure to their functions.

THE STUDY OF PLATELETS IN THE LABORATORY WITH THE LM

In living preparations of capillaries in which blood is circulating, platelets appear as oval, biconvex disks. However, in ordinary blood films, unless precautions are taken, platelets may aggregate and so be seen in clumps (labeled in Plate 11-1). With the oil-immersion objective single platelets generally have a flat rounded appearance (Fig. 10-7), because platelets tend to spread out on surfaces, where they reveal two ill-defined general regions. The outer part appears a fairly clear pale blue with a blood stain and is called its *hyalomere* (Gr. *hyalos*, glass; Gr. *meros*, part; Fig. 10-7). The more central part is called its *granulomere* because the colored material it contains (and by which it can be identified) is often in the form of granules (Fig. 10-7). Sometimes the granulomere appears as a solid clump of material which, in normal blood, may be due to a change having occurred before the platelet was fixed and stained. Sometimes platelets have spike-like pseudopodia extending from the periphery of the hyalomere. If blood is normal, this appearance also may be due to changes that occurred after the blood was drawn but before the platelets were fixed. Nevertheless, in abnormal conditions platelets may present different appearances. It has been suggested that younger platelets look bigger than older platelets because they spread better. However, the extent to which platelet morphology can be learned with the LM is not very great compared with what can be learned using the EM, as will become apparent shortly.

How Platelets Are Counted

To prevent platelets aggregating and in order that they may be counted as individual entities, the blood sample must be taken using tubes treated with an anticoagulant such as heparin, EDTA, or citrate. Platelets may be counted in any of three ways. First, the proportion of platelets to erythrocytes may be estimated, at least in terms of being normal, high, or low, from a blood film. The number of platelets in relation to the number of erythrocytes is determined in several areas of the film. For example, if representative areas show there is an average of 6 platelets to every 100 erythrocytes and a proper erythrocyte count is then made from fresh blood, the actual number of platelets per cubic millimeter of blood can be estimated; for example, if the erythrocyte count was 4,000,000 per cubic millimeter the platelet count would be 6/100 of 4,000,000 which is 240,000 per cubic millimeter.

The second method for counting platelets is to add to the blood sample an agent that will lyse the erythrocytes but leave the platelets intact. These may then be counted using a hemocytometer with a phase contrast microscope.

The third method, which is used in hospital hematology laboratories running large numbers of blood samples for platelet counts, is to count the platelets with an automatic electronic counting instrument. This, of course, is much quicker than either of the manual methods.

THE FINE STRUCTURE OF PLATELETS

EM sections of platelets are usually fixed in glutaraldehyde and stained with osmium tetroxide. However, other special methods can be used to demonstrate certain components more clearly, but only at the cost of obscuring certain others.

Seen with the EM, platelets are somewhat irregular in shape and vary in outline from being rounded to ovoid (Fig. 10-10). The difference probably depends on the plane in which each platelet is sectioned. Each is enclosed with plasmalemma, covered with cell coat (labeled in Figs. 10-10 and 10-11).

Microtubules and Filaments

The portion termed the *hyalomere* with the LM appears in the EM as a homogeneous, finely granular material containing near its periphery both microtubules (labeled in Figs. 10-10 and 10-11) and filaments. The former, seen in cross section, appear to advantage as compact bundles at opposite ends of a cross section of a platelet (Fig. 10-11); in longitudinal section they may be seen arching parallel to the cell membrane, just beneath it (Fig. 10-10). They probably function as a skeleton to maintain the platelet's ovoid shape. Filaments perhaps associated with the microtubules have also been described at the periphery of the platelet. Most seem to be of the actin-containing type and are thought to participate in clot retraction, as described in due course. Other features seen with the EM are as follows.

Two Systems of Tubules

The first system is termed the *surface-connecting canalicular system* because the tubules (seen in cross section as vesicles) belonging to it all communicate with the surface (Figs. 10-10, arrow, and 10-11). Furthermore, the inner surface of the membrane of vesicular profiles of this system (labeled scs in Fig. 10-10) reveals the same kind of carbohydrate-containing coat as is seen on the cell membrane surrounding the platelets (Figs. 10-10 and 10-11). Hence the surface-connecting canalicular system represents invaginations of the covering membrane of the platelet and it is concerned with taking substances into the interior and/or releasing substances from within the platelet to its exterior. The tubules of this system are relatively large and are most commonly cut in cross section as in Figure 10-10, *lower left*; hence they appear as membrane-bound vesicles which superficially appear as holes in platelets, as is obvious in Figure 10-10 (this is why they were first called vacuoles).

The second system of tubules is termed the *dense tubular system* because the membranous tubules of this system contain a material that is moderately electron-dense (Figs. 10-10, dts, and 10-11). It seems probable that the components of this system came from the Golgi apparatus of the megakaryocytes. It would be interesting to know the function of the components of this system.

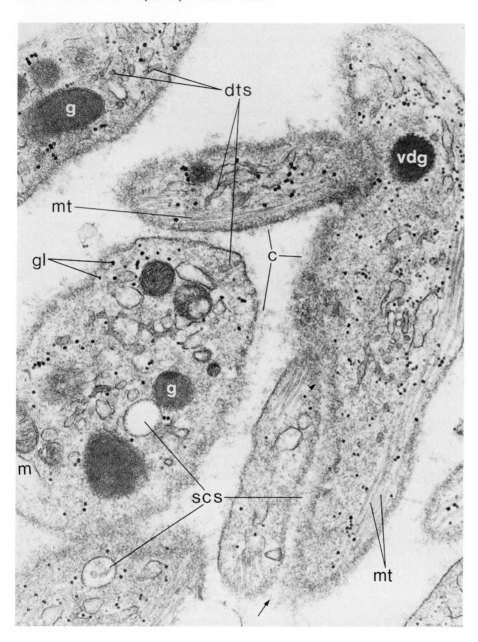

Fig. 10-10. Electron micrograph (×21,000) of a group of platelets. Note their cell coats (c) and channels of the surface-connecting canalicular system of tubules (scs) opening to the surface (arrow, *bottom center*). Some tubules of the dense tubular system (dts) are also present. Within the cytoplasm α granules (g), a very dense granule (vdg), glycogen particles (gl), and mitochrondria (m) are seen. Note the way the bundles of microtubules (mt) encircle the platelets parallel to their margins in such a way as to maintain their shape. (Courtesy of C. P. Leblond)

Mitochondria

Only one or two are seen in any given section of a platelet (Fig. 10-10).

Glycogen Particles

These appear in the form of single very small granules (Fig. 10-10, gl) distributed in small groups or sometimes in aggregates (Fig. 10-11).

Ribosomes

These are not common in platelets but when present are thought to indicate that the platelet was recently formed and hence carried away with it some ribosomes of the megakaryocyte cytoplasm.

Alpha Granules

These account for most of the colored granules seen with the LM. In the EM these granules are round to oval

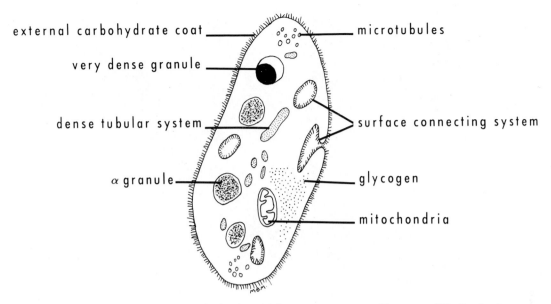

external carbohydrate coat ⎯⎯⎯⎯⎯⎯⎯⎯⎯ ⎯⎯⎯⎯⎯⎯⎯ microtubules

very dense granule ⎯⎯⎯⎯⎯⎯

dense tubular system ⎯⎯⎯⎯⎯⎯ ⎯⎯⎯⎯⎯ surface connecting system

α granule ⎯⎯⎯⎯ ⎯⎯⎯⎯⎯ glycogen

⎯⎯⎯⎯⎯ mitochondria

Fig. 10-11. Diagram of a rabbit platelet with its component parts. (Courtesy of H. Gardner)

and measure 0.2 to 0.3 μm. in diameter (Figs. 10-10, g, and 10-11). Their content of fine particulate matter sometimes appears slightly separated from the surrounding membrane. They contain many substances concerned in platelet function and, since they are membrane-bound and contain enzymes, are of the nature of secretory vesicles or lysosomes inherited from the cytoplasm of megakaryocytes from which platelets become detached. The α granules contain certain hydrolytic enzymes, including acid phosphatase, β-glucuronidase, and cathepsin.

Very Dense Granules

The content of this type of granule (labeled vdg in Fig. 10-10) is much more electron-dense than that of the other type of granule; hence this kind is termed the *very dense granule.* Sometimes the content of the very dense granule appears in electron micrographs to lie in an eccentric position (Fig. 10-11), leaving a wide, seemingly empty space between the content and the surrounding membrane. The relative number of very dense granules varies with species and in proportion to the serotonin content of the platelets. In rabbit platelets there are many very dense granules and the content of serotonin is correspondingly high, but in human platelets there are few and hence not much serotonin is present. Histochemical staining with the EM supports the view that serotonin is located in the very dense granules. Serotonin (5 hydroxytryptamine) is a pharmacologically potent substance that

in most parts of the body causes the muscle cells in blood vessels to contract.

In addition to serotonin, the dense granules have been shown to also contain calcium, ATP, and ADP. The significance of these findings will be mentioned presently.

ADHESION AND THE RELEASE REACTION

It has already been mentioned that circulating platelets do not normally adhere to the endothelium lining blood vessels. But if the continuity of the endothelial membrane is broken by physical injury or disease, platelets can come into contact with other tissues or tissue components. It has been known for some time that collagen has a very potent effect in causing platelets to adhere to it if it is exposed to flowing blood, as is shown in Figure 10-12. According to Weiss, basement membrane and the microfibrils associated with elastin in blood vessels, described in Chapter 19, also cause platelets to adhere to them when so exposed, but unlike collagen, this requires that calcium be available.

Next, it has been shown that what was termed the *release reaction* by Grette is set into motion by the adhesion of platelets, for example to collagen. This release reaction involves the release of the granules of platelets via the surface-conducting tubular system of the platelet that opens to its exterior (Figs. 10-10 and 10-11). The release reaction can be triggered by a variety of substances, including thrombin, collagen, ADP, and many

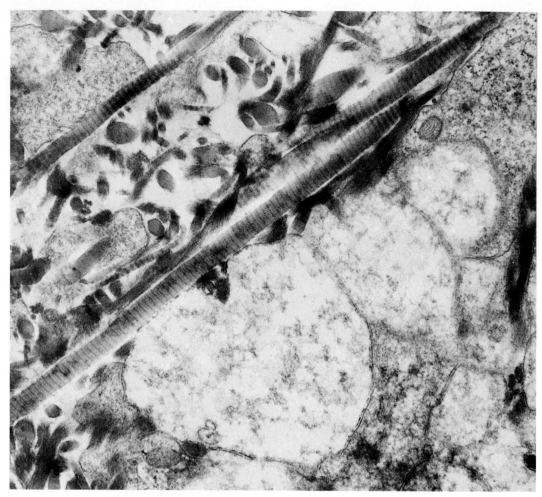

Fig. 10-12. Electron micrograph (×30,000) of platelets adhering to collagenic fibrils. Note the intimate association between the large platelet at *bottom center* and the fibril, which shows characteristic axial periodicity, just above it. Here the constituents of the platelets have disappeared, and the platelets are fusing into an amorphous mass. (Courtesy of J. F. Mustard)

other substances (see Weiss for details). These merely have to come into contact with the plasmalemma to initiate the release of granules through the portion of the plasmalemma that lines the surface-connecting tubular system.

The release reaction in which ADP is released from platelets that have, for example, adhered to collagen causes still more platelets to aggregate with those that have already accumulated; this explains how a platelet plug forms to block off a bleeding vessel. The platelets in a plug undergo degeneration and the final blocking of a cut blood vessel is due to fibroblasts and capillaries invading the plug and replacing it with connective tissue, which is termed *organization* of the thrombus.

THE ROLE OF PLATELETS IN CLOT RETRACTION

A process referred to as *clot retraction* soon occurs in a platelet plug forming in a cut vessel, a thrombus forming in an uncut vessel, or coagulated blood kept in a test tube. This retraction shrinks the clot down to as little as 10 per cent of its original volume and is dependent on there being both platelets and fibrin present.

To explain how platelets might bring about clot retraction requires that we describe how platelets change in form after aggregation and consequent thrombus formation. This change in their appearance is often referred to as *platelet activation*.

Platelet Activation

Before activation occurs, a platelet is the least deformable of all the circulating blood elements because it possesses such a well-developed skeleton of microtubules. As noted, however, there is in addition to the bundle of microtubules encircling the disk-shaped platelet along its margin a variable number of filaments, located just below the cell membrane. Activation is accompanied by a change of the disk-like shape to a spiny sphere and the granules move to a central position in the platelet. At the same time the marginal bundle of microtubules becomes disorganized, and numerous microfilaments now appear as a result of polymerization of soluble actin. Moreover, short myosin filaments are detectable amongst the microfilaments. The two types of filaments are thought to interact with one another so as to bring about retraction of the clot. Several hypotheses about how this is achieved have been proposed. One is based on the idea of the microfilament-rich spines of activated platelets making contact with fibrin threads and the whole platelet then functioning much as a sarcomere of striated muscle (Fig. 5-56), with the cell membrane at the tips of its spines, to which the microfilaments are attached, functioning more or less like Z lines, the microfilament-rich spines acting as an I band, and the body of the platelet as an A band. A further hypothesis is that the spines of activated platelets move in such a way as to pull on fibrin threads, alternately attaching and detaching by means of labile bonds, so as to pull the fibrin threads toward the center of the clot. This of course would require repeated cycles of contraction and relaxation to bring about retraction of the clot.

THE CONTROL OF PLATELET PRODUCTION—THROMBOPOIETIN

Experiments have shown that the serum (the component of blood plasma remaining after clotting has taken place) of animals that have suffered a severe blood loss will, if injected into normal animals, cause an increase in the platelet count. It is therefore visualized that, when such animals experience a severe hemorrhage, a substance is produced in them that enters the bloodstream and stimulates the formation of platelets. Sufficient work on this substance has been done to merit its being given the name *thrombopoietin*, and to indicate that it is probably a glycoprotein and closely related to erythropoietin. Its source has not been established and its action is not thoroughly understood; it probably results in increased numbers of megakaryocytes being produced and a speed-up in the maturation of platelets from megakaryocytes. It takes a few days for thrombopoietin to manifest its full effects.

ABNORMALITIES OF THE CLOTTING MECHANISM

Platelets have a life span of around 9 to 10 days, after which they are probably phagocytosed by macrophages. It follows that if there is a decreased rate of production of platelets, their number in blood gradually falls. Such a state of affairs occurs, for example, when the normal, functioning cells of bone marrow are crowded out by invasion or proliferation of tumor cells; for under these conditions there are not enough megakaryocytes to maintain normal numbers of platelets. There are other conditions in which the production of platelets is normal but they are removed too quickly from the circulation. To relieve this condition, the spleen, which is the most important site for the phagocytosis of platelets, may be removed surgically so that platelets can survive longer. A platelet deficiency, which is called *thrombocytopenia*, (Gr. *penia*, poverty), is associated with hemorrhages occurring for no apparent reason; these may appear in the skin, a mucous membrane, or other sites. As will be explained in more advanced courses, there are, in addition to the hemorrhagic diseases due to platelet deficiencies, a host of hemorrhagic diseases that result for one reason or another from an inability to form fibrin from fibrinogen. Since the formation of fibrin depends on a large number of factors, and since any of this large number may be implicated in a deficiency, there are several different bleeding diseases caused by an inability to form fibrin normally. Many have a genetic basis. Hemophilia is probably the best known example of a disease of this type.

REFERENCES AND OTHER READING

RED BLOOD CELLS

(*See also* Comprehensive General Reference listed for Chap. 11)

Bessis, M.: Corpuscles. Atlas of Red Blood Cell Shapes. Berlin, Springer-Verlag, 1974.

————: Blood Smears Reinterpreted. Berlin, Springer International, Springer-Verlag, 1977.

Bessis, M., Weed., R. I., and Leblond, P. F. (eds.): Red Cell Shape—Physiology, Pathology, Ultrastructure. New York, Springer-Verlag, 1973.

Surgenor, D.: The Red Blood Cell. ed. 2. vols 1 and 2. New York, Academic Press, 1974.

PLATELETS

Comprehensive General Reference

(*See also* Comprehensive General Reference listed for Chap. 11)

Weiss, J. H.: Platelet physiology and abnormalities of platelet function, Part I. N. Engl. J. Med., *293:*531, 1975.

Special References

Bak, I. J., Hassler, R., May, B., and Westerman, E.: Morphological and biochemical studies on the storage of serotonin and histamine in blood platelets of the rabbit. Life Sciences, *6*:1133, 1967.

Behnke, O.: Electron microscopic observations on the membrane systems of the rat blood platelet. Anat Rec., *158*:121, 1967.

Behnke, O., and Zelander, T.: Filamentous substructure of microtubules of the marginal bundle of mammalian blood platelets. J. Ultrastruc. Res., *19*:147, 1967.

Brass, L., and Bensusan, H.: The platelet: collagen interaction. Fed. Proc., *34*:241, 1975.

Brinkhaus, K. M., Shermer, R. W., and Mostofi, F. K. (eds.): The Platelet. International Academy of Pathology Monograph No. 11. Baltimore, Williams & Wilkins, 1971.

Hovig, T.: The ultrastructural basis of platelet function. *In* Baldini, M. G., and Ebbe, S. (eds.): Platelets: Production, Function, Transfusion and Storage. New York, Grune & Stratton, 1974.

Jørgensen, L., Rowsell, H. C., Hovig, T., and Mustard, J. F.: Resolution and organization of platelet-rich mural thrombi in carotid arteries of swine. Am. J. Pathol., *51*:681, 1967.

Miescher, P. A., and Jaffé, E. R. (eds.): Hemostasis and Thrombosis, Seminars in Hematology V. Nashville, Tenn., Henry M. Stratton, 1968.

Mustard, J. F., and Packham, M. A.: Factors influencing platelet function: adhesion, release and aggregation. Pharmacol. Rev., *22*:97, 1970.

Mustard, J. F., Glynn, M. F., Nishizawa, E. E., and Packham, M. A.: Platelet-surface interactions: relationship to thrombosis and hemostasis. Fed. Proc., *26*:106, 1967.

Nathaniel, E. J. H., and Chandler, A. B.: Electron microscopic study of adenosine diphosphate-induced platelet thrombi in the rat. J. Ultrastruct. Res., *22*:348, 1968.

Sandborn, E. B., LeBuis, J., and Bois, P.: Cytoplasmic microtubules in blood platelets. Blood, *27*:247, 1966.

Silver, M. D., and Gardner, H. A.: The very dense granule in rabbit platelets. J. Ultrastruct. Res., *23*:366, 1968.

Silver, M. D., and McKinstry, J. E.: Morphology of microtubules in rabbit platelets. Z. Zellforsch., *81*:12, 1967.

Stehbens, W. E., and Biscoe, T. J.: The ultrastructure of early platelet aggregation in vivo. Am. J. Pathol., *50*:219, 1967.

Ulutin, O. N., and Jones, J. V. (eds.): Platelets — Recent Advances in Basic Research and Clinical Aspects, International Symposium. Amsterdam, Excerpta Medica, 1975.

Walsh, P. N.: Platelet coagulant activities and hemostasis: a hypothesis. Blood, *43*:597, 1974.

Wright, J. H.: The histogenesis of the blood platelets. J. Morphol., *21*:263, 1910.

11 Blood Cells: Leukocytes

Like red blood cells, white blood cells (leukocytes) circulate in the bloodstream. However, unlike erythrocytes, which do their work in the bloodstream, leukocytes do their work by migrating through the walls of very small blood vessels into the tissues of the body. Furthermore, they are much less numerous than erythrocytes. Like erythrocytes they are commonly studied in stained blood films made as shown in Figure 10-1. Since leukocytes are all nucleated (in contrast to erythrocytes) they, although much less numerous than erythrocytes, appear to advantage in stained films because their nuclei are colored blue (Plates 11-1 and 11-2). Some kinds of leukocytes have a very short life span so there is a rapid turnover of these, with the older ones being removed from the circulation and new ones being added at the same rate. However, as we shall see, some kinds may have a relatively long life span in the circulatory system. Details on these and other aspects of leukocytes will be given here and in Chapter 12. But first we shall comment on two related properties they all possess—motility and the ability to form pseudopodia.

Motility and Pseudopodia

Leukocytes, as described in the next two chapters, develop in the blood-forming tissues. However, for them to enter the circulatory system they have to be able to move and somehow gain entrance to a blood vessel. Then, to leave the circulatory system again they have to penetrate the wall of a blood vessel in the reverse direction, a process called *diapedesis* (Gr. *dia*, through; *pedesis*, leaping), to enter the connective tissue where they mostly perform their functions. To penetrate a blood vessel a leukocyte commonly forms what is termed a *pseudopodium* (Gr. *pseudes*, false; *poux*, foot), a narrow bulge of cytoplasm extending from the main body of a cell in a manner suggesting the cell is forming an appendage, such as a foot. However, before the pseudopodium is formed the cell must adhere and become anchored to the endothelial lining of a very small blood vessel, commonly a venule. It can then poke a pseudopodium through the site where endothelial lining cells meet, as shown in Figure 11-5. The remainder of the leukocyte also proceeds to

work its way through the vessel wall and thus the leukocyte enters connective tissue and moves to the site of the action in which it subsequently participates. In order to do this the leukocyte requires a contractile apparatus, the nature of which has recently come to light.

The Contractile Apparatus

There is some indication that probably all cells contain the contractile proteins actin and myosin, proteins once conceived of as being confined to muscle cells. It seems, however, that in nonmuscle cells the actin-containing microfilaments are not permanent structures; soluble actin readily polymerizes into filaments probably capable of interacting with myosin and generating motile forces in the presence of ATP, but then these filaments rapidly disassemble again. Needless to say this instability of not only the actin-containing but also the myosin-containing filaments makes them much more difficult to study than their counterparts in muscle cells. The transitory nature of the filaments may in fact be necessary for rapid changes in both cell shape and direction of movement in nonmuscle cells. Thus cell motility is thought of as being due to a controlled sequential assembly, interactions, and disassembly of a contractile apparatus that is labile and not permanent as in striated muscle.

Many kinds of motility, including that of leukocytes, involve movement of the cell membrane; hence the action of the contractile apparatus seems to bring about movement at the cell surface. This is thought to be achieved by the actin-containing microfilaments being anchored directly or indirectly in the cell membrane, since this would allow forces generated by the interaction of actin and myosin to be translated directly into movements of the cell membrane. Hence it is not surprising that, as noted in Chapter 5, the region of cytoplasm just below the cell membrane is rich in microfilaments (Fig. 5-5). If the forces generated by filament interaction were to be utilized in cell motility, one kind of filament at least would have to be anchored somewhere and in most models proposed this site is considered to be the cell membrane. These models for nonmuscle cell motility are all basically extensions of the sliding filament model for striated muscle already briefly mentioned in Chapter 5 and explained in detail in Chapter 18. The main difference is that the cell membrane replaces the Z line as the attachment site for the actin-containing filaments.

Returning to the leukocyte, it could be envisaged how a local contraction in one part of the cell could change the cell's shape; moreover, contraction in the main body of the cell could cause a noncontracting part to be pushed out in the form of a pseudopodium. Sequential phases of attachment, pseudopodium formation, detachment, and so forth could bring about the sort of motility observed in many kinds of living leukocytes.

THE BASIS FOR CLASSIFYING LEUKOCYTES

Leukocytes can be studied in many ways. However, their structure was first studied extensively with the LM in blood films stained with blood stains of the Romanovsky type, of which there are several varieties. Since leukocytes are spread out thinly in films, their stained contents appear to better advantage than in sections. However, films cannot be examined by transmission electron microscopy, so EM studies have to be made on ultrathin sections.

Since leukocytes were first studied with the LM in stained films, the nomenclature used for distinguishing the different kinds was based chiefly on their appearances in this type of preparation. The five kinds thus distinguished were believed to represent only two main types, with one type being characterized by granular cytoplasm and the other by nongranular cytoplasm. Hence leukocytes were classed as either *granular* or *nongranular*. This terminology persists even though it is now known that nongranular leukocytes can have a few granules. It is important to be aware of the fact that this first step in classification is based on the LM appearance of the cytoplasm.

There are three kinds of granular leukocytes, so named because they differ with regard to the staining reaction of their cytoplasmic granules. Those with specific granules staining avidly with acid dyes are called *acidophilic* granular leukocytes, or, since eosin is the dye generally used, *eosinophilic* granular leukocytes. The short name now commonly used is *eosinophil* (Plate 11-1, *lower left*).

Those with granules staining intensely with basic dyes are termed *basophilic* granular leukocytes, or *basophils* (Plate 11-1, *lower right*).

Those with specific granules that are neither markedly acidophilic nor basophilic at normal pH are termed *neutrophilic* granular leukocytes or *neutrophils* (Plate 11-1, just above and between the eosinophil and the basophil). Neutrophils are also commonly referred to as *polymorphs*, an abbreviation of *polymorphonuclear leukocyte*, which term distinguishes neutrophils not by their cytoplasmic granules but by their nuclei, which exhibit many forms, consisting of anywhere from one to five lobes. The term *polymorph* is in turn often further abbreviated to *PMN*. We shall use all these terms (neutrophil, polymorph, and PMN) interchangeably. The cell labeled neutrophil in Plate 11-1 has three lobes.

There are two kinds of nongranular leukocytes. The more numerous and smaller ones are called *lymphocytes* (Plate 11-1, *middle and upper left*) because they are found in lymph as well as in blood. The larger and less numerous ones are called *monocytes* (Plate 11-1, *left, above center*).

To summarize, leukocytes are classified as follows:

Leukocytes
- Granular leukocytes
  - Neutrophils (Polymorphs, PMNs)
  - Eosinophils
  - Basophils
- Nongranular leukocytes
  - Lymphocytes
  - Monocytes

The preparation and study of blood films with the LM is a very common procedure in the practice of medicine for two main purposes. First, the presence of abnormal leukocytes is associated with various disease states. Second, a determination of the relative proportions of the different kinds of normal leukocytes in an individual's blood (called making a *differential count*) is important, because certain shifts in the relative proportions of the different kinds are of diagnostic significance.

LEUKOCYTE COUNTS

It is also very important to know whether the *total number* of leukocytes in a patient's blood is increased or decreased; this is determined by making a *leukocyte count* (often abbreviated to *WBC count*).

For this a known small volume of blood is mixed in a special pipet with a known large amount of leukocyte-counting fluid, which acts to destroy red cells and stain the nuclei of leukocytes. A little of the mixture is then placed over ruled squares on a special glass slide called a *hemocytometer* and a coverslip is placed on it so that there is a known depth of fluid over the squares. The number of leukocytes seen over a given number of squares (Fig. 11-1) is counted, and then, by knowing the dilution of the blood in counting fluid and the depth of the fluid over the squares, a calculation can be made of how many leukocytes are present in a cubic millimeter of blood.

Large numbers of routine leukocyte counts can be done with automatic electronic counting instruments, but since differential counts require the recognition of each individual kind of leukocyte, these must be done manually.

In normal adults total leukocyte counts vary from about 5,000 to 9,000 per cubic millimeter. There are variations within this range dependent on time of day and other factors. Leukocyte counts must be interpreted in relation to what is found in the differential count.

HOW TO FIND AND STUDY LEUKOCYTES IN A STAINED BLOOD FILM

In studying a normal blood film with the LM it should be realized that there are about 1,000 red cells to every leukocyte and, since both kinds of blood cells are spread over the slide, it may take some hunting around among red cells to find a leukocyte. However, it is easy to find one with the low-power objective because leukocytes, in contrast to red cells, have nuclei and these at this magnification appear as blue dots scattered around in a background of red cells.

Blood films are usually provided with a coverslip but sometimes not. A film with no coverslip can be seen fairly clearly with the low-power objective but not with the high-power (dry) objective. They can, however, be studied with the oil-immersion objective by putting a drop of oil directly on the film. A common procedure is to spot the nucleus of a leukocyte in a film with the low-power objective, then center it and switch to oil-immersion.

A film usually is thicker at the end from which it is spread (Figs. 10-1 and 10-4). Leukocytes are more numerous and easier to find in the thicker part. But wherever the film is thick (and this is indicated by red cells being superimposed on one another to a great degree) the leukocytes do not stain sharply and hence are difficult to study. They appear to much better advantage in the thinner part of the film, but here they are not as numerous as might be anticipated, because, being somewhat larger than erythrocytes, they tend to be drawn to the edges of the film as well as toward the very end of it. In either of these positions (the edge or the end), they may become distorted and their cytoplasm may be broken and scattered about them. Therefore it is best to learn the appearance of normal leukocytes from the regions where they are most difficult to find (the thinner part of the film except at its edges or end), and in order to find good examples of each kind the student may have to study not only one film but several.

The Differential Count. Since leukocytes are larger than red cells, and are of different sizes, they are distributed unevenly in a film. This creates a problem in attempting to ascertain the relative percentages of the different leukocytes present in a film. A proper sampling cannot be obtained from examining the leukocytes in only one small part of the film. A significant sample requires including in one's count the leukocytes from some of the poorer parts of the film as well as cells from the good parts.

In learning to distinguish the five different kinds of leukocytes in films, much time can be saved if the following traps are avoided:

(1) *Examining a Degenerating Leukocyte.* In every

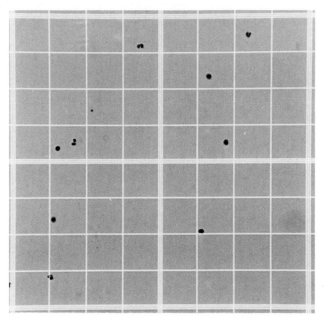

Fig. 11-1. Low-power photomicrograph of leukocytes in a hemocytometer prepared for a leukocyte count. The cells are counted in the large squares (1 mm. square) bounded by triple lines to give the average number per large square. Four such squares are seen in this illustration (the smaller ones are used for erythrocyte counts).

blood film there are many examples of partly broken-down leukocytes (Plate 11-1, *top right*), and it is a waste of time to try to identify their nature. So examine only well-formed and well-stained examples.

(2) *Confusing Clumps of Platelets With Leukocytes.* Unless special precautions are taken platelets commonly clump together (Plate 11-1, *center right*). Most of each platelet is pale blue, but its central part may contain dark-staining granules.

(3) *Examining Cells That Are Difficult to Classify.* At first the student should examine only leukocytes that are easily recognized and should disregard those that seem difficult to classify until he has more experience.

In the following description of the five kinds of leukocytes, the student will learn that both the nucleus and the cytoplasm give important information useful in identifying them.

THE GRANULAR LEUKOCYTES

NEUTROPHILS (POLYMORPHS)

As mentioned earlier the terms *neutrophil* and *polymorph* are both used for the same cell; we shall use them indiscriminately to encourage familiarity with both terms.

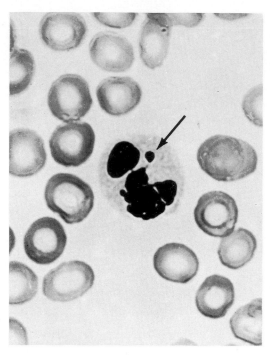

Fig. 11-2. Photomicrograph (×1,750) of blood cell film of a female. The neutrophil at *center* illustrates a characteristic "drumstick" appendage (*arrow*). (Davidson, W. M., and Smith, D. R.: Br. Med. J., *2:*6, 1954)

Numbers. Normally 50 to 70 per cent of the leukocytes are polymorphs. In absolute numbers, 3,000 to 6,000 per cubic millimeter of blood is considered normal. An individual with 5 liters of blood has 15 to 30 billion polymorphs in his circulation. Polymorphs are the commonest and usually the first kind of leukocyte seen in a normal film.

Appearance in Blood Films Seen With the LM

Polymorphs develop in myeloid tissue (bone marrow), where they go through many developmental changes before they finally assume their mature form, and then they are liberated into the bloodstream. In health only occasionally are polymorphs released into the bloodstream before they are mature. Under conditions of disease, however, more immature ones may be released and so are seen in films made from the peripheral blood. It is, therefore, necessary for the student to learn the appearance of both mature and immature polymorphs.

The average duration for the stay of granulocytes in the bloodstream is estimated at only 8 to 12 hours, after which they seem to leave the small blood vessels (venules) at random to enter the connective tissues.

Mature Polymorphs. These are from 10 to 12 μm. in di-

ameter; hence they are slightly less than half as wide again as erythrocytes in a film.

The nucleus is in the form of lobes that appear in a film to be either completely separated from one another or interconnected by no more than very delicate strands. The nucleus of a mature polymorph has from 2 to 5 (or even more) lobes (Plates 11-1 and 11-2). The substance of the lobes is made up of coarse chromatin that is rather densely packed (Plates 11-1 and 11-2). As a consequence, the nuclear material stains fairly deeply with basic dyes, being colored a blue or blue-purple in the usual preparation. The nucleoli cannot be distinguished.

Barr Bodies in Polymorphs. A few years after Barr and Bertram showed there was a sex difference in the chromatin of cells, Davidson and Smith demonstrated that it was possible to identify the chromosomal sex of an individual by the examination of blood films. The Barr body in a mature polymorph of a female is generally contained in one of the lobes of the nucleus, where it is very difficult, if not impossible, to identify because the chromatin is so packed; however, a Barr body sometimes appears as a separate tiny lobe which has the form of a *drumstick* (Fig. 11-2). According to Davidson and Smith, this happens in about 1 out of every 38 neutrophils of females. Somewhat similar little bodies very occasionally are seen in the neutrophils of males. But as many as 6 never are seen in a series of 500 neutrophils from males and at least 6 always can be seen in 500 neutrophils obtained from females.

Cytoplasm of Mature Polymorphs. This occupies more space than the nucleus and reveals little structural detail except that it is fairly heavily sprinkled with granules (Plate 11-2). There are two kinds of granules. The true neutrophilic granules in many preparations are so fine that they are difficult to resolve with the LM; hence all that may be seen is that the cytoplasm has a granular appearance. Commonly, these granules either have or impart to the cytoplasm a lavender (lilac) color. Granules larger than the specific neutrophilic granules are also seen; these are reddish-purple in color (Plate 11-1, neutrophil). Since this color is imparted to them by the methylene azure, which is one of the basic dyes in a blood stain, they are called *azurophilic granules.* As we shall see when we study the formation of granular leukocytes, the first granules that appear in cells of this lineage are of the azurophilic type; only later do true neutrophilic granules appear and, when they do appear, they are first seen in the Golgi region of the developing cells.

Immature Polymorphs. In the development of polymorphs, the nucleus at first has the form of an indented ovoid (Plate 11-2, at the 4 o'clock position). At this stage of development the cell is called a *neutrophilic metamyelocyte.* As it develops further the nucleus becomes increasingly indented so that it acquires a horseshoe shape, whereupon the cell is given the name *band* (or *stab*) *neu-*

Fig. 11-3. Electron micrograph of a mature neutrophil (from mouse bone marrow) reacted for the enzyme peroxidase. Peroxidase-positive electron-dense azurophilic granules (AG) corresponding to lysosomes, and peroxidase-negative and therefore lighter-staining specific granules (SG), can be seen in the cytoplasm. Several lobes of the nucleus (N) with condensed chromatin along its nuclear envelope are also visible. (Courtesy V. Kalnins)

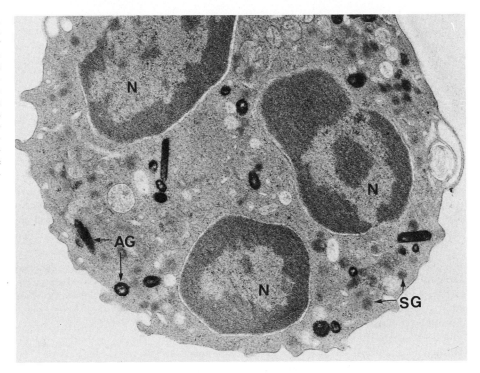

trophil (Plate 11-1, band neutrophil, and Plate 11-2, *top*). Under normal conditions the horseshoe-shaped nucleus of the band form becomes segmented to divide the nucleus into two or more lobes before the cell is released into the bloodstream from bone marrow; accordingly, under normal conditions not more than 1 or 2 per cent of band forms are seen in films. But if there is a great need for neutrophils in the blood (as will be explained under Inflammation and Functions of Polymorphs, below) some band forms and even some metamyelocytes are released into the bloodstream, and so these are seen in blood films.

The nuclei of neutrophilic metamyelocytes do not stain as deeply as those of band forms and those of band forms do not stain as deeply as those of mature forms. Both metamyelocytes and band neutrophils have cytoplasmic granules similar to those of mature neutrophils (Plate 11-2) and both may contain some azurophilic granules in addition to their specific (neutrophilic) granules.

From the above it is evident that the maturity of a polymorph is revealed chiefly by the shape of its nucleus and to a lesser extent by how heavily the nucleus stains.

The Fine Structure of Neutrophils

Representative leukocytes from bone marrow may be obtained for sectioning by obtaining tiny pieces of bone marrow from a sternal puncture; these are fixed and sectioned. In such sections there are, of course, many imma-

ture cells of various kinds, but normally there are always many mature polymorphs also. If whole blood is allowed to settle or if it is centrifuged, the erythrocytes are packed into a red layer in the bottom of the tube and the leukocytes form an extremely thin but just detectable whitish layer (called the *buffy coat*) just above them. Bits of this can be fixed and sectioned for electron microscopy. Still another way to see neutrophils in sections is to examine the tissues of an animal at the site of an injury that has caused neutrophils to migrate through the walls of venules into the tissues; this is the way in which the neutrophil in Figure 11-5 was obtained.

Nucleus. All ultrathin section cut through a mature neutrophil passes through only some of the lobes of its nucleus. Hence, in electron micrographs, neutrophils do not reveal as many lobes as they do in blood films, in which the whole cell is spread out in view. In sections observed with the EM the lobes of a nucleus are seen to have condensed chromatin distributed along the inner surface of the nuclear envelope (Fig. 11-3). In the more central part of a lobe the chromatin is extended, so the central parts of the lobes are in general pale (Fig. 11-3).

Cytoplasm. The cytoplasm of a mature polymorph does not contain a very good representation of the usual organelles. But a few mitochondria and a small Golgi apparatus can often be seen. Granules of glycogen are often scattered about. However, the salient feature of the cytoplasm is its great content of granules; it has been estimated that there may be from 50 to 200 in each cell. The granules are of two types, *azurophilic* and *specific*. The azurophilic granules are the larger (about 0.4 μm. in diameter) and amount to around 20 per cent of the total. They are round or oval in shape and denser in the EM than the specific granules. As is shown in Figure 11-3, in which the azurophilic granules are labeled AG, they are identified by testing them for peroxidases, enzymes they contain. As will be described in Chapter 12, they are formed at an earlier stage of development than the specific granules. The much more numerous smaller specific granules (Fig. 11-3) are up to 0.3 μm. in diameter and are found later as the cell develops.

Functions of the Granules. It has long been known that polymorphs contain enzymes concerned in the destruction of the bacteria they phagocytose. With the development of knowledge about lysosomes (discussed in Chap. 5) it soon became apparent that polymorphs were particularly rich in them. Bainton and Farquhar showed that the *azurophilic* granules are the *lysosomes* of polymorphs; they contain at least 6 hydrolytic enzymes as well as peroxidase (Farquhar and Bainton). In contrast the more numerous specific granules were found to contain no lysosomal enzymes but instead a bactericidal substance and also the enzyme alkaline phosphatase. It has been shown that, after a polymorph has phagocytosed certain bacteria (*E. coli*), a specific granule quickly fuses with the membranous sac containing the phagocytosed bacterium and empties its alkaline phosphatase into the sac. About 3 minutes later, azurophilic granules fuse with the sac and release their content of hydrolytic enzymes and peroxidase into it and this soon destroys the bacterium.

INFLAMMATION AND THE FUNCTIONS OF POLYMORPHS

Perspective. The process set in motion when living tissue is affected by an injurious agent is termed *inflammation*. This process operates to eliminate or neutralize the injurious agent and its effects and to repair the damaged tissue. It is sometimes described as having three phases — injury, reaction, and repair.

Polymorphs are of great importance in acute inflammation. When any of the body tissues is damaged, the reaction to injury tending to limit its spread and overcome it involves the leukocytes and plasma of blood, the cells and intercellular substances of connective tissue, and in particular what is called the *terminal vascular bed*, which includes the arterioles supplying the capillary bed and the venules that drain it, as will be described in more detail presently.

The kinds of injurious agents that can induce inflammation in a part of the body are many and varied. Body tissue may be invaded by bacteria, viruses, protozoa, or other kinds of pathogenic organisms. Inflammation can also occur when body tissue is injured by heat, radiation, cold, or chemicals. Furthermore, certain substances formed within the body can cause inflammation, as for example happens in gout (p. 59).

The classic signs and symptoms of inflammation in some part of the body, which are still often recited by professors, were listed as long ago as A.D. 200 as redness, heat, swelling, pain, and loss or impairment of function. We shall presently describe the microscopic changes in connective tissue that cause these signs and symptoms.

The presence of inflammation in any body part is denoted in medical language by adding the suffix *itis* to the part in which inflammation is diagnosed. Since almost any part of the body can be the seat of inflammation, a patient may be said to be suffering from (for example):

nasopharyngitis — inflammation of the lining of the nose and throat
sinusitis — inflammation of the lining of the nasal sinuses
tonsillitis — inflammation of the tonsils
laryngitis — inflammation of the larynx
arthritis — inflammation of joints
appendicitis — inflammation of the wall of the appendix
colitis — inflammation of the lining of the colon
cystitis — inflammation of the urinary bladder
cholecystitis — inflammation of the gallbladder
glomerulonephritis — inflammation of the glomeruli of the kidneys

The above examples illustrate that much illness in man involves inflammation in some parts of his body and hence an understanding of inflammation is of prime importance for the medical or paramedical student. The details of the process constitute a large part of a course of instruction in pathology. We shall here give only an elementary account of it. However, before doing this it should be mentioned that inflammation can be described as being *acute* or *chronic*. The classic symptoms and signs of inflammation refer to the acute type.

SOME HISTOLOGICAL FEATURES OF THE INFLAMMATORY REACTION

Almost everyone has run a dirty sliver through the protective epithelium of the skin into the connective tissue of a finger (Fig. 11-4, *top*) and found that unless it was properly treated the tissue around the sliver became inflamed. The presence of the inflammation is indicated by the area becoming red and swollen and by its feeling warm and painful, and, as a result, one would be disinclined to use the finger for playing the piano or typing a letter (impairment of function). The microscopic basis for these changes will now be described.

Fig. 11-4. Diagrams showing how neutrophils migrate from congested, dilated venules to combat bacteria introduced into the tissues through injury.

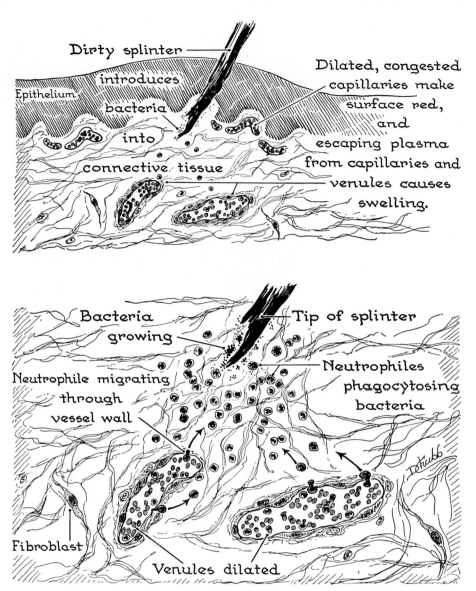

An ordinary sliver either carries pathogenic bacteria or pushes them from the surface of the skin into the connective tissue that lies beneath the epithelium (Fig. 11-4, *bottom*). In the nutritive wet intercellular substance the bacteria can at first multiply. They and any noxious substances they produce, together with the physical presence of a foreign object (the sliver) soon bring about changes in the vascular bed of the part. The mechanisms involved will be discussed presently.

Changes in Blood Flow Through the Vascular Bed. In previous discussions we have described capillary loops and mentioned that they are supplied by arterioles and drained by venules. Actually a vascular bed is complex because, as illustrated in Figure 19-23, arterioles are also connected to venules by thin-walled bypass channels, and it is from the proximal portions of these channels that many capillaries in a network arise (details are given in Chap. 19, p. 605). Smooth muscle cells are present in the walls of both the arterioles and the proximal portions of these channels, so both kinds of vessels are intimately involved in regulating blood flow through capillaries.

Following an injury the terminal vascular bed opens up and there is a temporarily increased blood flow, followed in turn by a slowing of the flow. At this stage the endothelium lining the venules becomes leaky and this allows plasma to escape into the surrounding intercellular

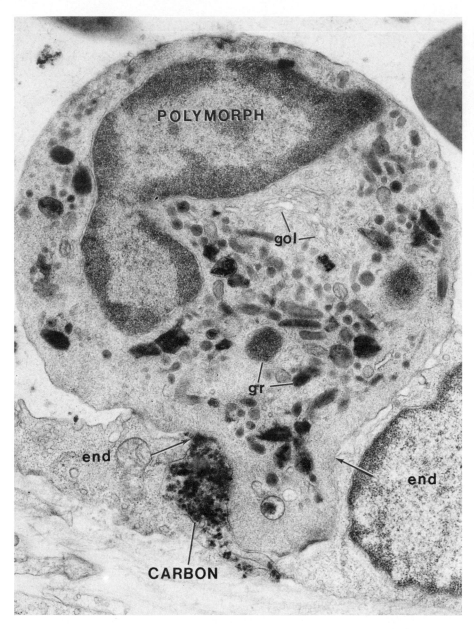

Fig. 11-5. Electron micrograph (×23,000) showing a polymorph beginning to migrate between two endothelial cells (end) in early inflammation. Note the Golgi apparatus (gol) and types of granules (gr). Inflammation was produced by injecting carbon particles intravenously; a clump of these can be seen to the left of the pseudopodium projecting through the site of attachment between endothelial cells lining this vessel. Note the variation in size of the granules of the neutrophil. (Movat, H. Z., and Fernando, N. V. P.: Lab. Invest., *12:*895, 1963)

substance. The leakage occurs between the edges of the contiguous endothelial cells, where they are not attached by fascia occludens (tight) junctions, but leakage can also occur through the damaged cytoplasm of the endothelial cells if the capillary walls have been directly damaged by the agent inducing the inflammation, as, for example, in thermal burns. Leakage through the walls of intact venules is to be explained, at least to some extent, by the local release of histamine (p. 248) and other vasoactive substances with similar effects. The leakage of plasma from venules into the intercellular substance is called fluid *exudation.*

Almost as soon as the blood flow becomes slowed, and exudation has occurred, polymorphs can be seen sticking to the endothelium lining the venules through which they were passing and, soon after, pseudopodia are inserted between the cell membranes of contiguous endothelial cells, as shown in Figure 11-5. Having made an opening with a pseudopodium, the rest of the polymorph then squeezes through to enter the intercellular substance outside the venule. From there the polymorphs, which of course are motile, migrate to the site of the injurious agent (which in this instance would be the site where bacteria were multiplying, as shown in Fig. 11-4). On reaching the bacteria they phagocytose and destroy them. Many mechanisms are, however, involved in this procedure, and for those interested, some are described below.

How Polymorphs Dispose of Infecting Bacteria

The question arises as to what attracts polymorphs and causes them to migrate through a venule and move toward the noxious agents they are to phagocytose. The attraction bacteria have for polymorphs has been ascribed to *chemotaxis*, that is, a chemical concentration gradient attracting polymorphs to the bacteria. Bacteria probably elaborate substances with this effect. But there is now much evidence indicating that polymorphs are also attracted to sites where antibodies have become fixed to antigens of the infective agent so as to form antigen-antibody complexes. But antigen-antibody complexes only attract polymorphs because they fix what is called *complement*, which will now be described briefly.

The term *complement* refers to a group of proteins present in normal plasma that become activated when an antibody combines with an antigen. The various components of complement combine with the antigen-antibody complex in an ordered sequence and, as they do so, various biological effects are produced.

The immunological mechanism of a given individual can identify only certain sites on foreign organisms or cells as antigenic, and these (termed *antigenic sites*) are the sites with which antibody combines. In those foreign cells where the antigenic sites lie spaced fairly closely together (as in bacteria and cells such as erythrocytes from donors of a different blood type) the combining of antibody also initiates the binding of complement to these sites. This in itself is sufficient to cause certain kinds of cells to lyse, an effect called *complement-mediated lysis*. But even if lysis does not ensue, several biologically active substances are formed and released from the various complement proteins during the process of complement fixation and activation. For example, it has been known for a long time that certain substances present in blood plasma can, by attaching to bacteria, make it easier for polymorphs to phagocytose them; such substances were therefore called *opsonins*, which is Greek for something to eat. It was already known that antibodies could be formed against bacterial antigens, so for a long time it was thought that antibodies themselves were responsible for the opsonizing effect. But now it is conceded that the opsonizing effect is due to split products released from complement when it becomes attached to the antigen-antibody complex. Complement is, therefore, of great importance in the inflammatory reaction and in facilitating the phagocytosis and hence the killing of bacteria. It should, perhaps, also be noted that viruses are inactivated by antibody alone, without complement having to be involved in the reaction.

If the injurious agent is a form of pathogenic bacteria that attracts polymorphs, the bacteria are engulfed by the cell membrane of the polymorph and so come to lie in a membranous sac within the cytoplasm, called a *phagosome*. As described a few pages back, the specific neutrophilic granules of the polymorph fuse with the sac containing the injurious agent and this is followed by the azurophilic granules fusing with it, and by this means the agent is destroyed by the hydrolytic enzymes of the azurophilic granules.

It is of interest that the action of the lysosomal enzymes from the azurophilic granules is not limited to destruction of phagocytosed bacteria. Under certain conditions these hydrolytic enzymes become liberated from polymorphs in quantity and may either cause or increase the severity of inflammatory reactions. For example in acute attacks of gout (described on p. 59) and the chronic disease rheumatoid arthritis, inflammation is elicited by substances produced in the body—urate crystals in gout and antibody complexes in rheumatoid arthritis. In both conditions there is extensive and continued phagocytosis of these substances, which is so vigorous that lysosomal hydrolytic enzymes are "spilt" to the exterior of the polymorph before each phagocytic vacuole has had time to close off completely and move down into the cytoplasm from the cell surface, as illustrated at *lower left* in Figure 5-38 on page 141.

THE CAUSES OF THE CLASSIC SIGNS AND SYMPTOMS OF ACUTE INFLAMMATION

The redness and increased local temperature noted at a site of acute inflammation is to be explained by an increased amount of blood flowing through the terminal vascular bed. This in turn is due to the dilation of the arterioles and venules that normally control the circulation through the bed. The swelling at the site of acute inflammation (unless severe enough to have caused local hemorrhage) is due to exudation of plasma out between the endothelial cells that line the dilated venules. The question arises as to how these changes occur in these vessels, which are not affected directly by the inflammatory agent itself.

Experiments have shown that if an animal is depleted of its leukocytes and infected at some site with bacteria, inflammation does not occur at the site where the bacteria were injected. (Under these conditions, however, the bacteria proliferate and eventually spread all through the body.) Hence it is obvious that the heat, redness, and swelling observed in a local inflammatory response is due to something produced by the body and not by the bacteria. The substances that act, for example, at a site of infection to produce the changes that account for heat, redness, and swelling are called *chemical mediators* of the acute inflammatory response. There are different kinds. One is referred to as the vasoactive amines; histamine is an amine released by mast cells in the vicinity. Another is serotonin; this is released from platelets but its role in man is uncertain. Other chemical mediators are also involved; their formation involves interactions between plasma peptides and proteins, a detailed description of which is far beyond the scope of this book. An important one is termed the kinin system. Complement is also involved. Inflammation is such an important condition and the subject of so much modern research, that up-to-date reviews and books on the subject are always available for those desiring in-depth information.

The pain involved in acute inflammation is due partly to the stretching of nerve endings by the swelling and partly to direct stimulation of nerve endings by pain-causing products of the inflammatory process.

The Role of Monocytes and Macrophages. The migration of polymorphs through the walls of venules is either accompanied by the migration of monocytes, or it is quickly followed by such a migration. The monocytes leave by the same means as the polymorphs. Monocytes, on entering the tissues, become macrophages. At first they participate with the polymorphs in phagocytic activities but soon they dominate the picture because the polymorphs have a very short life span and when their work is over they cease to enter the area. The macrophages remain longer. Polymorphs and macrophages seem to be attracted by different types of antigens; there are some forms of bacteria that do not attract polymorphs but do attract macrophages. Macrophages, moreover, are adapted to phagocytosing such debris as is left when inflammation subsides.

The phase of repair that ensues requires the formation of fibroblasts which in most areas are probably derived from the pericytes scattered along the smaller blood vessels. As was described in the previous chapter, fibroblasts synthesize and elaborate collagen and restore the intercellular substances of the part. New capillaries bud off from preexisting vessels to provide such blood supply as is needed. Epithelial membranes regenerate as was described in Chapter 7.

Pus and Pyrogens. Accumulations of dead polymorphs together with some breakdown products of infected tissue can account for the formation of a creamy-yellow semifluid material in infected wounds called *pus.* In infected wounds open to the surface pus can drain away or be absorbed into dressings. If, however, an accumulation forms in an area below (and not open to) the surface, it is called an *abscess* and surgical means may become necessary to drain it.

Certain products formed from the breakdown of polymorphs and bacterial toxins are termed *pyrogens* (Gr. *pyr,* fire; *gennan,* to produce) because if they are absorbed into the body and carried to the thermostat-like temperature control center in the brain, they affect it so that the body temperature is raised and the individual has a *fever.* The same or similar substances can also have an effect on the bone marrow, as will next be described.

Leukocytosis. Substances probably similar to those that induce fever somehow stimulate the release of mature polymorphs from the bone marrow so that severe infections of many types are associated with a rise in the total number of leukocytes per cubic millimeter of blood, which is called a *leukocytosis* (Gr. *osis,* a process, often one denoting an abnormal increase in something). Although there is a large pool of mature polymorphs in the bone marrow, bone marrow stimulation also results in increased numbers of *immature polymorphs* being released into the circulation. Accordingly, in patients suffering from many types of acute infections, the total leukocyte count rises, and a differential count made on a blood film reveals increased percentages of band neutrophils and neutrophilic metamyelocytes.

In tabulating the types of polymorphs seen in a film, it is customary to enter band and metamyelocyte forms on the left-hand side and more mature forms (with 2 to 5 lobes) on the right-hand side. Accordingly, if examination of regularly obtained blood films shows that the percentage of immature cells is *increasing,* it is said that a *shift to the left* is occurring. If, however, it is found regularly that the percentage of immature forms is *decreasing,* it is said that there is a *shift to the right.* So, in a general way, a shift to the *left* indicates that an infection is *progressing,* and a shift to the *right* indicates that it is *subsiding.*

EOSINOPHILS

Numbers. Eosinophils constitute from 1 to 4 per cent of the leukocytes seen in a normal blood film. In absolute figures, 120 to 350 eosinophils per cubic millimeter of blood is considered normal. However, the eosinophil counts of normal individuals tend to fluctuate; moreover, they show a diurnal (L. *diurnus,* daily) rhythm, being highest at night and lowest in the morning.

Appearance in Blood Films Seen With the LM. Eosinophils are from 12 to 15 μm. in diameter and hence are commonly slightly larger than neutrophils. Their nuclei are commonly composed of only *two lobes* (Plate 11-1), which may or may not be connected with a strand of nuclear material. Coarse clumps of chromatin are not so densely packed in the nuclei of eosinophils as they are in neutrophils; hence eosinophil nuclei do not stain as deeply (Plate 11-1).

The cytoplasm of eosinophils is somewhat irregular in outline because of occasional pseudopodia and is characteristically packed with large refractile granules that in well-stained blood films are colored red or orange (Plate 11-1). In poorly stained films their color may veer toward pink or a muddy blue. Even in poorly stained preparations they can be distinguished from the granules of neutrophils because they are more numerous—the cell seems to be packed with them—and because they are distinctly larger and more refractile (Plate 11-1).

Fine Structure. The EM reveals no special features in the bilobed nucleus except that, as in neutrophils, condensed chromatin is distributed peripherally on the inner surface of the nuclear envelope (Fig. 11-6). The chief feature of the cytoplasm is its content of *specific granules.* These ovoid membrane-bounded granules have a striking appearance and are 0.5 to 1.5 μm. long and 0.3 to 1 μm. wide (Fig. 11-6). In immature eosinophils they are composed of a homogeneous material of considerable density. In mature eosinophils some granules are seen to contain still denser bodies in their more central parts (Fig. 11-6) which are *crystalline* in structure and may have the form of rough rectangles. The shape of these central bodies differs with species. They sometimes occupy more and sometimes less then half the granule. The granules contain large amounts of peroxidase and most of the other enzymes found in the azurophilic granules of polymorphs;

Color Plates
11-1 to 11-2

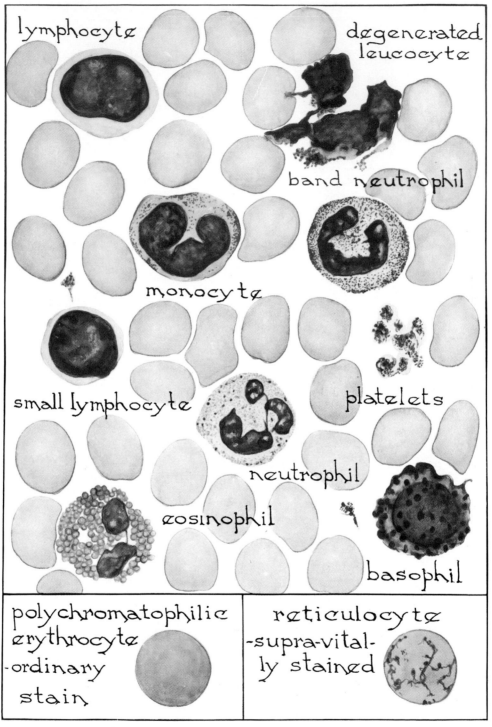

lymphocyte

degenerated
leucocyte

band neutrophil

monocyte

small lymphocyte

platelets

neutrophil

eosinophil

basophil

polychromatophilic
erythrocyte
-ordinary
stain

reticulocyte
-supra-vital-
ly stained

Plate 11-1. Illustration of erythrocytes, platelets, and the different kinds of leukocytes as they appear in a normal human blood film stained with Hastings' stain.

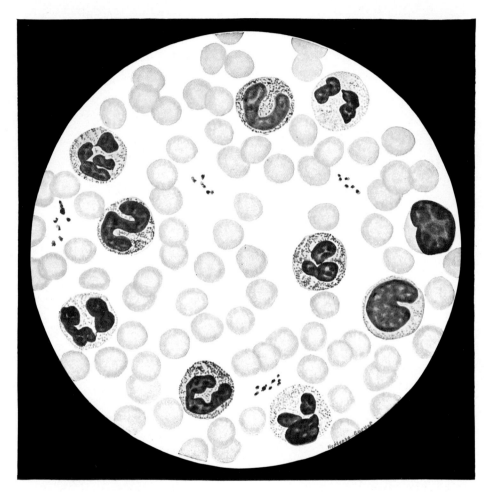

Plate 11-2. Illustration showing segmented and band neutrophils and neutrophilic metamye-locytes as they appear in a neutrophilic leukocytosis. A neutrophilic metamyelocyte can be seen at about 4 o'clock. Band neutrophils can be seen at 6:30, 9:30, and 12:30, respectively. With the exception of a lymphocyte at 3 o'clock, the remaining leukocytes are segmented neutrophils. Several of the neutrophils in this illustration show toxic granulation. (Kracke, R. R.: Diseases of the Blood. ed. 2. Philadelphia, J. B. Lippincott, 1941)

Fig. 11-6. Electron micrograph (×15,000) of eosinophil (mouse). Note the bilobed nucleus. Golgi saccules can be seen slightly *left of center,* as well as some free rounded vesicles filled with pale secretory material. The specific granules in the cytoplasm vary in size; many show the dark crystalline inclusion that characterizes the specific granules of eosinophils. A few mitochondria are visible. (Courtesy of A. Howatson)

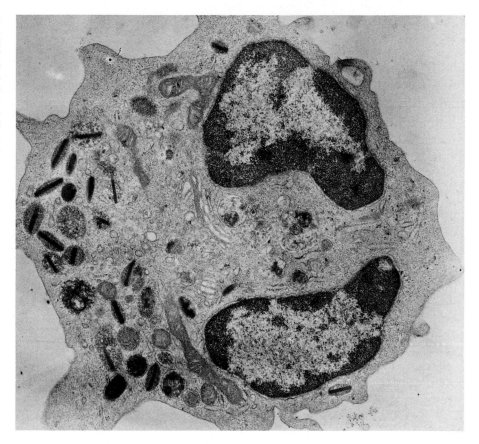

hence, in eosinophils the specific granules are regarded as lysosomes. Smaller granules, which are rounded and 0.1 to 0.5 μm. in diameter, have also been demonstrated in the cytoplasm. These have a homogeneous appearance and contain most of the arylsulfatases and acid phosphatase in the cell.

The Golgi and mitochondria are the only other organelles prominent in eosinophils, the remainder having minimal representation.

Functions of Eosinophils. After leaving the bone marrow where they are formed, eosinophils spend a few hours in the bloodstream (their half-life in the blood is 3 to 8 hours). Then, like polymorphs, they leave the circulating blood and enter the tissues, where they reside for a few days and perform their functions. They are normally found in the loose connective tissue layers of the intestine, lungs, and skin, and the superficial connective tissue of the external genitalia. Unlike polymorphs, they are not very phagocytic as far as bacteria are concerned, nor are they as motile. However, it has been recognized for a long time that eosinophils are somehow concerned in *anaphylactic* phenomena because they are more numerous both in sites of allergic reactions and in the blood

of individuals suffering from allergies. The hormone *hydrocortisone,* which depresses allergic reactions, also causes the number of eosinophils circulating in the blood to drop. Indeed, the diurnal variation in eosinophil counts in normal individuals is thought to be related to diurnal changes in the level of hydrocortisone secretion by the cortex of the adrenal glands. Eosinophils are commonly found in the nasal secretions of allergic individuals suffering from hay fever (allergic rhinitis) and in the sputum of patients with asthma. It is of interest that haptens (small molecules capable of conferring antigenic activity on otherwise nonantigenic proteins with which they combine), if injected into the lungs of experimental animals, can nonspecifically induce local accumulation of eosinophils. Moreover, it has been shown experimentally that eosinophils are attracted to free antigen-antibody complexes and can phagocytose them. However, although it is conceded they are involved in immunological responses, their precise role is not yet entirely clear.

It has been suggested that an important role of eosinophils is to diminish the deleterious effects of local allergic reactions. As noted in connection with mast cells (p. 252), eosinophils seem to play a part in confining and re-

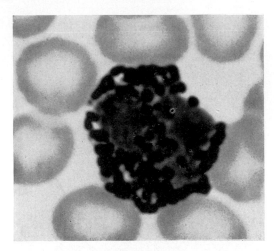

Fig. 11-7. Oil-immersion photomicrograph of a basophil from human blood. Its prominent granules are darker than the nucleus and tend to obscure it. (Courtesy of C. P. Leblond and Y. Clermont)

straining the localized inflammatory reactions associated with hypersensitivity reactions, for their specific granules contain many enzymes that degrade chemical mediators released by mast cells. Thus the slow-reacting substance of anaphylaxis released by mast cells is degraded by aryl-sulfatases in eosinophils, which also contain a histaminase capable of destroying histamine. Furthermore, eosinophils are attracted chemotactically toward a peptide, the *eosinophil chemotactic factor of anaphylaxis*, released by mast cells when they degranulate. Eosinophils also accumulate at sites of histamine release. When they arrive on the scene, they phagocytose and digest the granules liberated by mast cells. Hence it is now the general view that eosinophils play an important role in the control of local responses in allergic reactions.

Another finding of some diagnostic importance is that the relative number of eosinophils becomes increased in the blood of individuals infested with certain types of parasites. Hence eosinophils are thought to play an important role in defense against these parasites. In some instances there is evidence that eosinophils discharge lysosomal enzymes from their specific granules by exocytosis onto the surface of the parasite, but it is not known whether they are able to inflict direct damage on the parasite by this means. Further information about the functions of eosinophils will be found in the book by Beeson and Bass.

BASOPHILS

Numbers. Basophils comprise only about 0.5 per cent of the blood leukocytes; hence to find a good example of one, it may be necessary to examine several hundred leukocytes and perhaps even several different blood films. However, even if basophils constitute only one half of 1 per cent of the leukocytes in the blood (40 or so per cubic millimeter of blood), this still allows for there being enormous numbers of them in the body and so their possible role and importance deserve attention.

Appearance in Blood Films. Basophils are usually from 10 to 12 μm. in diameter; they are about the same size as neutrophils (Plate 11-1). Roughly half the cell consists of its nucleus, which may be bilobed or segmented but often presents an irregular shape. Although the nucleus stains less intensely than that of the neutrophil or eosinophil, in blood films stained with blood stains the nucleus is commonly obscured by the large, dark, blue-stained granules of the cytoplasm (Fig. 11-7). The granules of basophils are similar in many respects to those of mast cells and, like them, are metachromatic because they contain heparin. The EM has shown that the granules, which are large (up to 0.5 μm. in diameter), are enclosed by membrane.

Functions. The precise role of basophils has not been clearly established. Basophils are phagocytic and contain about half the histamine present in blood. Furthermore, basophils, like eosinophils, tend to leave the bloodstream under the influence of certain hormones, for example, hydrocortisone. They also tend to accumulate at sites of inflammation. There are indications that they are involved in allergic and inflammatory reactions.

Circulating immunoglobulin IgE (described in connection with allergy) readily becomes attached to the surface of basophils. Thus an encounter between basophils primed with IgE and the allergen that called forth the production of the IgE antibody can result in discharge of the granules from the basophils, with the release of histamine which, of course, affects blood vessels in a manner similar to that liberated by mast cells. If this reaction is of great magnitude and systemic, it can result in vascular collapse and death.

THE NONGRANULAR LEUKOCYTES

LYMPHOCYTES

Lymphocytes comprise one of the five kinds of blood cells. They were given their name because they are the only kind of blood cell found regularly and in quantity in lymph as well as blood.

Since their cytoplasm as seen with the LM revealed no obvious granules, they were classed as one of the two kinds of nongranular leukocytes. Monocytes, described below, are the other kind.

The Two Size Classes of Lymphocytes. In stained blood films two kinds of lymphocytes are found. First, what is termed a *small lymphocyte* (labeled on *left* of Plate 11-1) generally appears only slightly larger than an erythrocyte.

However, another type of lymphocyte is larger (*top left* in Plate 11-1). Those of the latter type are commonly termed *medium-sized* or *large lymphocytes*. (The reason for them being termed *medium-sized* lymphocytes is that it was usual in the past to describe a third type of lymphocyte which, however, was normally found only in lymphatic tissue and which was larger still and called a *large lymphocyte*. However, as far as blood cells are concerned there are two classes, *(1)* small lymphocytes and *(2)* a class of larger ones. Hence those of the second class are the large lymphocytes of the blood. But since it might be argued that there are still larger lymphocytes in lymphatic tissue it is still probably best to refer to the larger type in blood as *medium-sized* or *medium lymphocytes*, so we shall do this here.) In deciding whether some lymphocytes are larger than others, one must take into account the fact that the size of cells seen in films depends to a considerable extent on how thinly the cells are spread and this differs in different parts of a film. If two lymphocytes are found close together and one is obviously larger than the other, it may be correctly assumed that they have been spread to the same extent. However, the safest way to draw the conclusion that lymphocytes are of different sizes is to study them in sections and measure their nuclei. This will show that the nuclei of most lymphocytes are about 5 μm. in diameter whereas about 8 per cent of lymphocytes have nuclei that are about 7 μm. in diameter. However, if examples of these two types of cells were seen side by side in a blood film, the smaller would have an overall diameter of from 7 to 8 μm. and the larger a diameter of about 12 μm. The volume of the larger lymphocyte is calculated as being about 3 times that of the smaller. The smaller kind are termed *small lymphocytes* and the larger are now commonly termed *medium lymphocytes* for reasons given above.

Numbers. Next to neutrophils, lymphocytes are the commonest leukocytes in a normal blood film. In absolute numbers, there are 1,000 to 4,000 per cubic millimeter of blood. Hence about 20 to 40 per cent of all leukocytes seen in a normal blood film are lymphocytes. The percentage of lymphocytes in the blood of many experimental animals differs considerably from that in man; those engaged in experimental work can obtain detailed information about leukocytes of different species from Albritton's *Standard Values in Blood*.

Appearance in Blood Films and H and E Sections. The chromatin of small lymphocytes is mostly condensed so their nuclei are very small (Plate 11-1). Small lymphocytes have very little cytoplasm. Even in films where their cytoplasm is spread out, it is no more than a narrow rim of material exhibiting varying degrees of basophilia with blood stains (Plate 11-1, small lymphocyte). In sections the normal globular shape of the lymphocyte is preserved and the rim of unspread cytoplasm appears thinner still, staining so poorly with H and E that it can be seen only

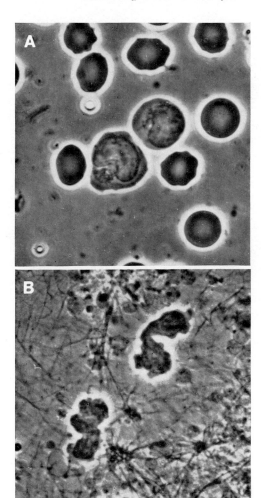

Fig. 11-8. Oil-immersion photomicrographs (phase contrast) of living lymphocytes in tissue cultures. (*A*) Two lymphocytes at the center are resting. (*B*) Two lymphocytes are seen here on the move. (Courtesy of D. Whitelaw)

with difficulty. The rounded or ovoid nucleus may exhibit a little indentation on one side.

Nucleoli are not visible in lymphocyte nuclei in films because they are obscured by the condensed chromatin. Even in routine sections they are not seen for the same reason. Nucleoli can only be seen in very thin sections of lymphocytes, where there is no chromatin above or below to obscure them.

Although lymphocytes lack any specific granules, the cytoplasm of about 10 per cent of lymphocytes is seen in stained films to contain a few reddish-purple azurophilic granules, which are probably lysosomes.

Living Lymphocytes. Living lymphocytes studied with the phase contrast microscope (Fig. 11-8) are seen to be very active, moving about at a relatively fast speed (their

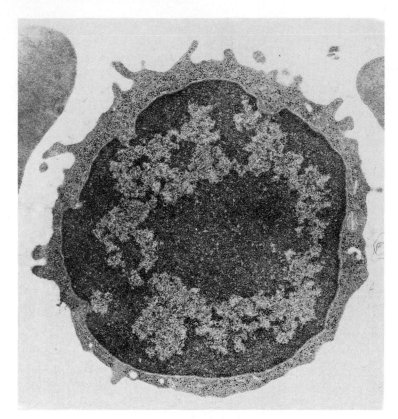

Fig. 11-9. Electron micrograph of a small lymphocyte. For description, *see* text. (Everett, N. B., and Perkins, W. D.: Hemopoietic stem cell migration. *In* Cairnie, A. B., Lala, P. K., and Osmond, D. G. (eds.): Stem Cells of Renewing Cell Populations. p. 228. New York, Academic Press, 1976)

speed, however, is magnified by the LM as much as their size). They can insinuate themselves between other cells and thus pass through endothelial linings and epithelial membranes. A moving lymphocyte has a head and a tail end; the head end consists of its nucleus, covered with a little cytoplasm, and its tail consists of drawn-out cytoplasm. In life a lymphocyte on the move thus has a shape like a tennis racquet.

The Fine Structure of Lymphocytes. This is very revealing both in terms of what it does and does not show. First, the nucleus of a small lymphocyte (Fig. 11-9), as might be expected from its appearance in the LM, contains a great deal of condensed chromatin and little extended chromatin. The cytoplasm reveals almost no organelles except free ribosomes which are indicated in Figure 11-9 by the fine stipling evident at this magnification. In other words, the small lymphocyte as it exists in blood is not equipped to perform any specialized function for it has not developed the organelle equipment required for performing specialized functions. It does, however, possess the organelle equipment (free ribosomes) essential for growth. The fine structure of a medium lymphocyte (Fig. 11-10) shows somewhat more evidence of differentiation than that of a small lymphocyte in that, in addition to free ribosomes, the cytoplasm also contains enough mitochon-

dria for occasional ones to be seen in sections. The medium lymphocyte shown in Figure 11-10 also reveals a little rER and a small Golgi (labeled in Fig. 11-10). Its nucleus, moreover, shows slightly more extended chromatin.

The fine structure of small lymphocytes is therefore suggestive of cells not differentiated for any special function, unlike the polymorphs, eosinophils, and basophils of the blood. Their fine structure is suggestive of an undifferentiated type of cell. Hence an important question that arises is what kind (or kinds) of cells lymphocytes can go on to form. As will be described in Chapter 13, which deals with the lymphatic tissues, there is clear evidence that lymphocytes develop into cells specialized to provide immunological defenses for the body. It will also be explained that there are two kinds of small lymphocytes, termed *B-* and *T-lymphocytes,* respectively. However, these two sub-types cannot, as once thought, be distinguished from one another by morphological criteria; but they can be distinguished by appropriate immunological methods. In man the B type of small lymphocyte is thought to originate in the bone marrow and the T type comes from the thymus gland. B- and T-lymphocytes cooperate in various ways in effecting immunological responses, as will be described in Chapter 13.

Fig. 11-10. Electron micrograph of a medium-sized lymphocyte. In its cytoplasm rough-surfaced endoplasmic reticulum (rER) and Golgi region (G) can be seen. For further description, *see* text. (Everett, N. B., and Perkins, W. D.: Hemopoietic stem cell migration. *In* Cairnie, A. B., Lala, P. K., and Osmond, D. G. (eds.): Stem Cells of Renewing Cell Populations. p. 229. New York, Academic Press, 1976)

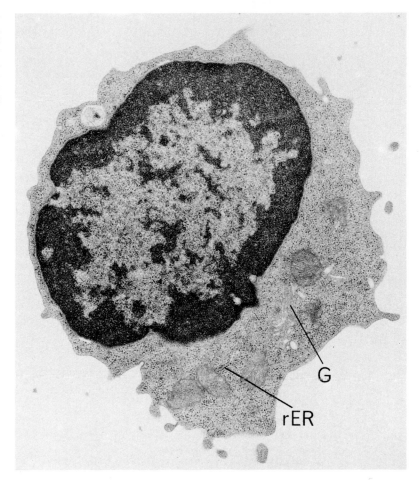

It is now difficult to imagine that only a few decades ago it was believed lymphocytes were end cells unable to reproduce themselves. Furthermore, their function was unknown. The development of knowledge in the last few decades about lymphocytes is one of the most fascinating stories in the history of medical research. Since most of the development of lymphocytes into functioning immunological cells occurs in lymphatic tissues, this aspect of lymphocytes and other pertinent facts of histological and medical interest are given in Chapter 13.

MONOCYTES

Numbers. Monocytes comprise from 2 to 8 per cent of the leukocytes of normal blood; in absolute figures they number 200 to 600 per cubic millimeter of blood. Hence a great many leukocytes may have to be examined before a good example of a monocyte is found. A typical monocyte can be distinguished without undue difficulty. However, in examining stained films of blood cells there are difficulties in deciding whether given cells are monocytes or medium lymphocytes and whether others are monocytes or neutrophilic metamyelocytes.

Appearance in Blood Films With the LM. The largest leukocytes seen in blood films are generally monocytes (labeled in Plate 11-1). They are from 12 to 15 μm. in diameter when suspended and assume a more or less spherical shape. When flattened in dried films, however, they are up to 20μm. in diameter.

Nucleus. As seen in stained films the nucleus is somewhat variable in shape; some are ovoid, some indented ovals, and others have an indentation large enough for the shape of the nucleus to be a thick horseshoe (Plate 11-1). Sometimes nuclei of the latter shape appear twisted or folded during preparation of the film. The chromatin of the nucleus is less condensed than in lymphocytes. It is stained a blue-violet shade in the usual preparation, and, since it is more spread out than that of lymphocytes, it does not stain as intensely. Nucleoli are not visible in the

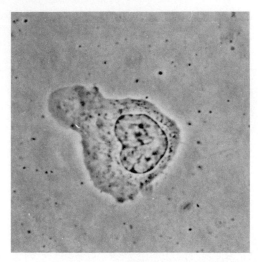

Fig. 11-11. Oil-immersion photomicrograph (phase contrast) of a monocyte in tissue culture. (Courtesy of D. Whitelaw)

usual stained film but can be seen in monocytes examined with the phase contrast microscope. There are often two in each nucleus.

Cytoplasm. This comprises the larger part of the cell. In stained blood films it is a pale blue-gray in color (Plate 11-1). Fine azurophilic granules can often be seen in it (Plate 11-1) but specific granules are, of course, lacking.

Motility. Monocytes can extend and withdraw pseudopodia (Fig. 11-11) and readily migrate through the endothelium lining capillaries or small venules to enter loose connective tissue and move through it.

Fine Structure. The nucleus of a monocyte is characteristically more indented than that of a lymphocyte (Figs. 11-12 and 11-13). There is a good deal of condensed peripheral chromatin (Figs. 11-12 and 11-13). More centrally there is some extended chromatin and two or more nucleoli may be seen.

The cytoplasm reveals a fairly well developed Golgi apparatus (G in Fig. 11-12). It also contains some free

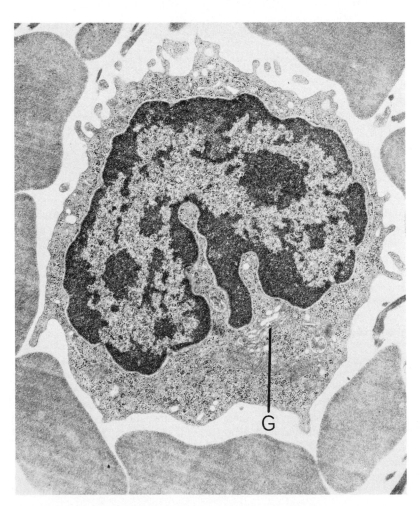

Fig. 11-12. Electron micrograph of a monocyte. Note the eccentric position of its bean-shaped nucleus, and its Golgi region (G). For further description, *see* text. (Everett, N. B., and Perkins, W. D.: Hemopoietic stem cell migration. *In* Cairnie, A. B., Lala, P. K., and Osmond, D. G. (eds.): Stem Cells of Renewing Cell Populations. p. 230. New York, Academic Press, 1976)

Fig. 11-13. Electron micrograph of part of a monocyte from bone marrow of a rabbit. This cell shows the features of a mature monocyte, including rER (see at *top*), several mitochondria (*upper right*), free ribosomes, and a group of lysosomes (*lower right*). (Nichols, B. A., Bainton, D. F., and Farquhar, M. G.: J. Cell Biol., *50:*498, 1971)

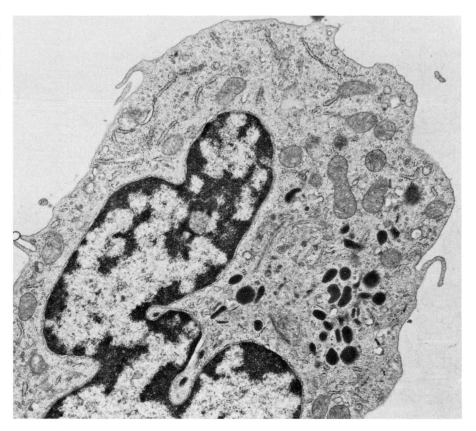

ribosomes and polyribosomes, a little rER, and some mitochondria (Fig. 11-13). Of interest is the presence of dense granules (Fig. 11-13) corresponding to the fine azurophilic granules seen with the LM; these are lysosomes. The cell border of monocytes tends to be ragged because of little pseudopodia projecting irregularly at many sites (Fig. 11-12).

Function. The function of monocytes is most easily summarized by stating that monocytes are the immediate precursors of macrophages of connective tissues (and the hematopoietic tissues too are considered to be one type of connective tissue). The function of monocytes is therefore not performed within the confines of the bloodstream. As already described, monocytes migrate in increased numbers from the bloodstream to the tissues in the inflammatory reaction (p. 285). Whether a monocyte as such can perform any of the functions of macrophages depends on how the two cells are defined. The easiest solution to this problem is to define monocytes as blood cells and macrophages as tissue cells and assume that any monocyte that leaves the bloodstream and enters the tissues for all practical purposes becomes a macrophage.

Life Span. Whitlaw showed by labeling experiments that under normal conditions monocytes leave the blood-stream in a random fashion with an average stay in the blood of about three days.

REFERENCES AND OTHER READING

Comprehensive General Reference for All Types of Blood Cells and Their Disorders

Williams, W. W., Beutler, E., Erslev, A. J., and Rundles, R. W.: Hematology. ed 2. New York, McGraw-Hill, 1977.

General

Bessis, M.: Living Blood Cells and Their Ultrastructure. New York, Springer-Verlag, 1973.
Cline, M. J.: The White Cell. Cambridge, Mass., Harvard University Press, 1975.
Low, F. N., and Freeman, J. A.: Electron Microscopic Atlas of Normal and Leukemic Human Blood. New York, Blakiston, 1958.
Metcalf, D., and Moore, M. A. S.: Haemopoietic Cells. Amsterdam, North-Holland Publishing Co., 1971.

Inflammation

Menaker, L. (ed.): The Biologic Basis of Wound Healing. New York, Harper & Row, 1975.

Movat, H. Z. (ed.): Inflammation, Immunity and Hypersensitivity. Molecular and Cellular Mechanisms. ed. 2. New York, Harper & Row, 1979.

Ryan, G. B., and Majno, G.: Acute Inflammation. Am. J. Pathol., *86:*183, 1977.

Zweifach, B. W., Grant, L., and McCluskey, R. T. (eds.): The Inflammatory Process. ed. 2, vols. 1 to 3. New York, Academic Press, 1974.

Granular Leukocytes

Ackerman, G. A.: Cytochemical properties of the blood basophilic granulocyte. Ann. N.Y. Acad. Sci., *103:*376, 1963.

Anderson, D. R.: Ultrastructure of normal leukemic leukocytes in human peripheral blood. J. Ultrastruct. Res., Suppl. 9, 1966.

Austen, K. F., and Orange, R. P.: Bronchial asthma: the possible role of the chemical mediators of immediate hypersensitivity in the pathogenesis of subacute chronic disease. Am. Rev. Respir. Dis., *112:*423, 1975.

Bainton, D. F., and Farquhar, M. C.: Origin of granules in polymorphonuclear leucocytes: two types derived from opposite faces of the Golgi apparatus in developing leucocytes. J. Cell Biol., *28:*277, 1966.

————: Differences in enzyme content of azurophil and specific granules of polymorphonuclear leucocytes: cytochemistry and electron microscopy of bone marrow cells. J. Cell Biol., *39:*299, 1968.

————: Segregation and packaging of granules in eosinophilic leucocytes. J. Cell Biol., *45:*54, 1970.

Bainton, D. F., Ullyot, J. L., and Farquhar, M. C.: The development of neutrophilic polymorphonuclear leucocytes in human bone marrow: origin and content of azurophil and specific granules. J. Exp. Med., *134:*907, 1971.

Beeson, P. B., and Bass, D. A.: The Eosinophil. Major Problems in Internal Medicine. vol. 14. Philadelphia, W. B. Saunders, 1977.

Cline, M. J.: The White Cell. Cambridge, Mass., Harvard University Press, 1975.

Davidson, W. M., and Smith, D. R.: A morphological sex difference in the polymorphonuclear neutrophil leucocytes. Br. Med. J., *2:*6, 1954.

De Castro, N. M.: Frequency variations of "drumsticks" of peripheral blood neutrophils in the rabbit in different alimentary conditions. Acta anat., *52:*341, 1963.

Farquhar, M. C., and Bainton, D. F.: Cytochemical Studies on Leucocyte Granules. Proc. 4th Internat. Congr. Histochemistry and Cytochemistry, Kyoto, Japan. pp. 25–26. Published by the Soc. Histochemistry and Cytochemistry, 1972.

Klebanoff, S. J., and Clark, R. A.: The Neutrophil: Function and Clinical Disorders. New York, Elsevier North-Holland, 1978.

Litt, M.: Eosinophils and antigen-antibody reaction. Ann. N.Y. Acad. Sci., *116.*964, 1964.

Zweifach, B. Z., Grant, L., and McCluskey, R. T. (eds.): The Inflammatory Process. ed. 2, vols. 1 to 3. New York, Academic Press, 1974.

Lymphocytes

(*See also* References listed for Chap. 13)

Dougherty, T. F.: Adrenal cortical control of lymphatic tissue mass. *In* Stohlman, F., Jr. (ed.): The Kinetic of Cellular Proliferation. p. 264. New York, Grune & Stratton, 1959.

Everett, N. B., and Caffrey, R. W.: Radioautographic studies of bone marrow and small lymphocytes. *In* Yoffey, J. M. (ed.): The Lymphocyte in Immunology and Haemopoiesis, p. 109. London, Edward Arnold, 1966.

Everett, N. B., and Perkins, W. D.: Hemopoietic stem cell migration. *In* Cairnie, A. B., Lala, P. K., and Osmond, D. G. (eds.): Stem Cells of Renewing Cell Populations. New York, Academic Press, 1976.

Everett, N. B., Caffrey, R. W., and Rieke, W. O.: The small lymphocyte of the rat: rate of formation, extent of recirculation and circulating life span. *In* Proc, IX Congr. International Soc. Hematology, Mexico City, vol. 3, p. 345, 1962.

Gowans, J. L.: Life span recirculation and transformation of lymphocytes. Int. Rev. Exp. Pathol., *5,* 1967.

Little, J. R., Brecher, G., Bradley, T. R., and Rose, S.: Determination of lymphocyte turnover by continuous infusion of tritiated thymidine. Blood, *19:*236, 1962.

Nowell, P. C.: Phytohemagglutinin: an initiator of mitosis in cultures of normal human leukocytes. Cancer Res., *20:*462, 1960.

Osmond, D. G., and Everett, N. B.: Radioautographic studies of bone marrow lymphocytes in vivo and in diffusion chamber cultures. Blood, *23:*1, 1964.

Trowell, O. A.: The sensitivity of lymphocytes to ionizing radiation. J. Pathol., Bact., *64:*687, 1952.

Yoffey, J. M. (ed.): The Lymphocyte in Immunology and Haemopoiesis. London, Edward Arnold, 1966. (This volume contains 43 reports by various investigators.)

Monocytes

Brahim, F., and Osmond, D. G.: Radioautographic studies on the production and fate of bone marrow lymphocytes and monocytes. Proc. Canad. Fed. Biol. Soc., *136:*1967.

Clark, E. R., and Clark, E. L.: Relation of monocytes of the blood to tissue macrophages. Am. J. Anat., *46:*149, 1930.

van Furth, R. (ed.): Mononuclear Phagocytes. Philadelphia, F. A. Davis, 1970.

Nichols, B. A., Bainton, D. F., and Farquhar, M. G.: Differentiation of monocytes. Origin, nature and fate of their azurophil granules. J. Cell Biol., *50:*498, 1971.

Tompkins, E. H.: The monocyte. Ann N.Y. Acad. Sci., *59:*732, 1955.

Volkman, A., and Gowans, J. H.: The origin of macrophages from bone marrow in the rat. Br. J. Exp. Pathol., *46:*62, 1965.

Whitelaw, D. M.: The intravascular lifespan of monocytes. Blood, *28:*455, 1966.

12 The Hematopoietic Tissues: Myeloid Tissue

PART 1: THE DEVELOPMENT OF THE MODERN CONCEPT OF THE ORIGIN OF BLOOD CELLS AND EARLY STAGES IN BLOOD CELL FORMATION

Not so long ago it was believed that the ancestral cell from which blood cells were derived could be specifically identified with the LM. It was also believed that the earliest stages through which cells passed in developing into the various kinds of blood cells could be recognized with the LM. This older view is no longer valid. Although the general features of the ancestral cell of blood cells and those of its more immediate progeny (such as their size) are known, their other features are not sufficiently distinctive for them to be distinguished by microscopy with certainty. How then do we know such relatively undifferentiated ancestral cells exist in the body? Before discussing how the existence of the ancestral cell and its immediate descendants was established without them having to be identified as such by microscopy, we must first provide some terminology.

Terminology. Blood cell formation is commonly referred to as *hematopoiesis* (Gr. *hemato*, blood; *poiein*, to make). Likewise the tissue in which blood cells are produced is termed *hematopoietic tissue* (this term, however, is usually shortened to *hemopoietic tissue,* and the former term, to *hemopoiesis*). There are two kinds of hematopoietic tissues, termed *myeloid* and *lymphatic tissue* respectively. The reason for one being termed *myeloid* (Gr. *myelos,* marrow) is that ever since blood cells and their immediate precursors could be distinguished with the LM it became evident that in man (*1*) erythrocytes and their immediate precursors, (*2*) granular leukocytes and their immediate precursors, and (*3*) platelets and the cells responsible for their formation were all housed in the marrow that fills the cavities of bones. Hence the tissue of bone marrow in which erythrocytes, granular leukocytes, and platelets are formed in man was termed *myeloid tissue.* It was also appreciated that lymphocytes and what were considered

to be their immediate precursors were so abundant in the thymus gland, lymph nodes, and spleen, that these tissues, so obviously rich in lymphocytes, should be termed *lymphatic tissue.*

At first it was assumed that all lymphocytes were formed in lymphatic tissue. But after it was discovered that there were two types, T and B, it was found that the latter type, even though they later constitute part of the population of lymphatic tissue, are apparently produced (in man) in myeloid tissue. It was also at first commonly thought that monocytes were derived from lymphocytes, but later it was established that they too were formed in myeloid tissue. Furthermore, it was realized that in prenatal life in man, and even in postnatal life in for example rats and mice, cells of the myeloid series are produced in the spleen—a lymphatic organ—as well as in myeloid tissue. So although classifying hematopoietic tissue into myeloid and lymphatic types is generally helpful, and indeed with respect to some parts of the lymphatic tissue essential, parts of lymphatic tissue in different species and at different times have some features in common with myeloid tissue.

Another basic point to establish here is that blood cells are free cells, which means they are not an integral part of a tissue structure, like fibroblasts, for example. Perhaps because it seemed inconceivable that there could be a self-renewing population of free cells, it was formerly believed that there were fixed cells with great mesenchymal potentiality (called primitive reticular cells) that persisted throughout life in myeloid and lymphatic tissue and gave rise to free cells. Radioautographic studies provided no evidence for this older view so it is no longer held. The blood cell population is now conceived of as a self-renewing population of free cells. How this concept evolved will now be described.

295

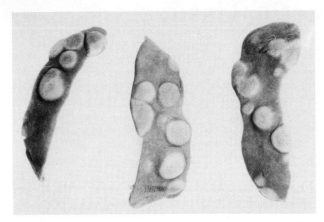

Fig. 12-1. Photograph of the spleens of three irradiated mice that were injected with bone marrow cells, removed 10 days after the injection, and fixed in Bouin's fixative. Each circular pale area is a colony of cells arising from a single pluripotential hematopoietic stem cell (CFU). (Courtesy of E. A. McCulloch)

DEVELOPMENT OF MODERN KNOWLEDGE ABOUT THE ANCESTRAL CELL OF ALL BLOOD CELLS AND ITS MORE IMMEDIATE DERIVATIVES

The story begins with research on the regeneration of blood cells in irradiated animals transfused with normal bone marrow cells. Following the advent of the atom bomb, increased research was devoted to the way in which exposure to sufficient amounts of radiation caused illness or death. Depending on the dose received, effects may be manifested quickly or slowly over a long term. The short-term effects can easily be investigated in small animals such as mice by exposing them to whole body x-radiation in the lethal range. As was described on page 56, the most important effect of radiation on cells is on their chromosomes, and the damage done in this way may not become apparent until a cell attempts to undergo mitosis, in which process the damage done is manifested by mitosis being abnormal and generally unsuccessful. As a result, the parts of the body most severely affected by total body radiation, such as might occur from severe atomic fallout, are those in which there is a rapid cell turnover. Since granular leukocytes on average circulate for only 9 hours, they must be produced in the bone marrow as rapidly as they are lost from the bloodstream if their numbers in blood are not to fall quickly. The same is true of platelets. Since erythrocytes live for four months, interference with their production after total body radiation does not become apparent immediately. Accordingly, after total body radiation in the lethal range, the polymorphs and platelets mostly disappear from the blood in a

few days. Likewise, the proliferation and development of lymphocytes is halted and hence the formation of plasma cells in response to antigens is quickly diminished. Primarily because of the failure of production of new polymorphs and new antibody-forming cells, the body becomes unable to resist infection. Finally, since the lining cells of the intestine are normally lost at a rapid rate and must be replaced at the same rapid rate, another serious immediate effect of total body radiation is that intestinal lining cells are not replaced as they are lost, so that patches of the intestine become denuded even though cells that persist stretch out and become relatively flat in an attempt to cover such areas. Denuded areas are soon invaded by bacteria and, since the body has lost its chief means for resisting infection and also its capacity to make platelets for preventing hemorrhages from infected denuded sites along the intestine, death soon occurs.

The Effects of Transfusion of Bone Marrow Cells. If, however, an irradiated mouse after receiving a lethal dose of whole body radiation is given an intravenous transfusion of marrow cells from another, preferably genetically identical, animal, it will recover. The reason for this is that certain cells in the transfused marrow settle out in the hematopoietic tissues of the host and repopulate them with new cells which, of course, are of the donor animal type. The grafted cells soon produce enough granular leukocytes and platelets to prevent the infection and hemorrhages that would ordinarily kill the animal. Furthermore, the ability of the animal for producing new antibody-forming cells is restored. It is assumed that enough lining cells of the intestine survive and are able to multiply and so provide a complete lining for the intestine again if the immunological defenses of the body are restored and if the remaining lining cells have enough time to do it.

The Spleen Colony Technic. An unexpected dividend of such proportions that it transformed future research on the stem cells responsible for the formation of blood cells emerged from a series of studies made by Till and McCulloch and McCulloch and Till on the biological effects of radiation. Mice that had received total body radiation in the lethal range were transfused with marrow cells from normal mice of the same pure strain. In the course of these experiments these investigators performed autopsies on animals in different stages of recovery and observed that the spleens of recovering animals developed little nodules that projected from the spleen surface (Fig. 12-1). Their histological studies with the LM indicated that these nodules were colonies of new cells of the erythrocyte and granulocyte series, sometimes with megakaryocytes. They termed the nodules *colonies* and immediately questioned whether each colony might be a clone, that is, whether it arose from a single cell with the potentiality to give rise to the cells of the erythrocyte, granulocyte, and megakaryocyte lines of differentiation. To determine this it was decided to employ marrow cells with radiation-induced chromosomal markers. This technic will next be described.

Chromosomal Markers. If cells with proliferative capacity are irradiated with doses insufficient to stop proliferation of all cells, some of the cells may suffer an injury to individual chromosomes that may involve their DNA, but not the DNA employed in that particular kind of cell for transcribing information necessary for the survival of the cell. Nevertheless the structure and hence appearance of some chromosomes may be sufficiently altered for them to be microscopically identifiable. Since breakage of chromosomes resulting from radiation and reassociation of broken fragments occur at random, the resulting chromosome configuration is unique, hence the term *chromosomal marker*. If a cell with a chromosome of this kind is allowed to proliferate, karyotypes of its progeny will reveal the chromosome abnormality that was created in the cell from which the clone originated.

Spleen Colonies Shown to Be Clones. Becker, McCulloch, and Till then prepared marrow suspensions that were irradiated enough to produce chromosomal markers in the marrow cells and used these to transfuse irradiated hosts. Nearly all of the dividing cells in each spleen colony that developed showed the same marker. So it was concluded that each colony originated from a single cell and hence represented a clone. This work, therefore, provided not conjecture but proof that there is a kind of cell in bone marrow that can give rise to cells of the erythrocyte series, cells of the granular leukocyte series, and megakaryocytes. They decided to term this pluripotential stem cell a *colony-forming unit* (CFU), a term that has now become well established.*

The Use of the Spleen Colony Method for Demonstrating the Circulation of Stem Cells. Until the spleen colony technic was evolved to demonstrate the presence and assay the numbers of stem cells in various hematopoietic tissues and in blood, little thought was given to the possibility that, under normal conditions, stem cells might circulate so that, having originated in one site, they could pass by the bloodstream to another site and seed it with stem cells. However, by means of the spleen colony technic, it was shown that CFUs could be recovered from circulating blood, although in relatively small numbers, and that although present in greater concentration in bone marrow they were also present, in adult mice, in certain other hematopoietic organs. Thus the spleen colony technic (by determining the numbers of colonies formed by the number of cells injected) provided a means for assaying the relative numbers of stem cells in any given cell preparation without having to know their morphology.

The development of a technic whereby the presence and numbers of the free stem cells giving rise to erythrocytes, granular leukocytes, and megakaryocytes could be determined—in other words, an assay technic for stem cells—was bound to facilitate research on finding out where and how these stem cells are formed in the body. Until this time it was still a common assumption that the free stem cells of marrow arose from reticular cells of marrow stroma. That this was highly improbable was shown by a series of extremely ingenious and informative experiments by Moore, Metcalf, and their associates, in which the spleen colony technic played a very important role. These investigators traced the origin of the free stem cells of hematopoietic tissues to free stem cells that develop in the yolk sac of the embryo. They postulated that the formation of blood cells in other sites in embryonic, fetal, and postnatal life is due to the stroma of these other hematopoietic tissues being seeded by free pluripotential stem cells originating in the yolk sac of the embryo. To explain this concept in more detail we first have to discuss the formation of blood cells in the embryo.

Blood Cell Formation in the Embryo. In Chapter 9 we described how mesenchymal cells become somewhat more flattened and connected with one another to surround a lumen and so become a primitive capillary (Fig. 9-3). The cells constituting the walls of such vessels differentiate into endothelial cells and proliferate so as to send out hollow buds that join up with other primitive vessels developing similarly in mesenchyme to form the circulatory system.

In the mesenchyme of the yolk sac of most mammalian embryos certain mesenchymal cells persist in what might otherwise become the empty lumen of a primitive capillary. The mesenchymal cells persisting in the lumen become free cells, and so a section cut across a developing blood vessel of this type will reveal a group of free cells lying in its lumen. This appearance gave rise to the name *blood island*. It was originally believed that the endothelium of the developing capillary gave rise to the blood cells in its lumen but it is now believed that the primitive blood cells within the island and the endothelium that surrounds the blood cells are independently derived from mesenchyme.

Hematopoiesis in Other Organs Traced to the Yolk Sac. The great many experiments involved in providing proof for the hypothesis that hematopoietic stem cells and hence all blood cells are derived from the yolk sac are brought together and described in a very informative book by Metcalf and Moore (*see* the general reference,

---

*The short form *CFU* is now often used in the plural as well as the singular. However, it is an abbreviation of three words and hence is properly written *C.F.U.* The plural form should therefore be C.F.U.s but since the periods are not really necessary they are commonly omitted and hence the plural form should be *CFUs*.

Newer Concepts, under References and Other Reading). Only a few will be mentioned here: these indicate that this hypothesis was proven by experimental methods and could not have been proven by purely morphological studies.

The hypothesis, in short, is that hematopoietic stem cells develop from mesenchymal cells in the blood islands of the yolk sac of the embryo, and that for a time the proliferation of the stem cells of blood cells occurs in the yolk sac. In the yolk sac there is, moreover, some differentiation that leads in particular to the formation of cells that synthesize hemoglobin (of the fetal type). Moore and Metcalf showed by means of the spleen colony technic that almost as soon as these cells appeared in the blood islands, CFUs were present among them. They also found that cells from the yolk sac could repopulate the hematopoietic tissues of a mouse given radiation in the lethal range. It was shown that hematopoiesis in the yolk sac was soon superseded by hematopoiesis occurring in the liver because of that organ having been seeded by stem cells from the yolk sac, and that subsequently the spleen and bone marrow of the embryo were seeded with stem cells from the liver. After birth the bone marrow and spleen have become the chief sites where the population of stem cells is maintained.

Whereas it was clear from the study of spleen colonies produced by CFUs with chromosomal markers that erythrocytes, granular leukocytes, and megakaryocytes were all formed by the CFU and that bone marrow cells would repopulate all of the hematopoietic tissues of an irradiated animal, it was not clear that the CFU was responsible for forming lymphocytes. A first step in establishing its role in this respect was showing that lymphocytes could be formed in myeloid tissue.

PART OF THE LYMPHOCYTE POPULATION FOUND TO BE PRODUCED IN MYELOID TISSUE

Since it was for so long commonly accepted that lymphocytes in man were produced in the lymphatic division of hematopoietic tissue and erythrocytes, granular leukocytes, and platelets in the myeloid division, little attention seems to have been paid to the presence of lymphocytes in myeloid tissue. It was not until Yoffey called attention to the fact that in normal laboratory animals there were large numbers of lymphocytes in bone marrow that interest was taken in this matter. With the rigid view held in the past, the presence of lymphocytes in marrow was at first explained as being due to large numbers of lymphocytes, formed in lymphatic tissue, being strained from circulating blood as it passed through the marrow. And indeed there is evidence that some lymphocytes may, in fact, be strained from the blood as it passes through mar-

row. However, as modern methods became available it was shown by ingenious labeling experiments that lymphocytes were indeed produced in the marrow of experimental animals in considerable numbers.

Osmond and Everett investigated the problem by preparing radioautographs of guinea pig marrow obtained at different times after having given the animals a dose of tritiated thymidine intravenously. They found that in the first four hours only about 0.4 per cent of the lymphocytes of marrow had become labeled, but after 3 days about 40 per cent of marrow lymphocytes were labeled, which, of course, suggested that some precursor cell of lymphocytes was dividing and taking up the label later found in the lymphocytes. They performed further experiments to show the labeled lymphocytes found in marrow had not been labeled elsewhere and strained out by the marrow; instead, they must have been formed in the marrow. Subsequently, Everett and Chaffrey, as well as Osmond, performed similar experiments on rats with much the same results.

Then Osmond, by injecting labeled thymidine directly into marrow, found the number of labeled lymphocytes appearing in blood to be at least 25 per cent of the very considerable number of labeled granular leukocytes appearing over the same period. Hence in the usual experimental animal the rate of production and entry of lymphocytes into the blood from marrow is very substantial.

When it was established that some lymphocytes were actually produced in myeloid tissue, the problem arose as to the type of stem cell from which they arose and what bearing a decision on this matter would have on whether or not the lymphocytes could originate from the CFU, which, if proven, would suggest it to be the ultimate source of all types of blood cells. Further work has indeed established this concept, as will be described below.

THE CFU AS THE ANCESTOR CELL OF LYMPHOCYTES

As described in the preceding, marrow cells injected into irradiated recipients bring about repopulation of all the hematopoietic tissues, both myeloid and lymphatic, and also cause spleen colonies to form in their hosts. Cytological studies of the colonies allow the cells of the erythrocyte and granulocyte cell lineages to be distinguished, as well as megakaryocytes. By using chromosomal markers it was shown that colonies are clones; thus all the cells mentioned above arise from a single stem cell. It has also been shown that yolk sac cells will bring about the formation of spleen colonies in their hosts. The question that then arose was whether CFUs are also responsible for bringing about the repopulation of the lymphatic tissues of the irradiated host, for if so, the formation of marrow lymphocytes could be attributed to them.

Very substantial evidence that cells of the lymphocyte series arise from the CFUs forming spleen colonies has been obtained. In 1962 Trentin and Fahlberg, by means of repeated transfers through irradiated animals, showed that cells obtained from an original single spleen colony could completely repopulate all the hematopoietic tissues of an irradiated mouse, which suggests that the CFU from which the original spleen colony developed had the potentiality to form cells of the lymphocyte series. Furthermore, Wu et al. showed that radiation-induced markers produced in CFUs could be traced into cells of the lymphatic division of the hematopoietic system. In order to show this, large numbers of CFUs with markers had to be obtained. This was done in an ingenious manner in a three-step experiment that, for the second step, utilized a special strain of mice with an inherited defect that prevents their own CFUs from forming colonies, but allows proliferation of CFUs from a related normal strain of mice in which markers have been produced by radiation. Thus this permits large numbers of CFUs with markers to multiply in their marrow, and the marrow cells thus obtained after some months contain many CFUs still with markers that can then be injected into irradiated normal mice. In due course the markers are found in the cells of the lymphatic tissues as well as in the myeloid tissue. The evidence from these experiments again strongly suggests that the CFU gives rise to cells of the lymphocyte series as well as the myeloid, and hence that the lymphocytes of marrow can be formed from CFUs.

If the CFU has the potentiality to form lymphocytes, it might be asked why this could not be established readily by examining spleen colonies and determining whether or not lymphocytes are present in them as well as cells of the erythrocyte and granulocyte series. This, however, presents several problems. With the LM it would be very difficult in ordinary sections to distinguish lymphocytes from certain of the cells of the erythrocyte series that may develop in a spleen colony. Secondly, since colonies develop in the spleen and since by the time they have formed there are lots of lymphocytes in the spleen stroma, the observer could not be certain that the presence of any lymphocyte identified in a colony was not due to its incorporation into a developing colony. Finally, chromosomal markers would be of no help in identifying a lymphocyte and proving it developed in a colony because chromosomal markers are detectable only at mitosis and small lymphocytes as such do not undergo mitosis. To see chromosomal markers in cells of the lymphocyte series small lymphocytes have to be stimulated, whereupon they develop into what are termed *activated lymphocytes*. It is not improbable that lymphocytes are indeed produced in spleen colonies, but it is difficult to prove this by morphological criteria.

There is, however, another way of determining whether lymphocytes appear in spleen colonies, namely by testing colony cells to see if any cells present possess any immunological properties. This also is difficult because, as will be explained in Chapter 13, both T- and B-lymphocytes usually must collaborate to produce immunologically active cells. Furthermore, the lymphocytes that function as T-lymphocytes can do so only after they have been processed in the thymus. Nevertheless, ingenious experiments have shown that some cells obtained from spleen colonies under the right circumstances do possess immunological properties.

In Chapter 13 we shall also describe the formation of T-lymphocytes in the thymus and why it is believed that this occurs because of CFUs (or perhaps a type of immediate progeny cell) settling out in the thymus and forming lymphocytes in this organ.

CONCLUSIONS

From all of the above-described experiments and others it seems established that all blood cells are derived from an ancestral cell type, which is the CFU. Furthermore, the ancestral cell type is a free cell and can be visualized as a pluripotential stem cell because the ancestry of all the various types of blood cells can be traced to it.

COMMENT ON OLDER CONCEPTS AND TERMINOLOGY

Those familiar with previous views about hematopoiesis are entitled to say that the concept of there being a single ancestral kind of free cell responsible for the formation of all types of blood cells is not new because this was a concept subscribed to for decades by the proponents of the monophyletic (Gr. *monos*, single; *phyle*, tribe) school of hematologists, who believed all blood cells were derived from a free ancestral cell type which they termed a *hemocytoblast*. Since the word *hemocytoblast* would seem an eminently proper term for the stem cell of all blood cells, it could be questioned why the CFU should not be termed a hemocytoblast. The reason for it not being so termed is that the monophyletic school had not only postulated the existence of a hemocytoblast, they also believed it to be a cell with morphological characteristics by which it could be recognized in stained films of bone marrow cells. In such preparations hemocytoblasts were postulated as being relatively large cells. The chromatin of their nuclei was described as being well dispersed and their cytoplasm as being extensive and staining a relatively pale blue color. Hence the name hemocytoblast became firmly tied to a relatively large cell with certain morphological characteristics that would permit it to be distinguished with the LM.

Although a CFU cannot be distinguished with certainty from certain other kinds of cells by its morphology, certain morphological features that it is known to possess indicate that it is very different from the type of cells described in the past as a hemocytoblast. For example, the CFU is known to be a small cell, not a large one. Furthermore, spleen colony assays show it is not as numerous in marrow as are the cells that were termed hemocytoblasts. Hence to term the CFU a hemocytoblast, a cell long ago described as having a particular morphology not possessed by the CFU, would cause endless confusion. Indeed many think that the sooner the term hemocytoblast is dropped from the literature, the better.

We shall now describe the evidence indicating the CFU does not possess the morphology attributed to the hemocytoblast.

How It Was Shown That CFUs Are Smaller and Less Numerous Than the Free Cells of Marrow Designated in the Past as Hemocytoblasts. Unit gravity sedimentation is a method by which it is possible to distinguish between cells (even if not distinguishable by other means) on the basis of differences in their size. The sizes of cells are obtained by this method from their rates of fall through a stationary liquid, since the rate of fall of a spherical body denser than its surrounding medium is known to be proportional to the square of its diameter. The principle on which this method is based is illustrated in reverse whenever one watches bubbles formed on the bottom of a glass of carbonated beverage rising to the surface, for the bubbles of larger diameter get to the surface before the smaller ones. Bubbles rise because their density is lower than that of their surrounding medium but their rates of rise are determined mainly by their diameters. The same happens in reverse with cells. Their density being greater than that of the surrounding medium makes them fall rather than rise. Here again, though, their rates of fall are determined mainly by their diameters. To carry out a determination, samples are taken at various depths throughout the length of the column of medium through which the cells have fallen in a fixed time.

The samples of cells obtained by unit gravity sedimentation can be assayed by the spleen colony technic. By this method the size of cells that gave rise to colonies was found to be too small for them to be equated with the cells described from morphological studies as hemocytoblasts.

STUDIES DIRECTED TOWARD DETERMINING THE FINE STRUCTURE OF THE CFU

It is to be appreciated that all that has been described about the CFU up to this point was determined without knowledge of its morphology except that it is a relatively small cell, and since it is a body cell it must have a nucleus and some cytoplasm. Its morphology has been difficult to establish because if there is only about one CFU to every 1,000 nucleated cells in marrow, how could anyone be sure they had found one to study? Furthermore, although a CFU has become committed to forming blood cells, it would not, as a pluripotential stem cell, have differentiated to any extent—so that theoretically it should not possess any special positive cytoplasmic features by which it could easily be distinguished. However, the problem has been attacked and progress has been made.

A logical first step in attempting to learn the appearance of CFUs would be to concentrate them in marrow preparations so that they might constitute a more substantial proportion of the cells and then see if they differed in morphology from the other cells present. Van Bekkum et al. were able to concentrate CFUs in a cell preparation by two successive steps. First they administered two different drugs to the mice from which they planned to obtain marrow cells. The drugs were of a type that were sometimes used in the treatment of cancer or leukemia and which act on cells as they attempt to enter or pass through mitosis by inhibiting the formation of microtubules, and hence spindles. Moreover, in sufficient dosage they kill cells that are regularly passing through cell cycles when they are administered. One interesting feature of stem cells is that they generally have relatively long resting periods (in the G_1 phase of the cell cycle) between division; hence they are relatively unaffected by the temporary use of the kinds of drugs mentioned above. But the destruction of other rapidly proliferating cells in their vicinity (which would be differentiating descendants of stem cells), perhaps by the removal of an inhibitor which ordinarily suppresses the proliferation of stem cells as suggested in Chapter 6, triggers the stem cells to proliferate at a time when the drug is no longer available. Hence after this drug treatment the relative proportion of stem cells in marrow is greatly increased and so it is possible to obtain cell preparations relatively rich in stem cells.

Next, by means of density gradient centrifugation it is possible to separate from cell preparations different fractions in which the cells are of slightly different densities. Following this procedure it is possible to test the different cell fractions obtained from marrow by the spleen colony method to find out which fraction contains most of the CFUs. By using this procedure after the one described above, van Bekkum et al. obtained from cell suspensions of bone marrow a fraction containing what they considered would constitute around 20 per cent stem cells. They studied cells from this fraction in stained films and with the EM. They found that around 20 per cent of the cells seen were of a morphological type that differed from the other cells present and fitted the concept of the kind of morphology a stem cell could be expected to possess, which will be described next.

As already mentioned, cells of different types can be identified with assurance if they possess cytoplasmic features that indicate they are specialized or are becoming specialized to perform some particular function. But a stem cell could be expected to reveal little more than mitochondria and free ribosomes, which organelles are essential for respiration and synthesizing protein for growth (multiplication), and only a very little rER and a small Golgi for producing and maintaining the cell membrane and cell coat. One further criterion that could be looked for in the stem cell of blood cells would be its size because, as already noted, the CFU is a relatively small cell.

These cells that van Bekkum et al. found to constitute about 20 per cent of the total were from 7 to 10 μm. in diameter and their cytoplasm revealed no organelles except free ribosomes and a few mitochrondria. An illustration provided by van Bekkum is shown in Figure 12-2. The cells they studied did not give a peroxidase reaction as did cells of the granulocyte and monocyte series present in the same preparations. A more important distinction, however, had to be made because the prospective stem cells bore a resemblance to lymphocytes. Small lymphocytes are in the same size range, being about 8 μm. in diameter (Fig. 11-9). Furthermore, the cytoplasm of a small lymphocyte, like that of the prospective stem cell, amounts to little more than a rim around its nucleus. However, van Bekkum et al. listed several differences they considered to exist between their prospective stem cells and lymphocytes. They noted that the prospective stem cells varied a little more in size and their nucleus, although roughly round, seemed more irregular in shape than that of lymphocytes and its indentations were not so deep. The chromatin was more finely dispersed than in lymphocytes, much of it in the latter being densely clumped. Although they could demonstrate a Golgi apparatus, some endoplasmic reticulum, and lysosomes in lymphocytes, they did not observe any of these organelles in the prospective stem cells. Mitochondria, although few in both types of cells, were more numerous but smaller in prospective stem cells than in lymphocytes. Finally, they observed that although some free ribosomes were present in lymphocytes, these were abundant in prospective stem cells, whereas clustered ribosomes seen in lymphocytes were few or absent in prospective stem cells.

PROBLEMS ARISING FROM THE ESTABLISHMENT OF THE MORPHOLOGY OF THE CFU

First, there would seem to be little doubt about the morphology described in the foregoing being that of the CFU and it is helpful to have this knowledge available.

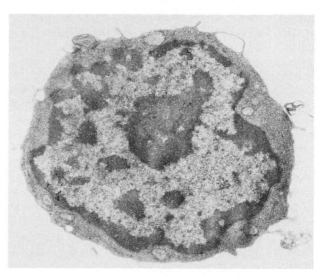

Fig. 12-2. Electron micrograph ($\times$21,000) of a presumed pluripotential hematopoietic stem cell obtained from rat bone marrow. For description, *see* text. (Van Bekkum, D. W.: The appearance of the multipotential hemopoietic stem cell. *In* Baum, S. J., and Ledney, G. D. (eds.): Experimental Hematology Today. New York, Springer-Verlag, 1977)

However, there is a danger in assuming that any cell with this sort of morphology is necessarily a CFU, since it leads to the misconceptions that CFUs can be distinguished from all other cells by their morphology and that their numbers can therefore be estimated in given cell suspensions by using the EM without resort to the spleen colony assay method. Whereas this latter method essentially assays cell potentiality, morphology does not always reveal true cell potentiality because it cannot disclose whether a cell is committed until that cell has become sufficiently differentiated for the nature of its commitment to be manifested.

Next, although it may be possible (but not easy) to distinguish CFUs from small lymphocytes by morphological criteria, it is doubtful whether the earliest progeny cells committed to differentiating into one or the other type of small lymphocyte could be distinguished morphologically from uncommitted CFUs with full potentiality for forming all kinds of blood cells. The appearance of early progeny cells of CFUs would be virtually identical to that of CFUs until there had been sufficient differentiation along a particular line for the cells to acquire new features. In other words, in studying the early stages of blood cell formation, morphology is not the right parameter to use for establishing cell potentiality; this must be done by utilizing spleen colony or in-vitro assay methods (soon to be described) to determine what kinds of progeny particular kinds of cells can or cannot go on to form.

A POSSIBLE UNFORTUNATE SIDE EFFECT OF ESTABLISHING THE MORPHOLOGY OF THE CFU

As noted above, before the CFU was discovered by means of the spleen colony assay technic, most members of the monophyletic school believed that the ancestral cell of all blood cells was a relatively large cell — the hemocytoblast. But there were also subscribers to the view that this ancestral cell was a small cell, in fact, the lymphocyte. So after it was established that the stem cells of blood were very similar in size range and morphology to small lymphocytes, and furthermore that cell suspensions prepared from the spleen (a lymphatic organ) would restore hematopoietic competence to irradiated animals, a certain toleration seems to have developed to the old view that the stem cells of blood are a type of small lymphocyte. In our opinion, such toleration could cause great confusion and is not justifiable for the following reasons.

First, it has been shown that relatively pure preparations of lymphocytes, obtained from the thymus gland or lymph nodes (both of which are heavily populated with lymphocytes) will not, when given to irradiated animals, restore their hematopoietic systems (Micklem and Ford; also Curry, Trentin, and Cheng). Moreover, they will not form spleen colonies. Cell preparations from the spleen, which is also heavily populated with lymphocytes, do, however, produce spleen colonies and restore hematopoietic function when injected into irradiated animals. However, this is to be explained not by lymphocytes serving as stem cells of blood but by the spleen, unlike lymph nodes or the thymus, acting as a huge filter for all kinds of circulating blood cells. As a result, a fair number of CFUs from circulating blood "home out" here at least temporarily so as to maintain within it a resident population of CFUs; indeed in the mouse and rat the spleen is a normal site of myeloid hematopoiesis. Thus it is the CFU content of spleen cell suspensions that accounts for their capacity for forming spleen colonies in irradiated animals and for restoring normal hematopoietic function.

THE CELLS CONCERNED IN THE REPOPULATION OF HEAVILY IRRADIATED HEMATOPOIETIC TISSUE

To consider this question we must distinguish between temporary restoration and the permanent reestablishment of a population of hematopoietic cells. It appears that both CFUs and their immediate descendants would be quite capable of migrating via the bloodstream from shielded marrow to the unshielded marrow of an irradiated animal. Furthermore, it would seem that both CFUs and their immediate descendants would possess sufficient proliferative capacity to go on proliferating once they reach the unshielded marrow. Hence both categories of cells could participate in repopulation. Blood samples taken from experimental animals under various conditions leading to repopulation of marrow and/or blood cell regeneration reveal, according to Everett and Perkins, an increased proportion of relatively undifferentiated blood cells. From their fine structure these were considered to be an assortment of the various kinds of immediate descendants of hematopoietic stem cells and also some of the hematopoietic stem cells themselves. It would seem that all of these could participate in repopulating depleted myeloid tissue. The immediate descendants of CFUs, that migrate for example from shielded to unshielded marrow, could help in the temporary restoration of the irradiated marrow by continuing to divide. But it is believed that such cells could not, with their diminished capacity for self-renewal, by themselves maintain a permanent blood cell population. The establishment and maintenance of a permanent repopulation of irradiated marrow is therefore thought to depend on migration into it of a sufficient number of CFUs.

A Note on Terminology

The only way a blood-forming cell can give rise to or form another kind of cell is by differentiating into it. Hence, for every more differentiated cell that is produced, a less differentiated one is lost. Furthermore, since the life spans of mature blood cells are limited (some being very short), there is a continuing requirement for less differentiated cells.

All kinds of blood cells are derived (stem) from the CFU, which is therefore called the *stem cell* of blood cells. But because CFUs are used up in the process of differentiation, they have to multiply in such a way as to maintain their own cell numbers, a process referred to as *self-renewal*. Indeed, CFUs are probably able to multiply indefinitely and this is why they persist as such all through life. However, the CFU does not have to multiply as extensively as might be thought, because along at least some of its lines of differentiation there are different orders of stem cells that can proliferate very extensively. Nevertheless, these orders of stem cells probably cannot maintain their numbers indefinitely and so they are thought to be replenished from time to time by sufficient differentiation of CFUs to supplement their population size.

Somewhere along each line of differentiation we begin to refer to progenitor cells instead of orders of stem cells. The term *progenitor cell* (L. for parent or ancestor) is generally used to denote a cell capable of further differentiation where no implication is intended about its necessarily having great capacity for self-renewal. Curiously enough, although the fertilized ovum is correctly described as the progenitor cell of all body cells, it should not be referred to as the stem cell of body cells because it obviously does not possess unlimited capacity for renewing itself as such, nor does it persist as such throughout adult life as do stem cells. Hence, the chief distinction drawn between stem cells and progenitor cells is that only the former possess virtually limitless capacity for renewing themselves as such throughout the life of an individual.

HOW BLOOD CELL LINEAGES CAN BE ASCERTAINED IN MICE AND HUMANS

In the foregoing it has been explained how methods such as the use of radiation and marrow transfusion, together with the detection of spleen colonies and the use of chromosomal markers and various inbred strains of mice, have been used to reveal which hematopoietic cells give rise to which kinds of blood cells in experimental animals. The results described have established that all types of blood cells in the animals used are members of clones, the mother cells of which are CFUs, and that the CFU is thus the pluripotential stem cell type of all kinds of blood cells. However, most methods essential for establishing this in experimental animals cannot be used in man. It can, of course, be assumed that the same situation exists in man as in these animals, but in the light of knowledge gained from experimental studies in animals it has been possible to investigate the situation in man directly by other methods now to be described. In this description we shall use the term *myeloid series* of cells to refer to those found in the lines of differentiation that result in the formation of erythrocytes, granular leukocytes, monocytes, and megakaryocytes.

As described on page 83, there is a neoplastic disease of man, termed *chronic myelogenous leukemia*, in which karyotypes of the neoplastic cells of the granular leukocyte series reveal the presence of the Philadelphia chromosome. This chromosomal anomaly develops at the somatic (not germ) cell level in a cell concerned with the formation of blood cells; hence it would be found in, and serve as a marker for, all the descendants of the cell in which the anomaly developed. Since it is detected in karyotypes of dividing cells of the granular leukocyte series, the anomaly must have developed in the cell that gives rise to these. But it is also found in dividing cells of the erythrocyte series and in megakaryocytes. There is even some preliminary indication that it may also be present in B-lymphocytes in patients with this type of leukemia. Accordingly, the Philadelphia chromosome serves as a marker that shows there is an order of stem cells that in man gives rise to granular leuko-

cytes, erythrocytes, megakaryocytes, and probably B-lymphocytes as well.

Another rewarding approach has been the study of blood cell lineages in women, since the enzyme glucose-6-phosphate dehydrogenase (G-6-PD) can be used as a marker. This particular enzyme occurs in two (equally effective) forms distinguishable from one another by electrophoresis. Its synthesis in a cell is coded for by a particular gene on an X chromosome. It will be recalled from Chapter 4 that whereas the body cells of males have only one X chromosome, those of females have two. Furthermore, only one of the two X chromosomes is active; the other remains condensed during the interphase as a Barr body. Next, in early embryonic life it is a matter of chance which of the two X chromosomes in any given body cell of a female will remain active, and when this decision is made it will be the same gene on this particular X chromosome that will code for one form of G-6-PD, not only in that cell but in all the descendants of that cell. Hence, as explained on page 94, a human female is a mosaic of two kinds of clones, with all the cells of one kind of clone having one particular X chromosome active and all the cells in the other having the other X chromosome active. What has proved to be of practical importance, however, is that in some black women one of the two X chromosomes codes for one form of the enzyme (G-6-PD) while the other one codes for the other form of the enzyme. So if all the blood cells of any given female heterozygous for this particular enzyme (Gr. *heteros*, other; *zygon*, yoke, meaning with alternative forms of the same gene in a given pair of homologous chromosomes) were derived from a single cell, they would all reveal the same form of the enzyme. Fialkow has observed that when a female heterozygous for G-6-PD develops chronic myelogenous leukemia, all the lines of blood cells except T-lymphocytes can reveal the same form of the enzyme. So except for T-lymphocytes they are all members of a clone that developed from a single ancestor.

Advantage has been taken of G-6-PD as a marker in studying the basis of another kind of blood disorder called *polycythemia* (Gr. *polys*, many; *kytos*, cell; *haima*, blood; and *ia*, a condition) *vera* (L. *vera*, true), a disease in which there is an overproduction of erythrocytes and to a lesser extent of leukocytes and platelets as well. It has been shown from studies on heterozygous females that this disease is clonal in nature with all the erythrocytes, granular leukocytes, and platelets revealing the same form of the enzyme. But it has also been shown that in this instance neither B- nor T-lymphocytes belong to this clone. Since from the preceding account the G-6-PD and Philadelphia chromosome studies have shown that in humans there is an order of stem cells that can give rise to erythrocytes, granular leukocytes, monocytes, platelets, and B-lymphocytes, the studies on polycythemia vera show there must also be an order of myeloid stem cells of lesser potentiality that give rise to erythrocytes, granular leukocytes, monocytes, and platelets.

Finally, studies utilizing the enzyme G-6-PD as a marker have been made on another type of blood cell disorder termed *sideroblastic anemia* (Gr. *sideros*, iron; *blastos*, germ) because certain precursor (blast) cells of erythrocytes contain demonstrable amounts of iron in the form of granules in their cytoplasm. In such a study Prchal et al. has shown that the same form of the enzyme is present in all lines of blood cells including T-lymphocytes, so that in man as well as in the mouse and rat there is a pluripotential stem cell that serves as the ancestral cell for all forms of blood cells. The previously described studies, however, also show there must be a second order of pluripotential stem cells that can give rise only to erythrocytes, granular leukocytes, monocytes, platelets, and B-lymphocytes. Then there must also be a third order of pluripotential stem cells that can give rise to only erythrocytes, granular leukocytes, monocytes, and platelets. The lineages are shown in the family tree of blood cells in man (Fig. 12-3). However, before describing this we must take into account findings that have been made from studying certain kinds of hematopoietic cells in vitro.

STUDIES ON HEMATOPOIETIC CELLS CULTIVATED IN VITRO

Since it was known that transfusing irradiated animals with untreated bone marrow cells led to cell colonies developing in their spleens, it was of interest to see if bone marrow cells would grow and form colonies outside the body. To ascertain this required the use of semisolid types of media so that if any cells proliferated they would not disperse but would remain close together. Experiments soon led to the finding that colonies of cells did indeed develop in such cultures provided the media also contained a specific regulatory factor, which was called *colony-stimulating factor* (CSF). Since it was not known which marrow cells multiplied to form these colonies, the cell from which they evolved was also designated a colony-forming unit (a CFU). However, since this term alone would confuse it with the cell that formed spleen colonies in irradiated animals it was called a CFU-C, the C indicating it formed a colony in a culture. Even so it was thought that adding a C did not distinguish it sufficiently from the CFU. So in an attempt to prevent confusion it was decided to term the CFU that forms colonies in the spleens of irradiated animals the *CFU-S*, the S indicating it forms colonies in the spleens of irradiated living animals. We think this is neither necessary nor helpful because soon after finding the CFU formed colonies in

the spleen it became known that it corresponds to the enormously important cell serving as the stem cell for all blood cells. As a result the term *CFU* (by itself) came to have a specific meaning, replacing the term *hemocytoblast*. In other words, the letters CFU became established as the specific symbol for the *stem cell of all blood cells*. Now that it also has this specific meaning it only causes confusion to use the term CFU-S to denote the stem cell of all blood cells because it relegates the letters CFU to being only a generic term for a whole class of cells that can form colonies. The fact that the CFU can form colonies in the spleens of irradiated hosts was, of course, important in leading to its discovery. But its importance in the body is not that it can form colonies but that it is the stem cell of all blood cells and moreover normally serves this function without forming a colony. Our view, therefore, is that the term CFU by itself is well enough established not to need any additional letter added to it to distinguish it from a long list of other cells able to form colonies.

CFU-C. As noted, the type of cell from which the first colonies were found to develop in cultures was termed the CFU-C. Microscopic studies of the cells in the colonies first showed that they were of the granular leukocyte series. Later it was found that cells of the monocyte-macrophage line also developed in colonies arising from the CFU-C. This was proven by experiments in which single bone marrow cells were selected and seeded separately in cultures. In some of these cultures single colonies developed. Each of these colonies must have grown from the single cell with which the culture was initially seeded. Yet in many instances the colony was found to contain both neutrophils and macrophages. The single cell from which the colony was derived — the CFU-C — must therefore have had the potentiality to differentiate along more than one line, the one leading to the formation of neutrophils and the other to macrophages, which are believed to be derived from monocytes.

Furthermore, Metcalf and Moore discovered a variety of leukemia that developed in certain strains of mice which showed an overproduction in the animals concerned of both granular leukocytes and monocytes. As a result of all these findings it became obvious that the CFU-C was the progenitor cell of both the neutrophil and the monocyte-macrophage lines of blood cells (*see* Fig. 12-3).

CFU-E. It was at first thought that only one kind of cell present in bone marrow formed colonies in culture and, as noted previously, because it formed them in culture it was termed the CFU-C. But then by using hematopoietic cells obtained from the livers of 13-day mouse embryos (which would contain CFUs and their various descendants) and by allowing the cells to become trapped in plasma that clotted in an appropriate medium containing the hormone erythropoietin, Stephenson, Axelrad, McLeod, and Shreeve were able to grow colonies of a different type.

These were small, rapidly developing colonies composed of cells that soon stained positively for hemoglobin. The cells differentiated and matured as the colony formed, leading finally to loss of the nucleus from each cell and the production of erythrocytes, apparently in much the same way as occurs during erythropoiesis in vivo, which is shown in Figure 12-6 (arrow, *lower right center*). Although the first successful erythrocytic cultures were grown from mouse fetal liver cells, it later became possible to grow colonies of erythropoietic cells from many sources, including human bone marrow.

It was evident both from the type of differentiation within the colonies and from the different nature of the factors required for their development that the progenitors of erythrocytic colonies were distinct from those of neutrophil-macrophage colonies, although both developed in culture. Stephenson et al. suggested that the erythropoietin-responsive entity from which each erythrocytic colony developed be termed the CFU-E (E originally stood for "that responds to erythropoietin" but more recently has come to mean "of the erythrocytic line of differentiation" or simply "erythrocytic"). The CFU-E has been formally shown by Cormack to be a single cell. He did this using time lapse cinemicrography with violet light. The fact that hemoglobin has an absorption maximum at the wavelength of violet light permitted him to trace the development of individual colonies of hemoglobin-containing cells backward to their origin from single cells.

After the discovery of the pluripotential hematopoietic stem cell, it was at first believed that erythropoietin (which was discovered much earlier) exerted its effect by inducing pluripotential stem cells to differentiate into morphologically recognizable erythrocytic precursor cells. Experiments in vivo in which variation in the level of erythropoietin was shown to have a profound effect on the rate of erythrocyte production had no immediate effect on the pluripotential hematopoietic stem cells. Consequently the idea was introduced of erythropoietin acting not on the pluripotential stem cells themselves but on cells forming from them that are committed so as to be responsive to erythropoietin. These exist, in a family tree, between the pluripotential stem cell and the morphologically recognizable erythrocytic precursor cell as shown in Figure 12-3 on page 306. Subsequent work in vitro has fully confirmed this notion and furthermore has shown that between the pluripotential stem cell and the cells recognizable with the LM there are cells at several levels of differentiation that are responsive to erythropoietin.

The CFU-E is a large, motile, proliferating cell, which does not appear to synthesize hemoglobin in detectable amounts until it is exposed to erythropoietin (to which it is exquisitely sensitive). Then it stops moving and its program of hemoglobin synthesis and morphological differentiation is turned on. From here on, no more than 5 or 6 cell divisions will take place before the cells in the colony lose their nuclei and become red blood cells.

BFU-E. Axelrad, McLeod, Shreeve, and Heath next showed there was an earlier colony-forming progenitor than the CFU-E along the erythrocytic line of differentiation. In culture it produced a striking picture, a large mass of mostly hemoglobin-containing cells in numerous colony-like groups either scattered about or fused together. This was called an *erythropoietic burst* and the kind of progenitor that gave rise to it was called a *BFU-E* (for "burst-forming unit responding to erythropoietin" or "burst-forming unit—erythropoietic"). The BFU-E is relatively small compared with the CFU-E (as shown by unit gravity sedimentation), with much greater proliferative capacity. Recently Gregory has provided evidence that BFU-Es constitute an early and a late type, with slightly different properties. It is believed that each BFU-E can give rise to a large number of CFU-Es, each of which in turn produces a number of red blood cells, thus achieving great amplification in cell number. Erythropoietin is known to act on the CFU-E to permit or induce its differentiation into morphologically recognizable erythrocytic precursors; its action is probably required continuously throughout this process. Whether erythropoietin or other regulatory factors act on BFU-E is still an open question.

BFU-Es circulate in peripheral blood, from which they can be readily cultured. CFU-Es do not seem to circulate under ordinary conditions. The number of BFU-Es in the circulation is high in the severe anemias associated with disorders of hemoglobin synthesis. BFU-Es under these conditions may be involved in the colonization and conversion of yellow to red marrow. There is evidence that the BFU-E is capable of differentiating along more than one line: it gives rise to the progenitors of megakaryocytic colonies as well as those of erythrocytic colonies in culture (*see* Fig. 12-3).

Recently Johnson and Metcalf, using mouse fetal liver cells, and Fauser and Messner, using human bone marrow cells, have been able to grow mixed colonies in culture in the presence of complex conditioned media. These colonies were composed of cells of the erythrocytic, granulocytic, and megakaryocytic lines of differentiation. Since each colony was a clone, its progenitor must have been at least tripotential. Thus, tissue culture methods that were originally confined to the assay of unipotential hematopoietic progenitors are now being extended in range to include hematopoietic cells that are less restricted in their potentiality.

Other Types of Colony-Forming Progenitors. A very important aspect of the development of cells along the vari-

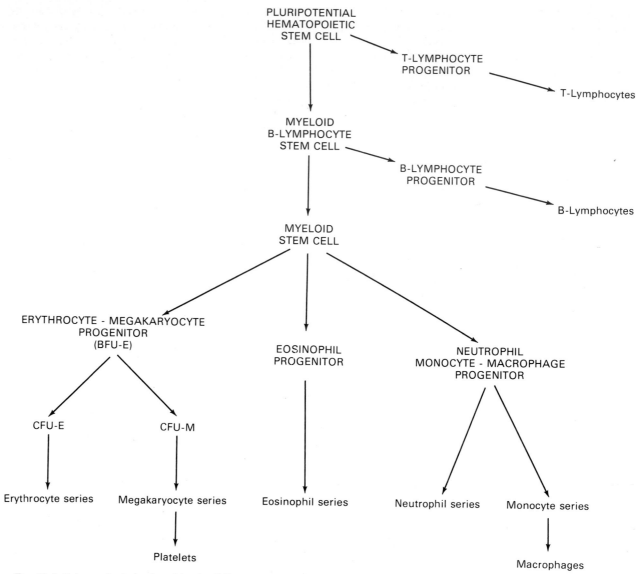

Fig. 12-3. Schema depicting how blood cell lineages originate from pluripotential hematopoietic stem cells. Very little is known about the origin of basophils, but they would presumably arise from the myeloid type of stem cell.

ous lines of hematopoietic differentiation has become clear as a result of research on hematopoietic colony formation in vitro. That is, a progenitor cell will only produce a colony of differentiating cells of a particular type if it is exposed to a specific factor. These factors are glycoproteins and they differ for the different types of colonies.

Thus it has now become possible, largely through the efforts of Metcalf and his group in Melbourne, to separate the factor responsible for eosinophilic colony formation from that responsible for neutrophil-macrophage colony formation. The progenitors of these colonies also seem to be different, so the entity that

used to be called CFU-C had to be subdivided still further. It is now possible to distinguish six distinct lines of differentiation in clonal colony culture under the influence of different regulatory factors: granulocyte-macrophage (with GM-CFC denoting the progenitor), erythropoietic (BFU-E and CFU-E), eosinophilic (EO-CFC), megakaryocytic (CFU-M), B-lymphocytic (BL CFC), and T-lymphocytic (TL-CFC). These culture methods also have the advantage of serving as assay methods for the specific regulatory factors responsible for the production of colonies along the different lines of hematopoietic differentiation. These assay methods in turn are being used to follow the purification and characterization of the individual factors—a very active area of research at the present time.

Since these regulatory factors influence cell differentiation they must somehow permanently affect gene expression in those cells in which they exert their effects.

Differentiation Pathways. In charts of the cells arising from the CFU that are insufficiently differentiated for them to be recognizable by microscopy, it is customary to designate the morphologically unrecognizable cells only by initials denoting the assay method by which they are studied and not to attempt to illustrate their appearance because of the uncertainty due to their low frequency and lack of distinguishing features. A tentative chart of the interrelationships and differentiation pathways of the cells discussed above would therefore appear as shown in Figure 12-3.

PART 2: THE HISTOLOGY OF MYELOID TISSUE AND THE STAGES OF BLOOD CELL FORMATION THAT CAN BE RECOGNIZED WITH THE LM

Basic Features. Myeloid tissue consists of two main components, a connective tissue *stroma* and *free blood cells* in various stages of formation. As already mentioned, stroma is a Greek word meaning anything laid out ready for sitting or lying on. However, free blood cells forming in myeloid tissue do not so much lie on the stroma as within it, for the stroma is a three-dimensional network of connective tissue cells and fibers (reticular and collagenic) with blood cells in all stages of development contained in its meshes.

In postnatal life myeloid tissue is found in man only in the cavities of bones. Myeloid tissue therefore constitutes the marrow of bones; this is why bone marrow is called *myeloid* (Gr. *myelos*, marrow) tissue.

Red and Yellow Marrow. In the adult there are two kinds of marrow, red and yellow. The color of red marrow is due to the vast number of red blood cells it is producing. Since yellow marrow is not producing red or any other kinds of blood cells, the space utilized in red marrow for producing blood cells is taken up by *fat cells*, and as fat is more or less yellow, the marrow too is yellow.

In the fetus the marrow of most bones is red. During the growing period in postnatal life the marrow of most bones becomes yellow, so that in adult man, red marrow is found only in the diploë of the bones of the vault of the skull, the ribs and sternum, the bodies of the vertebrae, the cancellous bone of some short bones, and at the ends of long bones. The marrow in the other sites is yellow.

It is often necessary to obtain a little red marrow for making films of marrow cells or for other kinds of tests. Marrow for these purposes is commonly obtained using a needle to extract some from the sternum. Red marrow can also be obtained from the crest of the ilium.

Under conditions of prolonged need for more blood cells a certain amount of yellow marrow may become replaced by red marrow. There is also some indication that temperature can influence whether marrow is yellow or red, for it has been reported that if the tail of a rat (the bones of which in adult rats ordinarily contain yellow marrow) is kept warmer than it would usually be, the marrow in the bones becomes red.

Why Is Myeloid Tissue, and Hence Formation of Blood Cells of the Myeloid Series, Confined in Adult Man to the Cavities of Bones? It helps in understanding the histology of bone marrow to be curious as to how a bony cavity could facilitate the formation of blood cells and promote their entry into the circulation. In the following we shall give some reasons.

First, a bony cavity is nonexpandable. If, for example, blood cell formation were to occur in the stroma of an expandable tissue like loose connective tissue, which of course is supplied with capillaries, the blood cells formed would merely be pushed farther and farther into the intercellular substance. There would be no inducement for them to migrate through the walls of capillaries or venules to enter the bloodstream. However, inside a bony cavity only a limited population of blood cells can be accommodated. As more are formed there is no place for them to go except into the bloodstream. In myeloid tissue this is made easy because of its being provided with wide, very thin-walled blood channels, called *sinusoids*, through whose walls the newly formed blood cells make their way into the bloodstream and are carried away by it.

THE HISTOLOGY OF SINUSOIDS

Sinusoids are not seen to advantage in ordinary H and E sections because the stroma in between the sinusoids is so packed with developing nucleated blood cells. With low power the stroma appears as a mass of blue nuclei (Fig. 12-4), which seem to impinge on, and squeeze, the sinusoids in their midst. However, here and there in this mass of forming blood cells, sinusoids can be dimly discerned as little patches of red blood cells surrounded by endothelial walls (Fig. 12-4). Sinusoids are seen to much better advantage in H and E sections of marrow taken from animals that have been given enough radiation to

endothelial   megakaryocyte
cells   sinusoids

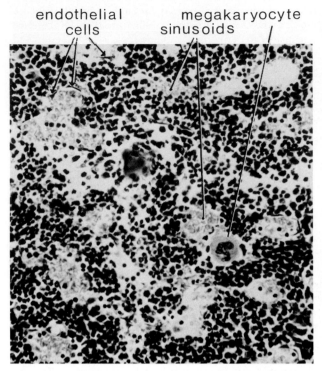

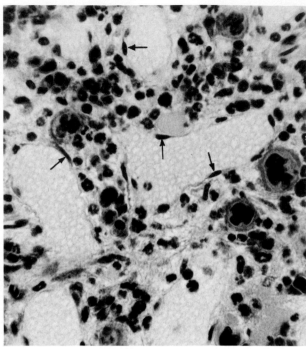

Fig. 12-4. Low-power photomicrograph of red bone marrow. This section shows numerous sinusoids, most of which contain red blood cells. Between them are innumerable cells of the erythrocytic and granular leukocytic series. A megakaryocyte is present at *lower middle right*. In a few sites the flat endothelial cells lining the sinusoids may be seen.

Fig. 12-5. Photomicrograph of bone marrow of a mouse 1 day after it was given a heavy dose of radiation. The cells between the sinusoids are undergoing pyknotic changes and the sinusoids are congested. The arrows point to nuclei of endothelial cells lining the sinusoids.

have arrested mitosis in the developing blood cells in the stroma between them. A cessation of mitosis prevents expansion of the mass of developing blood cells between the sinusoids; furthermore, many of the proliferating blood cell precursors die so that there is now enough space for the sinusoids to expand and for their shape and the lining of endothelial cells to be seen (Fig. 12-5).

The sinusoids have very weak walls that consist of endothelial cells supported only by delicate reticular fibers. It was believed a decade or so ago that the endothelial cells of sinusoids were of a special kind called reticuloendothelial cells, thicker than ordinary endothelial cells, and moreover phagocytic. The latter concept was based on the finding that if animals were given an intravenous injection of vital stain (described on page 253), it was picked up by what with the LM seemed to be the lining cells of sinusoids. The EM, however, has shown that the endothelium itself is not phagocytic. The impression that it was phagocytic was due, as the EM revealed, to pseudopodia of macrophages in the stroma extending in between the endothelial cells into the sinusoids, as shown

at *upper right* in Figure 12-6. So it is these pseudopodia that are responsible for phagocytosing vital stains from the bloodstream. It is therefore now believed that the endothelium lining the sinusoids is essentially similar to that elsewhere in that it lacks phagocytic properties. However, it does permit the exodus of newly formed blood cells of all types from the stroma into the lumina of the sinusoids. This appears to be achieved by the blood cells burrowing their way through temporary perforations in the endothelial cell cytoplasm. The migration pores are in all probability only present just as the newly formed cells are trying to get in, so access to the sinusoids seems to be an active process requiring motility in the newly formed blood cells.

Why Do Sinusoids Not Collapse? It might be thought that an expanding population of blood cells in the stroma might impinge upon the thin walls of a sinusoid to such an extent that it would cause the sinusoid to collapse and not be able to carry away the newly formed blood cells. Why this does not happen requires some explanation.

In bone marrow the sinusoids perform a function capil-

Fig. 12-6. Low-power electron micrograph (×1,700) showing the general appearance of myeloid tissue (rat), following intravenous injection of colloidal carbon so as to demonstrate macrophages (M). At *upper right* a macrophage is extending a large pseudopodium (indicated by arrow) up into the lumen of a sinusoid (S). Phagocytosed carbon particles are visible within this pseudopodium. Another macrophage (M), *left of center,* is phagocytosing a nucleus (indicated by an arrow) probably recently extruded from a normoblast in the island of developing erythroid cells (E) *above center.* Note the increasing electron density in the developing erythroid cells (E), due to accumulation of hemoglobin. A cell at the top of the island (indicated by asterisk) is in mitosis. Below the erythroid island, developing cells of the granulocytic series (My) may be seen. At *bottom,* a megakaryocyte (Meg) at *left* and a fat cell (F) at *right* are evident. Just above the fat cell a normoblast is extruding its nucleus (*arrow*). (Courtesy of S. Luk and G. Simon)

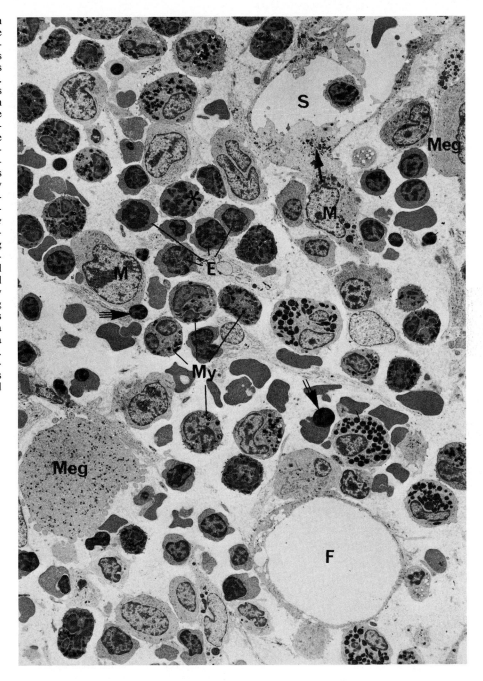

laries perform in most tissues, that of connecting the arterial side of the circulation with the venous side. As already noted, sinusoids have very weak walls. Accordingly, the only explanation for their not collapsing when the cell population increases outside them would be that they are kept open by the hydrostatic pressure within them equalling that outside them. The maintenance of this

hydrostatic pressure in sinusoids is to be explained by a special feature of the blood supply of bones: the chief arterial supply is brought through a bone to its marrow cavity and then the blood passes outwardly from the marrow cavity in vessels that drain through the bony walls of the cavity. Furthermore, as will be described in connection with the blood supply of bone in Chapter 15, the venous drainage of a bone is more restricted than that of most tissues (the nutrient vein of a bone being of smaller diameter than its companion artery), which suggests a somewhat elevated hydrostatic pressure might exist in marrow sinusoids. In other words, a condition could exist in sinusoids that would result in edema in other sites (*see* Fig. 8-7A). However, this pressure keeping the sinusoids open in marrow would not cause edema here because the marrow, being contained by bony walls, cannot swell.

It might be argued that since in certain animals some myeloid hematopoiesis occurs in postnatal life in the spleen, a bony cavity is not essential. However, it should be noted that the spleen possesses a tough capsule and that it is kept distended in life by hydrostatic pressure within it; at death it immediately collapses to a much smaller size. The spleen moreover is riddled with sinusoids that stay open and through whose walls blood cells, newly formed in the spleen, can pass. Hence where myeloid hematopoiesis occurs in the spleen it would seem to do so under much the same conditions of hydrostatic pressure as that occurring in bony cavities.

The next problem to consider is why circulating CFUs evidence a predilection for settling out in the stroma of the marrow of bony cavities and for forming blood cells of the myeloid series there. But to discuss this interesting problem we must first describe the stroma cells of bone marrow and, in particular, their origin.

THE CELLS OF THE STROMA OF MYELOID TISSUE

Fibroblasts. There are enough fibroblasts to form the collagenic fibers that support the arteries and arterioles bringing blood to the marrow and the venules and veins draining it away. The fibers associated with these vessels constitute the main basic support for marrow.

Reticular Cells. These are probably the most elusive cells of any tissue to delineate histologically. The name *reticular* is given to cells if they form a network of some kind. They can do this merely by sending out cytoplasmic processes that connect with those of adjacent cells so as to form a network of cell processes with spaces between them. Or, if cells produce fine fibers so as to produce a three-dimensional network of delicate fibers in which they lie either independently or connected by cytoplasmic processes, they too are termed reticular cells. The name *reticular*, however, is descriptive and does not signify origin. In the cortex of the thymus the reticulum is derived from epithelium. In bone marrow the reticulum consists of a three-dimensional network of delicate fibers produced by mesenchyme-derived reticular cells. Blood cell formation occurs in the interstices of this net.

The reticular cells of marrow are generally described as large irregularly shaped cells with pale cytoplasm and pale-staining nuclei. It has been shown by labeling experiments with tritiated thymidine that they have a very slow turnover time. Some at least may perform functions other than that of producing reticular fibers. It has been suggested that some may have phagocytic properties. Some, moreover, play an indirect role in immunological reactions that will be described in Chapter 13.

Macrophages. These are fairly numerous in marrow where they play a phagocytic role. As noted they account for the phagocytosis previously attributed to the endothelial cells of sinusoids (*see upper right* corner of Fig. 12-6). They are derived from monocytes.

Fat Cells. Fat cells full of fat (Fig. 12-6. F) are present here and there in red marrow. However, they constitute most of the cells of yellow marrow.

Endothelial Cells. These make up the walls of sinusoids (Fig. 12-5) as already described. They are not as effectively joined to one another in sinusoids as in capillaries, hence sinusoids probably leak plasma.

Osteogenic Cells. Osteogenic cells, as will be described in detail in Chapter 15, are stem cells of the skeletal tissues (cartilage and bone). Whereas their presence in bone marrow has been described for decades, it has been thought until very recently that their presence in myeloid tissue was merely incidental to the fact that the marrow was close to the bone they and their progeny had formed, and that their role in marrow was to provide for more bone formation when it was required, for example in the repair of a fracture. However, it now appears that their role in marrow may be of extraordinary importance in that they or their immediate progeny may be responsible for inducing the CFU to form cells of the myeloid series in myeloid tissue. This concept is best explained by describing the origin of osteogenic cells and the other cells involved in the formation of marrow stroma.

THE ORIGIN OF THE STROMAL CELLS OF BONE MARROW

For bone marrow to develop, there must first be a developing bone. As will be described in detail in Chapters 14 and 15, the first step in the formation of most bones is for a mass of closely packed mesenchymal cells (Fig. 15-36) to differentiate into a solid model of cartilage that has the form of the bone that will later take its place (Fig. 15-37). Because cartilage has no capillaries its cells are dependent on nutrients diffusing from outside the cartilage through its intercellular substance to supply its cells. But when the cartilage model increases in size its midsection is so far removed from its exterior from which nutrients are derived that its cells begin to die and the intercellular substance around them begins to become calcified and disintegrate, leaving large irregular holes in the central part of the cartilage model (Fig. 15-40). These holes constitute the beginning of a marrow cavity.

Concomitantly, all around the periphery of the cartilage model mesenchymal cells have become flattened to form a layered cellular membrane. This is at first called the *perichondrium* (Fig. 15-37, P) and later as the cartilage model begins to become replaced by bone it is called the *periosteum*. The deeper cells of this membrane are called *osteogenic* (or *osteoprogenitor*) cells and they can multiply and differentiate into either cartilage or bone-forming cells, depending on their microenvironment.

Soon osteogenic cells of the periosteum begin to form a layer of bone girdling the cartilage model. By this time capillaries from the adjacent mesenchyme have come close to the model. Then some capillaries and perivascular mesenchymal cells accompanying the capillaries burst through the cartilage model at some site and grow into the cavity that has formed in its midsection. Osteogenic cells from the periosteum accompany the capillaries and the perivascular mesenchymal cells in this invasion. These are the *three components* of what is termed the *periosteal bud* and it is from these that the stroma of marrow develops. The site of the periosteal bud later becomes the site of entry and exit of the nutrient artery and vein of the bone.

It is because the stromal cells of bone marrow are derived from the cells of the periosteal bud that one has to know something about bone before trying to understand the special nature of the stromal cells of marrow. The endothelial cells of the capillaries of the bud give rise to the endothelial cells of the arteries, arterioles, venules, and veins of the marrow and the walls of the sinusoids. The perivascular mesenchymal cells that accompany the capillaries give rise to the fibroblasts, reticular cells, and fat cells of the marrow stroma. The osteogenic cells of the bud, while comprising part of the stroma, also cover up all the dead cartilage and form bone on it so that in the early marrow cavity the developing marrow is riddled with bony trabeculae that have remnants of cartilage as their cores. An event then occurs which aroused little curiosity for decades: almost as soon as the marrow stroma begins to form as described above, blood cell formation commences in it. The probable reason for this event not seeming remarkable was that it was then believed that blood cell formation was due to an undifferentiated type of marrow stromal cell giving rise to the free stem cells of blood cells. But we now know that the reason for blood cell formation beginning in developing marrow is that CFUs, circulating in the bloodstream, are carried into the forming marrow via the capillaries of the periosteal bud, and here they settle out in the marrow stroma to give rise to cells of the myeloid series. There must, therefore, be some microenvironmental influence in a developing mar-

row cavity to cause them to do so. The osteogenic cells (and possibly also elevated hydrostatic pressure) are the most likely candidates for providing the signal to CFUs that this is the place to settle, proliferate, and differentiate. Evidence implicating osteogenic cells in this process will now be described.

It has always been of interest that occasionally little bits of bone will develop in ordinary connective tissues, far removed from any normal bony structure. Usually such pieces of bone develop in an old abdominal scar or in the wall of an old degenerated artery. What seems curious, however, is that often myeloid tissue develops in them. Recently it has been shown that bone formation can be experimentally induced in ordinary connective tissue by implanting specially prepared decalcified bone intercellular substance (Urist et al.; *see* references in Chap. 15). This induces osteogenic cells to develop from any cells present that have retained enough mesenchymal potentiality (presumably pericytes) to become osteogenic cells, and these can form both cartilage and bone. Hematopoiesis then begins in the cavity of the induced bone. Here again it would seem that osteogenic cells are the factor that induces CFUs to settle out from the blood.

Another finding indicating a close association between osteogenesis and blood cell formation is that in the repair of fractures, particularly of rabbit ribs, repair is associated with the formation of a great deal of cartilage in the callus that develops to connect the two fragments of rib together. This cartilage, as in the development of a bone, plays only a temporary supportive role and soon begins to become calcified and cavitate and, as occurs in the development of a bone, the cavities are invaded by capillaries and osteogenic cells. The latter proliferate, differentiate into osteoblasts, and form bone on the cartilage remnants. But as this occurs, hematopoiesis also begins in the spaces into which the osteogenic cells and capillaries have penetrated. Indeed this association between osteogenesis and blood cell formation is so striking in the repair of fractures that it should have suggested long ago that there might be some kind of a cause-and-effect relationship between the two processes of bone and blood cell formation.

It is significant in this connection that Friedenstein et al., having obtained pure cultures of marrow stromal cells and passaged them several times, found that when they transplanted cells from the cultures to sites beneath the capsule of kidneys in recipients immunologically compatible with the marrow donors, the transplanted stromal cells not only formed new bone, but hematopoiesis began in the newly formed bone. The blood cells that formed here were of host origin and so were not derived from the transplanted cells. From their findings, they concluded that the stromal cells, which they regarded as fibroblasts with osteogenic potentiality (cells that we would call osteogenic cells), were capable in their new site of providing the proper microenvironment for myeloid hematopoiesis.

From all the foregoing it seems reasonable to believe that CFUs are able to form the myeloid series of cells in bone marrow because marrow stromal cells with osteogenic potentialities, lining the surfaces of bone cavities and existing in its stroma, provide the right sort of microenvironment for facilitating localization of circulating CFUs in this tissue and promoting their proliferation and differentiation into the cells of the myeloid series. At any rate, we should no longer be content to accept that myeloid hematopoiesis in man is confined to bones without trying to find out why.

THE FORMATION OF ERYTHROCYTES (ERYTHROPOIESIS)

The immediate progenitor cell for this cell lineage seems to be the erythropoietin-sensitive CFU-E, provided we use this term in this instance to cover a population of cells that is moderately heterogeneous with respect to size and sensitivity to erythropoietin. The most mature of these cells probably corresponds to what is recognized microscopically as the proerythroblast. We shall, in the following, deal only with the cells of the erythrocytic lineage that can be identified by light microscopy in stained films of bone marrow. These are illustrated in Plate 12-1. We shall begin with the proerythroblast.

Morphologically Recognizable Stages

The *proerythroblast* is relatively large, ranging from 12 to 15 μm. in diameter. In stained films the chromatin of the nucleus is finely granular and the nucleus commonly reveals two prominent nucleoli. The cytoplasm is mildly basophilic (Plate 12-1). With the EM one important feature discerned in this type of cell and those that evolve from it is the relative lack of development of rER and Golgi. Another is that as the proerythroblast differentiates, more and more free ribosomes and polyribosomes appear; these become diffusely distributed throughout the cytoplasm. In the cytoplasm, moreover, there are some bundles of microtubules which are peripherally arranged more or less parallel with the cell surface.

The proerythroblast can proliferate, and on differentiation its progeny become what are termed *basophilic erythroblasts*. In stained films these are somewhat smaller than proerythroblasts. Their rounded nucleus is smaller and their chromatin is more condensed (Plate 12-1). Their cytoplasm is intensely basophilic.

With the EM the basophilia of the cytoplasm, noted with the LM, is seen to be due to its great content of polyribosomes (Fig. 12-7). The development of other organelles ordinarily seen in the cytoplasm is minimal.

The next step in differentiation along this line leads to the basophilic erythroblasts becoming *polychromatophilic erythroblasts* (Plate 12-1). The polychromatophilia observed in films stained with blood stains is due to the polyribosomes (which are basophilic) combining with the basic stains in the blood stain while the hemoglobin which is now being synthesized along polyribosomes is acidophilic and combines with the eosin of the blood stain. The net result is that the cytoplasm takes on a muddy-gray or bluish-pink color (Plate 12-1). The nucleus of the polychromatophilic erythroblast is somewhat smaller than that of the basophilic variety, and its chromatin is in the form of coarse granules which commonly are clumped so that the nucleus as a whole is very basophilic. No nucleoli can be seen in it. The polychromatophilic erythroblast is the last cell in the erythroid series capable of mitosis. Its nucleus soon becomes pyknotic and it is commonly extruded while the cytoplasm is still slightly polychromatophilic. This results in the formation of a *polychromatophilic erythrocyte,* as shown at *bottom left* in Plate 11-1.

As has been described already, the polychromatophilic erythrocyte is called a *reticulocyte* (*bottom right* in Plate 11-1) when it is stained by supravital technics because polyribosomes still present in its cytoplasm show up under these conditions as if they were in the form of a reticulum.

Another fate of polychromatophilic erythroblasts is for them, as they continue to divide, to lose evidence of their cytoplasmic basophilia. When this has happened, the cell is termed a *normoblast* (Plate 12-1) (also called orthochromatic erythroblast) because it is going to give rise to a normocytic erythrocyte. By this time a normoblast has a small spherical dark-staining pyknotic nucleus (Plate 12-1). This is lost by extrusion (Fig. 12-6). The many extruded nuclei of normoblasts are mostly phagocytosed by the macrophages of the stroma (Fig. 12-6). Occasionally, small particles of the nucleus are left behind in erythrocytes; these are called Howell-Jolly bodies.

The Fine Structure of Erythroblasts

Several erythroblasts are seen in Figure 12-7. Their most interesting feature is their great content of ribosomes and polyribosomes. Since basophilic erythroblasts multiply to some extent, their free ribosomes are essential for synthesizing more cell substance. However, their numbers of free ribosomes decrease as the cells mature. The polyribosomes represent sites where the globin chains of hemoglobin molecules are synthesized in the cytoplasm.

The increasing electron density of the cytoplasm of ma-

Fig. 12-7. Electron micrograph (×6,000) of an island of developing erythropoietic cells (in the liver of 5-day-old mouse). Three stages in maturation of red blood cells can be seen. Erythroblasts are lying in close apposition to liver cells. Their nuclear chromatin is clumped and their cytoplasm contains large numbers of free ribosomes. Right of *center* lies a reticulocyte. Its nucleus has been extruded and small mitochondria can still be seen in its cytoplasm. Ribosomes are present but the electron density of the cytoplasm is due to its content of hemoglobin. Above the reticulocyte is a mature erythrocyte. Its cytoplasm is very electron-dense owing to its high content of hemoglobin. No ribosomes or other organelles can be recognized in the cytoplasm of the mature erythrocyte. (Courtesy of K. Arakawa)

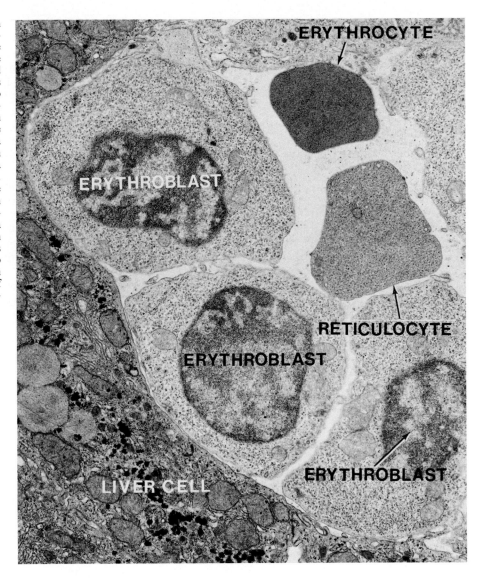

turing erythroblasts is to be explained by hemoglobin accumulating in their cytoplasm. Hemoglobin, of course, contains iron and for other reasons as well it is very electron-dense; this accounts for the fact that the next stage of the red cell series — the reticulocyte — is electron-dense (Fig. 12-7), as are erythrocytes themselves (Fig. 12-7). Under normal conditions, the body is very economical of iron and uses that obtained from old, worn-out red cells phagocytosed by macrophages of spleen and bone marrow for the synthesis of hemoglobin in new ones. But, under certain conditions, the body may suffer a deficiency of iron, and, as a result, an iron-deficiency anemia can occur. This is commonly of the hypochromic type (Fig. 10-5A).

The Regulation of Erythrocyte Production

A lack of proper supply of oxygen to the tissues stimulates the production of erythrocytes in the marrow and this effect is mediated by the glycoprotein hormone *erythropoietin*, which exerts its effect at the level of the BFU-E and the CFU-E. Erythrocyte production becomes greatly depressed if animals are transfused so as to raise their erythrocyte count far above normal. Under these circumstances the number of CFU-Es falls rapidly because their formation from BFU-Es, or perhaps their survival, depends on the availability of erythropoietin. In contrast, the number of BFU-Es does not fall so much; they remain available to give rise to new CFU-Es when

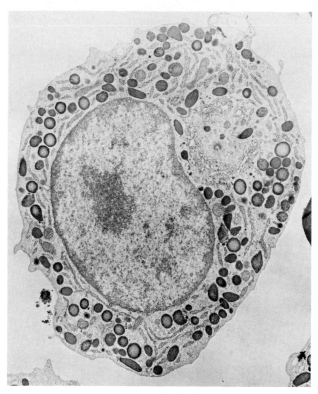

Fig. 12-8. Electron micrograph (×15,000) of a promyelocyte, reacted for the enzyme peroxidase. The only granules formed at this time are peroxidase-positive; these are lysosomes and correspond to the azurophilic granules seen with the LM. Note the well-developed Golgi at the indentation of the nucleus. (Bainton, D. F., Ullyot, J. L., and Farquhar, M. G.: J. Exp. Med., *134:*907, 1971)

erythropoietin production resumes. (Erythropoietin or its precursor is believed to be made mainly in the kidneys, but its precise source in these organs has not yet been clearly established.)

The Pathway by Which Erythrocytes Enter the Bloodstream

Different views have been held on this matter. It has been suggested that erythrocytes and the other types of newly formed blood cells pass through the cytoplasm of the endothelial cells of sinusoids by way of migration pores that appear only at the time of migration. When nucleated red cells (normoblasts) attempt passage through the vessel wall, their cytoplasm is elastic enough for the cytoplasmic portion to squeeze through but the nucleus is left behind, so that the erythrocyte that enters the circulation is enucleated. The naked nucleus is then promptly ingested by a macrophage. It should not, however, be concluded that red blood cells *must* lose their

nuclei in this way. In cultures where there are no sinusoids, developing erythrocytes nevertheless extrude their nuclei. It is also evident that reticulocytes are motile and thus have the capacity to enter sinusoids by active movement, without having to be squeezed through their walls passively.

THE FORMATION OF GRANULAR LEUKOCYTES (GRANULOPOIESIS)

The earliest stage in the granular leukocyte series that is usually considered readily distinguishable morphologically is the *promyelocyte* (Plate 12-1 and Fig. 12-8). However, since the granules first formed in cells of the granulocytic series are not of different specific types, it is impractical to attempt to distinguish different types of promyelocytes.

Morphologically Recognizable Stages of Formation of the Three Types of Granulocytes

The next step in differentiation along the granulocytic line is represented by the formation of *myelocytes* (Plate 12-1) from promyelocytes. This involves changes in the appearance of both the nucleus and the cytoplasm of the cells and a reduction in the size of the cells concerned (Plate 12-1). Whereas the nucleus of the promyelocyte is only slightly indented, the nucleus of the myelocyte begins to appear as an indented oval (Plate 12-1 and Fig. 12-9). Generally a cell is not called a myelocyte unless it has at least a dozen or so granules in its cytoplasm. However, more mature myelocytes may be loaded with granules. The granules that appear in the cell at this time may permit three different kinds of myelocytes to be distinguished. These mature to form the three kinds of granular leukocytes (Plate 12-1), and in the maturation process they pass through a *metamyelocyte* (Gr. *meta*, beyond) stage (Fig. 12-9), by which stage they have lost their capacity for mitosis.

EM STUDIES OF THE DEVELOPMENT OF POLYMORPHS

The fine structure of the cells leading to the formation of neutrophils has been investigated in detail by Bainton et al.

At the promyelocyte stage the granules of a polymorph are all of the azurophilic type (Figs. 12-8 and 12-9); these are either spherical or ovoid in shape. Rough ER can be seen scattered about in the cytoplasm and the Golgi is prominent close to the indentation in the nucleus in Figure 12-8. The azurophilic granules bud from Golgi sac-

Fig. 12-9. Diagram illustrating the development of neutrophil (pmn) leukocytes. Azurophilic granules (lysosomes) are represented in black and specific neutrophilic granules are depicted as circles. A description of the stages is given in the text. (Bainton, D. F., Ullyot, J. L., and Farquhar, M. G.: J. Exp. Med., *134*:907, 1971)

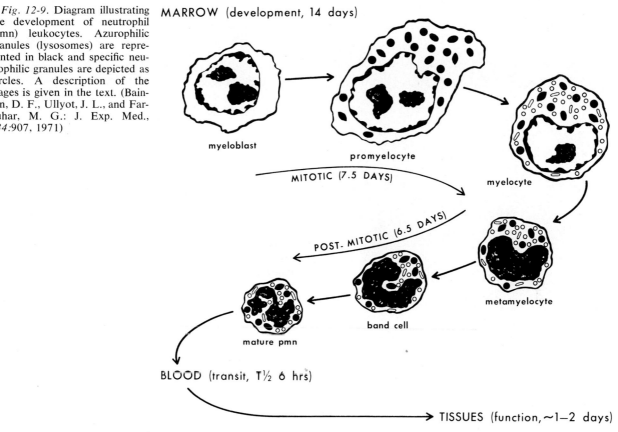

MARROW (development, 14 days)

myeloblast

promyelocyte

MITOTIC (7.5 DAYS)

myelocyte

POST-MITOTIC (6.5 DAYS)

metamyelocyte

band cell

mature pmn

BLOOD (transit, T½ 6 hrs)

TISSUES (function, ~1–2 days)

cules on the *concave* side of a stack; they are peroxidase-positive and represent lysosomes. The production of this kind of granule soon ends. The large number of them found at the promyelocyte stage decreases in the course of maturation toward the mature granulocyte. From the myelocyte stage on, granules of a new type begin to form, arising from the *convex* surface of the Golgi stack (Farquhar and Bainton). These granules are smaller and less dense than those produced earlier. They are the *specific neutrophilic granules* (appearing as circles in Fig. 12-9). The specific granules of developing neutrophils vary somewhat in size but are both smaller and rounder than the azurophilic granules (Fig. 11-3). They are not peroxidase-positive as are the azurophilic granules. Their function and that of the azurophilic granules was described on page 282.

The time course of the development and maturation of a polymorph is shown in Figure 12-9. The polymorph develops from a progenitor cell (labeled myeloblast in Figure 12-9), which some believe is a recognizable cell derived from a CFU-C and represents the immediate precursor of promyelocytes. At the promyelocyte stage the cell develops the azurophilic granules as already

described (black in Fig. 12-9). At the myelocyte stage it develops specific neutrophilic granules (circles in Fig. 12-9) and the azurophilic granules become more scarce. The cell then loses its ability to proliferate. Its subsequent maturation involves some reduction in size and the nucleus changing from the indented oval, through a kidney shape at the metamyelocyte stage, to the *band* (horseshoe) and finally to the lobed (*segmented*) shape (Fig. 12-9 and Plate 12-1). It then enters the bloodstream from which it enters the tissues where required. The times taken for the various stages are given in Figure 12-9.

The Development of Eosinophils

Leukocytes of this lineage are formed from a separate eosinophil progenitor, as indicated in Figure 12-3. The earliest stage that can be recognized morphologically in the eosinophil series is the myelocyte stage (Plate 12-1).

In forming an eosinophilic leukocyte the slightly indented nucleus of the eosinophilic myelocyte generally develops a deep constriction at the metamyelocyte stage of development (Plate 12-1, unlabeled). This deepens to divide the nucleus of the eosinophil into two lobes that

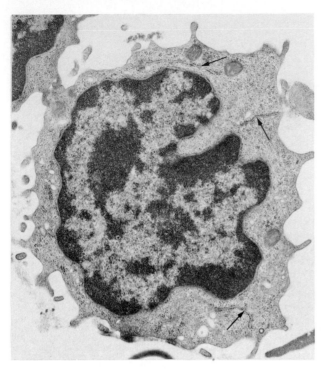

Fig. 12-10. Electron micrograph of a monocytoid cell. The nucleus is irregular in outline and reveals both condensed and extended chromatin. The cytoplasm contains numerous ribosomes and a few cisternae of rER (arrows). Some clear small vesicles are also apparent. (Everett, N. B., and Perkins, W. D.: Hemopoietic stem cell migration. *In* Cairnie, A. B., Lala, P. K., and Osmond, D. G. (eds.): Stem Cells of Renewing Cell Populations. New York, Academic Press, 1976)

usually remain joined together by a thin strand (*lower left* in Plate 11-1). As the constriction develops, the chromatin of the nucleus becomes more condensed and as a result the chromatin takes up a little more stain than the nucleus of a myelocyte. But the condensation of chromatin is not as great as in the neutrophil; hence the nuclei of eosinophils are paler than those of neutrophils (Plate 11-1).

The fine structure of the granules was illustrated in Figure 11-6. Bainton and Farquhar have studied the formation of the granules and shown they are lysosomal in nature and develop similarly to lysosomes in other kinds of cells.

The Development of Basophils

In forming a basophilic leukocyte the nucleus of a basophilic myelocyte undergoes less change than occurs in the formation of a neutrophil or eosinophil. Irregular constrictions may appear but it commonly becomes bilobular. Since its chromatin becomes only partly condensed, it

stains relatively lightly. In contrast, its granules stain deeply, and where spread over the nucleus tend to obscure it (Plate 12-1). The granules of the basophil, unlike those of the eosinophils and the azurophilic granules of neutrophils, are not lysosomal in nature. Since they contain heparin it could be assumed that they develop similarly to the secretory granules of other kinds of cells that secrete sulfated glycosaminoglycans.

THE FORMATION OF MONOCYTES

What could be learned with the LM about the origin and stages in the formation of monocytes was for decades rendered difficult by the realization that what appeared to be all stages of transition between medium-sized lymphocytes and monocytes could be seen in blood films. However, with the EM and tritiated thymidine labeling it became established that monocytes and lymphocytes represent two different lineages and, as described in Part 1 of this chapter, it was proved that monocytes are derived from CFU-C. It seems probable that the first step in differentiation of a CFU-C along the monocyte lineage involves the formation of a member of a class of cells which Everett and Perkins termed *monocytoid* (Fig. 12-10) because some of them, though relatively undifferentiated, possess features suggestive of those of identifiable cells found somewhat later along the monocyte line of differentiation. However, after this early stage in which clear-cut identification is not possible, cell types classed as *promonocytes* or *monoblasts* evolve. At this stage as well as in the preceding one, the cells can cycle but some leave the cycle to differentiate into monocytes. The monocyte itself is believed to be incapable of division. However, labeled thymidine is taken up by what would seem to be the monocyte's immediate precursor, for labeled monocytes appear shortly after labeled thymidine is available in marrow. Stages in the development of monocytes in marrow are not sufficiently clear-cut to be followed with the LM, as are stages in the formation of granulocytes. It is difficult enough as it is to distinguish mature monocytes with the LM in films of marrow cells. The features of fine structure by which they can be identified were described in Chapter 11 (p. 292).

STAGES SEEN WITH THE LM IN THE FORMATION OF LYMPHOCYTES IN MYELOID TISSUE

As mentioned earlier in this chapter, many lymphocytes are formed in marrow. Small lymphocytes do not take up labeled thymidine because small lymphocytes as such do not cycle. The fact that they become labeled in

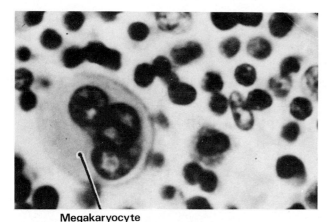

Megakaryocyte

Fig. 12-11. Photomicrograph showing a megakaryocyte in a section of red bone marrow obtained from an infant. The cells in this specimen are less tightly packed than is usual. Note the great size of the megakaryocyte compared with the other free cells of marrow. Three lobes of its multilobar nucleus appear in this plane of section.

due course suggests there must be some progenitor cell in marrow that undergoes mitosis and hence takes up label so that it is inherited by its progeny, small lymphocytes. Such a cell has been described on morphological grounds as existing in marrow, where it has been called a *transitional cell.* The size of this cell is somewhat larger than that of a small lymphocyte. It therefore seems probable that the cell lineage involved in the formation of lymphocytes in mouse marrow is as follows: a progenitor cell having the characteristics of a medium-sized lymphocyte or being somewhat larger proliferates, with its progeny differentiating into small lymphocytes that soon leave the marrow to be replaced by the new ones constantly being formed.

The small lymphocytes formed in the marrow of mammals are in all probability B-lymphocytes. They enter the blood and are filtered out mostly in the spleen but also in the other types of lymphatic tissue except the thymus, as will be explained in Chapter 13. In these tissues they are available for becoming activated by the specific antigens against which they are variously programmed to react. These antigens cause them to proliferate and differentiate into plasma cells producing specific antibodies, as described in the next chapter.

MEGAKARYOCYTES AND THE FORMATON OF PLATELETS

Megakaryocytes (Gr. *megas,* big; *karyon,* nut (nuclues); *kytos,* hollow vessel or cell) are so called because they are big cells with huge nuclei (Figs. 12-11 and 12-

12). The latter are the result of polyploidy, described in connection with Figure 3-17. As well as having a huge nucleus, a megakaryocyte has also a great deal of cytoplasm (Figs. 12-11 and 12-12). The function of the cell is to produce the platelets of the blood, which it does by liberating fragments of cytoplasm that enter the circulation as platelets. In H and E sections of red marrow, megakaryocytes are much larger than any other marrow cells (Figs. 12-4 and 12-11). The nucleus is colored a deep blue with hematoxylin. It may be ovoid in shape or lobulated. A megakaryocyte with a lobulated nucleus may, at the focus at which it is first examined, seem to be a multinucleated cell. But careful focusing of the microscope will show that what at first appear to be separate nuclei are in reality connected to one another. The only cell with which a megakaryocyte is sometimes confused is an osteoclast which is an equally large cell often seen on bone surfaces (Fig. 15-26). However, by focusing up and down, osteoclasts can be seen to be multinucleated cells with separate nuclei. So while osteoclasts and megakaryocytes can usually be distinguished by the fact that osteoclasts are seen on the surface of bone, focusing on nuclei permits osteoclasts seemingly within marrow to be distinguished from megakaryocytes.

Platelet Formation. In 1906 Wright discovered the origin of platelets. He devised a special stain (a variation of the polychrome methylene blue and eosin mixture) and used it to stain thin sections of red marrow, particularly

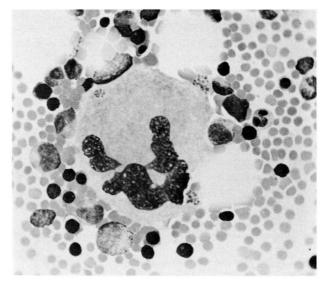

Fig. 12-12. Photomicrograph illustrating the appearance of a megakaryocyte in a stained smear of bone marrow cells. Note the appearance of its multilobar nucleus.

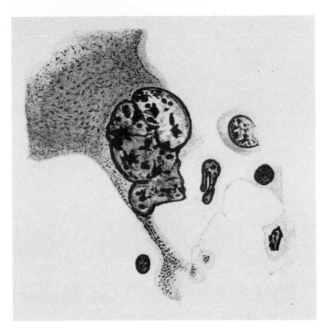

Fig. 12-13. Black-and-white version of one of Wright's colored illustrations of a megakaryocyte forming platelets in a section of kitten bone marrow, stained with Wright's own special blood stain. The picture shows a pseudopodium extending through a thin-walled blood vessel (sinusoid) at *bottom right* and liberating two platelets. (Wright, J. H.: J. Morphol., *21:*263, 1910)

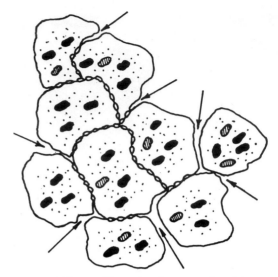

Fig. 12-14. Diagram illustrating the rows of vesicles seen in electron micrographs of mature megakaryocytes and along which the cytoplasm will separate into platelets.

that of kittens and puppies. Figure 12-13 shows his original colored drawing, but in black and white. He observed that megakaryocytes often extended cytoplasmic pseudopodia into the sinusoids of the marrow and, further, that the cytoplasmic pseudopodia stained identically with platelets in that the red granules with which the pseudopodia were stippled resembled the granulomere of a platelet and the remaining substance of the pseudopodia stained similarly to the hyalomere of a platelet (Fig. 12-13). Moreover, he pointed out that only those animals that possess megakaryocytes have platelets. The stippling of the cytoplasm of megakaryocyte cytoplasm can be seen in the low-power electron micrograph, Figure 12-6, where the cell is labeled Meg.

Confirmation that platelets are indeed derived from megakaryocyte cytoplasm came from EM studies. Yamada in 1957 described how the cytoplasm of mature megakaryocytes becomes completely subdivided by an anastomosing system of membranes so as to separate it into numerous compartments, each having its own limiting membrane. The cytoplasm first becomes divided up by the extensive development of membranous vesicles, arranged as shown in Figure 12-14. The size of the regions segregated from one another in this manner corresponds very roughly to that of platelets. The individual

vesicles fuse with adjacent ones (Fig. 12-14) and also with invaginations from the cell membrane, so that the cytoplasm appears riddled with anastomosing *platelet demarcation channels* (Fig. 12-15) and each future platelet becomes surrounded with membrane. It was proposed that by this mechanism platelets, each with its limiting membrane, would be able to separate from the megakaryocyte and still leave it covered with membrane.

It is not easy, however, to visualize a process as complex as platelet formation from sections. To investigate the matter directly, Cormack observed platelet formation by living megakaryocytes in plasma cultures, using time-lapse cinemicrography. Megakaryocytes under these conditions first go through an active amebalike stage, forming and retracting pseudopodia, and may then progressively fragment so as to produce a cloud of active fragments the size of platelets. However, if megakaryocytes adhere to a surface such as that of the culture vessel, they spread out (Fig. 12-16A), actively extending and retracting pseudopodia (Fig. 12-16B and C). Portions of these may detach from the cell (*bottom right* in Fig. 12-16B) and lead an independent existence. Scanning electron micrographs of the interiors of bone marrow sinusoids (such as those of Becker and De Bruyn) show structures termed *proplatelet processes (platelet ribbons)* extending from megakaryocytes into the lumina of sinusoids. Platelet ribbons can also form in vitro at the periphery of adherent megakaryocytes (a platelet ribbon is indicated by arrows in Fig. 12-16C). The bead-like segments in the ribbons forming in vitro are the same size

Color Plate
12-1

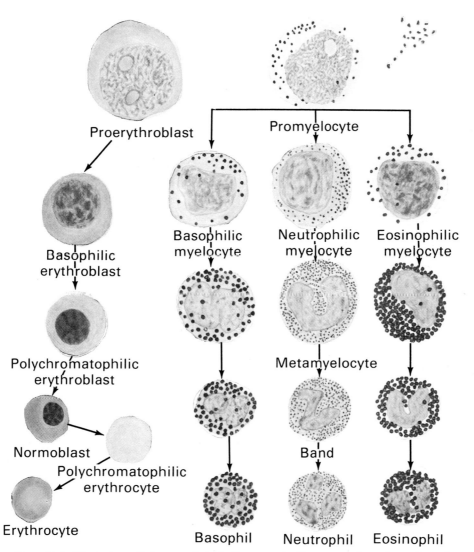

Proerythroblast

Promyelocyte

Basophilic
erythroblast

Basophilic
myelocyte

Neutrophilic
myelocyte

Eosinophilic
myelocyte

Polychromatophilic
erythroblast

Metamyelocyte

Normoblast

Polychromatophilic
erythrocyte

Band

Erythrocyte

Basophil

Neutrophil

Eosinophil

Plate 12-1. Illustration of the morphologically recognizable stages of erythrocytic and granular leukocytic differentiation in myeloid tissue. Normal human bone marrow cells as they appear in films stained with Hastings blood stain.

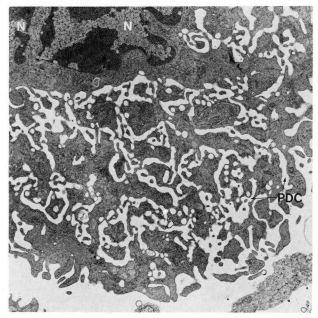

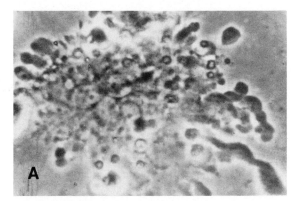

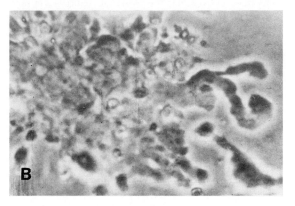

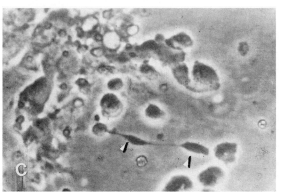

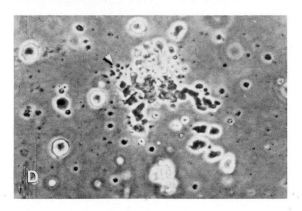

Fig. 12-15. Electron micrograph of a portion of a megakaryocyte (from mouse bone marrow) showing subdivision of its cytoplasm by a network of channels. These platelet demarcation channels (labeled PDC) originate by fusion of smaller vesicles as illustrated in Figure 12-14 and become continuous with the cell surface. Platelets form when fragments of cytoplasm detach from the cell and are released into the circulation. Part of the multilobar nucleus (N) is also shown. (Courtesy of V. Kalnins)

as free platelets and exhibit movement. Platelets may also pinch off a few at a time from the tips of pseudopodia of nonadherent megakaryocytes.

Following the release of its platelets in vitro, only an inactive remnant of the megakaryocyte remains, containing little more than its multilobar nucleus. Commonly this is phagocytosed by a macrophage. The liberation of

Fig. 12-16. Time-lapse photomicrographs showing stages involved in the formation of platelets by a mouse megakaryocyte (phase contrast). The first three photomicrographs (×2,000) illustrate stages in the formation of pseudopodia and a platelet ribbon (indicated by arrows in *C*) at the periphery of a mature megakaryocyte (note its multilobar nucleus, left of *center* in *A,* and its granular cytoplasm). The platelet ribbon (*C*) contains two bead-like segments, each ovoid in shape and about 4 μm. in length, the size of a platelet. These segments later become detached and move away from the body of the megakaryocyte. The same megakaryocyte is seen at a slightly later stage in (*D*) at lower magnification. Another group of recently formed platelets is indicated by the arrow at *upper left* in (*D*). (From the work of D. H. Cormack)

platelets thus appears to be the cell's terminal achievement. In life some platelets are probably liberated a few at a time from the tips of pseudopodia or platelet ribbons, but most would be formed terminally by fragmentation of the entire cytoplasm.

The Formation and Maturation of Megakaryocytes. Megakaryocytes are end cells that undergo mitosis without separation of their daughter chromosomes into separate nuclei and this results in their having a multilobar polyploid nucleus. The progenitor cell type giving rise to colonies of megakaryocytes in vitro, as noted, is called CFU-M. The way this progenitor is thought to arise from the myeloid stem cell is shown in Figure 12-3.

It has been shown that the enormous increase in size of the nucleus due to increasing ploidy is a prelude to the maturation of the cytoplasm permitting the cell to perform its special function of producing platelets.

As mentioned in connection with platelets in Chapter 10, there is some evidence that the production of platelets by megakaryocytes is stimulated by a humoral factor, which probably stimulates their maturation.

REFERENCES AND OTHER READING

THE FORMATION OF BLOOD CELLS IN MYELOID TISSUE

General: Older Concepts (Source book for the older literature)

Downey, H. (ed.): Downey's Handbook of Hematology. New York, Hoeber, 1938.

General: Newer Concepts

Cormack, D. H.: Blood Cell Formation. Film, slides and manual. Toronto, University of Toronto, 1978.
Metcalf, D., and Moore, M. A.: Haemopoietic Cells. Amsterdam, North Holland, 1971.

STEM CELLS AND EARLY PROGENITORS OF BLOOD CELLS

General

Haemopoietic Stem Cells. Ciba Foundation Symposium, 13, New Series. London, Elsevier, 1973.

Special

Adamson, J. W., Filakow, P. J., Murphy, S., Prchal, J. F., and Steinmann, L.: Polycythemia vera: stem cell and probable clonal origin of the disease. N. Engl. J. Med., *295:*913, 1976.
Axelrad, A. A., McLeod, D. L., Shreeve, M. M., and Heath, D. S.: Properties of cells that produce erythrocytic colonies in plasma culture. *In* Robinson, W. A. (ed.): Proceedings of the Second International Workshop of Hemopoiesis in Culture, Airlie, Virginia. p. 226. New York, Grune & Stratton, 1974.
Axelrad, A. A., McLeod, D. L., Suzuki, S., and Shreeve, M. M.: Regulation of the population size of erythropoietic progenitor cells. *In* Differentiation of Normal and Neoplastic Hemopoietic Cells. p. 155. Cold Spring Harbor Laboratory, 1978.
Becker, A. J., McCulloch, E. A., and Till, J. E.: Cytological demonstration of the clonal nature of spleen colonies derived from transplanted mouse marrow cells. Nature, *197:*452, 1963.
van Bekkum, D. W., and Dicke, K. A. (eds.): In Vitro Culture of Hemopoietic Cells. Rijswijk, The Radiobiological Institute TNO, 1972.
van Bekkum, D. W., van Noord, M. J., Maat, B., and Dicke, K. A.: Attempts at identification of hemopoietic stem cell in mouse. J. Hematol., *38:*547, 1971.
Cormack, D.: Time-lapse characterization of erythrocytic colony-forming cells in plasma cultures. Exp. Hematol., *4:*319, 1976.
Curry, J. L., Trentin, J. J., and Cheng, V.: Hemopoietic spleen colony studies III, Hemopoietic nature of spleen colonies induced by lymph node or thymus cells with or without phytohemagglutinin. J. Immunol., *99:*907, 1967.
Everett, N. B., and Perkins, W. D.: Hemopoietic stem cell migration. *In* Cairnie, A. B., Lala, P. K. and Osmond, D. G. (eds.): Stem Cells of Renewing Populations. New York, Academic Press, 1976.
Fauser, A. A., and Messner, H. A.: Identification of megakaryocytes, macrophages, and eosinophils in colonies of human bone marrow containing neutrophilic granulocytes and erythroblasts. Blood, *(in press).*
Fialkow, P. J., Jacobson, R. J., and Papayannopoulou, T.: Chronic myelocytic leukemia: clonal origin in a stem cell common to the granulocyte, erythrocyte, platelet and monocyte/macrophage. Am. J. Med., *63:*125, 1977.
Fowler, J. H., Wu, A. M., Till, J. E., McCulloch, E. A., and Siminovitch, L.: The cellular composition of hemopoietic spleen colonies. J. Cell Physiol., *69:*65, 1967.
Gregory, C. J.: Erythropoietin sensitivity as a differentiation marker in the hemopoietic system: studies of the three erythropoietic colony responses in culture. J. Cell. Physiol., *89:*289, 1976.
Heath , D. S., Axelrad, A. A., McLeod, D. L., and Shreeve, M. M.: Separation of the erythropoietin-responsive progenitors BFU-E and CFU-E in mouse bone marrow by unit gravity sedimentation. Blood, *47:*777, 1976.
Iscove, N. N., and Sieber, F.: Erythroid progenitors in mouse bone marrow detected by macroscopic colony formation in culture. Exp. Hematol., *3:*32, 1975.
Johnson, G. R., and Metcalf, D.: Pure and mixed erythroid colony formation in vitro stimulated by spleen conditioned medium with no detectable erythropoietin. Proc. Natl. Acad. Sci. U.S.A., *74:*3879, 1977.
McCulloch, E. A., and Till, J. E.: The sensitivity of cells from normal mouse bone marrow to gamma radiation in vitro and in vivo. Radiat. Res., *16:*822, 1962.
————: Stem cells in normal early haemopoiesis and certain clonal haemopathies. *In* Hoffbrand, A. V., Brain, M. C., and Hirsh, J. (eds.): Recent Advances in Haematology. p. 85. London, Churchill, 1977.
McCulloch, E. A., Mak, T. W., Price, G. B., and Till, J. E.: Organization and communication in populations of normal and leukemic hemopoietic cells. Biochim. Biophys. Acta., *355:*260, 1974.

McLeod, D. L., Shreeve, M., and Axelrad, A. A.: Improved plasma culture system for production of erythrocytic colonies in vitro: quantitative assay method for CFU-E. Blood, *44:*517, 1974.

Metcalf, D.: Hemopoietic colonies—in vitro cloning of normal and leukemic cells. Recent Results in Cancer Research. vol. 61. Berlin, Springer-Verlag, 1977.

Micklem, H. S., and Ford, C.: Proliferation of injected lymph node and thymus cells in lethally irradiated mice. Plast. Reconstr. Surg., *26:*436, 1960.

Micklem, H. S., Ford, C. E., Evans, E. P., and Gray, J.: Interrelationships of myeloid and lymphoid cells: studies with chromosome-marked cells transfused into lethally irradiated mice. Proc. R. Soc. (Biol.), *165:*78, 1966.

Miyake, T., Kung, C. K-H., and Goldwasser, E.: Purification of human erythropoietin. J. Biol. Chem., *252:*5558, 1977.

Moore, M. A. S., and Metcalf, D.: Ontogeny of the haemopoietic system: yolk sac origin of in vivo and in vitro colony-forming cells in the developing mouse embryo. Br. J. Haematol., *18:*279, 1970.

Prchal, J. F., Adamson, J. W., Steinmann, L., and Fialkow, P. J.: The single cell origin of human erythroid colonies. J. Cell. Physiol., *89:*489, 1976.

Prchal, J. T., Throckmorton, D. W., Carroll, A. J., Fuson, E. W., Gams, R. A., and Prchal, J. F.: A common progenitor for human myeloid and lymphoid cells. Nature, *274:*590, 1978.

Robinson, W. A. (ed.): Proceedings of the Second International Workshop on Hemopoiesis in Culture. New York, Grune & Stratton, 1974.

Stephenson, J. R., Axelrad, A. A., McLeod, D. L., and Shreeve, M. M.: Induction of colonies of hemoglobin-synthesizing cells by erythropoietin in vitro. Proc. Natl. Acad. Sci. U.S.A., *68:*1542, 1971.

Strome, J. E., McLeod, D. L., and Shreeve, M. M.: Evidence for the clonal nature of erythropoietic bursts: application of an in situ method for demonstrating centromeric heterochromatin in plasma cultures. Exp. Hematol., *6:*461, 1978.

Till, J. E., and McCulloch, E. A.: A direct measurement of the radiation sensitivity of normal mouse bone marrow cells. Radiat. Res., *14:*213, 1961.

Wu, A. M., Till, J. E., Siminovitch, L., and McCulloch, E. A.: A cytological study of the capacity for differentiation of normal hemopoietic colony-forming cells. J. Cell Physiol., *69:*177, 1967.

THE STROMA, BLOOD SUPPLY, AND SINUSOIDS OF MYELOID TISSUE

Becker, R. P., and De Bruyn, P. P. H.: The transmural passage of blood cells into myeloid sinusoids and the entry of platelets into the sinusoidal circulation; a scanning electron microscopic investigation. Am. J. Anat., *145:*183, 1976.

Weiss, L.: The structure of bone marrow. Functional interrelationships of vascular hematopoietic compartments in experimental hemolytic anemia: an electron microscope study. J. Morphol., *117:*467, 1965.

————: Histophysiology of bone marrow. Clin. Orthop., *52:*13, 1967.

Yoffey, J. M.: A note on the thick-walled and thin-walled arteries of bone marrow. J. Anat., *96:*425, 1962.

Zamboni, L., and Pease, D.: The vascular bed of the red bone marrow. J. Ultrastruct. Res., *5:*65, 1961.

BONE MARROW FORMATION AND OSTEOGENESIS

See also References under Bone Induction and Ectopic Bone in Chapter 15.

Friedenstein, A. J.: Precursor cells of mechanocytes. Int. Rev. Cytol., *47:*327, 1976.

Friedenstein, A. J., Chailakhyan, R. K., Latsinik, N. V., Panasyuk, A. F., and Keiliss-Borok, I. V.: Stromal cells responsible for transferring the microenvironment of the hemopoietic tissues. Transplantation, *17:*331, 1974.

For references and data on the osteogenic capacities of bone marrow *see* Ham, A. W., and Harris, W. R.: The repair and transplantation of bone. *In* Bourne, G. H. (ed.): The Biochemistry and Physiology of Bone. vol. 3, ed. 2. New York, Academic Press, 1971.

THE FORMATION OF ERYTHROCYTES

Krantz, S. B., and Jacobson, L. O. (eds.): Erythropoietin and the Regulation of Erythropoiesis. Chicago, University of Chicago Press, 1970.

Nienhuis, A. W., and Benz, E. J.: Regulation of hemoglobin synthesis during the development of the red cell. N. Engl. J. Med., *287:*1318, 1371, and 1430, 1977.

THE FORMATION OF GRANULAR LEUKOCYTES

Bainton, D. F., and Farquhar, M. C.: Origin of granules in polymorphonuclear leukocytes: two types derived from opposite faces of the Golgi apparatus in developing leukocytes. J. Cell Biol., *28:*277, 1966.

————: Differences in enzyme content of azurophil and specific granules of polymorphonuclear leukocytes: cytochemistry and electron microscopy of bone marrow cells. J. Cell Biol., *39:*299, 1968.

————: Segregation and packaging of granules in eosinophilic leukocytes. J. Cell Biol., *45:*54, 1970.

Bainton, D. F., Ullyot, J. L., and Farquhar, M. C.: The development of neutrophilic polymorphonuclear leukocytes in human bone marrow: origin and content of azurophil and specific granules. J. Exp. Med., *134:*907, 1971.

Farquhar, M. C., and Bainton, D. F.: Cytochemical Studies on Leukocyte Granules. Proc. 4th Internat. Congr. Histochemistry and Cytochemistry, Kyoto, Japan. p. 25. Published by the Soc. Histochemistry and Cytochemistry, 1972.

THE FORMATION OF MONOCYTES

Brahim, F., and Osmond, D. G.: Radioautographic studies of the production and fate of bone marrow lymphocytes and monocytes. Proc. Canad. Fed. Biol. Soc., pp. 136–137, 1967.

Osmond, D. G.: The origin of peritoneal macrophages from the bone marrow. Anat. Rec., *154:*397, 1966.

Nichols, B. A., Bainton, D. F., and Farquhar, M. G.: Differentiation of monocytes. Origin, nature and fate of their azurophilic granules. J. Cell Biol., *50:*498, 1971.

THE FORMATION OF LYMPHOCYTES IN MYELOID TISSUE

Osmond, D. G.: Potentials of bone marrow lymphocytes. *In* Cairnie, A. B., Lala, P. K., and Osmond, D. G. (eds.): Stem Cells of Renewing Cell Populations. New York, Academic Press, 1976.

Osmond, D. G., Miller, S. C., and Yoshida, Y.: Kinetic and hemopoietic properties of lymphoid cells in the bone marrow. *In* Haemopoietic Stem Cells. Ciba Foundation Symposium 13 (new series). Amsterdam, ASP (Elsevier. Excerpta Medica. North-Holland), 1973.

Yoffey, J. M., Hudson, G., and Osmond, D. G.: The lymphocyte in guinea pig bone marrow. J. Anat., *99:*841, 1965.

Yoshida, Y., and Osmond, D. G.: Identity and proliferation of small lymphocyte precursors in cultures of lymphocyte-rich fractions of guinea pig bone marrow. Blood, *37:*73, 1971.

MEGAKARYOCYTES AND THE FORMATION OF PLATELETS

Becker, R. P., and De Bruyn, P. P. H.: The transmural passage of blood cells into myeloid sinusoids and the entry of platelets into the sinusoidal circulation; a scanning electron microscopic investigation. Am. J. Anat., *145:*183, 1976.

Bentfeld-Barker, M. E., and Bainton, D. F.: Ultrastructure of rat megakaryocytes after prolonged thrombocytopenia. J. Ultrastruct. Res., *61:*201, 1977.

McLeod, D. L., Shreeve, M. M., and Axelrad, A. A.: Induction of megakaryocyte colonies with platelet formation in vitro. Nature, *261:*492, 1976.

Wright, J. H.: The histogenesis of the blood platelets. J. Morph., *21:*263, 1910.

Yamada, E.: The fine structure of the megakaryocyte in the mouse spleen. Acta Anat., *29:*267, 1957.

13 Lymphatic Tissue

The hematopoietic (blood cell-forming) tissues of the body, which represent a special kind of connective tissue, are of two types, *(1) myeloid*, dealt with in Chapter 12, and *(2) lymphatic*, which will be considered here.

Some General Considerations. Lymphatic tissue appears in four different forms in the body, and what these forms are and why they are all termed *lymphatic tissue* will now be explained.

It will be recalled that the body fluid called *lymph* originates as the excess tissue fluid forming from capillaries (Fig. 8-6, page 218) and that it is drained away from the intercellular substance in places where it is formed because it percolates into blind-ending lymphatic capillaries, whereupon it is termed *lymph*. These lymphatic capillaries pass inward in the body and in doing so those from various sites join with one another to form larger lymphatic vessels (called *lymphatics*) of various orders. Next, it was observed from anatomical dissections that there were little encapsulated structures of tissue distributed along the course of these lymphatic vessels, often in particular locations. These were at first termed *lymph glands* and, if they become swollen, they are still often referred to as swollen glands. However, they are not glands as we now understand them and so are more correctly termed *lymph nodes*. Studies showed that lymphatic vessels enter their convex surfaces (Fig. 13-11) and leave their concave ones, so lymph passes through them on the way to its final destination, which is the bloodstream. In reaching this destination, all the lymphatic vessels join to form two main trunks, respectively called the *thoracic duct* and the *right lymphatic duct*. Both continuously empty their contents of lymph into the venous side of the blood circulatory system, into which they open. So all the excess tissue fluid formed all over the body is returned to the bloodstream and on its way there it *passes through lymph nodes*.

Next, the LM showed that lymph nodes are heavily populated with the kind of cells normally found in lymph and which because of this had been called *lymphocytes*. Since there were so many of these cells in lymph nodes it was assumed that these nodes were the places where lymphocytes were produced, and therefore lymphatic tissue

became classified as a hematopoietic tissue. But since there were two other organs, the thymus and the spleen, that were heavily populated with lymphocytes and also believed to produce them, particularly the ones found in blood, the *thymus* and *spleen* also became classified as part of the lymphatic division of hematopoietic tissue, even though these organs were (curiously enough) singularly devoid of lymphatic vessels emptying into them. So what became known as the *lymphatic division* of hematopoietic tissue of the body comprised *(1) lymph nodes*, *(2)* the *thymus*, and *(3)* the *spleen*. In addition, since it was found that in several parts of the body there were little *nonencapsulated aggregations of lymphocytes* lying in the loose connective tissue, these aggregations too came to be considered a fourth part of the lymphatic tissue of the body. So lymphatic tissue was regarded as a hematopoietic tissue responsible for forming the blood cells known as lymphocytes because they were found in lymph that had passed through lymph nodes.

In reading further it should be realized that although histology is 160 years old, for 140 of these years the role of lymphocytes, one of the most numerous cell types in the body, remained very much of a mystery. However, in the last two decades there has been such a continuing explosion of knowledge about them and about the role of lymphatic tissue that it would now take many books to describe everything that is now known. One of the things learned (and related to the foregoing) is that there are *two types* of lymphocytes: *T-lymphocytes*, which originate in the thymus, and *B-lymphocytes*, which in man originate not in lymphatic tissue but in myeloid tissue. This to some extent confuses the concept of lymphatic tissue being the division of hematopoietic tissue that gives rise to the lymphocytes of the body, but we nevertheless have to live with this fact.

The Significance of the Distribution of Lymphatic Tissue. Although nearly everything of importance about lymphatic tissue has been ascertained relatively recently, one feature ascertained long ago still retains importance. The finding that lymph from every part of the body passes through lymph nodes before it is returned to the bloodstream suggested that *lymph nodes* might *act as filters* to remove particulate or foreign material from lymph before it was returned to the bloodstream. This suspicion was justified when it was found, for example, that the lymph nodes that drained lymph from the lungs of coal miners became literally loaded with particles of coal dust. Other more harmful dusts could be found in these nodes in individuals who breathed dusty air. Another characteristic of lymph nodes became obvious in individuals developing cancer (*see* Chap. 6), for it was found that cells from a primary malignant growth would in due course often gain entrance to lymphatics and then be filtered out in lymph nodes, where they could set up secondary malignant growths called *metastases* (Gr. *meta*, beyond; *stasis*, stand). It was also noted that the lymph nodes along lymphatic vessels that drained sites of infection would often become swollen and sometimes secondarily infected, which suggested they filtered, for example, bacteria from lymph and so prevented the bacteria from gaining entrance to the bloodstream. (Later it was discovered that what happens in lymph nodes under these circumstances is much more complicated, as will be explained.)

It was also noted that the *spleen* served a similar *filtering function* with regard to the bloodstream. Vast amounts of blood pass through it every day. It was noticed, for example, that in diseases in which erythrocytes did not live as long as usual, that iron-containing pigment resulting from destruction of hemoglobin accumulated in the spleen, and so it became accepted that an important function of the spleen was to serve as a perpetual graveyard for worn-out erythrocytes. However, the filtering function of lymph nodes and spleen is not performed by lymphocytes but by *macrophages*, as will be described shortly.

THE DEVELOPMENT OF KNOWLEDGE ABOUT LYMPHOCYTES

The Discovery of the Recirculation of Lymphocytes. When Yoffey and his associates counted the lymphocytes carried by the thoracic duct back to the bloodstream in experimental animals, they found that enormous numbers of lymphocytes were added to the bloodstream every day from the thoracic duct, so many in fact that it would be impossible for them to remain in the bloodstream without their numbers mounting rapidly. Instead their numbers remained relatively constant. What accounted for this?

At first it was thought that since lymphocytes are motile, they might continuously migrate from small blood vessels into tissues and even through the epithelium of the intestine to enter its lumen. Moreover, it was generally assumed they had a very short life span, so that after they entered tissues most would die, as would those that passed into the intestine. However, in 1959 Gowans

showed that if lymph (with its lymphocytes) was continuously drained from the thoracic duct, the lymphocytes in this lymph became fewer and fewer. Until this time it had been assumed that all these lymphocytes had been newly formed in the lymph nodes through which the lymph had drained. However, if this were true their numbers should not have diminished. Gowans' experiments indicated that the lymphocytes in lymph must therefore have come mostly from some other source; the most likely explanation was that they passed to the lymph from the bloodstream. He proved this by showing that if he injected the lymphocytes collected from the thoracic duct back into the bloodstream, the numbers in thoracic duct lymph returned to normal. Therefore, lymphocytes pass from blood to lymph. They do this in lymph nodes as will be described in detail later. Lymphocytes more or less continuously *recirculate* from the blood passing through lymph nodes into lymph; then they are carried by the thoracic and right lymphatic ducts back to the bloodstream again, and from there to blood vessels in lymph nodes, which they penetrate to enter the lymph again, and so on.

Until recirculation was demonstrated it had been assumed, as noted, that lymphocytes had a very short life span. When it was found that they recirculated, this assumption was put to the test. Radioactive tracers were by then available so the life span of lymphocytes could be investigated by labeling newly forming lymphocytes with tritiated thymidine. This required somewhat complicated experiments but showed that some lymphocytes have a *long life span*, (the length of this long life span varies) and that many of these lymphocytes *circulate back and forth between the lymph and the bloodstream.*

How It Was Established That Lymphocytes Are Immunologically Competent Cells. It is possible to inbreed mice, rats, or other experimental animals with conveniently short life spans by brother-to-sister matings through so many generations that for all practical purposes the animals of the inbred strain all have exactly the same genes. The proteins formed in their bodies are therefore all alike. Hence when some tissue, for example skin, is transplanted from one animal to another of the *same* inbred strain, the transplanted skin has no antigens foreign to the animal receiving the skin, and so the skin graft "takes" and readily becomes part of the host. Next, if an animal of one inbred strain is mated with an animal belonging to a *different* inbred strain, their offspring (called F_1 hybrids, F_1 indicating a *first filial* generation, from the L. *filius*, son, *filia*, daughter) will derive half their genes from their mother and half from their father. Since each of their body cells contains a set of chromosomes from their mother and also a set from their father, F_1 hybrids inherit the genes directing structural and enzymatic protein synthesis in both parents. These genes, of course, direct the formation of the same macromolecular components in F_1 hybrids as they do in the mother or father. So a tissue transplant from a parent to an F_1 hybrid does not contain any macromolecular components different from those already present in the hybrid. In other words, macromolecular substances such as proteins from the mother or the father of an F_1 hybrid would not be antigenic in that hybrid. (This statement holds true only for inbred animals and not for randomly bred individuals such as man.) But although an F_1 hybrid finds nothing antigenic in a transplant from either its father or its mother, any cells of the *transplant* able to react immunologically might find antigens in the hybrid host and react against it. For example, if the transplant were made from the father of an F_1 hybrid into that hybrid, any immunologically competent cells in the transplant, which would, of course, be father-derived, could find some of the mother-derived proteins of the hybrid sufficiently different to react against them. So whereas an F_1 hybrid, derived from crossing two pure strains, will find no antigens in a graft made to it from its father or mother, immunologically competent cells present in the graft could find antigens present in their host and react immunologically against them. This is called a *graft-versus-host* reaction. There is evidence that such a reaction is occurring when parental tissue is grafted to very young F_1 hybrids because these hybrids fail to grow and so become runts. Another phase or type of graft-versus-host reaction, which occurs in older F_1 hybrids, is what is called "wasting disease"; this is generally fatal. The question arises, of course, as to what kinds of cells in the graft were immunologically competent and reacted against the host.

To find out if lymphocytes were the cells that caused the graft-versus-host reaction, Gowans, in the early 1960s, collected lymphocytes from thoracic duct lymph of fathers or mothers of hybrid rats and injected these into the hybrids, whereupon the lymphocytes were found to cause wasting disease. Furthermore, if these lymphocytes are injected into young F_1 hybrids, runts develop (Fig. 13-1). Thus it was established that lymphocytes are the cells that can recognize foreign antigens and react immunologically to them. But to do this they go through certain changes; Gowans and also Gowans and McGregor found that under circumstances such as those described above small lymphocytes develop into larger cells with abundant free ribosomes in their cytoplasm (Fig. 13-2). Their content of cytoplasmic RNA is extensive enough to render the cytoplasm basophilic. These enlarged lymphocytes are able to divide repeatedly. Furthermore, it was shown by Nowell that addition of a substance known as *phytohemagglutinin* (PHA) to cultures of leukocytes stimulated small lymphocytes in the cultures to turn into larger cells that divided. The kind of cell into which small lymphocytes develop in vitro under these conditions is similar to the kind of large cell found in vivo that we have

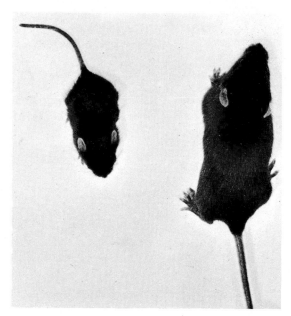

Fig. 13-1. Photograph of two F_1 hybrid mice, 13 days old, from the same litter, the result of mating a mouse of one inbred strain with one of another inbred strain. The mouse on the left is a runt. Within 1 day of birth it received 1×10^7 spleen cells from a mouse of one of the parental strains.

just described (illustrated in Fig. 13-2). We shall call both kinds *activated lymphocytes*. The name "blast cell" has also been used for the same type of cell because, like an embryonic cell, it generates further cells. However, the term "blast cell" has a particular connotation to hematologists managing patients with leukemia and so is best avoided in the present context. The name "lymphoblast" has also been used for this kind of cell but this term goes back to the days when small lymphocytes were considered the product of lymphoblasts, not as the cells from which blast cells could originate, so its use would be confusing. Accordingly, another name is indicated. The term "immunoblast" is commonly used but perhaps suggests greater knowledge than can be secured from morphological criteria alone. We shall therefore call these cells *activated lymphocytes*, a name sufficiently descriptive to be useful, yet noncommittal enough to avoid inaccuracy and furthermore sufficiently different from previously used terms to avoid confusion.

Next, it was discovered that if leukocytes from two unrelated individuals were mixed together in a culture, many lymphocytes would enlarge and divide without phytohemagglutinin being added. This was called the *mixed lymphocyte reaction* and was due to the lymphocytes of each individual finding those of the other individual antigenic. It was also noticed that when lymphocytes from identical twins were mixed, no mitosis occurred

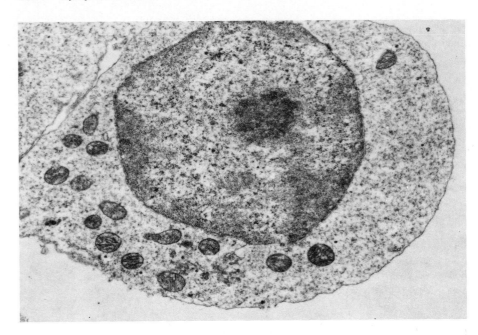

Fig. 13-2. Electron micrograph of an activated lymphocyte. This cell was obtained from the spleen of an irradiated mouse injected with small lymphocytes from a rat. Note that ribosomes are abundant in its wide rim of cytoplasm, but rER is absent. (Courtesy of J. Gowans)

unless phytohemagglutinin was added. Accordingly, it was established that lymphocytes in cell cultures could be stimulated, at least sometimes, to increase in size and divide (become *activated*) if they were *exposed to antigens.* So the concept that was held over most of this century—that lymphocytes were end-of-line cells—was finally dead and buried. Instead, when suitably exposed to the right antigen, lymphocytes become activated and *produce progeny cells.*

However, new information about lymphocytes did not stop here. It was found, for example, that when lymphocytes from a donor animal that had received a particular antigen were transferred to a host that had previously been given sufficient radiation to stop proliferation of the host's own immunologically competent cells, the host would exhibit an antibody response when exposed to this antigen even though it had not received this antigen before. Furthermore, this response was characterized by amplified production of antibody and was rapid in onset. This showed that new progeny cells were produced in response to antigen. The fact that the numbers of these transferred cells increased on re-exposure to antigen showed that the antigen-responsive cells were capable of proliferation in response to antigen, and the fact that they acquired the characteristics of plasma cells and became capable of producing specific antibody showed that they underwent differentiation. Similar experiments in which only a single functional cell was transferred to an irradiated host still generated a full immune response; furthermore, cells could repeatedly be transferred and immune responses would continue to be produced. This

demonstrated that the progenitor cell and its progeny were forming *clones* of identical cells in response to the antigen. It was in such experiments that cooperation between thymus-derived and bone marrow-derived lymphocytes was first discovered, as will be described below.

THE TWO MAIN KINDS OF SMALL LYMPHOCYTES

In the last decade it has become clear that there are two main classes of small lymphocytes. Those of one class, derived from the bursa of Fabricius in chickens and from the bone marrow in mammals, are termed *B-lymphocytes.* Those of the other, derived from the thymus, are referred to as *T-lymphocytes.* Two different types of immune reactions, *antibody production* and what are termed *cell-mediated responses* (which involve direct contact between T-lymphocytes and cells that they find foreign and hence antigenic) are carried out by these respective classes of lymphocytes. Both are essential for viability of the host.

B-LYMPHOCYTES AS THE SOURCE OF PLASMA CELLS

While plasma cells and lymphocytes have long been recognized, only recently were plasma cells shown to be derived from B-lymphocytes. When B-lymphocytes taking up residence in the lymphatic tissues are activated by their first contact with a given antigen, they undergo proliferation and differentiation; this is called a *primary immune response* and during the course of it some of them become antibody producers. The most active in this response develop into typical plasma cells (Figs. 9-18 and 9-19). When they do this they can be recognized easily by their great abundance of rER and a prominent Golgi (Fig. 9-20). However, activated B-lymphocytes not yet developed to this point can also produce some antibody.

Not all activated B-lymphocytes become active antibody producers. Some go back to having the appearance of unactivated, small lymphocytes. These (in contrast to B-lymphocytes in the peripheral blood, which have a short life span) may remain in lymphatic tissue for long periods. They are called *B memory cells* because they are descendants of B-lymphocytes that were activated by a particular antigen and hence they, as it were, lie in wait for the same antigen to come along again and if it does they immediately respond to it. Moreover, these cells can proliferate and so maintain or even amplify their numbers, so that there are enough of them to achieve immediate and extensive production of antibody to the antigen if they are again exposed to it. This kind of reaction is termed a *secondary response*. It differs from a primary response only in beginning more quickly and being more extensive. Both of these differences between secondary and primary responses can be explained by there being more B-lymphocytes to respond to a given antigen in secondary responses. After the first (primary) response *all* subsequent responses to the same antigen are termed *secondary* responses.

We next consider how there could be a primary response to any given antigen. How do B-lymphocytes recognize an antigen? How can a B-lymphocyte recognize a particular antigen if it has no memory of it?

ARE B-LYMPHOCYTES (AND ALSO T-LYMPHOCYTES) EACH ALREADY PROGRAMMED TO REACT WITH ONLY ONE PARTICULAR ANTIGEN WHEN FORMED?

After it was shown that lymphocytes could react to antigens, an intriguing question received much consideration. In discussing this we shall first consider B-lymphocytes. The question was whether a virgin B-lymphocyte (a B-lymphocyte born of a precursor cell that had not had contact with any antigen) has the potentiality to react to the first antigen it meets by going on to form plasma cells that produce the specific antibody capable of reacting with that particular antigen. In other words, can an antigen induce any virgin B-lymphocyte to differentiate into plasma cells producing the antibody specific for that antigen? This view, which was at first widely held,

would suggest that virgin B-lymphocytes are uncommitted but competent cells of such great potentiality that they can be induced to develop along a specialized differentiation pathway by the first antigen they encounter. An alternative concept, one that is now generally accepted, is that virgin B-lymphocytes are not all born alike; instead, each one is *programmed* so that it will only be able to *react to a particular antigen*.

Where Lymphocytes Are Programmed. According to the concept outlined above, B-lymphocytes are programmed in man as they are formed in myeloid tissue. T-lymphocytes are formed and programmed in the cortex of the thymus. The concept of lymphocytes being programmed before they enter the circulation is important since it means that all the lymphocytes (outside of these two sites where they are programmed), even though they look alike, are all especially programmed to react to a particular antigen and to this extent are all highly specialized cells. Furthermore, they are capable of being activated and producing more lymphocytes with the same program and it is these progeny cells that are responsible for immunological memory if they persist in the body. Since the virgin B- and T-lymphocytes of the body represent a wide assortment of lymphocytes already programmed to react with particular antigens, there are always at least a few in the general population that are programmed to react to an antigen should it gain access to the body. If an antigen does enter the body, the few can then quickly multiply.

HOW B-LYMPHOCYTES BECOME PROGRAMMED

The Structure of an Antibody Molecule

To understand how B-lymphocytes become programmed so that among the B-lymphocyte population there will be one or more already specialized to produce a specific antibody to any conceivable antigen that enters the body, something must be said about the structure of an antibody molecule and what determines its specificity. An antibody molecule is composed of four polypeptide chains; two are identical heavy chains and the other two are identical light chains. Each chain is made up of amino acids, the heavier chains having many more amino acids than the light ones. The molecule is symmetrical and Y-shaped. The stem of the Y consists only of parts of the two heavy chains. The arms each consist of the remainder of one heavy chain with a light chain lying alongside it.

There are two identical sites that can combine with antigen in each antibody molecule. These are at the free ends of the two arms of the Y. Thus each antigen combining (antigen recognition) site is constructed of the end of a heavy chain and the end of a light chain. The specificity of the antibody for a particular antigen resides in these combining sites and is determined by the particular amino acid sequences at the ends of the light and the heavy chains. Variations in amino acid sequence among antibody molecules of different specificities are confined to the regions of the chains that include these ends. Hence the name *variable region* for this part of the molecule. The remainder of the light and the heavy chains have constant amino acid sequences and comprise the *constant region* of the molecule.

As in all proteins, the amino acid sequences of constant and variable regions of antibody molecules are determined by structural genes. The genes determining the amino acid sequence in the variable region confer such diversity on antibody molecules that they are potentially capable of reacting with virtually all antigens with which we might ever come into contact. For those interested in how this could be achieved, we shall next explain how such diversity is accomplished.

The Genetic Basis of Antibody Diversity. As outlined above, it is generally accepted that the amino acid sequences of antibody (more commonly called *immunoglobulin*) molecules with different specificities, which of course are produced by different antibody-producing cells, vary only in the region of the molecule that combines with antigen; the remainder of the antibody molecule, even though made by different antibody-forming cells, is always the same. This suggests that the genes coding for the constant part of antibody molecules could have arisen from a single primitive gene that during evolution underwent reduplication. The fact that genetic markers in this region are inherited in simple Mendelian fashion indicates that there is only a single set of such genes coding for the constant region of immunoglobulin molecules. However, there seem to be a number of genes coding for the variable region of the immunoglobulin molecule. Since each polypeptide chain is known to be synthesized as a single unit, the genes responsible for the variable and constant regions of an immunoglobulin molecule must somehow join forces before they can code for a whole polypeptide chain. However, inheritance studies show that there is shuffling among the genes coding for the variable and constant regions, so this must take place before combination takes place.

The most widely held view of how antibody diversity is produced is that there are something like 50 to a few hundred or so genes coding for the variable region of the immunoglobulin molecule. These would be inherited through the germ cells. By recombination they would be capable of generating a wide variety of potential antibody specificities, and this variation could be broadened further by somatic mutation, thus accounting for the hundreds of thousands of different antibody specificities that reside in the different lymphocytes of each individual. Such a hypothesis would be consistent with the finding that certain strains of animals inherit in simple Mendelian fashion an inability to respond to certain synthetic or viral antigens, as if particular maternal or paternal genes are necessary for producing certain antibody specificities. This would also explain why amino acid sequences can vary in different antibodies from the same individual, in some instances by a single amino acid, as if these differences arose by mutation in somatic cells.

Each B-lymphocyte progenitor would thus become committed to expressing one gene coding for the variable region of a light chain and one gene coding for the variable region of a heavy chain. These two genes would participate with the genes responsible for the composition of the constant region of the molecule so that together they would all code for immunoglobulin molecules of a particular *specificity* (meaning capable of combining with antigenic molecules of one particular configuration). In developing B-lymphocytes it is a matter of chance which of the genes directing the amino acid sequence in the variable regions of the light and heavy chains combine with the genes coding for the composition of the constant region of the molecule. This random combination generates so many different kinds of antigen recognition sites in the variable regions of the immunoglobulin molecules that among the B-lymphocyte population there are always at least a few producing immunoglobulin molecules with combining sites to fit molecules of any antigen that might enter the body.

Programmed B-Lymphocytes

Once a particular gene combination is established, even though this happens by chance, the B-lymphocyte remains committed to producing immunoglobulin molecules of that one specificity. So the cell is now a *programmed B-lymphocyte.* An encounter with antigen of that specificity (and that specificity only) will activate the lymphocyte. Moreover, all the cells of the clone forming from it will be identically programmed and so will produce antibody molecules of the same specificity.

Each B-lymphocyte, after it becomes programmed but before it or its progeny ever develop into fully fledged antibody-producing plasma cells, makes a little of the specific immunoglobulin for which it is programmed so that this is present in small patches on its surface. These tiny surface patches of immunoglobulin are called *recognition sites* or *surface receptors,* and it is by means of these that a B-lymphocyte *recognizes* the particular antigen against which it is programmed to react. An encounter between specific antigen and receptor (under circumstances to be described below) activates that particular B-lymphocyte, causing clonal amplification and differentiation that results in the formation of a population of antibody-producing cells of the appropriate specificity.

The Activation of B-Lymphocytes and T Helper Factor

For a B-lymphocyte to be activated *two signals* appear to be necessary. The first of these is *contact of the appropriate antigen* with the immunoglobulin receptors on the surface of the B-lymphocyte as described above. The other signal requires *cooperation of T-lymphocytes* because even when the appropriate antigen contacts the B-lymphocyte, activation does not occur unless there is cooperation from T-lymphocytes; for this reason most antigens that activate B-lymphocytes are called *thymus-dependent antigens.*

Next, for a T-lymphocyte to be able to help in the activation of a B-lymphocyte, this T-lymphocyte must also be programmed to react specifically with the particular antigen that combines with the surface receptors of the B-lymphocyte it is going to help. When the antigen combines with the receptors on the surface of a T-lymphocyte programmed to react with that particular antigen, the T-lymphocyte releases what is termed a *T helper factor,* which thereupon must somehow come into contact with the B-lymphocyte to whose surface receptors the antigen concerned will specifically attach. With the arrival of the T helper factor as well as the antigen the B-lymphocyte becomes activated.

If an antigen of the thymus-dependent type were to combine with the B-lymphocyte's immunoglobulin surface receptors in the absence of T helper factor, no antibody production directed against that antigen would, of course, be initiated.

T-LYMPHOCYTES

T-lymphocytes originate and become programmed in the thymus. Most are long-lived and keep circulating back and forth between blood and lymph so that they are widely exposed to any antigens that might be present in any part of the body. Like B-lymphocytes, each T-lymphocyte is programmed to react with a specific antigen; however, although T-lymphocytes do not manufacture antibodies, their programming nevertheless serves different and very useful functions that we shall go on to describe. Moreover, like B-lymphocytes, T-lymphocytes have surface receptors by means of which they recognize the antigen to which they are programmed to react. Although the receptors on the surface of T-lymphocytes are not identical with the patches of immunoglobulin molecules serving as receptors on the surface of B-lymphocytes, there are some similarities, indicating that they too may be coded for by certain genes in similar fashion to the variable region of immunoglobulin molecules. However, less is known about the way immunological diversity is generated in T-lymphocytes than in B-lymphocytes.

On meeting antigen, T-lymphocytes programmed to recognize that antigen become *activated.* They enlarge, proliferate, and differentiate into any of several subtypes of T-lymphocytes: (*1*) *T killer cells* (*cytotoxic T-lymphocytes*) that, as will be described in detail presently, will react specifically with foreign cells that have gained entrance to the body and possess the antigen they recognize, (*2*) *T memory cells,* (*3*) *T helper cells,* (*4*) *T suppressor cells,* or (*5*) *T amplifier cells.* We shall first deal with killer cells. The other subtypes of T-lymphocytes will be described in due course.

A killer cell, to destroy a cell that bears the antigen it recognizes, must establish actual contact with the cell bearing that antigen. This type of immunological reaction involving *direct contact* between target cells and T killer cells is described as a *cell-mediated type* of immunological reaction. Because they are able to become killer cells, T-lymphocytes are the chief cause of rejection of transplants of tissues or organs made from one person to another.

The Mechanism of Action of T Killer Cells. Killing, as noted, requires contact between killer cells and target cells. There is no evidence of any release of soluble cytotoxic factors, nor is complement (described on page 285) required as would be the case if the killing were mediated by humoral antibody. Contact with killer cells differentiating from specifically activated T-lymphocytes induces selective *leakiness of the cell membrane* of the target cell as follows.

According to Allison, a motile killer cell makes contact by means of one of its cytoplasmic processes with a target cell, which it is able to recognize in a specific manner, and then after a period of contact it becomes detached again. However, in doing so it leaves behind a bit of its own cell membrane in the place where it was in contact. The piece of membrane it thus donates then proceeds to act very much like a gap junction in that it allows ions and small molecules to enter and leave the target cell. Potassium ions leak out of the cell and sodium ions (together with water) enter. Osmotic swelling also occurs, followed by lysis, release of cytoplasmic proteins, and death of the cell. Thus, although the recognition of a target cell by a killer cell is specific, its mechanism of killing is not, for all such target cells perish in the same manner no matter what kind they are.

The Role of Lymphocytes in Rejecting Transplants of Foreign Tissues or Organs

Tissue or organ transplants are commonly called *grafts.* Tissue transplantation (grafting) has been much studied in experimental animals, but before describing what has been learned about the conditions under which grafting is or is not successful, we should define some frequently used terms.

Terminology Used With Reference to Tissue Transplantation. A graft made from one part of an individual to another part of the same individual is called either an *autograft* (Gr. *autos,* self) or an *autochthonous* graft (Gr. *autochthon,* sprung from the earth itself, indigenous). A graft made from one animal of an inbred strain to another belonging to the same strain is termed either an *isograft* (Gr. *isos,* equal) or a *syngeneic* graft (Gr. *syn,* with, together; *gennan,* to produce). A graft attempted from one member of a given species to another member of the *same* species (but not between members of the same inbred strain) is called either a *homograft* (Gr. *homos,* same) or an *allograft* (Gr. *allos,* another), because it is being made to *another* member of the same species (hence it is also

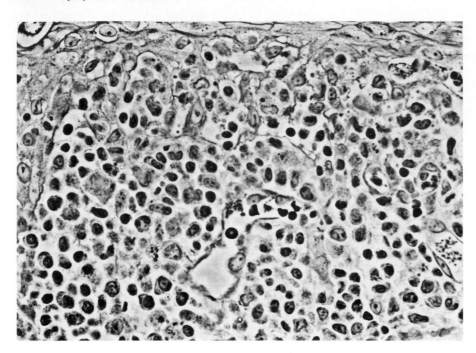

Fig. 13-3. Phase contrast photomicrograph of the site of transplantation of an allograft (homograft) of epidermis in a rabbit. The transplanted epidermis can be seen extending across the *top*. The bed of the transplant (host tissue) is heavily infiltrated with graft rejection cells. Some of the latter have infiltrated into the epidermal transplant at *top*. This is an example of what is known as a *homograft reaction*. (Weiner, J., Spiro, D., and Russel, P. S.: Am. J. Pathol., *44*:319, 1964)

sometimes referred to as being an *allogeneic* graft). A graft attempted between members of different species is called either a *heterograft* (Gr. *heteros*, other) or a *xenograft* (Gr. *xenos*, a stranger), and so may be referred to as being *xenogeneic*.

Allograft Rejection; the Homograft Reaction

In experimental studies skin is commonly used for studying whether grafts *take* or are rejected, since skin is easily transplanted and the surgical operation does not require, as transplanting organs does, that the blood vessels of the graft be surgically connected to those of the host. Skin is thin enough for its cells to be nourished by tissue fluid seeping into it from its graft bed and, if the transplanted skin is compatible with that of its host, blood vessels of the host will either grow into the graft or, as will soon be described, become connected with those of the graft to provide it with more permanent nourishment.

Skin autografts made from one part of an animal or person and transplanted to another part take readily. In animals belonging to pure strains skin grafts also take if made from one animal and transplanted to another (isografts). However, if skin is transplanted from one animal to another of the same species but not of the same strain (that is, a homograft), what is called a *homograft reaction* soon appears in the host at its site of contact with the graft. This can be seen to advantage if the graft is a very

thin shaving cut from the surface of the skin so that it consists almost entirely of epidermis (the epithelium) which, of course, is cellular. The connective tissue bed on which an epidermal graft is placed soon becomes infiltrated with what are generally termed *graft rejection cells* (Fig. 13-3); these are T-lymphocytes that have become activated to become killer cells, as will next be described. They make direct contact with the epidermal cells of the homograft (now usually referred to as an *allograft*), and kill them by the mechanism described above.

The Source and Nature of Graft Rejection Cells. The operative procedures involved even in transplanting skin incite some degree of inflammatory response in the site to which the graft is transplanted. There is dilation of small blood vessels in the graft bed and exudation and increased lymphatic drainage from it. In autografts and isografts the inflammatory reaction subsides in a few days. In allografts, however, inflammation persists because a new factor enters the picture to maintain the inflammatory process, as will now be explained.

Because of the early inflammation it would be quite possible for T-lymphocytes to leave small blood vessels of the graft bed and enter the tissues at the site of an allograft where they could meet an antigen to which they were programmed to react. These lymphocytes could then enter a lymphatic and pass to the nearest lymph node where they could settle out, develop into activated lymphocytes, and produce progeny. Another possibility is that antigens from the graft might seep into the host tissue of the graft bed and from there into the lymphatic capillaries draining it, and thus reach the nearest lymph node where they could encounter appropriately programmed T-lymphocytes, which they would of course activate. As noted, these activated lymphocytes are larger and have more basophilic cytoplasm (due to RNA) than ordinary lymphocytes. Some of these then go on to differentiate into *killer cells (cytotoxic T-lymphocytes).* From a lymph node killer cells would reach the graft bed by entering efferent lymphatics of the node and from lymph they would be delivered into the bloodstream. They need make only one circuit in the circulation before entering the loose connective tissues. Being motile, they wander randomly and those that encounter the allograft are able to adhere to and destroy its cells. However, many of the killer cells miss the allograft entirely; these are commonly found in the connective tissue under the lining of the intestine.

T-Lymphocytes as Memory Cells. As well as becoming killer cells, activated T-lymphocytes can take another pathway. They can stay within a lymph node and proliferate, with their progeny once more having the morphological appearance of small lymphocytes. Since this population of small lymphocytes is programmed to respond only to the antigens of the allograft, and since the numbers of these cells have been increased through mitosis of their progenitors, there are now many more of them than before the first exposure of the host to the allograft. These lymphocytes are accordingly termed *T memory cells* and many of them recirculate. Their persistence after a first allograft explains why a second allograft from the same donor is rejected much more quickly and energetically than the first graft.

When a first allograft is made there may be only very few T-lymphocytes in the regional lymph node programmed to react to the antigens it bears. So to mount a proper offensive against it, the few T-lymphocytes activated have to undergo numerous mitoses to produce enough killer cells to reject the graft, and all this takes time. However, with a second allograft there would be numerous memory cells ready to become activated, so, instead of beginning from few cells, the second response would begin from many cells; hence the production of killer cells would be greater and the rejection of the graft much quicker.

Relation of Blood Supply to the Taking or Rejection of Grafts. Immunological compatibility between animals has been much studied by skin grafts being made from one animal to another to see whether they would take. As noted, skin can generally be transferred from one part of the body to another without having to connect up blood vessels by surgical methods. It is assumed that for the first few days the transplanted skin lives due to diffusion from the tissue fluid of the graft bed keeping the cells of the graft alive. This gives time for new blood vessels to grow from the graft bed into the graft and thereafter maintain it. However, Ham and Cloutier made both autografts and allografts of skin every one or two days on a pig and at the end of the experiment injected the blood vascular system of the pig with the black material shown in Figure 13-4. They found, much to their surprise, that *autografts* were not revascularized by new arteries and veins growing into them to replace those previously existing, but instead the capillaries of the host soon became connected to capillaries of the autograft and in a few days the connections were sufficiently numerous for blood to again utilize the original arteries and veins of the autograft (Fig. 13-4B and C). Since there would not have been time for new arteries or veins to have grown into the graft, the only conclusion that could be drawn was that, after the capillaries of the host and the graft became connected, the previously existing arteries and veins of the graft soon became filled with blood that thereafter circulated through them. They also discovered that this observation had already been made and reported years before but had gone relatively unnoticed.

Of particular interest in this experiment, however, was that in *allografts* the capillaries of the host and those of the transplanted skin showed no indication whatsoever of becoming connected (Fig. 13-4D). As might be expected a typical homograft reaction also developed. But even so it is curious that before this occurred there would not have been any capillary connections established.

Why Humoral Antibodies Are Not the Cause of Graft Rejection. The antigens of allografts also incite the formation of some plasma cells from B-lymphocytes in their hosts. The plasma cells produce humoral antibodies that react specifically with these antigens. But this does not necessarily affect the transplanted tissue cells deleteriously. Antibody combining with antigen on body cells does damage to them only if it in turn fixes *complement* (p. 285). Only on a few kinds of body cells (erythrocytes and leukocytes, for instance) are antigenic sites close enough to fix complement under these conditions. On most body cells, however, antigens are not close enough for complement to be fixed when antibody combines with them; this is why antibody, even if formed in response to a foreign transplant, may not have any deleterious effect on the cells of the transplant. Indeed humoral antibody combining with antigens on the cells of a foreign transplant may have the reverse effect in that it may hide these antigens from the activated T-lymphocytes concerned with their destruction. Another possibility is that the antigen-antibody complex may have the effect of inhibiting immunological activity of the graft rejection cells. This

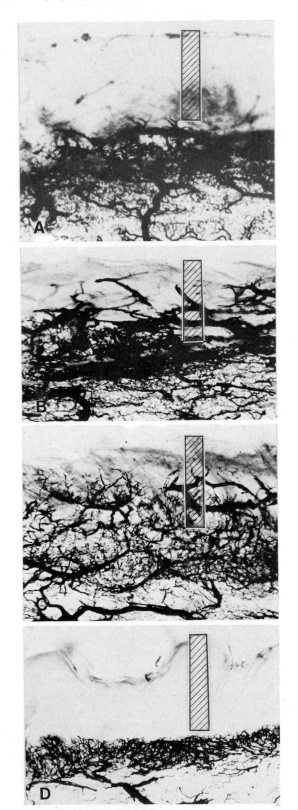

Fig. 13-4. These are all photomicrographs of sections of full-thickness skin transplants made at different times onto the same pig. The host's vascular system was perfused with India ink in warm gelatin. In each picture the transplant thickness is indicated by a striped band. (*A*) This shows an autograft after 3 days. Note the increased vascularity of the graft bed. Any black material in the graft itself is not India ink. (*B* and *C*) These two pictures are of autografts that have been in place for 7 and 10 days, respectively. The 7-day one shows that the former large vessels of the graft are now open to the circulation and the 10-day graft shows complete revascularization. (*D*) This is an allograft that has been in place for several days; no circulation whatsoever has been established in it.

opposite effect of humoral antibody is termed *enhancement* because antibody may actually enhance the survival of a foreign transplant.

Rationale of Measures Taken to Prevent the Allograft Rejection. The homograft reaction is, of course, the chief obstacle to be overcome in successfully transplanting tissues and organs from one person to another. One measure that can be taken is in the selection of the donor, since all individuals that are not identical twins have some different genes, so that their tissues contain different antigens; this is the inevitable result of random breeding. The selection of a suitable donor for a transplant therefore hinges on the use of laboratory tests that show the extent to which lymphocytes of the host will react with the antigens of the donor. Next, when the donor has been selected and transplantation effected, measures may be taken to suppress a homograft reaction. One method is to use *immunosuppressive drugs,* which act in various ways to inhibit formation of new lymphocytes. However, attempting to suppress allograft rejection with drugs is not without some danger, since these drugs may also suppress the ability of the host to combat all antigens, with the result that he may become unable to ward off infections.

SUBPOPULATIONS OF T-LYMPHOCYTES

It is now recognized that T-lymphocytes do not represent a single homogeneous population of thymus-derived cells but instead a number of subsets having different functions, locations, degrees of maturity, life spans, and surface markers by which they can be recognized despite their identical microscopic appearance. Of the several subclasses, one can act either as *killer cells* capable of destroying foreign cells on contact (as already described) or as *suppressor* cells (described below) capable of *interfering* with either humoral or cell-mediated immune responses. Another subclass of T-lymphocytes acts as *helper cells* by providing T helper factor to facilitate immune responses, as described in connection with the activation of B-lymphocytes. Another subclass would be the *T memory cells* already described. Whether the suppressor cells act by blocking T helper lymphocytes or in a more direct way by interfering with the proliferation or differentiation of B- or T-lymphocytes is not known. Mature T-lymphocytes, which recirculate, are characteristically long-lived. However, within the spleen and thymus there are less mature T-lymphocytes that do not recirculate, are short-lived, and take part in maintaining or broadening the base of the T-lymphocyte population; these are the so-called *amplifier* T cells.

Of Particular Interest to Those Interested in Research. Exposure of T-lymphocytes to antigens results in formation of a remarkable array of products. These include not only a factor facilitating humoral and cell-mediated immune responses (*T helper factor*), but also other factors inducing cell division (*mitogenic factor*), loss of macrophage mobility (*macrophage migration inhibition factor,* MIF), cell death (*cytotoxic factor*), inhibition of viral replication (*interferon*), and even sustained proliferation and differentiation of myeloid progenitor cells (*colony stimulating factors*). T-lymphocytes thus seem to play a central role in the regulation of a wide variety of cellular processes, including some that are not strictly immunological.

DISTINGUISHING BETWEEN B- AND T-LYMPHOCYTES

B- and T-lymphocytes cannot be distinguished from one another by scanning electron microscopy as was previously thought. Both have surfaces covered with short microvilli but their form is not static and responds rapidly to contact with other surfaces, which explains why they may have different appearances in the SEM.

B-lymphocytes may nevertheless be distinguished from T-lymphocytes because B-lymphocytes possess surface immunoglobulin and this is readily revealed by immunofluorescence. Moreover, their surface is studded with what are known as *Fc receptors,* which can combine with a particular site in the constant region of all immunoglobulin molecules. Other sites known as *complement receptors* also exist at the surface of B-lymphocytes; these can combine specifically with one component of complement (C3) in complexes composed of antigen, antibody, and complement, and there are specific technics for demonstrating the presence of the latter. Macrophages also have these two types of surface receptors but T-lymphocytes do not. *Human T-lymphocytes* moreover have the specific but unexplained property of forming *rosettes* with sheep red blood cells, which means that the red cells stick all over the surface of the lymphocyte, and they can be readily distinguished by this method.

Cells of the lymphocyte series not possessing surface markers characteristic of T- or B-lymphocytes are referred to as *null* (L. *nullus,* not any) *cells.* They may represent stages in the differentiation of T- or B-lymphocytes. Neoplasms developing from lymphocytes in man or animals can mostly be classified as being of either T cell or B cell origin; those that are of neither T nor B cell origin are referred to as *null cell* tumors.

WHAT PROTECTS THE MACROMOLECULES OF THE BODY FROM ATTACK BY THE BODY'S IMMUNOLOGICAL SYSTEM?

Natural and Acquired Immunological Tolerance

Natural Immunological Tolerance. Tissues such as skin can be transplanted successfully from one site to another in the same individual, from one identical twin to another, or from one animal of a pure inbred strain to another animal of the same strain without inciting a homograft reaction. But if tissue is transplanted from a donor to a genetically nonidentical host, it is rejected because as far as the lymphocytes of the host are concerned the macromolecules of the transplanted tissue are foreign antigens. Why then do the lymphocytes of the body not find the macromolecules of the body's own great variety of tissues antigenic and therefore react to them? The most probable answer is that no lymphocytes programmed to react to macromolecules of an individual's body ever survive long enough to do so. This would also explain why that individual's body will accept transplants from an identical twin or another individual of the same pure strain. Thus it is said that the body has a *natural immunological tolerance* to its own macromolecules. But how could this be so if the body develops lymphocytes programmed to react with every conceivable antigen?

It might be thought that since the macromolecules of all the cells of an individual's body, including those of its lymphocytes, are all synthesized under the direction of the genes of that individual's body, the lymphocytes forming in that body might somehow be unable to react against that body's macromolecules. But this is not the case, for if macromolecules produced in the body are kept secluded until later in life and then happen to gain entrance to the body where they become exposed to its lymphocytes, the lymphocytes will react to them as vigorously as they would to anyone else's macromolecules. For example, in males spermatozoa (germ cells) are not formed until puberty and even then they are formed inside tubes that shield them from contact with lymphocytes. But if taken from their seclusion and injected into the male in which they were formed, the lymphocytes find them antigenic and produce antibodies that react with them just as readily as if they were foreign spermatozoa. *Autoimmune diseases* are manifestations of immune responses in individuals to their own macromolecules; one immunological reaction that is the result of secluded antigen gaining entrance to the body from the thyroid gland is described in Chapter 25 (p. 807). So the reason for lymphocytes not reacting against self is not that they have the same genetic heritage. Hence there would be no reason for assuming that among the lymphocytes that develop in the body there would not be vast numbers programmed to react with the macromolecules of that body. But before inquiring into what might happen to lymphocytes programmed to react with self, we shall give some further background.

Induced Immunological Tolerance. To explain further why the body has a natural immunological tolerance of its own macromolecules, we can learn much from how *induced tolerance* develops. This term refers to the way experimental animals can be made tolerant of foreign antigens so that they do not react immunologically against these antigens.

As is well known, there are several blood types in man and this is why erythrocytes of donors and recipients must be typed and matched prior to doing blood transfusions; otherwise a recipient of mismatched blood could suffer immunological reactions that might be fatal. In 1945, Owen in studying *nonidentical* (dizygotic) twin calves found some examples of these unlike calf twins each having its own and also its twin's type of red blood cells in its circulation, with no ill effects being observed. The reason for the unlike twins sharing common blood cells is that nonidentical twins in cattle commonly share the same placenta in which their two bloodstreams become mixed. They end up having blood that contains macromolecules from both twins, yet neither twin seems to find the other's macromolecules antigenic. Both seem to accept the other's antigens as their own, without reacting against them. This is described by saying that each has an *induced tolerance* to the other's macromolecules. Billingham, Brent, and Medawar then found that skin could be transplanted successfully between nonidentical twin calves that had shared a common blood supply, and subsequently it was shown that it was possible to induce tolerance to any of a great variety of antigens merely by injecting the antigen into experimental animals *before or immediately after birth.*

All this led to the general concept that any antigen given an animal before or immediately after birth seems to be tolerated immunologically by that animal in the same way as the macromolecules of its own body. Furthermore, it was found that an animal remains tolerant to the antigen injected as long as some of it remains in its body.

Timing therefore became very important with regard to whether macromolecules would be regarded as part of self or as foreign. It would seem, generally speaking, that lymphocytes do not recognize any macromolecules as antigens until about the time of birth. This is compatible with the finding that plasma cells do not begin to appear until close to birth, and even then there are only a few. So a fetus is not making antibodies in anything but a minor way. In other words, a fetus has not yet produced a population of programmed lymphocytes with some among them to react to any conceivable antigen. It would therefore seem that the production of programmed T- and B-lymphocytes does not begin until around the time of birth. But when this happens we must ask why some of the lymphocytes then being programmed to react against a multitude of antigens do not come to react against the macromolecules of the body in which they exist. A plausible theory, sometimes called the *clonal abortion hypothesis,* has been suggested, namely that *premature contact* of an antigen with a lymphocyte that has just been programmed to react with that antigen, but that has not yet formed a clone of identically programmed cells, causes the lymphocyte's death. So that lymphocytes as they became programmed to react against any macromolecule present in the body would be abundantly and continuously exposed to such potential antigens and hence would be *killed.* Furthermore, throughout life every lymphocyte that subsequently became programmed to react to some kind of body macromolecule would similarly be killed. Likewise, any foreign antigen given just before or immediately after birth would have the same effect, and provided it was given before any lymphocytes programmed to react to it had been able to mature it would, as long as it lasted in the body, lead to the death of all lymphocytes subsequently being formed and programmed to react against it. Hence the theory that premature contact of antigen with lymphocytes that are being programmed causes their death would explain both *natural* and *induced* tolerance.

How then could the body react to foreign invaders such as bacteria and viruses and to tissue transplants from other individuals? The reason would be that, before the body was exposed to these (which would be after birth), a population of *matured* programmed lymphocytes that could react against any conceivable antigen (except those already present that had made premature contact with lymphocytes being programmed to react to them) would have been built up in the body. (Before this occurs a newborn baby would have received antibodies from its mother via the placenta and these would help tide it over until it could make its own.) Furthermore, no population of lymphocytes could subsequently be built up against body macromolecules or antigens to which tolerance had been induced because each new lymphocyte that was programmed to react against such antigens would have had premature contact with them and thus been destroyed. Moreover, later after birth when, for example, the body experienced an infection of some kind so that a new foreign antigen was present in it, each new lymphocyte just being programmed to react against that foreign antigen would also be destroyed by premature contact with it. But this would make no material difference with regard to the control of the infection because there would already have been *mature programmed lymphocytes formed before this antigen was present*. These would be activated as programmed lymphocytes, and since they can reproduce as programmed lymphocytes, they could overcome the infection. It would seem that the premature contact between lymphocytes and the respective antigen that causes death of the lymphocytes occurs around the time the lymphocyte is completing its programming process and before it has had time to reproduce.

Next, most foreign antigens to which the body can become exposed postnatally are of the thymus-dependent type. So even if B-lymphocytes were formed in later life that were programmed to react with outside antigens that gained entrance to the body, these programmed B-lymphocytes would not be able to produce antibody capable of reacting with these antigens without the help of similarly programmed T-lymphocytes. Thus the *production of programmed T-lymphocytes by the thymus* is of primary importance. T-lymphocytes, as will be described later, are produced in an environment within the thymus that during fetal life would have thorough exposure both to body macromolecules and to any foreign antigens reaching the fetus. But in postnatal life this environment becomes restricted to some extent with regard to the entry of foreign antigens. First, *no lymphatics drain into the thymus* and to this extent it is protected from antigens that might otherwise have gained entrance to it by this route. Second, the site in which T-lymphocytes are being produced and programmed in the thymus in postnatal life is protected to some extent from antigens present in blood by what has been described as a *barrier*, the effectiveness of which is controversial. It will be described later in connection with the thymus. It could be argued, however, that this "barrier," to some extent at least, shields the site from new antigens, so that there would be less probability of antigens that gained entrance to the body and bloodstream being able to make *premature contact* with T-lymphocytes that were being programmed in the thymus to react with these foreign antigens at any given time throughout life. There would, of course, be some T-lymphocytes in other parts of the body that had previously been programmed to react with any new antigen, but it would presumably be helpful to keep producing more. Nevertheless, in the site where the T-lymphocytes were being programmed there would be enough of the body's own macromolecules to eliminate by premature contact those that were being programmed to react against self. Further interesting aspects of the immunological role of the thymus will be mentioned in the following section, in which we discuss the histology of this organ.

Finally, it should be appreciated that clonal abortion still remains a hypothetical concept, but we consider it a reasonable one.

THE MICROSCOPIC STRUCTURE OF THE FOUR ARRANGEMENTS OF LYMPHATIC TISSUE IN THE BODY AND ITS RELATION TO THEIR RESPECTIVE FUNCTIONS

THE THYMUS

Understanding the cellular basis of immune processes began with experiments on the thymus. Until about 20 years ago it was assumed that the thymus was not essential to life, for removing the organ from mature animals seemed to have little effect on them. However, early in the 1960s, it was shown that if the thymus was removed from a *newborn* animal it subsequently did not develop immunological competence and soon died. In particular it was unable to reject transplants of foreign tissue, but its capacity to make antibodies was also diminished. Experimental evidence suggested that the thymus normally made an internal secretion that was essential if the other lymphatic organs were to function normally. However, it was later shown that the effects of removal of the thymus at birth were also due to the fact that the thymus normally makes a special kind of lymphocyte (*T-lymphocytes*) that it feeds into the body and that is vital for immunological reactions. So it is now accepted that the thymus is one of the keystones of the defense mechanisms of the body.

Gross Characteristics. The thymus is a lymphatic organ most of which lies in the thorax immediately beneath the upper part of the sternum (Fig. 13-5). It is a flattened pinkish-gray mass, roughly triangular in shape, with its apex extending up into the neck. Its shape probably reminded an early anatomist of a thyme leaf, hence its name. In most species it consists of two parts, one on each side, that are not actually fused. In man it is generally considered to be a bilobed single structure because its two lobes are in apposition along the midline.

Size in Relation to Age. The size of the thymus varies greatly in relation to age. It is largest, in relation to the remainder of the body, during fetal life and the first 2 years of postnatal life. From the 2nd year until the time of puberty it continues to increase in size but not so rapidly as the remainder of the body. After puberty it begins to involute (*L. involvere*, to roll up) and as a consequence it slowly becomes smaller as an individual ages.

For many years the size and weight of the thymus particularly in childhood were underestimated because

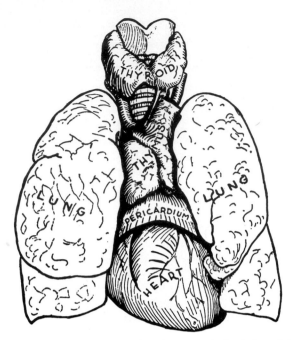

Fig. 13-5. Diagram illustrating the anatomical relation of the thymus to adjacent organs in a child. (Grant, J. C. B., and Basmajian, J. V.: Grant's Method of Anatomy. ed. 7. Baltimore, Williams & Wilkins, 1965)

serious diseases in childhood tend to bring about premature involution. Since so many people surveyed in the past had suffered communicable diseases of childhood (now largely preventable), the mean values compiled from them were not really normal. According to modern views the thymus gland weighs about 10 to 15 g. at birth and 30 to 40 g. at puberty. From then onward its weight slowly declines, but the gland still retains substantial identity in old individuals. However, its size in middle-aged and older people has probably been underestimated because the data are largely from autopsies made on people who died after long illnesses. In middle-aged and older people killed in accidents the thymus is larger than in patients of comparable age that died from disease.

The Development of the Epithelial Component of the Thymus. The thymus develops as a result of tubes of epithelial cells growing out into mesenchyme from the 3rd pharyngeal pouch on each side of the body. These tubes soon become solid cords, which in due course are pulled down into the thorax and lose connection with their points of origin. At this stage the thymus resembles an endocrine gland because it is composed of cords of epithelial cells. These proliferate and send out side branches each a forerunner of the core (medulla) of a lobule. The arrangement of cells then begins to change.

Groups of epithelial cells become arranged around a central point, much as football players pile up around and over a loose ball. These little groups of cells are known as *Hassall's corpuscles* (labeled Hc in Fig. 13-6B). The other cells of the epithelial cords become less densely arranged and tend to spread apart, but remain connected with one another because the processes of these cells adhere to one another. This makes a 3-dimensional sponge-like structure. This unusual shape and arrangement of the epithelial cells gave rise to the term *epithelial reticulum* (L. *rete,* net), so the cells of the reticulum are called *epithelial reticular cells.* This development of epithelium does not, of course, occur in a void but in mesenchyme, as will now be explained.

The Development of the Lymphatic Component of the Thymus. The epithelium grows in blunt protrusions into a mass of dough-like mesenchyme that later forms a thin capsule around the organ. In the regions between the epithelial protrusions, the mesenchyme remains and forms thin partitions (septa) that do not extend all the way to the center of the thymus but remain incomplete. The central epithelial part of the organ is thus continuous but it extends outward in all directions and peripherally it appears as the medulla of each lobule (Fig. 13-6A). Lymphocytes appear and soon fill the interstices between the epithelial cells to become the prominent cells in the thymus (dark in Fig. 13-6). It has now been established that these lymphocytes are derived from hematopoietic stem cells (CFUs), or perhaps a special type of immediate progeny cells with which the thymus is seeded, and that these cells develop into larger cells in the peripheral part of the cortex where they proliferate and differentiate to produce small lymphocytes; these are then found in the deep cortex, as will be described presently.

It should be mentioned that there is a very rapid turnover of the lymphocyte population of the thymus. If animals are given enough total body radiation the lymphocyte content of the thymus, as might be expected, mostly disappears, as do the leukocytes being produced in the bone marrow. However, an animal treated this way can generally be saved if it is immediately injected intravenously with a suspension of bone marrow cells obtained from a nonirradiated animal of the same strain. Certain of the injected bone marrow cells bring about the repopulation of the bone marrow of the host and also of the thymus. Moreover, by using chromosome markers it has been shown that the lymphocytes in the repopulated thymus of the irradiated animal are derived from the *donor* marrow cells, not from the host. Other evidence makes it clear that in postnatal life in normal unirradiated animals as well, there are cells from bone marrow (CFUs or a special type of immediate progeny) that circulate and take up residence in the thymus gland to serve as progenitor cells for lymphocytes.

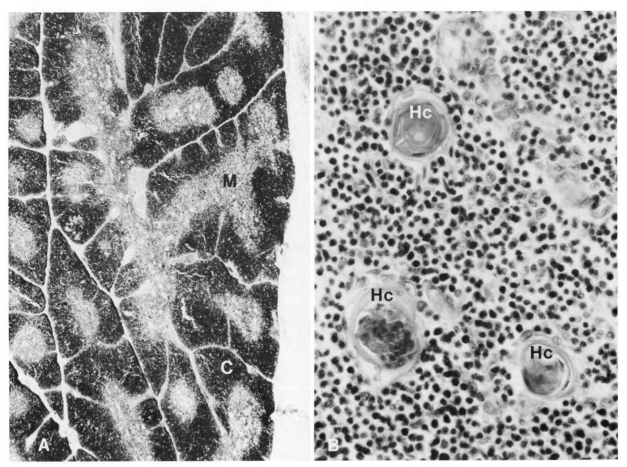

Fig. 13-6. (A) Very low power photomicrograph of the thymus gland of a child. The septa appear as clear lines. The cortex (C) of the lobules is dark; the medulla (M) is light. Observe that the medulla of one lobule is continuous with that of another. *(B)* High-power photomicrograph of an area of medulla. Three Hassall's corpuscles (Hc) are shown.

Microscopic Structure. Each *lobe* of the thymus is surrounded by a *capsule* of connective tissue. This extends into the substance of each lobe to form *septa* and divides the two lobes into incomplete *lobules,* which are usually from 1 to 2 mm. in width (Fig. 13-6A). The septa, although they penetrate deeply into the organ, do not partition the thymic tissue completely into lobules because in the central part of each lobe the thymic tissue of a given lobule is continuous with that of other lobules (Fig. 13-6A). If, however, a lobule is sectioned parallel to and near the surface, it may appear as if it were completely surrounded by septa. As the thymus involutes, fat cells accumulate in the septa.

Cortex and Medulla. Lymphocytes are not spread evenly throughout the substance of each lobule; instead, they tend to be concentrated toward borders that abut on the capsule or interlobular septa. The peripheral part of

each lobule, heavily infiltrated with lymphocytes, is termed its *cortex* (L. for bark or shell), which is labeled C in Figure 13-6A, while the more central, paler part of the lobule that does not contain so many lymphocytes is called its *medulla* (M in Fig. 13-6A). The cortex is covered by a connective tissue capsule; this is thin in the rat and mouse. The capsule may contain some small blood vessels that, although they may supply the cortex in some animals, do *not* do so in the mouse, as will be described later. An important point about the capsule of the thymus is that, unlike that of lymph nodes, *no lymphatics* enter it. *No lymph therefore drains into the thymus.*

The epithelial cells are arranged in a network, with spaces between the processes of the cells. These processes are linked by desmosomes. The interstices between the epithelial cells are packed with cells of the lymphocyte series; these and their nuclei are of three orders of size. The nuclei of the cells in the outer cortex are large; these cells may be considered *lymphoblasts.* Deeper in the cortex nuclei are somewhat smaller, and closer still to the medulla they are mostly of the size seen in small lymphocytes. Sainte-Marie and Leblond classified the cells of the lymphocyte series in the thymic cortex of rats into three groups on the basis of the size of their nucleus. By counting mitotic figures they estimated that each of the largest cells probably gave rise to 128 small lymphocytes, which would require six consecutive divisions. Mitosis occurs in the largest and the medium-sized cells. As the cells multiply and differentiate to form small lymphocytes, the latter move through the interstices of the epithelial network toward the medulla. The progenitor cells that give rise to the lymphocytes of the thymus would ordinarily enter the thymus in small numbers; they cannot be recognized. Thus the microscopic structure of the cortex as described above applies to what is seen after lymphoblasts have already been produced in large numbers. Morphological details of earlier events such as the entry of blood stem cells (which are smaller than lymphoblasts) into the thymus and the production of lymphoblasts from these cells are unknown.

THE BLOOD SUPPLY OF THE CORTEX AND THE POSSIBILITY OF A BARRIER TO ANTIGENS IN THE THYMIC CORTEX

How and When T-Lymphocytes Are Programmed

T-lymphocytes from the thymus circulate via the bloodstream and settle in certain areas of lymph nodes and spleen; in these lymphatic organs they are in a good position to come into contact with antigens that the variously programmed T-lymphocytes will recognize. Since there have to be as many kinds of differently programmed T-lymphocyte as there are potential antigens, the problem again arises as to how they become variously programmed. The way diversity is generated has been discussed with reference to B-lymphocytes, about which much more is known, mainly because their surface receptors are identical with antigen-combining sites of antibodies and this enables studies on specificity to be carried out. Until very recently T-lymphocyte receptors with specificity for antigen were unavailable, so very few studies could be done. However, it is now known that T-lymphocytes do not possess the immunoglobulin-like receptors that B-lymphocytes have on their surface. The T-lymphocyte receptors do nevertheless react specifically with antigen and so probably have a variable region like immunoglobulin molecules.

In attempting to visualize how T-lymphocytes each with specificity for a different antigen could be produced in the thymus, it is probably significant that the thymus is

a seat of enormous and continuous production of lymphocytes, a situation that would be likely to permit genetic variation. Next, a T-lymphocyte that has left the thymus to take up residence elsewhere in the body, on meeting the appropriate antigen, will become activated and give rise to a clone of cells all programmed in the same way; this indicates that the basis for its specificity is at the level of its genes. Thus, although T-lymphocytes do not become antibody-forming cells as do B-lymphocytes, they do develop specificity for particular antigens in much the same way as B-lymphocytes.

There were, however, complications that had to be thought of in connection with this concept. First, if lymphocytes are variously programmed in the thymus to react with every conceivable antigen, there is the same problem of why some of them do not become programmed to react with the macromolecules of the body in which they form. A concept that would explain why this does not happen was outlined in the earlier section on Natural and Acquired Immunological Tolerance (p. 333). In this connection it has been suggested that the large amount of lymphocyte death observed in the thymus could be accounted for by the destruction of T-lymphocytes programmed to react to body macromolecules that they encounter before they mature. Experiments have shown that an animal can be made tolerant to a foreign antigen by injecting the antigen into its thymus, but only if this is done before the thymus has had time to seed the other parts of the lymphatic system with programmed T-lymphocytes. Presumably when the thymus is injected with an antigen under these circumstances no T-lymphocytes programmed to react against that antigen would emerge from the thymus because they would be destroyed by premature contact with the antigen. So the animal would become tolerant to that antigen and remain tolerant to it for as long as the antigen persisted in the thymus.

The Blood Supply of the Thymus and Its Relation to the Thymic Barrier

It is therefore considered very probable that any T-lymphocytes being programmed in the thymus to react against body macromolecules would have adequate premature contact with these substances to prevent them from maturing and multiplying. Since T-lymphocytes are formed throughout life, the great amount of lymphocyte death in the thymus may be due to T-lymphocytes that are being programmed to react against self being killed by premature exposure to body macromolecules. However, if foreign antigens that gained entrance to the body were to have premature contact with T-lymphocytes that were being programmed throughout life to react to them they, too, would be destroyed. Hence it would be advantageous if lymphocytes being formed and programmed in the

Fig. 13-7. Electron micrograph (×12,000) of cortex of thymus (mouse). A capillary (CAP.) is cut in cross section. It is surrounded by a connective tissue space (SPACE), which at *right* contains a pericyte (PER.) and its processes. Surrounding this space is an epithelial membrane composed of cells (EP.) joined together by desmosomes. At *upper right* a lymphocyte (LY.) has been caught in the act of migrating between two epithelial cells of the barrier, presumably to enter the connective tissue space. (Clark, S. L., Jr.: Am. J. Anat., *112:1*, 1963)

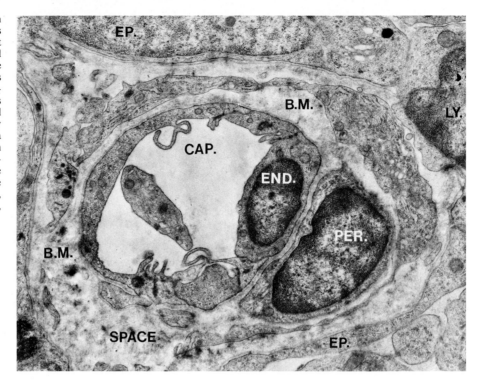

thymus to react against foreign antigens were not prematurely exposed to them.

It should be appreciated in this connection that the thymus may have already produced a full quota of T-lymphocytes that are programmed to react with any conceivable *foreign* antigen (and only foreign antigens) and that the other lymphatic tissues have been seeded with them before the offspring in any species are ever exposed to foreign antigens; this could be why tolerance to any foreign antigen can only be induced before or very shortly after birth. However, in later life, although the other lymphatic tissues could have already become seeded with T-lymphocytes programmed to react against all possible antigens, foreign antigens, if they were to enter the bloodstream and gain access to the cortex of the thymus, could stop the formation of any further T-lymphocytes programmed to react with them by having premature contact with them. This could happen if T-lymphocytes were produced in the thymus in an environment to which foreign antigens in the blood had ready access. However, there is reason to believe that the thymic cortex where T-lymphocytes are being programmed and formed in postnatal life is protected to some degree from foreign blood-borne antigens, at least from the concentrations in which these are present in the blood. One protection afforded the cortex is that it is not supplied by lymphatics, which would, of course, carry foreign antigens in even greater concentration than the blood. Second, for antigens to

move from the capillaries of the cortex to sites of T-lymphocyte production it would be necessary for them to pass through several membranes, as will soon be described. But first we have to describe the blood supply of the cortex.

The Blood Supply of the Cortex. The cortex of the thymus is supplied *only with capillaries.* In an extensive study, Raviola and Karnovsky showed by injecting the vascular bed of the thymus of mice that the capillaries originate from arterioles located at the cortico-medullary junction. From these they ascend into the cortex, where they form anastomosing capillary arcades from which capillaries return to the cortico-medullary junction to drain into the postcapillary venules of the medulla.

The Components of the Blood-Thymus Barrier in the Cortex. According to Clark, a continuous epithelium surrounds the capillaries of the cortex (Fig. 13-7, EP). Thus the reticular epithelial cells form a lining for narrow channels through which these capillaries are conducted. Between the capillaries (with their pericytes) on the one hand and the epithelial membrane on the other, a space may be seen (labeled in Fig. 13-7). Basement membrane material is associated with both the epithelial reticular cells and the endothelium of the capillaries. The space between a capillary and the epithelial cells lining the channel in which it lies may contain lymphocytes and macrophages. There are thus three components of the blood-thymus barrier through which an antigen in a capillary

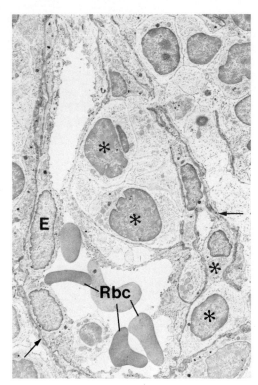

Fig. 13-8. Electron micrograph (×1,800) of thymic medulla showing several lymphocytes (marked by asterisks) migrating through the wall of a postcapillary venule. The lumen of the venule contains red blood cells (Rbc). The endothelium that lines the venule is labeled E and the basal lamina is indicated by arrows. The lymphocytes marked by asterisks have broken through the basal lamina but have still to pass between endothelial cells to gain entrance to the lumen of the venule. (Courtesy of W. Hwang and G. Simon)

would have to pass in order to reach lymphocytes forming in the cortex. First it would have to penetrate the wall of the capillary and its basement membrane. Second, it would enter the perivascular space (Fig. 13-7) which presumably would contain tissue fluid and macrophages. It is conceivable that the flow in this perivascular space might be toward the medulla so as to wash the antigen into the medulla. Moreover, macrophages in the space could take up antigen that gained access to it. Third, such macromolecules as did manage to get across the tissue fluid-filled space to reach the epithelial barrier would then have to penetrate this barrier to enter the regions where lymphocytes are forming.

There has been controversy as to whether the blood-thymus barrier is effective in postnatal life with regard to shielding forming lymphocytes from antigens. In considering this matter it should be realized that when foreign antigens gain entrance to the bloodstream, they become greatly diluted; this is in contrast to the concentration of antigens that can occur in the lymph that drains into a lymph node. However, Raviola and Karnovsky have shown in a most extensive study, using different antigens that they could trace, that some confusion about the effectiveness of the barrier stems from not limiting the barrier concept to the cortex. They found the barrier was effective in preventing antigens from reaching the interior of the cortex, but antigens were nevertheless able to reach the medulla. Their paper should be read for details.

HOW T-LYMPHOCYTES FORMED IN THE CORTEX LEAVE THE THYMUS

The thymic cortex is a very active site of lymphocyte production, particularly in fetal and early postnatal life. Unlike lymph nodes and spleen whose lymphatic tissue virtually disappears if an animal is deprived of exposure to antigens as in a germ-free environment, the thymus is a continuous producer of lymphocytes and its rate of production remains unaffected by levels of antigens in the environment or numbers of lymphocytes in the peripheral blood. The thymus is thus an *autonomous lymphocyte producer*. As might be expected, Sainte-Marie and Kostiuk found more lymphocytes in the blood leaving the thymus than in the blood entering it. The number of newly formed cells released from the thymus each day is so great that it is sufficient to replace the entire population of blood lymphocytes approximately four times over. It is difficult to ascertain what proportion of lymphocytes produced in the thymus die there. The concept outlined previously, to the effect that T-lymphocytes programmed so as to recognize macromolecules of the body as antigenic would all die in the thymus, may account for much cell death in the thymus. Furthermore, if variability of the programming of lymphocytes in the thymus is due to mutation occurring, cell death could be explained by some of the mutants not being viable.

To some extent the cortex and medulla of the thymus behave as separate entities. As the T-lymphocyte progenitors proliferate and differentiate behind the thymic barrier of the cortex, their progeny migrate from the outer to the inner cortex and the T-lymphocytes produced leave the thymus from the inner cortex without having entered the medulla of the gland. The T-lymphocytes in the thymic medulla, on the other hand, represent part of the recirculating pool of T-lymphocytes, so they exchange freely with the T-lymphocytes of other lymphatic organs. From the medulla it seems these lymphocytes are able to enter the blood circulation by migrating through the walls of venules with a characteristically high endothelium, known as *postcapillary venules* (Fig. 13-8).

Blood drains from the medulla by way of veins and these are associated with some perivascular connective tissue. There are also some lymphatics and these drain away such lymph as is formed; this probably reaches the lymphatics via connections with the perivascular spaces.

It should be noted that plasma cells are *not* normal constituents of the thymic cortex. There are two reasons for this: (*1*) T-lymphocytes cannot develop into plasma cells, and (*2*) if any B-lymphocyte should penetrate a capillary and enter the thymic cortex, it would find itself in an environment in which it would be most unlikely to encounter an antigen. However, some blood-borne B-lymphocytes may emerge in the thymic medulla and here there is no blood-thymus barrier to prevent blood-borne antigens from escaping into the perivascular tissue, so an occasional B-lymphocyte may here form a few plasma cells. Furthermore, if the thymus is damaged in such a way that parts of it become vascularized from the adjacent connective tissue, B-lymphocytes and antigens could both gain access to the injured area so that plasma cells could subsequently form.

THE THYMIC HORMONE AND ITS PRODUCTION

Development of Knowledge. A time-tested way for determining whether a given organ produces a hormone is to remove it from an experimental animal and see what happens. In 1961, Archer and Pierce and also Miller reported that removal of the thymus from a *newborn* animal resulted in impaired development of the immunological capacities of the animal.

In seeking an explanation, due consideration was given to the possibility of the lymphatic tissue of the body being cut off from the supply of lymphocytes it would receive from the thymus in early postnatal life. (At that time it was not known that there were B- and T-lymphocytes with different functions.) It was also assumed that if the thymus was not removed until later, enough time would have elapsed for it to have built up the lymphocyte population of the other lymphatic organs sufficiently for them to carry on independently.

However, evidence for another theory was soon forthcoming. It was found that if a thymus is transplanted from another animal into one thymectomized at birth, the thymectomized animal recovers most of its immunologic competence. It might be thought that this would be due to the transplanted thymus producing lymphocytes (of donor origin) and feeding them to the other lymphatic organs of the host. But even when a thymus gland is transplanted syngeneically, it takes several days for the capillaries of the host to re-establish a circulation. Since lymphocytes are sensitive cells, the lymphocytes of a thymic transplant that stay in the transplant (some migrate from it) commonly die before circulation is re-established. The cells that survive in the transplant are mostly the hardier epithelial reticular cells.

Evidence from transplantation experiments thus began to suggest that the thymus is necessary for animals to become immunologically competent in the first week or so of life because of some *humoral factor* (such as a hor-

mone) being secreted into the blood by the epithelial cells of the thymus. To test this, bits of thymus were placed in diffusion chambers and transplanted into animals thymectomized at birth. The pores of the chambers were too small to permit cells to leave but big enough to allow soluble substances to enter or leave. Thymic tissue in chambers transplanted into newborn thymectomized animals was found to partly prevent the usual effect of thymectomy. Sections made of thymic tissue from chambers left in place for some time show that all that remains of the tissue is a mass of cells of the epithelial reticular type. Accordingly, it seemed reasonable to conclude that the epithelial reticular cells of the thymus, through some humoral factor, influence lymphocytes far away from the thymus, an influence which in the first week or so of life is necessary for lymphocytes in the other lymphatic organs to proliferate, develop, and function immunologically in a normal way.

However, the production of a humoral factor is only part of the reason for early thymectomy causing impairment of the immunological system. In due course it was shown that the thymus produced T-lymphocytes, which as already explained perform particular roles. It was further shown that if animals are thymectomized at birth, the number of lymphocytes obtained from the thoracic duct is profoundly reduced. If animals several months old are thymectomized, the number of lymphocytes obtained from the thoracic duct is, with time, also substantially reduced. So with the development of knowledge that T-lymphocytes originate in the thymus only and, hence, if the thymus is removed at birth the other lymphatic tissues do not become properly seeded with them, it became obvious that the effects of thymectomy at birth could mostly be explained by a lack of production of T-lymphocytes. After a few weeks of life, the effect of thymectomy in a mouse would not be so severe because by then the other lymphatic organs would already have been seeded with T-lymphocytes. However, the role of the thymic hormone is also important because it is now known that *T-lymphocytes differentiate from their precursor cells under its influence.* One candidate for the hormone is a polypeptide known as *thymopoietin,* with 49 amino acids whose sequence is known. This acts rapidly to induce formation of T-lymphocyte surface marker on the precursors of T-lymphocytes, soon to be described.

THE EFFECTS OF CERTAIN HORMONES ON THE THYMUS

The growth hormone of the pars anterior of the pituitary gland and also thyroid hormone (Chap. 25) stimulate the growth of the thymus gland. Most steroid hormones (Chap. 25) on the other hand—if in sufficient quantity in the bloodstream—tend to bring about involution of the gland. Hence having substantial quantities of sex hormone in the circulation at the time of puberty is probably an important factor in causing the thymus gland to begin to involute at this time. Selye, from his studies on the effects of stress, believes that the premature involution of the gland observed in children who suffer from serious diseases or other forms of stress is caused by oversecretion of adrenal cortical steroid hormones as a result of the disease or stress condition. A deficiency of either adrenal cortical hormone or sex hormone in an animal, brought about by removing the endocrine glands responsible for secreting these hormones, is associated with apparent hypertrophy of the thymus or failure of the thymus to involute.

DISTINGUISHING A SECTION OF THYMUS FROM ONE OF A LYMPH NODE OR OTHER LYMPHATIC TISSUE

There are many ways to do this; however, since Hassal's corpuscles are seen only in the medulla of the thymus and not in other lymphatic tissues, their presence denotes a section of the thymus. EM studies have shown that the epithelial cells involved in forming Hassal's corpuscles pass through the same changes that are seen in the formation of keratinized epithelium, described in Chapter 7.

THE DIFFERENTIATION OF T-LYMPHOCYTES

The precursor cells of T-lymphocytes, as shown in Figure 12-3 (p. 306), are progeny of pluripotential hematopoietic stem cells (CFUs) and are cells restricted to differentiating along the T-lymphocyte pathway. They are potentially capable of migrating to the thymus and also of being influenced by it, but, because they have not yet responded to its influence, these precursor cells lack the surface markers that characterize T-lymphocytes. It is the influence of the thymus that brings about differentiation of these precursors into T-lymphocytes. This step in their differentiation is manifested by their acquiring the surface marker typical of T-lymphocytes.

It would seem that although T-lymphocytes all become variously programmed in the thymic cortex to react to individual antigens, they do not necessarily all become fully immunocompetent in this site. When the T-lymphocytes formed in the thymic cortex leave this part of the thymus they do not return to it, but recirculating T-lymphocytes, which have now attained their full measure of immunocompetence, do seem capable of entering the thymic medulla. The T-lymphocytes leaving the thymic cortex mature into the several subclasses already described, each kind bearing the surface markers typical of T-lymphocytes: (*1*) mature, immunologically competent T-lymphocytes, (*2*) helper T-lymphocytes, and (*3*) killer/suppressor T-lymphocytes. All of this maturation occurs

in the absence of antigen. Some of these programmed cells move from the thymus to lymph nodes and spleen; this migration seems to be involved in their maturation. The small, mature competent T-lymphocytes will recirculate from blood into lymphoid tissues and back to blood.

Finally, the development of knowledge and concepts with regard to T-lymphocytes has led to some striking practical results. Lymphoid progenitor cells of human fetal liver have been successfully transplanted into patients with severe immunodeficiency, an otherwise fatal disease. No graft-versus-host disease developed and furthermore functionally active T-lymphocytes were formed that were tolerant of their new host and yet were capable of rejecting cells that were foreign to their host.

THE NONENCAPSULATED LYMPHATIC NODULES OF LOOSE CONNECTIVE TISSUE

Antigens such as those of pollens, viruses, or bacteria may penetrate the wet epithelial membranes lining various tubes in the body that open to the outside world—in particular, the membranes lining the respiratory and digestive tract and the genitourinary tract. Little depots of lymphatic tissue called *lymphatic nodules* are variously scattered about in the loose connective tissue that lies beneath and supports such wet epithelial membranes, providing a further line of defense behind them. The association between lymphatic tissue and wet epithelium can be particularly intimate as in *tonsils,* which are paired structures disposed in 3 different sites (tongue, pharynx, and nasopharynx), or more remote as in the urinary bladder (Fig. 13-9). Although most prevalent beneath wet epithelial membranes, lymphatic nodules occasionally are seen in other sites.

Appearance in Sections. Most nonencapsulated lymphatic nodules in loose connective tissue are single but in some sites—for example, in tonsils or in the ileum—they become confluent. In the lower part of the small intestine, the confluent nodules form structures called *Peyer's patches* which are large enough to be seen with the naked eye. An isolated nodule in loose connective tissue is roughly spherical and up to a millimeter or so in diameter (Fig. 13-9). In an H and E section it appears under low power as a dark blue area. Under higher magnification the blue appearance is seen to be primarily due to small lymphocytes; since these cells have little cytoplasm, there is a great concentration of nuclei in the nodule so that the nodule is noticeable as a rounded blue area.

The periphery of a nodule is not sharply defined (Fig. 13-9, *left side*). Lymphocytes produced in the nodule may be pushed out from its periphery so that at this site the appearance gradually changes from a dense concentration of lymphocytes to decreasing concentration in the ad-

Fig. 13-9. A lymphatic nodule lying in loose connective tissue beneath a wet epithelial membrane (urinary bladder of a dog). The epithelium above the lymphatic nodule is of the transitional type.

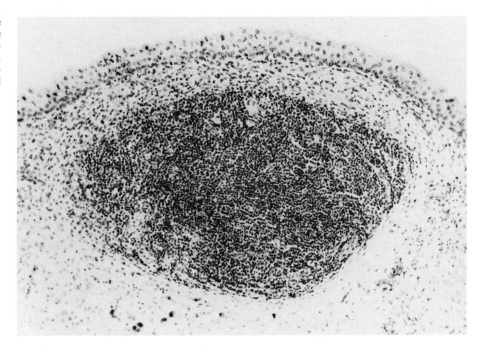

jacent tissue. Lymphatic nodules are *not encapsulated;* they lie naked in loose connective tissue. To avoid misunderstanding, it should be noted that the lymph nodes and the spleen are enclosed by connective tissue capsules.

The Development of Lymphatic Nodules in Loose Connective Tissue

Lymphatic nodules are not as common in loose connective tissue before birth as after birth. Furthermore, they do not develop nearly as extensively in germ-free animals after birth as they do in ordinary animals. It seems, therefore, that the presence and recognition of antigens have much to do with their development. An antigen that gained entrance to the intercellular substance beneath a wet epithelium would activate B-lymphocytes that had moved into the area, and by proliferation and differentiation these would give rise to the nodule.

Lymphatic nodules in loose connective tissue sometimes acquire what is termed a *germinal center,* which will be described in more detail in due course in connection with lymph nodes. They are pale-staining, rounded areas in the middle of lymphatic nodules that sometimes exhibit many mitotic figures.

The Functions of Lymphatic Nodules in Loose Connective Tissue

The functions of lymphatic nodules in loose connective tissue are not very clearly established; the nodules per-

haps serve much the same purpose as the lymphatic nodules of lymph nodes. Certainly they produce lymphocytes. Plasma cells often form in association with them, as, for example, in tonsils or in the alimentary tract. Indeed activated lymphocytes from lymphatic nodules may well be the source of the plasma cells scattered throughout the loose connective tissue beneath wet epithelial membranes such as that of the alimentary tract. The possibility has been suggested that some of the depots of confluent nodules in close association with the epithelium lining the intestine, as, for example, in the tonsil, appendix, or Peyer's patches, are a normal source of B-lymphocytes in mammals. (In birds, B-lymphocytes are formed in the bursa of Fabricius, which is somewhat similarly associated with an epithelial membrane.)

Difference Between Nonencapsulated Nodules and Lymphocytic Infiltration

Infiltrations of lymphocytes may occur in and around the site of damaged tissue. Such diffuse infiltrations are regarded as part of, or the end result of, an *inflammatory reaction* and differ from nodules in appearance because they are not round like isolated nodules, but of *irregular* shape. They differ also from confluent nodules because in the latter the outlines of the individual nodules that have fused are apparent on close scrutiny. Furthermore, lymphocytic infiltrations do not have any germinal centers as discrete or confluent nodules may have. Tissue infiltrations of cells of the lymphocyte series may be seen in

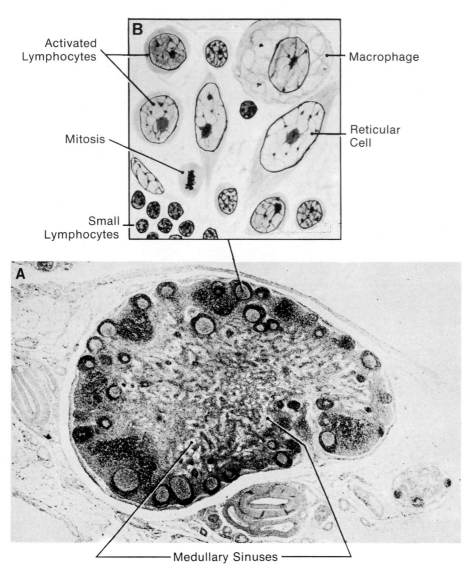

Activated Lymphocytes

Macrophage

Mitosis

Reticular Cell

Small Lymphocytes

Medullary Sinuses

Fig. 13-10. (*A*) Low-power photomicrograph of a lymph node. (*B*) High-power drawing of some cells of a germinal center.

homograft reactions and also in what are called *delayed hypersensitivity reactions.* Some other types of leukocytes are generally present along with lymphocytes in lymphocytic infiltrations.

LYMPH NODES

Lymph nodes and some of their functions were described briefly at the beginning of this chapter. We shall now give details.

Distribution. Many lymph nodes are situated in the axilla and groin. A great many are also distributed along the great vessels of the neck and a considerable number in the thorax and abdomen, particularly in association with the great vessels and mesentery. A few are associated with the popliteal vessels, and a few are at the elbow. In general, then, lymph nodes are distributed not where lymph originates (as are lymphatic nodules) but along the course of the main tributaries that flow into the thoracic and the right lymphatic ducts.

THE MICROSCOPIC STRUCTURE OF LYMPH NODES

Some Preliminary Considerations. A lymph node seen under low power in an H and E section is mostly stained deep blue (Fig. 13-10A) because it is densely packed with lymphocytes with dark blue nuclei. A lymph node has an

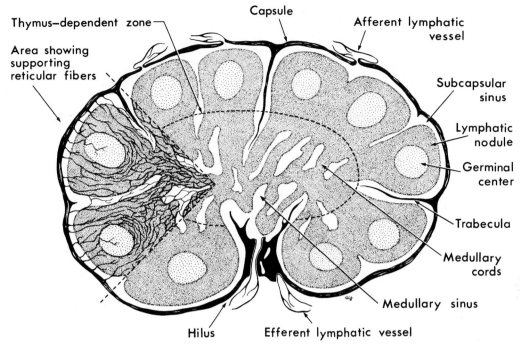

Fig. 13-11. Diagram of a lymph node. Note that the thymus-dependent zone extends for a variable distance to each side of the dotted line.

outer part called its *cortex* and an innermost part called its *medulla.* In general, lymphocytes are formed in the cortex and move to the medulla. The cortex of a lymph node, however, differs from that of the thymus because it is made up to a great extent of lymphatic nodules (Fig. 13-10A). Another difference is that there is no epithelial component in lymph nodes.

It is a mistake to approach the study of a lymph node with the impression that it is a static structure; indeed, it is a site of great activity. As noted, lymph drains through it and much phagocytosis by macrophages occurs in connection with any particulate matter that may be in lymph. Lymphocytes, both those produced in the node and those constantly being added from the bloodstream, pass into the lymph as it drains through the node. Killer cells and plasma cells that secrete antibodies are being formed in nodes (as needed) from activated T- and B-lymphocytes respectively. Furthermore, germinal centers form and then disappear again all the time. In other words, the study of a section of a lymph node suffers the same limitations as a snapshot of an ever changing scene. Frequent reference to Figures 13-10 and 13-11 in the following descriptions should help in visualizing the sites where various activities occur.

Size and Shape. Lymph nodes range in size from that of seeds to that of (shelled) almonds. Bean-shaped nodes are common and facilitate description because they possess convex and concave surfaces, so we shall describe the structure of a node of this shape.

The Capsule and Afferent and Efferent Lymphatics

A lymph node is surrounded by a connective tissue *capsule* (Fig. 13-11) that overlies its cortex. Since nodes commonly lie in fat tissue, some fat usually adheres to the outer aspect of the capsule when nodes are removed for sectioning. This may help in distinguishing a section of a lymph node from one of spleen, which has a smooth peritoneal surface. Lymphatic vessels penetrate the capsule covering the convex aspect of the node (Fig. 13-11) and others leave from the deepest part of the indentation, which is called the *hilus.* The lymphatic vessels that bring lymph *to* the node through the capsule are called *afferent lymphatics,* and those that carry it *away* from the hilus of the node are called *efferent lymphatics* (Fig. 13-11). Both kinds are provided with valves of the flap type so that lymph in them cannot pass backward toward its point of origin (Fig. 13-11).

The capsule (black in Fig. 13-11) is thicker at the hilus, where it gives off *trabeculae* (L. for little beams) of connective tissue that extend into the substance of the node to provide support and carry blood vessels (Fig. 13-11). Trabeculae also extend inward from the portion of the capsule that covers the convex aspect of the node (Fig. 13-11).

The Stroma of a Node

Like bone marrow, the substance of the node consists of a *stroma* in which free cells are loosely held in place. The stroma consists of cells and intercellular substance, which is mostly in the form of networks of reticular fibers associated with basement membrane material. These fibers connect with the capsule (Fig. 13-11, *left*) and also with the collagenic fibers of the trabeculae that extend into the node from both the capsule and the hilus to provide internal support (Fig. 13-11, *left*).

The reticular net in a node varies from being fairly closely woven to fairly open in texture. In the cortex there are rounded areas where the net is almost nonexistent (Fig. 13-11, *germinal center*). These rounded areas lie in more or less pyramidal areas of a looser mesh (gray in Fig. 13-11). The bases of these pyramidal areas face, but do not abut on, the capsule; they are however, connected to it by a few reticular or collagenic fibers. The spaces between adjacent pyramidal areas are crossed by a more open reticular net. Many such spaces contain a trabecula derived from the capsule (black in Fig. 13-11). The networks of reticular fibers of the pyramidal areas (gray in Fig. 13-11) continue into the medulla where the narrow ends of the pyramidal areas merge into structures called *medullary cords* (Fig. 13-11). The network in these often contains more plasma cells than lymphocytes. The medullary cords commonly branch and anastomose with one another as well as connecting with the pyramidal areas. The numbers of connective tissue trabeculae and the distribution of the mesh of reticular fibers seem to vary somewhat in different species. The density of the reticular mesh is generally greater around the blood vessels it supports. The sites where free cells, mostly lymphocytes, are held in the stroma are indicated in gray in Figure 13-11.

The Cells of the Stroma. It was generally believed in the past that the reticular fibers of the stroma were made by *reticular cells* and that these were mesenchymally derived, ill-defined pale cells (Fig. 13-10B) with cytoplasmic processes that extended irregularly from them, and that they were to some extent phagocytic. It was also believed that *fibroblasts* were present in the stroma in sites where there was a need for the kind of support provided by ordinary collagenic fibers, as for example where there were partitions or blood vessels, and that *macrophages* were present in the stroma, but as free cells in the interstices of the reticular net.

It has recently been found that the stromal cells differ in the various regions and it has been possible to classify them by morphological and cytochemical criteria. In B-lymphocyte-rich areas such as the lymphatic nodules, not only in lymph nodes but also in the spleen, what have been called *dendritic reticular cells* predominate; these were given their name because their cytoplasm branches to form many processes (Gr. *dendron,* tree). Although nonphagocytic, these cells can bind antigen on their surface. They have a thin rim of cytoplasm and are joined to each other by desmosomes. (They also stain for nonspecific esterase in their cytoplasm and for 5′ nucleotidase at their surface.) In T-lymphocyte-rich areas such as the deep cortex of lymph nodes (and periarteriolar lymphatic sheaths of spleen, which will be described in due course), the stromal cells have a polymorphic nucleus and finger-like processes that interdigitate between other cells. (They also have acid phosphatase in their Golgi regions and abundant ATPase at their surface.) Regions rich in both B- and T-lymphocytes have stromal cells with the characteristics of macrophages. (They possess the cytoplasmic enzymes nonspecific esterase and acid phosphatase, but neither 5′ nucleotidase nor ATPase at their surface.) Around blood and lymph vessels are stromal cells that appear to be fibroblasts (they show alkaline phosphatase at their surface). The first two types of stromal cells described here would seem to correspond to what in the past have been termed *reticular cells.*

The Sinuses of a Node

The word *sinus* is Latin for a *hollow space* and the term *sinusoid* is from the Latin *sinus* and the Greek *eidos* which means *form.* So a sinusoid is something that has the form of a hollow space. The word sinus is used in gross anatomy to denote a hollow space. In histology the word *sinusoid* is generally used to denote a thin-walled vessel with a relatively large lumen through which blood or lymph flows in life. In lymph nodes the subcapsular sinus is more of the order of a hollow space than a tube so it is termed a *sinus.*

As already mentioned, some reticular or collagenic fibers extend between the broad bases of the pyramidal areas of a lymph node and the parts of the capsule they face. A similar arrangement exists between the sides of adjacent pyramidal areas, in which space a trabecula may or may not be present (Fig. 13-11), and in the spaces between medullary cords (Fig. 13-11). These spaces that are crossed by a few reticular or collagenic fibers constitute what are called the *sinuses* of the node as will now be described.

The Lymphatic Sinuses. Afferent lymphatics empty lymph through the capsule of a node into a space between the capsule and the bases of the pyramidal areas that is

Fig. 13-12. Electron micrograph (×2,100) of the cortex of a lymph node. The thin capsule (Cs) is seen at *top*. Below this is the subcapsular sinus (S), which contains lymphocytes (Ly) and macrophages (Ma). The subcapsular sinus is lined with endothelial cells (E) and traversed by some fine trabeculae of collagenic fibers which are covered with endothelium (*see also* the next illustration). An asterisk indicates a gap in the endothelial lining of the sinus. In the lymphatic nodule that lies below the sinus some lymphocytes are labeled Ly and a reticular cell, RC. (Nopajaroonsri, C., Luk, S. C., and Simon, G. T.: Am. J. Pathol., *65:*1, 1971)

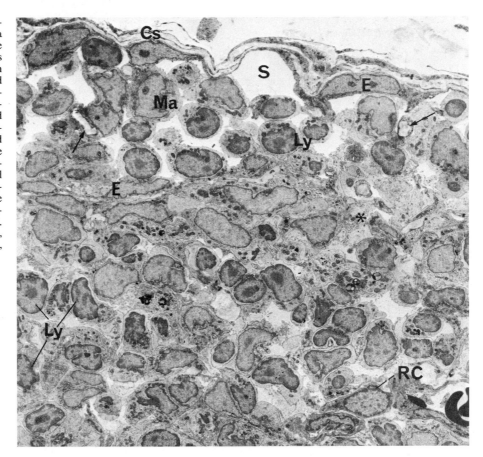

called the *subcapsular sinus* (Figs. 13-11 and 13-12, S). In the past this space, from studies with the LM, was generally described as containing phagocytic cells whose cytoplasmic processes connected with one another so that they formed a cobweb-like network through which lymph passed and was strained of particulate matter by the phagocytic action of the then-called "reticuloendothelial" cells of the cobweb.

The study of rat lymph nodes with the EM by Nopajaroonsri, Luk, and Simon, at relatively low magnifications, indicates a different type of structure. The subcapsular sinus (Fig. 13-12, S) proves to be a potential space but one that contains many *free cells.* It is lined by what they term *lymphatic endothelium* (Fig. 13-12, E), which consists of flattened cells not significantly different from the ordinary endothelium that lines lymphatic and blood vessels in general. They found, however, that while the endothelium lining the capsule was continuous, that lining the deeper side of the sinus was discontinuous. Neither endothelium had a basement membrane. They found that occasional collagenic or reticular trabeculae cross the subcapsular sinus (Fig. 13-13) and that these are covered with endothelium. The sinus contains a great many free cells, most of which are macrophages and lymphocytes (Fig. 13-12, Ma and Ly). Their findings therefore differ from older views about the structure of lymph sinuses but, since both concepts indicate the existence of many phagocytic cells in the sinuses, both support the concept of filtration occurring in them. According to the newer view both macrophages and lymphocytes in the pyramidal areas already described would have easy access to the sinuses via the discontinuous endothelium on this side of the sinus.

From the subcapsular sinus lymph continues through the node by way of the *cortical* and *subcortical sinuses,* which exist between the sides of the pyramidal areas previously described. Here further lymphocytes are added to the lymph. These channels in turn connect with the *medullary sinuses,* which exist between the medullary cords (Fig. 13-11) and deliver lymph to the efferent lymphatics that leave the node. All these sinuses were found, in the EM study mentioned above, to have the same type of structure as the subcapsular sinus in that they are lined with lymphatic endothelial cells but these are all discon-

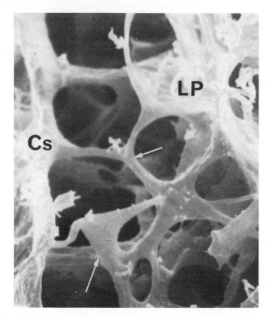

Fig. 13-13. Scanning electron micrograph (×1,900) of a subcapsular lymphatic sinus showing the meshwork of trabeculae (arrows) joining the capsule (Cs) to the stroma of the node (LP). These trabeculae correspond to the collagen bundles seen traversing the sinus with transmission electron microscopy. (Courtesy of S. Luk and G. Simon)

tinuous. Furthermore, as in the subcapsular sinus there is no definite basement membrane. Here also gaps between the lining cells would permit free entry or exit of cells from the pyramidal areas or the medullary cords. Lymphocytes and macrophages were the common types of cells seen in the various sinuses.

The Lymphatic Nodules of a Node

The areas of fine reticular mesh described above that provide a framework for the pyramidal areas and join with medullary cords are packed, except in their central parts (when germinal centers are present), with cells of the lymphocyte series; these are mostly small lymphocytes but larger progenitor cells are also present. The mesh of the medullary cords is likewise packed with free cells that vary from lymphocytes to cells in various stages of differentiation into plasma cells. Next, the roughly pyramidal areas packed with cells of the lymphocyte series have enough of a rounded appearance to have been termed *lymphatic nodules* and, indeed, if they contain germinal centers, as they do in Figure 13-10, the appearance of more or less rounded nodules is accentuated by the fact that densely packed lymphocytes form a ring around each germinal center (Fig. 13-10). These nodules,

however, have tails that continue down into the medullary cords, but this does not necessarily show in every section. It is therefore common to speak of the cortex of a lymph node such as the one illustrated in Figure 13-10A as containing lymphatic nodules (instead of pyramidal areas). These are often separated from one another but can become confluent as so many are in Figure 13-10.

The Thymus-Dependent Zone of a Node

Thymectomy performed at birth has a very characteristic and specific effect on the structure of an animal's lymph nodes. In the normal adult mouse the cortex consists of lymphatic nodules that are often confluent and may or may not have germinal centers. The zones of the node between the level of germinal centers and that of the medullary cords are termed the *mid* and *deep cortical zones;* these are not as densely packed with lymphocytes as the more superficial part of the cortex. Blood vessels of a special type called *postcapillary venules,* with walls characteristically consisting of more or less *cuboidal* endothelium through which lymphocytes commonly migrate from blood to lymph (Figs. 13-20 and 13-21) are present in these zones. (Ordinary venules are thin-walled, having a flattened endothelium consisting of cells with a *squamous* shape.)

As described by Parrott the effects of thymectomy at birth are manifested chiefly in the *mid* and *deep cortex* which become depleted of lymphocytes, and the postcapillary venules normally present become thin-walled like ordinary venules. This region was termed by Parrott, de Sousa, and East the *thymus-dependent zone* of a lymph node. In Figure 13-11 this zone extends for a variable distance *on either side* of the line labeled "thymus-dependent zone." It is now believed that the lymphocytes of this zone are chiefly T-lymphocytes and that this zone must be seeded from the thymus to develop and be maintained.

The thymus-dependent zone of a lymph node is the zone primarily involved when an allograft is placed in a region that drains into the node. Parrott showed that clusters of large free cells with basophilic cytoplasm appear in this region under such conditions within a few days. The clusters are often associated with postcapillary venules. However, in allografts made in mice thymectomized at birth, no early changes of this kind are seen in the lymph nodes along drainage routes and only later do a few free cells with basophilic cytoplasm appear. It has been shown, moreover, that when thymic transplants are made into mice thymectomized at birth, lymphocytes from the transplant migrate into the bloodstream and eventually take up a position in the thymus-dependent areas of lymph nodes.

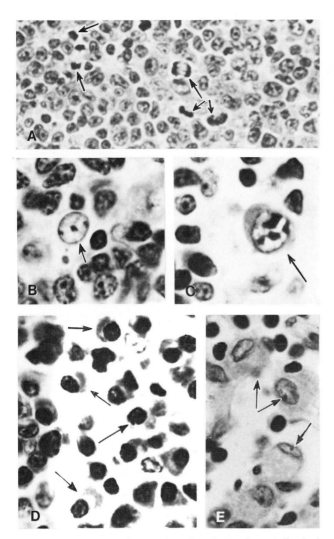

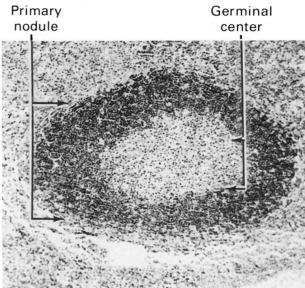

Fig. 13-15. Low-power photomicrograph of part of a lymph node (dog), showing a primary nodule. The central part of this contains a pale germinal center.

Fig. 13-14. Photomicrographs of regions of a mediastinal lymph node (rat). (*A*) Active germinal center. Arrows indicate cells in mitosis. (*B*) Germinal center. Arrow indicates the nucleus of a reticular cell. Note that its cytoplasm is very indistinct. (*C*) Edge of a germinal center. Arrow indicates a large cell with a ring of basophilic cytoplasm that has a sharp edge. This is a free, rounded cell, probably a plasmablast. (*D*) Medullary cord. Arrows indicate plasma cells. Note the negative Golgi areas in the cytoplasm, as seen at *bottom left*. (*E*) Medullary sinuses. Arrows indicate macrophages.

It therefore seems that inability of thymectomized mice to reject allografts is due to the fact that they lack T-lymphocytes in the parts of their lymph nodes that would be concerned with producing killer cells.

Immunofluorescence technics show that *B-lymphocytes*, on the other hand, are localized in the *lymphatic nodules* of the cortex, whereas T-lymphocytes are found

in the deep cortex. So in the diagram shown in Figure 13-11 the thymus-dependent zone of the node would be a zone that, as noted, extends for a short distance to either side of the dotted line labeled "thymus-dependent zone." Extending from a little bit above this line to the broad base of a pyramidal area, the lymphocytes would be primarily of the B type. However, there is much movement of lymphocytes of both kinds so there is a good deal of mixing of the two types. B-lymphocytes moreover are present in the tips of the pyramidal areas and along their sides. They are also present in the medullary cords, for the latter are the chief site of formation of plasma cells which, of course, are derived from B-lymphocytes.

Germinal Centers. These are rounded areas commonly seen in the middle of lymphatic nodules (often called *primary nodules*) of the cortex, so germinal centers are sometimes referred to as *secondary nodules*. The position of the germinal centers (secondary nodules) in relation to the pyramidal cortical areas is shown in Figure 13-11 and their appearance in a very low power view of a section of a lymph node is illustrated in Figure 13-10A. Individual germinal centers are also shown at slightly higher magnifications in Figures 13-14A, 13-15, and 13-16 and at high magnification in Figure 13-14B and C.

Significance of Germinal Centers. Some of the facts from which we can reason the significance of germinal centers are as follows. First, they do not develop in lymphatic nodules before birth, nor are they found postnat-

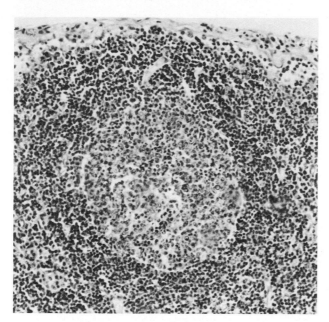

Fig. 13-16. Low-power photomicrograph of a primary nodule containing a germinal center that is not pale but basophilic. On close inspection it would be seen to contain many mitotic figures (*see* Figs. 13-14A, B, and C for higher-power views of this type of germinal center).

ally in animals raised in a germ-free environment. Other evidence also indicates that germinal centers only develop in the primary nodules of a lymph node because that node has been exposed to an antigen that in all probability has reached it via lymph originating in some body site where a foreign antigen was present. Commonly this occurs as a result of a bacterial infection in the part of the body from which the lymph draining through the node was derived. Next, whereas antibody can be produced in lymph nodes that have not developed germinal centers, these centers commonly appear during the course of prolonged exposure of a lymph node to an antigen. Hence the development of germinal centers in a primary response would seem to be an indication of there being a substantial and prolonged demand for antibody production.

What is of even greater interest, however, is the fact that germinal centers make their appearance in the primary nodules of a node much more rapidly when there is a secondary response to the same antigen—that is, when a node is exposed a second time to the same antigen and responds by producing specific antibody to that antigen. This shows that there is a basis for immunological memory in primary nodules. Two factors may be involved in this memory as will now be described.

One factor seems to be that in the sites where germinal

centers develop in primary nodules there are dendritic reticular cells with large pale nuclei (Fig. 13-14B, arrow) and cytoplasm that is relatively indistinct, often extending in the form of processes; hence these cells have an extensive surface. Nossal found that the surface of dendritic reticular cells in the vicinity of the lymphatic nodules of the cortex become studded with antibody molecules produced as a result of an individual's first exposure to a particular antigen. Hence, if the same antigen arrives in the lymph node as a result of a second exposure to it, much of the antigen could be trapped by the antibody on the surface of these dendritic reticular cells. In this way the second lot of antigen could be concentrated at a site where appropriately programmed lymphocytes in the nodule would be likely to encounter it and hence be activated.

A second way memory is involved in producing a heightened secondary response is that long-lived memory cells of both T- and B-varieties would have remained in the lymphatic tissues after the first exposure to an antigen. On re-exposure to the same antigen, even after a long time, these would rapidly become activated. Because there are so many of them to encounter the antigen, the secondary response is characterized by amplified production of antibody and the rapid formation of germinal centers.

Germinal centers, although consisting mostly of B-lymphocytes, also contain small numbers of T-lymphocytes. Furthermore, macrophages abound in these centers. T-lymphocytes, due to their role as helper cells, appear to be necessary for the formation of germinal centers and also for immunological memory, for congenitally athymic mice lack both germinal centers and immunological memory, and thymic grafts restore both, presumably by providing T helper cells.

INVESTIGATION OF PRIMARY AND SECONDARY RESPONSES BY MEANS OF IMMUNOFLUORESCENCE

Coons in 1958 used the immunofluoresence sandwich technic, which he devised (Fig. 9-21), to study these responses in lymph nodes. He found that by the fourth day in a primary response about 50 cells in any given section cut from a node revealed antibody, and that their numbers did not increase to any extent over the next four days. However, in a secondary response he found that by the second day after antigen was injected there were hundreds of cells making antibody in a comparable area. Furthermore he found that these cells were distributed irregularly enough (Fig. 13-17) to indicate that they did not belong to a single clone but instead had arisen independently.

To summarize: the difference between a primary and a secondary response (and also the relation of these re-

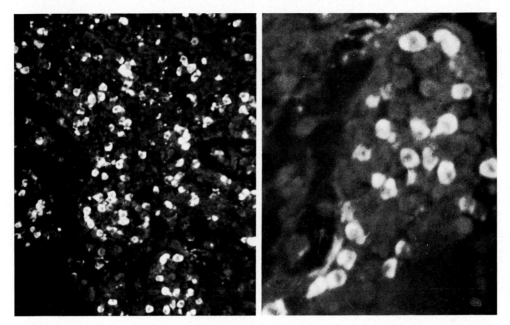

Fig. 13-17. Low-power and high-power fluorescence photomicrographs of a portion of a popliteal lymph node of a rabbit after a second injection of diphtheria toxoid. Sites where antibody is present appear as bright areas. Careful inspection of the picture on the right will show that antibody is present in the cytoplasm of cells with the characteristics of young plasma cells. (Courtesy of G. Sainte-Marie)

sponses to the formation of germinal centers) is essentially that on first exposure to an antigen, the number of B-lymphocytes programmed to react with that antigen in a nodule is relatively low. These few cells nevertheless become activated and proliferate, either differentiating into plasma cells or returning to the state of being small lymphocytes (memory cells) that tend to remain in the lymph node. Thus after a primary response there are many more B-lymphocytes, all of which are identical in being programmed similarly to the first. Since there are now many more of them to react on a second exposure to the same antigen, more antibody is now produced per unit time and thus higher antibody levels are reached in a shorter time. Microscopic evidence of their activation, namely formation of germinal centers (which indicates activation of a number of B-lymphocytes) also appears sooner.

Now that we have described the roles played by *lymphocytes* in primary and secondary responses, and also the role of the *dendritic reticular cells* present in the nodules, we should also add that *macrophages,* as well as serving a phagocytic filtering function in lymph nodes and other lymphatic tissues, also participate in a nonspecific way in the immune response. Macrophages remove excess antigen, partly degrade it, and even seem capable of presenting it to lymphocytes in a more immunogenic form. Since the microscopic appearance of dendritic reticular cells and macrophages is so similar, many do not attempt to distinguish between them.

THE CHANGES IN FINE STRUCTURE THAT OCCUR AS AN ACTIVATED B-LYMPHOCYTE BECOMES A PLASMA CELL

An *activated B-lymphocyte* typically has a larger nucleus than a small lymphocyte and the chromatin is not so condensed. It has a wide rim of basophilic cytoplasm as seen in sections with the LM. With the EM the nucleus of an activated lymphocyte is relatively pale-staining (labeled N in Fig. 13-18A). The cytoplasm is characterized by an abundance of free ribosomes and polysomes (ps in Fig. 13-18A). Cells of the B-lymphocyte type that differentiate into plasma cells are sometimes called *plasmablasts* or *immunoblasts.* As such a cell becomes a plasma cell it develops large cisternae of rER (labeled in Fig. 13-18B) and a larger Golgi so as to become a secretory cell that elaborates antibody. Activated B-lymphocytes customarily migrate to medullary cords, where they complete their development into plasma cells. Plasma cells are nonmotile and live for only a few days. As differentiation occurs, the nucleus of a plasma cell becomes smaller and its cytoplasm relatively more abundant.

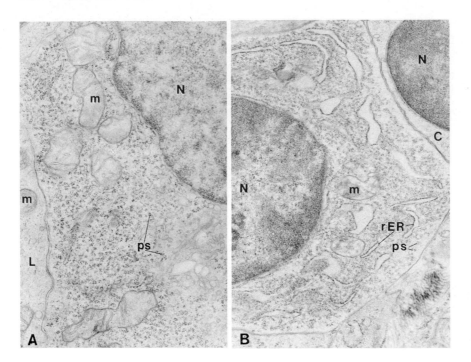

Fig. 13-18. Electron micrographs of cells of a lymph node taken a few days after an antigen was injected into the site that drained into it, showing changes in the appearance of a lymphocyte as it develops into a plasma cell. (*A*) At *lower left* the cytoplasm of a small (unactivated) lymphocyte (L) contains only a few ribosomes and few mitochondria (m). The remainder of this micrograph shows an activated lymphocyte, the cytoplasm of which shows abundant ribosomes and polysomes (PS). (*B*) This micrograph shows further development of an activated lymphocyte. As well as abundant free ribosomes and polysomes, this cell has a considerable content of rER, indicating its differentiation along the plasma cell series. At *upper right,* part of a small (unactivated) lymphocyte may be seen; compare the appearance of its nucleus (N) and cytoplasm (C) with that of the other cells illustrated in parts *A* and *B* of this figure. (Courtesy of H. Movat)

The Different Classes of Immunoglobulins

As mentioned in Chapter 9 in connection with mast cells and allergy, there are several different classes of antibody molecules. We have in this chapter discussed immune responses and where they occur, and to round out the account for those who would like more information at this time, we next briefly describe the different classes of immunoglobulins.

Based on their molecular size and composition, 5 classes of immunoglobulins are recognized. Enough is now known about these different classes to suggest that they perform different functions in the body and are synthesized in different locations.

IgG is the immunoglobulin present in highest concentration in normal serum; it represents about 75 per cent of the total immunoglobulin. It is the antibody that is usually referred to in connection with prolonged immunization procedures. Its sedimentation coefficient of 6 to 7S corresponds to a molecular weight of around 150,000. IgG molecules are relatively long-lived in the body and are capable of fixing complement. This class of immunoglobulin is produced by plasma cells and also by cells that look like activated B-lymphocytes but have developed some rER. Such cells lie free in loose connective tissue, in lymphatic nodules under wet epithelial surfaces, in the medulla of lymph nodes, and in the red pulp of the spleen. IgG is the *only* class of immunoglobulins that can cross the placenta; this allows a baby to be provided with antibodies from its mother to help it after it is born until it has had time to make its own.

Immunoglobulin molecules of the class known as *IgM* are much larger than those of IgG, with a molecular weight of about 900,000 and a sedimentation coefficient of 19S. Each molecule is a pentamer of 5 IgG subunits held together in a ring by disulfide bonds. This is the immunoglobulin characteristically produced early in a humoral antibody response to an antigen, by the same

kinds of cells that produce IgG and at the same sites. It is now clear that the same cells are capable of producing both classes of immunoglobulins. IgM is much more efficient than IgG in fixing and activating complement and therefore mediating cytotoxic reactions. IgM is less efficient than IgG, however, in neutralization reactions, that is, ones in which functional molecules (such as those of enzymes) are inactivated by combination with antibody. On interacting with an antigen, IgM is more likely than IgG to produce an antigen-antibody complex that precipitates.

IgA is another major class of immunoglobulins. It is characteristic of bodily secretions. It also occurs in serum, where its concentration is usually greater than that of IgM. It occurs in tears and milk but predominantly in the mucous secretions of the respiratory and gastrointestinal tracts. Its molecules have the general character of immunoglobulin molecules but they are composed of 1 to 4 immunoglobulin subunits. The IgA that appears in secretions (*secretory IgA*) is mainly in the form of a dimer, held together by a polypeptide component known as the *secretory component.* The molecular weight of secretory IgA is around 400,000. The precursor molecules for IgA are synthesized in plasma cells; the secretory component seems to be synthesized in epithelial cells so that the dimer and the secretory component are able to combine before the secretory IgA is secreted. Since molecules of secretory IgA possess antibody activity and are secreted onto wet epithelial surfaces, these molecules provide a first line of defense against potential invaders before the latter actually enter the body. IgA is believed to be especially active against viruses.

IgD is a minor immunoglobulin class that differs from IgG only in the detailed structure of its molecules. Its function is unknown but it may be related to the regulation of immune responses.

IgE, as mentioned in connection with mast cells in Chapter 9,

Fig. 13-19. Electron micrograph (×15,000) of a small post-capillary venule (about 8 μm. in diameter) in the cortex of a lymph node (rat). Note the characteristic tall endothelial cells lining the vessel. The one at *top left* shows vacuoles and prominent Golgi regions (G). The basal lamina (bl) surrounding the vessel is also indicated. (Courtesy of C. Nopajaroonsri and G. Simon)

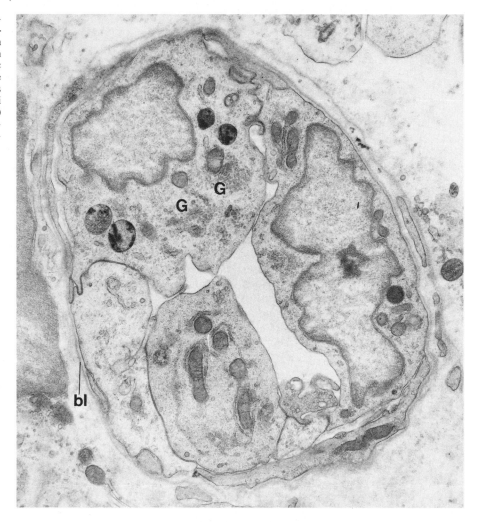

represents a minor class of immunoglobulins that has a special affinity for mast cells and basophils and it *mediates allergic reactions*. These molecules, whose production is stimulated by antigens like pollen and dusts, become attached to Fc receptors on the surface of mast cells by their Fc end, leaving their antigen combining sites free to interact with these antigens. The result of antigen binding is sudden release of mast cell granules, with the pharmacological consequences attendant upon exposure of blood vessels to histamine and the other vasoactive substances contained in mast cell granules. IgE is produced in plasma cells that are situated under wet epithelial surfaces, that is, in the same regions as those that produce IgA but in different locations from those that make IgG. IgE exists in the monomeric form and its molecules are of about the same size as those of IgG. The amino acid sequence in its heavy chains is, however, slightly different. IgE, like IgA and IgD, does not fix complement.

On exposure to any antigen, the production of immunoglobulins of all 5 classes is stimulated but complex regulatory mechanisms soon come into play so that, under different conditions, one or other of the immunoglobulins eventually predominates.

THE BLOOD SUPPLY OF LYMPH NODES AND HOW LYMPHOCYTES PASS FROM BLOOD TO LYMPH

A lymph node is supplied entirely (or almost entirely) from arteries that enter it at the hilus.

Arterioles from these arteries ascend into the substance of the node via the substance of both the trabeculae and the medullary cords. The arterioles reach as far as the cortex but, according to Menzies, the arterioles end in capillaries before germinal centers are approached. A germinal center and the area of cortex immediately surrounding it are thus supplied only with capillaries.

Many capillaries that descend in the cortex (toward the medulla) become postcapillary venules, which in many instances are relatively long and lined with cuboidal (or even taller) endothelium (Fig. 13-19). These venules are most numerous in the cortical area indicated roughly in Figure 13-11 as the thymus-dependent zone of the

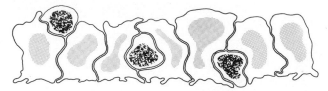

Fig. 13-20. Diagram showing how lymphocytes can migrate between the relatively tall endothelial cells that line postcapillary venules in such a manner that the endothelial cells remain sealed to one another at some level so as to prevent undue fluid loss. (Schoefl, G. I.: J. Exp. Med., *136:*568, 1972)

node. It is through the walls of these curious venules that lymphocytes chiefly migrate from blood to lymph in their recirculation. Different views have arisen about how lymphocytes pass through the endothelium of these vessels because of the problem of interpreting from sections what was really happening in three dimensions. The situation was studied by Schoefl who presents convincing evidence that lymphocytes migrate through the endothelium by passing *between* contiguous endothelial cells. Because the endothelial cells are tall in these vessels the endothelium remains as a seal as a lymphocyte passes between cells, because by the time a lymphocyte reaches the basement membrane the cells between which it passed have closed over the opening between them on the luminal side (Fig. 13-20). Figure 13-21 shows two lymphocytes migrating through the endothelium, which has closed over on the luminal side. One lymphocyte has broken through the basement membrane to enter the substance of the node, from which it will probably be carried away in the lymph, eventually to enter the thoracic duct and from there to return to the bloodstream again. The recirculation of lymphocytes was dealt with earlier in this chapter (p. 324).

Differences Between Various Nodes. There is some variation in the microscopic appearance between lymph nodes taken from different parts of the body. In some, the lymphatic nodules of the cortex are highly developed and little medulla is apparent. In a section of a node of this type, the student will have difficulty finding medullary cords and sinuses. In nodes taken from other parts of the body, the medulla rather than the cortex may be well developed. These nodes should be used to study medullary cords. It should always be remembered that a single slice cut through a node may not be truly representative of its overall microscopic structure.

HEMAL LYMPH NODES AND HEMAL NODES

Most mammals have, in addition to lymph nodes, a much smaller number of structures that are similar except that they are yellow or red instead of gray in color. On section, these structures resemble lymph nodes except that they have somewhat better defined channels in their

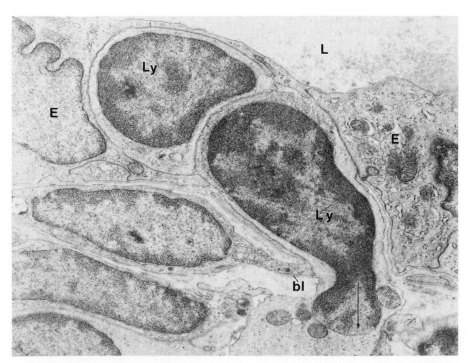

Fig. 13-21. Electron micrograph (×18,500) of part of the wall of a postcapillary venule of a lymph node (rat), showing two lymphocytes (Ly) passing down through the wall between two endothelial cells (E) lining the lumen (L). Part of one lymphocyte (indicated by arrow) has created a gap in the basal lamina (bl) and is escaping from the vessel. (Nopajaroonsri, C., Luk, S., and Simon, G. T.: Am. J. Pathol, *65:*1, 1971)

coarse mesh, and either some or all of these channels are filled with *blood* instead of lymph. If only some are filled with blood and others with lymph, the structure is called a *hemal lymph node.* If all the channels are filled with blood, it is called a *hemal node.*

There is some question as to whether hemal lymph nodes or hemal nodes are constant structures in man, but they have often been described as commonly occurring in the prevertebral peritoneal tissue, in the root of the mesentery, near the rim of the pelvis, and occasionally in other sites. There are not enough of them in man to filter very much blood, but it is important to know that they exist lest if discovered at operation or autopsy they be mistaken for pathologically altered tissue.

THE SPLEEN

The nonencapsulated lymphatic nodules, lymph nodes, and spleen are the important sites in the body in which lymphocytes become activated to form cells that either produce antibodies or mediate the cell-mediated type of immunological reaction. However, there is a division of labor among these three types of lymphatic tissue so that a suitable response to antigens may be present in any of the 3 main types of body fluids tissue fluid, lymph, or blood. The nonencapsulated lymphatic nodules are exposed to antigens that may be present in the tissue fluid in which they are bathed. Lymph nodes are arranged along lymphatic vessels and constructed in such a way that lymphocytes are efficiently exposed to the lymph that drains through them. Finally, the spleen is an organ isolated from the above-mentioned two types of body fluids, but designed to give antigens present in blood wide and reasonably prolonged exposure to variously programmed immunologically competent cells as the blood circulates through it.

Gross Characteristics. The spleen is an organ roughly the size and shape of a clenched fist. It lies in the abdomen in the shelter of the left 9th, 10th, and 11th ribs, with its long axis parallel with them. Its purple color is due to its great content of blood. It is soft in consistency and more friable than most organs. (The possibility of it being ruptured from severe crushing type injuries should always be taken into account.) Most of its surface is smooth and not attached by fat or loose connective tissue to the organs or structures with which it is in contact; such a surface is called a *serosa.* A long fissure may be seen close to its medial border; this is termed the *hilus.* On approaching this, the splenic artery divides into several branches that enter the substance of the spleen separately at different points along the elongated hilus. Veins and lymphatics leave the spleen in association with the arteries that enter it. The veins later unite to form the splenic vein.

No afferent lymphatics enter the free surface of the spleen as occurs in lymph nodes, the surfaces of which are of course attached to the tissue in which they lie. Such lymphatics as exist in the spleen are efferent and they are confined to the connective tissue sheaths of the blood vessels, as will be described presently. As noted, they leave the hilus.

Functions of the Spleen

First, as noted, the spleen serves as the site where antigens if present in the blood can activate suitably programmed lymphocytes to develop into immunologically functioning cells.

Second, in many animals but not normally in man, the spleen in postnatal life is a hematopoietic organ producing not only cells of the lymphocyte series but also those of the erythrocyte and granulocyte series as well as megakaryocytes and platelets. In man the spleen serves this function under normal conditions only in fetal life; however, the spleen retains the potentiality for blood cell formation even in adult life. Under certain pathological conditions it may again become a hematopoietic organ producing the cells ordinarily formed in bone marrow. This, when it occurs, is called *extramedullary hematopoiesis.*

Third, the spleen abounds in macrophages with ready access to the blood that circulates through it. The chief matter they phagocytose in filtering blood is old, worn-out erythrocytes but they also participate in the phagocytosis of worn-out leukocytes and platelets. Most of the iron they liberate from the hemoglobin of worn-out erythrocytes that they phagocytose they restore to the circulation, where it is used over again in the formation of new erythrocytes in the bone marrow. The macrophages of the spleen also produce the pigment bilirubin from the breakdown of hemoglobin; this circulates to the liver where it becomes a constituent of bile.

Fourth, the spleen can serve a mechanical function. In normal life it is more or less distended with blood that is circulating through it and in this sense it is more or less a storehouse for blood. Particularly in animals that are sometimes called upon for great bursts of activity, the spleen can release stored blood into the circulation so as to provide for a more efficient pumping action of the heart; in this sense the spleen can act as an automatic transfusion bank. The fact that it is normally somewhat distended with blood in life is apparent if the size of the spleen seen at a surgical operation is compared with its size seen at autopsy, because after death the spleen contracts and squeezes much of its blood into the splenic vein as the pressure within it falls.

Finally, it is believed the spleen permits blood cells to become concentrated by separating them to some extent

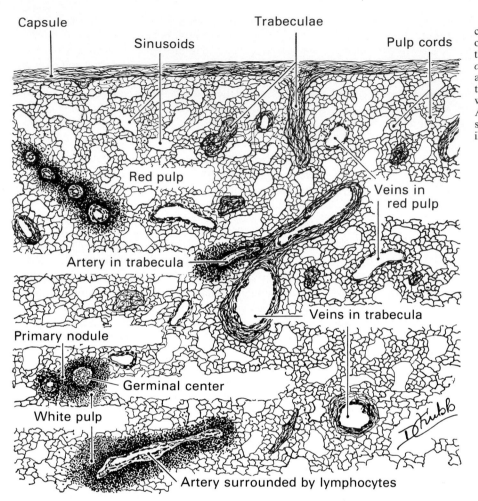

Capsule Sinusoids Trabeculae Pulp cords

Red pulp

Veins in red pulp

Artery in trabecula

Veins in trabecula

Primary nodule

Germinal center

White pulp

Artery surrounded by lymphocytes

Fig. 13-22. Diagram of section cut perpendicular to the surface of distended human spleen. Note that the white pulp (*left lower corner*) consists of nodules and aggregations of lymphocytes, and that the red pulp is an open mesh with sinusoids running through it. A trabecula with veins may be seen in the central part of the illustration.

from the plasma in which they are suspended. The concentrated cells may be retained in the spleen for varying periods and then released into the circulation. In addition to cells, platelets may be similarly held in the spleen, for a considerable proportion of the body's platelets are normally found in it.

White and Red Pulp

Much can be learned about the internal structure of the spleen by examining, with the naked eye or a magnifying glass, a slice cut through a spleen (this is commonly done at postmortem examinations). It will be seen to be surrounded by a connective tissue capsule (Figs. 13-22 and 13-23). The capsule has some smooth muscle fibers in it but these cannot be seen with the naked eye. The capsule is smooth because it is covered with a continuous layer of mesothelium. Trabeculae of connective tissue (Figs. 13-22 and 13-23) extend into the substance of the organ both

from the hilus and to a lesser extent from the capsule. The remainder of the interior of the spleen is filled with what is called *splenic pulp*. Two kinds of pulp can be seen with the naked eye: *white*, and *red*. The white pulp is distributed as tiny little firm gray islands (dark in Fig. 13-22) somewhat less than 1 mm. in diameter, among the soft red pulp that fills all the remaining space. The basic framework of the pulp is a network of reticular fibers (Fig. 13-22).

THE MICROSCOPIC STRUCTURE OF
THE HUMAN SPLEEN

If sections cut perpendicular to the capsule are examined with the LM, it will be obvious that the little nodules of gray pulp observed on the cut surface of the spleen with the naked eye are *lymphatic nodules* (Fig. 13-24). These, then, are the chief sites of lymphocyte production in the spleen. Moreover, it will be seen that the red pulp

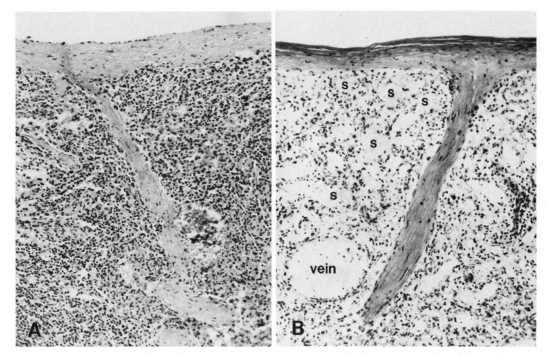

Fig. 13-23. Low-power photomicrographs of sections cut perpendicular to the capsule of the spleen. (*A*) Collapsed spleen. The capsule and also a trabecula extending in from the capsule may be seen. (*B*) Spleen distended with fixative through its veins. Note that the red pulp has been opened up by this procedure, and that the sinusoids (s) are patent.

Fig. 13-24. Low-power photomicrograph of a distended human spleen. In this section an artery that has left a trabecula and is passing through red pulp is cut longitudinally. Many lymphocytes, disposed in a fine reticular mesh, are seen above the artery. Toward the left-hand side the lymphatic tissue accompanying the artery is expanded into a primary nodule. The artery at the site of the primary nodule has given off a branch which has entered the nodule as a follicular artery. The border area between the white and red pulp is referred to as the marginal zone.

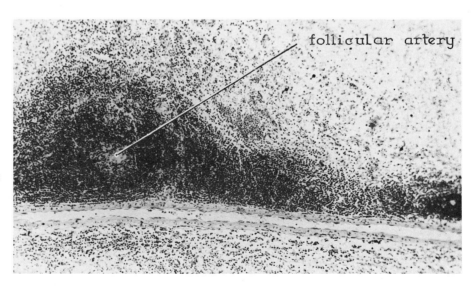

that surrounds the lymphatic nodules contains vast numbers of red blood cells in its mesh (these are not shown in Fig. 13-22) because the red pulp represents the part of the spleen that is designed to *filter blood.*

Some Problems Associated With the Study of the Spleen. Whereas in many laboratory animals the spleen serves the same functions as the spleen of man, in postnatal life the spleen of such animals commonly performs the addi-

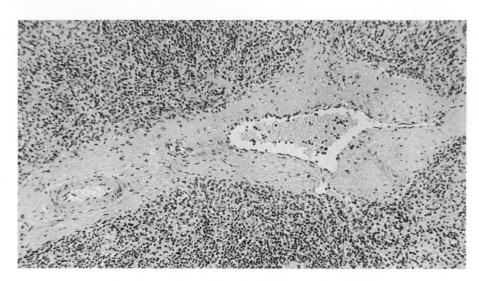

Fig. 13-25. Low-power photomicrograph of collapsed spleen, cut near its center. A large trabecula is seen extending across the middle of the field. It contains an artery (with relatively small lumen and thick wall) at *lower left* and a vein (with relatively large lumen and thin wall) at *right*.

tional functions of producing erythrocytes, granular leukocytes, and platelets, which functions are not performed by the spleen of man after birth. Accordingly, it is much simpler in many respects to limit our discussion of the microscopic structure and function of the spleen in postnatal life to the spleen of man. However, since the spleen in laboratory animals possesses many of the features seen in man, illustrations of animal spleen are often used in addition to those of human spleen.

Another factor is that so far as possible a histological description of any organ should relate to its structure as it is during life. Special measures must be taken if sections of the spleen are to serve this purpose, because the splenic vein drains into the portal vein in which blood, instead of only being under very slight pressure, as it is in the vena cava, is under somewhat higher pressure. This pressure is transmitted back along the splenic vein to its tributaries within the spleen and from them into the large passageways called *sinusoids* within the red pulp of the spleen. Because of the venous pressure the sinusoids are mostly congested and expanded with blood. A spleen removed at operation, as it sometimes is, will contract as soon as a clamp is taken from the splenic vein since this allows the blood in the sinusoids and veins under pressure to escape from the opened vein. Likewise, after death, pressure drops in the vascular system, including the portal system, so that the spleen contracts and forces blood out through its veins. Accordingly, unless special measures are taken, sections of spleen reveal the microscopic structure of a *collapsed spleen* and not the microscopic structure of the spleen distended as it was during life. The best procedure for obtaining sections of spleen that represent its structure during life is to perfuse the vein of a collapsed spleen with fixative under sufficient pressure to restore the organ to its normal size.

The Capsule. The relatively well-developed capsule (Fig. 13-23) consists of collagenic and elastic fibers in which fibroblasts and sometimes some smooth muscle cells are distributed. Some animal spleens have more smooth muscle cells in their capsule than in man, and its contraction can assist the smooth muscle of the trabeculae in contracting the spleen and so forcing blood into circulation in times of emergency. It is doubtful whether there is enough smooth muscle in the capsule of the spleen of man to function very efficiently in this respect.

The plentiful elastin content of the capsule allows it to be stretched in life; hence, in a collapsed spleen (so commonly used for preparing sections) the capsule appears even thicker than it is during life.

The capsule is covered with a serosal (peritoneal) coat of mesothelium; this consists of a single layer of squamous cells. The cytoplasm of these mesothelial cells is too scant to be seen in ordinary sections but their flat nuclei may be noticed.

The Trabeculae. These are scattered throughout the substance of the spleen (Figs. 13-22, 13-23, and 13-25). They extend in from the hilus like a branching tree, with its branches passing in various directions to connect often with trabeculae that extend in from the capsule. In any section trabeculae will be cut in almost every plane. Most, of course, will be cut obliquely. Like the capsule, they consist of dense connective tissue in which there is a fair amount of elastin. They also contain a few smooth muscle cells but, as in the capsule, the amount of smooth muscle in them is not as great in man as in certain animals.

The trabeculae from the hilus convey arteries, veins, and nerves. In general, the largest trabeculae are seen near the hilus, and these contain the largest vessels. The detailed microscopic structure of arteries and veins will not be considered until Chapter 19, but if the student cares to glance at Figure 19-11, he will see that arteries are ringed with a much thicker layer of smooth muscle cells than veins. By using these criteria the student can readily distinguish an artery from a vein in most trabeculae (Fig. 13-25). In Figure 13-25 the artery is on the left and the vein on the right. The wall of the vein is thin, but the vein here lies in a thick trabecula. Perhaps the most logical way to describe the microscopic structure and functions of the various parts of the spleen is to do this in the order in which they are supplied with blood. So we shall follow the blood from the arteries of the trabeculae out into the splenic pulp and back to the veins of the trabeculae, because in taking this journey through the spleen all significant components will be encountered.

The Relation of the Arteries to the White Pulp. The arteries that travel in from the hilus in the larger trabeculae branch into small branches that leave the trabeculae (the smaller trabeculae, therefore, contain only veins) to enter the pulp. To support the arteries, the reticular fibers of the stroma of the splenic pulp become condensed chiefly along one side of them (but also to some extent around them) to provide them with fairly substantial reticular *sheaths*. The reticular fibers in these hold lymphocytes in their meshes (Fig. 13-24). Although these sheaths, infiltrated with the lymphocytes, are not true lymphatic nodules along most of their course, they do become expanded in certain places (usually at one side) to form lymphatic nodules (Fig. 13-22, *lower left;* Fig. 13-24, *left*), which may contain germinal centers. The white pulp of the spleen, then, is *distributed along the arteries that leave the trabeculae.*

In each site where a sheath is expanded into a lymphatic nodule the artery gives off a branch to supply the nodule (Fig. 13-24, *left*). This is termed a *follicular artery* (in the spleen lymphatic nodules are often termed *lymphatic follicles*). A follicular artery gives off branches to supply the capillary beds of the lymphatic nodule and then emerges from the follicle into the surrounding red pulp as described below.

The Arterial Supply of Red Pulp. A follicular artery, on leaving white pulp and entering the adjacent red pulp, according to Solnitzky, divides into 2 to 6 branches that radiate in different directions from their origin. Since these arterial branches radiate like straight bristles from the handle of an artist's brush, they are called *penicillar arteries* (L. *penicillus,* painter's brush). Each of these, according to Solnitzky, divides into 2 or 3 arterioles, most of which soon enter curious little structures called *ellipsoids* (Fig. 13-26), whereupon they lose all their arteriolar characteristics (muscular and elastic walls) to become capillaries. Before considering the further course of the blood through the red pulp of the spleen, we should briefly

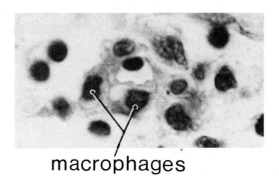
macrophages

Fig. 13-26. Oil-immersion photomicrograph showing an ellipsoid, cut in cross section, in distended human spleen. This consists of an arrangement of macrophages surrounding a capillary, the lumen of which contains a lymphocyte. The lumen appears as a white space between the macrophages.

discuss the role of the white pulp in immunological responses.

IMMUNOLOGICAL RESPONSES IN THE SPLEEN

In considering the immunological responses in the spleen it may help to compare its structure and functions with those of lymph nodes.

First, the spleen is concerned with antigens that are present in the bloodstream and, except in the relatively rare instances of septicemia (generalized infection of the blood), the concentration of antigen in the blood could not be expected to be nearly as great as that in lymph draining to a lymph node from a site of infection. Next, it seems likely that lymph nodes would be more concerned with cell-mediated reactions (because of antigens draining directly from, say, sites of foreign transplants via lymph to regional nodes) than the spleen which, because it receives blood from all over the body, receives only low concentrations of such antigens. There is therefore reason to think that the spleen is concerned mostly with the formation of humoral antibodies and we shall now discuss where the cells develop that form them.

Movat and Fernando studied spleens of rabbits after the latter were given an antigen intravenously. The first indication of an immunological response was the development of activated lymphocytes. These appeared between the second and the fourth day in the peripheral parts of primary nodules. By the sixth day both immature and mature plasma cells were found in the same sites. Moreover, some plasma cells by this time had spilled over from the white pulp into the red pulp.

Nine days after antigenic stimulation, it was found that the penicillar arteries radiating from the lymphatic nodules to deliver blood into the red pulp, though commonly ensheathed with lymphocytes, were now ensheathed mostly with plasma cells. Accordingly, it seems that certain lymphocytes of the white pulp of the spleen under the influence of antigenic stimulation become activated to form cells that in the EM are characterized by a great abundance of free ribosomes in their cytoplasm. Cells of this type forming in the spleen migrate toward the red pulp and serve as a source of cells that divide and differentiate to form the *plasma cells* seen in the red pulp.

The Respective Sites of T- and B-Lymphocytes

The above-mentioned study provided information about the sites at which the activated lymphocytes giving rise to the plasma cell series develop after administering antigen intravenously. However, when this study was made it was not known that there were two kinds of lymphocytes, T and B. When this became known it was of interest to investigate the respective locations of T- and B-lymphocytes in the spleen. It should, of course, be appreciated that the lymphocyte population in the spleen is by no means static; it changes from hour to hour and from day to day, so that determining where different kinds of lymphocytes are located is not so easy as determining where various cells are located in organs that contain a stable population.

One approach has been to remove the thymus at birth and determine which sites in the spleen were not properly populated. These experiments indicate that the population of lymphocytes in the perivascular lymphatic sheaths of the arteries and arterioles extending from trabeculae to lymphatic nodules (Fig. 13-24, *right side*) is greatly reduced, so it seems that the lymphocytes in these sheaths are mostly of the T type.

Other experiments utilizing immunofluorescence to localize T- and B-lymphocytes in sections of spleen have provided further information. It seems that the T-lymphocytes of the sheaths are not derived directly from the arterial vessels with which they are associated but instead take up their positions after the blood in which they were being carried has emptied from the termination of these vessels into what is called the *marginal zone* between the white and red pulp.

The Marginal Zone. To explain this it may help to consult Figure 13-24, which shows that the border between the white and red pulp is not sharply defined. Instead, there is a zone around the lymphatic follicle at the left, and also around the periarterial lymphatic sheath of the artery shown, where there are more lymphocytes than are present in red pulp but fewer than are seen in white pulp. Such a zone of transition between white and red pulp is called the *marginal zone;* it surrounds the periarterial sheaths and is continuous around the follicles to which the arteries lead.

It is mostly into this marginal zone that the blood vessels entering the nodule, after branching within it, empty their blood at various points around the periphery of the nodule. Whether this blood is emptied into the splenic pulp itself or into the sinusoids of the pulp will be discussed later in connection with the circulation through the red pulp.

The marginal zone is the region where circulating lymphocytes enter the substance of the spleen from the arteries that end here. T-lymphocytes from the circulation tend to accumulate in the periarteriolar sheaths, whereas B-lymphocytes tend to move back into the substance of the lymphatic nodules. Both kinds of lymphocytes can, however, move from the marginal zone into the red pulp so as to reach the bloodstream and again recirculate. Postcapillary venules of the special kind seen in other lymphatic organs have not been described in the white pulp of the spleen.

An antigen from the circulation could also enter the splenic pulp in the marginal zone, there to be phagocytosed by macrophages and/or become attached to the surface of dendritic reticular cells in the vicinity of lymphatic nodules. When programmed B-lymphocytes become activated by appropriate antigen, they proliferate and differentiate into antibody-producing cells that accumulate in the red pulp.

Since the topics discussed in the preceding paragraphs are the subject of much current research, with new findings becoming available all the time, further information, if desired, should be sought from the current literature.

THE SINUSOIDS OF THE RED PULP

The nonliving framework of the red pulp consists basically of a mesh of reticular fibers continuous with the collagenic fibers of the trabeculae and capsule (Fig. 13-22). The reticular mesh of red pulp, though of an open type itself, is permeated by passageways that measure from 12 to 40 μm. across. Since these passageways drain into veins, they are termed the *venous sinusoids* (or simply *sinusoids*) of the red pulp (Fig. 13-22). The walls of many (if not all) of these sinusoids are composed of long, narrow endothelial cells that are longitudinally disposed in the sinus wall (Fig. 13-27). These cells bulge into the lumen slightly where their nuclei are located, but their cytoplasm (which extends along a sinusoid in each direction from their nuclei) is not, in a distended spleen, very bulky. Cross sections of sinusoids revealing these cytoplasmic processes, which are slightly separated from each other in a distended spleen, are seen in Figure 13-27. Hence it is said there are longitudinal slits between the long endothelial cells that line sinusoids.

A sinusoid in life is therefore similar to an old leaky barrel whose longitudinal staves have shrunken away from one another to leave open slits between them. Like

Fig. 13-27. Oil-immersion phase contrast photomicrograph of distended spleen. Two sinusoids (S) are cut in cross section so that their longitudinally disposed, narrow stave-like lining cells are also cut in cross section. The cells are slightly separated from one another so as to leave slit-like spaces between them.

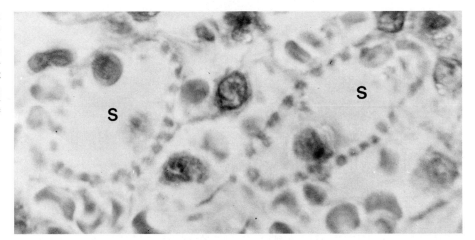

barrels that are encircled by iron hoops, the endothelial "staves" of the venous sinusoids are somewhat similarly surrounded and supported by hoops of reticular fibers, associated with basement membrane material, as will be described presently (Fig. 13-29).

The So-Called Pulp Cords. From the appearance seen in a single section, the red pulp between two adjacent sinusoids often resembles a cord; indeed, these areas were termed *Billroth* (or *pulp*) *cords* (Fig. 13-22, *top right*), However, the student who will have by now been trained to think in 3 dimensions will quickly realize that this name is annoyingly misleading. For anything to be a cord it should be surrounded on all sides by material different from itself—for example a fishing line dangling in water is a cord surrounded on all sides by water. A so-called pulp cord, although in a particular section it may be seen to have a sinusoidal space on either side of it, is not *surrounded* by a space, for sections taken below and above would show that the substance of the so-called cord was continuous with the substance of the red pulp. Thus the pulp between two sinusoids is no more in the form of a cord than the substance between 2 holes in a slice of Swiss cheese.

Robinson, in his studies on distended human spleens, examined thick sections with a binocular microscope arranged to give stereoscopic vision. He described the pulp between the sinusoids as consisting of a vast, delicate network of star-like cells having long, irregular cytoplasmic processes running in all directions and uniting one cell with another. He visualized the interstices of this cellular network as comprising a vast cavernous system of intercellular spaces that were in free communication with the venous sinusoids through the longitudinal slits in the walls of the latter (Fig. 13-27). Moreover, Robinson described blood from the follicular arteries as being emptied into the substance of the red pulp (and not directly

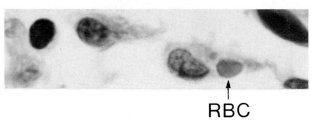

Fig. 13-28. Oil-immersion photomicrograph showing two macrophages in a human spleen (distended). This spleen was removed to alleviate excessive red blood cell destruction. Note that the macrophage at *right* has phagocytosed an erythrocyte (labeled RBC).

into the sinusoids, as will be described presently) and red blood cells, leukocytes, and platelets from the pulp entering sinusoids through the slits between their endothelial cells.

In a random section cut from a distended spleen, sinusoids and the so-called pulp cords are cut in various planes. In many of the planes in which sinusoids are cut they are not as distinct as when cut in cross section. So it is sometimes difficult to distinguish between sinusoids and the pulp between them, because both sinusoids and pulp contain erythrocytes and nucleated cells (in the instance of sinusoids these are mostly leukocytes). Macrophages are numerous in the pulp between sinusoids; one shown in Figure 13-28 has phagocytosed a red blood cell (labeled RBC).

THE FINE STRUCTURE OF THE RED PULP

In interpreting observations made with the EM it is of course important to know whether a given study was made on human spleen or the spleen of a laboratory

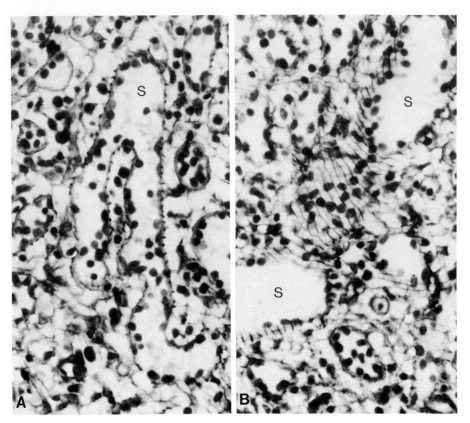

Fig. 13-29. Photomicrographs of distended spleen, stained by the PAS procedure to demonstrate the basement membrane material surrounding the sinusoids. (*A*) Sinusoids (S) are seen here cut in longitudinal section. Note that their scant basement membrane material is in the form of anastomosing rings that encircle the sinusoids. The rings in this plane of section appear as dark dots along the outside margin of the sinusoids, as may be seen just right of *center*. Note also the nuclei of endothelial cells bulging into the lumen, within which there are also a few blood cells. (*B*) A sinusoid is seen here in grazing section, disclosing the anastomosing rings of basement membrane material surrounding it (as seen at *center*). (Courtesy of B. H. Smith)

animal and whether the spleen was collapsed or distended to life size. The EM has confirmed that the basic structural framework of red pulp is a network of reticular fibers continuous with collagenic fibers of the trabeculae. Chen and Weiss in their EM studies of human spleen found that at the edges of sinusoids the reticular fibers are associated with basement membrane material and arranged in the form of rings around the sinusoids. Figure 13-29 is a photomicrograph that illustrates this unique distribution of the basement membrane material. Among other things, Chen and Weiss also describe two types of filaments in the endothelial cells of sinusoids, which cells they believe to be contractile and play a role in the removal of damaged blood cells. They also describe adventitial cells bordering on the endothelial cells of the sinusoids and associated with the basement membrane material encircling the sinusoids. In addition to reticular cells and macrophages the red pulp in life contains blood cells (both red and white) in relatively large numbers as well as many plasma cells. It is believed that erythrocytes are strained through the slits between the endothelial cells that line the sinusoids at sites not occluded by the anastomosing rings of basement membrane. It is probable that worn-out erythrocytes (or imperfect, fragile erythrocytes)

are not sufficiently elastic to pass undamaged through the slits and that once damaged they become phagocytosed by macrophages in the substance of the pulp. Leukocytes, being mobile, can pass through the slits fairly readily.

The macrophages of the pulp and the endothelial cells lining the sinusoids were once believed to be one and the same kind of cell, spoken of as "reticuloendothelial" cells. By using colloidal carbon Burke and Simon showed that the endothelial cells of the sinusoids have very little phagocytic capacity compared with macrophages within the pulp; so here, as in bone marrow, the cells lining sinusoids are not primarily phagocytic, as was once thought. The extensive phagocytosis seeming with the LM to occur along sinusoidal walls could be due to macrophages, for Burke and Simon found that these commonly protrude processes into the sinusoidal lumen between endothelial cells.

Summary of Functions of Red Pulp

In postnatal life in man the two most important functions of the red pulp are (*1*) to dispose of worn-out erythrocytes and other cellular material that might otherwise clutter up the bloodstream, and (*2*) to provide antibodies. The first function is performed by the macrophages of the red pulp and the second by the plasma cells which are also present in red pulp but whose origin can be traced to the white pulp. A third but less important function of the red pulp is to act as a storage reservoir for blood. Finally, in a sense it could be said that the spleen produces both iron and a bile pigment; these are formed by the breakdown of hemoglobin in macrophages that have phagocytosed erythrocytes.

THE FATE OF MACROPHAGES THAT ENTER THE SINUSOIDS

The splenic vein drains into the hepatic portal system and so the large number of macrophages that enter the sinusoids to leave the spleen via the splenic vein go into the liver, from which phagocytic cells of the same general type may be released into the circulation. It seems probable that these, being large cells, are unable to pass through the capillaries of the lungs so they make their way into the air spaces and are ultimately coughed up or swallowed and disintegrate in the stomach.

THEORIES ABOUT HOW BLOOD CIRCULATES THROUGH THE RED PULP

Studies of sections of spleen have in the past led to two main theories about the circulation through the red pulp. According to one—the open circulation theory—arterial blood from the ellipsoids is delivered directly into the substance of red pulp (Fig. 13-30) and only gains entrance to the sinusoids by percolating through the slits in sinusoidal walls. According to the other—the closed circulation theory—arterial blood is delivered via capillaries directly into sinusoids (Fig. 13-30), and the great content of erythrocytes in the red pulp between sinusoids is explained by the erythrocytes passing back and forth between the pulp and the sinusoids via the slits in the walls of the latter.

In evaluating these two theories we encounter again the problem of whether studies were made in human spleen or on the spleen of other mammals. Various animals reveal differences, for example, in the structure and size of ellipsoids; these, for example, are highly developed in cats. The spleens of mice and rats, as already noted, are hematopoietic. Then again, the question arises as to whether studies made on distended spleens would support the same theory as studies made on collapsed spleens. Indeed, there is a third theory to the effect that the circulation in a collapsed spleen is closed but in a distended spleen, open.

Robinson in his studies of human spleens which he distended through their veins concluded that blood from the ellipsoids empties into the substance of the red pulp and therefore has to pass from there through sinusoidal walls to gain entrance to the lumina of sinusoids. Chen and Weiss in their EM study of human spleens noted that all the terminal arterial vessels observed opened into red pulp between sinusoids. There is therefore substantial evidence for the open circulation theory in human spleen.

In EM studies on the spleens of rabbits Burke and Simon place emphasis on the existence of zones between areas of white pulp

and red pulp, which they term *transitional* zones, and where there is a large marginal sinus from which they believe the majority of other sinusoids arise, but they were unable to show any direct connection between capillaries and sinusoids or the substance of red pulp. In another study, however, they found that carbon injected intravenously appeared so quickly in the sinusoids that it suggested that they were in direct connection with capillaries.

In trying to decide whether the splenic circulation is open or closed it is often assumed that the beginning of a sinusoid is as definite a structure as it becomes farther along its course. However, in a distended spleen there are many areas where it is difficult (if not impossible) to distinguish sinusoids from interstices between cells of pulp cords and it would probably be a matter of opinion as to whether the terminations of capillaries were in pulp or sinusoids. This could be the basis for the theory that the circulation can be *either closed or open*, depending on circumstances. According to this view, the beginnings of the venous sinusoids, which appear as tubular structures in a contracted spleen, may exhibit in a distended spleen so many openings between the cells of their walls that they cease to be recognizable structures and become no more than fairly open passageways through a reticular mesh that abounds with communicating spaces. In other words, some consider that the first parts of the venous sinusoids, when these are distended, would be so leaky that they should not be considered structures, and hence that the circulation under these conditions is open. But when the spleen is contracted, the cells of the walls of the sinusoids come close enough together to justify the view that they are tubular structures; under these conditions, the circulation is closed.

Another approach to the problem was made by Knisely, who utilized a quartz-rod illuminator to study the passageways by which blood circulates between the arteries and the veins in the exposed spleen of living animals. Knisely found that the arterial capillaries branch after passing through the region of ellipsoids, and that some branches pass directly to the veins. These capillaries (Fig. 13-31, capillary shunts), which are controlled by sphincters, provide a *bypass* or *shunt* circulation so that blood can pass through the spleen without being emptied into either the red pulp or the sinusoids. Knisely found that the other set of capillary branches empty into the sinusoids; in this respect Knisely's findings seem to support the closed circulation theory. Knisely found, moreover, that there were sphincters at each end of the sinusoids, and that, depending on the degree of contraction or relaxation of these sphincters, sinusoids exhibit different states of form and function that he termed phases (Fig. 13-31). With both sphincters open, a sinusoid would be relatively narrow; in this state it would be said to be in a *conducting* phase. With the efferent sphincter contracted but the afferent one open, a sinusoid is said to be in a *filtration-filling* phase, with its walls retaining erythrocytes but allowing plasma to escape into the pulp cords. When the sinusoid becomes filled with erythrocytes, the afferent sphincter closes, and the sinusoid enters the *storage phase*. Then, when both sphincters open, it enters the *emptying phase*, and the red blood cells packed in it are washed into the circulation.

The study of the circulation of the living spleen by quartz-rod illuminator is a difficult technic to employ and cannot be expected to reveal the kind of tissue or cellular detail obtainable in sections studied with either the LM or the EM. In their use of this method, MacKenzie, Whipple, and Wintersteiner were unable to confirm many of Knisely's findings. However, Peck and Hoerr made a further study of both the method and the problem. Their work emphasized the necessity for very exacting precautions if the method is to yield information of value, and they

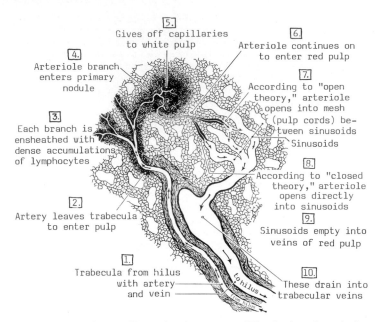

5. Gives off capillaries to white pulp

4. Arteriole branch enters primary nodule

6. Arteriole continues on to enter red pulp

7. According to "open theory," arteriole opens into mesh (pulp cords) between sinusoids

Sinusoids

3. Each branch is ensheathed with dense accumulations of lymphocytes

8. According to "closed theory," arteriole opens directly into sinusoids

2. Artery leaves trabecula to enter pulp

9. Sinusoids empty into veins of red pulp

1. Trabecula from hilus with artery and vein

10. These drain into trabecular veins

Fig. 13-30. Diagram illustrating the course of blood taken through the spleen according to the open and the closed theories of circulation. The captions should be read clockwise, by number.

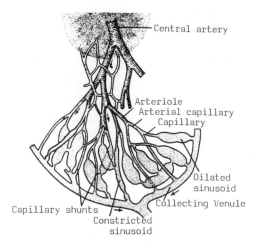

Central artery

Arteriole
Arterial capillary
Capillary

Dilated sinusoid

Capillary shunts
Constricted sinusoid
Collecting Venule

Fig. 13-31. Diagram of splenic circulation, according to Knisely. (Peck, H. M., and Hoerr, N. L.: Anat. Rec., *109:*447, 1951)

found, when these precautions were taken, that the intermediary circulation in the spleen is essentially as Knisely described it. However, while these studies on living spleen provided physiological information that would not be obtainable from studying sections, such as the existence of capillary bypasses and the same sinusoid existing in different phases, they could scarcely be expected to prove that there is always unbroken endothelial continuity between capillaries and the beginnings of sinusoids and hence settle the "open" versus "closed" circulation controversy.

REFERENCES AND OTHER READING

GENERAL REFERENCES

Fudenberg, H. H., Stites, D. P., Caldwell, J. L., and Wells, J. V. (eds.): Basic and Clinical Immunology. Los Altos, Lange, 1976.

Golub, E. S. (ed.): The Cellular Basis of the Immune Response. Sunderland, Mass., Sinauer Associates, 1977.

Humphrey, J. H., and White, R. G.: Immunology for Students of Medicine. ed. 3. Oxford, Blackwell Scientific Publications, 1970.

Metcalf, D., and Moore, M. A. S.: Haemopoietic Cells. Amsterdam, North-Holland, 1971.

Weiss, L.: The Cells and Tissues of the Immune System. Englewood Cliffs, N. J., Prentice-Hall, 1972.

SPECIAL REFERENCES

T- and B-Lymphocytes, Immune Responses, and Tolerance

Able, M. D., Lee, J. C., and Rosenau, W.: Lymphocyte-target cell interaction in vitro. Ultrastructural and cinematographic studies. Am. J. Pathol., *60:*421, 1970.

Allison, A. C.: The mechanism of lymphocyte-mediated cytotoxicity. *In* Clarkson, B. (ed.): Control of Proliferation in Animal Cells. p. 454. Cold Spring Harbor Laboratory, 1974.

Bach, M. K. (ed.): Immediate Hypersensitivity—Modern Concepts and Developments. Immunology Series, vol. 7. New York, Marcel Dekker, 1978.

Billingham, R. E.: Actively acquired tolerance and its role in development. *In* McElroy, W. D., and Glass, B. (eds.): The Chemical Basis of Development. p. 575. Baltimore, Johns Hopkins Press, 1958.

Billingham, R. E., Brent, L., and Medawar, P. B.: Quantitative studies on tissue transplantation immunity. III. Actively acquired tolerance. Philos. Trans. R. Soc. Lond [Biol. Sci.], *15:*357, 1956.

Bloom, B. R.: In vitro approaches to the mechanism of cell-mediated immune reactions. Adv. Immunol., *13:*101, 1971.

Boyse, E. A., and Cantor, H.: Surface characteristics of T-lymphocyte subpopulations. Hosp. Prac., *12:*81, 1977.

Burnet, Sir MacFarlane: The Clonal Selection Theory of Acquired Immunity. Nashville, Tenn., Vanderbilt University Press, and Cambridge, England, University Press, 1959.

Claman, H. N., and Chaperon, E. A.: Immunologic complementation between thymus and marrow cells—a model for the two cell theory of immunocompetence. Transplant. Rev., *1*:92, 1969.

Claman, H. N., and Mosier, D. E.: Cell-cell interactions in antibody production. Prog. Allergy, *16*:40, 1972.

Dresser, D. W. (ed.): Immunological Tolerance. Br. Med. Bull., *32* (No. 2):101, 1976.

Feldmann, M., and Nossal, G. V. V.: Cellular basis of antibody production. Q. Rev. Biol., *47*:269, 1972.

Gesner, B. M., and Gowans, J. L.: The fate of lethally irradiated mice given isologous and heterologous thoracic duct lymphocytes. Br. J. Exp. Pathol., *43*:431, 1962.

Goldschneider, I., and McGregor, D. D.: Anatomical distribution of T and B lymphocytes in the rat. J. Exp. Med., *138*:1443, 1973.

Gowans, J. L.: The recirculation of lymphocytes from blood to lymph in the rat. J. Physiol., *146*:54, 1959.

———: The fate of parental strain small lymphocytes in F₁ hybrid rats. Ann. N.Y. Acad. Sci., *99*:432, 1962.

Gowans, J. L., McGregor, D. D., and Cowen, D. M.: Initiation of immune response by small lymphocytes. Nature, *196*:651, 1962.

———: The role of small lymphocytes in the rejection of homografts of skin. *In* Wolstenholme, G. E., and Knight, Julie (eds.): The Immunologically Competent Cell. Ciba Foundation Study Group No. 16, p. 20. London, Churchill, 1963.

Gutman, G. A., and Weissman, I. L.: Lymphoid tissue architecture: Experimental analysis of the origin and distribution of T-cells and B-cells. Immunology, *23*:465, 1972.

Katz, D. H.: Lymphocyte Differentiation, Recognition and Regulation. New York, Academic Press, 1977.

Lucas, D. O. (ed.): Regulatory Mechanisms in Lymphocyte Activation. Proceedings of 11th Leukocyte Culture Conf. New York, Academic Press, 1977.

Mitchison, N. A.: Cell cooperation in the immune response: the hypothesis of an antigen preservation mechanism. Immunopathology, *6*:52, 1971.

Möller, G. (ed.): Lymphocyte immunoglobulin: synthesis and surface representation. Transplant. Rev., *14*, 1973.

Nelson, D. S. (ed.): Immunobiology of the Macrophage. New York, Academic Press, 1976.

Nossal, G. J. V.: B-lymphocyte receptors and lymphocyte activation. *In* Brinkley, B. R., and Porter, K. R. (eds.): International Cell Biology 1976-1977. p. 103. New York, Rockefeller University Press, 1977.

Owen, R. D.: Immunogenetic consequences of vascular anastomoses between bovine twins. Science, *102*:400, 1945; Fed. Proc., *16*:581, 1957.

Paul, W. E., and Benacerraf, B.: Functional specificity of thymus-dependent lymphocytes. Science, *195*:1293, 1977.

Raff, M. C.: T and B lymphocytes and immune responses. Nature, *242*:19, 1973.

Schlesinger, M. (ed.): Lymphocytes and Their Cell Membranes. New York, Academic Press, 1976.

Stuart, F. P. (ed.): Immunological Tolerance and Enhancement. Baltimore, University Park Press, 1978.

Stutman, O. (ed.): Contemporary Topics in Immunobiology. vol. 7. T Cells. New York, Plenum Press, 1977.

Waksman, B. H.: Tolerance, the thymus, and suppressor T cells. Clin. Exp. Immunol., *28*:363, 1977.

Yoffey, J. M. (ed.): The Lymphocyte in Immunology and Haemopoiesis. London, Edward Arnold, 1966.

The Thymus

Alapper, C.: Morphogenesis of the thymus. Am. J. Anat., *78*:139, 1946.

Archer, O. K., and Pierce, J. C.: Role of the thymus in development of the immune response. Fed. Proc., *20*:26, 1961.

Clark, S. L., Jr.: The penetration of proteins and colloidal materials into the thymus from the bloodstream. *In* Defendi, V., and Metcalf, D. (eds.): A Wistar Institute Symposium Monograph No. 2. p. 9. Philadelphia, Wistar Inst. Press, 1964.

Osoba, D.: Thymic function, immunologic deficiency and autoimmunity. Med. Clin. North. Am., *56*:319, 1972.

Raviola, E., and Karnovsky, M. J.: Evidence for a blood-thymus barrier using electron-opaque tracers. J. Exp. Med., *136*:466, 1972.

Smith, C.: Studies on the thymus of the mammal. VIII. Intrathymic lymphatic vessels. Anat. Rec., *122*:173, 1955.

Lymphatic Nodules and Lymph Nodes

Bailey, R. P., and Weiss, L.: Light and electron microscopic studies of postcapillary venules in developing human fetal lymph nodes. Am. J. Anat., *143*:43, 1975.

Brahim, F., and Osmond, D. G.: Migration of newly formed small lymphocytes from bone marrow to lymph nodes during primary immune responses. Clin. Exp. Immunol., *24*:515, 1976.

Everett, N. B., and Tyler (Caffrey), R. W.: Lymphopoiesis in the thymus and other tissues: functional implications. Int. Rev. Cytol., *22*:205, 1967.

Farr, A. G., and De Bruyn, P. P. H.: The mode of lymphocyte migration through post-capillary venule endothelium in lymph node. Am. J. Anat., *143*:59, 1975.

Herman, P. G., Yamamoto, I., and Mellins, H. Z.: Blood microcirculation in the lymph node during the primary immune response. J. Exp. Med., *136*:697, 1972.

Leduc, E. H., Coons, A. H., and Connolly, J. M.: Studies on antibody production. II. The primary and secondary responses in the popliteal lymph node of the rabbit. J. Exp. Med., *102*:61, 1955.

Menzies, D. W.: The blood supply of the para-aortic lymph node of the rat. *In* Further Studies in Pathology. p. 176. Melbourne, Australia, University Press, 1965.

Micklem, H. S., Ford, C. E., Evans, E. P., and Gray, J. G.: Interrelationships of myeloid and lymphoid cells. Studies with chromosome-marked cells transfused into lethally irradiated mice. Proc. Roy. Soc. (Biol.), *165*:78, 1966.

Nopajaroonsri, C., Luk, S. C., and Simon, G. T.: Ultrastructure of the normal lymph node. Am. J. Pathol., *65*:1, 1971.

———: The passage of intravenously injected colloidal carbon into lymph node parenchyma. Lab. Invest., *30*:533, 1974.

Parrott, D. M. V.: The response of draining lymph nodes to immunological stimulation in intact and thymectomized animals. J. Clin. Pathol., *20* (Symp. Tissue Org. Transplant., Suppl.):456, 1967.

Sainte-Marie, G.: Labelling of lymphoid organs by repeated injections of ³H-thymidine. Rev. Can. Biol., *32*:251, 1973.

Schoefl, G. I.: The migration of lymphocytes across the vascular endothelium in lymphoid tissue, a reexamination. J. Exp. Med., *136*:568, 1972.

Weller, C. V.: The hemolymph nodes. *In* Downey's Handbook of Hematology. p. 1759. New York, Hoeber, 1938.

Yoffey, J. M., and Courtice, F. C.: Lymphatics, Lymph and the Lymphomyeloid Complex. New York, Academic Press, 1971.

Spleen

Barnhart, M. I., Baechler, C. A., and Lusher, J. M.: Arteriovenous shunts in the human spleen. Am. J. Hematology, *1:*105, 1976.

Barnhart, M. I., and Lusher, J. M.: The human spleen as revealed by scanning electron microscopy. Am. J. Hematology *1:*243, 1976.

Bradfield, J. W., and Born, G. V. R.: The migration of rat thoracic duct lymphocytes through the spleen in vivo. Br. J. Exp. Pathol., *54:*509, 1973.

Burke, J. S., and Simon, G. T.: Electron microscopy of the spleen. I. Anatomy and microcirculation. Am. J. Pathol., *58:*127, 1970.

————: Electron microscopy of the spleen. II. Phagocytosis of colloidal carbon. Am. J. Pathol., *58:*157, 1970.

Chen, L-T., and Weiss, L.: Electron microscopy of the red pulp of human spleen. Am. J. Anat., *134:*425, 1972.

Doggett, T. H.: The capillary system of the dog's spleen. Anat. Rec., *110:*65, 1951.

Ford, W. L.: The kinetics of lymphocyte recirculation within the rat spleen. Cell Tissue Kinet., *2:*171, 1969.

Knisley, M. H.: Spleen studies: I. Microscopic observations of the circulatory system of living unstimulated mammalian spleens. Anat. Rec., *65:*23, 1936.

————: Spleen studies: II. Microscopic observations of the circulatory system of living traumatized, and of drying spleens. Anat. Rec., *65:*131, 1936.

Lewis, O. J.: The blood vessels of the adult mammalian spleen. J. Anat., *91:*245, 1957.

Robinson, W. L.: Some points on the mechanism of filtration by the spleen. Am. J. Pathol., *4:*309, 1928.

————: The vascular mechanism of the spleen. Am. J. Pathol., *2:*341, 1926.

————: The venous drainage of the cat spleen. Am. J. Pathol., *6:*19, 1930.

Solnitzky, O.: The Schweigger-Seidel sheath (ellipsoid) of the spleen. Anat. Rec., *69:*55, 1937.

Weiss, L.: A study of the structure of splenic sinuses in man and in the albino rat, with the light microscope and the electron microscope. J. Biophys. Biochem. Cytol., *3:*599, 1957.

14 Tendons, Ligaments, and Cartilage

INTRODUCTION TO THE STUDY OF THE SKELETAL TISSUES

With tendons and cartilage, we begin the study of the skeletal connective tissues. This subject will be covered not only in the remainder of this chapter but also in the next two chapters, which deal with bones and joints respectively.

The histology of the skeletal tissues involves far more than just cell biology, for it is the nonliving intercellular substances of these tissues that serve the important roles they play in the body. For example, their supportive, weight-bearing function is due to their intercellular substances. Furthermore, it is the matrix of bone that serves as the calcium storehouse for the body and the intercellular substance (matrix) of cartilage that provides the smooth, polished surfaces of moveable joints, lubricated by yet another (fluid) type of intercellular substance.

Cells, of course, are important here as elsewhere, for they are responsible for producing and maintaining the intercellular substances in which they come to be housed. This raises two very important points about studying cartilage and bone: (*1*) understanding how the constituent cells of cartilage and bone receive their oxygen and nutrients, and (*2*) appreciating that the mechanisms whereby this is accomplished is different in these two tissues.

Finally, a thorough knowledge of the histology of the skeletal tissues is of the greatest importance in several branches of surgery, medicine, and dentistry. In particular, in contrast to those diseases that have been brought under control in civilized societies, the widespread use of motor vehicles and even some modern industrial activities have increased greatly the incidence of damage to the skeleton. This has led to greatly increased efforts in fundamental research on cartilage and bone, witnessed by the considerable growth in the literature on *orthopedics* (Gr. *orthos*, straight; *pais*, child), the specialty concerned with preservation and restoration of normal structure and function of bones and joints. Since bones act as *calcium reservoirs* for the body and certain hormones affect calcium metabolism, the role of bones and the effects on the skeleton of several metabolic diseases is another important medical topic. *Arthritis*, which has such an effect on joints, is also still with us, as is *periodontal disease*, in which the attachment of teeth to bone by the periodontal ligament is affected. Investigation into such afflictions involving the skeletal tissues is now an active area of research.

DENSE ORDINARY CONNECTIVE TISSUE

In this chapter we deal first with dense ordinary connective tissue (the tissue of which tendons and ligaments are composed) and then with cartilage, which will be considered further in Chapters 15 and 16.

Classification. Dense ordinary connective tissue is commonly classified into two main types, that *regularly arranged,* and that *irregularly arranged.* In the regularly arranged kind, the collagenic fibers all run more or less in the same plane and the same direction. Hence structures built of it have great tensile strength and can withstand tremendous pulls exerted in the plane and direction of their fibers, without stretching. Obviously, dense regularly arranged connective tissue is ideal for tendons and ligaments, which join muscles to bones and bones to bones, and for other sites where pull is exerted in one general direction (Fig. 14-1). The cells in the dense regularly arranged kind are nearly all *fibrocytes* and are located between the parallel bundles of collagenic fibers (Fig. 14-1).

In the irregularly arranged type, the collagenic fibers run either in different directions in the same plane or in every direction. In the sheets of dense irregularly arranged connective tissue that comprise aponeuroses and sheaths of various sorts, the fibers are more or less in the same plane but may run in different directions. Such sheets can withstand stretching in those directions in which their fibers run. In other body sites, however, such as in the reticular layer of dermis of the skin (which comprises most of the substance of the skin) the collagenic fibers run both in different directions and in different planes, and hence dermis can withstand stretching in any direction.

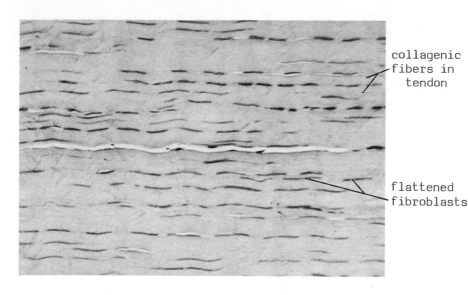

Fig. 14-1. Low-power photomicrograph of a longitudinal section of a tendon. Tendons consist chiefly of bundles of collagenic fibers which run in one direction, with rows of flattened fibroblasts between them. Note that this tissue consists almost entirely of intercellular substance.

The *capsules* of many organs—for example, lymph nodes and spleen—are composed of thin, dense, irregularly arranged connective tissue, and this type of connective tissue often extends from the capsule into organs as *septa* or *trabeculae.* Dense connective tissue often forms an outer wrapping for tubes of various sorts in the body, as well as for muscles and nerves. It forms a sheath in which the central nervous sytem (brain and spinal cord) is enclosed. In short, it is a very common tissue and will be seen in many sections studied in the laboratory. Here we shall study only one example—the dense, regularly arranged connective tissue of tendons.

TENDONS

Development. Tendons appear in the embryo as dense bundles of fibroblasts oriented in the same plane and packed closely together. The fibroblasts proliferate to permit growth of the tendon. But, as development proceeds, the fibroblasts become arranged in rows and secrete more and more collagen between the rows to form the type of arrangement shown in Figure 14-1. The character of the structure thus changes from being primarily cellular to being *primarily intercellular substance.*

Blood Supply. During development, when tendons are cellular, they have a reasonably good blood supply, necessary for collagen to be synthesized and secreted. But when the fiber bundles have been built up, the capillary blood supply within the tendon bundles almost disappears.

Tendon Sheaths. Some tendons in certain sites where they otherwise might rub against bone or other friction-generating surfaces are enclosed in sheaths. Actually a

tendon sheath comprises two sheaths. The outer one is a connective tissue tube and its exterior is attached to the structures that surround it. The inner sheath directly encloses the tendon and is firmly attached to it. There is a space between the inner and the outer sheath, filled with a slippery solution containing hyaluronic acid and rather similar to *synovial fluid,* which will be described in connection with joints in Chapter 16.

The inner surface of the outer tendon sheath and the outer surface of the inner sheath do not possess a continuous lining of cells, so the surfaces that glide over one another are mostly those of intercellular substances, chiefly collagen, along which, however, some cells are scattered as in synovial membranes of joints (p. 474). The synovial fluid between the two sheaths is an excellent lubricant.

Regeneration of Tendons. Tendons may be severed in accidents. With proper surgical treatment they heal excellently and in due course become as strong as before. Repair is effected by fibroblasts from the inner tendon sheath or, if the tendon has no proper sheath, from the loose connective tissue around its periphery. These grow into the site where the cut ends are apposed, proliferating all the while. Gradually the fibroblasts become oriented along the axis of the tendon. Then they re-enact the same scene witnessed when a tendon develops. At first the fibroblasts have a good capillary blood supply and produce much collagen, which becomes deposited in bundles between them and arranged along the long axis of the tendon. Some of the cells grow into the cut ends of the tendon, where the new collagen being formed unites with the old. As more and more collagen is deposited between the fibroblasts, the capillary blood supply diminishes, and the site of the repair eventually becomes almost free of capillaries. It is not generally believed that the old fibrocytes between the fiber bundles of the original tendon contribute very much, if anything, to the repair process; these old fibroblasts (fibrocytes) have probably lost their reproductive powers. Furthermore, it could be assumed that the young fibroblasts bringing about the repair would mostly be derived from pericytes.

An interesting factor in regard to the repair of tendons is described by Peacock and Van Winkle, whose publications should be read for details by students inclined toward surgical careers. They point out that the problem of achieving successful repair of a severed tendon more or less hinges on the same factors that could cause adhesions of the tendon, so that its subsequent gliding functions might suffer. Isolating the connected ends of a severed tendon from adjacent connective tissue, so that adhesions between the healing tendon and adjacent connective tissue will not occur, prevents the tendon ends from becoming united, because repair of the severed ends depends on connective tissue cells and blood vessels reaching the severed ends from outside the tendon. However here, as in bone, natural remodeling of the healing structure can be extraordinarily efficient in aiding the restoration of function. In addition to pointing out the best ways to obtain good functional results, these authors describe the difference in procedures that should be used for repairing extensor and flexor tendons so as to obtain the best results.

Grafts of Tendons. It was once thought that grafts of dense connective tissue structures such as tendons and fasciae continue to live on autologous transplantation. Indeed sutures of fascia were sometimes used in repairing wounds and were termed *living sutures.* It seems probable that the basis for this belief was an uncritical attitude that viewed everything in the body as being alive. Actually most of the substance of dense connective tissue is nonliving material. The relatively few cells in these dense tissues that are transplanted probably all die, but the intercellular substances of which the transplants mostly consist (and which are of course nonliving materials) persist long enough for new cells to invade and replace those of the transplant. In due course they replace much of its intercellular substance with newly formed tissue. Such autologous grafts are useful, not because their cells live, but because their *intercellular substance persists* long enough to provide a suitable model for replacement by new cells that invade the transplant from host tissue and produce new intercellular substance as needed.

How Tendons Are Attached. Tendons connect muscles to bone or cartilage so that the contraction of a muscle can pull on the bony or cartilaginous structure into which the tendon is said to be *inserted.* The manner in which the tendon is attached to the muscle will be described in Chapter 18.

It is perhaps somewhat misleading to say that the other end of the tendon is inserted into bone or cartilage because it makes it sound as if this end were somehow poked in so as to gain some sort of firm attachment. Actually what happens is that the cells forming the collagenic fibers at this end of the tendon are not ordinary fibroblasts; they are of the type found in the coverings of bones or cartilages and such cells can produce the intercellular substances of bone or cartilage. Since these tissues both contain much collagen, cartilage- or bone-forming cells are capable of making the collagen of the tendon at the site where it is inserted. But they also produce the amorphous intercellular substances characteristic of bone or cartilage. So where tendon insertions are forming at the surface of a bony or cartilaginous structure, the cells produce a mixture of (*1*) the intercellular substance of tendon and (*2*) the intercellular substances of bone or cartilage. Accordingly there is a gradual transition along the tendon near its insertion from being pure dense connective tissue to being a mixture of dense connective tissue and either bone or cartilage. Where this is cartilage, the tissue is said to be *fibrocartilage* (Fig. 14-6).

Furthermore, during growth, the bones to which tendons are inserted grow by bone being added to their surface. Thus a tendon insertion into what began as a small bone eventually becomes an insertion into a large bone. This requires constant rebuilding of the tendon insertion during the growth of the bone. Hence as a result of the growth of the bone the early attachment of the tendon becomes buried deeper and deeper within its substance. Where the collagen bundles of the tendon insertion lie buried in the new bone they are termed *Sharpey's fibers;* these will be described later after we have considered the development and growth of bones. Tendon insertions into growing cartilages would have to undergo similar rebuilding as the cartilages increased in size.

Elastic Ligaments. It should be noted that certain of the ligaments, for example the *ligamenta flava* and the *ligamentum nuchae,* are composed primarily of *elastin.* Here the elastin is formed by fibroblasts. The formation of elastin was described on page 235.

CARTILAGE

The reader will find it helpful to realize at the outset that one problem in connection with describing cartilage in a textbook is to avoid unnecessary duplication. Moreover, since cartilage therefore has to be dealt with in three separate chapters (Chaps. 14, 15, and 16), all three need to be read in order to cover the subject completely.

Cartilage is a relatively solid type of connective tissue that unlike dense ordinary connective tissue does not bend and so it can bear weight to some extent. However, it is not nearly as strong as bone.

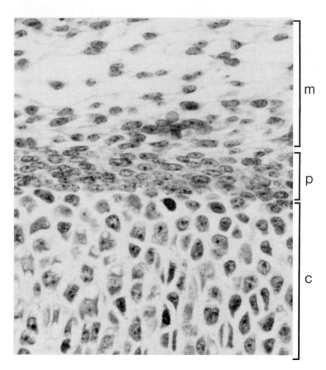

Fig. 14-2. Photomicrograph of the periphery of a cartilage model (mouse embryo). The lower part of the illustration shows developing hyaline cartilage (c). The top third contains loose mesenchyme (m). Between the two the mesenchyme is condensed and is forming the future perichondrium (p).

Sites in the Body. Cartilage is found in only two kinds of sites after growth is over in postnatal life. First, some extraskeletal cartilaginous structures exist in the body. For example, there are horseshoe-shaped rings of cartilage in the wall of the trachea (windpipe). The role of these is to prevent the wall of the trachea, which otherwise consists chiefly of ordinary (flexible) connective tissue, from collapsing when air is drawn into the lungs. Irregular cartilaginous structures are also present in the walls' of the larger air tubes leading into the lungs. Moreover, plates of cartilage are found in the larynx, nose, and in one part of the eustachian tube (which connects the middle ear with the nasopharynx and so permits the air pressure to be equalized between the two cavities). Cartilage also remains in the costal cartilages (which connect the anterior ends of the ribs to the sternum) where it provides a firm connection between the ribs and the sternum that nevertheless is flexible enough to permit the rib cage to expand in respiratory movements.

The second site where cartilage remains and performs its function through life is in moveable joints. In freely moveable joints the ends of bones are capped with cartilage. In this instance the cartilage is termed *articular*

cartilage and provides smooth slippery surfaces on the ends of bones where they meet in the joint, so that friction is minimized. We shall deal with articular cartilage, a very important subject, at some length in Chapter 15. Cartilage also persists in some joints that are not freely moveable.

Most of the cartilage developing in the body, however, appears in prenatal life and has only a temporary existence because its fate is to be replaced by bone. Nevertheless, its development and presence are essential for bones to develop and grow in length. Since bone growth continues after birth, some of it persists postnatally until longitudinal growth of bones is over. The life story of this cartilage will be given in Chapter 15, which deals with the development, growth, and structure of bones.

General Features. In this chapter we shall describe only some general features of cartilage, such as that existing in the walls of the trachea.

Pure cartilage is termed *hyaline* (Gr. *hyalos,* glass) because it is a pearly white material that is somewhat translucent; this appearance is due to its particular intercellular substance. In certain sites such as the ear, however, the cartilage is called *elastic* because there is some elastin in its intercellular substance, and in other sites cartilage may contain so much collagen that it is termed *fibrocartilage.* We give examples of elastic and fibrocartilage at the end of this chapter. But it is important to learn here the general properties and structure of *hyaline cartilage,* for this is the type of cartilage that constitutes the articular cartilages forming in connection with the development and growth of bones.

HYALINE CARTILAGE AND ITS PROPERTIES

Gross Appearance. Those students who have dissected moveable joints where hyaline cartilage covers the ends of the bones that *articulate* (L. *articulatus,* jointed) with one another as *articular cartilage* will already be familiar with the gross appearance of hyaline cartilage. Other students can and quickly should remedy their deficiency by a visit to a market where soup bones are sold. The latter generally include the articulating ends of fresh bones. Among these there will probably be some that participated in moveable joints and whose free ends are capped with a layer of material exhibiting a glistening, smooth, glass-like surface, *hyaline cartilage.* Beneath its surface the layer of cartilage capping an end of a bone appears as a pearly white material, due to its distinctive intercellular substance.

The Development of Hyaline Cartilage. Since this subject will be dealt with in detail later when we study the development of bone, we comment on it here only to explain

Fig. 14-3. Semidiagrammatic drawing of a section of uncalcified hyaline cartilage covered with perichondrium, illustrating the processes of appositional and interstitial growth.

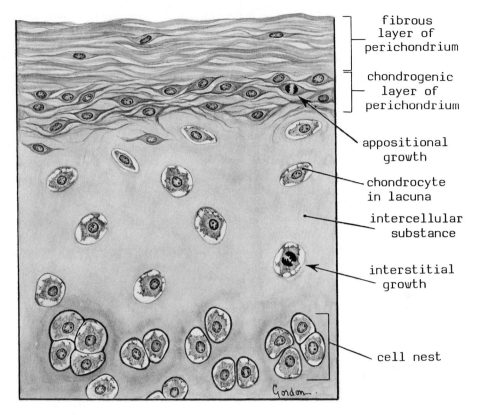

fibrous layer of perichondrium

chondrogenic layer of perichondrium

appositional growth

chondrocyte in lacuna

intercellular substance

interstitial growth

cell nest

what existed beforehand at sites where cartilage such as that illustrated in Figure 14-3 subsequently develops.

In the embryo, cartilage develops from *mesenchyme*. At the site where cartilage is to develop, the mesenchymal cells becomes very closely packed together (*condensed*), so much so that individual cells cannot be distinguished with the low-power objective. The site of the packed mesenchymal cells constitutes a *model* having the form of the cartilaginous structure that will later develop from it.

If after such a model continued to develop we were to remove a piece of tissue from one side, a piece extending into its central part, and cut a section from the piece of tissue it would appear as shown in Figure 14-2. This shows that in the more central part of the model the previously packed mesenchymal cells have begun to differentiate into cartilage cells, indicated histologically by their forming a pale intercellular substance that separates the differentiated cells from one another (Fig. 14-2,c). Surrounding this developing cartilage, the mesenchymal cells remain closely packed (Fig. 14-2, p). They will soon form a relatively thick membrane, called the *perichondrium* (Gr. *peri*, around; *chondros*, cartilage) because it surrounds the cartilage. The cells of the inner layer of this

membrane remain relatively undifferentiated, constituting what is called the *chondrogenic layer* of the perichondrium (Fig. 14-3). The cells of this layer can proliferate and differentiate into cartilage cells and so form more cartilage on the exterior of that already formed. The mesenchymal cells of the outer layer of the membrane differentiate into fibroblasts that form collagen, and so the whole structure becomes surrounded with a fibrous membrane termed the *fibrous layer* of the perichondrium (Fig. 14-3). Cartilage that developed as described above can be seen in the drawing of a young tracheal cartilage (Fig. 14-3), which we now describe.

The LM Appearance of a Growing Tracheal Cartilage

The perichondrium, as shown at the *top* of Figure 14-3, consists of two layers. The outermost is composed of ordinary, dense, regularly arranged connective tissue and consists chiefly of collagenic fibers, among which are a few flattened fibroblasts or fibrocytes. The deeper layer of the perichondrium consists of plumper cells that are *chondrogenic* (labeled *chondrogenic layer of perichondrium* in Fig. 14-3), which means that as well as being able to proliferate, as shown by the presence of a mitotic figure, labeled *appositional growth* in Figure 14-3, they are able to differentiate into *chondrocytes*. The chondrocytes in turn add intercellular substance to the surface of the cartilage and this accounts for the cartilage growing along this surface. The chondrogenic layer of the perichondrium of tracheal cartilages eventually disappears, so that in older individuals it ultimately consists of only a fibrous layer that can no longer add new layers of cartilage to the surface it covers.

The cells of cartilage are called *chondrocytes* and, whether they form directly from the mesenchyme of the original model of a cartilaginous structure or as a result of the differentiation of cells of the chondrogenic layer, they secrete intercellular substance around themselves and so subsequently reside in little cavities called *lacunae* (L. for small pits or cavities) in the intercellular substance they have secreted. When a chondrocyte has finished secreting intercellular substance around itself, the lacuna in which it resides is termed a *primary lacuna*. However, such a chondrocyte may still be able to divide a few times more (mitotic figure, labeled *interstitial growth* in Fig. 14-3) and, if so, the tendency is for daughter cells to reside in the same lacuna, with only a thin partition of intercellular substance being formed between them. Sometimes each of these divide again so that there may now be four cells in the primary lacuna (labeled *cell nest* in Fig. 14-3). Since each chondrocyte secretes enough intercellular substance to form a thin wall between itself and its sister cell, it lives in what is termed a *secondary lacuna* and the secondary lacunae of a *cell nest* are therefore all within the original primary lacuna. Cartilage cells seen in a cell nest represent clones because they are the progeny of the original cartilage cell occupying the primary lacuna. Typically, chondrocytes have a rounded nucleus with one or more nucleoli. In life their cytoplasm fills the lacuna in which the cell resides. However, in stained sections the cytoplasm is commonly shrunken away from the borders of the lacuna because of shrinkage artifact. Glycogen and fat may be present in the cytoplasm of large chondrocytes. Chondrocytes vary in size and shape; generally this reflects their degree of maturation. Young chondrocytes instead of being spherical are commonly flattened (Fig. 14-3). Old or, more precisely, *mature* cartilage cells tend to be large and rounded (Fig. 14-3). Size, then, is an important indication of the extent to which any given chondrocyte has differentiated and matured.

The Two Growth Mechanisms of Cartilage

One point to establish from the foregoing that is of great importance in understanding the development and growth of bones (described in Chap. 15) is that young cartilage can *grow by an interstitial growth mechanism,* that is, as a result of young cartilage cells already surrounded by intercellular substance (Fig. 14-3, *interstitial growth*), and therefore lying in its interstices, undergoing division. Furthermore, the intercellular substance of young cartilage is sufficiently malleable to expand from within when interstitial growth occurs.

A given cartilaginous structure can also become larger by having new cartilage deposited on one of its surfaces, a mechanism termed *appositional growth* (Fig. 14-3). This mechanism depends on the relatively undifferentiated cells at the surface of cartilage proliferating and differentiating into young cartilage cells.

Perichondrial Transplants. Advantage can sometimes be taken of the appositional growth mechanism of cartilage by transplanting autologous perichondrium to sites where cartilage has been mostly destroyed. Where this is successful, the transplanted piece of perichondrium produces new cartilage to repair the defect (*see* references to Skoog et al. at the end of Chap. 16).

The Fine Structure of Chondrocytes

Good preparations show that chondrocytes fill their lacunae completely (Fig. 14-4). They exhibit several somewhat pyramidal processes (often called *cytoplasmic footlets*) that extend into the surrounding matrix at various points around their periphery. The nucleus is irregularly ovoid and reveals both condensed and extended chromatin; the former is distributed along the inner surface of the nuclear envelope and in island-like clumps scattered about in the extended chromatin (Fig. 14-4). The nuclear envelope is irregular and clearly reveals pores (arrows in Fig. 14-4). A portion of a nucleolus is indicated by N in Figure 14-4.

The cytoplasm of a chondrocyte reveals the same assortment of organelles that characterizes epithelial secretory cells but they are not arranged in such a polarized manner. The most impressive cytoplasmic constituent is rER (Fig. 14-4), responsible for the synthesis of protein components of the organic intercellular substances the cell secretes. Many cisternae of the rER are dilated by their contents (Fig. 14-4). The Golgi apparatus is generally localized close to the nucleus where it is more or less indented (Fig. 14-4). Secretory vesicles can also be identified in this region. Relatively few mitochondria are present (*lower left,* Fig. 14-4), which supports the concept of chondrocytes depending to a considerable extent on deriving their energy from glycolysis (described on p. 119). In general, the organelles of chondrocytes are similar to those of fibroblasts (p. 233, Fig. 9-8), which also synthesize and secrete the components of fibrous and amorphous types of intercellular substance. However, there are certain special features about the fibrous and amorphous types of intercellular substance in cartilage, as will be described below.

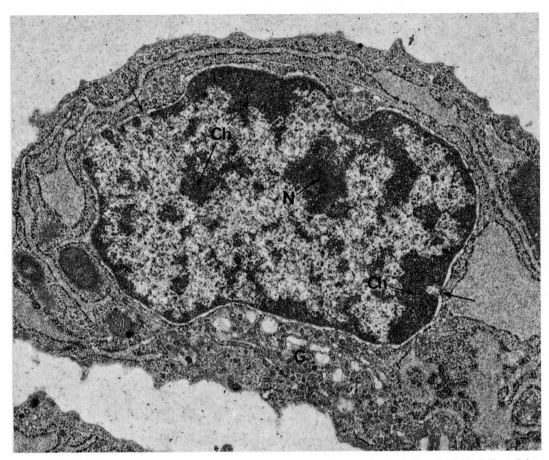

Fig. 14-4. Electron micrograph of a chondrocyte in its lacuna in a tracheal cartilage (chick). Pale-staining cartilage matrix may be seen at *top* and *bottom* external to the lacuna, which is entirely filled with the chondrocyte. The nucleus shows extended and condensed chromatin and nuclear pores (arrows at *top left* and *bottom right* of nucleus); a nucleolus is labeled N. The cytoplasm contains distended cisternae of rER above and on either side of the nucleus. The Golgi region (G) is located close to the indentation on the lower side of the nucleus. Mitochondria are seen at *lower left.* (Courtesy of V. Kalnins)

The Intercellular Substance (Matrix) of Hyaline Cartilage

The organic intercellular substance of cartilage (and also bone) is commonly referred to as its *matrix* (L. meaning the groundwork on which something is cast or develops), probably because it is the groundwork into which calcium salts can be deposited.

Chemical Composition. Estimates of the collagen content of cartilage matrix range from about 50 to 70 per cent of the dry weight, depending on the source of the cartilage. The remainder of the matrix consists primarily of glycosaminoglycans, with some noncollagenic proteins and glycoproteins. The glycosaminoglycans are mostly sulfated and include chondroitin 4- and 6-sulfates and keratan sulfate, but hyaluronic acid is present as well.

The sulfated glycosaminoglycans are attached to noncollagenic proteins to form proteoglycans.

It should also be mentioned that about 75 per cent of the wet weight of cartilage matrix is due to tissue fluid held in its gel structure; this tissue fluid is of the greatest importance in maintaining the viability of the chondrocytes and hence the form and function of cartilage.

Staining Reactions. The matrix of cartilage in H and E sections may appear colorless or blue, depending on the type of hematoxylin used. The staining is mainly due to the sulfated glycosaminoglycans in the proteoglycan of the matrix. Lacunae are lined with a thin layer of matrix that is particularly rich in proteoglycan, and this can frequently be distinguished in H and E sections because it stains more intensely than the matrix between the la-

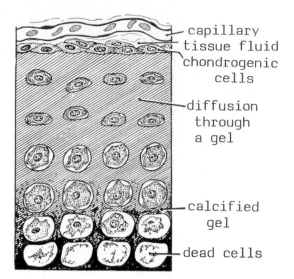

capillary
tissue fluid
chondrogenic
    cells

diffusion
  through
  a gel

calcified
    gel

dead cells

Fig. 14-5. Diagram of a section of hyaline cartilage. A capillary, forming tissue fluid, is shown outside the limits of the cartilage. For the chondrocytes to be nourished, substances dissolved in tissue fluid must diffuse through the gelled intercellular substances of the cartilage to reach the deeply buried cells. If the intercellular substance becomes calcified, as indicated in the lower part of the diagram (black), diffusion cannot occur so the cells die. (Ham, A. W.: J. Bone Joint Surg. [Am.], *34-A:*701, 1952)

cunae; it is shown as dark lines encircling the lacunae in Figure 14-3.

Stains such as toluidine blue may be used to advantage for staining cartilage since glycosaminoglycans stain metachromatically (p. 216). Certain other cationic stains (safranin O and ruthenium red) are particularly useful for staining cartilage matrix as they are suitable for both the LM and EM (Shephard). Finally, the PAS procedure is also useful for staining cartilage because it stains the glycoprotein in the matrix.

The Fine Structure of Cartilage Matrix. This differs somewhat in cartilage occupying various positions in which it serves different functions. Most studies have been done on articular cartilage, so we shall postpone describing the fine structure of cartilage in detail until we deal with articular cartilage (Chap. 16), where it is of much greater importance than in, for instance, tracheal cartilages. However, we shall mention some of its general features here.

Most of the collagenic fibrils in cartilage are narrower than in ordinary connective tissue or bone. In general they range from 10 nm. to 100 nm. in diameter. Moreover, they have a somewhat different molecular constitution from collagen found elsewhere. Whereas in ordinary

connective tissues and bone tropocollagen molecules are in the form of a triple helix consisting of two alpha 1 chains and a single alpha 2 chain (Type I collagen), those of cartilage matrix comprise three identical alpha 1 chains (Type II collagen). Their amino acid constitution is also somewhat different from that of the collagen found elsewhere.

As already noted, about 75 per cent of the wet weight of cartilage matrix represents the tissue fluid held in place by an intricate network of macromolecules consisting mostly of sulfated glycosaminoglycans attached to noncollagenous proteins to form proteoglycans.

Whereas the collagenic fibrils provide a scaffolding that internally supports the matrix, the intricate macromolecular network mentioned above has the capacity for holding a relatively vast amount of tissue fluid in its interstices and this is held so firmly that cartilage intercellular substance, though mostly fluid in content, constitutes a firm material than can bear weight.

The Mechanism of Nutrition in Cartilage

The curious student may have wondered why no capillaries appear in illustrations of cartilage. This is because capillaries are not present in the condensed mesenchyme from which cartilage develops and hence are not present in the cartilage. Cartilage is thus a *nonvascular* tissue, which means that it contains no capillaries to supply it with oxygen and nutrients. How then do the cartilage cells situated in their lacunae within their intercellular substance receive nutrients and how do they rid themselves of their waste products? As noted, 75 per cent of the intercellular substance of cartilage is tissue fluid, held in position by a macromolecular mesh consisting chiefly of proteoglycans. It is this remarkably great fluid content of cartilage matrix that permits gases, nutrients, and waste products to diffuse back and forth between the capillaries *outside the cartilage* and the chondrocytes residing in the lacunae within the cartilage matrix (Fig. 14-5).

Another very important point to understand about skeletal tissues is that the kind of diffusion mechanism that operates in cartilage matrix cannot function if the cartilage matrix becomes impregnated with calcium salts. Hence, *if cartilage becomes calcified it dies* (Fig. 14-5). As we shall see this does not happen in bone because in bone (but not in cartilage) there is an arrangement whereby the matrix becomes calcified without curtailing or even interfering with the life processes of the cells buried within its calcified intercellular substance.

It is not unusual to see some calcification of cartilage matrix in the more central parts of the tracheal cartilages of older people and this is associated with death of chondrocytes where the calcification occurs.

The Grafting of Cartilage—Absence of the Homograft Reaction

Two tissues commonly transplanted by plastic surgeons are skin and cartilage. When skin is transplanted from one person to another (a *homograft* or an *allograft*) it is almost invariably rejected, so for a permanent "take" it is necessary to use skin autografts. (Fortunately, this can usually be done in such a way that an individual ends up with skin both in the site from which the skin for grafting was removed and also in the site to which it was transplanted, as will be described in Chap. 20.)

The grafting of cartilage is rendered difficult because there is not much extraskeletal cartilage from which to obtain autografts. So if the nose or an ear has to be reconstructed there is not much autologous material that can be spared. This led, many years ago, to attempts at using cartilage obtained from people who had just died as grafts for those patients who needed reconstructive surgery. It might be thought that such grafts, being homografts, would be promptly destroyed by a homograft reaction. However, it was found that some cartilage homografts survived in their new hosts as living tissue.

Before considering why homografts of cartilage, in contrast to skin grafts, can survive, we should point out that for any kind of cartilage graft to persist without being gradually resorbed, *its cells must continue to live.* Grafts of dead cartilage eventually become resorbed probably because they are invaded by capillaries and fibroblasts. The matrix of living cartilage seems to act as a barrier to such invasion. Even autografts of cartilage sometimes become resorbed in part; it is thought that this is due to the graft bed furnishing an insufficient supply of nutrients to keep the chondrocytes of the graft alive. Cartilage grafts must be placed in beds that will ensure an adequate supply of nutrients for continued viability of the chondrocytes of the graft. Provided this is done, even homografts of cartilage will survive for long periods.

The unique feature that permits a cartilage homograft to survive is that for the most part the cells in the graft are entirely surrounded with a substantial amount of matrix that permits only very limited diffusion of substances with high molecular weights. This of course restricts disclosure of foreign antigens of the chondrocytes in the homograft to the immunologically responsive cells of the host and furthermore would prevent any killer cells formed from establishing effective contact with their target foreign cells, the chondrocytes in the homograft.

The repair of hyaline cartilage will be discussed when we describe articular cartilage in Chapter 16 (pp. 469–473).

Besides hyaline cartilage there are two other kinds of cartilage in the body, *fibrocartilage* and *elastic cartilage.* These will be briefly described below.

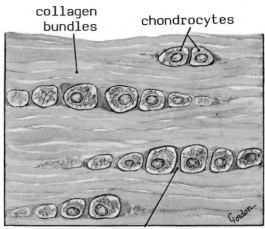

Fig. 14-6. High-power drawing of fibrocartilage taken from a tendon close to its point of insertion.

FIBROCARTILAGE

Although present in several places in the body, fibrocartilage is most easily studied in tendon insertions, particularly where the insertion is into cartilage . On approaching such an insertion a tendon takes on a different appearance, as shown in Figure 14-6. It was noted earlier in this chapter that where a tendon inserts into cartilage it is formed by chondrogenic cells instead of ordinary fibroblasts. These are larger and more rounded (Fig. 14-6) than fibroblasts and lie in rows or layers, between which there are bundles of collagenic fibers. In between the individual rounded cells in these rows there is a basophilic nonfibrous intercellular substance (Fig. 14-6) reminiscent of the matrix lying close to chondrocytes in hyaline cartilage (Fig. 14-3); its basophilia is due to sulfated glycosaminoglycans.

The properties and position of fibrocartilage both suggest that it would develop from mesenchymal cells at the border between the developing fibrous and chondrogenic layers of the perichondrium. In early development the cells here would have the potentiality to differentiate into either fibroblasts or chondrocytes and in this instance they seem to retain an ability to exploit both capacities, but in sequence, producing first the collagen and then the nonfibrous intercellular material. In addition to forming tendon insertions, fibrocartilage is also found in the symphysis pubis (p. 477) and in intervertebral disks (pp. 477–479).

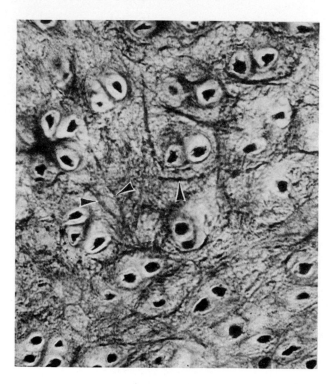

Fig. 14-7. Photomicrograph of elastic cartilage from external ear. Elastic fibers (indicated by arrows) are seen as dark lines crisscrossing the matrix.

ELASTIC CARTILAGE

Although hyaline cartilage is elastic to some degree, it is not as elastic as cartilage that contains considerable numbers of elastic fibers in its intercellular substance. In some sites, for example, the external ear and the epiglottis, a tissue that is firm and yet very elastic is required. In these sites *elastic cartilage* is found. It is basically similar to hyaline cartilage, but its chondrocytes can produce *elastic fibers* as well as collagen fibrils and nonfibrous intercellular substance, so it contains elastic fibers scattered throughout its substance (Fig.14-7).

REFERENCES AND OTHER READING

Cartilage

See references at end of Chapter 16.

Tendons

Buck, R. C.: Regeneration of tendon. J. Pathol., *66:*1, 1953.
Peacock, E. E., and van Winkle, W.: Surgery and Biology of Wound Repair. Philadelphia, W. B. Saunders, 1970.

15 Bone and Bones

In this chapter we have to deal not only with bone as a special kind of connective tissue but also with how bone tissue is arranged to form the structures called bones. These structures (bones) live, grow, and are remodeled, and are repaired if they are broken. However, the two aspects of the problem—bone as a tissue and bones as individual structures—cannot be conveniently separated, so that in describing bone as a tissue we will sometimes have to discuss particular bones, and in describing bones we may also have to discuss further points about the nature of bone tissue.

SIMILARITIES BETWEEN CARTILAGE AND BONE

The easiest way to begin the study of bone tissue is to compare and contrast it with that of its sister tissue, cartilage, described in Chapter 14. Like cartilage, bone consists of cells and an organic intercellular substance (called its *matrix*) which, as in cartilage, consists of collagenic fibrils embedded in an amorphous component. However, the ratio of fibrous to amorphous component in the matrix is much higher in bone than in cartilage, and both the collagen and the amorphous component are somewhat different in composition in the two tissues.

Next, it may be useful at the outset to compare Figure 14-3 with Figure 15-1. As is illustrated in Figure 15-1, the cells of bone (labeled Oc) like those of cartilage live in lacunae within a matrix (M in Fig. 15-1). In bone these cells are called *osteocytes* (Gr. *osteon*, bone). Furthermore, just as cartilaginous structures (except at articular surfaces) are covered with perichondrium, the outer surfaces of bones are covered with a membrane called *periosteum* (Gr. *peri*, around) (Fig. 15-1, P). Finally, bone tissue, like cartilage, develops from mesenchyme. However, the microenvironment in which it develops is different from that in which cartilage develops; as pointed out in Chapter 14, cartilage develops where there are no capillaries. Bone, as we shall see, develops from mesenchyme where there are capillaries present.

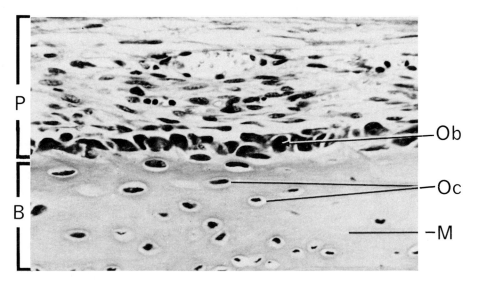

Fig. 15-1. Photomicrograph of one side of a growing bone (decalcified section, stained H and E). The periosteum (P) is seen at *top*. Its deepest layer consists of osteoblasts (Ob) apposed to the surface of the bone (B). Osteocytes (Oc) lie within their lacunae in the bone matrix (M).

SOME IMPORTANT DIFFERENCES BETWEEN CARTILAGE AND BONE

(1) Different Methods Must Be Employed in the Study of Bone. Bone is much stronger than cartilage because normal cartilage persisting in the body is not calcified and hence cartilaginous structures of any great dimension would bend if called upon to bear weight. But the matrix of bone is calcified and hence stone-like, so it resists bending and can bear much weight. However, when we attempt to study bone in the histology or pathology laboratory, its stone-like character presents a problem because it cannot, as it is, be sliced in paraffin to prepare H and E sections. To overcome this difficulty, pieces of bone, after being fixed, can be placed in a decalcifying solution to dissolve the mineral from them. Acids were commonly used in the past for this purpose but they have been largely superseded by chelating (Gr. *chele,* claw) agents, which have the ability to combine with the calcium ions of the deposit and "claw" them out by converting them to soluble compounds. These compounds wash out from the matrix without damaging its organic components or the cells of bone as much as older decalcifying methods did. The common one used is EDTA (ethylenediamine tetra-acetic acid). Following decalcification a block of bone can be dehydrated, cleared, embedded in paraffin, sectioned, and stained. Sections so prepared are called *decalcified sections* or, more properly, sections of *decalcified bone.* One is shown in Figure 15-1. They reveal only the organic components of bone—the osteocytes and the organic matrix, which consists of collagen and amorphous intercellular substance in which the osteocytes are buried.

An important point to make here is that even though the mineral is removed by the decalcification procedure, bone substance still retains its form. Even a whole bone can be decalcified and still look the same (Fig. 15-2, *bottom*). However, as is also shown in Figure 15-2, *top,* it

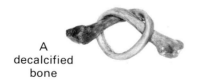

A
decalcified
bone

Fig. 15-2. A simple demonstration of the flexibility of a decalcified bone.

cannot now bear weight; indeed it is so flexible it can even be tied up in a knot. So bone differs from normal cartilage in that it must usually be studied in decalcified sections.

A second important point to make about sections of decalcified bone is that due to difficulty in obtaining ideal fixation of calcified bone, and also due to side effects of the decalcifying procedure, the cells of bone (*osteocytes*) are generally shrunken away from the walls of the lacunae they inhabit (Figs. 15-1 and 15-3A). Accordingly, the cytoplasm of osteocytes appears to poor advantage in H and E sections of decalcified bone. The presence of bone cells in lacunae can, however, be deduced from the fact that the nuclei of osteocytes are well stained and obvious (Figs. 15-1 and 15-3A). It should be noted here that the method of preparing bone sections for EM studies preserves osteocytes much better, as will be illustrated later.

(2) The Mechanism for Nutrition in Bone Is Different From That of Cartilage. If the organic matrix of bone in which osteocytes live were solidly calcified, no diffusion of nutrients could occur through it and its osteocytes would die just as chondrocytes die when the matrix surrounding them becomes calcified. However, by studying bone by another method, early investigators obtained the clue as to how nutrients reached osteocytes when the matrix surrounding them became calcified. They cut thin little pieces of a calcified bone with a saw and ground these down on an abrasive surface until they were thin enough to transmit light (though still remaining very thick as compared to paraffin sections). When examined with the LM, these sections (called *ground bone sections*) disclosed something not seen in a decalcified section, namely that the osteocytes in calcified bone are connected both to each other and to a canal (Fig. 15-3B), or to some other surface where there is tissue fluid, by what appear as fine lines (Fig. 15-3B). (The vast numbers of these fine lines seen in such a section are due to its thickness.) Eventually these lines were shown to be tiny tubular passageways through the calcified matrix and were called *canaliculi* (L. dim. of *canalis,* tubular passageway or channel); they were found to contain tissue fluid and hair-like cytoplasmic processes of osteocytes that connected osteocytes together. It is now known that canaliculi provide the means for nutrients to reach osteocytes, thus keeping them alive even though they exist within a calcified matrix. How canaliculi are formed and function will be discussed shortly. Here, however, it should be mentioned that the main reason canaliculi are indistinct or hardly seen at all in H and E sections of decalcified bone (as in Fig. 15-3A) is that when the mineral deposit is removed there is nothing left to keep the matrix rigid enough for them to stay open, so they are mostly obliterated. However, with the more refined methods of fixation used for electron microscopy, canaliculi can be seen in EM sections even in decalcified material (Fig. 15-4, *see* legend). Furthermore,

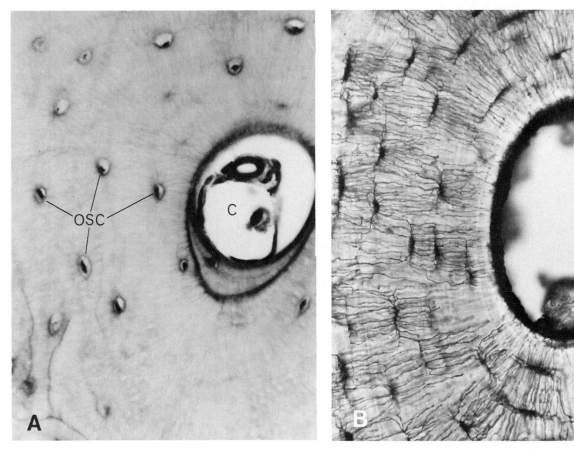

Fig. 15-3. Photomicrographs illustrating the appearance of bone in decalcified and undecalcified sections. (*A*) Decalcified bone stained with H and E. The osteocytes (OSC) in their lacunae are visible (though imperfectly fixed) but the canaliculi between the lacunae are indistinct. The canal (C) to the right contains blood vessels that in life supply the osteocytes with tissue fluid via the canaliculi. (*B*) Comparable field in unstained section made by grinding down undecalcified bone. Here the lacunae appear as dark flattened ovals but the osteocytes they contain are not preserved. The fine lines (canaliculi) connecting lacunae to each other and to the canal at *right* are seen to advantage, but the contents of the canal have not been preserved.

by using special heavy microtomes and special knives it is possible to cut sections of bone that has not been decalcified thin enough for the EM, particularly from embryos or young animals, the bones of which have not become as dense and stone-like as bones of adults. Some illustrations of these will be given later.

(3) Unlike Cartilage, Bone Is a Vascular Tissue. As already noted, normal cartilage does not contain any capillaries, so that the capillaries supplying the nutrients for chondrocytes always lie outside the substance of the cartilage. But since the matrix of cartilage readily permits the diffusion of nutrients and waste products over relatively great distances, chondrocytes can live even though far away from capillaries. However, the situation is different in bone tissue. The canaliculi permitting the passage of nutrients from capillaries to osteocytes are of very

fine caliber (as shown in Fig. 15-4, toward the upper left corner); thus it could not be expected that any mechanism for transmitting nutrients would be able to operate effectively over very long distances. Indeed, Ham in 1952 reported that osteocytes almost always lay within 0.1 to 0.2 mm. of a free surface or a canal where there were capillaries. This means that what in the gross may seem to be dense bone substance is seen under the microscope to be permeated with capillaries lying in canals. (Two small blood vessels that would be associated with capillaries can be seen in the canal labeled C in Fig. 15-3A.) Furthermore, since capillaries do not burrow into dense bone to take up their position, bone must be built up around capillaries in such a way that osteocytes will be no farther away than 0.1 to 0.2 mm. from a source of fresh tissue fluid. How this is done will soon be described. This dis-

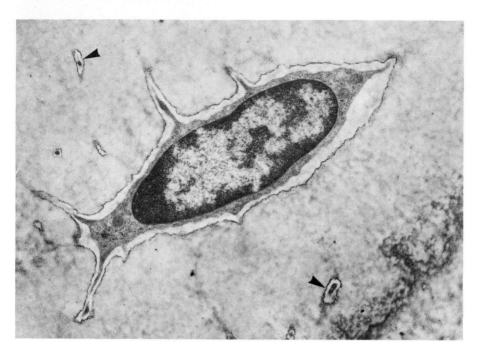

Fig. 15-4. Electron micrograph of part of a decalcified section of bone, showing an osteocyte in its lacuna with the proximal parts of four of its cytoplasmic processes extending into canaliculi. Two canaliculi with processes cut in cross section are indicated by arrows. (Courtesy of S. Luk and G. Simon)

tance would seem to be approximately the limit over which the canalicular mechanism providing nutrients to osteocytes in calcified bone can operate.

(4) Unlike Cartilage, Bone Grows Only by the Appositional Mechanism. It should now be apparent why the study of the formation and growth of bone is quite a fascinating subject. However, one more factor to be considered that makes it even more interesting is that bone, unlike cartilage, can grow only by the *appositional* mechanism. Cartilage can grow by both interstitial and appositional mechanisms, but since bone matrix begins to become calcified almost as soon as it is formed, bone tissue cannot expand from within its substance. Hence all bone growth must occur on some preexisting surface. So the only way any given bony structure can be changed in size or shape is by new bone forming on one or more of its surfaces or older bone being removed from one or more of its other surfaces. The cells involved in the formation or removal of bone at such surfaces will be described shortly.

With the above introduction we can now begin the study of the development of bone in the embryo, which is basic to what comes later.

THE DEVELOPMENT OF BONE

The development of bone is described as being due to *osteogenesis* (Gr. *gennan,* to produce). Another term for the process by which bone develops is *ossification.* A knowledge of how, where, and when this process occurs in embryonic life is fundamental to understanding subse-

quent growth and maintenance of the skeleton. Unfortunately, however, the terminology commonly used in connection with osteogenesis can be misleading.

Terminology. It was long ago noticed that osteogenesis (ossification) began in the body in two general sites, (*1*) in areas of ordinary mesenchyme and (*2*) within the more or less central disintegrating parts of cartilage models of bones-to-be. Since some of the sites in which osteogenesis began in mesenchymal areas (in which there was no preexisting cartilage) were somewhat membranous in appearance, ossification in these sites was described as *intramembranous ossification.* Ossification seen to begin in disintegrating central parts of cartilage models of bone-to-be, however, was termed *endochondral ossification.* It is to be emphasized that these two terms refer only to the environment in which ossification occurs. They have no significance whatsoever about the nature of the process of ossification or the kind of bone that results from it, which as we shall see is always the same. However, this is not always appreciated and as a result the terms are sometimes used as if they referred to two different kinds of ossification. But what is worse is that bones resulting from ossification in an intramembranous environment are commonly termed "membrane bones" and those resulting from ossification in a cartilaginous environment are commonly termed "cartilage bones." This terminology tends to suggest that the bone tissue developing in these two sites is different, whereas it is the same. Furthermore, to the uninitiated student these two terms unfortunately may suggest that the bones that form in the two different environments do so as a result of membrane or cartilage actually changing into bone. It should be emphasized that no kind of adult fully differentiated tissue *ever* changes into another kind. We now begin an account of intramembranous ossification with the assertion that this term is merely descriptive of the environment in which ossification begins in certain parts of the body and that ossification here results in the formation of the same kind of bone as forms in endochondral ossification, which will be described later.

INTRAMEMBRANOUS OSSIFICATION

Intramembranous ossification is most easily studied in the development of the skull. We shall use for our example of intramembranous ossification the development, followed by growth and remodeling, of a parietal bone. In the site where each parietal bone forms there is first a layer of loose mesenchyme that fills the space between the developing skin of the scalp and the developing brain below. Since the mesenchyme here is in the form of a layer it was at first regarded as a membrane; this is why the ossification beginning in it was called *intramembranous* ossification. Before ossification begins here the mesenchyme consists of widely separated, more or less triangular or star-shaped pale cells with processes that often connect with those of adjacent mesenchymal cells (shown at periphery in Fig. 15-5A). Then, in one or two sites in the mesenchyme where a parietal bone will begin to form and where some blood capillaries are present, a slight change occurs that represents the initiation of formation of what is called a *center of osteogenesis*. This begins with a few of the mesenchymal cells in a given site becoming more rounded and their cytoplasm staining more deeply with hematoxylin; four are shown in the center of Figure 15-5A. At the same time their processes become thicker (Fig. 15-5B) and connect with processes of other cells of the same kind developing here. The cells undergoing this change in appearance represent mesenchymal cells that quickly and imperceptibly pass through an *osteogenic cell* stage (as will be described later) to differentiate into *osteoblasts* (Gr. *blastos*, germ), so-called because they will soon "generate" the organic matrix of bone. These will then surround themselves with matrix to become *osteocytes,* and so come to be situated in lacunae completely surrounded by bone matrix that almost immediately begins to absorb calcium salts, thus becoming *calcified.* However, calcification does not cause the death of the osteocytes, because of the formation of canaliculi.

How Canaliculi Are Formed. The way osteoblasts cause canaliculi to form is shown diagrammatically in Figure 15-5C. First, the cytoplasmic processes of the four osteoblasts developing in Figure 15-5B connect with one another. When these osteoblasts secrete the organic matrix of bone around themselves (gray in Fig. 15-5C) their

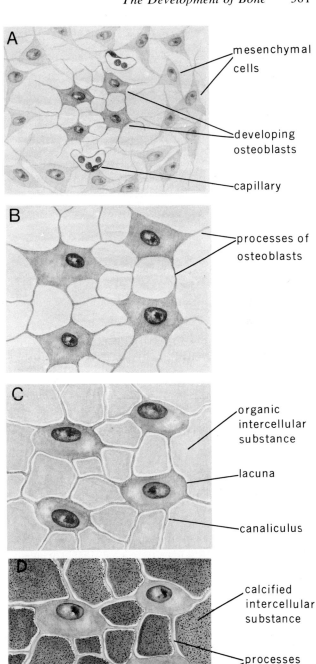

mesenchymal cells

developing osteoblasts

capillary

processes of osteoblasts

organic intercellular substance

lacuna

canaliculus

calcified intercellular substance

processes in canaliculi

Fig. 15-5. Diagrams illustrating how bone forms in an intramembranous environment. (*A*) Mesenchymal cells begin to differentiate in the presence of capillaries. (*B*) They become recognizable as osteoblasts. (*C*) They secrete the organic intercellular substance of bone and their processes act as molds for the formation of canaliculi. (*D*) They eventually become buried in intercellular substance as osteocytes and the bone matrix becomes impregnated with calcium salts.

bone
intercellular
substance

osteocytes

basophilic
cytoplasm

blood
vessels

osteoblasts

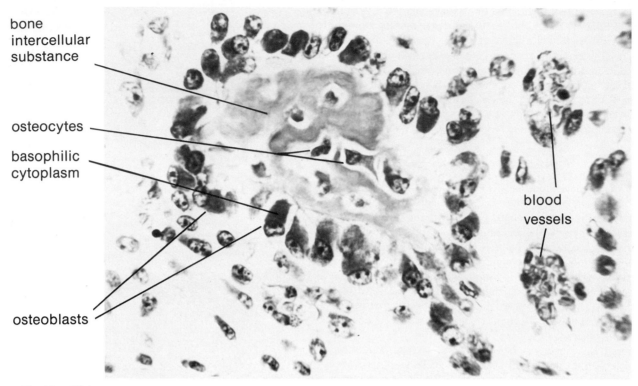

Fig. 15-6. High-power photomicrograph of a transverse section of a forming trabecula of bone, in the developing skull of a pig embryo. Osteoblasts arranged around its periphery are laying down intercellular substance of bone. Some bone cells have entirely surrounded themselves with intercellular substance so as to become buried as osteocytes in it; these reside in lacunae.

cytoplasmic processes act as molds around which the organic matrix is, as it were, poured. When the organic matrix "sets" it soon becomes impregnated with calcium salts (dark in Fig. 15-5D) and hence becomes stone-like and impermeable, but it remains riddled with the processes of osteoblasts, which now lie in their canaliculi. Such spaces as exist between the osteoblast processes and the walls of the canaliculi in which they lie become filled with tissue fluid derived from capillaries just outside the island of forming bone. Osteoblasts buried in the intercellular substance they have secreted (Fig. 15-5D) have thus become *osteocytes*. Tissue fluid also fills the tiny spaces between them and the walls of the lacunae in which they now live (Fig. 15-5D).

What Is Seen at This Stage in a Decalcified Section. The first little mass of bone is probably in the form of a little irregular bar, which in Figure 15-6 is cut in cross section. A little bar of bone is called a *trabecula* (L. dim. of *trabs*, a beam) or a *spicule*.

The cells at the periphery of Figure 15-6 are mesenchymal cells; only their nuclei are seen to advantage because their cytoplasm stains only faintly. The dark-staining intercellular material in the central area, labeled *bone intercellular substance*, has just been formed by osteoblasts

that became surrounded as they produced it and so have now become *osteocytes*. Canaliculi, as already noted, are not usually evident in H and E sections. The bony trabecula, cut in cross section, is ringed with *osteoblasts,* labeled in Figure 15-6. Typically these are relatively large cells with the nucleus having an eccentric position and the cytoplasm being so basophilic (and hence such a dark blue in an H and E section) that it is difficult sometimes to distinguish nucleus from cytoplasm. Note that two wide capillaries are present on the right, labeled *blood vessels;* their presence shows that osteogenesis is occurring here, as always, in a vascular environment.

The Formation of Cancellous Bone. After a small mass of bone has formed in each site from which a parietal bone will develop, further growth is not due to its becoming evenly enlarged, but by trabeculae (spicules) extending out from it in a radial fashion. These are probably formed by other mesenchymal cells differentiating into osteoblasts and osteocytes in the sites where the new trabeculae form. Next, continued growth of the trabeculae, brought about in the same manner, causes them to join one another so as to form a network of connecting trabeculae (Fig. 15-7); such an anastomosing network of bone trabeculae is called *cancellous* (L. *cancellus*, a lattice)

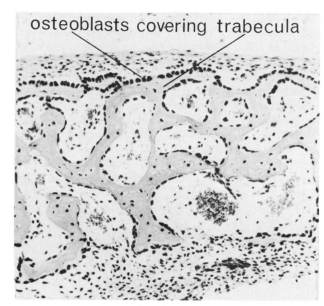

osteoblasts covering trabecula

Fig. 15-7. Low-power photomicrograph of a skull bone of a pig embryo (later stage than in Fig. 15-6). This is trabecular (*cancellous*) bone with its trabeculae enclosing spaces. Note the basophilic osteoblasts covering the trabeculae and lining the spaces.

bone (Fig. 15-7). By the time this forms it would seem that few mesenchymal cells of the area remain in an undifferentiated state. But before they disappear from the scene they leave a heritage of what are termed *osteogenic cells* that take up positions so as to cover or line all the surfaces of trabeculae not occupied by osteoblasts forming bone on the surface.

Summary to This Point in the Intramembranous Ossification Process. The following has so far happened in the development of a parietal bone. At first mesenchymal cells differentiate into osteoblasts that form bony trabeculae; these anastomose with one another to form cancellous bone. Before the mesenchymal cells are all "used up," some differentiate to a limited extent into *osteogenic cells.* Osteogenic cells are thin, flattened cells that cover or line bone surfaces. They are committed to forming either bone or cartilage and serve as stem cells to maintain a population of themselves on all bone surfaces, where there are always enough to develop into further osteoblasts or chondrocytes and form more bone or cartilage by appositional growth. Whether they differentiate into osteoblasts or chondroblasts depends on their microenvironment. If capillaries are present they differentiate into osteoblasts and so form bone. In the absence of capillaries they differentiate into chondrocytes and form cartilage. We shall now describe the mechanism of appositional growth in more detail in order to comment further on the development of a parietal bone.

The Appositional Growth of Bone on an Isolated Trabecula. To keep this description as simple as possible we shall assume that a trabecula in a capillary-rich environment is covered on all surfaces with an even layer of more or less flattened osteogenic cells, as shown in Figure 15-8A. The first step in appositional growth is for the osteogenic cells to divide to increase their numbers so that some can differentiate into osteoblasts without exhausting their supply. For the sake of simplicity this is shown in Figure 15-8B by them dividing so as to form two layers of osteogenic cells. Then, as shown in Figure 15-8C, the osteogenic cells of the deeper layer differentiate into osteoblasts which secrete matrix around their cell bodies and processes so as to form a new layer of bone, appropriately provided with canaliculi, on the bone surfaces;

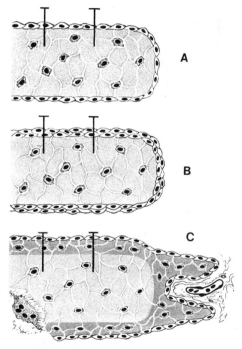

A

B

C

Fig. 15-8. Diagrams illustrating that bone grows by apposition but not by the interstitial mechanism. The positions of two pins driven into a bone are indicated in (*A*), (*B*), and (*C*). Note that they stay the same distance apart, indicating that bone does not grow by the interstitial mechanism, but only by apposition, which requires that new layers of bone be deposited on surfaces. (*A*) A trabecula of bone is covered on all surfaces with a layer of osteogenic cells. (*B*) These cells proliferate. (*C*) The cells of the innermost layer differentiate into osteoblasts and form a new layer of bone by secreting organic intercellular substance. The surface still remains covered by osteogenic cells except at sites of resorption where osteoclasts are present (*lower left corner*). At *right*, this diagram illustrates how new bone can be laid down on surfaces, extending the length of a trabecula to surround a capillary, so that the cells of the newly formed bone will have a source of nutrition. (Ham, A. W.: J. Bone Joint Surg., *34-A:*701, 1952)

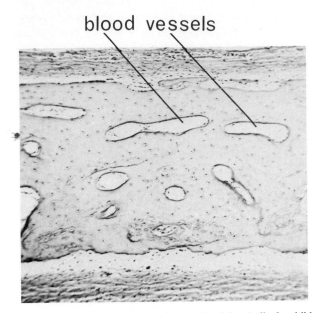

blood vessels

Fig. 15-9. Low-power photomicrograph of the skull of a child. Cancellous bone (as shown in Fig. 15-7) has become filled in by appositional growth to constitute a plate of compact (dense) bone. Figure 15-10 shows how this is achieved. Former spaces in the cancellous bone are reduced to canals containing blood vessels.

moreover, this is done with the new bone surfaces still being covered with osteogenic cells so that further layers of bone can be formed with same way.

The next point to make about appositional growth is that as each successive layer of osteoblasts develops from osteogenic cells on a surface, the osteoblasts develop processes. On the sides of the osteoblasts the processes of adjacent cells connect with each other by cell junctions. On the deep side of each osteoblast (its side apposed to bone), its processes somehow connect with the processes of those extending to the surface from the most recently formed osteocytes now in lacunae just beneath the surface. So when the osteoblasts lay down matrix on the surface and along their sides, their processes are connected both with those of osteoblasts beside them and those of osteocytes beneath them in the most recently formed layer of bone. Accordingly, by the time the osteoblasts have secreted a new layer of matrix their processes have served as molds for canaliculi that connect each osteocyte in the newly formed layer of bone both with canaliculi of osteocytes below them and with the surface above them.

The thoughtful reader will now question how many new layers can be added this way without the osteocytes in the middle of the trabecula becoming too far away from a supply of fresh tissue fluid (which comes from outside the trabecula). Actually, most trabeculae do not become

thick enough for this to happen. If, however, they do become sufficiently thick for their central regions to be more than about 0.1 to 0.2 mm. from a surface, it will be found that they contain a central blood vessel that provides the deeply located osteocytes with tissue fluid (Ham). Since blood vessels do not bore into bone, they must attain this central position by having bone built around them. The way this can be achieved is shown at the right side of Figure 15-8C. The capillary shown here would in due course become enclosed by bone forming by appositional growth so that the trabecula here could become much thicker without the osteocytes dying in its core.

THE PROCESSES BY WHICH BONE IS REMODELED

Two independent processes are involved in the remodeling of bone. They are (*1*) addition of bone tissue to the surface of preexisting bone by appositional growth and (*2*) resorption of bone from surfaces. It is by the addition of newly formed bone to surfaces that a trabecula can grow in size. The resorption of bone from surfaces is accomplished by large multinucleated cells called *osteoclasts* (Gr. *klan,* to break) that appear on bone surfaces. One is shown at the lower left corner of the trabecula shown in Figure 15-8C, where it has eroded a cavity which it now occupies. As a result of new bone having been formed at some sites by appositional growth, and older bone having been resorbed at another site by an osteoclast, the trabecula has been *remodeled.* These two processes, appositional growth and bone resorption from surfaces, are the only ways the shape and size of a bone can change during pre- and postnatal life.

We shall now describe how appositional growth accounts for cancellous bone being converted into compact bone.

HOW CANCELLOUS BONE IS CONVERTED INTO COMPACT (DENSE) BONE

The development of a parietal bone provides an example of how *cancellous* bone (Fig. 15-7) becomes converted to *compact (dense)* bone (Fig. 15-9).

Cancellous bone is characterized by possessing more space occupied by loose connective tissue and blood vessels than by bone substance. Compact bone (Fig. 15-9), however, is characterized by possessing more bone than space occupied by soft tissue and blood vessels. This is only a general working rule for distinguishing between the two types; there is no precise method. To understand how cancellous bone (such as that shown in Fig. 15-7)

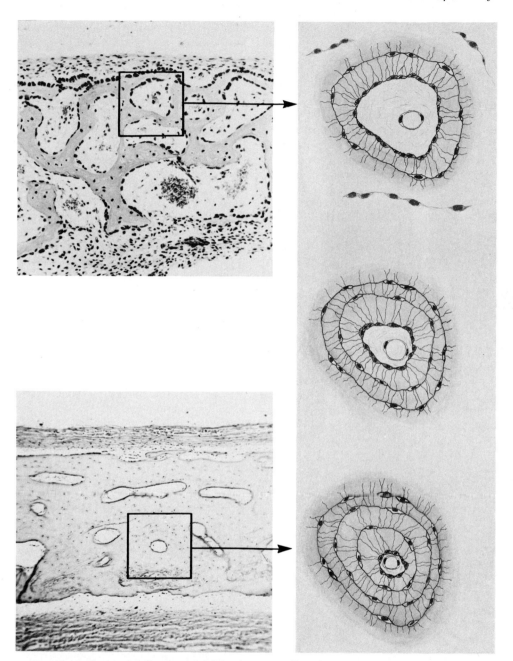

Fig. 15-10. Composite diagram explaining how cancellous bone becomes converted into dense (compact) bone. For details, *see* text.

can be converted into compact bone (Fig. 15-9), it is necessary to appreciate how appositional growth alters the microscopic appearance of the trabeculae of a cancellous network.

The Effects of Appositional Growth in a Cancellous Network. The anastomosing trabeculae of a cancellous net-

work are all covered with osteogenic cells. Hence all the spaces in cancellous bone are lined with osteogenic cells. If the osteogenic cells surrounding a space multiply, like the osteogenic cells lining the spaces in Figure 15-10, *right side,* and then those in the deeper layers differentiate into osteoblasts so as to form a new layer of bone on the trabecular surface, the trabeculae surrounding any given space in a cancellous network become thicker and the space they surround becomes correspondingly smaller, as shown in Figure 15-10, *right side,* reading from *top to bottom.* Every time this process is repeated the trabeculae become thicker and the individual spaces surrounded by trabeculae become correspondingly smaller. Finally, if this process were to occur in all the spaces surrounded by trabeculae in a cancellous network, as is shown from *top* to *bottom* on the right side of Figure 15-10, there would eventually be more bone than space present; so what would have been cancellous bone (Fig. 15-10, *top left*) would have been thus converted into dense (compact) bone like that shown in Figure 15-10, *lower left.*

Next, each layer of bone formed on the trabecula would have its canaliculi connected to those of the layer it covered, as shown in Figure 15-10, *right,* fine dark lines. Furthermore, the spaces in the cancellous network containing the blood vessels would now be so small that the vessel would be housed in no more than a canal, in the center of what was formerly a space. This vessel would supply tissue fluid and nutrients to all the cells of the bone now surrounding it, via their anastomosing canaliculi.

Haversian Systems (Osteons). The layered structure, built up by successive layers of bone being added to the bony walls of spaces in cancellous bone, with the layers appearing as successive rings in cross section (Fig. 15-10, *right*) around a small central space only large enough to contain one or two vessels and a lining of osteogenic cells, is called a *haversian system* (after Havers who first described it) or *osteon.* Osteons are the usual units of structure of compact bone. Because they are mostly less

than around 0.4 mm. or so in diameter, they permit compact bone to exist with its osteocytes being no farther away than around 0.1 to 0.2 mm. from the central blood vessels of each system, which were formerly the blood vessels in the spaces of the cancellous network in which the haversian systems were built. Hence the distance over which the canalicular system operates effectively would seem to be the factor that limits the diameter of osteons. Since the layers of each system are laid down consecutively, the processes of osteoblasts in each new layer must continue to connect with those of osteocytes in the previous layer if tissue fluid from the vessel in the canal is to reach osteocytes in the outermost layers.

The length of haversian systems (osteons) developing in parietal bones is small compared with those in long bones. As a consequence, those in parietal bones are called *primitive* osteons.

When the spaces in the network of cancellous bone have become filled in with osteons, a parietal bone consists of a simple plate of dense (compact) bone (Fig. 15-10, *bottom pictures*). But in order to accommodate the enlarging brain of the *fetus* (L. for unborn offspring fed by a placenta until birth), each developing parietal bone has both to enlarge, so as to cover a greater area, and undergo a change in its curvature, as illustrated in Figure 15-11. Furthermore, these processes have to continue into postnatal life until the head reaches its adult size.

The Growth and Remodeling of a Plate of Compact Bone. After the cancellous bone of a developing parietal bone has become a curved plate of compact bone it continues to grow until it reaches its adult size. This process depends on continuous appositional growth, but the question arises as to just where this appositional growth occurs. To delve into this matter it should first be mentioned that the two parietal bones (one on each side) throughout their growth are separated from each other and from the other skull bones they meet by what are termed *sutures* (L. *sutura,* a seam). During the growing period these sutures contain loose connective tissue, blood vessels, and osteogenic cells; hence they permit appositional growth at the edges of the bones meeting in a suture. With regard to accommodating the enlarging brain, there have been different views about the extent to which enlargement of the skull is due to appositional growth in sutures and/or on the convex surface of bones such as the parietal bones. Probably what happens is a combination of both processes, as we shall now outline. Figure 15-11A shows that appositional growth alone in sutures could explain enlargement of the vault of the skull. However, this enlargement could also be explained solely by appositional growth on the convex surfaces of the bones concerned, as shown in Figure 15-11B.

Remodeling. Furthermore, as the skull enlarges (as a result of growth in sutures and/or appositional growth on

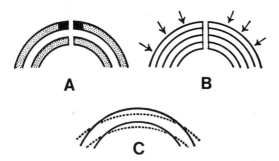

Fig. 15-11. Diagrams illustrating possible ways in which bones forming the vault of the cranium could grow and change in curvature. (*A*) By appositional growth in the sutures (new bone shown in black). (*B*) By appositional growth on the convex surface, accompanied by resorption (not indicated) along the concave surface. (*C*) By appositional growth at certain sites on the convex surface with resorption along the concave surface at the same sites, so as to change in curvature from that depicted in solid lines to that indicated in dotted lines.

the outer surfaces) the *curvature* of the parietal bone has to change as shown in Figure 15-11C. This requires appositional growth on the convex surface at certain sites (Fig. 15-11C) and resorption from the concave surface at the same sites.

Fontanelles. At birth ossification has advanced far enough for the adjacent bones of the skull to have approached one another so closely that they are separated from one another only by narrow sutures. However, at the sites where *more* than two bones meet, the suture space remains larger and such areas are termed *fontanelles* (soft spots). There are six of these soft areas not yet filled with bone in the skull of the newborn infant. The most prominent, the *anterior* or *frontal* fontanelle, is situated at the point where the two parietal bones and the bone advancing from dual centers of ossification of the frontal bone meet. Manual inspection of this fontanelle (by gently feeling it) in an infant can give a physician valuable information as to whether ossification is proceeding normally.

The parietal bones as they grow are, for some time after birth, composed of only a single plate of bone which, however, contains some spaces filled with loose connective tissue and thin-walled veins (Fig. 15-9). As growth of the skull continues, the remodeling process (appositional growth in some sites and resorption in others) gradually converts these single plates of bone over most of the skull into double plates of compact bone between which there is some cancellous bone and a considerable amount of marrow.

Since cancellous bone and the bone marrow it contains in its spaces separate two plates of compact bone at this stage, this arrangement of two plates of bone is termed the *diploë* (Gr. *diploë*, fold) and the many large, thin-walled veins present in the marrow between the two plates are correspondingly called the *diploetic veins*. The double-plate arrangement of the diploë over most of the skull is attained in childhood (at about the age of 8 years). Later on, in adult life, the bones meeting at the various sutures fuse and it becomes possible for diploetic veins to pass from one skull bone to another.

IMMATURE AND MATURE BONE

Kinds of Bone

It has already been emphasized that bone forming as a result of intramembranous ossification is no different from that forming by endochondral ossification, and hence if the terms *membrane bone* and *cartilage bone* are ever used, they do not signify different kinds of bone but only that the bone was in these two instances formed in different tissue environments in the embryo. However, as just described there are two kinds of bone characterized

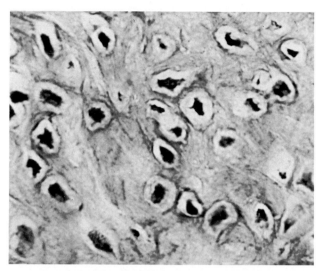

Fig. 15-12. High-power photomicrograph of immature bone, as seen in a decalcified H and E section.

by whether they consist chiefly of trabeculae, with relatively large spaces between them (*cancellous bone*), or primarily of bone substance, with small spaces (*compact* or *dense bone*). We shall now describe how in addition to bone being classified as cancellous or compact, it can be classified as either *immature* or *mature*. These two types of bone are distinguished from one another by the arrangement and relative amounts of the various components of their intercellular substance and also by the relative numbers of osteocytes they possess in relation to their content of intercellular substance. By these morphological criteria Pritchard describes three types: (*1*) bundle bone, (*2*) woven bone, and (*3*) fine-fibered bone.

Bone is classified as immature and mature because bundle bone and woven bone are for the most part the types of bone that are the first to develop in embryonic life—for example the bone in Figure 15-12 is immature. Later fine-fibered bone is the kind formed and so it is referred to as mature bone. For the most part the immature types of bone have only a temporary existence in the body, being replaced as growth continues with mature bone.

Immature Bone. Immature bone (Fig. 15-12) has proportionately more cells than mature bone. Immature bone is of two types, *woven bone* or *coarsely bundled* bone. In the former the bundles of collagen fibers of its matrix run in various directions; this accounts for the term *woven*. The intercellular substance, moreover, appears to have a greater proportion of proteoglycan and/or glycoprotein than mature bone because it is colored blue in H and E sections. It is reported as having a greater calcium content than other types of bone. Bundle bone differs from

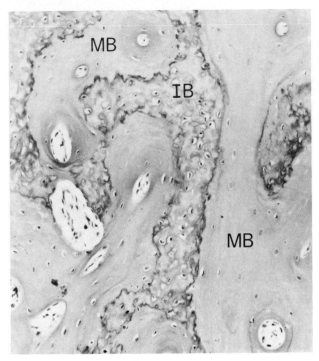

Fig. 15-13. Low-power photomicrograph showing immature bone (IB) and mature bone (MB) in an H and E section of decalcified bone. Regions of immature bone have been surrounded or otherwise encroached upon by mature bone forming later.

woven by having thick bundles of collagen fibers which may lie parallel to each other with osteocytes between them.

Although the matrix of immature bone stains very unevenly it so often demonstrates basophilia that areas of immature bone that have become surrounded by mature bone may be spotted easily on low-power examination (IB in Fig. 15-13). Unless it is appreciated that bits of immature bone can become surrounded by, and hence incorporated into, dense mature bone as seen in Figure 15-13, its presence might be *mistakenly interpreted as being due to some degenerative change* having occurred in mature bone.

Almost all immature bone forming during embryonic life is in due course replaced with mature bone, which will be described next. According to Pritchard, who gives an excellent and comprehensive account of types of bone, some immature bone persists in tooth sockets, near cranial sutures, in the osseous labyrinth, and near tendon and ligament attachments; in these sites, however, it usually is mixed with mature bone. It should be mentioned also that immature bone often appears in postnatal life in the repair of fractures and in rapidly growing tumors of bone that arise from osteogenic cells.

Mature Bone. The formation and growth of *mature* (also called *lamellar*) *bone* is characterized by new layers being added to bony surfaces in an orderly way. Each layer is from 4 to 12 μm. thick. The osteoblasts responsible for producing the successive layers of mature bone become incorporated as osteocytes within or between the layers of bone matrix that they form. In general, the direction of the collagenic fibrils in any given layer is usually at an angle to that of the fibrils in immediately adjacent layers. Sometimes the direction of the fibrils in one layer is at right angles to the direction of those in the next. Since the direction of the fibrils in immediately adjacent layers is not the same, adjacent layers may appear optically different.

Mature bone can be distinguished from immature bone by the way its *matrix stains evenly and lightly* (MB in Fig. 15-13), the regularity of its lamellae, the fact that the direction of fibrils in immediately adjacent lamellae is different, and by its fewer cells, which are more regularly arranged and in flatter lacunae than in immature bone (Fig. 15-13).

DETAILS OF CELLS AND THE INTERCELLULAR SUBSTANCE OF BONE

It would seem logical to follow the description of intramembranous ossification and the growth and structure of a bone that develops in a membranous environment with a description of endochondral ossification and the growth and structure of a bone that develops in a cartilaginous environment. But as we shall see, in order to deal adequately with bones that develop in a cartilaginous environment, it is essential to know more about the cells and intercellular substance of bone than has so far been described, so discussion of endochondral ossification will be postponed until we have dealt with the following.

OSTEOGENIC CELLS

Distribution and Some Terminology. Osteogenic cells lie on bone surfaces as constituents of two membranes, (*1*) as the deepest layer of the *periosteum* (Gr. *peri,* around), the membrane that *covers the outer surface* of any given bone, and (*2*) the *endosteum* (Gr. *endon,* within) that *lines the internal surfaces* of all cavities within bones. The bony walls of bone cavities are said to be lined with endosteum (these cavities would include the marrow cavities, all the haversian canals of compact bone, and all the spaces in cancellous bone). But since some trabeculae of cancellous bone in a given section may appear not to be continuous with one another, and hence may seem not to surround cavities, such trabeculae should be said to be *covered* with endosteum, not *lined* with it.

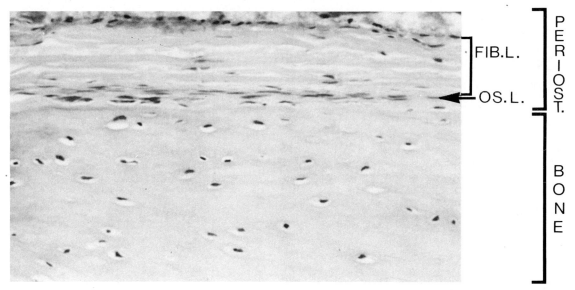

Fig. 15-14. Photomicrograph showing resting periosteum covering a bone (rib of rabbit). The fibrous layer (FIB.L.) is the thicker of the two layers of the periosteum; the osteogenic layer (OS.L.) is not prominent.

Osteogenic cells are also present scattered about within the tissue framework of the marrow that fills the cavities of bones.

The Periosteum. This membrane covers the outer surface of a bone except where it articulates with other bones in joints. It has: (*1*) an outer *fibrous* layer and (*2*) an inner *osteogenic* layer (labeled FIB.L. and OS.L., respectively, in Fig. 15-14). When neither appositional growth nor resorption is occurring it is referred to as *resting periosteum* and its outer layer, which consists of collagenic fibers and a few fibroblasts, is the thicker. There are also some elastic fibers in the periosteum. Murakamin and Emory suggested that these are neither part of the fibrous layer nor produced by the fibroblasts of that layer. Their findings suggested that the elastin is produced by the outermost osteogenic cells of the deep layer; hence it would in a sense constitute a middle (third) layer.

The deep (osteogenic) layer of *resting* periosteum is not prominent. However, close inspection of an external surface of a bone with the LM will show at least the nuclei of thin, pale, flattened, more or less spindle-shaped but otherwise nondescript cells lying on the outer surface of a bone. These are resting osteogenic cells. Their position is indicated in Figure 15-14 by the label OS.L.

Experiments have shown that if periosteum is stripped from a bone at an operation and transplanted to soft tissue, it will not usually form bone in its new location. This is because periosteum, stripped from living bone, consists chiefly of the fibrous layer, because the osteogenic cells

remain tightly attached to the bone surface. However, if periosteum is carefully dissected from a bone so as to remove the deep layer as well as the fibrous layer and then transplanted to soft tissue, it will form some bone in its new location. So the experiments with "stripped" periosteum indicated not that the periosteum was not osteogenic (as was once suggested) but that the fibrous layer is not osteogenic.

The periosteum contains blood vessels, some of which enter and leave bone. The periosteum provides anchorage for these as they leave or enter the soft tissues outside the bone. Smaller blood vessels serve the periosteum itself; in resting periosteum these can be seen occasionally in the fibrous layer. In active periosteum, in which the osteogenic layer becomes thickened, they are also seen amongst the osteogenic cells.

The Importance of Periosteum. As will be described later, the cells of the osteogenic layer of the periosteum account for nearly all the bone formation that occurs in the development and growth of the bones of the body.

The Endosteum. This membrane that lines the spaces in cancellous bone, the marrow cavity, and the haversian canals of compact (dense) bone is composed essentially in resting bone of a continuous layer of inactive osteogenic cells, in which state they appear as rather nondescript flattened cells. But the endosteum of a bone is probably never resting over its entire extent. During the growth of a long bone the marrow cavity is constantly being widened. As a result the otherwise continuous layer of os-

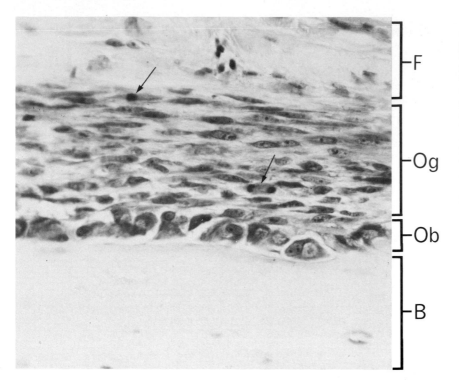

Fig. 15-15. Photomicrograph showing the periosteum shortly after, and close to, a fracture. The fibrous layer (F) has become lifted away from the bone (B) by the greatly thickened osteogenic layer (Og) in which osteogenic cells are proliferating. Mitotic figures are indicated by arrows. At the bone surface osteogenic cells have differentiated into osteoblasts (Ob) which will soon form a new layer of bone on the surface on which they lie. (Ham, A. W., and Harris, W. R.: *In* Bourne, G. H. (ed.): The Biochemistry and Physiology of Bone. ed. 2, vol. 3. New York, Academic Press, 1971)

teogenic cells of the endosteum is often interrupted by osteoclasts, which act to resorb bone matrix from the inside of the wall of a tubular bone to make the marrow cavity wider. Even when growth is over, the demands of the body for calcium may necessitate osteoclastic resorption from the inner surface of a bone. Moreover, if a bone becomes broken the presence of the osteogenic lining cells is manifested by their proliferation and differentiation into new bone to help repair the injury. The osteogenic cells in haversian canals, moreover, serve as a new source of cells to form new haversian systems when old ones are resorbed, as will be described in detail later.

Why Osteogenic Cells in Resting Periosteum Cannot Be Identified by Their Morphology

Distinguishing different kinds of body cells by their morphology, whether with the LM or the EM, depends on their possessing some feature (or features) related to their particular specialized function. But relatively undifferentiated cells have seldom acquired morphological features by which they can be identified with certainty. Hence resting osteogenic cells, as described in periosteum and endosteum, are identified not because they exhibit particular morphological features but by the positions they occupy (Fig. 15-14). That the thin, flattened, nondescript cells on bone surfaces are osteogenic cells is

proven only when they become activated by being subjected to some stimulus that causes their multiplication and differentiation into cell types identifiable as osteoblasts or chondroblasts. To use a perhaps familiar quotation, it is a case of "by their works ye shall know them."

The Morphology of Activated Osteogenic Cells as Seen in Appositional Growth. It is one thing to know there is such a thing as appositional growth (as described in the foregoing) but another for a histologist or histopathologist to be able to recognize in a routine H and E section that appositional growth was occurring in a bone from which a section was obtained. Although appositional growth may be studied histologically in sections of growing bones, more informative histological preparations may be obtained by preparing longitudinal sections of a rabbit's rib that has been fractured and allowed to heal for a few days. Examination of the rib in the regions on either side of the fracture will reveal that active appositional growth is occurring beneath the fibrous layer of the periosteum (this is an early step in the repair of a rib fracture). By examining sites at different distances from the fracture and several fractures in which healing has been allowed to progress for different periods of time, various stages of appositional growth, and also the capacity of osteogenic cells for differentiating into either cartilage or bone cells, can readily be observed.

First, as shown in Figure 15-15, the fibrous layer (F) of

Fig. 15-16. Photomicrograph of a longitudinal section of a rib at a site close to a fracture that has been healing a few days longer than the one seen in Figure 15-15. Osteogenic cells of the periosteum have proliferated and some have differentiated into osteoblasts that have laid down a layer of new bone on the old. Note the fibrous layer (FIB. L.) and osteogenic layer (OS. L.) of the periosteum, and the osteoblasts (OB.) along the inner border of the periosteum. Intercellular substance of bone is labeled I.S., osteocytes in lacunae, O.S. in LAC., and a blood vessel in a canal, B.V. Note also the cementing line (C.L.) between the new and old bone.

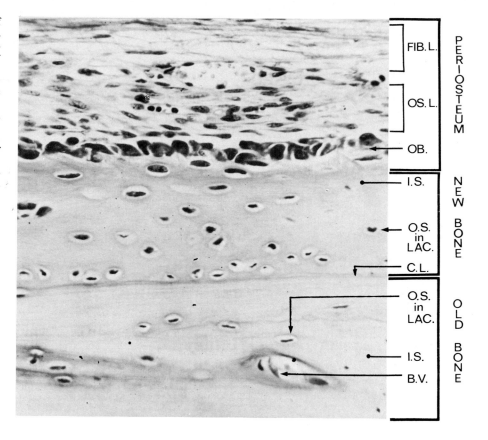

the periosteum becomes lifted away from bone (B) below by extensive proliferation of osteogenic cells taking place in the osteogenic layer (Og) after the bone was broken. The most recently formed osteogenic cells lie closest to the fibrous layer and the oldest ones, which have already differentiated into osteoblasts (Ob), lie against the bone surface, where, had they been left in place a little longer, they would have formed a new layer of bone on that surface. Between them and the fibrous layer of the periosteum, the activated osteogenic cells differ from resting osteogenic cells in being both plumper and longer, though still spindle-shaped. Both nuclei and cytoplasm have become more basophilic, indicating an increase in their content of RNA. Two mitotic figures (arrows) are evidence that much cell division is occurring amongst them. The fine structure of the cytoplasm of the osteogenic cells would differ in relation to the extent of their differentiation into osteoblasts. In general, the basophilia of the cytoplasm of the least differentiated osteogenic cells could be expected to be due chiefly to free ribosomes related to growth. But then as the osteogenic cells differentiate into osteoblasts the basophilia would be due more and more to rER for the synthesis of protein for secretion, as will be described shortly.

We next refer to Figure 15-16, which shows many interesting features of bone in a later stage in the repair process. Here there has been time for many of the osteogenic cells, so numerous at the previous stage, to have differentiated into osteoblasts. The deeper osteoblasts have now become osteocytes after forming new bone (labeled in Fig. 15-16) on the preexisting old bone (also labeled in Fig. 15-16). Between the old and the recently formed new bone a blue line called a *cementing line* (Fig. 15-16, C.L.) or *watermark* is found. This new bone has formed since the periosteum was activated. The layer of osteoblasts (OB.) is ready at this point to form more bone on the new bone already formed. The osteogenic layer of the periosteum (OS.L.) is now thinner than in Figure 15-15 (Og) and the cells of this layer seem to be returning to the inactive type. Unlike what is seen in Figure 15-15, there are transitional cells here between osteoblasts and osteocytes; these are obvious in between the layer of osteoblasts (Fig. 15-16, OB.) and the surface of the new bone. Note that the size of the newly formed osteocytes varies with their age. Those formed first (the deepest) are now smaller than those formed more recently. Note also that the osteocytes are farther apart than the osteoblasts in the layer above them. We shall comment on this later.

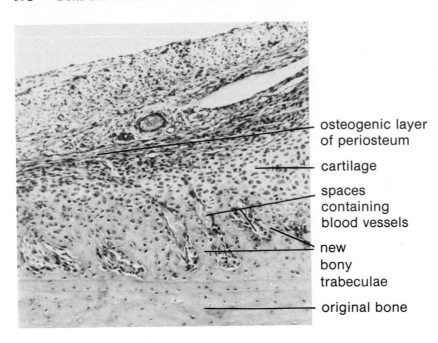

osteogenic layer
of periosteum

cartilage

spaces
containing
blood vessels

new
bony
trabeculae

original bone

Fig. 15-17. Photomicrograph of a longitudinal section of a rabbit's rib close to a fracture (that is to the *right*) after healing for 5 days. The osteogenic cell proliferation shown in Figure 15-15 has continued, and along the bone osteogenic cells have differentiated into osteocytes and formed bony trabeculae cemented to the bone. This area is vascular (*see* blood vessels between trabeculae). Toward the *right* the osteogenic cells have differentiated into chondrocytes, forming a mass of cartilage which has no blood vessels in it. (Ham, A. W., and Harris, W. R.: *In* Bourne, G. H. (ed.): The Biochemistry and Physiology of Bone. ed. 2, vol. 3. New York, Academic Press, 1971)

The Basis for Classifying Osteogenic Cells as Stem Cells

For any cell to be classified as a stem cell requires that the cell should have an extensive capacity for reproducing itself throughout life. Also, the term *stem cell* usually, but not always, implies that the ancestry of more than one kind of cell formed in postnatal life can be traced to it; this means it is a *pluripotential* cell, a potentiality not implied by the terms *precursor* or *progenitor* cell. As will be described later in connection with endochondral ossification, the prenatal formation of both bone and cartilage can be traced to a common pluripotential ancestral cell, and the particular tissue that develops at any given site depends on the ancestral (osteogenic) cells differentiating in different microenvironments. However, to satisfy the requirements for being considered pluripotential stem cells, osteogenic cells should be shown to retain pluripotential capacity and the capacity for extensive proliferation throughout postnatal life. That they do so is also readily demonstrated in the repair of fractures, as follows.

From studies on fracture healing, Ham in 1930 found that whether osteogenic cells of the periosteum differentiated to form bone or cartilage depended on whether differentiation occurred in the presence or absence of capillaries. In other words, close to capillaries they differentiated into osteoblasts but away from capillaries they differentiated into chondrocytes. It is to be noted in Figure 15-17 that close to the rib, where new bony trabeculae are forming, there are spaces between the trabeculae and these spaces contain a blood supply. But at the

right side of the illustration it can be seen that the cartilage that has developed in the reparative tissue (called *callus*) is farther away from the blood supply provided by vessels close to the surface of the original bone. The relative distribution of bone and cartilage would seem to indicate that where osteogenic cells grow more rapidly than capillaries, the osteogenic cells differentiate into chondrocytes. But where the growth of capillaries keeps up with the growth of osteogenic cells, the osteogenic cells differentiate into osteoblasts and osteocytes. Tissue culture experiments by Bassett and Herrmann in 1961 showed that oxygen tension was the determining factor with regard to whether certain cells they were growing in vitro formed bone or cartilage. Since a capillary blood supply would be the important factor in supplying oxygen to rapidly growing and differentiating osteogenic cells in a callus, it would seem that whether new growth of capillaries can keep up with the rapid growth of osteogenic cells so as to provide a good supply of oxygen is the determining factor that affects their differentiation in vivo. There may, of course, be other subsidiary factors involved such as pressure or other physical conditions such as movement of the forming tissue.

The factors involved in the induction of differentiation of stem cells in general seem to be so complicated that it is of interest that at least in the instance of osteogenic cells the cause of induction seems to be relatively simple. Also of practical interest is the fact that conceiving of osteogenic cells as stem cells and understanding the nature of the microenvironment that affects their differentiation enormously facilitate understanding how and why both cartilage and bone are involved in endochondral ossification and the development and growth of long bones.

Secondary Cartilage. In view of the foregoing, and since we have previously described intramembranous ossification, we can now comment on the formation of *"second-ary" cartilage.* This term refers to cartilage that develops in association with certain bones after they have been formed as a result of intramembranous ossification. If it were not for the formation of secondary cartilage, bones forming intramembranously would have no articular cartilage should they be called upon to participate in freely moveable joints—which some must do. Secondary cartilage develops later than the bone with which it is associated, which is the reverse of what happens in endochondral ossification, in which process (to be described presently) cartilage develops first and is only later replaced by bone, except for articular cartilage, which persists from the original cartilage of the cartilaginous model of a bone-to-be.

The secondary cartilage forming the articular cartilages of a bone that develops by intramembranous ossification originates from mesenchymal cells. These occupy a position where a moveable joint will form and thus they are subjected in prenatal life (after the bone has formed) to physical forces such as pressure or other mechanical stress. It would not be surprising if one way in which that pressure acted would be to prevent low-pressure capillaries from growing into the mesenchyme, thus preserving a nonvascular environment in which cartilage would develop from the packed mesenchymal cells present at such sites.

For a detailed consideration of secondary cartilage *see* papers by Hall (listed at the end of Chap. 16).

Demonstration by Radioautography of Osteogenic Cells and the Fate of Their Progeny. One reason for osteogenic cells receiving limited attention for several decades was that it was commonly assumed that osteoblasts themselves could divide and so provide for the growth, maintenance, and repair of bone. It was not until it became possible to study bone formation by radioautography that widespread interest was aroused in what we term the *osteogenic* cell. Beginning in 1960, the formation of bone was studied by this method by several investigators (*see* References on Osteogenic (Osteoprogenitor) Cells. Osteoblasts, and Osteocytes). These studies indicated that label only appeared in osteoblasts after enough time had elapsed for labeled precursor cells to have differentiated into osteoblasts. Label, moreover, only appeared in osteocytes where there had been enough time for osteocytes to have developed from labeled osteoblasts. The general consensus of opinion from radioautographic studies seemed to be that the cell taking up the label, and hence capable of proliferation and differentiation into

osteoblasts, was a special kind of cell that possessed a more limited spectrum of possibilities for differentiation than a true mesenchymal cell, being limited to evolving into cells of the kind ordinarily found in bone. Perhaps because some of the newer generations of investigators using radioautography to demonstrate the existence of this cell were unaware its existence and capabilities had already been appreciated and described several decades before radioautography became available and that it had already been given a name, the *osteogenic cell,* they termed it the *osteoprogenitor* (Gr. *osteon,* bone; L. *progenitor,* parent or ancestor) cell. We think *osteogenic* is the better term because (*1*) this was the name given to the layer of the periosteum that long ago was established as the source of cells responsible for growth and much of the repair of bone; (*2*) it would be awkward to have to describe the osteogenic layer of the periosteum as the osteoprogenitor cell layer; (*3*) since it is thought that osteogenic sarcomas arise from osteogenic cells it would be awkward to have to refer to them as osteoprogenitor cell sarcomas; and finally (*4*) the term *osteogenic cell* has for decades before the advent of radioautography been described as a cell that can differentiate into either bone cells or cartilage cells. As yet the term *osteoprogenitor cell* does not seem to have acquired this latter breadth of meaning.

Ectopic Osteogenesis

The term *ectopic* (Gr. *ektopos,* displaced) refers to ossification occurring somewhere in the body where bone does not belong, that is, in some soft tissue not forming part of the skeleton. In man ectopic bone is not very common. However, in routine autopsies small amounts are occasionally observed in the walls of arteries of older people, in old operation scars, and in kidneys that have been the seat of some long-continued disease process. In itself, ectopic ossification does not constitute a pathological problem of any consequence because it is so rare and probably does no harm when it occurs. Ectopic bone formation, however, is of importance because it has aroused the curiosity of the investigative-minded about the kind of cells in ordinary connective tissue that could produce it, and also about the factors that could induce these cells to form bone in such strange places. Furthermore, in the minds of those investigating the problem would be the thought that if all the factors involved in ectopic bone formation could be ascertained, it might be possible to apply this knowledge to facilitate the healing of bones in situations where the normal supply of osteogenic cells is deficient or where their response to bone injuries has not been adequate to achieve proper repair.

Development of Knowledge. Experimental attempts directed toward producing ectopic bone were frustrating for a long time. For example, it would seem logical to try transplanting dead calcified bone into various soft tissues to see if it could induce ectopic bone formation beside it. Various claims were made about the success of following this procedure but the end result was that dead bone, transplanted to muscle or into ordinary connective tissue, only occasionally induced ectopic ossification beside it and then only after a relatively long period of time. Attempts to produce ossification by injecting calcium salts into tissue likewise did not prove to be very successful. In effect, the presence of calcified material did not seem to be the answer to how to incite ectopic bone formation. However, one experimental finding aroused a great deal of interest several decades ago: Huggins showed that transplanting the mucous membrane lining the urinary bladder to the abdominal wall of animals would induce ectopic ossification at its new site. This method (and modifications of it) has since been used to induce bone formation in more elaborate experiments, and it showed that there could be such a thing as a factor that induced osteogenesis in ordinary connective tissue. But the next and most interesting finding about induction of ectopic osteogenesis came from the work of Urist and his associates when they showed that transplanting bone fragments *that had been decalcified,* fast-frozen, and dehydrated, into ordinary connective tissue, would in the majority of instances induce ectopic osteogenesis. Reddi and his coworkers have also investigated ectopic bone formation. They used demineralized powders (of a certain particle size) made from dehydrated shafts of bones and showed that these induced bone formation.

There are many aspects of bone induction to intrigue those interested in how microenvironment can affect the differentiation of competent cells. Superficially, it might be thought that if bone or dentin would induce bone formation, it would be because of their mineral content. But as noted, if calcified bone intercellular substance is transplanted, the inductive effect seldom occurs, whereas transplanted demineralized matrix of bone or dentin commonly exerts the inductive effect. Next, it seems that the collagen of dense ordinary connective tissue from tendon or skin is ineffective in this respect. So at least at first, it was concluded that it was the unmasked collagen of bone or dentin that was responsible for bone induction, and this view is still entertained. However, Urist and his associates (*see* References) have described evidence indicating that a noncollagenous protein in bone or dentin matrix is responsible for the inductive effect. They have termed this component *BMP* for *bone morphogenic protein.* They believe that BMP is a small polypeptide that exists as a component of bone matrix; they have moreover shown that BMP can be produced by neoplastic osteogenic cells (*see* References under Urist).

We shall now consider what kind of cell found in soft tissues possesses the potentiality to respond to the inductive effect of the bone-inducing substances.

The Origin of the Osteogenic Cells. The concept of some type of cell in ordinary connective tissue (including the endomysium of muscle) retaining considerable mesenchymal potentiality is by no means new. It should be clearly understood that the concept of there being some particular kind of cell in connective tissue that retains *mesenchymal potentiality* is a very different concept from that of conceiving of fibroblasts, macrophages, or any of the other types of *specialized* connective tissue cells being able to *transform* into a variety of other cell types. As already noted in Chapter 9, the one cell type found in ordinary connective tissue that has attracted most attention as being the most likely candidate for being relatively undifferentiated, and hence possessing mesenchymal potentiality, is the type originally termed *adventitial cells* by Marchand, probably because this word can be used with reference to something that is "added to from outside," and the cells he described were seen along the side of capillaries. Subsequently this cell became known as a *perivascular cell* or *pericyte.* It is described in more detail on page 228. It is found along the sides of the smaller arterioles and venules as well as beside capillaries.

Urist and his associates, in their studies on osteogenesis in response to implanted decalcified bone matrix, observed that osteoblasts appeared after the ingrowth of new small blood vessels. They consider (we believe with good reason) that the cells growing in with the capillaries were cells with sufficient mesenchymal potentiality to account for the osteogenesis observed. Although they referred to these cells as mesenchymal cells, they could have been pericytes. Finally, it is of interest that cartilage sometimes develops along with bone in ectopic osteogenesis, which could be expected because any cells that could form bone would have to pass through an osteogenic cell stage, from which they could differentiate into either cartilage or bone.

Büring, in an interesting study in 1975 utilizing parabiosis, radiation, and tritiated thymidine labeling, concluded that whereas blood-derived cells might be involved in releasing the inductive factor from transplanted decalcified lyophilized transplants of bone matrix, the cells that developed and were responsible for bone formation were derived from the host—in particular, they were progeny of their perivascular mesenchymal cells. We would term such cells pericytes on the understanding that pericytes possess a good deal of mesenchymal potentiality.

It is also of interest that ectopic bone formation is followed by hematopoiesis in the stroma of any cavity forming in the ectopic bone. As described in Chapter 12, it was once believed that blood cells and bone were produced locally from a common ancestral cell. The fact that hematopoiesis follows ossification is now explained by circulating CFUs settling out and differentiating into blood cells, probably because osteogenic cells provide the proper microenvironment in the bony cavity that has formed.

OSTEOBLASTS

Functions. Osteoblasts do not divide. Their primary function is to synthesize and secrete the organic matrix of bone and to do this around their processes so as to cause the formation of canaliculi. A subsidiary function of osteoblasts may be to participate in the process by which the matrix becomes calcified, as will be described shortly.

Morphology Seen in H and E Sections

Osteoblasts (Ob in Fig. 15-15) are relatively large and either more or less rounded to polygonal, or roughly columnar in shape. Their single nuclei are commonly eccentrically situated in the part of the cell farthest away from a bone surface. The cytoplasm is deeply basophilic except where, as is shown in the osteoblast at the right hand end of the row Ob in Figure 15-15, it reveals a pale area due to a well-developed negative Golgi image. Several such images are also obvious in the numerous osteoblasts in Figure 5-28 (p. 130) where the reason for this "negative" appearance is explained. The cytoplasmic processes of osteoblasts are not seen in H and E sections, but from other types of preparations it is believed (as already noted) that those of adjacent cells on a surface are in contact with one another and also with the processes of the osteocytes in lacunae immediately below the surface. Hence when rows or groups of osteoblasts finish forming intercellular substance about themselves and become osteocytes, their processes remain in contact not only with the surface but also with one another and with the processes of the deeper osteocytes.

Osteoblasts in H and E sections resemble plasma cells (Fig. 9-19); this is because both types of cells synthesize much protein, which requires extensive cytoplasm containing much rER and a well-developed Golgi. Hence, at the level of the LM the position of osteoblasts on bone surfaces is helpful in distinguishing them from plasma cells. However, their fine structure differs from that of plasma cells.

The Fine Structure of Osteoblasts and Its Relation to Their Function

The osteoblast has the fine structure of a secretory cell. The chief product it secretes is procollagen but it also secretes the amorphous components of bone matrix and

some enzymes. As might be expected of a secretory cell, it contains an abundance of rER (Fig. 15-18). However, the organelles of the cytoplasm of an osteoblast (Fig. 15-18) are not arranged in such a polarized a manner as those of an epithelial gland cell (Fig. 5-21), which secretes only through its apex. In the latter type of cell the rER is mostly near the base of the cell and the Golgi is located above the nucleus. The secretory vesicles budding from it travel to the apical region where their contents are secreted by exocytosis. However, in an osteoblast the rER is very widely distributed in a somewhat disorderly way (Fig. 15-18). The Golgi lies near the side of the nucleus facing the bulk of the cytoplasm. Although it does not generally appear as a parallel array of wide flattened saccules, short sections of saccules cut longitudinally may be seen. Three orders of secretory vesicles containing procollagen are shown in Figure 15-19. The saccules first formed (SS in Fig. 15-19) contain filaments of procollagen in random array. Next, cylindrical saccules (CS) contain slender filaments disposed longitudinally elong the long axis of the saccule. Finally, elongated saccules (secretory granules) labeled Sg and containing procollagen are shown at *upper left* in Figure 15-19. Their contents are delivered to the surface where the procollagen becomes organized into collagenic fibrils as occurs in association with fibroblasts (described on p. 233). Collagenic fibrils formed as a result of the secretion of osteoblasts are seen in the region labeled o in the middle of Figure 15-20.

A possible reason for the organelles of osteoblasts not being arranged in as orderly a way as in an epithelial gland cell that secretes through its apex could be that an osteoblast has to be able to secrete through almost any part of its surface. The first osteoblasts forming from mesenchymal cells in intramembranous ossification have no preexisting bone surface on which to secrete matrix, so they have to somehow surround themselves with it (Fig. 15-5) to become osteocytes, suggesting they secrete all around their circumference. Then in the appositional growth of bone where there is a bone surface on which to secrete, they subsequently become buried in the matrix they secrete which would again seem to require secreting over their whole surface. It is to be noted in Figure 15-16 that the osteocytes into which osteoblasts differentiate, and which are seen just below the layer of osteoblasts, are much more widely separated from each other than the osteoblasts in the row above them because matrix has been secreted between them. Odontoblasts (dentin-forming cells of teeth) are rather similar in function to osteoblasts but differ from them in being polarized so as to secrete through one of their ends. For this reason they lend themselves to the study of the formation and secretion of matrix and its subsequent calcification to much better advantage than osteoblasts, as will be apparent in Chapter 21.

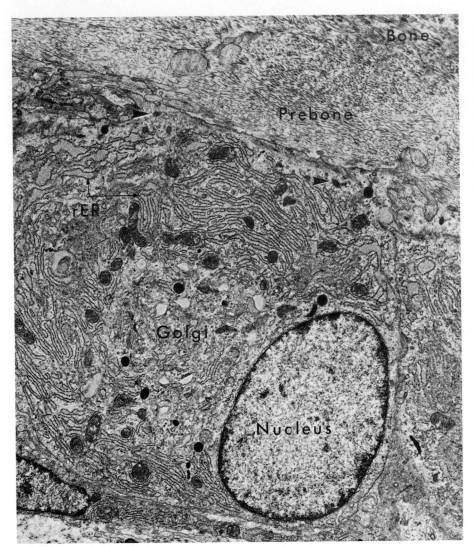

Fig. 15-18. Electron micrograph (×9,000) of an osteoblast (from decalcified rat bone). Note the numerous collagen fibers in the bone (*top right*) and prebone beneath it, bordering on the cell. These are formed from procollagen secreted by the cell. The procollagen is carried in secretory vesicles (indicated by arrows close to upper border of cell) originating from the Golgi saccules (*see also* Fig. 15-19) and is released by fusion of these vesicles with the cell membrane. (Courtesy of M. Weinstock)

Filaments in the Cell Bodies and Processes of Osteoblasts. It was observed some time ago (Cameron) that the peripheral cytoplasm in osteoblasts commonly contained few organelles but did possess bundles of very fine filaments (now termed *microfilaments*). Then Hancox and Boothroy noted that the filaments extended into the processes of osteoblasts. Recently King and Holtrop showed that microfilaments were 5 to 7 nm. wide and very numerous in the processes (p in Fig. 15-20) and, furthermore, they are actin-like because they bind heavy meromyosin. Possible functions of the microfilaments of osteoblasts will be considered in due course.

Having dealt with the osteoblasts that secrete the components of bone matrix, we can now deal with the matrix and its subsequent calcification.

THE ORGANIC INTERCELLULAR SUBSTANCE OF BONE (BONE MATRIX)

Comparison With Cartilage. The chief differences between the matrix of bone and the matrix of cartilage are related to their respective functions. The matrix of cartilage has to serve as a means for diffusion of nutrients over long distances, which requires a substantial amorphous component. Furthermore, it is not called upon to provide great tensile strength as in bone, so it does not have to possess as great a content of collagenic fibrils as bone. Since bone has canaliculi it does not have to depend on diffusion through its intercellular substance to keep its cells alive. It might therefore be thought bone matrix would not require any amorphous organic component;

Fig. 15-19. Electron micrograph of the Golgi region of an osteoblast (×30,000), showing spherical saccules (SS) containing fine filaments in random array, cylindrical saccules (CS) containing slender filaments aligned parallel with the long axis of the saccule, and elongated secretory granules (Sg). Cisternae of rough-surfaced endoplasmic reticulum (rER) are also present in close proximity to the Golgi region. (Leblond, C. P., and Weinstock, M.: *In* Bourne, G. H. (ed.): The Biochemistry and Physiology of Bone, ed. 2, vol. 4. New York, Academic Press, 1976)

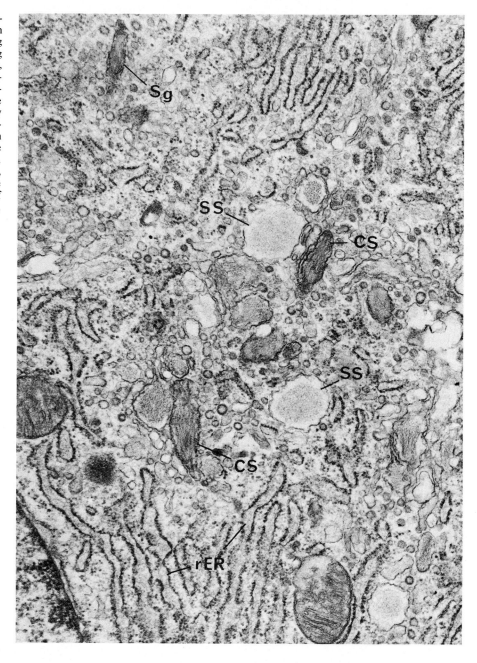

however, there is *some* amorphous organic content in the matrix of adult bone. Although in adult bone the matrix stains pink to red because of its great collagen content, it is also to some extent PAS-positive, which indicates the presence of some glycoprotein. It has also been shown to take up radioactive sulfur while forming, which indicates some content of sulfated glycosaminoglycan. Further-

more, chemical analysis of mature bone indicates the presence of some noncollagenous protein, some of which could be accounted for by the presence of glycoprotein and proteoglycan. Forming bone matrix also has been shown to take up albumin from tissue fluid (Owen and Triffit, and Owen et al.). This is not secreted by osteoblasts but derived from the blood via tissue fluid. Like-

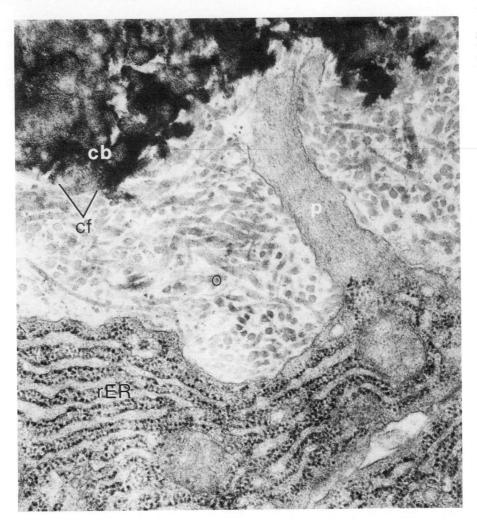

Fig. 15-20. Electron micrograph (×36,000) of one edge of an osteoblast. Between it and the dark-staining calcified bone matrix (cb) above lies a wide zone of osteoid tissue (prebone), labeled o, that contains an abundance of newly formed collagenic fibrils. The boundary between the uncalcified osteoid tissue (pale) and the calcified bone (electron-dense) is the calcification front, labeled cf. Note the abundant rER in the osteoblast. At *right* a cytoplasmic process (p) extends into the matrix where it would enter a canaliculus; note that it is packed with microfilaments. (Courtesy of M. Holtrop)

wise, it is believed that some glycoprotein incorporated in bone matrix may be derived from blood. In order to discuss the possible roles of any of these amorphous components of bone matrix we might first consider whether their functions are served (*1*) in mature bone or (*2*) as bone becomes calcified. To go into this problem we first have to deal with the difference between *ossification* and *calcification.*

Ossification and Calcification

The term *ossification* is used surprisingly often in the literature as if it were a synonym for *calcification,* thus causing confusion. Calcification often occurs in degenerating soft tissues; this, however, is not ossification. Since bone is normally calcified, ossification can be defined as a process which includes both the secretion of

the organic matrix of bone by specific cells and its subsequent calcification. However, the term *ossification* can also be used to denote only the processes involved in the formation of bone-forming cells and their subsequent elaboration of organic matrix. In other words, it is possible to have calcification without ossification and ossification without calcification. The product in the latter case is called *osteoid* (bone-like) *tissue* or *prebone.* Ossification without calcification can occur, for example, if the concentration of calcium and/or phosphate ions in the bloodstream is sufficiently reduced by dietary procedures so there are too few of these ions to form a precipitate of $Ca_3(PO_4)_2$ in sites where calcification would normally occur, as in newly forming bone. Under these conditions osteogenesis occurs but results in the formation of only uncalcified bone matrix (osteoid tissue). This occurs in the dietary deficiency diseases called *rickets* in young children and *osteomalacia* in adults (both conditions will be described later). It is of interest to medical and dental students that osteoid tissue cannot be counted on to show up in x-rays, for x-rays outline bone only if it is calcified or at least has taken up enough mineral to be detected by x-rays. X-rays, for example, do not reveal whether or not a fracture is healing unless the reparative tissue (called a *callus*) is becoming calcified as it is formed. For example, Ham et al. showed that if fractures produced in rats were allowed to heal for several weeks under conditions of dietary deficiency of the kind that produces rickets, x-rays showed little if any evidence of callus. However, histological studies showed that a healing callus was present, but it consisted of osteoid tissue and cartilage. Restoring a normal diet to such animals resulted in the calluses already formed becoming apparent on x-ray in four days because of the preexisting osteoid tissue of the callus absorbing calcium salts.

Calcification Fronts. The formation of osteoid tissue (prebone) is a normal event in all bone formation, just as the formation of predentin is a normal event in connection with the formation of calcified dentin in developing teeth (to be described on p. 654). The first step in osteogenesis is for osteoblasts to secrete the organic component of matrix. In a micrograph this appears as collagenic fibrils separated from one another fairly widely by a pale amorphous material (*middle* of Fig. 15-20). The layer of this matrix closest to the osteoblast normally remains uncalcified, or only slightly calcified, at least for some time. In other words, newly formed bone matrix first exists as *osteoid tissue* (labeled o in Fig. 15-20). Farther away from the osteoblast the osteoid tissue (prebone) begins to become calcified and the site at which this occurs is termed a *calcification front* (cf in Fig. 15-20). We shall now comment on how calcification is thought to occur here.

The Calcification of Bone

The aspects of the process that begins at a calcification front and results in the organic matrix of bone just formed by osteoblasts becoming thoroughly impregnated with calcium salts are not yet all thoroughly understood. The problem, however, has attracted a great deal of investigation and much has been learned about it. We shall endeavor to give a simple account of the present status of the problem and its background, but in the reverse order, so that we start with the deposition of calcium salts and then go on to consider possible mechanisms.

Background. Calcification in forming bone requires that calcium salts be laid down in the newly formed matrix. These salts must be obtained from the tissue fluid in which the newly formed organic matrix is bathed and the

mineral salts in tissue fluid are in turn derived from circulating blood. Whereas it is known that the eventual deposit of mineral in bone is crystalline in form, with the crystals being very similar to those of hydroxyapatite, $Ca_{10}(PO_4)_6(OH)_2$, it is now believed the first deposit of mineral is amorphous $Ca_3(PO_4)_2$. Hence, while the study of crystalline structure of mineral in bone is of importance for several reasons, the problem of crystal formation is not the same as that of calcification if calcium is first deposited in matrix in the form of amorphous $Ca_3(PO_4)_2$. How crystals form from the latter is a different problem from why the calcium salts just mentioned are deposited in newly formed bone matrix.

Since the mineral of bone must come to it from blood via tissue fluid, we must begin by considering how calcium and phosphate are carried in blood. The greater part of the calcium in blood is bound to protein and does not directly combine with phosphate ions. The remainder of the calcium in blood is, however, ionized or can combine with phosphate ions. Since $Ca_3(PO_4)_2$ is not very soluble, it follows that regulatory mechanisms must operate in the body to prevent an increase in the product of calcium and phosphate ions (generally referred to as the *Ca × P product*) sufficient to precipitate $Ca_3(PO_4)_2$ in the blood, because this would cause trouble. However, under certain circumstances, for example, after administrating a huge dose of vitamin D or a great deal of parathyroid hormone, both of which procedures cause an increase in the plasma level of calcium in experimental animals, there is such an increase in the Ca × P product that calcium salts precipitate into soft tissue, in particular the proximal part of the aorta, the heart, and the kidneys. On the other hand other conditions, for example, a lack of vitamin D or calcium in the diet, may lower the concentration of Ca ions in the blood so much that the Ca × P product is insufficient to permit normal calcification to occur in growing bones.

Since too great a product of Ca × P ions causes calcification to occur in sites other than bone, whereas an insufficient Ca × P product does not permit normal calcification of growing bones, it would seem that under normal conditions (*1*) there would have to be some mechanism operating in calcifying bone to increase the local concentration of Ca × P product in the tissue fluid, so that $Ca_3(PO_4)_2$ would precipitate locally, or (*2*) newly formed matrix would possess some special physical or chemical quality causing it to take up calcium phosphate selectively from a solution in which calcium and phosphate ordinarily stay in solution. Hypotheses were advanced with regard to both possibilities as follows.

A Theory That Could Explain a Local Concentration in the Ca × P Product. First, a very plausible theory with regard to a mechanism that would cause local increase in the Ca

× P product in newly formed matrix was advanced in the early 1930's by Robison and his coworkers. It was based on the finding that osteoblasts secrete the enzyme alkaline phosphatase, which could act locally on substrates such as hexosephosphates or glycerophosphates to set free more phosphate ions sufficient to raise the Ca × P product to the point where calcium phosphate would precipitate the adjacent newly formed matrix. Even though there is a striking association between the production of alkaline phosphatase and sites of calcification (for example, when a bone is broken and osteogenic cells multiply and form large numbers of osteoblasts to repair the injury, the alkaline phosphatase content of blood becomes increased), there were enough flaws in the theory for it to have become generally discarded. Nevertheless, for some of us a suspicion lingered that this theory was somehow of significance—a suspicion that recently seems to have been justified, as will soon be explained.

Theories as to How the Organic Matrix Could Attract a Mineral Deposit.

With regard to a possible mechanism whereby newly formed matrix could possess some physical or chemical activity that would remove calcium and/or phosphate ions from tissue fluid, even without a local increase in the level of the Ca × P product, two theories have received much consideration.

The first of these theories would seem to be based primarily on the fact that the apatite crystals of mineral that form in bone matrix are very closely associated with bone collagen. It is very difficult to investigate crystals in mature bone with the EM because it requires cutting ultrathin sections of very dense material. The crystals have been variously described as being rod-like or tubular, from 15 to 150 nm. long and from 2 to 8 nm. wide. When tubular, their widths are said to relate to their lengths. They have been described as being diposed within collagenic fibrils and/or lying along their surfaces. It has been suggested that if they are inside fibrils, they occupy the holes—the gap regions between the ends of molecules arranged in fibrils (Fig. 9-11, p. 234). If they lie along fibrils their position is thought to bear some relation to the cross banding of the fibrils. There has been much interest in the association of crystals with collagen because of the concept that collagen initiates the deposition of mineral or crystal formation. However, as already mentioned, the formation of crystals is probably not the first step in calcification, for it is now generally conceded that mineral is first deposited as amorphous calcium phosphate and that the apatite crystals subsequently evolve from the amorphous form. Moreover, since the collagen of bone is the same type of collagen as that in the soft tissues, it might be thought that if the ability of collagen to initiate calcification were so important, collagen elsewhere would also initiate calcification or crystal formation. Furthermore, when calcification occurs in cartilage matrix, in

which collagen fibrils are not as abundant as in bone (as will be described later), the process of calcification does not appear to begin in association with collagen but instead with the amorphous component of the matrix with which we deal next.

Possible Relation of the Amorphous Component of Matrix to Calcification.

It has been shown by chemical analysis (*see* Herring) that osteoid tissue (prebone; Figs. 15-18 and 15-20) contains many times more *noncollagenous protein* and about twice as much glycosaminoglycan as calcified bone. This suggests that much of the organic amorphous component of bone matrix is in the form of proteoglycans and glycoproteins that may serve to help initiate or further the calcification process, after which much of this amorphous component is lost. In this connection it must be taken into account that on becoming calcified the organic intercellular substance of bone must somehow absorb a great amount of mineral, and unless it did so without swelling greatly in size, it would require that something previously in the organic matrix be displaced. Most of this would be water (as tissue fluid) held in place by the proteoglycans and the glycoproteins, some of which might themselves be lost along with the fluid with which they were associated.

In the foregoing we have dealt with concepts more or less based on the belief that concentrations of Ca^{2+} and PO_4^{2-} ions in tissue fluid were such that it would require either (*1*) some special mechanism to raise the concentration of one or the other type of ion in the matrix or (*2*) some special affinity of bone collagen or bone amorphous intercellular substance for them to bring about calcification of newly formed bone matrix. However, Termine and Eanes, by mixing modified tissue culture solutions, each of which contained physiological concentrations of salts, in such a way as to achieve a range of Ca × P products, found that at physiological concentrations of these two ions calcium phosphate would precipitate. In the light of these findings the problem of determining why calcification occurs in the newly formed organic matrix of bone did not seem as formidable as before. However, these findings presented a further problem—that of determining why the intercellular substances of ordinary connective tissue do not also become calcified.

Calcification Inhibitors.

The reason for calcification not occurring more commonly in the intercellular substances of ordinary connective tissue is now believed to be the presence in such tissue of *calcification inhibitors* that act normally to prevent calcium deposits from forming in soft tissues. Perhaps the most potent inhibitors are those constituting a family of inorganic compounds comprising the pyrophosphates, phosphonates, and diphosphonates. The last mentioned are particularly effective and are undergoing clinical trials to see if they will stop pathological calcification from occurring.

The finding of a category of calcification inhibitors immediately influenced thinking about normal calcification in bone, raising the question whether local removal or inactivation of inhibitors could be a factor in its occurrence. And indeed it now seems from a recent further finding that a concurrent situation occurs at calcification fronts in which there is both a factor operating to cause a local increase in the concentration of PO_4^{2-} ions and also an enzyme that destroys inorganic pyrophosphate, an inhibitor of calcification. To explain this in more detail requires that we describe matrix vesicles.

Matrix Vesicles and Calcification. Matrix vesicles are minute, more or less rounded structures that range from 30 nm. to 1 μm. in size and that have been seen in the matrix of cartilage and osteoid tissue and at other sites underoing calcification. They were identified in cartilage matrix in 1967 by Anderson and subsequently he and others provided substantial evidence that they play a role in initiating calcification. (For relevant details, *see* References and Other Reading).

Matrix vesicles are each surrounded with a membrane identical with the cell membrane (Fig. 15-21). Three possible origins have been suggested: that they are (*1*) structures that bud off from the plasmalemma of chondrocytes or osteoblasts; (*2*) a kind of lysosome extruded by chondrocytes or osteoblasts; or (*3*) structures derived from mitochondria that have accumulated calcium (a function mitochondria are known to possess) and subsequently been extruded from the cell in the form of tiny bodies. The most probable view at the moment is that they are special structures that bud off from the cell membrane of chondroblasts or osteoblasts. Studies also show that they bud off from odontoblasts to initiate the mineralization of dentin. Matrix vesicles are known to contain lipid and accumulate calcium. They also exhibit certain enzyme activities. Of particular interest is that they have a relatively high alkaline phosphatase activity. They would seem able to serve several roles in initiating calcification. First, they accumulate calcium. Second, their phosphatase acts to bring about enzymatic hydrolysis of ester phosphate to yield orthophosphate, which could react with the calcium provided by the vesicles so as to bring about a precipitation. This, of course, would provide a mechanism by which a local increase in the Ca × P product could bring about precipitation with the local increase in free phosphate ions becoming available in the way proposed long ago by Robison, previously described. But in addition they provide pyrophosphatase, an enzyme that destroys inorganic pyrophosphate, which would otherwise act as an inhibitor of calcification. Hence because matrix vesicles are found where calcification occurs, and since they have several actions that would promote the process, it seems they could provide the marginal factor needed to set off and maintain the process by which calcification oc-

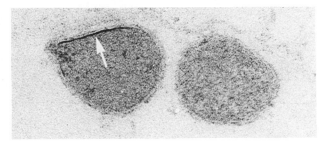

Fig. 15-21. Electron micrograph (×117,000) of two matrix vesicles at high magnification. The one at *left* contains a needle-like electron-dense mineral deposit (indicated by arrow) closely associated with the inner aspect of its membrane that has caused it to flatten. (Anderson, H. C.: *In* Bourne, G. H. (ed.): The Biochemistry and Physiology of Bone. ed. 2, vol. 4. New York, Academic Press, 1976)

curs at calcification fronts in forming bone and also in cartilage, as will be described shortly in connection with the development and longitudinal growth of bones.

OSTEOCYTES

In ordinary H and E sections of decalcified bone the cytoplasm of osteocytes is not seen to advantage. It is not nearly as extensive or basophilic as that of osteoblasts on bone surfaces (Fig. 15-16). The lacunae in which osteocytes come to be housed near the surface of bone shortly after they have formed are relatively rounded, but older ones are generally ovoid, as are the osteocytes they contain (Fig. 15-16).

Fine Structure. In lacunae in undecalcified sections osteocytes are seen with the EM to be generally separated from the calcified matrix that surrounds them by a layer of osteoid tissue (o in Fig. 15-22). The line of demarcation (b) between the plasmalemma of the osteocyte and the layer of osteoid (o) is not always easy to distinguish. In Figure 15-22 the layer of osteoid is about as wide as the layer of cytoplasm seen between the plasmalemma and the nucleus. The collagenic fibrils of the osteoid show characteristic cross banding where cut longitudinally and in general are randomly arranged. In some osteocytes, however, the cytoplasm approaches the calcified matrix closely (as in Fig. 15-23).

It is to be appreciated that only occasionally, in the ultrathin sections used in the EM, would a section "catch" a process leading off from the osteocyte into a canaliculus and furthermore the chances against following it for any distance in any given section would be slim. A process leaving an osteocyte can be seen in Figure 15-23.

Holtrop and Weinger, however, obtained sections in

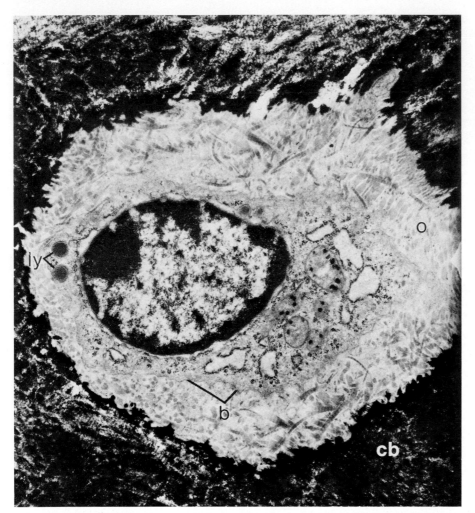

Fig. 15-22. Electron micrograph (×25,000) of an osteocyte in its lacuna. The wall of the lacuna consists of uncalcified osteoid tissue (prebone), labeled o, containing abundant collagenic fibrils; peripheral to this is calcified bone (cb). The border (b) between the osteocyte and the osteoid tissue is not easy to discern. Two dense bodies representing lysosomes (ly) are seen at *center left.* (Holtrop, M. E., and Weinger, J. M.: Ultrastructural evidence for a transport system in bone. Proc. 4th Parathyroid Conference. Amsterdam, Excerpta Medica, 1971)

which osteocyte processes in their canaliculi could be followed for considerable distances. These disclosed that the processes of adjacent osteocytes were in contact with one another over an extensive area by means of side-by-side junctions, probably of the gap type (Fig. 15-24). Since electrolytes or even small molecules could pass from one osteocyte to another by this means, the possibility of an intracellular transport mechanism between osteocytes and bone surfaces where there are capillaries has been suggested by Holtrop and Weinger. Other possible transport mechanisms will be considered shortly.

The cell bodies of osteocytes also were observed to contain filaments of the type seen in the processes, but only in the region close to the plasmalemma. Microtubules are found in the cell bodies of osteocytes but not in their processes. The extent to which other organelles are found in osteocytes varies in relation to their age. Those of young osteocytes are much like those of os-

teoblasts, but as osteocytes become mature their content of rER and Golgi components, which of course are concerned with the synthesis and secretion of matrix components, becomes greatly reduced. Various bodies such as the two dense bodies seen in Figure 15-22, believed to be of the general nature of lysosomes or their end-products, have been described particularly in older osteocytes; the possible significance of these will be described in a following section.

Possible Mechanisms by Which Nutrients Are Supplied to Osteocytes and Waste Products Removed From Them

As already emphasized, the fact that osteocytes are no more than 0.1 to 0.2 mm. from a capillary that could serve as a source of nutrients for osteocytes adjacent to it suggests that the canalicular mechanism by which the os-

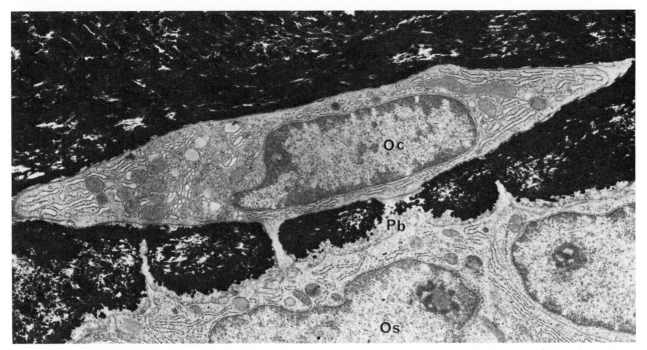

Fig. 15-23. Electron micrograph of a young and relatively flat osteocyte (Oc) in its lacuna in calcified bone. Below it are osteoblasts (Os). A process from the osteocyte connects with an osteoblast in the plane of section. Parts of processes of osteoblasts are also seen. Some osteoid tissue (prebone), labeled Pb, is present between the osteoblasts and the calcified bone but very little of it can be discerned between the osteocyte and the wall of its lacuna. (Courtesy of M. Weinstock)

teocytes are nourished and rid themselves of waste products has a very limited capacity for transporting nutrients and waste products. There are three possible ways it could function but these are not mutually exclusive.

First, the fact that the cytoplasmic processes of osteocytes are connected to one another by gap junctions, as shown by Holtrop, and that these are of a side-to-side type enabling them to connect one process to another over substantial areas, raises the possibility of there being direct passage of certain ions and small molecules from the cytoplasm of one osteocyte to that of the next; such components would have derived originally from the capillary that serves units of osteocytes as, for example, in a haversian system.

Second, it is generally agreed that tissue fluid must be present between the cell bodies of osteocytes and the walls of the lacunae they inhabit and also between the processes of osteocytes and their surrounding canaliculi. Osteocytes are a type of connective tissue cell, and connective tissue cells of all kinds must be bathed in tissue fluid. The only question here is how much tissue fluid lies around them and whether only a little of it is free while most is contained by the amorphous component of osteoid tissue so often seen between osteocytes and cal-

cified matrix, as for example in Figure 15-22. However, the fact that tissue fluid exists in lacunae and canaliculi, either free or in osteoid tissue, indicates the possibility of diffusion via this tissue fluid between osteocytes and the capillaries in the canals of haversian systems of dense bone or spaces of cancellous bone.

A third possible mechanism should be mentioned by which tissue fluid could provide nutrients to osteocytes and this is that there could be a circulation of tissue fluid in a lacunar-canalicular system. Doty and Schofield showed that if horseradish peroxidase (the molecules of which are small enough for some to escape through capillary walls into tissue fluid) is injected intravenously into rats, it can be detected in the lacunae and canaliculi of rat bones within 30 minutes. Since this marker makes its appearance between osteocytes and the walls of their lacunae and canaliculi, the marker must be in the tissue fluid. The question therefore arises whether the marker molecules reach this position so quickly because of (*1*) *circulation* of tissue fluid or (*2*) *diffusion* through tissue fluid that is free and at rest or bound and at rest in osteoid tissue.

As was explained in Chapter 8 (p. 219), for tissue fluid to circulate it must be formed at one site and reabsorbed

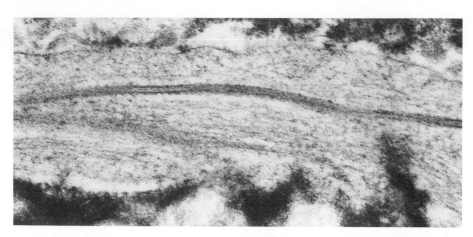

Fig. 15-24. Electron micrograph (×135,00) of a cell junction between two osteocytic processes that overlap each other within a canaliculus. Dark-staining bone may be seen at *top* and *bottom*, bordering on the canaliculus. Note the abundant microfilaments in the two gray-staining processes extending across the middle of the micrograph, one above the other. The side-by-side contact of the two cell membranes (each of which can be discerned *left of center* and at extreme *right*) along the junction provides an extensive area of contact between the adjacent osteocytes. In all probability, this represents a gap junction. (Holtrop, M. E.: The ultrastructure of bone. Ann. Clin. Lab. Sci., 5:264, 1975)

at another, which requires that the hydrostatic pressure in a capillary be higher at the point where the tissue fluid is formed than at the site where it is absorbed back into capillaries. Furthermore, the protein content of blood must have become more concentrated at the site where tissue fluid is resorbed because of fluid loss along the course of the capillary. This increased concentration of protein (colloid) molecules exerts enough osmotic pressure to draw tissue fluid back into the capillary at sites where hydrostatic pressure has diminished. Could such an arrangement exist in bone?

Experiments in which circulation of tissue fluid in the lacunar-canalicular system is thought to have occurred have been performed on small animals. Here, where bones are not well developed and in general are of the cancellous type, it could be reasoned that, as was explained in Chapter 12 (Myeloid Tissue) on page 309, because of the outflow of blood from a bone being somewhat restricted, the hydrostatic pressure in the marrow cavities (into which blood is delivered by arteries) could be higher than outside the bone. It could be reasoned further that tissue fluid formed in or close to the marrow cavity would tend to pass outwardly through such passageways that exist, to reach the exterior of the bone. But in cancellous bones there would be exit routes through soft tissue that would be easier for tissue fluid to follow than routes through bone trabeculae. However, because of the possibility of a hydrostatic pressure gradient between the interior and exterior of a bone, it is possible there could

be slight circulation of tissue fluid through the lacunar-canalicular systems of the developing shafts of a bone in young small animals where bone is as yet of the cancellous type (Fig. 15-25A).

When we consider, however, the compact bone that makes up the shafts of bones of larger animals and man (Fig. 15-25B), where the marrow cavity is separated from the bone exterior by a vast number of haversian systems solidly packed together (as will be described in detail shortly) with the osteocytes of each haversian system being nourished from capillaries in the central canal of each system, there would seem to be no way of explaining how hydrostatic pressure could be high or low enough in any site to bring about formation and absorption of tissue fluid and hence account for circulation of tissue fluid through a haversian system. Thus there would seem to be no way to explain how tissue fluid formed along haversian canals could be driven by hydrostatic pressure to the exterior of a given haversian system and then drawn back through a return system to a site of lower hydrostatic and greater osmotic pressure. As far as the dense bone of larger animals and man is concerned there is therefore no basis for conceiving of a frank circulation of tissue fluid in the lacunar-canalicular system dependent on differences in hydrostatic and osmotic pressures in different sites. However, there is another possibility to be considered.

The Possible Role of the Filaments of Osteocyte Processes. The discovery that the processes of osteoblasts and osteocytes are composed essentially of longitudinally dis-

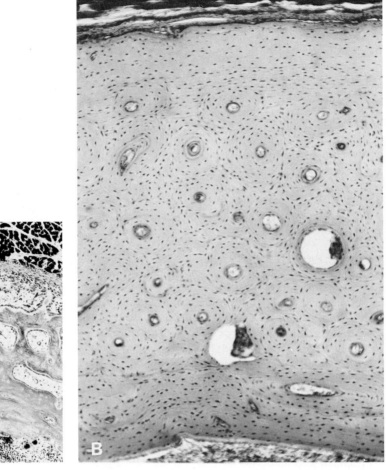

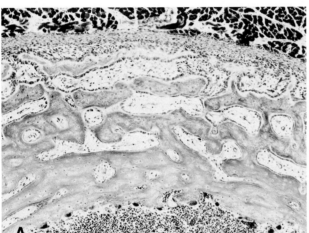

Fig. 15-25. (*A*) Photomicrograph of part of a cross section through a growing femur of a kitten. The dark-staining tissue at *top* is muscle (outside the bone). Below this the periosteum of the developing shaft is seen. The shaft at this stage consists essentially of cancellous bone. Note the osteoblasts covering trabeculae in the outer region of the shaft. The bone near the inside of the shaft at *bottom* is more compact in nature and along its inner surface is undergoing resorption by osteoclasts, which are visible as dark-staining, large cells along the bone surface. They are eroding the bone to enlarge its marrow cavity, the myeloid tissue of which is seen below.

In the shaft of a growing bone there is much loose connective tissue where tissue fluid could be formed and through which it might circulate. Tissue fluid formed in the interior of the bone might move through this soft tissue, and perhaps also through canaliculi, to reach the exterior of the bone. (Courtesy of M. Weinstock)

(*B*) Photomicrograph of part of a cross section through the shaft of a large, mature bone. This illustration may be compared with the diagram of dense bone shown in Figure 15-56. Below the periosteum (near *top*) there are several layers of bone comprising outer circumferential lamellae, which are formed by the periosteum. At *bottom,* the inner surface of the shaft is lined by inner circumferential lamellae. Between the outer and the inner circumferential lamellae the bone substance consists of haversian systems, each with a central canal surrounded by concentric layers of bone. The parts between adjacent haversian systems are filled with interstitial lamellae. In compact (dense) bone it seems unlikely that tissue fluid formed in the marrow cavity could reach the exterior of the bone through canaliculi. (Courtesy of M. Weinstock)

posed actin-containing filaments (Figs. 15-20 and 15-24) suggests that these processes may be capable of movement. If so, we could visualize various sections of the processes shortening and lengthening so as to keep the tissue fluid in canaliculi "stirred up"; this might maintain fairly constant concentrations of diffusible substances along canaliculi and lacunae and could conceivably even account for a possible very limited type of circulation. If so, an incredible amount of microactivity would be taking place in our living bones.

Possible Functions of Osteocytes

There is no reason to believe that osteocytes *in vivo* serve any proliferative function. Unlike cartilage, where two or more chondrocytes can sometimes be seen in a single lacuna, the lacunae of bone, with very few exceptions, contain only a single osteocyte.

There are two main theories about osteocyte function, that (*1*) they preserve the integrity of the matrix they inhabit and (*2*) they function so as to release calcium from bone when there is an increased demand for it. Details follow:

(*1*) The first theory is more or less based on the idea that osteocytes are in a sense grown-up osteoblasts. Hence, as older versions of the cells that produce the matrix in which osteocytes live, they as osteocytes continue, but to a lesser degree, the same osteoblastic type of function to keep the organic matrix in good repair and also, possibly by secreting enzymes and perhaps even matrix vesicles, help maintain its mineral content. However, they perhaps also play some less obvious role in preserving bone structure because it now seems apparent that unless bone contains living osteocytes, it is recognized as a foreign body and resorbed by osteoclasts. How osteocytes provide information to prevent this from happening would be a very interesting problem for investigation.

(*2*) The second theory about the function of osteocytes is that they can serve as agents to resorb bone, thereby liberating calcium to the blood. This concept, fathered primarily by Bélanger and his associates, is generally referred to as *osteocytic osteolysis*. In order to discuss it, we must first describe certain factors concerned in the regulation of blood calcium levels and also consider what is generally referred to as the role of bone as a calcium storehouse.

THE HORMONAL REGULATION OF BLOOD CALCIUM LEVELS

It is of the utmost importance that the blood calcium level be maintained within normal limits. Should the level fall too low, a condition called *tetany* develops. This is characterized by severe muscle spasms, caused by increased neuromuscular irritability due to insufficiency of calcium ions in the body tissues. These spasms can be severe enough to cause death. On the other side of the coin, elevated blood calcium levels can cause calcium salts to precipitate into soft tissues.

The function of maintaining a normal blood calcium level is allotted to the parathyroid glands. Removal of these from an animal causes tetany and, eventually, death. Tumors of a parathyroid gland (which occasionally occur in man), by secreting hormone in an uncontrolled way, can cause persistent high levels of calcium in the

blood, accompanied by precipitation of calcium salts into soft tissues.

Under normal conditions, the cells of the parathyroid glands monitor the level of calcium in the blood flowing through the capillaries of the glands. If the level is too low, the cells of the glands secrete more hormone. If the level is too high, they cease secreting until the calcium level falls.

The *parathyroid hormone,* commonly referred to as *PTH,* can raise the blood calcium level by exerting several minor and one major effect. For example, it acts on the kidneys to decrease calcium excretion and on the intestine to increase calcium absorption. But the major effect it exerts to keep the blood calcium level from falling to undesirable levels is that it activates cellular processes in bone which cause calcium to be liberated from its calcified matrix in such a way that the liberated calcium can reach the bloodstream and so raise the blood calcium level. It is because calcium can be made available from bone under such circumstances that bone is often referred to as the *calcium storehouse* of the body. The question then arises as to whether the PTH effect which results in calcium release from bone is mediated by osteoclasts, osteocytes, or both.

Background. It has long been accepted that the function of osteoclasts is to resorb calcified bone, and that they are responsible for the resorption of bone required for bone remodeling. It is also accepted that the calcium they liberate from bone in remodeling must be dissolved and carried away from the resorption site by blood or lymphatic vessels. Furthermore, as we shall see, it has been established since 1956 that osteoclasts resorbing bone are equipped with a specialized region termed a *ruffled border* which is responsible for them serving their resorptive function. We might, therefore, be puzzled as to why anyone would think of investigating osteocytes to see if they, too, were instrumental in bone resorption. One reason would seem to be that after PTH became available as a research tool, it was questioned by some investigators whether there were enough osteoclasts present to account for the increase in blood calcium level that occurred after PTH was administered to experimental animals. Or, even if there were enough osteoclasts, it was questioned whether these cells could respond to PTH administration soon enough to account for the blood calcium level rising as quickly as it does. However, it was shown with the EM, in 1978 using cultures of bone (King, Holtrop, and Raisz) and in 1979 using young thyroparathyroidectomized rats (Holtrop, King, Cox, and Reit), that changes in the fine structure of osteoclasts indicating increased resorptive activity occurred very quickly in response to PTH, and also that these changes were followed by an increase in numbers of osteoclasts. Further details will be given after we have described osteoclasts in the next section. Here it is enough to say that it can now be questioned whether it is necessary to visualize any other mechanism besides resorption by osteoclasts to explain liberation of calcium into the blood after PTH administration. It therefore seems pertinent to review the question of whether available histological evidence is sufficient to support the view that osteocytic osteolysis is a normal physiological process in the body.

First, in considering the osteocytic osteolysis hypothesis we should point out that calcified bone matrix is an odd kind of storehouse. The usual concept of a storehouse is that goods are stored there in rooms or lockers and removed at a later date with no damage being done to the storehouse. But to remove calcium from the bone storehouse requires, as far as we know, that the storehouse containing it be virtually destroyed. This is shown to advantage in connection with osteoclasts which, when they remove calcium from the storehouse, destroy the organic matrix in which the calcium is stored. Then, when the storehouse is to be rebuilt and restocked with calcium, different cells (osteoblasts) are called upon to build a *new* storehouse of organic matrix (which promptly becomes calcified).

The histological evidence pertinent to osteocytic osteolysis seems to us to be indefinite as to whether osteocytes would be (*1*) able to remove calcium salts from their lacunar walls without destroying the organic matrix, and later able to redeposit calcium in the old matrix, or (*2*) only able to resorb calcified matrix as osteoclasts do, with the result that their lacunae would become larger and larger. The LM studies, moreover, give little information about how any of these actions might be accomplished. However, the problem has also been investigated with the EM and studies of normal bone by this method have been described as indicating that osteocytes variously exist in any of three stages of a life cycle. First, the young ones have a fine structure commensurate with their synthesizing and secreting organic matrix. In the second stage, the amount of rER is diminished and lysosomes are more prominent in their cytoplasm. Then, in the third stage, they die. It has been reported that the administration of PTH greatly increases the proportion existing in the second stage, in which stage they are postulated to exert their resorptive effect.

Since ruffled borders are not present on osteocytes to provide an acidic microenvironment (as will be described in the following section on Osteoclasts), it is difficult to understand how osteocytes could exert rapid resorptive effects. Lysosome-derived enzymes could only be expected to affect the organic matrix. Of course, when osteocytes died, sufficient acidic products might result from their degradation to dissolve bone mineral and thus enlarge the size of their lacunae, and indeed empty lacunae often do appear enlarged.

However, generally speaking, the EM studies made on osteocytic osteolysis, while they provide interesting information on the life history of osteocytes, do not suggest to us that osteocytic osteolysis would or could be a rapid-acting normal physiological mechanism invoked by PTH to restore lowered blood calcium levels to normal. It is, of course, conceivable that PTH could speed up the life cycle of osteocytes so that they would die sooner than would be the case under normal conditions. Finally, since osteocytes and osteoclasts have now been shown to be derived from different cell lineages (as will be described in the following section), it would be surprising if it turned out that PTH exerted the same effect on osteocytes, which are derived from bone-building cells (osteoblasts), as it exerted on osteoclasts and their blood cell-derived precursors of the monocyte-macrophage line, which are specialized to destroy, not build.

OSTEOCLASTS

A hundred years have passed since Kolliker gave the name *osteoclasts* to large multinucleated cells he observed scattered along bone surfaces (Fig. 15-26) and ascribed to them the function of bone resorption. Since then there has been controversy about their origin, function, life span, and fate. The basic problem of their origin and relationship to other cells found in bone seems only recently to have been settled, with results that are likely to require a good deal of readjustment in the thinking of many of those interested in skeletal tissues. But first, some preliminary basic information.

The Study of Osteoclasts in the Laboratory With the LM

The Sites Where Osteoclasts Are Numerous. In looking for osteoclasts in sections of bone it saves time to know where they are relatively abundant. Such sites are those in which active bone resorption occurs as an essential part of the constant remodeling process by which, for example, a bone grows in length and width (described in detail later). Here we mention some sites where resorption occurs, so as to facilitate finding osteoclasts for laboratory study.

Perhaps the best kind of section in which to search for them is a longitudinal section of an end of a growing bone. A diagram of such a section will be found in Figure 15-52. The site to which an arrow points on the left side and which is labeled "1. resorbed here" is a good site for finding osteoclasts along the bone surface, as is also the site labeled "3. resorbed here," at the lower left side of the diagram and indicated by an arrow. A third good site for finding osteoclasts is indicated by the inner arrow which

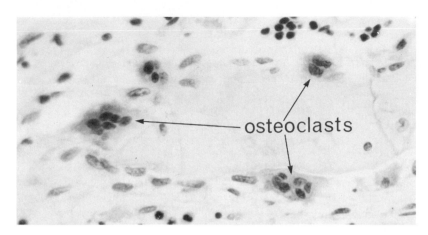

Fig. 15-26. High-power photomicrograph of part of a bony trabecula in the marrow cavity of a bone (dog). This trabecula is covered with osteogenic cells except for sites where osteoclasts are present. The large multinucleated osteoclasts lie in the shallow cavities (Howship's lacunae) they have eroded into the bone. The dark-staining nuclei at the periphery belong to myeloid cells. (Ham, A. W.: *In* Cowdry's Special Cytology, ed. 2, vol. 2. New York, Hoeber, 1932)

leads off from the words "replaced by bone here" on the right side of the diagram. All these sites are seats of active bone resorption in the constant remodeling of a bone as it grows in length and width.

The General Appearance of Osteoclasts in H and E Sections. Osteoclasts are large, multinucleated cells seen on bone surfaces where resorption is occurring. Histological evidence of their resorptive activity is provided by their often being located in little pits or declivities they have apparently eroded (as seen on the *left* in Fig. 15-26 and in Figs. 15-32A, B, and C); these are termed *Howship's lacunae* or *resorption bays*. Because of fixation artifact osteoclasts may be pulled away from the surface on which they were lying during life (Fig. 15-32A, B, and C). If this is an endosteal surface on which red bone marrow abuts, osteoclasts thus detached may be confused with megakaryocytes of marrow because the latter cells at one plane of focus may seem to be multinucleated. However, on focusing the microscope up and down it will be seen that what might appear to be separate nuclei in megakaryocytes are connected to each other (and are therefore lobes of a single nucleus), whereas those of osteoclasts are not.

Nuclei. There may be from two to a hundred or more nuclei in an osteoclast; commonly five or ten are seen. But since osteoclasts are as thick as they are wide, there may have been further nuclei above or below those in the section being examined. Serial sections generally show between ten and twenty. There is nothing special about most of the nuclei. However, dark, shrunken, and sometimes irregularly shaped nuclei, or even pyknotic nuclei, are sometimes seen in them and it is assumed that such osteoclasts are old and dying.

Cytoplasm. Depending on the functional state and age of the cell, the cytoplasm may be somewhat basophilic or acidophilic. Commonly that on the side of the cell closest to the bone contains fewer nuclei than on the side farther away. Close to the bone surface the cytoplasm of most osteoclasts is pale, foamy (vacuolated), or fuzzy.

Brush Borders. Between an osteoclast and a bone surface, particularly if the osteoclast is in a Howship's lacuna, an osteoclast may appear to be connected to the bone by innumerable straight, relatively stout hair-like structures (Fig. 15-27). Since these resemble the bristles

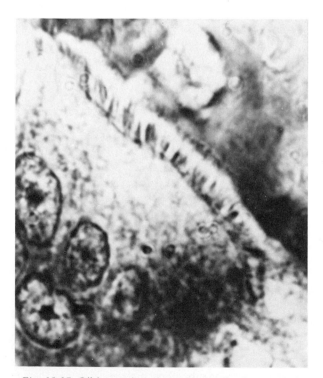

Fig. 15-27. Oil-immersion photomicrograph of an osteoclast with a well-developed brush border along its margin. The bone it is resorbing lies at *top right;* some of its nuclei are seen at *bottom left.* (Courtesy of W. Wilson)

of a brush, this kind of border was originally termed the *brush* or *striated border* of the osteoclast. Indeed, it was once suggested that the bristle-like structures, like cilia, might be motile and exert a scrubbing effect to wear away bone.

There are two common misconceptions about brush borders. The first is that they are a common feature of osteoclasts, whereas brush borders are not often seen for reasons to be explained later. So, if a student fails to find one in the first sections he examines, he should neither question his eyesight nor assume that any kind of border he sees between an osteoclast and bone must be a brush border. The second misconception is that the brush border seen with the LM is the same structure as what is termed the *ruffled border* of the osteoclast seen in the same position with the EM (and soon to be described). We shall, when discussing the fine structure of osteoclasts, explain why we think otherwise, namely that the brush border of light microscopy is actually part of the bone disclosed as it is being eroded.

THE ORIGIN OF OSTEOCLASTS

Since mitotic figures have almost never been observed in osteoclasts, it is conceded that they must arise from the fusion of uninucleated cells. However, the kind of cells that fuse to form osteoclasts has long been a matter of controversy. Since osteoclasts are the only kind of multinucleated giant cells found regularly and abundantly in the normal body and since they form in association with bone, most histologists have attributed their origin to cells of the bone cell lineage—to fusions of osteogenic cells and/or osteoblasts. However, many pathologists have expressed a different opinion. Since the latter, unlike histologists, are called upon to study the various kinds of disease processes, they become familiar with the fact that multinucleated giant cells form in many parts of the body in defense reactions to foreign invaders, such as the bacillus that causes tuberculosis (Fig. 9-29, *left*). They also form very commonly in association with nonliving materials that are foreign to the body but that may gain entrance to it, and so such multinucleated cells have in general been referred to as *foreign body giant cells* (Fig. 9-29, *right*). Hence a histopathologist might easily and logically look on osteoclasts as a type, perhaps a special type, of foreign body giant cell with some "foreign body" inciting their formation. In the instance of the osteoclast, the foreign body could be dead cartilage or bone. Since ordinary foreign body giant cells were believed to form as a result of the fusion of macrophages or monocytes, it is not surprising that many distinguished pathologists long ago attributed the origin of osteoclasts to the kind of leukocytes that were then called endothelial leukocytes

(and are now termed *monocytes*). Nevertheless, until recently histologists generally considered at least most osteoclasts to be cells of the bone cell series and to develop from fusions of cells of this lineage, generally osteogenic cells and osteoblasts.

There were, however, occasional findings that were disturbing to this view. For example, in 1952 Ham and Gordon compared the results of transplanting fresh living autologous cancellous bone chips into muscle with the results observed when similar material that before being transplanted was repeatedly frozen and thawed 3 times to kill all its constituent cells. They found that the covering and lining cells (osteogenic cells) of the untreated chips of cancellous bone lived, proliferated, and formed new bone. But no bone formed in association with the dead bone chips, which possessed no living cells of the bone cell lineage. However, they noted that osteoclasts still formed in association with both kinds of chips. In 1962, after thymidine labeling and radioautography had become available, Fischman and Hay in an ingenious experiment used this labeling technic to trace the origin of the nuclei of osteoclasts in regenerating newt limbs. They showed most convincingly that the label seen in osteoclast nuclei could be traced to leukocytes, in all likelihood to monocytes.

Around the same time, however, several other investigators were also using labeled thymidine in an attempt to trace the origin of osteoblasts, osteocytes, and osteoclasts in bone growth. Since label was seen first in osteogenic (osteoprogenitor) cells and then later in osteoblasts and still later in osteocytes and osteoclasts, it was assumed that labeled osteogenic cells and osteoblasts had fused to become osteoclasts and hence that osteoclasts were members of the bone cell lineage. But the work of Fischman and Hay had raised the possibility that the label appearing in osteoclasts had been taken up by a type of cell different from osteogenic cells, for example monocytes or their precursors, which could also have been labeled along with the osteogenic cells. Scott, in an EM study of forming bone in animals given labeled thymidine one hour previously, pointed out that label was seen in two types of cells. The fine structure of these cells suggested one type was of the bone cell lineage, but the other type revealed a fine structure more like that of phagocytic cells. The latter type was thought to be a precursor of osteoclasts. Luk et al. in an EM study of endosteum of growing bone reached similar conclusions.

Experiments Using Vital Staining. Meanwhile, evidence of another sort was obtained that indicated osteoclasts were not members of the bone cell lineage, but instead developed from the fusion of macrophages, as will now be described.

When the method of vital staining (described on p. 253) was first developed, many experiments were performed, not to determine the origin of osteoclasts but to see if they were phagocytic. Whereas it was shown readily that the cells we now term macrophages would take up vital stains such as trypan blue or particulate matter such as India ink, osteoclasts examined in the same animals showed no significant uptake. Since at that time osteoclasts were generally believed to develop from osteogenic cells or osteoblasts and since neither of these cell types was shown to be phagocytic, it caused little surprise that osteoclasts evidenced no phagocytic abilities when tested by this method. However, as uncertainty developed about the origin of osteoclasts in the 1960s, with the suspicion that osteoclasts might be derived from macrophages, it was natural that the thought would arise that if osteoclasts developed from phagocytic macrophages, they too should be phagocytic. So they were tested again by vital staining technics. But in short-term experiments the results were the same as before—there was no significant uptake of vital stain or particulate matter by osteoclasts. However, in 1963 Jee and Nolan, using bone charcoal as suitable particulate matter for vital staining, showed that this material could be found in osteoclasts, but only *after enough time* had elapsed for macrophages that had taken up the marker by phagocytosis to have fused and formed osteoclasts. This provided some proof for two concepts; first, that osteoclasts were derived from macrophages, and second, that osteoclasts themselves were not phagocytic.

How It Was Established That Osteoclasts Originate From a Type of Cell That Circulates in the Blood

In the 1970's a new approach to solving the problem of the origin of osteoclasts appeared as a result of Walker's outstanding experimental studies on the condition *osteopetrosis* (Gr. *petra*, stone; *osis*, a process) in mice and rats. This name was given to the condition because those suffering from it develop unusually dense bone. The reason for this is that while bone continues to form, the concurrent process of resorption necessary for bones to assume their proper shapes and densities is retarded. The retardation of resorption is due to osteoclasts not forming and functioning properly. The condition is congenital to certain strains of mice and rats, where it can lead to death. Since it became known that parathyroid hormone, thyrocalcitonin, and other hormones could affect the formation and activity of osteoclasts, the disease was first conceived of as probably being due to some inherited hormonal imbalance. But after investigating many aspects of osteopetrosis, Walker tried the expedient of connecting each member of a litter that was developing the condition to a normal littermate by vascular *parabiosis* (Gr. *para*, beyond; *biōsis*, living), so that the members of each pair shared a common blood supply.

Under these conditions the osteopetrotic littermates recovered. At first it was difficult to know why blood from the normal animals cured their osteopetrotic littermates. There was, of course, the possibility that hormones produced by the normal littermates were responsible. But the breakthrough came when Walker found that the parabiosis did not need to be permanent to keep the osteopetrotic littermates healthy. Even after a relatively short exposure to the blood of its normal littermate, the one inheriting the malady would thereafter be free of the disease. The only likely explanation for this latter finding would be that some type of cell circulating in the bloodstream of the normal littermate had taken up residence in the osteopetrotic animal, where it continued to produce the cells that fused to become normal osteoclasts and these soon replaced the defective ones previously made. Since it was known that the stem cell of blood, the CFU of Till and McCulloch (p. 297), could be isolated from blood, the CFU seemed to be the logical candidate for the cell that became established in the affected animal. In its new host it became the ancestral cell of normal monocytes that on entering the tissues developed into macrophages that fused to form normal osteoclasts. It could then even be reasoned that osteopetrosis was caused by a genetic defect in the hematopoietic stem cells of strains of mice and rats that developed the disease, a defect that was manifested in the monocyte-macrophage series.

The next kind of experiment undertaken involved giving sufficient radiation to osteopetrotic animals to destroy their capacity for producing their own blood cells and developing an immune response to foreign cells, but not enough to destroy the growth of cartilage and bone during the subsequent lifespan of the animals. Osteopetrotic mice treated this way were injected with suspensions of bone marrow cells from normal animals and this led to recovery from their osteopetrosis. However, it might be argued that suspensions of bone marrow cells could contain osteogenic cells that could become established in the irradiated host and form normal osteoclasts. But it was found that injections of spleen cells (which contain hematopoietic stem cells but not osteogenic cells) also cured the condition in irradiated osteopetrotic hosts.

Finally, it was shown that injecting cells obtained from the spleens of osteopetrotic mice into irradiated normal mice would cause the hitherto normal mice to develop osteopetrosis. This reinforced the hypothesis that a circulating blood cell must serve as the progenitor cell of osteoclasts. Since there is excellent evidence that macrophages are the cells that fuse to form osteoclasts and that monocytes are the blood cells that enter tissue to become macrophages, it would seem that it is the monocytes of osteopetrotic animals that are defective. However, if only normal monocyte progenitors (monoblasts) were transfused into an osteopetrotic animal, they would have no capacity for self renewal and so would not provide a permanent cure for the condition. So it would seem that the permanent cure obtained would require the osteopetrotic animals to be seeded with enough CFUs to serve as future stem cells of the blood cell series. As explained in Chapter 12, it has been established that the CFU has the capacity to go into cycle at any time throughout life and so maintain a supply of cells for differentiating into all forms of blood cells.

Studies on the Origin of Osteoclasts Utilizing the Nuclei of Quail Cells as Markers

As was described on page 334, embryos are immunologically tolerant to transplants of tissues of other species; hence if quail tissue is transplanted into chick embryos it is not rejected. Le Douarin showed that the nuclei of quail cells are sufficiently different from those of chicks and other species to serve as markers by which quail cells growing in chick embryos can be distinguished from cells of the chick. The recognizable "marker" that interphase quail cells possess is an extensive amount of nucleolus-associated chromatin. Feulgen preparations (which demonstrate the DNA in chromatin, p. 36) reveal so much nucleolus-associated chromatin in quail cells that they can be easily distinguished from chick cells, in which the chromatin is in general widely dispersed. Hence transplanting embryonic quail tissue of different kinds into chick embryos permits the embryonic origin of given tissues to be established.

The first investigators to use this method in an attempt to determine the origin of osteoclasts were Kahn and Simmons. They transplanted bone rudiments from quail embryos onto the chorioallantoic membranes of chick embryos (Fig. 15-28) and found that whereas the nuclei of the cells of the new bone forming were mostly, if not all, of the quail type (Q in Fig. 15-28A), those of most osteoclasts that had formed were of the chick type (C in Fig. 15-28B). These osteoclasts were therefore derived from the host, presumably from blood cells that became available when the quail transplant was vascularized by vessels from the chick host. But some osteoclasts seemed to reveal a mixture of the two types of nuclei and a few were composed solely (as far as could be determined from a single section) of nuclei of the quail type. The latter, it might be thought, could be explained if hematopoiesis had already begun in the quail transplant before it was transplanted and became vascularized by the chick host.

A second and very extensive study into the origin of osteoclasts, utilizing this technic, has been recently reported by Jotereau and Le Douarin. They point out a fact which might influence the interpretation of the findings in this kind of experiment: whereas the nuclei of chick os-

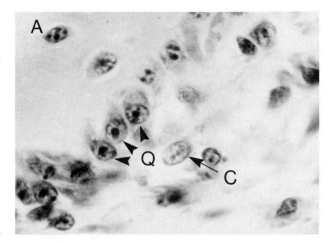

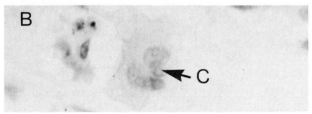

Fig. 15-28. (*A*) Oil-immersion photomicrograph of part of an epiphyseal cartilage of a bone rudiment of a quail embryo that has been transplanted to a chick chorioallantoic membrane. Its cells disclose the "marker" (described in the text) characteristic of quail cell nuclei (Q). Note that the chick cell nuclei (C) lack this marker. (*B*) Oil-immersion photomicrograph of an osteoclast from a quail bone rudiment transplanted to chick chorioallantoic membrane. Its nuclei are all of the chick type (C), indicating that this cell was derived not from quail cells but from host (chick) cells. The cytoplasm and outline of the osteoclast are not very distinct because the Feulgen technic was used to stain the nuclear DNA. (Courtesy of A. Kahn and D. Simmons)

teoclasts are always of the dispersed chromatin type, roughly one quarter to a third of the nuclei of the osteoclasts in normal quail do not reveal the mass of nucleolus-associated chromatin that would enable them to be distinguished from chick nuclei.

Moreover, in their experiment Jotereau and Le Douarin not only transplanted quail rudiments into chicks but also chick rudiments into quail embryos. In the latter the interpretation of the results was made very difficult by the fact that, as they point out, the nuclei in around a quarter to a third of the osteoclasts, even of a normal quail, do not possess the chromatin marker by which quail cells can be distinguished. But when quail limb buds were transplanted into chick embryos they found first that bone formation proceeded normally, with all the cells of the cartilage and bone that developed being of the quail type. But the blood and endothelial cells of the developing vascular system were all of the chick type. Moreover, the nuclei of the osteoclasts that developed were *all* of the chick type. They could not find a single example of a quail-type nucleus in any of the osteoclasts seen. Since an origin of osteoclasts from endothelial cells could be ruled out by Walker's experiments, the quail-chick experiments confirm that osteoclasts develop from some type of blood cell.

Studies With Labeled Thymidine

As already described, the earlier studies using labeled thymidine to mark osteoclast precursors were misinterpreted because it was not realized that blood cells as well as osteogenic cells were being labeled. Since then more sophisticated studies utilizing tritiated thymidine have been done. For example, Göthlin and Ericsson performed an elaborate experiment using parabiotic rats in which one of each pair was shielded while radiation was administered to the other. The cross circulation in each pair was shut off while tritiated thymidine was then given to the shielded animal, with the other (irradiated) rat of each pair being given unlabeled thymidine so that when the cross circulation was restored its cells would be unlikely to take up any labeled thymidine that might still come from its mate. They used repairing fractures for their study. They found that the cells of the bone cell lineage forming in the shielded animals were all labeled, but those of its mate were not. However, the monocytes and osteoclasts of both animals were labeled, which indicates the origin of the osteoclasts forming in the nonshielded animal as being from circulating labeled monocytes from the shielded rats of each pair.

Implications of These Studies

One very important sequel to this recently acquired evidence to the effect that osteoclasts are not members of the bone cell lineage is as follows. Under the impression that osteoclasts were members of the bone cell lineage, there were proponents of the view that they were not end cells but instead could, in the growth and remodeling of bone, become disassembled into osteoprogenitor cells and osteoblasts and so provide a source of these cells for further bone growth. A view of this nature, propounded in particular by Rasmussen and Bordier, gained wide acceptance in orthopedic and other clinical areas and also to some extent in histological circles. In view of all the foregoing evidence, it should be obvious that if an osteoclast were to become disassembled into the cells from which it was formed (a concept which would be very difficult to imagine from its fine structure), it would, in any case, only form a cluster of macrophages or monocytes, and from all the foregoing evidence there is no indication whatsoever that these cells form bone.

THE FINE STRUCTURE OF OSTEOCLASTS

The Four Regions of the Cytoplasm

In studying micrographs of functioning osteoclasts it is helpful to visualize the osteoclast as a more or less polarized cell made up of four regions of cytoplasm that merge more or less imperceptibly with one another. These regions and their locations in relation to the bone surface will now be described briefly for purposes of orientation. Their structure and functions will be dealt with in detail later.

The bone on which the osteoclast abuts is shown in the lower left corner of Figure 15-29, where it is labeled b. It is mostly pale because the material from which this section was cut was decalcified. However, a little mineral residue may remain to cause the dark spots seen in the otherwise pale decalcified bone matrix. The four regions of the cell cytoplasm are located as follows:

(1) The Ruffled Border. The region of specialized cytoplasm of a functioning osteoclast that abuts directly on the bone surface where resorption is occurring is termed its *ruffled border*. This name was given it because as seen in Figure 15-29, where it is labeled rb, and also in Figures 15-30 and 15-33, it is ruffled in the sense that the plasmalemma at this site is thrown into folds and villus-like processes whose tips reach and sometimes even project into the bone surface. The processes vary in diameter along their lengths and frequently branch and anastomose with one another. There are clefts between the processes, which in life would contain tissue fluid. The ruffled border in Figure 15-29 extends over somewhat more than the middle half of the bone surface visible and it is bordered on each edge by the next region of the cytoplasm to be described.

(2) The Clear Zone. The clear zone also abuts on the bone and, like a girdle, surrounds the site of ruffled border so that in a section some of the clear zone is seen on each side of the ruffled border. This is labeled cz in Figure 15-29. It differs profoundly from the ruffled border in that its plasmalemma is *not* thrown into villus-like processes but follows the contours of the bone surface. The cytoplasm of the clear zone will be described in detail presently.

(3) The Region of Vesicles and Vacuoles. The deep portion of the ruffled border merges into a cytoplasmic region characterized by the presence of what appear to be many membrane-bound vesicles of various sizes (Fig. 15-30). The larger ones are sometimes designated *vacuoles*, but they, like the vesicles, are lined by membrane and hence are structures, not just holes in the cytoplasm as suggested by the word *vacuole*. The clefts between villus-like processes of the ruffled border are continuous with at least many of the various-sized "vesicles" of the vesicular region, for example those indicated by arrows in Figure 15-30. Hence many of the so-called "vesicles" represent

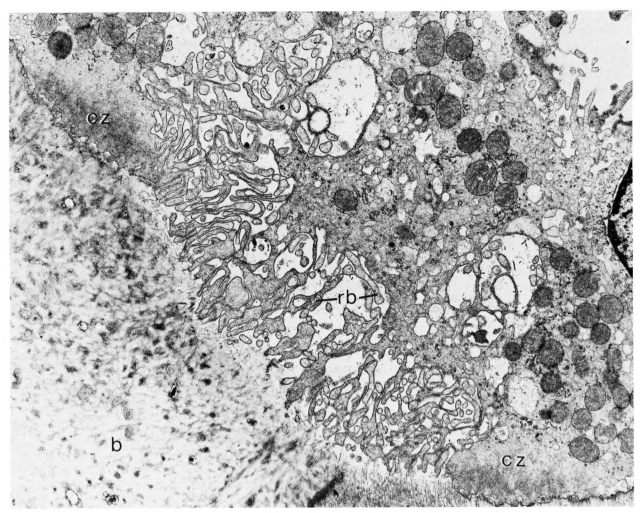

Fig. 15-29. Electron micrograph (×8,500) of ruffled border (rb) of an osteoclast, showing also its clear zone (cz). For details, *see* text. The bone (b) it is erroding is seen as a light area at the *lower left* corner. The basal part of the cell, seen at *upper right* extending to *lower right*, contains numerous mitochondria. Note also the vesicular region between the ruffled border and the basal region. (Holtrop, M. E., and King, G. J.: Clin. Orthop., *123:*177, 1977)

deep clefts extending in more or less tubular fashion from the ruffled border into the vesicular layer. When cut in oblique or cross section, these appear as vesicles.

(4) The Basal Part of the Cell. Only a portion of the basal part of the osteoclast is shown in Figure 15-29, where it may be seen at *upper right* and extends to the lower right-hand corner. We shall describe it in detail later in connection with Figure 15-35. Here it is enough to note that it contains the several nuclei of the cell. A portion of one nucleus is seen in Figure 15-35, *top right*. The cytoplasm associated with the nuclei contains a great many mitochondria; several are seen in Figures 15-29 and 15-35. As will be illustrated later, the cytoplasm here may reveal centrioles, a fair number of ribosomes and polyribosomes, some rER, and a good many Golgi saccules. The

cytoplasm of the basal region of the cell thus stands out in contrast to the other regions of the cytoplasm, which are singularly free of organelles except for microtubules and microfilaments.

We shall now deal with these various cytoplasmic regions of the osteoclast in more detail and in relation to their functions.

The Ruffled Border

Terminology. The discovery of the ruffled border had to await the use of the EM, so it was not observed and named until around the middle 1950's. The term "ruffled" is somewhat misleading here because ruffles in general are thought of as decorative pleats and hence the ruffled

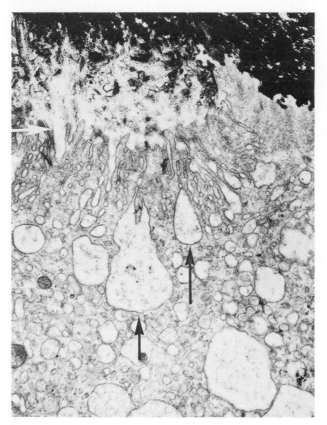

Fig. 15-30. Electron micrograph (×13,000) of ruffled border of an osteoclast, showing the apposed bone surface undergoing demineralization and resorption. Calcified bone (electron-dense) is seen at *top*. Adjacent to the ruffled border (extending from *left* to *right* just above the middle of the micrograph) the bone matrix appears pale because it has been demineralized by the osteoclast. The ruffled border consists of complex folds and projections, the tips of which are apposed to the bone substance. Electron-dense fragments of mineral are present in some of the large vesicles (vertical arrows) in the vesicular region beneath the ruffled border. Such vesicles open into crypts of the ruffled border and represent the bottoms of clefts extending down into the vesicular layer. Collagenic fibrils commonly extend down into clefts such as the one indicated by the horizontal arrow at *upper left* (*see* Fig. 15-34). (Courtesy of B. Boothroyd and N. Hancox)

border might be thought to be composed of adjacent parallel rows of pleat-like folds of the plasmalemma. Actually most sections of ruffled borders, supposedly cut at right angles to a bone surface, are sufficiently oblique to show that instead of consisting chiefly of parallel ruffles, the border is made up of a vast number of very irregular villus-like processes of the plasmalemma that vary in diameter along their lengths and branch and anastomose with one another. Hence a ruffled border is really a tangled web of what might be considered to be ruffles and villus-like tubular processes, with deep clefts in between them (Figs. 15-29; 15-33).

The plasmalemma that covers the processes and lines the vesicles seen in the cytoplasm beneath the border was closely studied by Kallio, Garant, and Minkin. They described the inner (cytoplasmic) surface of the plasmalemma of the ruffled border as being coated with fine, bristle-like structures about 15 to 20 nm. long, with a center-to-center spacing of 20 to 25 nm. The same type of coating was found in vesicles immediately below the ruffled border.

Effects of Parathyroid Hormone, Calcitonin, and Colchicine on Ruffled Borders. As already described, the hormone (PTH) of the parathyroid glands, administered in sufficient quantities to animals, stimulates bone resorption by increasing the numbers and resorptive activities of osteoclasts. PTH will, for example, increase the extent of ruffled borders of osteoclasts in cultured bone. It has also been shown that calcitonin, a hormone produced by certain cells of the thyroid gland (Chap. 25), will slow bone resorption on administration to animals. Furthermore, it was found more recently that in bone cultures calcitonin will reduce the number and extent of ruffled borders of osteoclasts previously stimulated by PTH. It was also shown that colchicine likewise reduces the extent of ruffled borders of osteoclasts; this effect is probably related to the action of colchicine in inhibiting assembly of microtubules, as described on page 59. For references, *see* Kallio et al., 1972; Raisz et al., 1973; King et al., 1978; and Holtrop et al., 1979.

Where Ruffled Borders Are Found. According to Holtrop, ruffled borders are not seen on osteoclasts unless they abut on bone. If osteoclasts leave a bone surface, both the ruffled border and the clear zone disappear. Osteoclasts may demonstrate more than one ruffled border if they abut on bone at more than one site, but they do not necessarily reveal a ruffled border at the sites where they abut on bone (Fig. 15-31). However, since sections used for the EM are so very thin, it is distinctly possible that such osteoclasts, if sectioned at another level, might demonstrate a ruffled border.

Factors Concerned in the Formation of Osteoclasts and Ruffled Borders. Presumably macrophages are attracted to naked calcified surfaces. Since osteoclasts do not form in association with osteoid tissue, it is assumed that it is the mineral in the matrix, freely exposed to tissue fluid, that attracts macrophages. Normally, all exposed bone surfaces are covered or lined with osteogenic cells and as such do not elicit the formation of osteoclasts. The precise site at which macrophages actually congregate and fuse to form osteoclasts is not entirely clear. It would seem most probable that it would be in association with a naked calcified bone surface. Regarding the way they fuse, although specific studies are still required on this matter, one way macrophages fuse to form giant cells may be by their first extending leaf-like pseudopodia toward one another, with those of one macrophage interdigitating

Fig. 15-31. Electron micrograph (×2,400) of an osteoclast (Oc) situated on the endosteal surface of a rabbit femur. Two nuclei and abundant mitochondria can be discerned. Note that in this particular plane of section no ruffled border is observed where the osteoclast is apposed to the bone surface above. (Luk, S. C., Nopajaroonsri, C., and Simon, G. T.: J. Ultrastruct. Res., *46:*165, 1974)

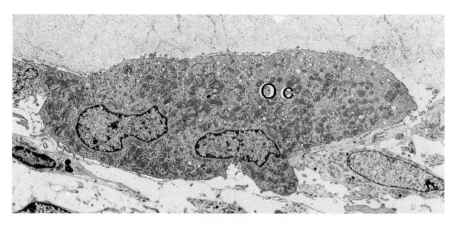

with those of another as shown in Figure 9-30, which electron micrograph was taken of macrophages gathering around agar (a foreign body) that had been injected at this site. The similarity of such pseudopodia to those of a ruffled border was noted by Scott and Pease in 1956 in their original description of ruffled borders.

The Relation of the Brush Border of Light Microscopy to the Ruffled Border of Electron Microscopy. According to Hancox the brush border of osteoclasts (Figs. 15-27 and 15-32A, B, and C) was first described in 1873 by Kolliker, who regarded it as part of the osteoclast. Hancox, however, mentions that since the early days there has been lively debate about its origin because in 1883 Pommer described the brush border as part of the bone instead of being part of the osteoclast because, in his opinion, the bristles of the "brush" were fibrils that projected from the bone surface after the mineralized substance of the bone between the fibrils had been dissolved. Furthermore, he noted the projecting fibrils could be traced microscopically into the bone substance. Nevertheless, in later years Kolliker's concept of the brush border seems to have prevailed, probably because most histologists of this century were unaware of Pommer's study and conclusions. At least one histologist was, for in 1952 Ham, blithely unaware of Pommer's concept, reported on a study he had made on osteoclasts, using phase contrast microscopy, in which he proposed the same thesis that Pommer had nearly 70 years before, namely that the bristles of a brush border are (collagenic) fibrils that project from the bone surface after the mineralized matrix between them is dissolved away. Illustrations from Ham's paper are shown in Figure 15-32. It should be mentioned that a better contrast can be achieved between the collagenic fibrils and whatever surrounds them with the phase contrast microscrope than can be obtained with the ordinary LM. Figure 15-32A illustrates an osteoclast that had shrunken from the bone because of fixation artifact. The brush border in this instance adheres to the osteoclast. However, in Figure 15-

32B the brush border has remained with the bone. In Figure 15-32C the bristles of the border can be seen to continue on into the bone substance, indicating that the bristles of the border are fibrils of bone substance that become freed when the mineral between them, and presumably other matrix components with which it was associated, are dissolved away. Figure 15-32D shows that the ends of bone chips, in the absence of osteoclasts but from which mineral is presumably dissolving, can present, without the help of osteoclasts, a brush-like, fringed border. Ham concluded that the brush border of osteoclasts really belonged to the bone. Furthermore, the reason for it not being seen in association with most osteoclasts was that it would only be apparent in sites where the collagenic fibrils of bone were disposed more or less at right angles to the surface on which the osteoclast abutted. Note that even where no osteoclast is present, as in Figure 15-32D, a brush-like border is seen only where the fibrils approach the surface more or less at right angles to it.

Next, it should be emphasized that up to this time the existence of a ruffled border on osteoclasts had not been established; this had to await the use of the EM in histology. It was not until 1956 that Scott and Pease made the first thorough EM study of osteoclasts. A side effect of this was to reopen the controversy about the brush border. They described the ruffled border of the osteoclast, pointing out that plasmalemma of the osteoclast, at sites where it abutted on bone and where resorption was occurring, presented an area of intricate infolding which they stated probably corresponds with Kolliker's brush border. It is to be noted that they used the word *probably.* Nevertheless, this view subsequently became widely accepted, but we think, uncritically, for two reasons.

First, because of Kolliker's concept it was believed that the brush border of light microscopy must play some role in resorption. It would be tempting, when the ruffled border was discovered with the EM in the same site and its

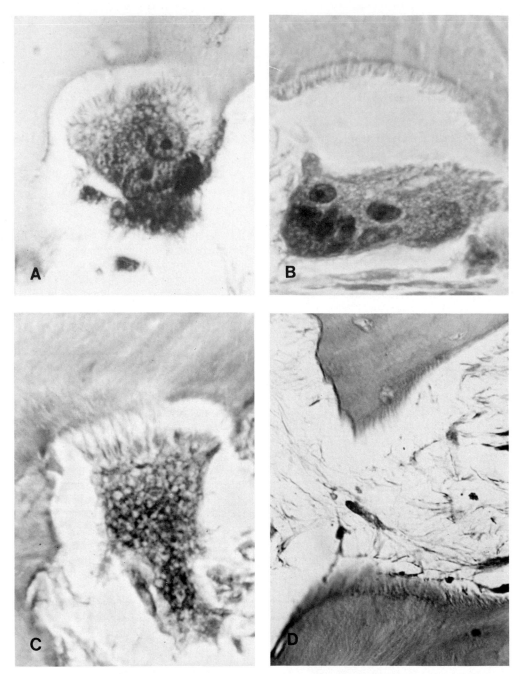

Fig. 15-32. (*A*) Photomicrograph (×1,250) of an osteoclast in a Howship's lacuna. Note that the top surface of the cell exhibits a brush border where it was apposed to the bone. (*B*) Photomicrograph (×1,250) of an osteoclast which has shrunken away from the bone to which it was apposed; note that the brush border here is seen on the bone surface instead of on the osteoclast. (*C*) Oil-immersion phase-contrast photomicrograph of an osteoclast, showing that the "bristles" of the brush border continue on into the bone matrix as collagenic fibrils. (*D*) Photomicrograph (×1,250) of brush borders on resorbing borders of bone chips where no osteoclasts are present. (Ham, A. W.: J. Bone Joint Surg., *34-A:*701, 1952)

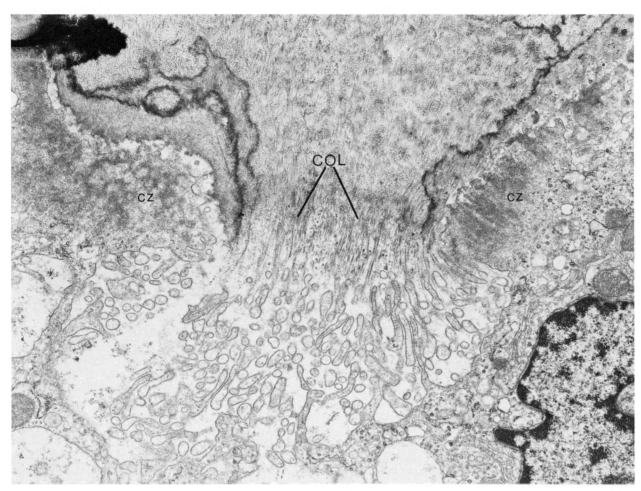

Fig. 15-33. Electron micrograph (×11,000) of an osteoclast (which lies *below*) wrapped around the bottom tip of a trabecula of partly calcified cartilage (which is seen at *top*). This trabecula extends down from an epiphyseal plate into the shaft of a developing bone. At such sites resorption of cartilaginous trabeculae proceeds at their free ends, as will be explained later. Note that at *center* the osteoclast is removing the calcified amorphous component of the cartilage more rapidly than the straight collagenic fibrils (COL) in the cartilage matrix. The remaining fibrils would appear in the LM as a brush border. Note also the clear zone (cz) seen on each side of the ruffled border, which occupies most of the lower part of the micrograph. A nucleus is seen at *lower right.* (Courtesy of M. Holtrop)

obvious involvement in bone resorption was appreciated, to assume that since the ruffled border obviously had the function postulated by Kolliker for the brush border, that they were one and the same structure. However, another interpretation would be that the *ruffled border is a cause of resorption* and the *brush border an effect* of resorption. This interpretation, which we believe to be correct, would explain them both being observed in the same site.

Second, now that countless micrographs of ruffled borders have become available for study, it seems *inconceivable* that any histologist familiar with both light and electron microscopy could believe that the irregular, anastomosing network of villus-like structures of which a ruffled border is composed could possibly appear as separated, relatively *thick straight bristles* (Fig. 15-27) in the thicker sections used for the LM. The only structures that could appear as straight bristles with the LM and which have now been demonstrated in electron micrographs as shown in Figure 15-33 (Holtrop) and Figure 15-34 (Bonucci) are the straight collagenic fibrils of calcified bone or cartilage at sites where they are disposed more or less at right angles to a surface undergoing resorption, in which process the mineral between the fibrils is removed so that they are freed from it and hence readily seen with the LM. The site where they thus become obvious (and appear with the LM as the bristles of a brush) extends just

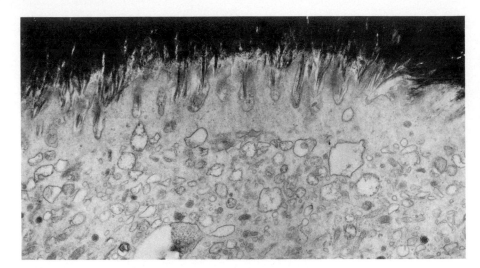

Fig. 15-34. Electron micrograph of a ruffled border of an osteoclast (which lies *below*) apposed to electron-dense calcified bone (*above*) in which the collagenic fibrils are oriented at right angles to the bone surface. This illustrates how the ends of such fibrils project down into the clefts of the ruffled border so that in the LM they would appear as the "bristles" of a brush border. (Courtesy of E. Bonucci)

above the edge of the ruffled border. Below, the fibrils extend for a short distance into the interstices of the ruffled border (Figs. 15-33 and 15-34).

We therefore conclude that Pommer and not Kolliker was right about the brush border. In order to discuss the possible roles of the ruffled border in bone resorption we first have to describe the other parts of the osteoclast.

The Clear Zone of the Osteoclast and Its Relation to the Ruffled Border.

As described by Holtrop, this zone has been referred to by many names, but the term *clear zone* has now become the most popular. This is because (*1*) its cytoplasm is pale and contains few (if any) organelles except filaments, and (*2*) it is properly termed a *zone* (Gr. *zōnē,* belt or girdle) because it encircles the site at which the ruffled border abuts on bone; hence in a section a clear zone (labeled cz in Figs. 15-29 and 15-33) can be seen on either side of a ruffled border.

Whereas the clear zone was first considered to be structureless and composed entirely of light granular material, it has now been shown that there are some denser bands in it, oriented perpendicular to the cell surface. These bands are composed of microfilaments that contain actin because they bind heavy meromyosin (King and Holtrop). It is known from studies of other types of cells that actin-containing filaments reaching a surface may act in some manner to hold a cell to a surface. So one theory of the role of the clear zone was that it might hold osteoclasts firmly against the bone all around the circumference of their ruffled borders, so that these borders were held in position at the site of their work. However, as reviewed by Holtrop, there is evidence indicating that marker molecules in tissue fluid can pass between the bone and the site of a clear zone (Lucht).

Another possibility is that the actin-containing filaments in the clear zone account for the agitation of the borders of osteoclasts observed with the LM in bone cultures. Osteoclasts have also been observed to move about in such preparations, but since the clear zone as such disappears when an osteoclast leaves a bone surface, this movement if due to the microfilaments might entail their becoming more dispersed.

The Vesicular Region

As shown in Figure 15-30 there is an ill-defined junction between the base of the ruffled border and a region of cytoplasm that exhibits many different-sized, membrane-bound spaces, the smaller of which are termed *vesicles* and the large ones *vacuoles* (even though the latter are bounded by membrane and hence not holes in the cytoplasm). The cytoplasm surrounding them is pale and relatively free of organelles. It merges in turn with the cytoplasm of the basal part of the cell, in which mitochondria are abundant as seen along the right-hand side of Figure 15-29.

The Possible Nature and Significance of the Vesicles. The origin and nature of vesicles is crucial to the problem of how osteoclasts function, as will become apparent in the next section. There are three possible origins.

(*1*) The membrane-bound structures that appear as vesicles or vacuoles in any given section may be no more than extensions of the clefts between the villus-like processes of the ruffled border that, because they pursue somewhat devious courses beneath the ruffled border, are commonly cut in cross or oblique sections so that they appear as vesicles. If this concept is correct, their lumina would all be continuous with the clefts of the ruffled border like those indicated by arrows in Figure 15-30. Furthermore, they would all be filled with tissue fluid and

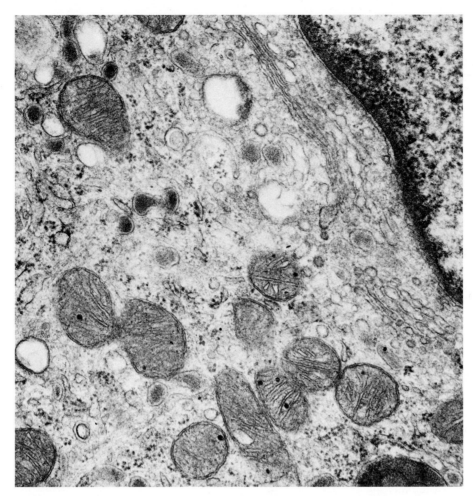

Fig. 15-35. Electron micrograph of part of the basal cytoplasm of an osteoclast close to a nucleus (*upper right*). To the left of this nucleus there are flattened Golgi saccules with some secretory vesicles leaving them. Some of the vesicles are lysosomes. Free ribosomes and polyribosomes are also present, but there is little rER. Note that mitochondria are abundant in this region of the cytoplasm. (Cameron, D. A.: The ultrastructure of bone. *In* Bourne, G. H. (ed.): The Biochemistry and Physiology of Bone. ed. 2, vol. 1. New York, Academic Press, 1972.

anything dissolved in this would have ready access to the clefts between villus-like processes (and vice versa).

(2) Vesicles may originate as described above but may then become pinched off from the ends of the clefts from which they were derived; hence their contents would no longer be continuous with the tissue fluid in the clefts of the border.

(3) The vesicles may be phagosomes derived from the plasmalemma lining the clefts between the villus-like processes of the ruffled border. This concept raises the possibility that they contain phagocytosed material and that they will fuse with primary lysosomes to become secondary lysosomes in which their phagocytosed contents will be digested.

Before discussing these three possibilities, however, we must first comment further on the basal portion of the osteoclast.

The Basal Cytoplasm

The basal portion of the osteoclast is the energy-producing portion of the cell and houses the cytoplasmic equipment by which the energy is mostly put to use. As shown in Figure 15-35, the mitochondria of the cell are found in this region and they are very abundant. To the left of the nucleus seen at the upper right corner of Figure 15-35 there are numerous Golgi stacks. There is, however, relatively little rER, but the amount of it is said to vary. There are fair numbers of ribosomes and polyribosomes.

The basal region would seem to account for the production and maintenance of the cytoplasm of the other three regions of the cytoplasm. Moreover, the numerous Golgi stacks suggest the formation and budding of many secretory vesicles from the stacks. Some of these secretory vesicles (*center left* in Fig. 15-35) contain dark rounded bodies with a narrow space between the surrounding membrane and the contained dark body. Other small vesicles are less distinct; however, these are all secretory vesicles of one kind or another. The question is whether they are all primary lysosomes destined to fuse with phagosomes to form secondary lysosomes or whether they or some of them, like the secretory granules of cells such as the acinar cells of the pancreas, are destined to fuse with the plasmalemma of the cell and empty their lytic contents extracellularly. This will be discussed in the next section.

HOW OSTEOCLASTS FUNCTION IN RESORBING BONE

Although a great deal of information available about the fine structure of different parts of the osteoclast could be correlated with their function, it is not usual to fit these two aspects together so as to allow visualization of a working model of the cell in action. This leaves the door open for assuming that certain of its parts perform functions for which they do not possess the proper organelle equipment. Accordingly, we shall here attempt to construct a working model of the osteoclast that would be dependent on the four parts of the cell performing functions for which they have the required organelle content and we shall then attempt to show how these functions could be coordinated so as to enable the osteoclast to resorb bone. We shall first describe what certain of the parts of the cell could, or could not, do.

(1) The Ruffled Border. The ruffled border is characterized by a vast expanse of plasmalemma arranged so as to fit into a relatively small space. To inquire into its function we must consider briefly the role of the cell membrane. This serves two important functions, absorption and excretion. There could be confusion about its function because it might be assumed lytic enzymes could be secreted by the tips of its villous processes. The only way what is defined as *secretion* occurs through a cell membrane is by Golgi-derived vesicles being delivered to the cell membrane and their membranous walls fusing with the plasmalemma, whereupon the fused membranes open up so that the contents of the secretory vesicle are emptied outside the cell (p. 134). Unless it could be shown that Golgi-derived secretory vesicles migrate up the villous processes of the ruffled border and empty their

contents through the plasmalemma of the processes close to the bone, it must be concluded that the villous processes do not serve a secretory function. Hence the functions that the plasmalemma of the villous processes close to the bone would serve would be absorption and/or excretion. More will be said about this later.

(2) The Clear Zone. As already described, there is a possibility that the clear zone provides a ring-like attachment of the osteoclast to the bone around the ruffled border. Even if it does not serve this purpose, it is at least closely apposed to the bone surface and hence it could be expected that it would restrict any circulation of tissue fluid into and out of the area occupied by the villous processes and the apposed bone surface.

(3) The Basal Part of the Osteoclast. This is a very important part of the osteoclast because it is the principal site of energy production in the cell. Moreover, it houses the numerous nuclei it obtained from the cells that fused to form the osteoclast. But in particular it has a *large number of Golgi stacks* for the same reason, because it has those of all the cells from which it was assembled. It also has a *very substantial content of mitochondria* because almost all the mitochondria seem to be gathered together in the basal part of the osteoclast. Obviously this is the part of the cell where the energy requirements are the greatest.

The extensive Golgi is the clue to the osteoclast being a secretory cell. The secretions it produces are budded off from the Golgi in the basal part of the cell and the secretory vesicles then move toward the vesicle region. As described in connection with the Golgi on page 135, two "kinds" of secretory vesicles can be liberated from the Golgi. One kind move to the plasmalemma, fuse with it, and empty their secretion outside the cell into tissue fluid. The other kind remain in the cell as lysosomes. There is no good reason to believe that the Golgi of an osteoclast does not form both types. Doty and Schofield found hydrolytic enzyme activity between the villous processes of the ruffled border. They concluded that this was due to enzymes being released via vesicles connected with the crypts of the border. Enzymes liberated extracellularly in this site could of course diffuse through the tissue fluid in the crypts directly to the bone surface.

The function of the enzymes liberated into the tissue fluid of the crypts on reaching the bone would seem to be concerned with the digestion of the noncollagenic organic components of bone matrix with which the inorganic compound is associated, as was suggested by Bonucci. Such an action would lead to fragmentation of the calcified matrix associated with the collagenic fibrils which, before being completely digested, could persist long enough to constitute a brush border at places where they are disposed more or less at right angles to the surface and lie in crypts of the ruffled border (where they would be undergoing degradation). The question that remains is how the osteoclast disposes of the fragmented mineral.

The Concept of Bone Salts Being Dissolved Because They Buffer Acid Excretions of the Ruffled Border

After it became known that living cells absorbed oxygen and excreted carbon dioxide, it seemed possible to those interested in bone that osteoclasts might be able to dissolve bone mineral because of their excreting CO_2 into the tissue fluid at the site where they contacted bone. It was assumed that this would result in local acidity which would act to dissolve the calcified salts contained in bone matrix. Later, when it became appreciated that the surfaces of living bone are always covered with osteogenic cells, and that the only noticeable place where this covering or lining membrane was missing was where osteoclasts were present, this old view seemed more acceptable because the finding that all living bone surfaces were covered elsewhere by a membrane suggested that retention of mineral by bone matrix could only be achieved if it was not in direct contact with tissue fluid. When the ruffled border of the osteoclast was discovered with the EM and was shown to possess villous processes that projected directly into the site where resorption was occurring, the concept of an excretion of some kind through the extensive surface of plasmalemma coming into contact with the bone made it seem even more possible that some excretory product could act to bring bone salt into solution. This seemed to be particularly true after it was shown that enzyme activity could degrade the organic constituents of bone matrix and so permit fragmentation of crystalline bone salt.

Next, in considering fine structure in relation to function, it must be remembered that the area to which the ruffled border is localized is, as just described, to a considerable extent walled off by the clear zone. It might therefore be thought that continued excretion of CO_2 into the localized tissue fluid in which both the villous processes of the ruffled border and the fragmenting bone are bathed would soon raise the concentration of CO_2 in this tissue fluid so that there would no longer be a diffusion gradient for CO_2 to be excreted from the cytoplasm of the villous processes into the tissue fluid at this site. However, it must be remembered that bone mineral consists mostly of relatively insoluble calcium salts that would act to buffer any increase in acidity by themselves being converted to acid salts which are much more soluble. Hence it could be reasoned that in this relatively tightly enclosed pool of tissue fluid the continued secretion of CO_2 would not increase the acidity to the point of suppressing continued diffusion of CO_2 into it; yet at the same time continued excretion of CO_2 would result in the calcium salts being converted into more soluble ones that would pass into solution. In keeping with the concept of a local acidic environment being involved in the removal of bone mineral is the finding that carbonic anhydrase, an enzyme that facilitates the production of H_2CO_3, is present in the area. Citric acid too is present in this region and hence could contribute to its acidity.

Whereas CO_2 was the excretory product first thought of as the causative factor in this process, it is of course not ruled out that other acid products of metabolism could be excreted by the membrane in this area. In discussing the liberation of acid it is not inappropriate to think of how the parietal cells of the gastric mucosa (to be described in Chap. 21) produce HCl. These cells are equipped with intracellular canaliculi with numerous microvilli, indicating that a very large surface area may be required for the formation and liberation of the acid. It is, of course, obvious that a large surface area is the outstanding feature of the ruffled border. In any event, whatever the cause, it has been shown that the pH is lowered in the region of the ruffled border, which suggests the liberation of acid of some sort. The point we wish to emphasize is that the relatively insoluble bone salts would buffer this acidity and so keep the acidity within certain limits. At the same time these bone salts because of their action in buffering acidity would become converted into acid salts, which because they are more soluble would pass steadily into solution.

It is obvious that bone mineral must be dissolved at the osteoclast-bone interface in the resorption process, for otherwise it would take days instead of hours for parathyroid hormone, acting through osteoclasts, to elevate the blood calcium level. Furthermore, the amount of mineral previously present in a site becoming a Howship's lacuna would represent a mass approximately half that of the osteoclast that erodes the lacuna. If this relatively huge amount of mineral had to be phagocytosed by the osteoclast and subsequently dissolved in phagosomes that fused with primary lysosomes, the EM would certainly disclose a vast number of mineral-containing phagosomes in undecalcified sections; in fact, the vesicle region would have to be so enormously expanded that an osteoclast would have a very different fine structure than the kind it discloses. The fact that a few fragments of mineral are sometimes seen in what appear to be vesicles is not necessarily proof that it is intracellular in phagosomes because, as already noted, what appear as vesicles can be invaginations of clefts. Moreover, even if occasional bits of mineral sometimes appear in what could perhaps be true phagosomes, this provides no evidence that this is the usual route by which mineral is disposed of, as sometimes seems to be assumed. Thus there appears to be no tenable alternative to the concept of bone mineral being dissolved through its buffering action on local acidity.

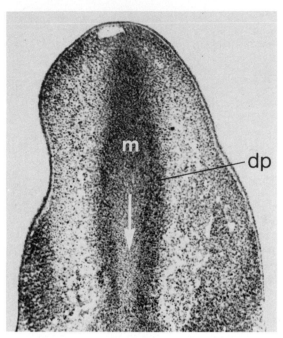

Fig. 15-36. Low-power photomicrograph of a developing toe of an embryo (rabbit). The darkly staining mass of mesenchyme (m) is beginning to differentiate in its middle (arrow) into the cartilage model of the terminal phalanx, and at its periphery into developing perichondrium (dp).

THE DEVELOPMENT, GROWTH IN LENGTH AND WIDTH, AND REMODELING OF LONG BONES

As mentioned on page 380, bone tissue normally develops in two different environments, (*1*) *intramembranous* and (*2*) *endochondral* (Gr. *endon,* within; *chondros,* cartilage). These two terms do *not* imply there are two kinds of bone tissue, membrane bone and cartilage bone—they refer merely to the environments in which bone of the same kind develops. Intramembranous ossification has already been described. We shall now describe endochondral ossification, from which most of the skeleton develops.

ENDOCHONDRAL OSSIFICATION

The Development of Cartilage Models of Future Bones

The process of endochondral ossification can be understood readily by observing the successive histological changes occurring as limb buds develop in the embryo.

As the mammalian embryo develops, little appendages push out from its trunk at the sites where its limbs will later appear; these are called *limb buds* and are essen-

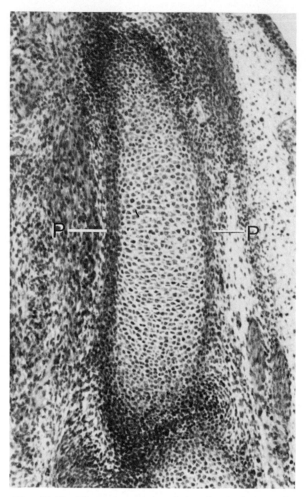

Fig. 15-37. Photomicrograph of the developing cartilage model of a metatarsal bone (mouse embryo) at a slightly later stage than in Figure 15-36. The middle region of developing cartilage is now readily distinguishable from the surrounding perichondrium (P).

tially mesodermal outgrowths covered with ectoderm. At their ends they form fingers and toes respectively. A longitudinal section of a developing toe of a rabbit embryo is shown in Figure 15-36.

The first sign of bone formation in limb buds or their appendages is in the mesenchyme of the site where a bone will develop. The mesenchymal cells here become very numerous and so packed together that they form a very rough outline of the bone-to-be (Fig. 15-36). Next, in the central core of this packed mesenchyme (m in Fig. 15-36) the cells become increasingly separated from one another because they begin to differentiate into chondrocytes, and the cartilage matrix they secrete, of course, separates them to an increasing extent (note the lighter central part of the mesenchyme indicated by an arrow in Fig. 15-36). This stage is more obvious in the development of a larger bone such as that shown in Figure 15-37, where an obvious cartilage model of the bone-to-be is seen.

The Formation of Perichondrium Around Cartilage Models. The mesenchyme immediately beside each developing cartilage model becomes condensed to form a surrounding membrane for it, called the *perichondrium* (Fig. 15-36, dp, and Fig. 15-37, P). It eventually develops two layers. The cells in its outer part (*fibrous layer*) differentiate into fibroblasts and form collagen; the outer part of the perichondrium thus becomes a connective tissue sheath. The mesenchymal cells in its inner part (between its fibrous layer and the cartilage model) remain relatively undifferentiated, retaining almost all the potentiality of the cells from which they are derived. They constitute the *chondrogenic layer* of the perichondrium.

The Growth of Cartilage Models of Bones-to-Be

Cartilage models increase in size by both interstitial growth (p. 372) and appositional growth (p. 372). Their growth in length is due to interstitial growth (Fig. 14-3); this involves both the division and enlargement of chondrocytes and the formation of additional intercellular substance by the chondrocytes. The models also grow in width. Although at first interstitial growth may be a factor in this, most of the later growth in width is accomplished by the appositional mechanism; that is, new layers of cartilage are added to the surface of the sides of the model by the proliferation and the differentiation of the cells of the chondrogenic layer of the perichondrium (Fig. 14-3, appositional growth).

Most of the cell division responsible for the interstitial growth in length of a model occurs near its ends rather than in its midsection. Hence, as growth continues, the chondrocytes left in the midsection of the model have time to mature. As they become larger, the intercellular substance about them becomes somewhat thinned out (Fig. 15-38). When the chondrocytes have become sufficiently hypertrophied and mature in this central region (hc in Fig. 15-38), the matrix surrounding them becomes calcified. This prevents the matrix from serving any longer as a means for diffusion of nutrients to the chondrocytes, so they die. With their death the lacunae appear mostly empty (Fig. 15-38), and seen afterward the lacunae combine to form cavities.

During the period in which the changes described above are taking place in the midsection of a cartilage model, the progressive development of the vascular system of the embryo leads to the perichondrium of the model being invaded by capillaries. Before their appearance, the relatively undifferentiated cells of the inner (chondrogenic) layer of the perichondrium, by prolifer-

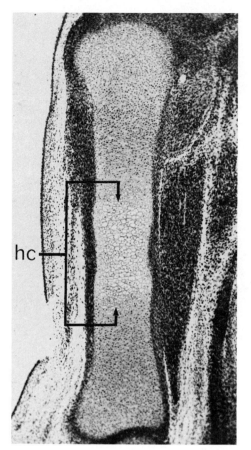

Fig. 15-38. Low-power photomicrograph of part of a leg of a rabbit embryo. This cartilage model is at a more advanced stage than in Figure 15-37 and the future form of the bone-to-be is well outlined. Note the hypertrophied chondrocytes (hc) in the middle region of the model.

ation and differentiation into cartilage cells, have been adding new layers of cartilage to the sides of the model (appositional growth) as shown in Figure 14-3. However, the appearance of capillaries in the perichondrium is associated with a changing differentiation pattern in the relatively undifferentiated cells of what up to now has been called the chondrogenic layer of the perichondrium. These cells, instead of continuing to differentiate into chondrocytes, begin to differentiate in the presence of capillaries into osteoblasts and osteocytes, with the result that a thin layer or shell of bone matrix is soon laid down around the shaft of the model (Fig. 15-39B). Since the membrane previously termed *perichondrium* now covers a shell of bone (*see* details in Fig. 15-39B) that has been laid down around the cartilage model, this membrane is now referred to as the *periosteum*.

The fact that the proliferating cells in the deep chon-

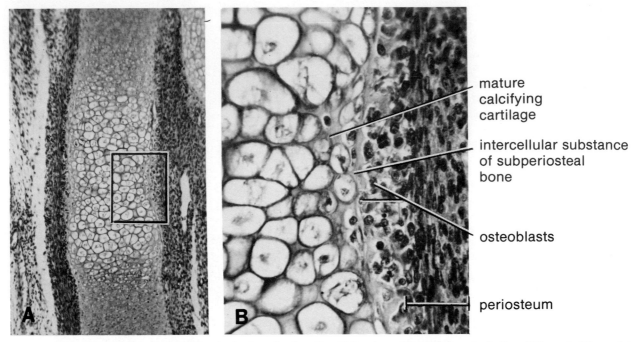

Fig. 15-39. (*A*) Photomicrograph of a developing bone in a leg of a rabbit embryo. The chondrocytes in the middle part of the model have hypertrophied and the matrix around them has calcified. (*B*) High-power photomicrograph of the area indicated in (*A*). The osteogenic cells of the former perichondrium (now the periosteum) have differentiated into osteoblasts and these have laid down a thin shell of intercellular substance of bone (subperiosteal bone) around the midsection of the model.

drogenic layer of the perichondrium now begin to differentiate into osteoblasts instead of cartilage cells should not be interpreted as indicating a change in the nature of these cells but should be attributed to a change in their microenvironment. The important factor here is probably more oxygen brought to them by the invading capillaries. The cells of the inner layer of the perichondrium, which at this stage becomes the periosteum, are osteogenic cells, and as described on page 392 they still retain their ability to differentiate into chondrocytes and form cartilage even into adult life, which ability they manifest in the repair of broken bones (Fig. 15-17). As already explained, these cells are best termed *osteogenic cells* and they are the pluripotential stem cells of the bone cell lineage, since they are able to differentiate into either cartilage- or bone-forming cells, depending on their microenvironment.

The Further Development of the Model

At this stage of development, the thinned out and calcified cartilage in the midsection of the model is beginning to weaken (Figs. 15-38 and 15-39) and the shaft of the model has gained a surrounding shell of supportive bone laid down by the recently vascularized perichondrium, now termed the *periosteum* (Fig. 15-39). Since the bone

formed here lies beneath the periosteum, between it and the cartilage model, it is called *subperiosteal bone*. It is of course, the same kind of bone that forms in so-called membranous areas, in cartilage, or anywhere else.

As development proceeds the cells of the condensed mesenchyme external to the osteogenic cells have differentiated into fibroblasts and produced collagenic fibers, so the periosteum now has two fairly distinct layers, an outer *fibrous* layer and an inner *osteogenic* one. The periosteum, however, unlike the former perichondrium, has a capillary blood supply, so it provides the vascular environment required for further bone formation.

The Formation of a Periosteal Bud. As the calcified cartilage in the midsection of the model begins to disintegrate, a bud of osteogenic cells, capillaries, and pericytes derived from the periosteum penetrates the breaking-down calcified cartilage at some site, usually near the middle of the model, and enters the interior of the cartilage model (Fig. 15-40, arrow). The invading osteogenic cells, capillaries, and pericytes constitute what is called the *periosteal bud* of a developing long bone. In some bones there may be more than one periosteal bud.

When the osteogenic cells and capillaries of the periosteal bud reach the interior of the midsection of the cartilage model, they are said to constitute a *center of ossifica-*

Fig. 15-40. Photomicrograph of a developing metatarsal bone (mouse embryo) at a stage where the calcified cartilage in the central part of the model is breaking down, resulting in the formation of spaces. The intercellular substance of the subperiosteal bone forming here around the midsection of the model stains more darkly than the cartilage it is covering. Osteogenic cells and blood vessels have grown into this central region at the site of the periosteal bud (arrow). In their vascular environment the osteogenic cells are beginning to differentiate into osteoblasts; these will lay down intercellular substance of bone on the remnants of the calcified cartilage.

Spaces in breaking-down calcified cartilage

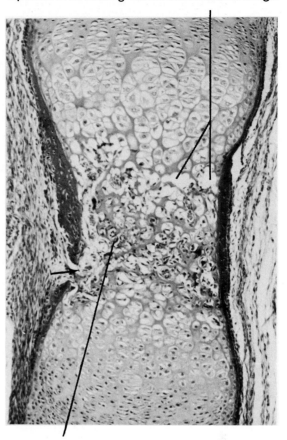

being invaded by blood vessels and osteo-blasts of periosteal bud (arrow).

tion; this means that bone formation beginning here will spread out to replace most of the cartilage model. In this process proliferating osteogenic cells gather round the remaining remnants of calcified cartilage and differentiate into osteoblasts that lay down bone intercellular substance over them (Fig. 15-41). The calcified cartilage still remaining in this part of the model is in the form of an irregular network riddled with spaces. The first bone formed in this area, since it is deposited on the cartilage remnants, is cancellous and its trabeculae have cores of calcified cartilage. In a good H and E section, this makes a pretty picture because the cores of calcified cartilage matrix are blue, while the bone covering them is pink or red (Fig. 15-41). The osteoblasts covering the trabeculae are blue.

The Development of the Stroma of Myeloid Tissue and Blood Cell Formation in It. As the subperiosteal bone becomes thicker (the process by which the bony shaft

grows in width will be described in detail shortly), there is no further need for the support provided by the first cancellous bone forming in the central part of the shaft, so it is gradually resorbed by osteoclasts. As this is taking place the stroma of myeloid tissue is formed from the components of the periosteal bud, as described on page 311, and the stroma is in turn seeded by circulating CFUs that begin multiplying in this environment and forming the different lines of blood cells described in Chapter 12. However, as noted in Chapter 12, some osteogenic cells persist in the stroma of the developing marrow.

The Terms Diaphysis and Epiphysis. At this stage of development the middle part of what was previously a solid cartilage model is now different from the two cartilaginous ends of the model. The midsection (the shaft of the future bone) is now essentially bony, consisting of a shell of subperiosteal bone, with a diminishing amount of

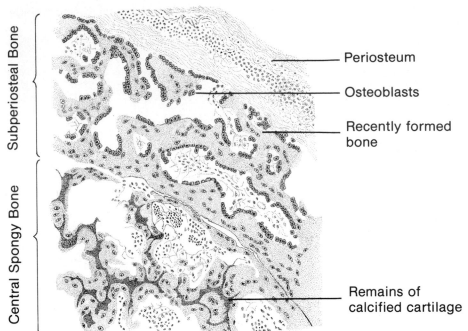

Subperiosteal Bone

Central Spongy Bone

— Periosteum

— Osteoblasts

— Recently formed bone

— Remains of calcified cartilage

Fig. 15-41. Diagrammatic drawing of a growing long bone (humerus) of sheep fetus, in cross section. Note the trabeculae of the central spongy (cancellous) bone show cores of calcified cartilage; these cores stain blue in contrast to the bone, which stains pink or red with H and E. (After Addison, W. H. F.: Piersol's Normal Histology. ed. 15. Philadelphia, J. B. Lippincott, 1932)

cancellous bone and an increasing amount of myeloid tissue in its interior. This portion of a bone is termed its *diaphysis,* a Greek word meaning something between and separating two other things. The two things thus separated are the cartilaginous ends of the model (Fig. 15-42). These are called *epiphyses* (Gr. *epiphysis,* outgrowth or excrescence) because the two epiphyses are in a sense excrescences, one on each end of the diaphysis. The common synonym for *diaphysis* is *shaft.* So at this point of development there is a bony diaphysis (shaft) with a cartilaginous epiphysis at each end.

The Diaphyseal Center of Ossification. Since the first center of ossification appears in a developing long bone as a result of the invasion of the middle part of the cartilage model by the cells of the periosteal bud, and since the middle part of the model becomes the diaphysis of the bone, the first center of ossification in a long bone is termed the *primary* or *diaphyseal center of ossification.*

The Further Growth of the Model

The models of all long bones are only able to grow in length because of *interstitial growth occurring in their cartilaginous epiphyses.* As a result, the epiphyses of a model would constantly elongate were it not for the fact that the epiphyseal cartilage abutting on the ends of the bony shaft (diaphysis) matures and calcifies, and as it dies it becomes replaced by bone forming from osteogenic

cells that invade it from the diaphysis. (To avoid duplication we postpone giving an account and illustrations of this process until we have described another stage in bone growth.) But first, when short bones (carpals of the hands and most of the tarsals of the feet) finish growing during their development, their large cartilaginous epiphyses eventually become replaced almost entirely with bone from the diaphysis; only a thin rim persists to serve as an articular cartilage. Immediately beneath each articular cartilage the bone trabeculae, instead of persisting as isolated trabeculae, form a supportive plate-like structure for the cartilage. The cartilage above it remains alive and is nourished by the synovial (joint) fluid (to be described presently). We shall now describe what happens in the development of longer bones since this differs in certain respects from that of short bones.

Epiphyseal Centers of Ossification. The development of the long bones of the body is complicated by the additional development of *epiphyseal centers of ossification.* In the simplest kind of long bone (shown in Fig. 15-43) a center of ossification develops in each of the two cartilaginous epiphyses. Each of these in due course gives rise to a bony epiphysis which, however, retains a covering of articular cartilage if it participates in a joint. The development of an epiphyseal center of ossification is heralded by maturation of chondrocytes in and near the middle of a cartilaginous end of a model. The chondrocytes here hypertrophy and the intercellular substance

cartilaginous epiphysis

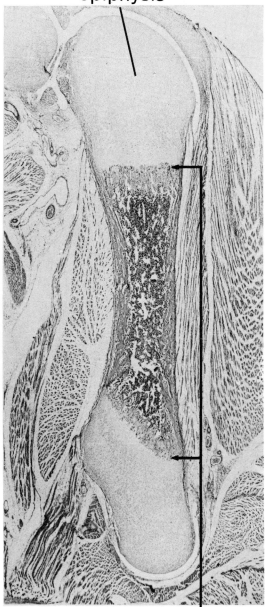

bony diaphysis

Fig. 15-42. Very low power photomicrograph of a developing femur of a rabbit. At this stage the cartilage of the model has been replaced by bone except at its ends. The bone formed by the periosteum and the periosteal bud constitutes the diaphysis; the cartilage left at the ends of the bone constitutes the epiphyses.

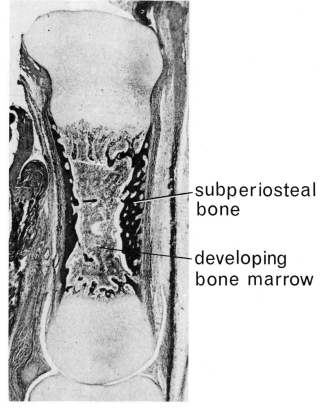

subperiosteal bone

developing bone marrow

Fig. 15-43. Low-power photomicrograph of a developing long bone. At this stage there is a substantial layer of subperiosteal bone around its midsection, and cartilage has disappeared from this central part of the model, which now contains myeloid tissue. Bone formation is advancing toward the ends of the bone but the epiphyses are still wholly cartilaginous; they will eventually develop epiphyseal centers of ossification and become replaced by bone, except for their very ends which will remain as the articular cartilages of the bone.

about them becomes thinned out and calcified so that the chondrocytes die. Cavities soon form and become invaded (presumably from the side of the model) by counterparts of the periosteal bud that grew into the diaphysis. The invading tissue consists of capillaries and osteogenic cells. The latter form osteoblasts that lay down bone on the remnants of calcified cartilage matrix just as in the diaphyseal center (Fig. 15-44). Meanwhile, the living chondrocytes immediately surrounding this area also begin to mature and die; the process of ossification then spreads out from the epiphyseal center in all directions (Fig. 15-44). However, ossification stops short of replacing all the cartilage in the end of a model. Enough is

epiphyseal   developing ossification
disk   center in epiphysis

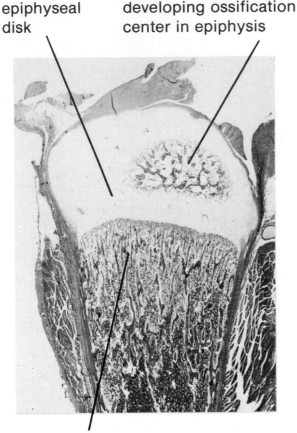

trabeculae on diaphyseal
side of epiphyseal disk

Fig. 15-44. Low-power photomicrograph of the upper end of a tibia (kitten) shortly after appearance of a center of ossification in the epiphysis. The cartilage that remains between the bone forming from the epiphyseal center of ossification and that forming from the diaphyseal center constitutes the epiphyseal disk.

left at articulating ends to constitute an articular cartilage (labeled in Fig. 15-45A). Furthermore, a transverse disk (plate) of cartilage extending right across the bone is retained between the bone derived from each epiphyseal center of ossification and that derived from the diaphyseal center. This transverse disk (plate) of cartilage separating the epiphyseal bone from the diaphyseal bone is termed the *epiphyseal disk* or *plate* (Figs. 15-44 and 15-45A). It persists until postnatal longitudinal growth of the bone has been completed; only then is it replaced by bone. It is of tremendous importance, for, as we shall soon explain, it alone is responsible for allowing the shaft of the long bone to lengthen until full growth is obtained.

The route by which capillaries and osteogenic cells gain entrance to the central part of an epiphysis probably is indicated later by the course of the larger blood vessels supplying that epiphysis. The blood supply of epiphyses will be described later in connection with the blood supply of bones.

The Growth of Models in Which Epiphyseal Centers of Ossification Have Appeared

The further longitudinal growth of the shaft of a long bone is accounted for by continuance of interstitial growth of cartilage cells in the epiphyseal disk. Since epiphyseal disks separate the bone-containing epiphyses from the bony diaphysis, interstitial growth of the cartilage of the epiphyseal plate (Fig. 15-46) constantly tends to thicken the plate and hence displace the bone of the epiphysis away from that of the diaphysis. The result is that the length of the model becomes increased. Actually, however, the thickness of the epiphyseal disk does not become increased even though interstitial growth occurs in it. This is because of the continuing maturation, calcification, and death of cartilage followed by replacement with newly formed bone on the diaphyseal side of the disk (Fig. 15-46).

A common error made in connection with describing what happens in an epiphyseal plate is to think of the chondrocytes, which are situated in rows, as moving down the plate toward the diaphysis as they become older. Actually the older cells that might be thought to have moved down the plate have, in relation to a fixed point in the cartilage matrix beside them, stayed exactly where they were (*see* the markers A and B in Fig. 15-46) and the multiplication of young chondrocytes above them has thickened the plate above them and moved the upper part of the epiphysis farther away from them and the diaphysis. If chondrocytes merely moved down their rows in the plate there would, of course, be no elongation of the bone.

There is then, as shown in Figure 15-46, a persistent race between two (in a sense opposing) processes in an epiphyseal plate: (*1*) interstitial growth, which tends to *thicken* it, and (*2*) calcification and consequent death of chondrocytes on the diaphyseal side of the plate; here the plate is being constantly *thinned* because of it being continuously replaced by bone. The latter process increases the length of the bony shaft. The race is eventually won by the latter process, but only after full growth in length has been attained in postnatal life. At this stage interstitial growth ceases in the plate and in man (but not in certain rodents) the cartilaginous plate becomes entirely replaced with bone from the diaphysis.

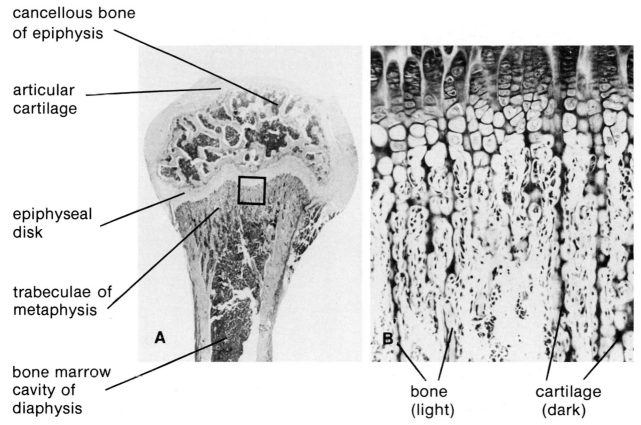

cancellous bone
of epiphysis

articular
cartilage

epiphyseal
disk

trabeculae of
metaphysis

bone marrow
cavity of
diaphysis

A

B

bone
(light)

cartilage
(dark)

Fig. 15-45. (*A*). Low-power photomicrograph of one end of a growing long bone (rat). Osteogenesis has now spread from the epiphyseal center of ossification so that only the articular cartilage above and the epiphyseal disk below remain cartilaginous. On the diaphyseal side of the epiphyseal plate (disk), metaphyseal trabeculae extend down into the diaphysis. (*B*) Medium-power photomicrograph of the area indicated in (*A*), showing trabeculae on the diaphyseal side of the epiphyseal plate (disk). These have cores of calcified cartilage on which bone has been deposited. The cartilaginous cores of the trabeculae were formerly partitions between columns of chondrocytes in the epiphyseal plate (disk).

The Light Microscopic Structure of an Epiphyseal Plate

If a longitudinal section of a growing bone is examined with the LM so as to allow the eye to sweep across the full thickness of the epiphyseal disk from its epiphyseal to its diaphyseal aspect (Fig. 15-47), the cartilage of the plate presents four successively different appearances. From the epiphysis to the diaphysis these regions, each of which merges imperceptibly into the next, are: (*1*) the *zone of resting cartilage,* (*2*) the *zone of proliferating young cartilage,* (*3*) the *zone of maturing cartilage,* and (*4*) the *zone of calcifying cartilage.* These four zones are labeled in Figure 15-47. Their special characteristics and functions will now be described.

(*1*) The zone of resting cartilage lies immediately adjacent to the bone of the epiphysis. Chondrocytes of moderate size are scattered irregularly throughout its intercellular substance. In some sites the cartilage of this zone is separated from the bone of the epiphysis by spaces containing blood vessels (Fig. 15-47). This zone of cartilage does not participate in the growth of the epiphyseal plate. It serves, first, to *anchor the plate* to the bone of the epiphysis; second, the capillaries in the spaces between it and the bone (Fig. 15-47) have been shown to be the source of the nutrients that by diffusion *nourish the cells in the other zones of the plate.*

(*2*) The second zone is composed of young proliferating cartilage cells. These are commonly thin and many are wedge-shaped. The cells in this zone are piled on top of one another like stacks of coins so that they form columns perpendicular to the plate (Fig. 15-47). In a growing bone, mitotic figures can be found among these cells. The plane

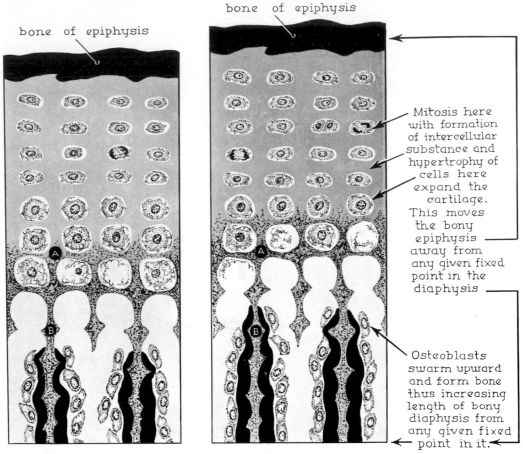

Fig. 15-46. Diagrams of two longitudinal sections cut through the same epiphyseal plate and part of the diaphysis of a growing long bone. The diagram on the right illustrates the changes that occur in what is represented in the left over a short period of time. Cartilage is gray, calcified cartilage is stippled, and bone is black. The sites labeled A and B are fixed points and remain at the same level in both diagrams. Note, however, that the "bone of epiphysis" has moved upward in the diagram on the right, and that the level of calcified cartilage and bone is also higher in the diagram on the right. (Ham, A. W.: J. Bone Joint Surg., *34-A:*701, 1952)

in which mitosis occurs exhibits considerable variability. It seems likely that the column arrangement is maintained because the bundles of collagenic fibrils in the partitions of intercellular substance between the columns run longitudinally (Ham). The function of this zone is *cell proliferation.* This is the site where a sufficient number of new cells must be produced to replace those that die at the diaphyseal surface of the disk, as will be described.

(*3*) The third zone contains cartilage cells in various stages of *maturation.* These, too, are arranged in columns. Those nearest the zone of proliferating cartilage are the least mature, and those nearest the diaphysis are the oldest and most mature (Fig. 15-47).

The cells of this zone were originally in the proliferating zone but were left behind as their neighbors on the epiphyseal side continued to proliferate and so drew away from them. The cells left behind in this zone gradually mature. In this process they become larger and accumulate glycogen in their cytoplasm. In becoming larger they take up more space and hence expand the epiphyseal disk longitudinally. The epiphyseal plate is therefore expanded in the long axis of the bone both by proliferation of cells in the second zone and by maturation of cells in the third zone. Moreover, the cells of this zone produce alkaline phosphatase, as may be demonstrated in sections by histochemical methods (Fig. 15-48). As this zone

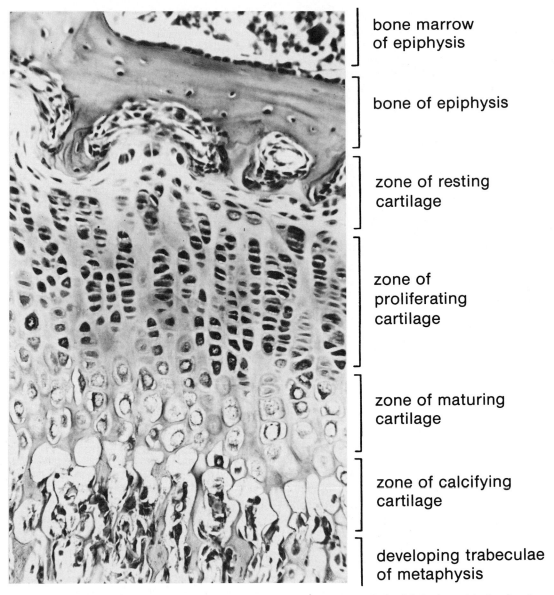

bone marrow
of epiphysis

bone of epiphysis

zone of resting
cartilage

zone of
proliferating
cartilage

zone of maturing
cartilage

zone of calcifying
cartilage

developing trabeculae
of metaphysis

Fig. 15-47. Photomicrograph of the epiphyseal plate (disk) at the upper end of a tibia (guinea pig), showing the various zones of cartilage in the plate.

merges into the next the intercellular substance around the cartilage cells becomes *increasingly calcified.* With the occurrence of calcification in the cartilage the third zone becomes the fourth zone.

(4) The fourth zone is very thin, being only one or a few cartilage cells thick. This zone abuts directly on the diaphysis so that it is invaded by both capillaries and osteogenic cells from the diaphysis.

Factors Involved in the Calcification of the Cartilage in Zone 4

First it is to be appreciated that although there may be some variations in different species, the chondrocytes in an epiphyseal plate in the common laboratory animals studied are supplied with nutrients that diffuse *"down" the plate* from the capillaries in zone 1. This is shown by

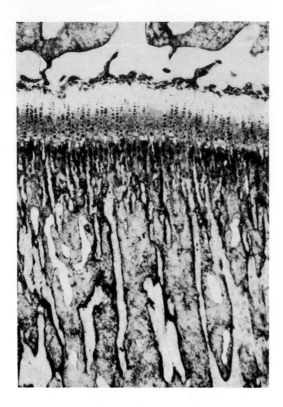

Fig. 15-48. Photomicrograph of an epiphyseal plate (disk) and metaphyseal trabeculae of a tibia (rat) stained histochemically for alkaline phosphatase. Note there is a dark band of phosphatase activity in the region of hypertrophied chondrocytes in the plate and another in the region of the osteoblasts invading the diaphyseal side of the plate. The zone of calcified cartilage is relatively free from phosphatase (it contains few living cells). (Morse, A., and Greep, R. O.: Anat. Rec., *111:*193, 1951)

the fact that if the plate becomes separated at the border between zones 3 and 4 from the diaphysis, the plate continues to grow in thickness, though separated from the diaphysis; indeed, as shown by Dale and Harris, the plate becomes even thicker than it would have been had it still been connected to the diaphysis (Fig. 15-64).

Second, the reason for a plate (connected to the diaphysis) remaining of a more or less constant thickness is that if it is connected to the diaphysis the cartilage matrix becomes calcified in zone 4 and its cells die (Fig. 15-47). The calcified cartilage matrix left behind is in part dissolved away by osteoclasts and in part covered with bone, as will be described shortly.

What Causes the Cartilage in Zone 4 to Become Calcified? There would seem to be three important factors.

(*1*) The hypertrophied cartilage cells secrete alkaline phosphatase (Fig. 15-48).

(*2*) Matrix vesicles (MV in Fig. 15-49) are liberated from the chondrocytes into the cartilage matrix between adjacent rows of chondrocytes at this site.

(*3*) Calcium and phosphate ions from the blood become abundant for the calcification process in zone 4 of the plate because blood capillaries from the diaphysis grow into any available interstices in the cartilage at the bottom of the plate (Fig. 15-50). It will now be explained how the calcified cartilage of zone 4 is invaded by capillaries and osteogenic cells.

The Process by Which the Calcified Cartilage Matrix Is Replaced by Bone in Zone 4

The calcified cartilage matrix exposed to the diaphysis in zone 4 begins to break up in a special way as it is invaded from the diaphysis by osteogenic cells and capillaries. To explain this we have to distinguish between two kinds of partitions of matrix in the plate. First, there are very thin partitions between the chondrocytes in any given column (Figs. 15-47 and 15-50). Second, as seen in longitudinal sections, there are thicker partitions of matrix between adjacent columns (Fig. 15-47).

The Invasion of Capillaries. As shown in Figure 15-50, the capillaries from the diaphysis invade the columns of chondrocytes from the diaphyseal side when the chondrocytes in zone 4 die and the partitions between their now empty lacunae disintegrate. The capillaries (the red blood cells of which are darkly stained in Fig. 15-50) grow in as loops. They sometimes rupture as they penetrate newly vacated lacunae so that blood cells may escape into lacunae. An example is indicated by an arrow in Figure 15-50.

Blood leakage at this site probably explains why this is where a disease process termed the juvenile type of *osteomyelitis* (Gr. *osteon,* bone; *myelos,* marrow), which means inflammation of the bone marrow, commonly begins. This condition can arise in a child that has had an

Fig. 15-49. Electron micrograph showing matrix vesicles (MV) liberated from chondrocytes (Ch) into cartilage matrix. Note also the collagenic fibrils in the cartilage matrix. (Anderson, H. C.: *In* Bourne, G. H. (ed.): The Biochemistry and Physiology of Bone. ed. 2, vol. 4. New York, Academic Press, 1976)

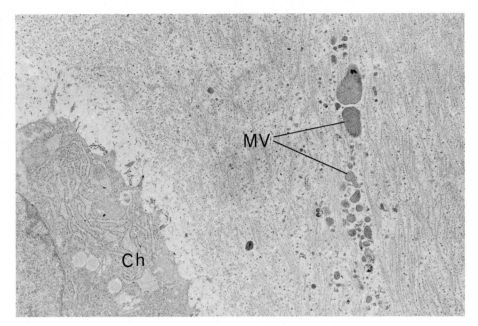

infection somewhere else in his body from which bacteria are to some extent gaining entrance into his bloodstream. This site on the diaphyseal side of the epiphyseal plate of a growing bone where capillaries are leaking blood seems to be a particularly vulnerable site where bacteria gaining entrance to the bloodstream escape again and set up an infection in this area.

The Invasion of Osteogenic Cells and Osteoblasts. As shown in Figure 15-46, some of the partitions of calcified matrix between rows of cartilage cells also disappear. Those that remain are soon covered with bone (Fig. 15-46). This occurs because osteogenic cells multiply and move into the area, where they differentiate into osteoblasts that arrange themselves along the remnants of the cartilaginous trabeculae and cover them with a layer of bone (Fig. 15-47). This results, on the diaphyseal side of the epiphyseal disk, in the formation of what appear in longitudinal sections (Fig. 15-45B) as longitudinally disposed bone *trabeculae* with cartilaginous cores, the cartilage cores of which are continuous with the as yet uncalcified cartilaginous intercellular substance of the disk (partitions between columns), and by this means the newly formed bony trabeculae are united firmly with the substance of the cartilaginous disk.

Summary of the Mechanism by Which a Bone Grows in Length

Interstitial growth of cartilage in the epiphyseal side of an epiphyseal plate pushes the epiphysis farther away

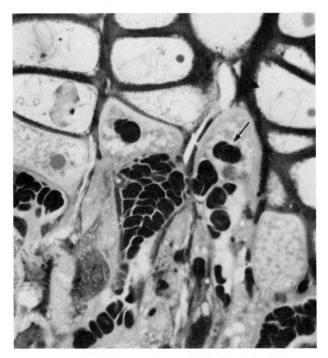

Fig. 15-50. Photomicrograph (×500) of part of the diaphyseal side of an epiphyseal plate, stained with toluidine blue. Capillaries, filled with dark-staining erythrocytes, loop up at *center* toward the plate from the metaphysis below. Some of these capillary loops may rupture (*see* text) and release their erythrocytes into lacunae of the disk, as indicated by arrow. (Serafini-Fracassini, A., and Smith, J. W.: The Structure and Biochemistry of Cartilage. Edinburgh, Churchill-Livingstone, 1974)

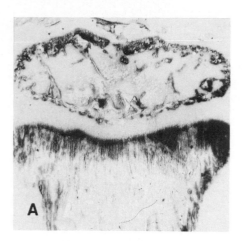

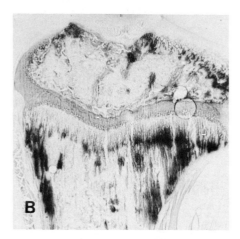

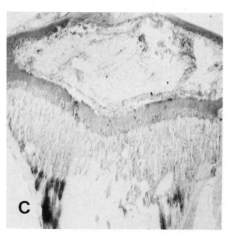

Fig. 15-51. (*A*) Radioautograph of the end of a tibia of a rat, 5 minutes after injection of radiophosphorus. (*B*) Similar preparation from rat 2 days after injection. (*C*) Similar preparation from rat 8 days after injection. For description, *see* text. (Leblond, C. P., Wilkinson, G. W., Bélanger, L. F., and Robichon, J.: Am. J. Anat., 86:289, 1950)

from the diaphysis. But the epiphyseal plate does not become thicker because it is just as constantly resorbed and replaced by bone on its diaphyseal aspect. This new bone, which is in the form of what seem to be longitudinally disposed bony trabeculae with cartilaginous cores (Figs. 15-45 and 15-46), makes the diaphysis longer.

The growth mechanism described above is the *only* mechanism by which the diaphysis can become lengthened. Bone cannot undergo interstitial growth. It can grow only by the appositional mechanism, and, as is shown in Figure 15-46, the new bone that is "apposed" and accounts for the growth in length of the diaphysis is added *to the ends of the prolongations of bone that extend into the cartilage;* this increases the penetration of the cartilage and makes the metaphysis longer (Fig. 15-46).

Resorption at the Diaphyseal Ends of Trabeculae

Since the epiphyseal ends of the bony trabeculae in this zone are constantly being elongated by the mechanism described above, it might be thought that the zone of trabeculated bone in the metaphysis would become increasingly elongated during the growing period. Instead, however, except at the periphery of the bone, this zone of trabeculated bone stays about the same length (Fig. 15-45A). This can only mean that as rapidly as bone is added to the (epiphyseal) ends of the metaphyseal trabeculae in the zone of calcification, bone is resorbed from their free (diaphyseal) ends that project toward the marrow cavity of the diaphysis. Osteoclasts commonly are seen here; often they are wrapped around the free ends of trabeculae as shown in Figure 15-33.

That the trabeculae present under the more central part of an epiphyseal disk of a growing animal at any given time are not the same ones that are present several days later is illustrated convincingly by means of radioautographs. As is shown in Figure 15-51A, a single injection of radioactive phosphorus given an animal will be taken up and hence will label the bone that is forming and calcifying at this time. However, the bone continues to grow in length and so the new bone that is added continuously (after the radioactive phosphorus is "used up") to the epiphyseal ends of the trabeculae—the ends that extend into the epiphyseal disk—is not labeled. So a considerable band of new unlabeled bone has already been formed there 2 days after the administration of the radiophosphorus (Fig. 15-51B). Meanwhile, the labeled bone of the trabeculae has been resorbed from the free (diaphyseal) ends of the trabeculae, so that the average total length of labeled bone in the trabeculae is shorter than it was 2 days previously. After 8 days all the labeled bone has been eroded from the trabeculae under the central part of the disk (Fig. 15-51C). Hence, the trabeculae present at this time (8 days after the radiophosphorus was administered) are composed of bone that has formed and calcified during the 8 days; therefore they are not the same trabeculae that were present 8 days before. However, it is to be noted that Figure 15-51C shows the persistence of some of the labeled bone in the developing shaft, some distance below the epiphyseal disk; why some of the bone that formed 8 days before under the periphery of the epiphyseal disk has persisted and has now become part of the shaft will be explained in the next section.

Under the *periphery of the epiphyseal disk,* the fate of the trabeculae is different from that described for the trabeculae under its more central part. However, an explanation of what happens to these involves a discussion of how a long bone *as a whole* changes in size and histological appearance during the growing period, and so we shall discuss this matter first.

THE GROWTH OF A BONE AS A WHOLE

Speaking generally, the growth in length of bones that develop in cartilage is fundamentally dependent on the ability of the cartilage that persists in them as epiphyseal disks or at their ends to grow by the interstitial mechanism, while at one of its aspects it is replaced by bone growing by the appositional mechanism at the same rate.

(*1*) Short bones such as the carpals do not develop epiphyseal centers of ossification and hence they depend for longitudinal growth on the interstitial growth of cartilage at their ends. This is replaced by bone from the diaphyseal center of ossification in the same way that cartilage is replaced on the diaphyseal side of an epiphyseal plate. What is left of it when growth in length is over becomes the articular cartilage of a joint.

(*2*) In long bones in which epiphyseal centers of ossification develop, and hence which have epiphyseal disks, interstitial growth of the cartilage of the part of the epiphyses that becomes the articular cartilage provides only for growth in size of the epiphyses and not for growth of the diaphysis. Articular cartilage may provide for growth in width of the epiphysis as well as for its growth in length, as will be described in the next chapter.

(*3*) In long bones that have epiphyseal disks, the interstitial growth of cartilage in the disks does not assist in the growth of the epiphysis after the bony epiphyses are reasonably well developed. After an epiphysis is well developed, the cartilage of an epiphyseal disk is no longer replaced with bone on its epiphyseal side, but only on its diaphyseal side (Fig. 15-47). With these facts established we can now consider some further points about the growth of a long bone as a whole.

The diaphyses of many long bones funnel outward as they approach their epiphyses (Fig. 15-52); hence, many bones are of a much greater diameter in their metaphyseal regions (the *metaphysis* is the part of the shaft that in a growing bone is composed of bony trabeculae that have cores of cartilage and is directly adjacent to the diaphyseal side of an epiphyseal disk) than in their midsections (Fig. 15-52). As may be seen by comparing the left and the right sides of Figure 15-52, the site, along the longitudinal axis of a bone, that is occupied by the flared metaphyseal portion of the diaphysis will, as the bone continues to elongate, be occupied later by the tubular and considerably narrower portion of the shaft. This means that as growth in length continues, the diameter of the portion of the shaft that is flared at any given time subsequently must become decreased. This requires that bone be resorbed continuously from the exterior of the flared portion (and osteoclasts are numerous here), and built up continuously on its inner aspect so that it can become a narrower shaft. We shall now consider how bone is built up on the inner aspect of the flared portion so that bone can be resorbed from its outer aspect without weakening the bone.

Why What Appear as Isolated Trabeculae Are Really the Walls of Tunnels. It is easy to get the impression from longitudinal sections of growing bone that the trabeculae of the metaphysis are like stalactites, hanging down from the diaphyseal side of the plate. However, if cross sections are cut of the metaphyses of larger mammals close to the plate, it will be found that only the free ends of the trabeculae are stalactite-like. Closer to the plate, the structures that in longitudinal sections appear as stalactite-like trabeculae are revealed in cross sections to be connected together to constitute a network honeycombed with spaces that are the lumina of tunnels (Fig. 15-53). Why the newly formed bony trabeculae (which have cartilaginous cores) appear to be isolated from one another in longitudinal sections and should appear, when seen in cross section, to comprise a cancellous network will now be explained.

In the zone of maturing cartilage the cartilage cells are arranged in longitudinal rows separated from one another by partitions of intercellular substance. If this area is visualized in 3 dimensions, it will be obvious that the rows of cells are contained in longitudinal tunnels, and that the partitions of intercellular substance between the rows of cells are the walls of these longitudinally disposed tunnels. As the cartilage cells in a tunnel mature and die at its diaphyseal end, the thinner partitions between tunnels tend to disintegrate, and by this means tunnels only one cartilage cell wide fuse with others of the same size to become relatively large tunnels, as shown in longitudinal section in Figure 15-46. These are invaded from the diaphysis by osteogenic cells, osteoblasts, and capillaries.

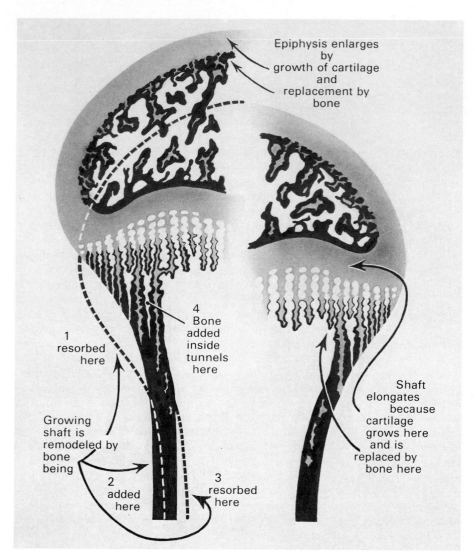

Epiphysis enlarges
by
growth of cartilage
and
replacement by
bone

1
resorbed
here

4
Bone
added
inside
tunnels
here

Growing
shaft is
remodeled by
bone
being

2
added
here

3
resorbed
here

Shaft
elongates
because
cartilage
grows here
and is
replaced by
bone here

Fig. 15-52. Diagram illustrating the surfaces where bone is deposited or resorbed during remodeling at the ends of growing long bones with flared extremities. (Ham, A. W.: J. Bone Joint Surg., *34-A:*701, 1952)

The osteoblasts line up along the sides of the tunnels and deposit bone on the tunnel surfaces (Fig. 15-46). Hence, in a longitudinal section, the wall between two adjacent tunnels will appear as a trabecula with a cartilage core that is covered on each side by a layer of bone (Fig. 15-53A and B). In other words, the bone seen *covering* the cartilaginous cores of the trabeculae in longitudinal sections is the bone that in cross section is seen to *line* the tunnels in cartilage (Fig. 15-53B). The osteoblasts that cover the trabeculae of longitudinal sections similarly are the osteoblasts that line the insides of the tunnels that are seen in cross sections. And the capillaries and the osteogenic cells that fill the spaces between the trabeculae of longitudinal sections are the contents of the tunnels seen in cross section.

How a Shaft of Compact Bone With Haversian Systems Forms Under the Periphery of the Plate. On the diaphyseal side of the more central part of the epiphyseal disk only a single layer of bone is commonly deposited inside the cartilaginous tunnels. Hence, the trabeculae seen in a longitudinal section of this area are narrow. However, at the periphery of the disk successive layers of bone are deposited inside the larger tunnels that have formed by the coalescence of a few smaller tunnels (Fig. 15-52). This narrows the lumina of these larger tunnels, and the several layers of bone laid down in them imparts a layered appearance to their thickened walls. The successive layers of bone deposited inside the tunnels are due to successive waves of appositional growth resulting from the osteogenic cells lining the tunnel undergoing proliferation

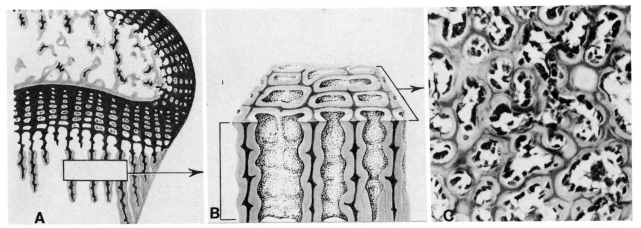

Fig. 15-53. (*A*) Diagram illustrating the way the trabeculae in a longitudinal section of an end of a growing bone appear like stalactites. (*B*) Seen in three dimensions, the so-called trabeculae near the epiphyseal plate represent walls of tunnels. (*C*) This photomicrograph shows a metaphysis of a growing bone in cross section, close to the epiphyseal plate. Here it can be seen that the so-called trabeculae are indeed the walls of tunnels and that they have cores of calcified cartilage (dark). The tunnels become filled in under the periphery of the plate to form haversian systems (the compact bone of the metaphysis).

and differentiation into the osteoblasts; these then form successive new layers of bone inside the tunnel. Finally, after several layers have been deposited, the tunnel is reduced to a narrow canal, which contains at least one blood vessel, some osteoblasts or osteogenic cells, and sometimes a lymphatic. This arrangement of a canal with concentric layers of bone surrounding it is, as noted earlier, called a *haversian system* or *osteon* (Fig. 15-56). Haversian systems represent the basic units of structure of compact (dense) bone. Each has one or two blood vessels in its canal, providing tissue fluid to nourish the osteocytes in the surrounding lamellae. As already explained, haversian systems are limited in the number of lamellae they can contain by the distance over which the canalicular mechanism can nourish osteocytes. This, of course, is not very great; hence, commonly a haversian canal is surrounded by less than half a dozen concentric lamellae (Fig. 15-56).

A haversian system (osteon) can develop only by means of a tunnel being filled in from its inside with concentric layers of bone. A haversian system, then, is in the nature of a bony tube with thick walls and a very narrow lumen. However, if ordinary tubes are bundled together side by side, crevices are left between them. Compact bone, though generally composed of longitudinally disposed tubular haversian systems, does not exhibit such crevices. With what are they filled?

Since the first compact bone forming under the periphery of a disk is the result of a cartilaginous tunnel being filled in with bone, the crevices between the haversian systems that form in this manner are at first filled with cartilage (Fig. 15-53B and C). Hence, in the shaft of a

very young growing bone, irregular bits of cartilage commonly will be seen (Fig. 15-52). It should be kept in mind by any student who wishes to understand bone growth well, that each of these bits of cartilage seen incorporated into the shaft of bone and situated between haversian systems was once part of a partition between rows of cartilage cells in the epiphyseal plate, and somewhat later became the cartilaginous core of a metaphyseal trabecula under the periphery of the plate. In the shafts of older bones, the crevices between adjacent haversian systems come to be filled with what are termed *interstitial lamellae* of bone. Why there is no cartilage between haversian systems in older bone (Fig. 15-56) will be made clear when we study how shafts of bones grow in width—our next subject.

HOW SHAFTS OF BONES GROW IN WIDTH

A long bone grows in width by new layers of bone being added to the outer aspect of the shaft by the appositional growth mechanism, while at the same time bone is eroded away from the inner aspect of the shaft. The net result of these two processes proceeding simultaneously is that, although the shaft as a whole becomes wider, its walls do not become unduly thick, and the width of the marrow cavity gradually increases. It also means that the bone of the shaft of an adult is not the same bone that made up the shaft of that bone when he was a young child which bone has all been resorbed from the inside as new bone was added to the exterior of the shaft during the growing period.

periosteal surface

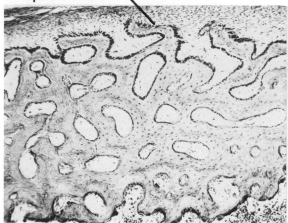

Fig. 15-54. Low-power photomicrograph of a radius of a growing puppy (cross section). Note the longitudinal ridges and grooves in the periosteal surface (*top*). The ridges are covered with osteoblasts, and the grooves lined with them. Haversian systems are developing throughout the thickness of the shaft.

The shaft of a bone grows in width by the appositional mechanism (Figs. 15-15 and 15-16). New bone is laid down beneath the periosteum by the osteogenic layer of that membrane. However, if a cross section through the shaft of a young bone growing in width is examined, it will be seen that much of the new bone of which it is composed is in the form of haversian systems. It has been explained that haversian systems always are formed as a result of tunnels (not necessarily cartilaginous ones) being filled in from the inside. How, then, can bony tunnels, to be subsequently filled in from the inside, be formed under the periosteum of a young growing bone?

A brief study of the periphery of a cross section of an actively growing shaft of a young animal will reveal how this occurs. The surface of such a shaft is not smooth; instead, it demonstrates a series of longitudinal ridges with grooves between them (Figs. 15-54 and 15-55). The osteogenic cells and the osteoblasts of the periosteum cover the tops of ridges and extend down to the bottoms of the grooves between them. The periosteum here also contains blood vessels (Fig. 15-55, 1). Longitudinal tunnels form from this arrangement as follows: the osteogenic cells of the periosteum covering the ridges proliferate, and some differentiate into osteoblasts which lay down bone so as gradually to extend the ridges over toward one another (Fig. 15-55, 2) till they meet (Fig. 15-55, 3). This converts the groove that formerly existed between 2 ridges into a tunnel. Since the groove was lined with periosteum containing osteogenic cells, osteoblasts, and

blood vessels, the tunnel now contains a lining of osteogenic cells and osteoblasts with a blood vessel somewhere in its lumen. As is shown in Figure 15-55 (4, 5, and 6), the continued proliferation of the osteogenic cells lining the tunnel, with their subsequent differentiation into osteoblasts and osteocytes, results in the tunnel being converted into a haversian system. It is in this manner that new haversian systems are added beneath the periosteum to the periphery of a young actively growing shaft.

As the growth in width of a bone slows down, the surface of the shaft becomes smoother. Appositional growth occurring under the periosteum, then, tends to add smooth, even layers to the surface of the shaft (Fig. 15-56). These are called *circumferential lamellae* because they tend to surround the whole shaft. However, if growth in width continues after they have formed, haversian systems can replace them by means of longitudinal troughs being eroded on the surface of the shaft by osteoclasts. When a longitudinal trough becomes sufficiently deep, the osteogenic cells and the osteoblasts of the periosteum line it and those at the surface roof over the trough and convert it into a tunnel. This thereupon is filled up from its interior by osteoblasts derived from osteogenic cells laying down successive lamellae of bone. By this means, bone consisting originally of circumferential lamellae or bone in almost any kind of arrangement can be replaced by bone consisting of haversian systems. In this instance, the crevices between the haversian systems filled with what are called interstitial lamellae would be the remains of the former circumferential lamellae.

The Incorporation of Periosteum-Derived Blood Vessels Into Growing Shafts of Bone—The Nature of Volkmann's Canals. As the two processes of bone deposition and bone resorption, on the outer and inner surfaces of a shaft respectively, continue through the growth period, the bone of the original shaft all eventually becomes resorbed, so that the shaft comes to be composed entirely of bone that has been deposited under the periosteum during the growing period. Since each haversian system forming under the periosteum is built around a periosteal vessel (Fig. 15-55), the blood vessels of the shaft, as growth in width continues, would seem to be vessels that were once in the periosteum and became incorporated into bone as the troughs they were in became roofed over. However, the roof forming over each trough is not quite complete. A hole is left in it at the site at which the periosteal vessel descends into the trough. As the successive haversian systems are added to the surface, the first-formed ones become more deeply buried, and so what were originally only holes in the roofs of troughs become elongated to constitute canals running at wide angles, often even right angles, to the haversian systems from the periosteum. These canals that thus come to convey periosteal vessels into the haversian canals of the compact bone shaft are

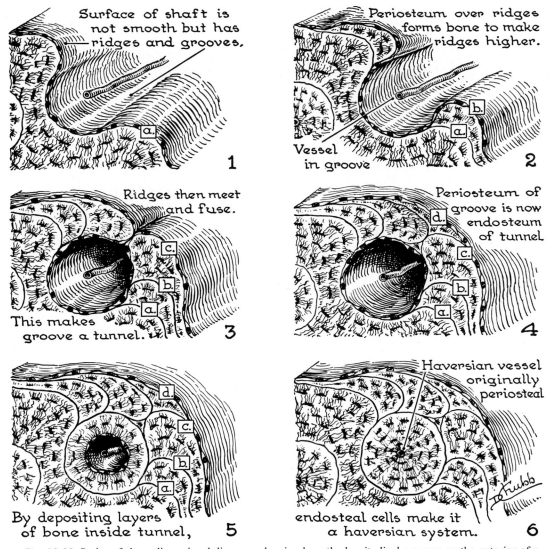

Fig. 15-55. Series of three-dimensional diagrams showing how the longitudinal grooves on the exterior of a growing bone shaft become roofed over to form tunnels, and how these are filled in with haversian systems and become incorporated so as to contribute bone substance to the periphery of the shaft. Note the way periosteal blood vessels too are incorporated so as to contribute blood supply to the shaft.

called *Volkmann's canals* (Fig. 15-56). Because of the way they are formed, they, unlike haversian canals, are not surrounded by concentric lamellae.

From the foregoing account of how a bone grows in width, it may seem that most of the blood supply of the cortex of the diaphysis of a fully grown bone would be derived from the periosteum. However, the circulation is more complicated than it seems, as will be described presently.

Circumferential, Haversian, and Interstitial Lamellae. As a bone attains its full width, it is usual for the osteoblasts

covering its outer surface and lining its inner surface to smooth these out by adding a few more or less final circumferential lamellae. These are called the *outer* and the *inner circumferential lamellae* (Figs. 15-25 and 15-56). In a sense they are like the finishing coats a plasterer applies to the walls of a room as he completes his work. Between the outer and the inner circumferential lamellae, the shaft of a bone consists of haversian systems made of haversian lamellae (Figs. 15-25B and 15-56). The crevices between these (interstitial lamellae) are either the remaining parts of old outer circumferential lamellae or old haver-

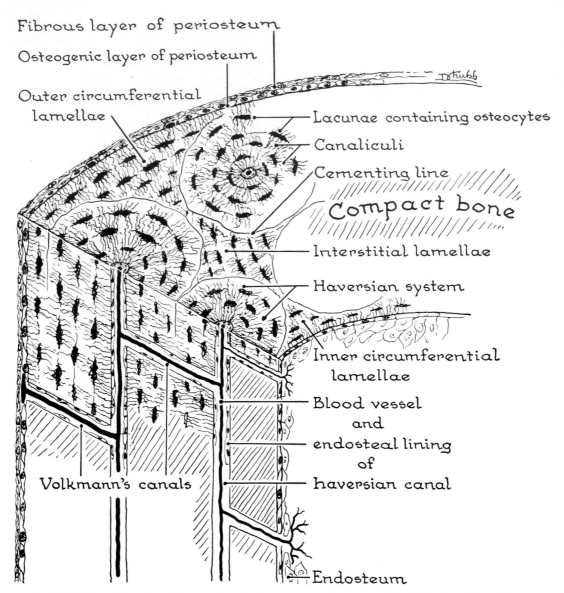

Fibrous layer of periosteum

Osteogenic layer of periosteum

Outer circumferential lamellae

Lacunae containing osteocytes

Canaliculi

Cementing line

Compact bone

Interstitial lamellae

Haversian system

Inner circumferential lamellae

Blood vessel and endosteal lining of haversian canal

Volkmann's canals

Endosteum

Fig. 15-56. Three-dimensional diagram showing the appearance in cross and longitudinal section of the components that enter into the structure of the cortex of the shaft of a long bone. There would be many more haversian systems in the cortex than shown here. The diagram shows the different kinds of lamellae and the relation between the blood vessels of the periosteum, Volkmann's canals, haversian canals, and the marrow cavity. As used here, the term blood vessels would include arteries, veins, and capillaries. Volkmann's canals extend at wide angles (sometimes virtually at right angles) to haversian systems.

sian systems (Figs. 15-25B and 15-56). There would be, of course, infinitely more haversian systems in the wall of a shaft than shown in the simplified diagram (Fig. 15-56). For this reason the actual photomicrograph of a cross section of the cortex of a long bone (Fig. 15-25B) should be studied carefully.

THE REMODELING OF BONE

The remodeling of bone can only be achieved by bone being resorbed from surfaces and added to surfaces.

Remodeling occurs under different circumstances. We have already described one kind that occurs as long bones grow in length and width. This kind ends up with a bone having its adult form and size. As already explained, the bone tissue in the bone of an adult is not the same as that present in the bone of the child because during growth the child's bone tissue is all resorbed. This type of remodeling is sometimes called *structural remodeling.*

Structural remodeling also occurs in connection with increased use or changed use of a particular bone. The formation of new extra bone, or a changed alignment of the trabeculae of cancellous bone or even of the compact (dense) bone of the shaft can occur so as to improve the ability of the bony structure to bear weight or stand up better to some new type of stress. How the need for increased or altered function can bring about resorption in some areas and new bone formation in others is not understood. What is known, however, is that the function of a bone has a great deal to do with determining its microscopic structure. For example, if a bone that is much used is put to rest, the amount of bone tissue in it becomes considerably reduced; this is termed *atrophy of disuse.*

In addition to structural remodeling there is another type sometimes termed *internal remodeling.* This is required because the haversian systems in compact bone or the trabeculae of cancellous bone do not last throughout the lifetime of an adult. Some haversian systems, or parts of them, are always being resorbed, with new ones being built in the tunnels caused by resorption. Internal remodeling occurs because bone does not last throughout life; it, like so many other tissues, must be constantly renewed, but not nearly so rapidly as other tissues.

There are many reasons for bone tissue not lasting as long as might be expected from its gross appearance. First, the canalicular mechanism by which the cells of compact bone are nourished is not a very efficient system. Anyone who understands the histology of bone and how osteocytes are nourished would expect that parts of haversian systems, particularly those farthest from haversian canals, might suffer nutritional deficiencies and hence the osteocytes in these more remote parts of systems would die. This brings up the problem of what happens to *dead bone,* that is, calcified bone in which the lacunae are empty because the osteocytes they formerly contained have died and lysed or in which lacunae contain only the pyknotic remains of dead osteocytes.

Parts of haversian systems in which osteocytes have died may persist for a long time if they are completely surrounded by haversian systems in which the bone is still alive. Hence it is not unusual in compact bone to see empty lacunae, particularly in interstitial lamellae. The probable reason for the persistence of dead bone in such locations is that any mechanisms that could bring about its resorption have no access to it. But if dead bone is exposed to the contents of a haversian canal, that is, capillaries and the blood cells they contain, in particular

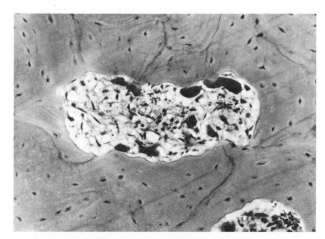

Fig. 15-57. Photomicrograph of a bone resorption cavity, probably in oblique section. The large dark cells are osteoclasts; their activity explains the etched-out borders of the cavity. (Courtesy of C. P. Leblond)

monocytes, the latter can form osteoclasts and the dead bone is resorbed. By this means what is termed a *resorption cavity* (Fig. 15-57) is formed within the bone substance. These are generally elongated tubular cavities and their normal fate in a healthy adult is that after they have been tidied up by osteoclasts in much the same way that a dentist tidies up a cavity in a tooth before he fills it (Fig. 15-57), the osteogenic cells line up around the inner surface of the cavity and form osteoblasts. The way a resorption cavity appears as it is being filled in by successive new layers of bone is shown in Figures 15-58 and 15-59.

The border between the edge of a resorption cavity, that thus becomes the boundary of a new haversian system, and the new bone of the system can be distinguished in most ordinary sections by a *cementing line* (Fig. 15-59). There is moreover another line that can be detected which is called a *frontier line* or *calcification front* (Fig. 15-59, not labeled); this line is seen between what appears to be the last layer of organic intercellular substance formed in the new haversian system and the layer that was formed previously and has become calcified. (Refer back to Fig. 15-20.) The reason for this line is that, in forming a haversian system, it takes some time for each layer of organic intercellular substance deposited to become calcified; hence in a new system the last layer to be formed, which is the layer that abuts on the lumen of the system, remains for an undetermined time in an uncalcified state and so during this period is referred to as *osteoid tissue* or *prebone.*

Although it is relatively easy from studying cross sections of bone to see resorptive cavities developing and new haversian systems being formed, it is difficult to gain

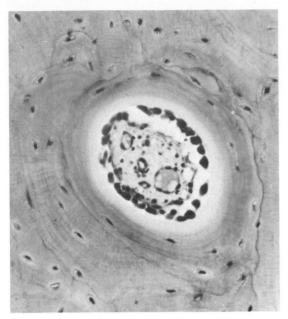

Fig. 15-58. Photomicrograph of a former resorption cavity being filled in to form a new haversian system. The dark cells encircling the cavity are osteoblasts. For details *see* right-hand side of Figure 15-59. (Courtesy of C. P. Leblond)

any appreciation of how long these systems last or how long it takes for new ones to form; in other words, ordinary studies give little information about the rate of turnover of haversian systems. There are, however, labeling methods available that allow new bone to be demonstrated as it is formed or calcified, and these can be used to determine how much new bone is formed during the time the label is available in the circulation. Radioactive calcium or phosphorus can be used to label bone mineral that is deposited when either is present in the circulation. A labeled amino acid, for example, proline, can be used to label newly forming organic matrix. It was also found that certain fluorescent substances could be injected into animals to label sites where calcification was occurring; tetracyclines have been much used for this purpose. This requires examining the sections by means of fluorescence microscopy. The various results obtained by these methods indicate that remodeling occurs to different extents in different bones and also to different extents in the same bone. From studies on dogs made by the newer methods, it appears that the annual rate at which the bone of the cortex of a long bone is replaced is somewhere between 5 and 10 per cent per year. (For details *see* Harris and Heaney.)

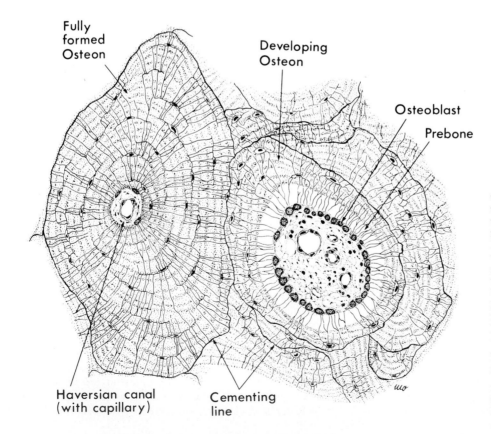

Fully formed Osteon

Developing Osteon

Osteoblast

Prebone

Haversian canal (with capillary)

Cementing line

Fig. 15-59. Diagram illustrating the way an osteon (haversian system) forms and explaining why the ring of osteoblasts lining the former resorption cavity seen in Figure 15-58 is separated from the bone by a layer of pale-staining material. As shown at *right*, this material is osteoid tissue (prebone), so called because its matrix has not yet calcified. At the periphery of this pale layer a frontier line (calcification front) marks the site where mineral is first being deposited. Farther out, cementing lines indicate where new layers of bone began to be laid down on the remains of older bone. A fully formed osteon is shown at *left*. (Courtesy of C. P. Leblond)

HOW CERTAIN NUTRITIONAL AND METABOLIC FACTORS CAN AFFECT GROWING BONES AND THE STRUCTURE OF BONES IN THE ADULT

The growing zone of a long bone is the segment of it including the epiphyseal plate that is being replaced by bone and the region of trabeculae forming beneath the plate that have cores of calcified cartilage. Thus metaphyses of growing bones are the site of great *anabolic activity*. The proliferation of osteogenic cells, their differentiation into osteoblasts, and the synthesis of organic matrix of bone at this site all involve a great deal of collagen synthesis as well as synthesis of proteoglycans and glycoproteins. With all this anabolic activity taking place, it should be obvious that any nutritional deficiencies or metabolic alterations that affect protein or even carbohydrate synthesis may be quickly reflected in some alteration of the growth pattern in this region.

Also, the growing zone is a site where calcium salts are being deposited into newly formed organic matrix at a very rapid rate. The normal growth of bone depends here on calcification occurring normally, just as it depends on protein synthesis occurring normally. Normally the two processes, (*1*) the synthesis of organic materials and (*2*) the calcification of organic intercellular substance, are synchronized. It is important to realize that the normal growth of bone depends on *two different processes* that generally operate in harmony with one another and that the factors that affect the anabolic processes are not the same factors that affect the calcification process, and vice versa. Next, because the growing zone is the site of such great activity it is very sensitive to any metabolic disturbance that may develop in a growing individual, and as a result of a metabolic disturbance its histological picture may quickly alter. The first question to ask is which process is primarily affected, the synthesis of the organic components of bone or the calcification of the organic intercellular substance?

To illustrate that interference with each of these processes is reflected in a different kind of histological picture in the metaphysis, we next describe briefly an example of interference (*1*) with the synthesis of the organic components of bone and (*2*) with the calcification of the organic intercellular substance of bone.

(*1*) *Scurvy.* Perhaps the most dramatic demonstration of interference with the synthesis of organic materials in a metaphysis is seen in *scurvy*, a disease that can affect adults as well as growing children, although in adults, in whom growth is no longer occurring in metaphyses, its manifestations in bone appear more slowly and in relation to bone maintenance and the maintenance of other connective tissues. The disease results basically from inability of connective tissue cells to produce their intercellular

substances. It was once the greatest threat to the life and welfare of sailors on long voyages (where it was noted that the disease often appeared after they ran out of potatoes). The possibility of an outbreak of scurvy always hung heavily over the heads of those engaged in polar exploration and indeed, in the early days of the settlement of the northern part of North America, scurvy became so widespread and serious in the long winters that it is a wonder anyone stayed here unless he was obliged to.

In due course it became fairly well established that scurvy did not develop in children and adults whose diets contained a supply of fresh fruits and vegetables and that a dietary supplement of lemon juice would prevent the disease from occurring. However, for a long time it was believed that the disease was caused by a *positive agent* of some sort (for example, poor air or tainted food) and therefore it was assumed that fresh fruits and vegetables somehow prevented this elusive unknown agent from exerting its evil effects. It was not until the present century that it became clear that diseases could be caused by a *lack of something*—for example, the essential food factors that we now term vitamins—and that scurvy was caused by a lack of vitamin C.

Although a vitamin C deficiency affects the metabolism of various types of cells in the body, its effects are particularly noticeable in the growing zone of a long bone. In particular, osteoblasts are unable to synthesize and secrete the organic constituents of normal bone matrix. The net result is that on a diet inadequate but not completely deficient in vitamin C, the metaphysis of, for example, the upper end of the tibia of a guinea pig (guinea pigs, like man, are sensitive to dietary deficiencies of vitamin C; many animals can make their own) shows very little anabolic activity (Fig. 15-60). Growth in the epiphyseal plate is slowed, and almost no new bone formation occurs on the diaphyseal plate (Fig. 15-60). The almost complete cessation of the formation of bone intercellular substance results in the shaft of the bone being very thin (Fig. 15-60). As a consequence, both the epiphyseal plate, lacking support by bone trabeculae beneath it, and the shaft are easily fractured.

The process of calcification, however, is *not* interfered with by scurvy. The little organic matrix that is formed becomes heavily calcified. Scurvy, therefore, represents a condition in which the defect lies in anabolic activities concerned with the *synthesis of organic intercellular substances*.

(*2*) *Rickets.* The mechanism of calcification is dependent on the Ca $\times$ P product in blood and tissue fluid in the vicinity of calcifying bone or cartilage being sufficient to permit the calcification process to proceed. It has been shown that calcification does not proceed normally in the growing zone of the bones of an infant if the product obtained by multiplying the number of milligrams of calcium

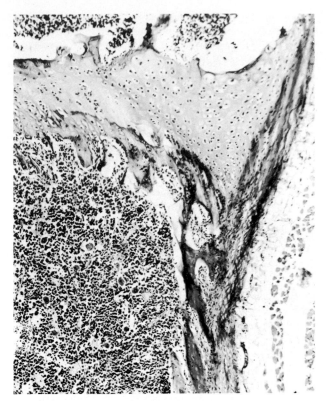

Fig. 15-60. Low-power photomicrograph of part of the upper end of a tibia (guinea pig), from an animal maintained for some weeks on a diet deficient in vitamin C so that it would develop scurvy. Note the inadequate formation of proper trabeculae on the diaphyseal side of the epiphyseal plate (just above *middle*), as a result, the plate is not supported by the proper number of trabeculae. Bone building for the shaft has almost ceased at the metaphysis so that it is very thin (*lower right*) and breaks easily. (Ham, A. W., and Elliott, H. C.: Am. J. Pathol., *14:*323, 1938)

per 100 ml. of serum by the number of milligrams of phosphorus per 100 ml. of blood falls below a certain value. It is to be noted that a reduced level of either calcium or phosphorus in the blood does not necessarily interfere with calcification; it is the product of the two concentrations that determines whether calcification will continue.

In a baby the growing skeleton normally absorbs large amounts of calcium phosphate which requires that the infant's diet contain an adequate amount of calcium and phosphorus. Further, for these minerals to be absorbed into the bloodstream an adequate supply of vitamin D is required. If an infant's diet is deficient in any or all of these essentials, the $Ca \times P$ product of the blood may fall below the minimum level required for calcification in the growing zone, with the result that a condition known as *rickets* develops. The earliest change noted is that al-

though growth continues and organic matrix continues to be synthesized, the calcification of cartilage almost ceases in the epiphyseal disks. If the intercellular substance surrounding the mature cells in this zone fails to become impregnated with mineral, the cells of this zone are not shut off from nutrition. Hence they do not die as they do under normal conditions, but continue to live. The result is that, since growth continues in the growing zone of the disks, the epiphyseal disks become thicker than normal (Fig. 15-61). Inasmuch as calcification is not entirely arrested but occurs in a few sites on the diaphyseal sides of the disk, the thickening of the disks tends to be irregular (Fig. 15-61). In the meantime, osteoblasts continue to lay down the organic intercellular substance of bone in the metaphysis, but this does not become calcified either because of the low $Ca \times P$ product. Instead, it exists in an uncalcified state until the diet is remedied. This new tissue, during the time it remains uncalcified, remains as *osteoid tissue* (Fig. 15-61). Furthermore, it seems as if the osteoblasts of the periosteum in the region of metaphyses somehow sense that calcification is not proceeding normally, for they increase their activities and lay down large amounts of osteoid tissue in the metaphyseal region just beneath the periosteum (Fig. 15-61, subperiosteal osteoid). This makes the metaphyseal regions knobby. The knobs so produced at the growing ends of the ribs are responsible in a rachitic child's chest for what is termed the "rachitic rosary,"

It is to be kept in mind that the changes occurring in the growing zones of bone in rickets are the result of *growth continuing while calcification fails.* For this reason, a disturbed mineral metabolism will cause more severe rickets in a child who is actively growing than in one who is not. The poorly calcified intercellular substance of bone characterizing rickets may bend with weight-bearing. Hence, rachitic children may be bowlegged.

A deficiency of vitamin D in the diet is the usual cause of rickets. The condition is more common in cold countries and where there is little sunshine and exposure to it. In humans vitamin D is made by the effects of sunshine on their skin, as will be explained in Chapter 20.

Effects of Disturbances of Metabolism on the Bones of Adults

Nutritional and metabolic defects show up in the metaphyses of growing bones much more quickly than they do in the bones of adults. However, as has been described, there is a turnover of both cancellous and compact bone throughout life. As noted, parts of old haversian systems die, resorption tunnels develop, and new haversian systems form in them so as to occupy the tunnels. In some individuals the skeleton is not properly maintained. As in children this can be due to conditions

Fig. 15-61. Low-power photomicrograph of part of the upper end of a tibia (rat), from an animal maintained on a diet with low Ca × P product so that it would develop rickets. Since calcification cannot proceed properly, the chondrocytes in the epiphyseal plate live longer, with the result that the plate becomes thick (darkly stained, just above *middle*). Irregular trabeculae of osteoid tissue are evident below the cartilage (under the epiphyseal plate), and much subperiosteal osteoid tissue is seen in the metaphysis, at *left*. (This is an example of severe low-phosphorus rickets.)

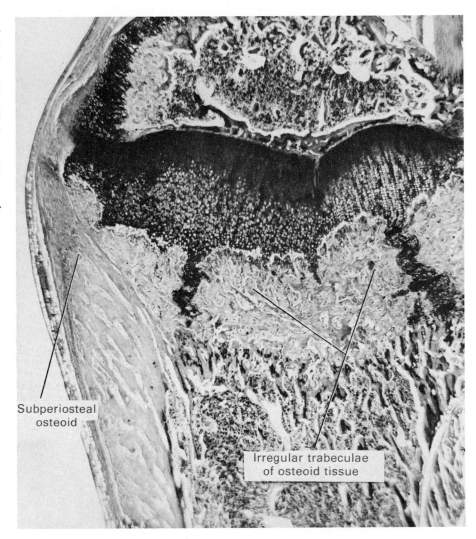

Subperiosteal osteoid

Irregular trabeculae of osteoid tissue

that do not permit the proper calcification of newly formed (maintenance) bone, or it can be due to a failure in the formation of organic bone matrix. Two examples to illustrate this will be briefly considered.

Osteomalacia. This condition which develops in adults is sometimes referred to as "adult rickets." In this condition the bone that forms to maintain the skeleton does not become properly calcified. In some populations of people living on poor diets, particularly those that are deficient in calcium or vitamin D, the condition may be prevalent. However, the condition can also develop in populations where the diet is reasonably good, because of individuals having metabolic defects that interfere with the absorption or excretion of minerals or because of vitamin D not exerting its normal metabolic effects for one reason or another.

Osteoporosis. This is a relatively common disorder of

the skeleton that develops as people grow older. In this instance the defect is not that newly formed bone is not properly calcified; it is primarily that not enough new bone matrix is produced to keep up with the increased rate of bone resorption that occurs in this condition. As a result the total bone mass in the body becomes less and less. An important histological method for investigating both conditions will now be described.

Microradiography. Determining the concentration of haversian systems in the cortex of a bone, the extent to which the different lamellae in a given haversian system are calcified, and the extent to which different haversian systems in a given section of bone are calcified, has been made possible by the development of the technic of microradiography. Undecalcified sections must, of course, be employed; these have been variously prepared by grinding or by special embedding of calcified bone and

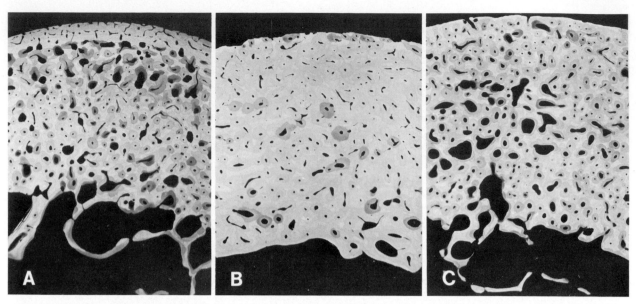

Fig. 15-62. Microradiographs of undecalcified sections of midshaft of a femur from people of different ages. (*A*) A 7-year-old. This indicates the relatively rapid turnover of bone normal for this age; it shows many resorption tunnels and newly formed haversian systems (the bone of which shows darker than that of the older, and hence more heavily calcified, systems, which, being denser, are whiter in the illustration). (*B*) A 25-year-old. There is little indication here of turnover of systems. There are almost no resorption tunnels, and most of the systems are well calcified and of similar density. (*C*) An 85-year-old. This shows two features characteristic of bone of people this age: (*1*) there are many resorption tunnels, which indicates increased resorption, and (*2*) the new layers of bone beginning to fill in some of the tunnels are poorly calcified (darker than well-calcified bone). Hence bones of the old have a higher content of bone of low density than bones of young adults. (Courtesy of J. Jowsey)

cutting it into sections with special heavy microtomes. Even more elaborate methods can be employed. Sections are placed over and in direct contact with a film or plate covered with fine-grain photographic emulsion. The preparation is then exposed (section side up) to very soft x-rays from a special source. The soft x-rays penetrate the section in relation to the amount of calcium present in its different parts. The developed film or plate constitutes a *microradiograph* of the section and shows the numbers and sizes of its haversian systems and the extent to which its different parts are calcified. The microradiograph can be compared with the actual section under the microscope. By this means histological appearances can be correlated with the sites of different densities indicated in the microradioautograph. Three microradiographs of cross sections of cortical bone from people of different ages are seen in Figure 15-62. The interpretation appears in the caption, which should be read carefully.

THE BLOOD SUPPLY OF A LONG BONE

We shall first consider a long bone whose growth is over. In such a bone the epiphyseal plates have finished their work and have become resorbed so there is no barrier between the marrow cavity of the diaphysis and that of the epiphyses.

How Do Three Sets of Blood Vessels Become Incorporated Into a Bone? Our study of the development of a long bone makes it easy to understand there are three ways blood vessels become incorporated into a long bone as it develops.

(*1*) *The Nutrient Artery and Vein.* First, it will be recalled that after the osteogenic cells along the side of a cartilage model of a bone-to-be are beginning to form a shell of bone around it (Fig. 15-39) a *periosteal bud* (Fig. 15-40) breaks through into the substance of the cartilage to enter it at the site where it is cavitating. The blood vessels of the bud become increasingly larger as the bone continues to grow and in due course become the *nutrient artery* and *vein* of that particular bone. In some bones (for example, the femur) nutrient arteries form at more than one site in this manner but in other bones (for example, the tibia) there is only one.

As was described in connection with myeloid tissue, the nutrient artery (or arteries) provide the blood supply for bone marrow. In addition the branches of the artery, besides serving the marrow, supply much of the shaft of the bone. Then, when the growth of a long bone is over and the epiphyseal plates have been resorbed, there is no

Fig. 15-63. Diagram illustrating that where an epiphysis is entirely covered by articular cartilage (*A*) (*right side*), its blood vessels must enter it by traversing the perichondrium at the periphery of the epiphyseal plate. This makes them vulnerable to rupture on epiphyseal displacement. In contrast, where an epiphysis is only partly covered by articular cartilage (*B*) (*left side*), its blood vessels enter in such a way that separation could occur without serious damage to them. (Dale, G. G., and Harris, W. R.: J. Bone Joint Surg., *40-B:*116, 1958)

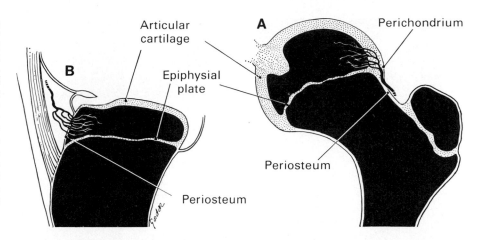

cartilaginous barrier between the marrow of the diaphysis and the epiphyses of a long bone so the blood vessels of the diaphysis can anastomose with those of the marrow of the epiphyses, the origin of which will next be described.

(2) The Metaphyseal Vessels. To understand how these vessels obtain access to the marrow cavity of a bone it will be helpful to glance again at Figure 15-52. It is to be noted here that around the flared end of the bone the spaces between the trabeculae just below the periphery of the epiphyseal plate extend out to the periosteum covering the flared portion of the diaphysis. Blood vessels from the periosteum are present in these canals and they extend to the epiphyseal plate. But when growth is over and the epiphyseal plate is resorbed, these blood vessels can pass directly into the marrow cavity of the epiphysis, which is now in free communication with the marrow cavity of the diaphysis, and so they are able to anastomose with vessels from the nutrient vessels.

(3) The Periosteal Vessels. In connection with our description of how the shaft of a bone grows in width, we pointed out that capillaries from the periosteum become successively buried in each new haversian system added to the exterior of a shaft and that, as successive systems are buried, their vessels retain their connection with periosteal vessels by way of Volkmann's canals (Figs. 15-55 and 15-56). From the way these vessels are incorporated into the shaft of a bone it might be assumed that they would provide the chief blood supply for the cortex of the shaft. But this does not seem to be what happens. Suspicion that the compact bone of a shaft is not supplied with blood primarily from the periosteal vessels might be aroused from the fact noted by De Haas and Macnab that a *nutrient vein* is generally *smaller than its companion nutrient artery,* which leads to the thought that much of the blood that enters a bone by way of the nutrient artery must leave by some route other than the nutrient vein. The studies of Brooks indicate that, instead of the blood

flowing inward from the periosteum through the cortex of a bone, the circulation is in the other direction—that is, that blood from the nutrient artery is fed by means of anastomoses into the system of vessels that lie in the haversian canals of the cortex of a long bone; blood flows out through these vessels to be drained away from the bone by way of periosteal vessels. It now seems generally accepted that under normal conditions at least the *inner two thirds of the cortex receives its blood supply from the nutrient artery* and that only in some sites do the periosteal vessels contribute significant amounts of blood to the haversian systems of the cortex. However, should the medullary supply be injured, as might occur in some fractures or in certain operative procedures such as when some of the marrow cavity is reamed out, it seems probable that periosteal vessels can then supply more of the cortex than they do under ordinary circumstances.

It should be very clear, from the above discussion, that a thorough knowledge about the blood supply of a long bone is a matter of profound importance to those involved in orthopedic or reconstructive surgery and that further investigation as to what happens as a result of different types of injury or operative procedures is warranted.

The Blood Supply of the Epiphyses of Long Bones. The blood supply of epiphyses and epiphyseal plates is of great interest with regard to certain problems in growing children. Dale and Harris distinguish two kinds of epiphyses in growing bones. In one kind the articular cartilage is continuous with that of the epiphyseal plate (Fig. 15-63A) and in the other it is not (Fig. 15-63B). In the first kind (Fig. 15-63A) the blood vessels supplying the epiphysis have to travel through the site where the cartilage of the epiphyseal plate is continuous with articular cartilage in order to reach the marrow cavity of the epiphysis. In the second kind of arrangement, shown in Figure 15-63B, the blood vessels do not have to pass through either articular or epiphyseal plate cartilage to enter the

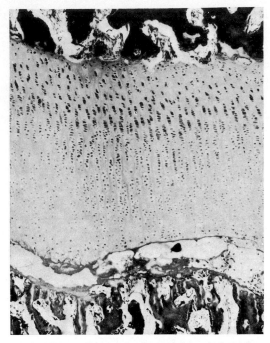

Fig. 15-64. Photomicrograph of an epiphyseal plate of a radius (rabbit) 10 days after the epiphysis, together with the epiphyseal plate, was separated from the diaphysis. Note that the line of separation (near *bottom*) occurs across the zone of hypertrophied cells. During the period following separation, the plate has grown greatly in thickness; this shows that its source of nutrition was provided from the epiphysis by the vessels illustrated in Figure 15-65. (Dale, G. G., and Harris, W. R.: J. Bone Joint Surg., *40-B:*116, 1958)

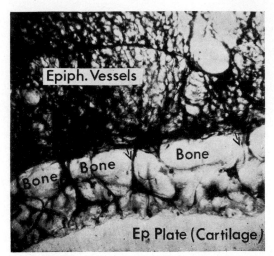

Fig. 15-65. Photomicrograph of longitudinal section through an epiphyseal plate and part of an epiphysis of a growing long bone of a rabbit. The arteries supplying this epiphysis were injected with opaque material. This illustration shows that vessels from the epiphysis penetrate the bone lying between the marrow of the epiphysis and the epiphyseal plate, to supply nutriment to the epiphyseal border of the epiphyseal plate. As shown in Figure 15-64, these vessels can support viability and growth of the plate if it is separated from the diaphysis. (Salter, R. M., and Harris, W. R.: J. Bone Joint Surg., *45-A:*587, 1963)

epiphysis; instead they pierce the perichondrium-like tissue that covers one side of the epiphysis. These two types of epiphysis behave differently if an epiphyseal separation occurs.

Epiphyseal separations sometimes occur in children as a result of an accident. If some shearing or other force causes such a separation, it generally occurs in the zone of mature, hypertrophied cartilage cells of the plate, as is shown in Figure 15-64, for this is the weakest part of the plate. If this happens in an epiphysis of the type illustrated on the right side (A) of Figure 15-63, the blood vessels passing through the cartilage at the end of the plate are likely to be ruptured. However, if a separation occurs in the type illustrated on the left (B) in Figure 15-63, the epiphysis still retains its blood supply. Harris and Hobson showed that the upper femoral epiphysis is of the type illustrated on the right in Figure 15-63 and that separation of an epiphysis of this type, by experimental means, leads to the death of the detached fragment. Dale and Harris, however, have shown that an epiphysis of the type illustrated on the left in Figure 15-63 may be detached without death of the epiphyseal plate occurring (Fig. 15-

64). Furthermore, experimental detachment of this type of epiphysis gave valuable information about the source from which the proliferating cells of an epiphyseal plate receive their nourishment, as will next be described.

The Blood Supply of the Epiphyseal Plate. Since the diaphyseal side of an epiphyseal plate abounds in capillary loops disposed between the forming trabeculae of bone in that region, and which penetrate into the zone of calcifying cartilage of the plate, it might at first be thought that these capillaries of diaphyseal (nutrient artery) origin might be able to provide the nourishment necessary for the cell division that occurs toward the epiphyseal side of the plate and for the synthesis of such intercellular substance as occurs in association with the chondrocytes in a growing plate. However, as has been stressed, the calcification of the intercellular substance of cartilage makes it much less able to serve as a medium for diffusion, and hence nourishment would have great difficulty in penetrating from diaphyseal capillaries through the zone of calcified cartilage to reach the zone of proliferating cells. Moreover, inspection of Figure 15-47 will show that there are on the diaphyseal side of the layer of epiphyseal bone that abuts on the epiphyseal plate, in the zone labeled *resting cartilage,* canals that contain capillaries. These have been studied by injection methods by Salter and Harris, one of whose preparations is seen in Figure 15-65; this shows branches from epiphyseal vessels penetrating the bone of the epiphysis to supply the zone of "resting" cartilage cells of the plate. That nourishment from these capillaries diffuses through the remainder of the plate to nourish the cells of its various living layers was shown by Dale and Harris; for, as noted, they found that if the blood supply of the epiphysis remained intact, epiphyseal plates could be separated from the metaphysis (and hence from metaphyseal blood vessels), and yet the separated plates would continue to grow in thickness (Fig. 15-64). These experiments and others show clearly that the cartilage of the epiphyseal plate, at least in the animals used in these experiments, obtains the nutrients it requires for growth *from its epiphyseal side,* and probably principally from the small vessels seen in the canals immediately on the diaphyseal side of the bone of the epiphysis illustrated in Figures 15-47 and 15-65. Some nourishment may also diffuse in from the periphery of the plate. Kember and Sissons, however, have suggested from their studies in the epiphyseal plates of children, that the mechanism of nutrition here may be somewhat different from that in the usual experimental animals used to study this subject.

The Blood Vessels of Haversian Systems (Osteons) of Compact Bone. The arrangement of haversian systems in compact bone is very complex as new ones are substituted for old ones in the slow remodeling that takes place during life. Cohen and Harris made a 3-dimensional study of haversian systems and their anastomoses in compact bone, and provide details about their sizes and the courses they pursue. The blood vessels of adjacent haversian systems, because of the way they are incorporated within new systems added to the exterior of a bone (namely by vessels derived from the periosteum being surrounded with successive layers of new bone), would constitute an anastomosing network connected both to vessels of the medulla and vessels of the periosteum. In general, the vessels in haversian systems run more or less parallel to the shaft of the bone. Depending on how close they are to the larger vessels from which they originate or into which they drain, they vary in number and size. In some both an arteriole and a venule are present (Fig. 15-66). In this illustration the wall of the canal is also seen to be lined with osteogenic cells. However, in other instances only a single capillary is seen in a haversian system (Fig. 15-67). (In such a site it could be expected that the haversian canal here again would be lined with the cytoplasm of osteogenic cells, but this does not show in Fig. 15-67, probably because the type of fixation and decalcification used in preparing ordinary bone sections for light microscopy is not good enough to preserve such detail. As is to be observed, the procedures used for preparing sections for the EM (Fig. 15-66) preserve much more detail.)

Since vessels in haversian systems run more or less

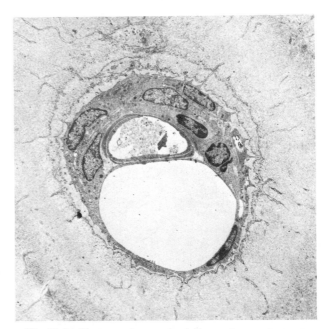

Fig. 15-66. Electron micrograph of a haversian canal, showing that the canal is lined by cells of the bone cell series. Some of these are osteogenic cells; others are differentiating into osteoblasts (note their cytoplasmic processes extending into canaliculi). An arteriole (*upper center*) and a venule (*center*) are also evident in the canal. (Courtesy of S. C. Luk and G. T. Simon)

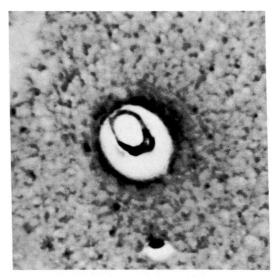

Fig. 15-67. Photomicrograph (×800) of a haversian canal (radius of dog) containing a single large capillary. The stippled appearance of the bone matrix is due to osteocyte processes in canaliculi having been cut in cross and oblique section. (Ham, A. W.: J. Bone Joint Surg., *34-A:*701, 1952)

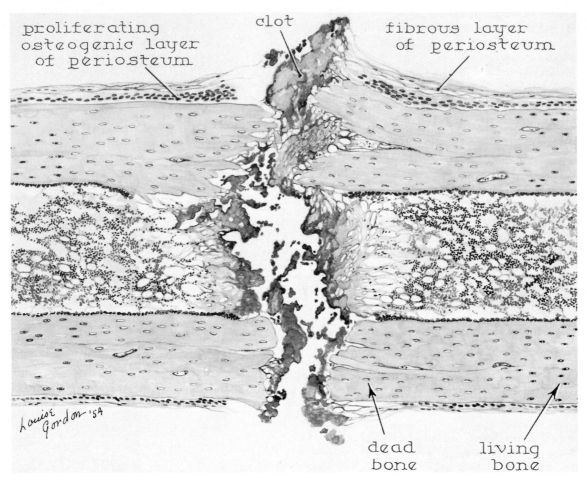

proliferating osteogenic layer of periosteum

clot

fibrous layer of periosteum

Louise Gordon '5A

dead bone

living bone

Fig. 15-68. Drawing of a longitudinal section of a rabbit's rib in which a fracture has been healing for 2 days. *See* text for explanation. (Ham, A. W., and Harris, W. R.: *In* Bourne, G. H. (ed.): The Biochemistry and Physiology of Bone. ed. 2, vol. 3, p. 338. New York, Academic Press, 1971)

parallel with the shaft of a long bone their severance, when a fracture occurs, leads to their open ends soon becoming sealed off by hemostatic mechanisms and so circulation through them ceases back to some site where they anastomose. Between this site and the fracture the osteocytes in the compact bone have no source of nutrition and so they die. This means there is dead bone on either side of a fracture back to where haversian vessels anastomose with one another, as will be mentioned further as we discuss fractures.

THE HEALING OF A SIMPLE FRACTURE OF A LONG BONE

In a simple fracture a bone is broken into two parts, each of which is termed a *fragment*. Further, the periosteum is usually torn and the fragments are displaced so that their ends are not in perfect apposition to one another. Hence it is usually necessary for fractures to be reduced; that is, the fragments are led back, usually by manipulation, so that their broken ends are in apposition to one another, and the line of the bone is restored. The bone is then immobilized to keep things in place, usually by means of a cast.

For one reason or another a fracture may need to be reduced at an open operation and the two fragments joined by a metallic device. Under these conditions the healing process, as will be described later, may be somewhat different from the one we shall describe first.

Immediate Effects of the Injury. There is both direct and indirect injury to tissue, for not only is the bone broken, the soft tissues associated with the bone are also torn (Fig. 15-68). Both the blood vessels that cross the line of the fracture and those of the adjacent soft tissue are torn.

Fig. 15-69. Drawings illustrating how periosteal collars form, approach one another, and fuse in the repair of a fracture. Also illustrated is the formation of internal callus and the way trabeculae become cemented to the original bone fragments. Living bone of the original fragments is depicted in light gray, dead portions in dark gray, and new bone of the external and internal callus in black. In the external callus, cartilage is stippled lightly, and proliferating osteogenic cells are stippled darkly. For further details, *see* text.

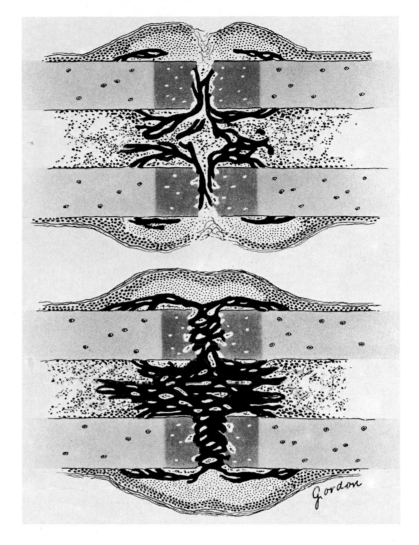

The more displacement there is, the more blood vessels are torn and bleed into and around the fracture area. This blood soon coagulates to form a clot in and about the site of the fracture (Fig. 15-68). The second type of injury caused by a fracture is indirect. As noted, haversian blood vessels run more or less longitudinally in bone, so the vessels in haversian systems are all torn at the fracture line and circulation in them stops back to sites where they anastomose with other haversian vessels. Since anastomoses between vessels of adjacent haversian systems are probably not overly abundant, this means that circulation ceases in haversian vessels for some distance each side of the fracture line. This results in *the death of the osteocytes of the haversian systems for a certain distance on each side of the fracture line;* this is shown by empty lacunae (Fig. 15-68, dead bone).

Injury to blood vessels also accounts for death of both some periosteal and some marrow tissue on each side of the fracture line. However, since both of these tissues have a better blood supply than the bone itself, the periosteal tissue and the marrow tissue do not die for as great a distance from each side of the fracture line as does the bone (Fig. 15-68).

Dead bone is generally recognized because dead osteocytes undergo lysis; hence, in most dead bone the lacunae, at least after some days, appear empty (Figs. 15-68, 15-69, and 15-70). However, the osteocytes sometimes become pyknotic (dark and rounded). After 2 days, the irregular line of demarcation between dead bone (with empty lacunae), which extends from both sides of the fracture line, and living bone (the lacunae of which contain normal osteocytes) farther away from the fracture line generally can be recognized as in Figures 15-68, 15-69, and 15-70. The distance from a fracture line over which

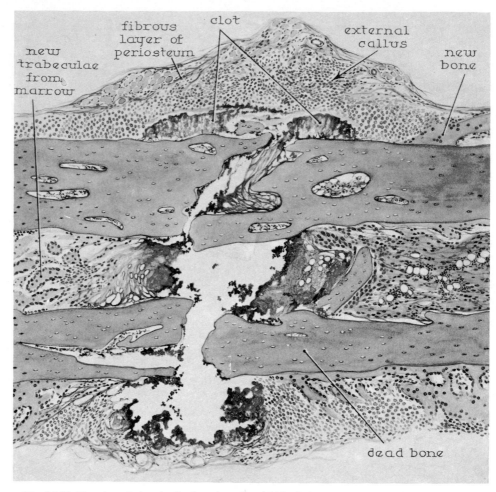

Fig. 15-70. Drawing of a longitudinal section of a rabbit's rib in which a fracture has been healing for 1 week. For details, *see* text. (Ham, A. W., and Harris, W. R.: *In* Bourne, G. H. (ed.): The Biochemistry and Physiology of Bone, ed. 2, vol. 3, p. 338. New York, Academic Press, 1971)

bone dies as a result of its blood supply being interrupted differs, depending on the site of the fracture and the particular bone fractured.

Early Stages of Repair

The Term Callus. A fracture is repaired by a growth of new tissue that develops around and between the ends of the fragments; this new tissue, which sooner or later forms a bridge between the fragments so that they are united (Figs. 15-68, 15-69, and 15-70), is termed a *callus.* Some accounts of fracture healing are unnecessarily complicated by using names such as *provisional callus, temporary callus, bridging callus,* and *permanent callus.* These terms suggest that different calluses exist at dif-

ferent times, each being replaced by another. Actually, what happens is that only one callus develops and, like any bony structure, it is remodeled as it grows. However, there is one classification that is helpful in describing callus formation; that is to speak of the callus that forms *around* the opposing ends of the bone fragments as the *external callus* and that which forms *between* the ends of the bone fragments and between the marrow cavities as the *internal callus* (Fig. 15-71).

The Cellular Origin of Callus. An informative method for investigating the cellular origin of callus tissue is to study sections of healing fractures in ribs. A rib can be fractured in an anesthetized rabbit with the fingers (without any incision being necessary) and during healing the adjacent ribs act as a splint for the one that is fractured. By using a group of rabbits and preparing sections of a fractured rib at representative days over a period of a couple of weeks, day to day repair of the fracture can be followed.

Sections taken over the first two days following the fracture show that the cells responsible for bringing about eventual bony repair of the fracture have already begun to proliferate. The greatest proliferation seen this early is in the deep layer of the periosteum close to, but not directly at, the site of the fracture. This layer becomes thicker (Fig. 15-68) because of active cell proliferation occurring among the osteogenic cells (Fig. 15-15). The thickening of the osteogenic cells lifts the fibrous layer of the periosteum farther away from the bone. Over the first few days the osteogenic cells lining the marrow cavity also begin to proliferate but the thickening of this layer is not as great as that of the osteogenic layer of the periosteum (Fig. 15-68).

Over the next few days the proliferation of osteogenic cells continues in both periosteal and endosteal regions, but those cells in the deep layer of the periosteum show the greater activity. They proliferate so rapidly that they soon form a distinct collar around each fragment close to the line of the fracture (Figs. 15-69, *top*, and 15-70). In addition to proliferating, these cells now manifest signs of differentiation. When the osteogenic cells begin to proliferate after a fracture, the capillaries among them also proliferate, but they do not seem to grow as quickly as the osteogenic cells. As a result, the osteogenic cells more deeply disposed in the collars (those closest to the bone) differentiate in the presence of a blood supply; consequently, they become osteoblasts and form new bony trabeculae in this region (Figs. 15-17, 15-69, and 15-70). The new trabeculae that develop are cemented firmly to the bone matrix of the fragment, even though the bone of the fragment may be dead (Fig. 15-69). Those osteogenic cells in the more superficial parts of the collar (those farther away from the bone) seem to grow so quickly that the capillaries from the periosteum cannot keep up with them. When these osteogenic cells differentiate, they must do so in a nonvascular environment, so they tend to differentiate into chondrocytes, and as a result cartilage develops in the outer parts of the collars (Figs. 15-17, 15-69, and 15-70). The amount of cartilage forming in a callus is, we think, dependent on how quickly the callus tissue grows; if it grows very rapidly, capillaries seem unable to keep up with it, so its outer parts become nonvascular and cartilaginous. However, if callus tissue develops more slowly, new capillaries can keep pace with the osteogenic cells, so the osteogenic cells in such a callus differentiate in a vascular environment and so form bone. However, there also may be other factors that influence the amount of cartilage that forms—for example, species and movement.

When the collars resulting from growth and differentia-

tion of osteogenic cells of the deep layer of the periosteum are well developed, they generally exhibit 3 layers that merge into one another (Figs. 15-69 and 15-70). The layer closest to the fragment consists of bony trabeculae cemented to the bone; the next (intermediate) layer consists of cartilage which merges imperceptibly into the outer parts of the bony trabeculae on one side and into the outer layer of the callus on the other. The third (outer) layer consists of proliferating osteogenic cells. The merging of these layers into one another is shown to advantage in Figure 15-17.

The collars continue to grow chiefly because of the proliferation of osteogenic cells in their outer layer and to a lesser extent because of the interstitial growth of cartilage in their middle layers. Such growth as occurs in the collars makes them thicker and makes them bulge toward each other. Sooner or later the collars from the two fragments meet and fuse (Figs. 15-69 and 15-70); when this occurs, union of the fragments has been achieved. Union is also achieved in the marrow cavity by developing trabeculae there forming a bridge (Fig. 15-69, *bottom*). Soon the histological picture of the healing fracture comes to resemble that illustrated in Figure 15-71.

The Fate of the Cartilage. The cartilage developing in a callus normally has a temporary existence only; like that in embryonic models of bones-to-be, it is eventually replaced with bone. Those cartilage cells closest to the newly formed bone mature and the intercellular substance around them becomes calcified, and this causes their death. The region in which this occurs is seen as a V-shaped line in a longitudinal section of a fracture at this stage of healing (Fig. 15-71). As the cartilage becomes calcified it is replaced progressively with bone; this makes the angle of the V increasingly acute. Finally the cartilage is all replaced with bone of the cancellous type. It is to be observed that the trabeculae of bone that replace the calcified cartilage have cores of cartilage on the diaphyseal side of an epiphyseal plate. Furthermore, hematopoiesis begins in the spaces of this cancellous bone from circulating CFUs.

The Remodeling of the Callus. To understand the remodeling process it is important to realize that those trabeculae of bone that form close to the original fragments become firmly cemented to them. Since they also connect with one another, the two fragments are bridged by a cancellous network (Fig. 15-69, *bottom*). Moreover, it is important to realize that osteoblasts in building new trabeculae can lay down their matrix *on dead regions* of the fragments (as well as on living portions of them), so that by this means new trabeculae of bone become firmly cemented here and there to dead bone. However, between these trabeculae there are capillary-containing spaces, and the matrix of the dead bone is slowly etched away by osteoclasts (except where new trabeculae fasten

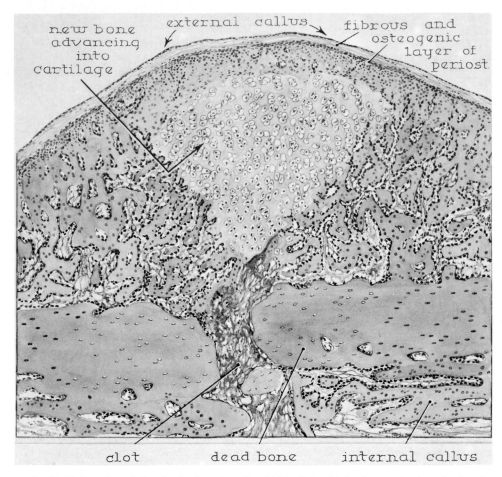

Fig. 15-71. Drawing of a longitudinal section of a rabbit's rib in which a fracture has been healing for 2 weeks. For explanation, *see* text. (Ham, A. W., and Harris, W. R.: *In* Bourne, G. H. (ed.): The Biochemistry and Physiology of Bone. ed. 2, vol. 3, p. 338. New York, Academic Press, 1971)

onto it). Next, osteoblasts move into the spaces that have been deepened into the matrix of the dead bone by this process and lay down new living bone in them. By this means the matrix of the dead bone eventually is almost all replaced with new living bone.

At this stage the external callus constitutes a fusiform mass of cancellous bone around the two fragments from which much of the dead bone has been resorbed. By this time an internal callus has also developed (Fig. 15-69). This has two parts that are continuous with one another. First, in the marrow of each fragment, new trabeculae of bone develop from both the endosteum that lines the marrow cavity and the osteogenic cells of the marrow itself. As shown in Figure 15-69 trabeculae from one fragment connect with those of the other. Second, internal callus forms also between the ends of the fragments. In a rabbit's rib, which has a very thin cortex, this originates from

osteogenic cells from the external surfaces of the bone growing down into the space between the two fragments and also from endosteal cells from the marrow growing outward in the space between the two ends of the bone, to form cancellous bone between the ends of the broken bone (Fig. 15-69, *top* and *bottom*).

As the cartilage of the callus is being replaced with bone, and continuing afterward, when the callus consists of cancellous bone, the callus is gradually remodeled. We have already described how cancellous bone can be converted into compact bone. The same process occurs in the cancellous bone between the two fragments and around their immediate periphery. This makes the bone strong in this site and as a consequence the trabeculae in the periphery of the callus are no longer necessary to provide strength, so they are gradually resorbed. Eventually, the original line of the bone may be so well restored by this process that the site of the fracture can no longer be felt or seen on x-ray as a bony thickening.

The Healing of Fractures of Bones With Thick Cortices. While the study of the healing of fractures in rabbits' ribs provides superb material for observing the principal stages in the repair of a fracture, the cortex of a rabbit's rib is so thin that it does not disclose properly the participation of the osteogenic cells of the haversian canals (Fig. 15-66) that occurs in the healing of thick bones containing large numbers of haversian systems. Hence to appreciate what happens in the healing of fractures of the larger long bones of man, studies should also be made of the healing of fractures of bones in man or larger experimental animals. If these are treated without operation by means of a cast, an external callus develops and healing is much the same as in a rabbit's rib except that in due course osteogenic cells and capillaries grow out into the gap between the exposed ends of the fragments from the haversian canals and make a contribution to the part of the internal callus that develops between the cortices of the fragments. However, with rigid fixation of a fracture, obtained by fixing the fragments firmly together at open operation, the haversian canals become a more important source of callus.

The Healing of Fractures of Bones With Thick Cortices Under Conditions of Rigid Fixation. Experimental studies on dogs and large animals, in which the shaft of a bone with a substantial cortex was cut across by a method that would permit the ends of the two fragments to be smooth and even enough to be brought into direct apposition and held rigidly in close apposition through the healing period, showed that little external callus developed. Nevertheless, as already described, the osteogenic cells and endothelial cells of capillaries all die for some distance back from the fracture line because circulation in the capillaries is interrupted back to the site where the capillaries in the canals anastomose with functioning vessels. Likewise, the osteocytes in the bone surrounding the haversian canals close to the fracture line also die, so that the fracture line is faced on both its side by dead bone. But on both sides of the fracture line, back at the sites where osteogenic cells and capillaries are still alive in the haversian canals, there is proliferation and, as a result, osteogenic cells and capillaries grow toward the fracture line. Osteoclasts appear here and ream out the canals to make them larger; further, the osteogenic cells, which continue to proliferate, differentiate into osteoblasts and begin to rebuild new haversian systems within the widening canals. This dual process advances to the fracture line and under the best of circumstances newly forming osteons from one fragment may cross the line and extend into the fragment on the other side of the line so that new osteons cross the fracture line. The process is much the same as the ordinary remodeling of the shaft of a bone, in

which old osteons are replaced by new ones. The process, however, is believed to be more rapid because of its being stimulated by the injury. For a detailed account of what happens in experiments of this nature, the reader is referred to Schenk and Willengger.

Fractures, however, as they occur in man, do not often lead to the ends of the fragments being smooth and even so that they can be fitted together in close apposition. Indeed, in a study by Grant in which fractures were produced by the same kind of force that would operate in an accident, the two ends of the fragments were not sufficiently smooth or even for them to be fitted at open operation so as to achieve direct contact with one another except at a few sites. Hence, when they were joined together by mechanical means so as to approach each other as closely as possible, some space still remained in many places between their ends. In the healing process Grant observed that although haversian canals on each side of the fracture line became reamed out by osteoclasts, and osteogenic cells and capillaries grew along these to reach the fracture site, before there could be any attempt to cross the line they first had to fill the spaces between the fragments with bone, which they did. The bone formed here was commonly of the immature type. Thus the first union achieved between the two fragments is that they are joined only by *immature bone* and not by osteons crossing from one fragment to the other to provide pegs of living bone (new osteons) inserting into each fragment like dowel pins joining pieces of wood in furniture, as may occur later. Moreover, at this time the fracture line previously seen on x-ray may no longer be apparent, and thus give an impression that substantial healing has been achieved. Substantial union does not occur until the whole area of bone encompassing the fracture area is remodeled, in which process new haversian systems are built which extend across the fracture line to peg one fragment directly into the other. This takes a long time, not being complete even after a year.

Grant found, moreover, that in fractures treated with less stable fixation so that an external callus developed, the external callus had mostly disappeared after $4^{1/2}$ months or so. The histological changes occurring from then on were much the same as those observed in the animals in which rigid fixation had been obtained. It is obvious therefore that the healing of a fracture under conditions of close apposition and rigid fixation is not a different type of healing, and that rigid fixation merely substitutes, as it were, for an external callus, which under ordinary circumstances forms quickly enough to provide the support required for extensive remodeling of bone in the region encompassing the ends of the two fragments. The internal callus from the endosteum and marrow helps in providing some new bone from the remodeling process.

It is a fascinating question why the osteogenic cells of

HISTORY OF A COMPACT BONE GRAFT

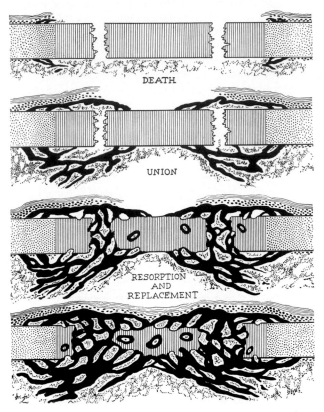

DEATH

UNION

RESORPTION
AND
REPLACEMENT

Fig. 15-72. Series of diagrams illustrating what happens to a block of bone cortex cut free from its blood supply and placed back into the defect caused by its removal. The periosteal surface lies above, and the marrow surface below, in each picture. Viable preexisting bone is depicted in medium stipple, dead bone is cross-hatched, and new bone is shown in black. (Ham, A. W.: J. Bone Joint Surg., *34-A:*701, 1952)

the periosteum are not sufficiently activated to produce a substantial external callus when rigid fixation of the fragments is achieved. As one investigator remarked, "they behave as if they did not know the bone was broken." Somehow restoration of the rigidity of the bone seems to prevent sending of the message that would ordinarily result in the local proliferation of the osteogenic cells of the periosteum, whereas even slight movement between the fragments somehow indicates to the osteogenic cells that the function of bone in bearing weight—its chief function—has been impaired. But since this function depends on mass and since an external callus provides more mass, the question arises as to whether a message is ordinarily sent as a result of a loss of mass or a lack of function being detected.

THE TRANSPLANTATION OF BONE

Bone transplants are often used when fractured bones fail to heal or substantial parts of a bone are destroyed by accident or disease. They are also useful in permitting certain reconstructions of the face by plastic surgeons and are sometimes employed to bring about bony union between two bones separated by a joint that has become diseased. Indeed, transplantation of bone is a common surgical operation. The transplanting of bone is also referred to as bone grafting, but this is not a very accurate term to use with regard to the transplantation of bone.

Bone transplants can be classified into two types in two different ways. First, there are *autologous transplants* (*autografts*), in which bone is transplanted from one site to another in the *same individual,* and *homologous transplants* (*homografts* or *allografts*), in which bone is transplanted from *one individual to another.* Second, transplants may be made of either *compact* or *cancellous* bone.

Transplants of Autologous Bone. In explaining the problems associated with successfully transplanting bone it is best to begin with what happens when a piece of compact bone is cut from one bone and transplanted to a bed cut for it in some other bone in the same individual.

Decades ago it was believed by many surgeons that transplanted compact bone continued to live on in its new site. Now it is known that the osteocytes of a piece of compact bone that is transplanted die, and that sooner or later in a successful "transplant" the *dead transplanted bone is replaced by new bone.*

When a graft of compact bone is cut, it is, of course, severed from its blood supply (Fig. 15-72). When it is fitted into its new position its osteocytes, if they were to live, would have to obtain all their oxygen and nourishment through canaliculi. Hence, the only osteocytes that survive after a piece of compact bone is transplanted are the very few close enough to functioning capillaries in the bed of the host bone to permit the canalicular mechanism to function. This means that at best only a few osteocytes very close to a surface where there is tissue fluid can survive in transplanted bone.

However, osteogenic cells of the periosteum and such endosteal cells as are present on a transplant, being situated at surfaces, are more likely to be sufficiently well bathed in tissue fluid to survive than osteocytes within the transplant. Indeed, some of the covering and lining cells of compact bone do survive and grow if they are in a suitable environment, and they may contribute a little toward osteogenesis, which, however, comes mostly from the covering and lining cells of the bone into which the transplant is inserted (Fig. 15-72).

If most of the osteocytes of transplanted compact bone

Fig. 15-73. Photomicrograph showing the appearance of a homograft reaction to a compact bone allograft. A piece of compact bone from a donor rat was transplanted, together with its periosteal connective tissue, into a genetically unrelated rat. Note that the periosteal connective tissue (middle third of picture) and many of the spaces in the bone (which extends along the lower margin) have become infiltrated with large numbers of cells having the morphology of small lymphocytes. These are graft rejection (killer) cells derived from T-lymphocytes of the host. (Courtesy of F. Langer and K. Pritzker)

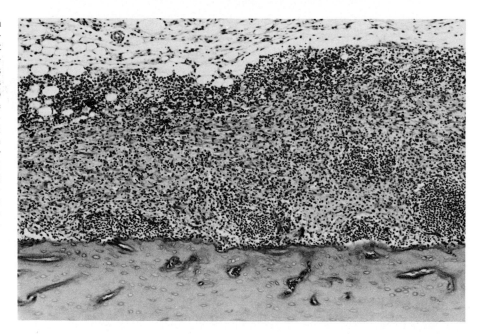

die, it might be thought that a transplant of compact bone would be of little use; but a transplant can be of the greatest use even though most of its constituent cells do die. Bone transplants are placed so that each end extends well into living bone tissue of the two fragments they bridge. Cells from the osteogenic layer of the periosteum, endosteum, and marrow of the host bone proliferate and, together with capillaries, push out toward the transplant to form new trabeculae of bone (Fig. 15-72). After a time the bony trabeculae, increasing in length and breadth by new bone being deposited on their surfaces, reach the transplant and unite with it (Fig. 15-72). It is to be understood that new bone deposited on dead bone becomes firmly cemented to it, just as the new bone deposited on the calcified cartilage on the diaphyseal side of the epiphyseal plate becomes firmly cemented to the cartilage. This step in the history of a compact bone transplant is illustrated in Figure 15-72, which shows that new trabeculae from the host have firmly united with the dead bone of the transplant. It is also evident in this illustration that the osteogenic cells and the osteoblasts from which these new trabeculae arose came from some little distance behind the dead edge of the graft bed.

After the transplant is united to host bone, it must be resorbed slowly and replaced with new bone. Resorption occurs in two general sites: (*1*) on the outer surfaces of the transplant in between areas where trabeculae of new bone have become cemented to it, and (*2*) on the inner surface of haversian canals (Fig. 15-72, *bottom*).

It is to be understood that functioning blood vessels are as necessary for resorption of bone as for deposition and maintenance of viability of bone. Accordingly, little resorption can occur from the inner surfaces of the haversian canals of a transplant until there are functioning blood vessels in these haversian canals. Commonly it takes many weeks for new blood vessels to grow into the haversian canals of a compact bone graft.

The growth of new blood vessels and osteogenic cells into the haversian canals of the transplant is associated both with the resorption of dead bone from the canals by osteoclasts, which widens them (Fig. 15-72), and also with the deposition of new bone on the sides of the canals, which narrows them again (Fig. 15-72). The same two processes operate simultaneously on the exterior of the transplant and also at the dead edges of the graft bed, so before long the transplant and the edge of the bed both become a conglomerate of living, host-derived bone and dead bone (Fig. 15-72, *bottom*). Eventually nearly all (if not all) the dead bone is resorbed with new bone being substituted for it, but this takes time.

THE TRANSPLANTATION OF HOMOLOGOUS COMPACT BONE

As pointed out in connection with the fate of transplanted autologous bone, the value of a transplant of compact bone does not depend upon the survival of any of its cells but upon the ability of its calcified intercellular substance to somehow stimulate osteogenesis from the bed of host tissue into which it is placed. The osteogenesis

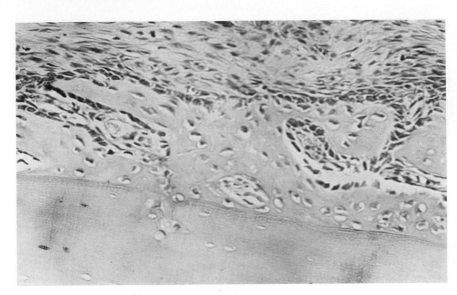

Fig. 15-74. Photomicrograph of part of an autologous cancellous bone chip, 10 days after transplantation to muscle tissue of the host. The original bone of the transplant extends across the *bottom*. New bone (of the immature type) has formed above from the osteogenic cells that covered its surface. (Chalmers, J.: J. Bone Joint Surg. Brit., *41:*160, 1959)

that an autologous transplant incites will in due course replace the bone of the transplant (Fig. 15-72). It might therefore seem that homologous transplants of compact bone would serve this purpose as well as autologous bone.

In Chapter 13 the homograft reaction was described. The question therefore arises here as to whether homologous bone would incite a homograft reaction that would prevent its serving the purpose outlined. The evidence indicates that it does incite a homograft reaction, but nevertheless homologous grafts are sometimes just as successful as autologous ones of compact bone. The many factors involved have been described by Langer et al., whose photomicrograph in Figure 15-73 shows a homograft reaction developing in association with a homologous transplant of compact bone in an experimental animal.

THE TRANSPLANTATION OF FRAGMENTS OF CANCELLOUS BONE

Autologous Transplants. Cancellous fragments (often termed cancellous chips) of autologous bone can be obtained, for example, from the crest of the ilium. These are used for an entirely different purpose.

Early observations on the transplantation of cancellous chips suggested that the osteocytes of small chips received enough nutrient in their new location to survive. But more critical studies showed that when cancellous chips were transplanted, for example, into muscle, the osteocytes of the chips died. However, the osteogenic cells that covered and/or lined the cancellous bone from which the chips were obtained continued to live and quickly

gave rise to new bone on some surface of the otherwise dead fragment of cancellous bone that had been transplanted, as shown in Figure 15-74. From experiments such as this it became evident that autologous cancellous fragments could be used to set up little centers of osteogenesis in sites where new bone formation was required and they are now much used for this purpose.

Some confusion about their effects arose because the possibility was raised that they acted by virtue of their being able to induce bone formation from some type of cell in the site to which they were transplanted. This idea led to the concept that chips of compact bone might serve the same purpose as cancellous chips. However, in 1952, Ham and Gordon showed that if autologous chips of cancellous bone were frozen and thawed three times to kill all their cells and then transplanted into muscle, no new bone formed on any of their surfaces. Similar cancellous chips not frozen and thawed, and similarly transplanted, showed new bone forming on their surfaces. They concluded from their work that the bone seen in association with transplanted cancellous chips was not induced bone but bone formed from the osteogenic cells that covered or lined the chips.

Cancellous bone is rich in covering and lining cells (osteogenic cells) in relation to its bulk. Chips of compact bone, however, would hardly ever have covering or lining cells on their surfaces. Hence since the bone that forms in association with transplanted cancellous bone chips is not induced bone but arises from their covering or lining osteogenic cells, transplants of autologous cancellous bone, and not chips of compact bone, should be used to set up centers of osteogenesis when these are needed to enhance bone formation.

Fig. 15-75. Photomicrograph of a homologous cancellous bone chip, 10 days after transplantation to muscle tissue. The transplanted bone was lamellar. It can be seen (*left* of *center*) that some immature bone has formed at its periphery from its covering osteogenic cells. There is at this stage a well-developed homograft reaction, which is resulting in death of the cells associated with the new bone. Note the large number of small lymphocytes that have infiltrated between the two main fragments of cancellous bone. The large dark-stained cells at *left* and *center* are osteoclasts. (Chalmers, J.: J. Bone Joint Surg. Brit., *41:*160, 1959)

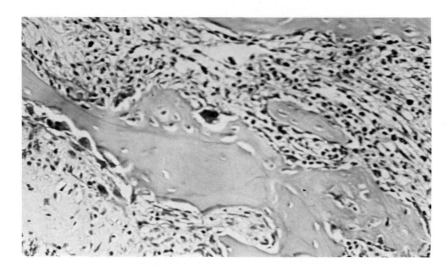

Transplants of Homologous Chips of Cancellous Bone. Chambers has shown that chips of homologous cancellous bone, for the first few days, act similarly to transplanted autologous chips in that the covering or lining cells of the chips proliferate and begin forming new bone on the surface of the chips transplanted. But, as shown in Figure 15-75, by 10 days a homograft reaction sets in and destroys the cells of the new bone formed, and many osteoclasts resorb both the bone of the transplanted chips and the new bone formed from the covering and lining cells.

Since the new bone that begins to form in association with transplanted homologous chips is by 10 days being destroyed by a homograft reaction, it is obvious that the new bone must have developed from the osteogenic cells of the transplanted homologous bone. If it were induced bone of host origin it would not incite a homograft reaction. (It should, however, be mentioned that very occasionally homologous bone chips left in position for months may reveal a little bone formation beside them; this, it is believed, is an example of transplanted bone inducing bone formation from some type of host cell, in all likelihood pericytes.)

REFERENCES AND OTHER READING

Bone histology is important to many disciplines and so current research involving bone is published in various journals dealing with general and cell biology, anatomy, biochemistry, endocrinology, and, in particular, orthopedics. It is an enormous project to provide a comprehensive bibliography, but one particular source deserves special mention since each of its many chapters has a very comprehensive list of references:

COMPREHENSIVE GENERAL REFERENCE

Bourne, G. H. (ed.): The Biochemistry and Physiology of Bone. ed. 2, vols. 1 to 4. New York, Academic Press, 1971 to 1976.

The following references are arranged in an order which as far as possible follows that in which various aspects of bone are dealt with in the text.

GENERAL BIOLOGY OF BONE

Hancox, N. M.: Biology of Bone. New York, Cambridge University Press, 1972.
Pritchard, J. J.: General histology of bone. *In* Bourne, G. H. (ed.): The Biochemistry and Physiology of Bone. ed. 2, vol. 1, p. 1. New York, Academic Press, 1972.

SPECIAL REFERENCES

Prenatal Development of Bone

Ascenzi, A., and Bendetti, L.: An electron microscope study of the foetal membranous ossification. Acta Anat. (Basel), *37:*370, 1962.
Bassett, A. L.: Current concepts of bone formation. J. Bone Joint Surg., *44-A:*1217, 1962.
Bernard, G. W., and Pease, D. C.: An electron microscope study of initial intramembranous osteogenesis. Am. J. Anat., *125:*271, 1969.
Decker, J. D.: An electron microscope investigation of osteogenesis in the embryonic chick. Am. J. Anat., *118:*591, 1966.
Fell, H. B.: Skeletal development in tissue culture. *In* Bourne, G. H. (ed.): The Biochemistry and Physiology of Bone. ed. 1. New York, Academic Press, 1956.
Gardner, E.: Osteogenesis in the human embryo and fetus. *In* Bourne, G. H. (ed.): The Biochemistry and Physiology of Bone. ed. 2, vol. 3, p. 77. New York, Academic Press, 1971.

Hall, B. K.: Histogenesis and morphogenesis of bone. Clin. Orthop., *71*:249, 1971.
———: Cellular differentiation in skeletal tissues. Biol. Rev., *45*:455, 1970.

Osteogenic (Osteoprogenitor) Cells, Osteoblasts, and Osteocytes

Bassett, C. A. L., and Herrmann, I.: Influence of oxygen concentration and mechanical factors on differentiation of connective tissues in vitro. Nature, *190*:460, 1961.
Cameron, D. A.: The ultrastructure of bone. *In* Bourne, G. H. (ed.): The Biochemistry and Physiology of Bone. ed. 2, vol. 1, p. 191. New York, Academic Press, 1972.
Ham, A. W.: Cartilage and bone. *In* Cowdry, E. V. (ed.): Special Cytology. ed. 2, vol. 2, p. 980. New York, Hoeber, 1932.
Holtrop, M. E.: The ultrastructure of bone. Ann. Clin. Lab. Sci., *5*:264, 1975.
Holtrop, M. E., and Weinger, J. M.: Ultrastructural evidence for a transport system in bone. *In* Talmage, R. V., and Munson, P. L. (eds.): Calcium, Parathyroid Hormone and the Calcitonins. p. 365. Amsterdam, Excerpta Medica, 1970.
King, G. J., and Holtrop, M. E.: Actin-like filaments in bone cells of cultured mouse calvaria as demonstrated by binding to heavy meromyosin. J. Cell Biol., *66*:445, 1975.
Owen, M.: Cell population kinetics of an osteogenic tissue. J. Cell Biol., *19*:19, 1963.
———: Uptake of ³H-uridine into precursor pools and RNA in osteogenic cells. J. Cell Sci., *2*:39, 1967.
———: The origin of bone cells. Int. Rev. Cytol., *28*:213, 1970.
———: Cellular dynamics of bone. *In* Bourne, G. H. (ed.): The Biochemistry and Physiology of Bone. ed. 2, vol. 3, p. 271. New York, Academic Press, 1971.
Pritchard, J. J.: The osteoblast. *In* Bourne, G. H. (ed.): The Biochemistry and Physiology of Bone. ed. 2, vol. 1, p. 21. New York, Academic Press, 1972.
Tonna, E. A., and Cronkite, E. P.: Autoradiographic studies of cell proliferation in the periosteum of intact and fractured femora of mice utilizing DNA labeling with ³H-thymidine. Proc. Soc. Exp. Biol. Med., *107*:719, 1961.
———: An autographic study of periosteal cell proliferation with tritiated thymidine. Lab. Invest., *11*:455, 1962.
———: The periosteum: autoradiographic studies on cellular proliferation and transformation, utilizing tritiated thymidine. Clin. Orthop., *30*:218, 1963.
Tonna, E. A., and Pentel, L. P.: Chondrogenic cell formation via osteogenic cell progeny transformation. Lab Invest., *27*:418, 1972.

Effects of Hormones on Bone

See references for Chapter 25.

Secondary Cartilage

See references for Chapter 16.

Bone Induction and Ectopic Bone

Büring, K.: On the origin of cells in heterotopic bone formation. Clinical Orthop., *110*:293, 1975.
Reddi, A. H.: Collagen and cell differentiation. *In* Ramachandran, G. N., and Reddi, A. H. (eds.): Biochemistry of Collagen. New York, Plenum, 1976.

Reddi, A. H., and Anderson, W. A.: Collagenous bone matrix induced endochondral ossification and hemopoiesis. J. Cell Biol., *69*:557, 1976.
Reddi, A. H., Gay, R., Gay, S., and Miller, E. J.: Transitions in collagen types during matrix-induced cartilage, bone and bone marrow formation. Proc. Natl. Acad. Sci., *74*:5589, 1977.
Urist, M. R.: Bone: formation by autoinduction. Science, *150*:893, 1965.
Urist, M. R., Felser, J. M., Hanamura, H., and Finerman, G. A. M.: An osteosarcoma cell and matrix retained morphogen for normal bone formation. Clin. Orthop. *124*:251, 1977.
Urist, M. R., Granstein, R., Nogami, H., Svenson, L., and Murphy, R.: Transmembrane bone morphogenesis across multiple-walled diffusion chambers. Arch. Surg., *112*:612, 1977.
Urist, M. R., Silverman, B. F., Büring, K., Dubuc, F. L., and Rosenberg, J. M.: The bone induction principle. Clin Orthop., *53*:243, 1967.
Urist, M. R., Hay, P. H., Dubuc, F. L., and Büring, K.: Osteogenic competence. Clin. Orthop., *64*:194, 1969.

The Organic Matrix of Bone and Its Calcification

Anderson, H. C.: Calcification of rachitic cartilage to study matrix vesicle function. Fed. Proc., *35*:147, 1976.
———: Matrix vesicles of cartilage and bone. *In* Bourne, G. H. (ed.): The Biochemistry and Physiology of Bone. ed. 2, vol. 4, p. 135. New York, Academic Press, 1976.
Bowness, J. M.: Present concepts of the role of ground substance in calcification. Clin. Orthop., *59*:233, 1968.
Eanes, E. D., and Posner, A. S.: Structure and chemistry of bone collagen. *In* Schraer, H. (ed.): Biological Calcification. Cellular and Molecular Aspects. pp. 1-26. 1970.
Fernandez-Madrid, F.: Collagen biosynthesis. A review. Clin. Orthop., *68*:103, 1970.
Herring, G. M.: The organic matrix of bone. *In* Bourne, G. H. (ed.): The Biochemistry and Physiology of Bone. ed. 2, vol. 1, p. 128. New York, Academic Press, 1972.
Howell, D. S.: Calcification mechanisms. Isr. J. Med. Sci., *12*:91, 1976.
Leblond, C. P., and Weinstock, M.: Radioautographic studies of bone formation. *In* Bourne, G. H. (ed.): The Biochemistry and Physiology of Bone. ed. 2, vol. 3, p. 181. New York, Academic Press, 1971.
Owen, M., and Triffitt, J. T.: Extravascular albumin in bone tissue. J. Physiol., *257*:293, 1976.
———: Plasma glycoproteins and bone. *In* Talmage, R. V., and Munson, P. L. (eds.): Calcium, Parathyroid Hormone and the Calcitonins. Amsterdam, Excerpta Medica, 1970.
Russell, R. G. G., and Fleisch, H.: Pyrophosphate and diphosphonates. *In* Bourne, G. H. (ed.): The Biochemistry and Physiology of Bone. ed. 2, vol. 4, p. 61. New York, Academic Press, 1976.
Tanes, D. R.: Mechanisms of calcification. Clin. Orthop., *42*:207, 1965.
Triffitt, J. T., and Owen, M.: Studies on bone matrix glycoproteins. Biochem. J., *136*:125, 1973.
Urist, M. R.: Biochemistry of calcification. *In* Bourne, G. H. (ed.): The Biochemistry and Physiology of Bone. ed. 2, vol. 4, p. 2. New York, Academic Press, 1976.

Mechanisms of Nutrition in Bone

Doty, S. B., and Schofield, B. H.: Metabolic and structural changes within osteocytes of rat bone. *In* Talmage, R. V., and

Munson, P. L. (eds.): Calcium, Parathyroid Hormone and Calcitonins. Amsterdam, Excerpta Medica, 1971.

Ham, A. W.: Some histophysiological problems peculiar to calcified tissues. J. Bone Joint Surg., *34-A:*701, 1952.

Harris, W. R., and Ham, A. W.: The mechanism of nutrition in bone and how it affects its structure, repair and transplantation. *In* Ciba Foundation Symposium on Bone Structure and Metabolism. p. 135. London, J. & A. Churchill, 1956.

Holtrop, M. E., and Weinger, J. M.: Ultrastructural evidence for a transport system in bone. *In* Talmage, R. V., and Munson, P. L. (eds.): Calcium, Parathyroid Hormone and the Calcitonins. p. 365. Amsterdam, Excerpta Medica, 1970.

Owen, M., Howlett, C. R., and Triffett, J. T.: Movement of [125]albumin and [125]polyvinyl-pyrrolidone through bone tissue fluid. Calcif. Tissue Res., *23:*103, 1977.

Osteocytic Osteolysis

Baud, C. A.: The Fine Structure of Normal and Parathormone Treated Bone. Proc. 4th Europ. Symp. on Calcified Tissues. Excerpta med. (Leiden), *120:*4, 1966.

Bélanger, L. F., Migicovsky, B. B., Copp, D. H., and Vincent, J.: Resorption without osteoclasts (osteolysis). *In* Sognnaes, R. F. (ed.): Mechanisms of Hard Tissue Destruction. p. 531. Washington, Am. Assoc. Adv. Sci., 1965.

Bélanger, L. F., and Robichon, J.: Parathormone-induced osteolysis in dogs. J. Bone Joint Surg., *46-A:*1008, 1964.

Bélanger, L. F., Semba, T., Tolnai, S., Copp, D. H., Krook, L., and Gries, C.: The two faces of resorption. Third European Symposium on Calcified Tissues. New York, Springer-Verlag, 1966.

Bélanger, L. F.: Osteocytic osteolysis. Calcif. Tissue Res., *4:*1, 1969.

————: Osteocytic Resorption. *In* Bourne, G. H. (ed.): The Biochemistry and Physiology of Bone. ed. 2, vol. 3, p. 240. New York, Academic Press, 1971.

Bonucci, E., Gherardi, G., and Faraggiana, T.: Bone changes in hemodialyzed uremic subjects. Virchows Arch. A. Pathol. Anat. Histol., *371:*183, 1976.

Cameron, D. A., Parshall, H. A., and Robinson, R. A.: Changes in the fine structure of bone cells after the administration of parathyroid extract. J. Cell Biol., *33:*1, 1967.

Jande, S. S.: Effects of parathormone on osteocytes and their surrounding bone matrix. An electron microscopic study. Z. Zellforsch. Mikrosk. Anat., *130:*463, 1972.

Jande, S. S., and Bélanger, J. F.: The life-cycle of the osteocyte. Clin. Orthop., *94:*281, 1973.

Marks, S. C., and Walker, D. G.: Mammalian osteopetrosis—a model for studying cellular and humoral factors in bone resorption. *In* Bourne, G. H. (ed.): The Biochemistry and Physiology of Bone. ed. 2, vol. 4, p. 227. New York, Academic Press, 1976.

Osteoclasts

Bonucci, E.: The organic-inorganic relationships in bone matrix undergoing osteoclastic resorption. Calcif. Tissue Res., *16:*13, 1974.

Cameron, D. A.: The ultrastructure of bone. *In* Bourne, G. H. (ed.): The Biochemistry and Physiology of Bone. ed. 2, vol. 1, p. 191. New York, Academic Press, 1972.

Doty, S. B., and Schofield, B. H.: Electron microscopic localization of hydrolytic enzymes in osteoclasts. Histochem. J., *4:*245, 1972.

Fischman, D. A., and Hay, E. D.: Origin of osteoclasts from mononuclear leukocytes in regenerating newt limbs. Anat. Rec., *143:*329, 1962.

Gonzales, F.: Electron microscopy of osteoclasts. Anat. Rec., *139:*330, 1961.

Gonzales, F., and Karnovsky, M. J.: Electron microscopy of osteoclasts in healing fractures of rat bone. J. Biophy. Biochem. Cytol., *9:*299, 1961.

Göthlin, G., and Ericsson, J. L. E.: The osteoclast. Clin. Orthop., *120:*201, 1976.

Hall, B. K.: The origin and fate of osteoclasts. Anat. Rec., *183:*1, 1975.

Ham, A. W.: Some histophysiological problems peculiar to calcified tissues. J. Bone Joint Surg., *36-A:*701, 1952.

Ham, A. W., and Gordon, S.: The origin of bone that forms in association with cancellous chips transplanted into muscle. Br. J. Plastic Surg., *5:*154, 1952.

Hancox, N. M.: Motion picture studies of osteoclasts. *In* Rose, G. G. (ed.): Cinemicrography in Cell Biology. p. 141. New York, Academic Press, 1963.

————: The osteoclast. *In* Bourne, G. H. (ed.): The Biochemistry and Physiology of Bone. ed. 2, vol. 1, p. 45. New York, Academic Press, 1972.

Hancox, N. M., and Boothroyd, B.: Structure-function relationships in the osteoclast. *In* Sognnaes, R. F. (ed.): Mechanisms of Hard Tissue Destruction. Washington, D.C., Am. Assoc. Adv. Science, 1963.

Holtrop, M. E.: The ultrastructure of bone. Ann. Clin. Lab. Sci., *5:*264, 1975.

————: The ultrastructure of osteoclasts during stimulation and inhibition of bone resorption. *In* Scow, R. O., Ebling, F. J. G., and Henderson, I. W. (eds.): Proc. 4th International Congr. of Endocrinology. p. 462. Amsterdam, Excerpta Medica, 1973.

Holtrop, M. E., and King, G. J.: The ultrastructure of the osteoclast and its functional implications. Clin. Orthop., *123:*177, 1977.

Holtrop, M. E., King, G. J., Cox, K. A., and Reit, B.: Time related changes in the ultrastructure of osteoclasts after injection of parathyroid hormone in young rats. Calcif. Tissue Res., *in press.*

Irving, J. T., and Handelman, C. S.: Bone destruction by multinucleated giant cells. *In* Sognnaes, R. F. (ed.): Mechanisms of Hard Tissue Destruction. Washington, D. C., Am. Assoc. Adv. Science Pub. No. 75, p. 515, 1963.

Jee, W. S. S., and Nolan, P. D.: Origin of osteoclasts from the fusion of phagocytes. Nature, *200:*225, 1963.

Jotereau, F. V., and Le Douarin, N. M.: The developmental relationship between osteocytes and osteoclasts: a study using the quail-chick nuclear marker in endochondral ossification. Dev. Biol., *63:*253, 1978.

Kahn, A. J., and Simmons, D. J.: Investigation of cell lineages in bone using a chimaera of chick and quail embryonic tissue. Nature, *258:*325, 1975.

Kallio, D. M., Garant, P. R., and Minkin, C.: Evidence of coated membranes in the ruffled border of the osteoclast. J. Ultrastruct. Res., *37:*169, 1971.

————: Ultrastructural effects of calcitonin on osteoclasts in tissue culture. J. Ultrastruct. Res., *39:*305, 1972.

King, G. J., Holtrop, M. E., and Raisz, L. G.: The relation of ultrastructural changes in osteoclasts to resorption in bone cultures stimulated with parathyroid hormone. Metabolic Bone Diseases and Related Research, *1:*67, 1978.

Loutit, J. F., and Sanson, J. M.: Osteopetrosis of microphthalmic mice—a defect of the hemopoietic stem cell? Calcif. Tissue Res., *20:*251, 1976.

Lucht, V., and Norgaard, J. O.: Uptake of peroxidase by calcitonin in inhibited osteoclasts. Histochemistry, *54:*143, 1977.

Luk, S. C., Nopajaroonsri, C., and Simon, G. T.: The ultrastructure of endosteum: a topographic study in young adult rabbits. J. Ultrastruct. Res., *46:*165, 1974.

Marks, S. C., and Walker, D. G.: Mammalian osteopetrosis—a model for studying cellular and humoral factors in bone resorption. *In* Bourne, G. H. (ed.): The Biochemistry and Physiology of Bone. ed. 2, vol. 4, p. 227. New York, Academic Press, 1976.

Mundy, G. R., Varani, J., Orr, W., Gondek, M. D., and Ward, P. A.: Resorbing bone is chemotactic for monocytes. Nature, *275:*132, 1978.

Raisz, L. G., Holtrop, M. E., and Simmons, H. A.: Inhibition of bone resorption by colchicine in organ culture. Endocrinology, *92:*556, 1973.

Rasmussen, H., and Bordier, P.: The cellular basis of metabolic bone disease. N. Engl. J. Med., *289:*25, 1973.

———: The Physiological and Cellular Basis of Metabolic Bone Disease. Baltimore, Williams & Wilkins, 1974.

Scott, B. L., and Pease, D. C.: Electron microscopy of the epiphyseal apparatus. Anat. Rec., *126:*465, 1956.

———: Thymidine-³H electron microscope radioautography of osteogenic cells in the fetal rat. J. Cell Biol., *35:*1967.

Walker, D. G.: Experimental osteopetrosis. Clin. Orthop., *97:*158, 1973.

———: Bone resorption restored in osteopetrotic mice by transplants of normal bone marrow and spleen cells. Science, *190:*784, 1975.

———: Spleen cells transmit osteopetrosis in mice. Science, *190:*785, 1975.

———: Control of bone resorption by hematopoietic tissue. The induction and reversal of congenital osteopetrosis in mice through use of bone marrow and splenic transplants. J. Exp. Med., *142:*651, 1975.

Effects of Nutritional and Metabolic Disturbances on Bone Growth and Remodeling

Amprino, R.: Bone histophysiology. Guys Hosp. Rep., *116:*51, 1967.

Barer, M., and Jowsey, J.: Bone formation and resorption in normal human ribs. Clin. Orthop., *52:*241, 1967.

Burkhart, J. M., and Jowsey, J.: Parathyroid and thyroid hormones in the development of immobilization osteoporosis. Endocrinology, *81:*1053, 1967.

Frost, H. M.: Tetracycline-based histological analysis of bone remodelling. Calcif. Tissue Res., *3:*211, 1969.

Ham, A. W., and Elliott, H. C.: The bone and cartilage lesions of protracted moderate scurvy. Am. J. Pathol., *14:*323, 1938.

Harris, W. H., and Heaney, R. P.: Skeletal renewal and metabolic bone disease. N. Engl. J. Med., *280:*193-253, 303, 1969.

Jowsey, J., and Gordan, G.: Bone turnover and osteoporosis. *In* Bourne, G. H. (ed.): The Biochemistry and Physiology of Bone. ed. 2, vol. 3, p. 202. New York, Academic Press, 1971.

Jowsey, J., and Riggs, B. L.: Assessment of bone turnover by microradiography and autoradiography. Semin. Nucl. Med., *2:*3, 1972.

Silberberg, M., and Silberberg, R.: Steroid hormones and bone. *In* Bourne, G. H. (ed.): The Biochemistry and Physiology of Bone. ed. 2, vol. 3, p. 401. New York, Academic Press, 1971.

The Blood Supply of Bones

Brookes, M.: Femoral growth after occlusion of the principal nutrient canal in day-old rabbits. J. Bone Joint Surg., *39:*563, 1957.

———: Sequelae of experimental parietal ischemia in long bones of the rabbit. J. Anat., *94:*552, 1960.

Brookes, M., and Harrison, R. G.: The vascularization of the rabbit femur and tibiofibula. J. Anat., *91:*61, 1957.

Cohen, J., and Harris, W. H.: The three-dimensional anatomy of haversian systems, J. Bone Joint Surg., *49-A:*419, 1958.

Dale, G. G., and Harris, W. R.: Prognosis of epiphyseal separation. J. Bone Joint Surg., *40-B:*116, 1958.

Harris, W. R., and Bobechko, W. P.: The radiographic density of avascular bone. J. Bone Joint Surg., *42-B:*626, 1960.

Harris, W. R., and Ham, A. W.: The mechanism of nutrition in bone and how it affects its structure, repair and transplantation. *In* Ciba Foundation Symposium on Bone Structure and Metabolism. p. 135. London, J. & A. Churchill, 1956.

Harrison, R. C., and Gámez, F. N.: Hormonal effects on the vascularization of bone. Symp. Zool. Soc. London, *II:*I, 1964.

Irving, M. H.: The blood supply of the growth cartilage in young rats. J. Anat., *98:*631, 1964.

Johnson, R. W.: A physiological study of the blood supply of the diaphysis. J. Bone Joint Surg., *9:*153, 1927.

Kember, N. F., and Sissons, H. A.: Quantitative histology of the human growth plate. J. Bone Joint Surg., *58-B:*426, 1976.

Rhinelander, F. W.: Circulation of Bone. *In* Bourne, G. H. (ed.): The Biochemistry and Physiology of Bone. ed. 2, vol. 2, p. 1. New York, Academic Press, 1972.

Salter, R. B., and Harris, W. R.: Injuries involving the epiphyseal plate. J. Bone Joint Surg., *45-A:*587, 1963.

Trueta, J., and Harrison, M. H. M.: The normal vascular anatomy of the femoral head in adult man. J. Bone Joint Surg., *35:*442, 1953.

The Repair and Transplantation of Bone

Chalmers, J.: Bone transplantation. Symp. on Tissue and Organ Transplantation. J. Clin. Pathol., *20*[Suppl.]:540, 1967.

Crelin, E. S., White, A. A., Panjabi, M. M., and Southwick, W.: Microscopic changes in fractured rabbit tibias. Conn. Med., *42:*561, 1978.

Gordon, S., and Ham, A. W.: The fate of transplanted cancellous bone. *In* The Gallie Addresses. p. 296. Toronto, University of Toronto Press, 1950.

Grant, C. G.: An investigation of the mechanical aspects of long-term fracture healing following rigid fixation. Ph.D. Thesis, Institute of Medical Science, University of Toronto, 1973.

Ham, A. W.: An histologic study of the early phases of bone repair. J. Bone Joint Surg., *12:*827, 1930.

Ham, A. W., and Harris, W. R.: Repair and transplantation of bone. *In* Bourne, G. H. (ed.): The Biochemistry and Physiology of Bone. ed. 2, vol. 3, pp. 338 and 379. New York, Academic Press, 1971.

Ham, A. W., Tisdall, F. F., and Drake, T. G. H.: Experimental noncalcification of callus simulating nonunion. J. Bone Joint Surg., *20:*345, 1938.

Langer, F., Czitrom, A., Pritzker, K. P., and Gross, A. E.: The immunogenicity of fresh and frozen allogeneic bone. J. Bone Joint Surg., *57-A:*216, 1975.

Schenk, R., and Willenegger, H.: Morphological findings in primary fracture healing. Symp. Biol. Hung., *7:*75, 1967.

Wilkinson, G. W., and Leblond, C. P.: The deposition of radiophosphorus in fractured bones in rats. Surg. Gynecol. Obstet., *97:*143, 1953.

16 Joints

Joint afflictions are probably the greatest single cause of disability seen by members of the medical profession, and it is therefore important that the student become familiar with the structure of joints and learn as much about them as possible.

Definition and Function. The words *articulation* (L. *articulatio,* the place of union or junction between two or more bones) and *joint* (L. *junctio,* a joining, connection) are used synonymously to refer to structural arrangements that connect two or more bones together at their site of meeting. Although many joints permit movement between the bones they connect, this is not essential for a connecting structure to be termed a *joint;* indeed some joints become as solid as the bones they connect. Another

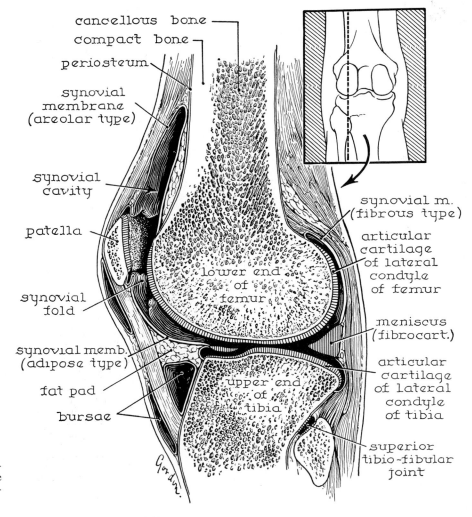

cancellous bone
compact bone
periosteum
synovial membrane (areolar type)
synovial cavity
patella
synovial fold
synovial memb. (adipose type)
fat pad
bursae

synovial m. (fibrous type)
articular cartilage of lateral condyle of femur
meniscus (fibrocart.)
articular cartilage of lateral condyle of tibia
superior tibio-fibular joint

lower end of femur
upper end of tibia

Fig. 16-1. Drawing of a longitudinal section of a human knee joint. The plane of section is indicated in the inset.

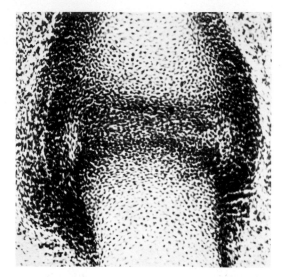

Fig. 16-2. Low-power photomicrograph of a longitudinal section of a developing interphalangeal joint (20-mm. human embryo). The developing cartilaginous ends of the bones-to-be appear pale. The dark-staining material at *center* is condensed mesenchyme of the articular disk; the dark-staining stripes on each side of the ends of the developing cartilage models represent condensed mesenchyme destined to form the capsule of the joint. The small clear areas seen in the dark-staining, otherwise condensed mesenchyme of the disk represent the beginnings of the synovial cavity.

function of some joints is to allow the structures they connect to grow.

Classification. Joints may be classified in several ways. Since there are only two kinds that give much trouble, termed *synovial joints* and *symphyses,* we shall describe these two clinically important kinds first.

SYNOVIAL JOINTS

In order to describe *synovial joints* (Gr. *syn,* together; L. *ovum,* egg), it must be noted that for free movement to occur between two bones meeting in a joint, the two surfaces moving on each other must be lubricated. The lubricant is called *synovial fluid* (black in Fig. 16-1) because it reminded whoever named these joints of the white of an egg. Furthermore, for movement to occur in such a joint with little friction, the surfaces moving on each other must be smooth and slippery. This is achieved by the ends of the bones being capped with hyaline cartilage, so that the free surfaces that move on each other consist of naked noncalcified intercellular substance of *articular cartilage* (cross-striped in Fig. 16-1).

Next, a synovial joint is ensheathed by a *joint capsule.* This does not impede movement because it blends with the periosteum of the bones meeting in the joint at some distance away from their articulating ends (Fig. 16-1). The capsule is lined with a special layer called the *synovial membrane* (Fig. 16-1), which both forms and resorbs synovial fluid, as described presently.

In order to understand the details of a synovial joint it is important to learn first how it develops.

Development. It was explained in Chapter 15 that central mesenchyme in embryonic limb buds differentiates into cartilage so that cartilage models of bones-to-be are formed. The mesenchyme immediately surrounding the shaft of a cartilage model becomes arranged into an indistinctly 2-layered membrane, the *perichondrium.* The outer layer of this membrane assumes a fibrous nature and the inner one remains cellular and chondrogenic, so that by appositional growth it can add further layers of cartilage to the sides of the shaft, causing it to grow in width. We shall now consider the series of events that occur in regions where the ends of cartilage models approach one another (Fig. 16-2) and a synovial joint develops.

The mesenchyme between the ill-defined ends of two developing models becomes condensed (the dark area between the ends of the two cartilage models of bones-to-be in Fig. 16-2); this is called the *articular disk of mesenchyme* or the *primitive joint plate* (Fig. 16-2). In a manner similar to that in which perichondrium forms around shafts of cartilage models, mesenchyme that surrounds the whole region where the two ends of the cartilage models are developing also becomes condensed to form the counterpart of the perichondrium in this region (Fig. 16-2); this is the forerunner of the *capsule* of the joint. This fits like a sleeve over the end of each cartilage model and extends for some distance to become continuous with the perichondrium covering the shafts of the models.

As development proceeds, the amorphous intercellular substance and tissue fluid between mesenchymal cells of the articular disk increase and, as a result, the cells become widely separated from one another in certain areas. This soon leads to the appearance of fluid-filled clefts in the substance of the disk. These spaces gradually fuse with one another so that a continuous cavity, the *synovial cavity,* comes to occupy the site formerly occupied by the bulk of the disk. This permits the ends of the two cartilage models to come into contact and articulate with each other.

The process by which a synovial cavity is formed is not confined to the region between the two ends of the models; the same process causes the cavity to extend along the sides of the two models for some distance (the final result is shown in Fig. 16-1). The outer part of the condensed mesenchyme that surrounds the joint area, and which is the counterpart of the fibrous layer of the perichondrium of the shafts of the models, is thereby more or less split away from deeper layers of perichon-drium (that still cover the sides of the ends of the models). This outer part develops into the joint capsule. However, the developing joint capsule remains continuous with the tightly attached perichondrium (or periosteum, as the case may be) that covers the shafts of the models some little distance back from their ends (Fig. 16-1).

As development continues, differentiation occurs in the forming joint capsule. The mesenchyme comprising its outer, thicker layer differentiates into dense fibrous tissue, which becomes the stronger and thicker part of the joint capsule, while that of its inner layer forms its synovial layer, commonly termed the *synovial membrane,* the microscopic structure of which will be described presently.

THE MICROSCOPIC STRUCTURE OF ARTICULAR CARTILAGE

Articular cartilage is an example of hyaline cartilage (as described in Chap. 14 and illustrated in Fig. 14-3) except that its free surface as shown in Figure 16-3 is *not covered with perichondrium.* Hence articular cartilage is unique in that the surface it presents in a synovial joint to articulate with another articular cartilage is that of naked cartilage matrix.

The Cells of Articular Cartilage. The cells of articular cartilage are all descendants of chondrocytes that were located in the end portions of cartilaginous models of bones-to-be. In postnatal life articular cartilage of long bones must continue to grow in order for an epiphysis to enlarge to its adult size. During growth the articular cartilage thus plays the same growth role for an epiphysis of a long bone as the epiphyseal plate does for the diaphysis; in short bones it serves for growth of the bone as a whole.

In the epiphysis of a growing bone, proliferation occurs in the chondrocytes close to the articular surface. As is evident in Figure 16-3, in growing animals the cells close to the articular surface are more scattered than those deeper in the cartilage. Mitosis during growth has been observed mostly in those chondrocytes lying in about the third ill-defined row of cells parallel to the surface.

Deeper in the cartilage, chondrocytes are arranged in longitudinal rows perpendicular to the surface, and for the most part lie in longitudinally disposed cell nests (Fig. 16-3). This arrangement suggests that as they divided it was easier for the two cells forming from a mitosis to separate longitudinally, probably because most of the collagenic fibrils of the intercellular substance lie more or less at right angles to the surface. So the arrangement of cell nests in articular cartilage is probably determined by the orientation of the collagenic fibrils in much the same way

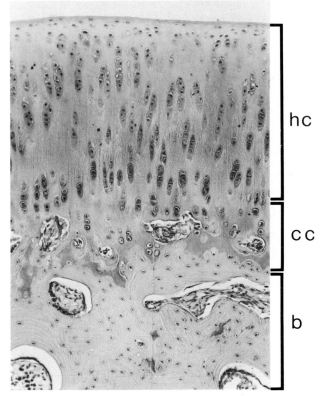

Fig. 16-3. Photomicrograph showing articular cartilage and subchondral bone (b) of a knee joint of a rabbit. The articular cartilage consists of three ill-defined zones. In the superficial zone the chondrocytes are small and flattened. In the middle zone the cells are arranged in columns lying perpendicular to the surface. Both the superficial and the middle zones are typical hyaline cartilage (labeled hc). The deep zone of the articular cartilage consists of calcified cartilage (cc) and contains small chondrocytes. Note the absence of blood vessels in the uncalcified zones (hc) of articular cartilage. (Courtesy of R. Salter and E. Bogoch)

as it is in epiphyseal plates, where the cell nests also are arranged in longitudinal columns. Furthermore, it seems that the mitoses producing the cell nests during growth normally occur only in the zone of the columns close to the articular surface. Deeper down in the columns, the chondrocytes can develop into larger cells and, of course, continue to produce intercellular substance.

In the deepest part of the articular cartilage the intercellular substance becomes calcified (cc in Fig. 16-3) and stains somewhat more deeply, even in decalcified H and E sections, than the intercellular substance surrounding the cells in the outer part of this layer (hc in Fig. 16-3). During the period of growth this layer of calcified cartilage is more or less continuously replaced by new bone in the same manner as occurs on the diaphyseal side of an epiphyseal plate. But the replacement process here is much more irregular. In Figure 16-3, the bone matrix (b) is more lightly stained than the calcified cartilage to which it is firmly attached. The bone fits against the calcified cartilage to form a bony plate which supports the articular cartilage. The bone here is a mixture of compact and cancellous in that a substantial amount of compact bone is present, but there are also many fairly wide canals of the haversian type, which contain osteogenic cells and blood vessels (Fig. 16-3).

The Fine Structure of Chondrocytes. This was described in Chapter 14 and illustrated in Figure 14-4, so only brief comment will be made here.

During the growth period, chondrocytes of articular cartilage are synthesizing and secreting both the protein (tropocollagen) and the proteoglycan components of the intercellular substance of cartilage. As might be expected, chondrocytes engaged in this activity demonstrate the usual features of cells synthesizing protein and carbohydrate required for intercellular substances in that their cytoplasm reveals abundant cisternae of rER and a well-developed Golgi apparatus (Fig. 14-4). The borders of chondrocytes appear very ragged because their cytoplasm extends for short distances in the form of processes much like microvilli but generally termed *cytoplasmic footlets*.

As chondrocytes become older the organelles associated with protein synthesis and secretion (rER and Golgi apparatus) become less prominent and glycogen and lipid may accumulate in the cytoplasm. Silberberg and Silberberg believe that chondrocytes that die in the substance of the cartilage after growth is over are replaced by fibrillar scars.

The Source of Nutrients for Articular Cartilage. Since articular cartilage contains no capillaries, nutrients must diffuse to its cells from outside its substance. Calcification of intercellular substance in its deeper layers probably shuts off nutrients derived from capillaries of the cancellous bone that underlies it; it is said, however, that there are certain sites where a little nourishment may percolate through to it by this route. Around its periphery articular cartilage probably obtains some nourishment from vessels of the synovial membrane in a manner to be described presently. But the greater part of an articular cartilage obtains its nourishment from the synovial fluid. It has been demonstrated repeatedly that fragments of cartilage, detached by injury and floating freely in the synovial fluid, not only survive but also in some instances grow in size. Furthermore, in experimentally produced fractures of necks of femurs of dogs, in which the heads of the bones are separated completely from all blood supply and then pinned in place, the articular cartilages of the

heads, as seen in sections, appear generally to survive over the succeeding months. When good results are obtained in such fractures, the dead bone (and marrow) of the head is all replaced, as has been described in connection with the healing of a fracture, and new bone develops to support the living articular cartilage that has survived the whole procedure. Since a head of a femur has no blood supply until it is revascularized, and since the region directly beneath the articular cartilage is the last part of the head to be revascularized, it seems evident that synovial fluid is capable of supporting viability of chondrocytes of articular cartilage. This shows that synovial fluid even under normal circumstances would provide nutrients for most of the cells of articular cartilage.

Growth and Maintenance. Articular cartilage, as noted, provides for growth of a bony epiphysis in the same way as an epiphyseal disk provides for growth in length of a bony diaphysis; indeed, in short bones without epiphyseal disks (Fig. 15-43), the articular cartilages serve as the sites wherein the bone as a whole grows in length. During the growing period, mitotic figures are observed among the chondrocytes of articular cartilage, not in the most superficial layer of flat cells (which might otherwise be assumed to be the youngest cells in the cartilage), but somewhat deeper, in about the third or fourth layer below the surface. Deep to this layer the chondrocytes of articular cartilage are more mature, and still deeper, next to the bone, they are hypertrophied and the intercellular substance surrounding them is calcified. During the period of active growth this zone of calcified cartilage is continuously being replaced by bone, which forms from the osteogenic cells and osteoblasts that invade this layer of cartilage from the marrow cavity of the epiphysis. However, when the epiphysis has grown to its full size these two processes—the growth of the cartilage and its replacement by bone—appear to cease. Elliott could not find mitotic figures in the articular cartilages of adult animals even if they were specifically exercised.

If mitosis does not occur in the articular cartilage of an adult, it must be assumed that its chondrocytes, for the most part, have a very long life span and that they compensate for wear and tear by producing more intercellular substance throughout life. Indeed Rosenthal and his associates have shown that the numbers of cells in articular cartilage decrease in relation to the amount of intercellular substance throughout life.

THE MATRIX OF ARTICULAR CARTILAGE

Diffusion Mechanisms Accounting for Nutrition Within Articular Cartilage. As emphasized in the two preceding chapters, there are no capillaries within cartilage; hence chondrocytes must obtain nourishment from nutrients that diffuse into it via its intercellular substance. They also must rid themselves of waste products of metabolism by diffusion through it in the opposite direction. Furthermore, the source of the nutrients diffusing into articular cartilage is synovial fluid and the nutrients in it are in turn derived from capillaries close to the inner surface of the synovial membrane. It is important to realize that this is a *very long pathway for nutrients and waste products to have to take.*

Next, if diffusion mechanisms are to operate effectively through the matrix of articular cartilage it must, of course, contain sufficient water (tissue fluid). Actually, articular cartilage contains about 75 to 80 per cent water. But although this explains why its intercellular substance serves as an effective medium for diffusion, it also raises a question: what makes it possible for the matrix to be firm and somewhat elastic in composition, instead of being semifluid in consistency? Further, how is it possible for articular cartilage to withstand pressure as, for example, in the knee joints when a person is standing and these joints are bearing the weight of almost all the body, without the articular cartilages being squeezed out of shape or rendered functionless? The chemical composition of articular cartilage has been much studied in recent years in order to try to answer these questions and to establish why articular cartilage possesses its unique physical properties and yet holds so much water. However, this has proved to be a complex subject and it would go beyond the scope of this book to provide more than an elementary account of it (however, in-depth studies are listed in References and Other Reading).

It is known that roughly 80 per cent of articular cartilage is water because its dry weight is only about 20 to 25 per cent of its wet weight. Of its dry weight about half is due to collagen, so that collagen actually only constitutes about 10 per cent of the substance of living articular cartilage. The remaining 10 per cent of its wet weight consists of noncollagenic substances, mostly proteoglycan complexes of one sort or another. The secret of its physical properties seems to lie in the association between its collagen and proteoglycans. Before attempting to discuss this association, however, we shall first comment further on collagen, already described on page 231.

Some Biochemical Features of Collagen: the Collagen Molecule. In recent years the biochemistry of collagen, the principal fibrous protein in the intercellular substance of connective tissues, has been much investigated.

As described in connection with intercellular substances on page 231, the collagen molecule is composed of a triple helix of polypeptide chains. These have a repeating glycine residue in every third position, except at the N and C terminals, where telopeptides give the molecule its antigenic specificity. Each chain has more than 1,000 amino acid residues; the collagen triple helix, or tropocollagen molecule, has a molecular weight of approximately 100,000. As described on page 234 and illustrated in Figure 9-11, molecules of collagen are oriented in a quarter-stagger overlap to form collagenic fibrils. Intramolecular and intermolecular chemical cross links between chains within a molecule and between molecules within a fibril stabilize the structural unit—the fibril.

Minor variations in primary amino acid sequence alter the chemical properties of the collagen molecule so that the fibrils composed of them are different. There are four types of collagen (*see* p. 231). Of interest to us here is that Type I collagen is characteristically found in ordinary connective tissue (including tendon, fascia, and the fibrocartilage of menisci of joints) and also in the special type of connective tissue bone, but the collagen of hyaline cartilage (including articular cartilage) is of the Type II kind described on page 231. We shall refer to this type again in connection with the nucleus pulposus, described later in connection with joints between vertebrae.

Collagenic Fibrils in the Matrix of Articular Cartilage. The collagen in articular cartilage exists in the form of fibrils, the formation and fine structure of which are described on page 233. In *fibrocartilage*, however, as mentioned in Chapter 14, the fibrils are bundled together to form coarse collagenic fibers. The fibrils in *articular cartilage* vary in diameter, apparently in relation to the position they occupy, as shown in the electron micrograph in Figure 16-4. In examining this, there are parts of two chondrocytes, labeled C, which may be used for landmarks.

The thin zone lining a lacuna, that appears as a dark line in an H and E section (Fig. 14-3), is very pale in an electron micrograph (Fig. 16-4, where it is labeled H) and is termed a *pericellular halo*. It contains only *very fine* collagenic fibrils and presumably relatively more proteoglycan and glycoprotein; the latter substances are not dense enough to show up well in micrographs but they account for the heavy staining of the halo observed with light microscopy. A little farther away from the cell more mature collagenic fibrils (labeled TF) are numerous and disposed so as to encircle lacunae. These surrounding fibrils characterize what are termed *territorial zones*. Farther away, the collagen between the territorial zones of lacunae is termed the *interterritorial matrix* (labeled IT). Here the fibrils are larger and their cross banding is readily seen. The fibrils here are randomly arranged.

The interstices between fibrils contain some glycoprotein and a variety of proteoglycans (for an account of the structure of these proteoglycans, *see* Rosenberg). It has been suggested that the protein moiety of the proteoglycans is anchored to the collagenic fibrils and that

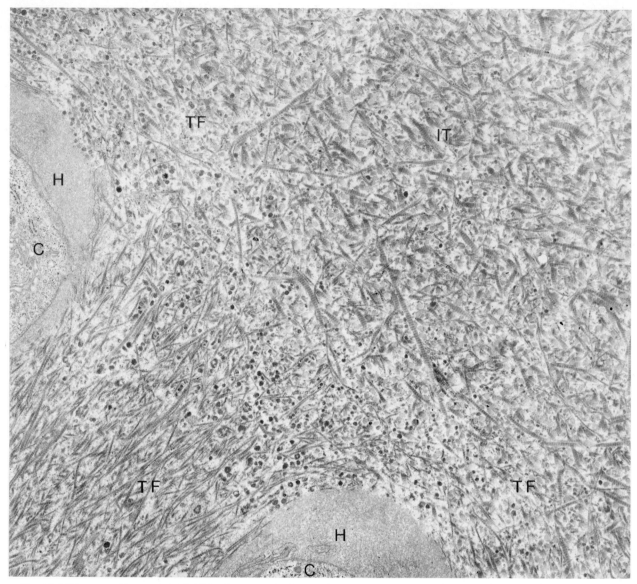

Fig. 16-4. Electron micrograph (×15,000) of human articular cartilage, showing the appearance of collagenic fibrils in its matrix. At *left,* and also *bottom center,* portions of chondrocytes (C) filling their lacunae are seen. Surrounding each chondrocyte is a relatively homogeneous looking region termed a pericellular halo (H) containing extremely fine collagenic fibrils (only 4 to 10 nm. in diameter). External to this (*left of center* and also *lower right* in this micrograph) fibrils of the territorial zone are seen; these are labeled TF. Note their orientation around the lacunae. At *upper right* the wide mature fibrils (30 to 200 nm. in diameter) characteristic of the interterritorial matrix (IT) may be seen to have a random arrangement. (Lane, J. M., and Weiss, C.: Review of articular cartilage collagen research. Arthritis Rheum., *18:*553, 1975)

this interaction is essential if the cartilage matrix is to behave like a gel and hold water. The stiffness of the gel is attributed to the water-holding capacity of the glycosaminoglycan molecules of the proteoglycan aggregates. These glycosaminoglycan molecules have a huge surface area and, since they are negatively charged, great affinity for polar water molecules. The cartilage matrix is therefore kept extensively hydrated and so serves as an efficient medium for diffusion for the solutes required for the maintenance of chondrocytes.

THE HEALING OF DAMAGED ARTICULAR CARTILAGE

This is a challenging area for research because the prospects of satisfactory repair or regeneration of articular cartilage after injury have in the past been dismal. First, it has been generally acknowledged that wounds of articular cartilage that do not involve its underlying bone do not heal, and that at best all that can be expected is that there may be some molding of the matrix around their edges that perhaps involves production of a little new matrix by chondrocytes adjacent to the wound. Failure to heal is of course attributed to the seeming inability of chondrocytes of full-grown articular cartilage to undergo mitosis. Second, it has also been generally conceded that, if a fracture involves both an articular cartilage and the bone plate supporting it, healing can occur. However, this healing of cartilage is not due to proliferation of chondrocytes of articular cartilage. Instead it is a side effect of damage done to underlying tissue, including repair of the fracture of the underlying bone. As described in the previous chapter, the healing of a bone fracture involves formation of an external callus, which forms through proliferation of osteogenic cells and subsequent differentiation of these cells into both bone and cartilage cells. So the repair of articular cartilage that occurs when the underlying bone is fractured can be due in part to callus tissue that forms from the repair of the bone extending up through the fracture site into the defect in the articular cartilage and at best repairing it with a mixture of new bone and new cartilage. The latter tissue, however, is generally mixed with ordinary connective tissue that forms from pericytes and fibroblasts. However, since the bony component of the repair tissue would become calcified, the mixture does not provide a smooth surface for the articular cartilage and so this type of repair generally ends up causing an arthritic joint.

One very interesting aspect of the problem of healing of articular cartilage has been explored by Salter and his associates (*see* References and Other Reading), which is the effect of continuous passive motion of a joint on the healing process. This approach is based in part on the concept that since joints are specifically designed to permit motion, such healing as might occur after injury to a joint would not be as effective if the joint were put to rest as it might be if the movement for which the joint was designed continued to occur. In support of this concept is the knowledge that if motion is prevented in the joints of developing embryos, these joints do not develop normally. For example, Drachman and others have reported that paralysis of chick embryos induced by administering curare via the chorioallantoic membrane causes abnormalities in the developing joints of these chicks, one feature of which is that the articular cartilages do not develop properly. It has also been noted that motion seems to be related to the formation of cartilage. In the repair of bone fractures, for example, continued motion between the two fragments may result in excessive formation of cartilage in the callus or even in the development of what is termed a *pseudarthrosis*, where so much cartilage is formed between the two ends of the bony fragments that a "false joint" allowing movement to occur forms between the broken ends of the bone. In addition, the fact that cartilage-containing joints develop from condensed mesenchyme between bones that have developed as a result of "intramembranous ossification" strongly suggests that physical stress such as motion or pressure can somehow influence the formation of cartilage from mesenchymal cells. So there would seem to be several reasons for thinking that if formation of cartilage were to be encouraged in joint injuries, this would best be achieved by subjecting the joint to motion.

There is also a histophysiological reason for believing that motion could permit better repair, or at least cause less damage, than would occur with the injured cartilage at rest. We have already explained that for nutrients to reach the chondrocytes they first have to diffuse from the synovial membrane into the synovial fluid, then diffuse through the latter to the surface of the articular cartilage, and finally pass through the intercellular substance of the cartilage to the chondrocytes. Since there is only a thin film of synovial fluid between two apposed articular cartilages, any nutrients present in this film in a stationary joint would soon be absorbed into the cartilage and metabolized. Moreover, if a joint were kept at rest there would be *no circulation* of synovial fluid in the film. For fresh films of synovial fluid to keep replacing older ones so as to provide fresh nutrients to the articular surface, there would have to be movement. In other words there has to be *circulation* of synovial fluid if old films of synovial fluid are to be replaced with fresh ones.

An Experimental Approach

In order to investigate the effects of movement on the repair of joint injuries, Salter and his associates devised an apparatus by which a knee joint of a nearly full-grown rabbit could be comfortably maintained under conditions of continuous passive motion while the animal recovered from experimental operative injuries of different sorts. Hence they were able to determine the extent, rate, and character of the repair process (*1*) under conditions of continuous passive motion, and compare them with results obtained with joints subjected to identical injuries but (*2*) kept immobilized or (*3*) allowed to heal in animals with cage freedom (these animals moved their affected

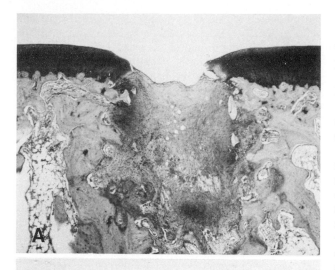

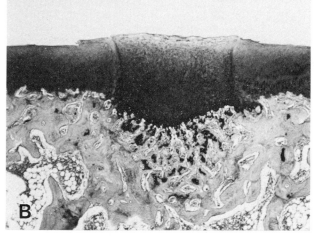

Fig. 16-5. Low-power photomicrographs (toluidine blue stain) showing articular cartilage in a rabbit knee joint, healing under different conditions, after a surgical defect was created by drilling a hole through the cartilage down into the subchondral bone beneath the cartilage. (*A*) This type of healing is obtained after three weeks if the joint is immobilized. Note the inadequate healing of the defect in the cartilage with loose ordinary connective tissue. (*B*) This type of healing is obtained after three weeks of continuous passive motion of the joint. Note that the defect in this case has become filled with newly formed hyaline cartilage. The source of this cartilage is illustrated in Figure 16-6. (Courtesy of R. Salter and E. Bogoch)

joints only when they felt inclined, and usually not before a week after operation, presumably because of pain). One of us (Ham) was privileged in being allowed to examine the sections and photomicrographs obtained and had the opportunity of conferring with the investigators so as to be able to provide the following account of their study.

The first type of injury, the healing of which was stud-

ied under the 3 conditions mentioned above, was that of a 1-mm. drill hole that extended from the articular surface through the articular cartilage and into its underlying supportive bone. The common type of healing observed after 3 weeks in rabbits in which the injured knee was immobilized or in animals allowed cage freedom is illustrated in Figure 16-5A, which is a photomicrograph of a section stained with toluidine blue, which colors cartilage matrix a deep blue (black in Fig. 16-5). As is evident in Figure 16-5A, the gap created by the drill hole is not in this instance filled with cartilage but only with a loose arrangement of ordinary connective tissue. It would seem, however, that deeper down a fair amount of new bone has formed as a result of the injury to the subchondral bone made by the drill. However, as is shown in Figure 16-5B, which is representative of what was found in the majority of the rabbits in which the knee joint was subjected to continuous passive motion, the gap in the articular cartilage is filled with a mass of new cartilage that appears to have arisen from the depths of the drill hole.

The source of this new cartilage is indicated in Figure 16-6, which shows photomicrographs of H and E sections of the identical site shown in Figure 16-5B, and taken after the same length of time. Particularly in the illustration on the right (Fig. 16-6) it can be seen that the source of the cartilage that filled the defect in the articular cartilage was the reparative tissue that formed as a result of the healing of the fracture of the subchondral bone. So we next have to explain why cells participating in the repair of bone should extend up into the drill hole and differentiate only into cartilage in this site. To understand this, several factors have to be taken into consideration. First, although termed osteogenic cells, the cells that cover and line bone surfaces, and also constitute one type of marrow stromal cell, are equally chondrogenic. As those who have read the preceding chapter on bone, and in particular the parts about its development and the repair of fractures, will realize, these osteochondrogenic cells differentiate into chondrocytes or osteoblasts, and hence form cartilage or bone, depending on the environment in which they differentiate. As noted, if it is vascular (and hence relatively rich in oxygen) they form bone, but if the environment is nonvascular they form cartilage (Ham). Next, what seems to happen here is that the reparative tissue, which would extend from the bone to the bottom of the gap in the cartilage, would in general be the reparative tissue farthest away from the bone and hence farthest away from the capillaries that in early repair are close to the bone. In this relatively nonvascular site the osteogenic cells would be differentiating into cartilage. When this new reparative tissue closed the gap it would begin to receive nutrients from the synovial fluid that would have filled the gap. Hence the newly forming tissue at the bottom of the gap would then be receiving

Fig. 16-6. Photomicrographs (H and E stain) showing cartilaginous repair of articular cartilage in a rabbit knee joint after a defect was created by a drill hole. The knee joint was subjected to continuous passive motion for three weeks. Note that in the region of the articular cartilage the reparative tissue, which originated from the bone below, is entirely cartilaginous and that the intercellular substance of the reparative tissue seems to be fusing with the edges of the original articular cartilage. The cell nests visible in and close to the edges of the original cartilage are probably to be explained by the fact that the rabbits used were not quite full grown and hence a few mitoses could have occurred in chondrocytes close to the site of the injury. (Courtesy of R. Salter, D. Simmonds, B. Malcolm, and E. Rumble)

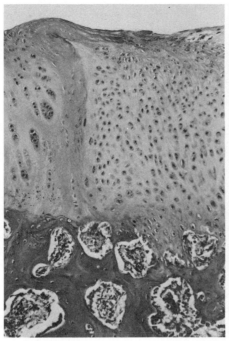
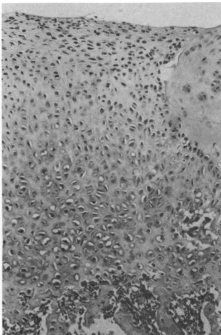

nutrients from above and would be in a relatively oxygen-poor, nonvascular environment that would cause the tissue to continue to differentiate into cartilage cells. Moreover, since young cartilage cells proliferate readily, as a consequence of the stimulus of continuous passive motion the young cartilage cells would continue to proliferate until they had filled the gap. Hence the repair of a drill hole in articular cartilage is brought about not by cartilage cells derived from articular cartilage but from young cartilage cells forming from the "osteochondrogenic" cells that cover and line the underlying bone and which are present also in the stroma of marrow. The reasons for bone not being formed in the defect under conditions of continuous passive motion would seem to be first that the motion maintains a fresh supply of synovial fluid in the gap to supply adequate nutrition for growing cartilage in a nonvascular environment, and second that continuous passive motion provides the stimulus for complete cartilage repair. It would therefore seem that continuous passive motion provides the necessary fresh conditions for the repair of articular cartilage if cartilage cells are available to proliferate and provide the new cells that are required. What is also emphasized by this experiment, however, is the seeming inability of the cells of articular cartilage themselves to proliferate and repair an injury, a matter to be discussed later.

In view of the interesting results obtained in this experiment, the investigators decided to study the healing of experimental fractures of the lateral condyle of a rabbit femur, produced by driving a scalpel not only through the articular cartilage, subchondral bone, and epiphyseal plate, but far enough to split off the lateral condyle from the femur. This condyle was then fixed, by means of a tiny compression screw, in juxtaposition with the site on the femur from which it had been separated.

A typical example of what was observed after 4 weeks of healing of such a fracture under conditions of immobilization is shown in Figure 16-7A, and an example of healing under continuous passive motion is shown in Figure 16-7B. In 80 per cent of the latter group the gap in the cartilage was closed and the underlying bone plate was continuous. However, there was little evidence that the gap in the articular cartilage in this instance was filled from below by a growth of osteogenic cells providing new young cartilage cells to fill it, as occurs in the repair of a drill hole. What seems to happen here is that under conditions of continuous passive motion enough interstitial growth of cartilage (p. 372) may occur on each side of the gap to close it. This would probably require mitosis of some of the chondrocytes adjacent to the gap, and a few examples of this were observed (Harris). But most of the interstitial growth was probably due to increased formation of intercellular substance by the chondrocytes of the articular cartilage, particularly by those adjacent to the gap.

It is of interest that further experiments indicated that it is mostly during the first week after the fracture has been produced that continuous passive motion produces ef-

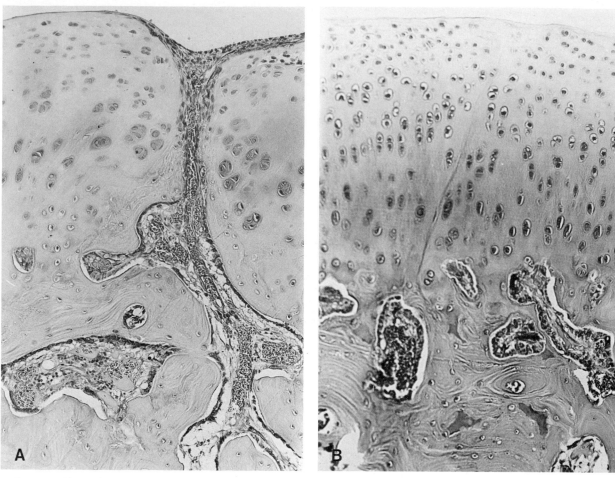

Fig. 16-7. Photomicrographs (safranin O stain) showing experimentally induced fracture sites of lateral condyle of a rabbit femur healing under different conditions. (*A*) Healing obtained after four weeks of immobilization. Note that the gap in the cartilage has become invaded from below by loose ordinary connective tissue with blood vessels. (*B*) Healing obtained after four weeks of continuous passive motion. The gap in the cartilage has closed, apparently without any new tissue having invaded it from below. (Courtesy of R. Salter and D. Harris)

fects that lead to effective healing. Here again there could be two factors involved. First, unlike what could happen in immobilized joints, there would be neither starvation of chondrocytes because of lack of circulation of synovial fluid nor undue accumulation of waste products in them and their surrounding matrix to cause them damage. Second, there could be the stimulus of continuous motion to institute such growth as is possible in articular cartilage.

Finally, the results of these experiments of Salter and his associates, outlined briefly above, should have important implications in the treatment of injured joints. But we are nevertheless left with the conclusion that after growth of the body is over, the reparative capacity retained by cells of articular cartilage seems meager. Unlike cartilage that is covered with a perichondrium, which still contains

chondrogenic cells, or bone that is covered with a periosteum or endosteum containing osteogenic cells, there *seems* to be no provision in articular cartilage after full growth is attained for the persistence of cells that could serve as a substantial source of new cells for either maintenance or repair purposes. Such a situation arouses curiosity, because during the growth of short bones the chondrocytes near the articular surface proliferate sufficiently for the articular cartilage to serve the same purpose as the epiphyseal plates of longer bones (Fig. 15-45) and because these cells, unlike those of the epiphyseal plate, persist and their morphology does not suggest that they have become as highly specialized as those deeper down in the articular cartilage. So it might be thought that they should be able to resume proliferative activities under

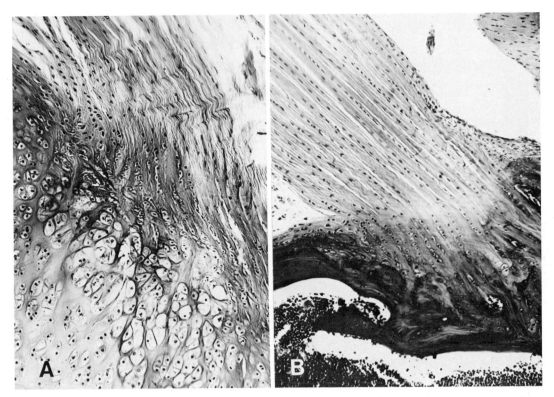

Fig. 16-8. (*A*) Photomicrograph of the site of insertion of a patellar tendon (rat). (*B*) Photomicrograph of the site of insertion of an anterior cruciate ligament (rat). Note the bundles of collagenic fibers in bone ((Sharpey's fibers) at the bottom of each illustration.

conditions in which repair was required. Hence, in the light of some of the matters discussed in Chapter 6, one might be inclined to speculate as follows. Since articular cartilages are anatomically *locked in a compartment* by a joint capsule, and, *after growth is over*, by bony plates beneath them, and since their chondrocytes subsequently exist in an excellent diffusion medium, the possibility of proliferation of the less differentiated cells being continuously restrained by a specific (chalone-like) inhibitor released by the much more numerous differentiated chondrocytes that inhabit the same compartment (a type of mechanism discussed in Chap. 6) might be visualized as a possible explanation for the *seeming inability* of less differentiated chondrocytes to undergo division.

THE JOINT CAPSULE AND SYNOVIAL MEMBRANE

The joint capsule consists of 2 layers: an outer fibrous layer, commonly called the *fibrous capsule* of the joint, and an inner one called the *synovial membrane* (Fig. 16-1).

The *fibrous capsule* of a joint is continuous with the fibrous layer of periosteum of the bones that meet at the joint (Fig. 16-1). It is composed of sheets of collagenic fibers that run from the periosteum of one bone to that of the other. It is relatively inelastic and hence makes a contribution to the stability of the joint. Occasionally, gaps are present in fibrous capsules; if so, the synovial membrane rests on muscles or other structures surrounding the joint. The *ligaments* of a joint represent cord-like thickenings of the capsule. These may be incorporated in the capsule or may be separated from it by *bursae* formed by outpouchings of the synovial lining (Fig. 16-1, bursae). Near their attachments ligaments undergo a transition into fibrocartilage (Fig. 16-8); the collagenic fibers become associated with increased amounts of amorphous intercellular substance, and the fibroblasts become encapsulated and resemble chondrocytes (Fig. 16-8).

Sharpey's Fibers. The collagenic fibers extend into the substance of the bone to which they are attached as typical *Sharpey's fibers* (Fig. 16-8B). It is to be remembered that bundles of collagenic fibers can become buried in bone as Sharpey's fibers (to serve as an anchorage for tendons, muscles, or the periodontal membrane) only when

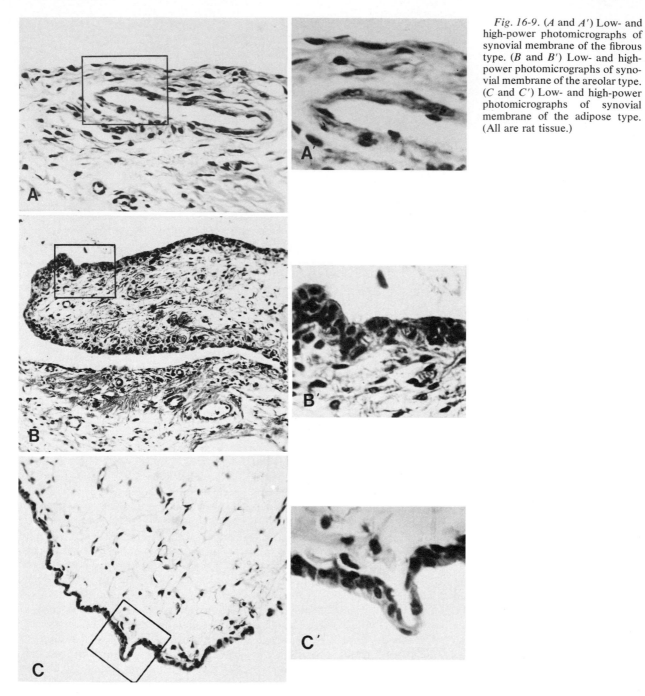

Fig. 16-9. (*A* and *A'*) Low- and high-power photomicrographs of synovial membrane of the fibrous type. (*B* and *B'*) Low- and high-power photomicrographs of synovial membrane of the areolar type. (*C* and *C'*) Low- and high-power photomicrographs of synovial membrane of the adipose type. (All are rat tissue.)

the fibers are formed before, or as, bone intercellular substance is deposited around them and onto the surface of the bone (appositional growth) by the osteoblasts lying between the fiber bundles close to the bone. In this sense, a tendon serves as the periosteum of a bone at the site of its insertion (see Sharpey's fibers, Fig. 16-8B).

Synovial Membrane. The *synovial membrane,* the inner layer of the joint capsule, lines the joint everywhere except over the articular cartilages (Fig. 16-1). The inner surface of the synovial membrane is usually smooth and glistening and it may be thrown into numerous processes; some of these are termed *villi.* It is abundantly supplied with blood vessels, nerves, and lymphatics, as will be described presently.

The cells in this membrane are called *synovial cells.* They are relatively undifferentiated and tend to be concentrated along the inner border of the membrane; indeed, in some instances they may be so concentrated as to give the appearance of forming a continuous cellular membrane. However, careful microscopic study of such a membrane will show that the cells disposed along its inner surface lie *in among* rather than *on* the collagenic fibers which also participate in forming the inner lining of the membrane.

The inner lining of the joint capsule, which contains the synovial cells, may lie directly on the fibrous capsule of the joint or may be separated from the fibrous capsule by a layer of areolar tissue or a layer of adipose tissue (Fig. 16-1). Accordingly, Key distinguishes three morphologic types of synovial membrane: (*1*) fibrous, (*2*) areolar, and (*3*) adipose. These are illustrated in Figure 16-9 and will now be described.

The fibrous type is found over ligaments and tendons and in other areas where the synovial lining is subjected to pressure (Fig. 16-1). The surface cells are characteristically widely separated from one another (Fig. 16-9A and A'), and although they are slightly larger and more numerous than the fibroblasts that are farther removed from the surface, it is often difficult to distinguish them from ordinary fibroblasts in sections. Since intercellular substance, rather than cells, comprises most of the lining of this type of synovial membrane, this type of membrane provides strong evidence in favor of the concept that synovial cavities are of the nature of connective tissue spaces.

The areolar type of synovial membrane is found where the membrane is required to move freely over the fibrous capsule of the joint, as, for example, in the suprapatellar pouch of the knee joint (Fig. 16-1). The surface cells are grouped fairly closely together in this type of lining (Fig. 16-9B and B'), usually in 3 or 4 rows, and are embedded in a layer of collagenic fibers that blend smoothly into those of the areolar tissue. Usually many elastic fibers are present in this type of lining; these usually are arranged in a lamina and probably serve to keep synovial projections from being nipped between the articular cartilages (Davies).

The adipose type of synovial lining covers the intra-articular fat pads (Fig. 16-1) and most closely resembles a true cellular lining membrane in appearance. The surface cells are usually formed into a single layer, which appears to rest on the adipose tissue (Fig. 16-9C and C'). However, careful inspection will reveal that the surface cells are more or less embedded in a thin layer of collagenic fibers, as are the surface cells in the other two types of lining membrane.

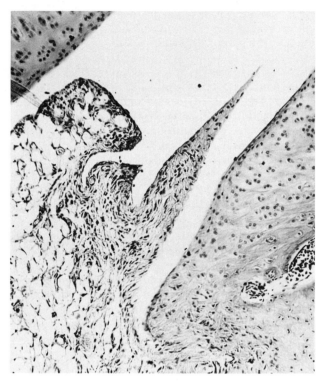

Fig. 16-10. Low-power photomicrograph of the border of a patella (rat), showing the synovial fold (*center*), which is wedge-shaped in this plane of section. A small portion of the patella is seen at *top left* and articular cartilage at *lower right.*

Synovial cells vary quite a bit in appearance and there are numerous mast cells in synovial membranes.

Transition Zone. At the site of attachment of the synovial membrane to the periphery of the articular cartilage, a transition is observed between synovial cells and chondrocytes; this region is known as the *transition zone.* In this site a fold or fringe of synovial tissue overlies the articular cartilage for a short distance. The fold, when cut in cross section in a longitudinal section of a joint, appears wedge-shaped (Fig. 16-10). The tip of the wedge is relatively noncellular and the base cellular. The areolar tissue that underlies the base undergoes an abrupt change into fibrous tissue as it nears the articular cartilage and in turn merges with the articular cartilage.

Repair of the Synovial Membrane. Since synovial cells are relatively undifferentiated, synovial tissues are capable of rapid and complete repair. It is helpful to know this because synovial tissues must be removed in certain types of operations on joints. Key found that following removal of a portion of the synovial lining from knee joints of rabbits there was rapid deposition of fibrin in the wounded area, and this quickly became organized by young connective tissue cells that grew in from the fibrous capsule. These soon differentiated into synovial cells, so that within 2 months the newly formed synovial lining could not be distinguished from undamaged adjacent areas.

Intra-articular Menisci. These structures (Fig. 16-1) develop from portions of the articular disk of mesenchyme (Fig. 16-2) that formerly occupied the space between the developing articular cartilages of the joint concerned. In menisci the mesenchyme tends to differentiate into fibrocartilage. Menisci may have a free inner border (as in the knee joint) or they may traverse the joint, dividing it into two separate synovial cavities (as in the sternoclavicular joint).

The menisci of the knee joint may be torn as the result of an injury, and it is common practice to excise an affected meniscus. Following the removal of a meniscus a new one sometimes forms, growing in from the fibrous capsule of the joint. The new structure that forms in this fashion is an almost complete duplicate of the former meniscus, but it consists of dense fibrous tissue rather than fibrocartilage. New menisci that form in this fashion may themselves become injured and require removal; indeed, it was because of this that it was found that intra-articular menisci can regenerate (Smillie).

Blood Vessels and Lymphatics. Synovial joints have a relatively rich blood supply. The branches of arteries that approach a joint commonly supply three structures: one branch goes to the epiphyses, the second to the joint capsule, and the third to the synovial membrane. In these sites they supply capillary beds. There are arteriovenous anastomoses in joints but their significance has not yet been determined.

The synovial membrane has a very rich supply of capillaries and in many sites these approach the inner surface of the membrane very closely. As a result blood may escape into the synovial fluid from a relatively minor injury to the joint. Blood vessels are arranged in a circular network at the periphery of the articular cartilage in the transition zone; this arrangement constitutes the *circulus articuli vasculosus* of Hunter. Gardner's papers should be consulted for details regarding the blood supply of joints.

The lymphatic plexus lies somewhat more deeply from the synovial surface than do the blood capillaries. The lymphatic capillaries begin as blind tubes; these are often enlarged at their blind ends. After piercing the elastic lamina of the synovial lining they converge into larger vessels passing in the general direction of the flexor aspect of the joint. Here they anastomose freely with periosteal lymphatics and then empty into the main lymphatic vessels of the limb (*see* Davies).

Nerve Supply. Students will find this rather easier to understand if they remember to return to it after reading the chapters on muscle and nervous tissue. Hilton's law,

enunciated by John Hilton in 1863, continues to be the fundamental statement about the nerve supply of joints: "The same trunks of nerves whose branches supply the muscles moving a joint also furnish a distribution of nerves to the skin over the insertions of the same muscles, and . . . the interior of the joint receives its nerves from the same source."

Articular cartilage contains no nerve endings. The capsular structures, however, contain several different kinds of afferent endings, those of the joint capsule being mostly of the Ruffini type. The different kinds of endings in synovial joints will be described in connection with afferent endings in the junctions between tendons and muscles and in tendons themselves, under the headings Tendon Organs and Joint Receptors in Chapter 18. In addition it should be mentioned that small myelinated fibers pass to the joint capsule and ligaments of the joint, where they end in free endings. These fibers are concerned with the sense of pain. There are very few of these free endings in the connective tissue of the synovial membrane; hence it would seem not very sensitive to pain. That the synovial membrane is indeed not very sensitive to pain has been confirmed at operations in which joints have been opened under local anesthesia. The free endings in the capsule and ligaments of joints seem to be stimulated most easily by stretching or twisting these structures. Small myelinated fibers also form free endings in the adventitia of blood vessels; these are probably vasosensory, and at least some probably are concerned with the sense of pain. Endings of this type in the adventitia of blood vessels are probably the only kind of free afferent endings in synovial membranes.

Nonmyelinated sympathetic fibers (which are efferent) end in the smooth muscle of blood vessels of joints to regulate the flow of blood.

Fibers reach larger joints from many spinal nerves, and any given nerve may supply more than one joint. Joint pain is generally poorly localized.

Gardner has made extensive studies on the nerve supply of joints and his papers provide detailed information on this subject.

Synovial Fluid. Since the synovial cavity develops as a connective tissue space, it should contain a ground substance and be perfused with tissue fluid. This concept of the cavity and its contents has been supported by the investigations of Bauer and his colleagues, who showed that synovial fluid was an ultrafiltrate or dialysate of blood (as is tissue fluid), together with what they termed *mucin*, which Meyer identified as *hyaluronic acid*. In synovial fluid (in contrast to the aqueous humor of the eye) hyaluronic acid is highly polymerized and this accounts for the high viscosity and lubricating quality of synovial fluid.

The various projections of synovial membrane that extend into the synovial cavity and the closeness of capillaries to the surface of the cavity make it easy to understand how tissue fluid could gain ready access to the cavity. The hyaluronic acid in synovial fluid is produced by the synovial cells; it constitutes the ground substance of the synovial membrane and also gains entrance to the synovial fluid.

The cell content of synovial fluid varies considerably from joint to joint and from species to species, and it tends to become increased after death. Counts of from 80 to several thousand cells per cubic millimeter have been found by different investigators. Key found a typical differential count to be 58 per cent monocytes, 15 per cent macrophages, 14 per cent ill-defined types of phagocytes, 1 per cent "primitive cells," 3 per cent synovial cells, and 5 per cent other types of blood leukocytes.

The passage of substances into and out of the synovial fluid depends upon their molecular weight. Crystalloids diffuse readily in both directions. This is of importance in the treatment of joint diseases, for soluble drugs given an individual can quickly enter the synovial fluid. Gases also diffuse readily in both directions. Hence, in caisson disease (the bends), nitrogen bubbles commonly appear in joint cavities. This disease occurs when divers or other people working under high atmospheric pressure return too quickly to normal atmospheric pressure. The sudden decompression of the individual causes too sudden a release of gases dissolved in the bloodstream and other fluids, just as carbon dioxide bubbles from soda water when the cap is removed from a bottle.

Proteins (large colloidal molecules) leave synovial fluid by way of lymphatics but particulate matter must be removed from synovial fluid by phagocytosis. Although synovial cells have some phagocytic capacity, most phagocytosis of particulate matter introduced into synovial fluid is brought about by macrophages. Removal of particulate matter from joints is a slow process and phagocytes containing hemosiderin may be seen in the synovial tissues of joints months after blood has escaped into the synovial fluid.

Changes Associated With Aging. A condition called *osteoarthritis* tends to develop in joints as individuals age. This condition is so common that its development to some degree is considered by some investigators to be a normal consequence of the aging process. As noted, cells of articular cartilage seem unable to divide to maintain articular cartilage in the same way as many other body tissues are maintained. Should the condition develop prematurely or in severe form it is, of course, considered to be pathological. It consists essentially of a curious combination of degenerative and proliferative processes.

The *degenerative* changes are seen to best advantage in the more central parts of articular cartilages. The noncollagenic component of the matrix appears to change in character. As a result, the collagenic fibrils of the matrix become unmasked and visible in sections. As the condition progresses, collagenic fibers become freely exposed on the articular surface; this gives the surface an appearance like the "pile" of a carpet, and the condition is termed *fibrillation* of the cartilage.

The *proliferation* changes occur around the periphery of the articular cartilage, particularly in the transition zone and at sites of attachment of tendons and ligaments. Cartilage proliferates in these regions and is replaced by bone in such a fashion that bony spurs, termed *osteophytes*, grow so as to form lips around the joint. It may be that these outgrowths represent an attempt to restrain movement to the joint.

This combination of degenerative and proliferative changes, although it occurs commonly in the aged, may also occur in younger individuals, particularly if the direction of a stress borne by a joint has been altered by some kind of injury. Hence to some extent the condition appears to be the consequence of joints having to perform too much or the wrong kind of work.

SYMPHYSES

Symphysis is a Greek word that denotes a *growing together*. It is used in relation to joints in which individual bones are separated, but held together, by combinations of hyaline cartilage and fibrocartilage. It is probable that this name was coined because cartilage is so commonly concerned in growth of bones that symphyses were conceived of as joints in which individual bones had grown together by means of their cartilaginous caps, and enough fibrocartilage formed between or around the hyaline cartilage to hold the two bones together. Because of flexibility in the fibrocartilage such a joint would permit a slight amount of movement.

The *symphysis pubis* is an example of such a joint. In it the tissue between the cartilage caps of the bones concerned consists almost entirely of *fibrocartilage*. A tiny slit-like space exists in this fibrocartilage, and in women during pregnancy this space becomes larger, thus allowing for greater movement between the pubic bones during passage of the fetus through the birth canal. In some lower animals the pubic bones actually become separated during pregnancy. Hall and her associates have studied the process in pregnant mice and have investigated the effects of hormones on the process (*see* References and Other Reading).

As mentioned at the beginning of this chapter, there are two kinds of joints that are commonly affected so as to require a vast amount of medical and surgical attention. Synovial joints (described above) are one kind and a modified type of symphysis, the *intervertebral joint,* is the

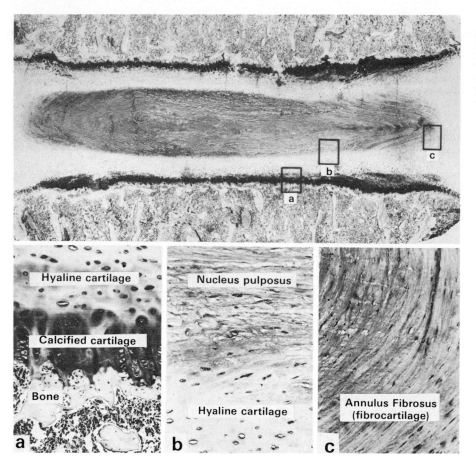

Fig. 16-11. (*Top*) Very low-power and (*bottom*) medium-power photomicrographs of an intervertebral disk of a young child. The areas marked a, b, and c in the top picture are shown at higher magnifications in the bottom three pictures.

other. Back pain (although sometimes due to other causes) can result from alterations from the normal in the vertebral column and is so common in our society that it constitutes a major health problem; hence it is desirable that students should also learn as much as possible about intervertebral joints.

In evolution a semirigid, rod-like structure called the *notochord* was the forerunner of the vertebral column. In the course of evolution, with the advent of segmentation in vertebrates, the notochord became replaced by rigid bony vertebrae the bodies of which were joined together by a modification of a symphysis, as shown in Figure 16-11 which illustrates the microscopic structure of the different parts of an intervertebral joint (disk) at different magnifications. As can be seen in the top low-power photomicrograph, the surface of the bone of each vertebra is covered with a layer of uncalcified hyaline cartilage (light in *top* picture and in part a). Between the bone and the uncalcified cartilage there is a dark layer of calcified cartilage (labeled in Fig. 16-11, part a). Next, running across most of the middle of the top illustration is a flattened

oval. This is where the section passed through the *nucleus pulposus* of the intervertebral disk. This is believed to be the evolutionary heritage of the notochord that first formed the axial skeleton of vertebrates. At least in the young it contains some cells, but most of it consists of intercellular substance with some of the characteristics of hyaline cartilage. It has been demonstrated recently that its central portion (which is loaded in compression) contains mostly Type II collagen, as does articular cartilage. However, the peripheral part of the nucleus pulposus and the *annulus fibrosus* (Fig. 16-11, part c), which is composed of fibrocartilage and encircles the nucleus pulposus, are both loaded in tension and contain primarily Type I collagen, the type found in tendons.

The combination of the semifluid nucleus pulposus, situated in the middle of the hyaline cartilage between the bodies of two vertebrae, with the annulus fibrosus at its periphery (Fig. 16-11, part c) provides a cushion between the two vertebral bodies and permits slight movement between them.

Unfortunately, for reasons described in later medical

courses, intervertebral disks can suffer degenerative changes that interfere with their normal supportive function. Furthermore, a nucleus pulposus may herniate (break) through the structures that normally confine it if these become weakened and pressure is still put upon it. If it herniates through the calcified cartilage and bone into the marrow of the body of a vertebra, as is shown in Figure 16-12C, it does not seem to occasion any distress. Examples of such permeations are often found at autopsies and are known as Schmorl's nodules. If, however, the nucleus pulposus herniates through the annulus fibrosus the condition, termed a *ruptured disk,* can have painful disabling consequences. This is primarily due to material from the nucleus pulposus being extruded under pressure into a very confined space through which, as will be described in Chapter 18, the spinal nerves emerge from the spinal cord by passing through the intervertebral canals on each side of the vertebral column to enter the body tissues of a body segment (refer to Fig. 17-34). Hence a ruptured intervertebral disk can interfere with the functions of the nerves that leave or enter at the foramen associated with the site of disk rupture.

As will be learned later, although a disk degeneration or rupture can cause severe pain and hopefully only temporary disability, surgical treatment is sometimes required. However, even severe strains without rupture can cause disabilities. Furthermore, the other joint that connects the posterior facets of adjacent vertebrae is of the synovial type and can be strained and cause problems.

OTHER TYPES OF JOINTS

In addition to synovial joints and symphyses, there are three other kinds of joints; syndesmoses, synchondroses, and synostoses. These will be described very briefly.

SYNDESMOSES

The prefix *syn* is used with reference to joints because it means *together* (Gr.), while *desmos* is the Greek word for *band* or *bond;* in connection with joints it has become restricted to imply bands or bonds of *dense connective tissue. Syndesmoses,* then, are joints wherein bones, at their site of meeting, are held together by bands of dense fibrous tissue. It is important to understand that in a syndesmosis the bands of dense connective tissue extend from one *bare* bony surface to another.

The sutures of the skull during the period when the skull is growing in size provide good examples of syndesmoses. The flat bones of the skull develop from separate centers of ossification and thereafter increase in extent because new bone is continuously added to their edges in

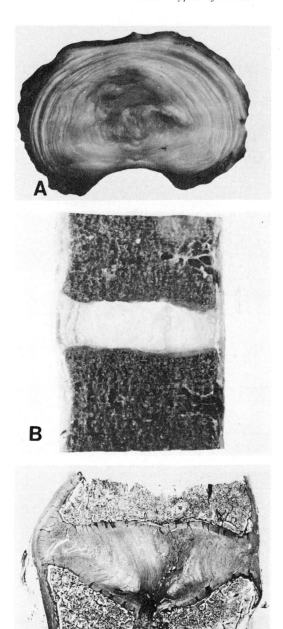

Fig. 16-12. Very low power photomicrographs showing (*A*) a horizontal section of an intervertebral disk. The circularly disposed fibers in the annulus fibrosus may be seen in the periphery; the central dark area is the nucleus pulposus. (*B*) A vertical section of the bodies of two vertebrae and the intervertebral disk between them. The fibers of the annulus fibrosus may just be seen near the edges of the disk; the paler material is the nucleus pulposus. (*C*) A vertical section of two vertebrae and the intervertebral disk between them. Note that in this case the nucleus pulposus has ruptured into the substance of the body of the vertebra below. (Courtesy of W. Donohue)

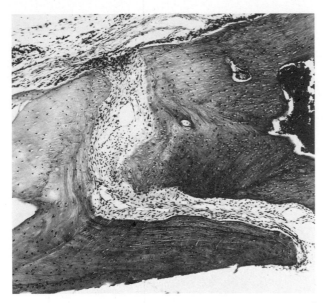

Fig. 16-13. Low-power photomicrograph of parietotemporal joint of a rat. This is an example of a suture (syndesmosis).

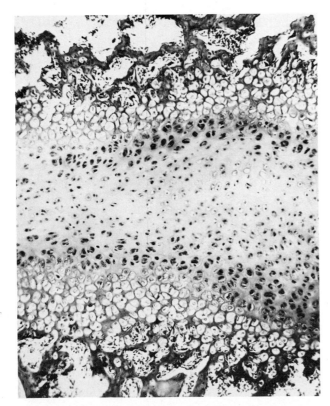

Fig. 16-14. Low-power photomicrograph of basisphenoid joint (rat). Notice that the cartilage is being replaced by bone on both its sides.

sutures by appositional growth. As a result the young connective tissue that at first exists between the edges of two adjacent bones becomes reduced eventually to a narrow band (Fig. 16-13) which joins the edges of the two bones together; hence, a suture is a syndesmosis. Osteogenic cells between the two bones in the suture can still proliferate and differentiate into bone cells. By this means layers of new bone can be added to the edges of the bones in the suture, and this permits the bones meeting at the suture to grow in extent as the skull increases in size. Thus a syndesmosis permits bones to increase in extent by the appositional growth mechanism. When growth is over, the connective tissue in a suture may be replaced by bone; thus the syndesmosis becomes converted into a synostosis, soon to be described. Once this happens the two bones that meet at the joint can no longer grow in extent.

Suture lines are commonly irregular; the edges of the bones concerned may be serrated, or they may interlock by means of toothlike processes. When a suture is cut in cross section, the suture line is usually seen to be oblique (Fig. 16-13). Not uncommonly an isolated ossicle, called a Wormian bone, may be seen in the connective tissue of a suture; such a bone forms as a result of detachment of a little group of osteoblasts or a little bone spicule from the edge of one of the bones that meet in the suture.

SYNCHONDROSES

During the growing period, epiphyseal disks are examples of *synchondroses* (joints in which bones are connected by *cartilage*) because they consist of hyaline cartilage and connect the bony epiphyses arising from epiphyseal centers of ossification with the bony diaphysis arising from the diaphyseal centers of ossification. It is to be understood that in most epiphyseal plates any substantial growth of bone occurs only on the diaphyseal side of the plate. However, the synchondrosis between the basioccipital and the basisphenoid bones is unlike an epiphyseal plate in this respect, since it provides for the growth of both of the bones that meet at this joint; in sections it therefore appears as a "double-sided" epiphyseal disk (Fig. 16-14).

SYNOSTOSES

When growth is over, most syndesmoses and synchondroses become *synostoses* (joints in which one bone is cemented to another). This is emphatic evidence that the chief function of syndesmoses and synchondroses is to permit *growth* rather than movement. It is of interest that operative procedures (including the use of bone transplants) are sometimes used to convert synovial joints into synostoses when pathological conditions make movement undesirable.

REFERENCES AND OTHER READING
(FOR CHAPS. 14 AND 16)

Cartilage, Including Secondary (Adventitial) Cartilage

General References: Books

Serafini-Fracassini, A., and Smith, J. W.: The Structure and Biochemistry of Cartilage. Edinburgh, Churchill-Livingstone, 1974.

General References: Articles and Reviews

Fell, H. B.: Skeletal development in tissue culture. *In* Bourne, G. H. (ed.): The Biochemistry and Physiology of Bone. p. 401. New York, Academic Press, 1956.
Gibson, T.: The transplantation of cartilage. *In* Porter, K. A. (ed.): The College of Pathologists Symposium on Tissue and Organ Transplantation. London, British Medical Association, 1967.
Hall, B. K.: *In vitro* studies on the mechanical evocation of adventitious cartilage in the chick. J. Exp. Zool., *168:*283, 1968.
———: Hypoxia and differentiation of cartilage and bone from common germinal cells *in vitro.* Life Sci., *8:*553, 1969.
———: Differentiation of cartilage and bone from common germinal cells, 1. The role of acid mucopolysaccharides and collagen. J. Exp. Zool., *173:*383, 1970.
———: Cellular differentiation in skeletal tissues. Biol. Rev., *45:*455, 1970.
———: Calcification of cartilage formed on avian membrane bones. Clin. Orthop., *78:*182, 1971.
Laskin, D. M., Sarnat, B. G., and Bain, J. A.: Respiration and anaerobic glycolysis of transplanted cartilage. Proc. Soc. Exp. Biol. Med., *79:*474, 1952.
Murray, P. D. F., and Smiles, M.: Factors in the evolution of adventitious (secondary) cartilage in the chick embryo. Aust. J. Zool., *13:*351, 1965.
Pritchard, J. J.: A cytological and histochemical study of bone and cartilage formation in the rat. J. Anat., *86:*259, 1952.
Revel, J. P.: Role of the Golgi apparatus of cartilage cells in the elaboration of matrix glycosaminoglycans. *In* Balasz, E. A. (ed.): Chemistry and Molecular Biology of the Intercellular Matrix. p. 1485. New York, Academic Press, 1970.
Rosenberg, L.: Structure of cartilage proteoglycans. *In* Burleigh, P. M. C., and Poole, A. R. (eds.): Dynamics of Connective Tissue Macromolecules. p. 105. Amsterdam, North-Holland, 1975.
Sanzone, C. F., and Reith, E. J.: The development of the elastic cartilage of the mouse pinna. Am. J. Anat., *146:*31, 1976.
Shaw, J. C., and Bassett, C. A. L.: The effects of varying oxygen concentration on osteogenesis and embryonic cartilage in vitro. J. Bone Joint Surg., *49-A:*73, 1967.
Shepard, N., and Mitchell, N.: The localization of articular cartilage proteoglycan by electron microscopy. Anat. Rec., *187:*463, 1977.
Skoog, T., Ohlsén, L., and Sohn, A.: Perichondrial potential for cartilaginous regeneration. Scand. J. Reconstr. Surg., *6:*123, 1972.

Joints, General

Davies, D. V.: The anatomy and physiology of joints. *In* Copeman's Textbook of the Rheumatic Diseases. ed. 2, p. 40. Edinburgh, E. & S. Livingstone, 1955.
Gardner, E.: The anatomy of the joints. Instruc. Lect. Am. Acad. Orthop. Surg. vol. 9. Ann Arbor, Edwards, 1952.
———: Blood and nerve supply of joints. Stanford Med. Bull., *11:*203, 1953.
———: The innervation of the elbow joint. Anat. Rec., *102:*161, 1948.
———: The innervation of the hip joint. Anat. Rec., *101:*353, 1948.
———: The innervation of the knee joint. Anat. Rec., *101:*109, 1948.
———: The innervation of the shoulder joint. Anat. Rec., *102:*1, 1948.
———: The nerve supply of diarthrodial joints. Stanford Med. Bull., *6:*367, 1948.
———: Physiology of movable joints. Physiol. Rev., *30:*127, 1950.
Gardner, E., and Gray, D. J.: Prenatal development of the human hip joint. Am. J. Anat., *87:*163, 1950.
Grant, J. C. B.: Interarticular synovial folds. Br. J. Surg., *18:*636, 1931.
Haines, R. W.: The development of joints. J. Anat., *81:*33, 1947.
Sokoloff, L. (ed.): The Joints and Synovial Fluid. New York, Academic Press, 1978.

Synovial Joints and Articular Cartilage

Barnett, C. H., Davies, D. V., and MacConaill, M. A.: Synovial Joints. London, Longmans, Green, 1961.
Crelin, E. S., and Southwick, W. O.: Changes induced by sustained pressure in the knee joint articular cartilage of adult rabbits. Anat. Rec., *149:*113, 1964.
Elliott, H. C.: Studies on articular cartilage. I. Growth Mechanisms. Am. J. Anat., *58:*127, 1936.
Enneking, W. F., and Horowitz, M.: The intra-articular effects of immobilized human knees. J. Bone Joint Surg., *54-A:*973, 1972.
Field, P. L., and Hueston, J. T.: Articular cartilage loss in longstanding immobilization of interphalangeal joints. Br. J. Plast. Surg., *23:*186, 1970.
Finterbush, A., and Friedmann, B.: Reversibility of joint changes produced by immobilization in rabbits, Clin. Orthop., *111:*290, 1975.
Glucksmann, A.: The role of mechanical stresses in vitro: II. The role of tension and pressure in chondrogenesis. Anat. Rec., *73:*39, 1939.
Greenwald, A. S.: A pathway for nutrients from the medullary cavity to the articular cartilage of the human femoral head. J. Bone Joint Surg., *51-B:*797, 1969.
Hall, B. K.: Differentiation and maintenance of articular (secondary) cartilage on avian membrane bones. Conference on Articular Cartilage, Supplement to Ann. Rheum. Dis., p. 34, 1975.
Hall, M. C.: Articular changes in the knee of the adult rat after prolonged immobilization in extension. Clin. Orthop., *34:*184, 1964.
Harris, D. J.: The Healing of Intra-articular Fractures with Continuous Passive Motion. M.Sc. Thesis, University of Toronto, 1978.
Hjertquist, S., and Lemperg, R.: Histological, autoradiographic and microchemical studies of spontaneously healing os-

teochondral articular defects in adult rabbits. Calcif. Tissue Res., *8:*54, 1971.

Honner, R., and Thompson, R. C.: The nutritional pathways of articular cartilage. J. Bone Joint Surg., *53-A:*4, 1971.

Key, J. A.: The reformation of synovial membrane in the knees of rabbits after synovectomy. J. Bone Joint Surg. (N.S.), *7:*793, 1925.

———: The synovial membrane of joints and bursae. *In* Cowdrey's Special Cytology. ed. 2, p. 1053. New York, Hoeber, 1932.

Lane, J. M., and Weiss, C.: Review of articular cartilage collagen research. Arthritis Rheum., *18:*553, 1975.

Lanier, R. R.: The effects of exercise on the knee-joints of inbred mice. Anat. Rec., *94:*311, 1946.

Lever, J. D., and Ford, E. H. R.: Histological, histochemical and electron microscopic observations on synovial membrane. Anat. Rec., *132:*525, 1958.

Mankin, H. J.: The reaction of articular cartilage to injury and osteoarthritis. Part I. N. Engl. J. Med., *291:*1285, 1974; and Part II, ibid., *291:*1355, 1974.

Rosenthal, O., Bowie, M. A., and Wagoner, G.: Studies in the metabolism of articular cartilage. I. Respiration and glycolysis of cartilage in relation to its age. J. Cell. Comp. Physiol., *17:*221, 1941.

Salter, R. B., and Field, P.: The effects of continuous compression on living articular cartilage. J. Bone Joint Surg., *42-A:*31, 1960.

Salter, R. B., Harris, D. J., and Clements, N. D.: The healing of bone and cartilage in transarticular fractures with continuous passive motion. Orthop. Trans., *2:*77, 1978.

Salter, R. B., Bogoch, E. R., and Harris, D. J.: Further studies in continuous passive motion. Orthop. Trans., *in press.*

Silberberg, M., Silberberg, R., and Hasler, M.: Ultrastructure of articular cartilage of mice treated with somatotrophin. J. Bone Joint Surg., *46-A:*766, 1964.

Silberberg, R., Silberberg, M., and Feir, D.: Life cycle of articular cartilage cells: an electron microscopic study of the hip joint of the mouse. Am. J. Anat., *114:*17, 1964.

Skoog, T., and Johansson, S. H.: The formation of articular cartilage from free periochondrial grafts. Plast. Reconstr. Surg., *57:*1, 1976.

Walmsley, R., and Bruce, J.: The early stages of replacement of the semilunar cartilages of the knee joint in rabbits after operative excision. J. Anat., *72:*260, 1938.

Whillis, J.: The development of synovial joints. J. Anat., *74:*277, 1940.

Symphyses

Adams, P., Eyre, D. R., and Muir, H.: Biochemical aspects of development and ageing of human lumbar intervertebral disc. Rheumatol. Rehab., *16:*22, 1977.

Bradford, F. K., and Spurling, R. G.: The Intervertebral Disc. Springfield, Ill., Charles C Thomas, 1941.

Crelin, E. S., and Koch, W. E.: Development of mouse pubic joint in vivo following initial differentiation in vitro. Anat. Rec., *153:*161, 1965.

Hall, K.: The effect of hysterectomy on the action of oestrone on the symphysis pubis of ovariectomized mice. J. Endocrinol., *7:*299, 1951.

———: The effect of oestrone and progesterone on the histologic structure of the symphysis pubis of the castrated female mouse. J. Endocrinol., *7:*54, 1950.

Hall, K., and Newton, W. H.: The action of "Relaxin" in the mouse. Lancet, *1:*54, 1946.

———: The effect of oestrone and relaxin on the x-ray appearance of the pelvis of the mouse. J. Physiol., *106:*18, 1947.

———: The normal course of separation of the pubes in pregnant mice. J. Physiol., *104:*346, 1946.

17 Nervous Tissue

In this chapter our main purpose is to deal with the structure and function of the third of the four basic tissues, nervous tissue. However, the reader will find that this chapter serves also as an introduction to one of the systems of the body, the *nervous system*. *Systems* are groups of organs or structures, made up of tissues, that work together to carry out special functions for the body. Part 4 of this book consists of an orderly description of each of the organ systems — with one exception, the nervous system, since this is dealt with in the present chapter.

Since the organization of nervous tissue within the nervous system is to a large extent determined by the way it evolved, it is logical to describe the organization of nervous tissue in relation to the evolutionary development of the nervous system. Therefore, after briefly describing the two subdivisions of the system and the basic shapes of nerve cells we go on to describe the ways they evolved and became organized to constitute the nervous system.

Central and Peripheral Divisions of the Nervous System. The first division, the *central nervous system* or CNS, lies deep in the body, surrounded and protected by bone. It consists of the *brain,* which is encased by the skull, and the *spinal cord,* which extends down the canal of the vertebral column to a position between the first and second lumbar vertebrae (Fig. 17-1).

The second broad division of the nervous system, the *peripheral nervous system* or PNS, is represented primarily by cord-like *nerves* leading off from the brain and spinal cord. Nerves leave the CNS in pairs, with one of each pair supplying each side of the body (Fig. 17-1). Those that emerge from the brain are termed *cranial nerves,* and they pass out through small canals (*foramina*) in the skull; those that leave the spinal cord bilaterally through canals (intervertebral foramina) located between adjacent vertebrae of the vertebral column constitute the *spinal nerves.*

Neurons. The structural and functional unit of nervous tissue and hence of the nervous system is, of course, the nerve cell. Nerve cells, which are called *neurons* (Gr.

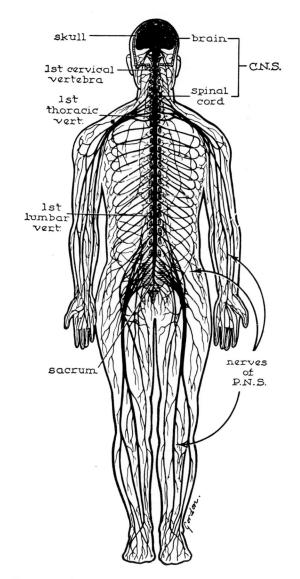

Fig. 17-1. Diagram of the CNS and PNS, showing the continuity between them.

483

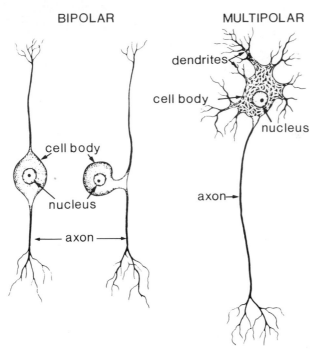

Fig. 17-2. Basic shapes of neurons.

neuron, nerve), are structurally unique in that cytoplasmic processes extend from them as delicate strands of cytoplasm called *nerve fibers,* some of which can be as long as a leg. Neurons are commonly classified according to the number of these cytoplasmic processes. Those with only one process are termed *unipolar* neurons, those with two, *bipolar* neurons (Fig. 17-2), and those with more than two, *multipolar* neurons (Fig. 17-2). Unipolar neurons are relatively rare and multipolar ones are very common in nervous tissue.

A neuron thus has two characteristic features. First, it has a *cell body* (Fig. 17-2). This consists of its nucleus and what is usually a large amount of cytoplasm that encloses the nucleus and is therefore sometimes called the *perikaryon* (Gr. *peri,* around; *karyon,* nut or nucleus). It houses most of the organelles that maintain structural and functional integrity of the fine cytoplasmic processes (termed *nerve fibers*) extending from it; the latter constitute the second characteristic feature of a neuron.

It is important to realize that neurons do not divide. Furthermore, from shortly after birth, new ones do not develop from precursor cells.

How Nerve Cell Processes Are Classified—Axon and Dendrites. Neurons have one (and only one) process known as an *axon* (Gr. for axle or axis), probably so called because the axon tends to be straight. Thus only one of the two fibers of a bipolar neuron and one of the many fibers of a multipolar neuron is an axon (Fig. 17-2). The other fiber of a bipolar neuron, like the one at *left* in Figure 17-2, and all the remaining ones of a multipolar neuron, like the one at *right* in Figure 17-2, are called *dendrites* (Gr. *dendron,* tree) because they branch like trees (Fig. 17-2, *right*).

Nerve impulses are propagated by a neuron along its axon to its destination, whereas impulses picked up by dendrites are transmitted toward the cell body. So in general, axons propagate impulses away from the cell body of a neuron and dendrites transmit impulses toward it. (There are, however, exceptions to this general rule in that certain fibers which would be considered to be axons because of their structural and functional characteristics transmit impulses toward the cell body. Nevertheless the general rule is useful.) Axons and dendrites will be considered in detail later.

Interneuronal Transmission of Impulses. Neurons, while remaining individual cells, are functionally linked together by their fibers. These fibers are often remarkably long but their length is limited by their having to be maintained by the cell body. The longest, however, reach several feet in length. Impulses can nonetheless be conducted over much longer distances by passing from one neuron to another, as between relays in long-distance telephone transmission. The junctions allowing impulses to pass from one neuron to another are called *synapses* (Gr. *synapsis,* a conjunction, connection) and are commonly placed where the axon of one neuron ends in a special structural arrangement on part of another neuron. When impulses arrive at a synapse, they either trigger or inhibit initiation of impulses in the second neuron.

In the next section we shall consider how neurons are linked together so as to constitute the *nervous system* of the body.

THE ORGANIZATION OF NERVOUS TISSUE

The organization of nervous tissue within the nervous system is most easily explained by briefly tracing some of the stages of evolution of the nervous system.

The Evolution of Neurons. Cells of multicellular animals gradually became increasingly specialized to do different kinds of work. Muscle cells (specialized for contractility) probably appeared before nerve cells because certain sponges, though vegetable-like, possess cells specialized for contractility around their pores. These muscle-like cells are in direct contact with sea water and, should it contain a noxious substance, they are directly stimulated to contract so as to close the pores.

As multicellular organisms evolved further and were composed of more and more different kinds of cells, muscle cells came to be located more deeply in the body.

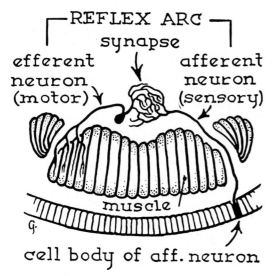

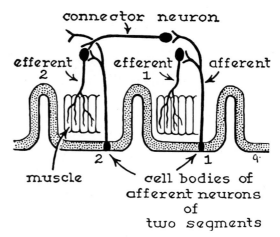

Fig. 17-4. Diagram of a portion of a hypothetical segmented organism, showing a connector neuron between segments.

Fig. 17-3. Diagram of an afferent and an efferent neuron arranged to constitute a reflex arc in the earthworm. (Redrawn from Parker, G. H.: The Elementary Nervous System. Philadelphia, J. B. Lippincott, 1919)

This development required that irritable cells be exposed to surface stimulation and arranged so that they could conduct excitation to the deeply situated muscle cells. In one of the first arrangements to evolve, the cell bodies of neurons were located at the body surface, with the axon of each in direct contact with a more deeply located muscle cell.

Further evolution of nervous tissue hinged on the development of pathways consisting of two or more neurons. In such pathways a process of a neuron comes into contact with either the cell body or a process of another neuron at a synapse. An arrangement of two or more neurons is required in all but very simple multicellular animals if a stimulus is to evoke a response in a muscle or gland. An example of such an arrangement of two neurons is seen in each segment of an earthworm (Fig. 17-3).

Afferent and Efferent Neurons in Reflex Arcs. The first neuron in such a pathway, which in the earthworm (but not in man) has its cell body at the surface, carries impulses deep into the body and is therefore called an *afferent* (L. *ad,* to; and *ferre,* to carry) *neuron.* The second neuron, however, carries impulses away from the deeper part of the body, toward the muscle cells, and is therefore termed an *efferent* (L. *ex,* out; and *ferre,* to carry) *neuron.* Together these two neurons constitute the simplest form of *reflex arc* (L. *reflectere,* to bend back; *arcus,* bow or curved line). Through evolution, as animals became elongated by reduplication of their basic units of body structure (*segments*), each segment contained both afferent

and efferent neurons so as to permit reflex activity in each segment. Because the human body is also segmented, each body segment contains its own afferent and efferent neurons.

Connector Neurons in Segmented Animals. With the evolution of segmented animals came a further type of neuron that permitted communication *between segments,* thereby allowing their activities to be coordinated in the interests of the animal as a whole. Hence, each body segment has, in addition to afferent and efferent neurons, intersegmental *connector neurons.* From Figure 17-4 it can be seen how these connector neurons could enable a stimulus received in one segment to elicit an effect in the next. Intersegmental connector neurons thus serve an *integrative function* and broaden the base of reflex arcs from one to many segments.

Spinal Cord and Brain. As further evolution continued, there was an increase in the number of connector neurons, some extending for short distances and others extending farther. Moreover, connector neurons became bundled together along the axis of the animal in a more or less central position and evolved into a structure known as the *spinal cord.* In the head region this became expanded to form the *brain,* which houses countless connector neurons, including those for integrating sensory inputs from special receptors in the nose, eyes, ears, and mouth.

From the foregoing it will be appreciated that *connector neurons all lie within the CNS.* Furthermore, *portions of afferent and efferent neurons* of each body segment also *lie within the CNS.* As we shall see, the other parts of the afferent and efferent neurons, because they lie outside the CNS, constitute the PNS. In order to explain this we

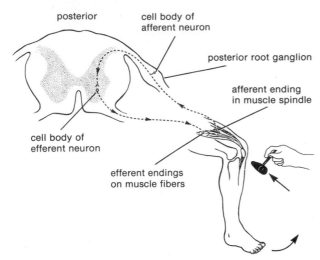

Fig. 17-5. Diagram illustrating a simple two-neuron reflex in man, the knee jerk or stretch reflex. Note that the cell body of the afferent neuron lies in a posterior root ganglion, outside the CNS.

now describe how the position of the cell bodies of afferent neurons changed as evolution continued.

Posterior Root and Cranial Ganglia. The first afferent neurons to evolve, as noted, had their cell bodies at the surface of the animal (Fig. 17-3). However, the body surface was not a suitable place because the cell bodies of these neurons were far too easily injured there. Damage to the cell body of a neuron is particularly serious since nerve cells are not replaced (*see* p. 42). Nevertheless, the cell body of a viable nerve cell can, under suitable circumstances, *regenerate new fibers* if fibers are damaged. It is therefore better to have cell bodies of afferent neurons located more deeply (out of harm's way), with a long fiber reaching from each to the surface to pick up stimuli; then if this fiber is damaged it can be regenerated from the protected cell body. This arrangement is general in the sensory neurons of higher animals.

In man, the nerve cell bodies of almost all afferent neurons lie extremely close to the CNS without becoming part of it. As shown in Figure 17-5, the cell bodies of such neurons are housed in small rounded nodules termed *ganglia* (meaning a lump). The ganglia housing cell bodies of afferent neurons of body segments are called *spinal* or *posterior* (*dorsal*) *root ganglia.* There are two ganglia for each segment, with one lying on each side of the vertebral column. However, it should be borne in mind that although segmentation of the body is indicated by vertebrae of the vertebral column, each segment corresponds to adjacent halves of vertebrae. Figure 17-34 shows the cross-sectional appearance of the vertebral column at a level where two intervertebral foramina extend from the ver-

tebral canal, one on each side; such foramina lie between contiguous vertebrae and mark the middle of a segment. As can be seen at *left* in Figure 17-34, spinal ganglia lie protected within these intervertebral foramina.

Other afferent fibers enter the brain by way of certain cranial nerves. The cell bodies of these afferent neurons are also situated in ganglia (termed *cranial ganglia*) close to the brain, but not actually inside it. The term *cerebrospinal* ganglia is sometimes used to refer to both cranial and spinal ganglia. All the *cell bodies of the afferent neurons* entering the CNS from body segments are therefore *housed in either spinal or cranial ganglia.*

Afferent Neurons. The afferent neurons are essentially bipolar cells. In evolution they began by having one fiber that reached to the surface and brought impulses toward the cell body and another that passed inward, conducting impulses toward the spinal cord. This type of bipolar afferent neuron is shown at *left* in Figure 17-2. During evolution the two fibers moved, as it were, toward one another like the hands of a clock until they fused together, so that except in a few places such bipolar cells *appear to have only one pole* and are therefore sometimes called *pseudounipolar* or even *unipolar.* It is interesting that the two fibers also move together and fuse to form a common proximal segment during embryological development of afferent neurons in the posterior root ganglia. As can be seen at *center* in Figure 17-2, the common proximal process branches at a position close to the cell body to form a T-shaped junction with two fibers extending in opposite directions from it. The longer of the two branches (the *peripheral fiber*) extends to a sensory ending while the shorter one (the *central fiber*) enters the spinal cord. Except for the termination of the peripheral fiber at the sensory ending, which receives impulses locally and is therefore dendritic, both the central and the peripheral fibers have the structure of an axon. Furthermore, they both actively propagate impulses toward the spinal cord. So in this special instance both fibers are generally regarded as constituting the axon, with the cell body being attached, as it were, to one side of the axon. Alternatively, these fibers may be referred to as the central and peripheral branches, respectively, of an afferent fiber.

The fibers of afferent neurons enter the spinal cord posterolaterally and within the cord may synapse directly with efferent neurons of the same segment (as in Fig. 17-5) or with intersegmental connector neurons. However, some also pass for short distances down the cord, or for longer distances up the cord, to synapse with efferent neurons of other segments or other connector neurons.

Efferent Neurons. The cell bodies of efferent neurons are multipolar and, except for certain autonomic neurons (described later), all lie *within the CNS.* The axons of spinal efferent neurons in general leave the spinal cord by way of the anterior roots of spinal nerves of the same segment as that in which the cell bodies lie (as in Fig. 17-5). They terminate at efferent endings in the muscles. Muscle cells of viscera, however, are innervated by efferent fibers from autonomic neurons that lie outside the CNS. We shall describe the efferent endings on muscle cells in the next chapter.

Actions Involving Reflex Arcs. Medical and paramedical students will soon be testing reflexes to learn whether various parts of the nervous system are functioning properly. One reflex that is frequently tested is the *knee jerk.* A patient crosses his knees and relaxes his leg muscles, and the knee that is on top is given a sharp tap just below the patella as shown in Figure 17-5. The stretch on the tendon pulls on the quadriceps femoris muscle, stimulating stretch receptors (described in Chap. 18) in the muscle. This causes impulses to be generated in afferent neurons that conduct them toward the spinal cord. Here, these afferent neurons synapse with efferent ones, the axons of which extend to muscle fibers in the same muscle as shown in Figure 17-5. It is common for both afferent and efferent fibers of a given segment to travel in the same peripheral nerve. The contraction elicited in the muscle by the efferent impulses causes the foot to kick forward. The knee jerk is an example of the simplest kind of reflex found in the body, involving only two neurons. Most other reflexes are more complex and involve more neurons.

Reflexes, of course, are basic to human behavior. Nevertheless, as discovered by Pavlov in his classic experiments on dogs, reflex behavior can undergo modification by conditioning. Although synapses between afferent and efferent neurons exist in the spinal cord, afferent impulses commonly pass to the brain before they activate an efferent response. Because of its association neurons the brain contains countless alternative circuits, so that once afferent impulses reach the brain, they can elicit any of a host of different efferent responses, depending on the particular circuit employed. Conditioning procedures influence which of these circuits is preferred and extend the range of possible responses to given stimuli. All in all, it is understandable why a particular stimulus does not evoke the same response in every one; indeed, what is distinctly enjoyable for one individual may be quite unpleasant for another.

The Segmental Basis of Innervation. In order to understand the nerve supply and reflexes of the various parts of the body, it is important to appreciate that the organization of the nervous system reflects the *basic segmental plan* of the body. Spinal nerves, for instance, contain the afferent and efferent fibers of an individual body segment and supply only tissues that develop from that segment. However, muscle fibers in any given segment commonly blend with those of other segments to form muscles that traverse many segments. Muscle fibers arising from a given segment nevertheless retain their efferent innervation from that segment, so that large muscles may have efferent innervation from several segments.

The importance of the foregoing becomes obvious when a site of injury of the spinal cord is being investigated, for if the injury destroys afferent or efferent neurons (or their fibers) in a segment, the site of the lesion may be determined by locating the region from which sensation has been lost or investigating which particular muscles have lost their function.

Summary The cell bodies of the afferent neurons lie within spinal or cerebral ganglia just outside the CNS. However, cell bodies of all connector neurons and of all efferent neurons (except some belonging to the autonomic nervous system) lie within the CNS. The skin and muscles developing from a given body segment are innervated by nerves from that segment.

THE DEVELOPMENT OF THE CENTRAL NERVOUS SYSTEM

In order to understand the histology of the nervous system it is also necessary to know something about how it develops in the embryo. A brief account follows.

The early development of the neural tube and neural crests from ectoderm was described in Chapter 6 and illustrated in Figure 6-3, which shows how the tube develops into the spinal cord and brain. The cells of the neural tube and crests constitute *neuroectoderm.* We shall first consider how the neuroectodermal cells of the neural tube develop into the CNS and then discuss how the neural crests participate in the formation of peripheral and autonomic nervous tissue.

The Development of the Spinal Cord

As a result of cell proliferation, the wall of the neural tube becomes thickened and in due course its lumen becomes small (Fig. 6-3, *bottom left*). The developing vertebral column elongates much more than the spinal cord contained in its canal, and this has two important effects. First, since the cord remains connected to the brain, its end in the adult does not reach the termination of the vertebral canal but only as far as the level of the first or second lumbar vertebrae (Fig. 17-1). Second, the various segmental regions of the cord, originally in line with the segments they innervate, gradually assume levels that are higher than their respective body segments; hence the afferent and efferent fibers that pass out from each segment of the cord to reach their body segments must first pass down along the sides of the cord to reach their corresponding intervertebral foramina. This arrangement is particularly evident toward the caudal end of the cord and explains why the caudal portion of the vertebral canal does not contain any spinal cord but instead contains afferent and efferent fibers reaching down from lower segments of the cord to reach their proper intervertebral foramina.

The Development of the Brain

The following account is intended for students who have not yet learned about the brain from other courses.

It is not uncommon for a student examining a brain for the first time to wonder how such a complex organ (Fig. 17-6) could have developed from anything as simple as a neural tube. Two underlying growth mechanisms are involved: (*1*) dissimilar growth rates of different parts of the wall of the neural tube so that it becomes thicker in some parts than in others, and (*2*) longitudinal growth of the neural tube where the brain will develop, which results in its becoming too long to fit lengthwise into the space it occupies; as a result it becomes flexed.

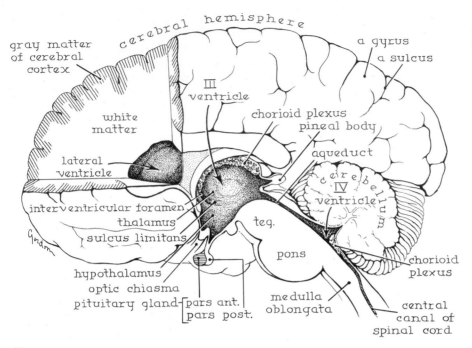

Fig. 17-6. A median sagittal section of the brain of man. A portion of frontal lobe has been cut out (*upper left*) to disclose that lateral ventricle. What was originally the lumen of the neural tube is shown in dark stipple. In following the text the student should begin at the right lower corner and follow the central canal of the cord into the various ventricles of the brain, and visualize how the main parts of the brain have developed from the parts of the wall of the neural tube.

The cranial end of the tube then develops three swellings separated by constrictions. These swellings (*vesicles*) are called the *forebrain, midbrain,* and *hindbrain,* respectively. We first describe the hindbrain (the part continuous with the spinal cord) and then work forward.

The Hindbrain. If, for example, a rubber tube is bent upon itself the region of the bend does not remain tubular but is broad and flattened and the lumen is distorted into a transverse slit. Similarly, when the neural tube is bent in the hindbrain at what is called the pontine flexure, its lateral walls diverge and the form described for the rubber tube is assumed. The thin roof stretches more than the floor and becomes a thin cover over the widened lumen at this site. The floor, however, becomes thick in the hindbrain and constitutes the *medulla* and *pons* (Fig. 17-6). The sides of the tube form large swellings that fuse together and constitute the *cerebellum* (Fig. 17-6). The lumen of the neural tube persists in the hindbrain as a cavity (Fig. 17-6), called the fourth *ventricle* (from the L., meaning a cavity in a hollow organ). As will be explained in due course, this contains cerebrospinal fluid and communicates with the other ventricles of the brain.

The Midbrain. This retains its tubular structure and its lumen is reduced to a small *aqueduct* (Fig. 17-6) that connects the ventricles of the forebrain with that of the hindbrain.

The medulla, pons, and midbrain all contain important groups of cell bodies of neurons; the regions containing such aggregates of nerve cell bodies are termed *nuclei*. Ascending and descending fibers may synapse in these regions or pass uninterrupted through them.

The Forebrain. The cephalic flexure developing between the midbrain and forebrain does not produce the rubber-tube effect as in the pontine flexure, so the lumen here does not become flattened. It is helpful to regard the forebrain as consisting of two portions. In the hind or caudal (L. *cauda,* tail) part of the forebrain, thickenings of the walls of the tube form the *thalamus* and *hypothalamus*. The rostral part (from the L. for beak, meaning situated at the snout end) consists of two *cerebral hemispheres* (Fig. 17-6).

The thalamus is concerned primarily with relaying afferent impulses from lower levels of the brain and cord to higher centers in the cerebral hemispheres. The hypothalamus regulates and integrates many important body functions, mainly by way of the autonomic nervous system, which will be described later. It also produces neurosecretions and controls the release of many hormones, as will be described in connection with endocrine glands in Chapter 22. The lumen of the neural tube persists here as a vertical slit known as the *third ventricle* (Fig. 17-6).

In the rostral part of the forebrain the dorsolateral walls of the neural tube form two huge evaginations known as the *cerebral hemispheres* (Fig. 17-6). Their cavities, the *lateral ventricles,* connect with the third ventricle through interventricular foramina. The surface of the cerebral hemispheres is deeply corrugated, with the deeper grooves being termed *fissures* and the shallower ones *sulci*. The latter separate ridges of tissue called *gyri* (Fig. 17-6) from one another.

Within the *cerebrum* (comprising the two cerebral hemispheres), sensory information, particularly from organs of special sense, is integrated and voluntary motor responses are initiated and coordinated. This is, moreover, the part of the brain where complex thought processes such as learning, memorization, and the acquisition and use of language—processes in all likelihood going on now in the mind of the reader—take place.

The nervous tissue of the CNS develops from the cells of the wall of the neural tube. Neuroectodermal (neuroepithelial) cells forming the tube can differentiate as shown in Figure 17-7 along three separate pathways to form (*1*) neurons, (*2*) cells termed oligodendrocytes and astrocytes, to be described in the following, and (*3*) ependymal cells that line the lumen of the tube and later the ventricles of the brain. The way these three kinds of cells are arranged in the CNS is described in the following.

Fig. 17-7. Diagram illustrating the main lines along which neuroectodermal cells of the neural tube differentiate in forming the CNS.

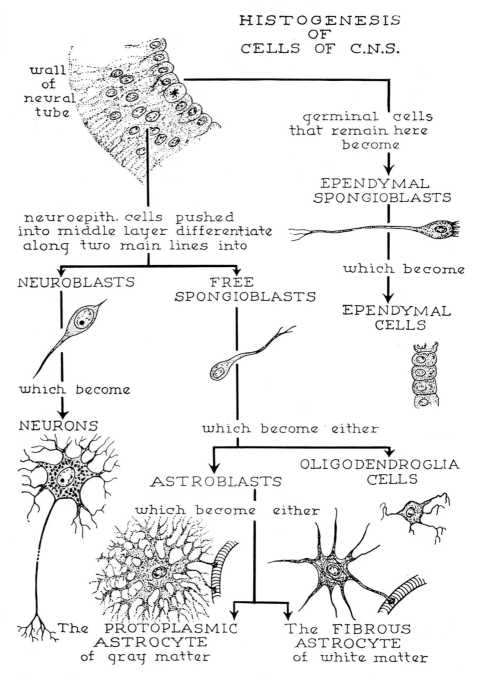

HISTOGENESIS OF CELLS OF C.N.S.

wall of neural tube

germinal cells that remain here become

EPENDYMAL SPONGIOBLASTS

which become

EPENDYMAL CELLS

neuroepith. cells pushed into middle layer differentiate along two main lines into

NEUROBLASTS

FREE SPONGIOBLASTS

which become

NEURONS

which become either

ASTROBLASTS

OLIGODENDROGLIA CELLS

which become either

The PROTOPLASMIC ASTROCYTE of gray matter

The FIBROUS ASTROCYTE of white matter

THE CELLS OF THE CNS AND THEIR ORIGINS

Two important features of the tissue of the CNS should be emphasized before its detailed histological study is begun.

First, unlike the arrangements that exist in the body, whereby, for example, the functioning cells of epithelial or muscle tissue are supported by the intercellular substances of connective tissue, in the CNS the functioning cells of nervous tissue (neurons and their processes) are not directly supported by connective tissue cells or its intercellular substances but by cells derived from the same progenitor cells as neurons (Fig. 17-7). These cells are of a type termed *neuroglia* (Gr. *glia,* glue) because in their supportive role they seem to "glue" neurons together by

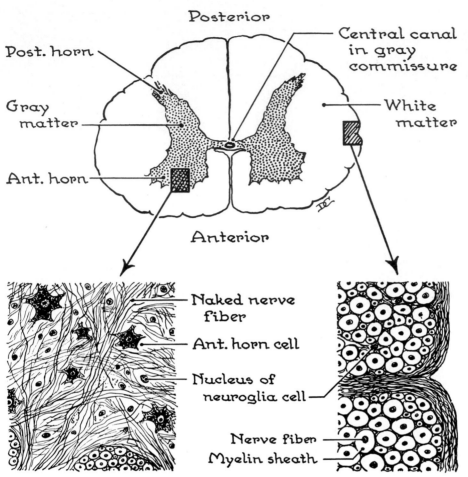

being present between neuronal cell bodies and fibers, holding them in place. Hence *within* the CNS, connective tissue is found only in association with blood vessels penetrating it to supply it with nutrients. As a consequence the tissue of the CNS is soft and structurally weak.

Second, the cells of one kind of neuroglia are called *oligodendrocytes* (Gr. *oligos*, little; *dendron*, tree) because they are small cells with only a few processes branching off from them (Fig. 17-7). They are responsible in the CNS for elaborating a fatty material termed *myelin* (Gr. *myelos*, marrow) in such a way as to form a coat for most of the individual axons of the CNS over most of their lengths. Such axons are termed *myelinated fibers*. The myelin coating of these fibers serves primarily for electrical insulation.

Another kind of neuroglial cell is termed an *astrocyte* (Gr. *astron*, star) because it has many processes extending out in star-like fashion from its cell body (Fig. 17-7).

Still another variety of cells seen in the CNS and origi-

nally classed as a further type of neuroglia are the *microglia*, so named because of their small size. It is now known, however, that they are not derived from the progenitor cells of neurons as are true neuroglia, but instead develop from monocytes and hence are tiny macrophages.

With the understanding that neurons and their supporting cells both are derived from common progenitor cells of the neural tube and that oligodendrocytes produce the myelin coating of myelinated fibers, we can now describe the differences in microscopic structure between the gray and white matter of the CNS, which is commonly one of the first laboratory exercises engaged in by students beginning to study the histology of the CNS.

THE GRAY AND WHITE MATTER OF THE CNS

The two main components of the CNS were long ago called *gray* and *white matter* from their gross appearance. The reason for this distinction will now be described.

Gray Matter. As a result of proliferation in the inner part of the wall of the neural tube (Fig. 17-7) cells are pushed into the middle layers of the wall. Most of these cells differentiate into neuroblasts and eventually neurons (Fig. 17-7). A few, however, differentiate into *neuroglia.* The *cell bodies of neurons* and their various associated supporting (glial) cells are the principal components of *gray matter.* The cell bodies of neurons lie surrounded by tangled masses of fibers representing the beginnings and endings of nerve fibers that lead to or from the neuronal cell bodies. Due to its matted appearance in the LM, this component of gray matter is called *neuropil* (Gr. *pilos,* felt). The axons in the neuropil are not heavily myelinated and the dendrites lack myelin altogether.

In the spinal cord the gray matter roughly resembles an "H" in shape when seen in cross section (Fig. 17-8). Hence the gray matter is said to have two *posterior horns* and two *anterior horns.* Actually, the horns are continuous columns that extend up and down the cord. In some parts of the cord there is a lateral column on each side as well. Cell bodies of neurons are seen to advantage in the anterior horns (Fig. 17-8, *lower left*). Gray matter is gray because it contains *a lot of cells* and *not very much myelin.*

White Matter. In the spinal cord the white matter, which surrounds the H shaped region of gray matter (Fig. 17-8), contains a vast number of nerve fibers extending up and down the cord. It is white because the majority of fibers are ensheathed with the white fatty material *myelin.* Hence myelin makes up most of the substance of white matter.

White matter *does not contain any cell bodies of neurons.* The fibers it contains originate from cell bodies lying either in the gray matter of the brain or spinal cord or in the spinal ganglia. The fibers are organized into tracts, each of which contains fibers from neurons with similar roles, so that there are separate motor and sensory tracts.

Although white matter contains no cell bodies of neurons it does contain many glial cells. In the developing spinal cord, spongioblasts from the developing middle layer differentiate into astrocytes and oligodendrocytes (Fig. 17-7). These two types of glial cells (chiefly oligodendrocytes) fit into the crevices between the axons (Fig. 17-8, *right*) and send out their processes among them. Oligodendrocytes are commonly arranged in rows between myelinated axons and, as noted, are responsible for laying down myelin in the CNS. Since myelin is a lipid-protein complex containing cholesterol, phospholipids, and glycolipids, as well as proteins, it is mostly dissolved away by fat solvents. Hence, when ordinary paraffin sections of nervous tissue are prepared, the lipid component of the myelin is extracted. When such sections are then stained with H and E, each site where myelin was present

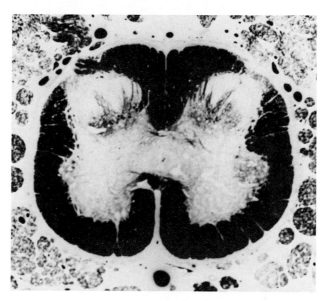

Fig. 17-9. Low-power photomicrograph of a cross section of spinal cord (sacral region) fixed in osmic acid. The white matter appears black due to the myelin of the sheaths of the nerve fibers

appears as a round space that seems empty apart for a little round dot representing a cross section of the axon that in life was surrounded by the myelin (Fig. 17-8, *lower right*). Occasional nuclei are seen in white matter between the empty round spaces; these belong to glial cells.

By utilizing fixatives that render myelin insoluble, it is possible to demonstrate myelin with suitable special stains, even in paraffin sections. Osmic acid fixes myelin so that it does not dissolve away in paraffin sections and moreover stains myelin black, so that in sections of spinal cord fixed in osmic acid the white matter of the cord appears black (Fig. 17-9).

Myelination in the CNS. In the CNS, myelin is formed by *oligodendrocytes,* chiefly those lying between nerve fibers of white matter. However, some myelin is also formed (though to a much lesser extent) by oligodendrocytes in the grey matter. Each oligodendrocyte participates in forming a myelin sheath by wrapping a segment of a nerve fiber in spiral fashion with successive layers of one of its processes, as shown in Figure 17-10. The cytoplasm of the process becomes squeezed back into the cell body so that the wrapping material (Fig. 17-10) comes to consist of little more than double layers of cell membrane, which supply the lipids, phospholipids, and cholesterol for the myelin. The process of myelination here is in some ways similar to that occurring in the PNS in the myelination of peripheral nerve fibers, but in other ways it is more complicated. After myelination in the PNS has been

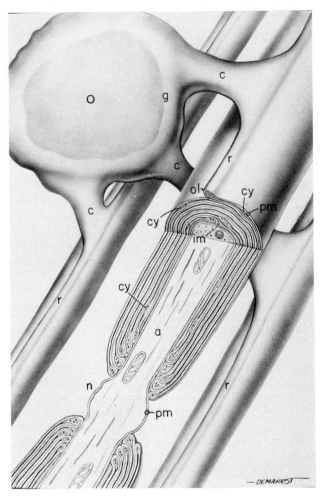

Fig. 17-10. Diagrammatic drawing illustrating how oligodendrocytes are related to nerve fibers in white matter and how myelin is formed around the fibers by means of wide, flattened processes wrapping fibers with successive layers that become converted to myelin. Note that an oligodendrocyte (O) sends processes (c) to more than one nerve fiber, so oligodendrocytes are involved in myelinating parts of more than one nerve fiber. The junction between the part of a fiber myelinated by the process of one oligodendrocyte and the part myelinated by the next oligodendrocyte is a node of Ranvier (n). (Bunge, M. L., Bunge, R. P., and Ris, H.: J. Biophys. Biochem. Cytol., *10*:67, 1961)

read about later in this chapter, myelination in the CNS will be easier to visualize.

The process of myelination in the CNS begins in the gray matter, close to the cell body of a neuron, and advances along the axon into the white matter. This process begins early in the fourth month of fetal life, and is incomplete at birth, so that some fibers only become myelinated during the first year of life. The total amount of myelin in the CNS increases from birth to maturity and individual fibers become more heavily myelinated during the growth period. In both the CNS and PNS, the myelin sheath is interrupted at *nodes of Ranvier* (n in Fig. 17-10). (The structure and significance of these nodes will be explained when we discuss the conduction of nerve impulses.) The segments of a nerve fiber between consecutive nodes are called *internodes*.

THE DISTRIBUTION OF GRAY AND WHITE MATTER IN THE BRAIN

In the brain the formation of gray and white matter initially follows a pattern similar to that in the spinal cord, where gray matter forms from the middle layers and white matter from the outer layer of the neural tube. In the medulla, pons, midbrain, and parts of the forebrain, gray matter develops in positions corresponding roughly to those in the spinal cord, and the gray matter becomes covered by white matter, as in the cord. In certain other parts of the brain, however, neuroblasts from the middle layers of the neural tube migrate out through the outer layer of the wall (where white matter will develop) and so take up a position on the very outside of the tube. Because of this the cerebral hemispheres and the cerebellum acquire a covering (*cortex*) of *gray matter* (Fig. 17-6). Hence in these two parts of the brain the gray matter exists not only deep to the white matter but also superficial to it. This explains why the outer region of the spinal cord consists of white matter whereas that of the cerebrum and cerebellum is gray matter.

Having explained how nervous tissue is arranged to form the gray and white matter of the CNS, we now go on to describe nerve cells of the CNS in detail.

THE NEURONS OF THE CNS

Most neurons of the CNS are multipolar and most possess many dichotomously branching dendrites (Fig. 17-2, *right*). They have a single axon which also may have branches. The branches of axons, however, come off more or less at right angles and are termed *collaterals* (indicated by arrows in Fig. 17-11). At their terminations, axons break up into tree-like branches (arborizations).

THE CELL BODIES OF NEURONS

The cell bodies of neurons are commonly large but a few are small (4 μm. in diameter). Indeed the larger ones (up to 135 μm. in diameter) are among the largest cells in the body. The cell bodies of different kinds of neurons may be rounded, flattened, ovoid, or pyramidal. As

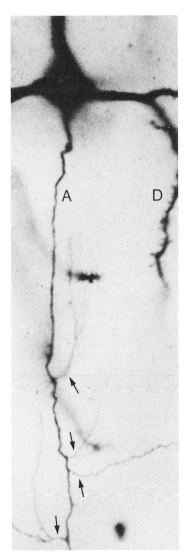

Fig. 17-11. Medium-power photomicrograph of a pyramidal cell of the cerebral cortex of a cat, showing its axon (A) and one of its dendrites (D). Note the spines on the dendrite. Collateral branches of the axon are indicated by arrows. Modified Golgi stain. (Courtesy of E. G. Bertram)

noted, the cell bodies of neurons of the CNS are all located in gray matter.

Nucleus. The nucleus of most neurons has a central position in the cell body but, as we shall see, in autonomic neurons of the PNS it is commonly somewhat eccentric in position. In general, the nucleus is large and spherical (Figs. 17-12 and 17-13). The nucleus in small neurons, though smaller, is even larger in relation to the cell body than in larger neurons. The chromatin of the nucleus of many kinds of neurons is almost entirely of the extended

type (Figs. 17-12 and 17-13), so that chromatin granules are very small or not seen at all with the LM. As a result, the single large central nucleolus in the center of the nucleus is typically very prominent. Its somewhat striking LM appearance (Figs. 17-12 and 17-14) has been described as resembling an owl's eye, possibly by a student who studied at night. In electron micrographs some peripheral chromatin can be seen on the inner aspect of the nuclear envelope (Fig. 17-13). Certain types of neurons with large cell bodies are characteristically tetraploid.

Nissl Substance. With the LM clumps of basophilic material are commonly seen in the cell body and larger dendrites of nerve cells (Fig. 17-12). These are termed *Nissl bodies,* after the German neurologist Franz Nissl who first described them at the turn of the century. Seen with the EM, Nissl substance consists of regions of cytoplasm rich in flattened cisternae of rER with numerous free and attached ribosomes and polysomes scattered between adjacent cisternae (Fig. 17-13). The abundant rRNA of free and attached ribosomes is, of course, the cause of the basophilia of Nissl bodies seen with the LM. In large motor neurons the Nissl bodies are large and the flattened cisternae are commonly arranged more or less parallel with one another, but in other types of nerve cells they are disposed in a more irregular fashion in the cytoplasm, as in Figure 17-13.

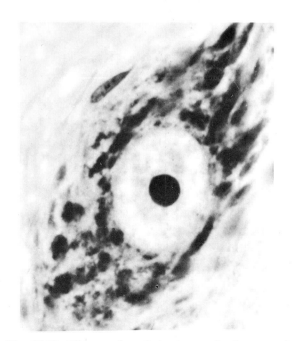

Fig. 17-12. Oil-immersion photomicrograph of an anterior horn cell of the spinal cord of a cat (cresyl violet stain). Nissl substance is seen to advantage. (Barr, M. L., Bertram, L. F., and Lindsay, H. A.: Anat. Rec., *107*:283, 1950)

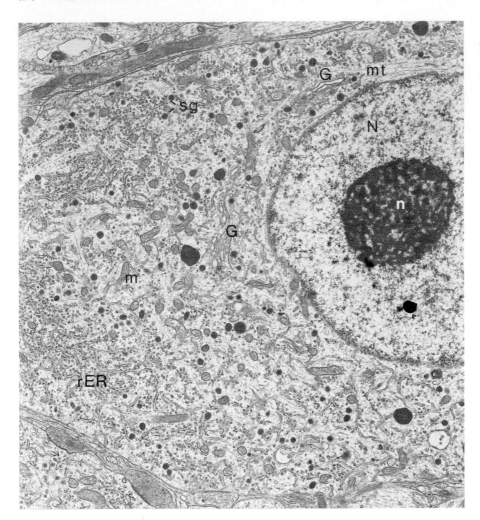

Fig. 17-13. Electron micrograph (×15,000) of part of the cell body of a neuron of the supraoptic nucleus (rat). Note that the nucleus (N) at *right* contains only a small amount of condensed chromatin, arranged peripherally along the inner membrane of the nuclear envelope, and that most of its chromatin is extended. The nucleolus (n) is very prominent. In the cytoplasm, flattened cisternae of rER are visible at *upper left* and *lower left,* with abundant polysomes scattered about between them. Golgi stacks (G) are present near the nucleus. Some microtubules (mt) and many mitochondria (m) may also be seen. Since this type of neuron is also a neurosecretory cell, secretory granules (sg) are present in the cytoplasm. (Paterson, J. A., and Leblond, C. P.: J. Comp. Neurol., *175*:373, 1977)

The abundant free ribosomes in the cell body (Fig. 17-13) continuously synthesize new cytoplasmic proteins that flow along the axon (and the dendrites too) to replace proteins used up in metabolism.

If the axon is accidentally severed, a change known as the *axon reaction* ensues; the Nissl substance disappears temporarily from the cell body (this is termed *chromatolysis*) and the nucleus moves over to one side (Fig. 17-14). In the event that the axon is regenerated the Nissl substance reappears.

Neurofilaments. The LM showed what at first were thought to be fibrils in nerve cells, so these were called *neurofibrils.* The EM showed, however, that the so-called fibrils were bundles of filaments, termed *neurofilaments* (labeled F in Fig. 17-15). They are about 10 nm. in diameter and hence correspond to what are now called *intermediate filaments.* Their composition has not been established except for the fact that they consist of protein.

Neurotubules. These are typical microtubules, 24 nm. in diameter (labeled in Figs. 17-13 and 17-15). Their role is to maintain the shape of the neuron and in particular that of its processes (Figs. 17-16 and 17-19).

The Other Cytoplasmic Components. It was in the cell bodies of neurons that Golgi first demonstrated the apparatus that bears his name. The location of the Golgi saccules varies in different kinds of nerve cells. In some, Golgi stacks are scattered all around the nucleus and, as described on page 130, it is now believed these are all connected with one another. The common distribution of the Golgi stacks is indicated by the regions labeled G in Figures 17-13 and 17-15. Mitochondria are abundant and distributed fairly evenly throughout the cytoplasm of the cell body (m in Figs. 17-13 and 17-15). Lysosomes also are present.

Two pigments may also be present in the cell bodies of nerve cells. The first, *lipofuscin,* is a yellow-brown pig-

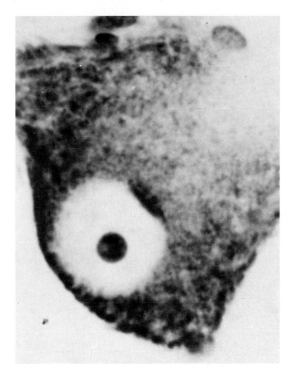

Fig. 17-14. High-power photomicrograph of a neuron, showing severe chromatolysis during an axon reaction. The axon hillock is at *upper right,* and chromatolysis is typically most severe between the nucleus and the axon hillock. The nucleus has taken up an eccentric position. (Barr, M. L., and Hamilton, J. D.: J. Comp. Neurol., *89:*93, 1948)

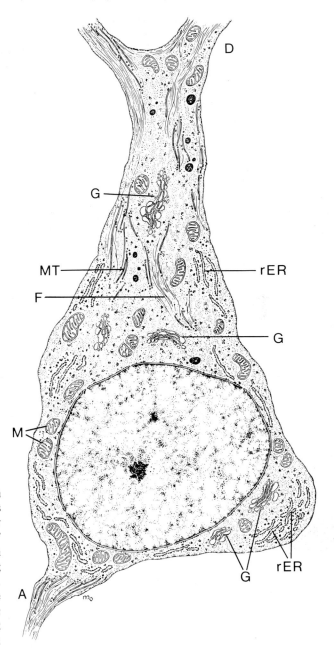

Fig. 17-15. Diagram illustrating the fine structure of the cell body of a neuron. A, axon hillock; D, dendrites; rER, rough-surfaced endoplasmic reticulum; G, Golgi stacks; MT, microtubules; M, mitochondria; and F, filaments. (Courtesy of C. P. Leblond)

ment that appears during postnatal life, first in ganglion cells (Fig. 5-62) and later in neurons of the CNS. Its amount increases with age but its significance is not really understood. It is believed to represent a "wear and tear" product that cannot be eliminated by lysosomal digestion and hence accumulates in residual bodies over the long lifetime of the cell (our nerve cells are as old as we are). The dark brown pigment *melanin* also occurs in nerve cells in a few parts of the CNS, notably the *substantia nigra* (L. *nigra,* black), a landmark in the midbrain that will probably be noticed in gross anatomy when the brain is dissected. However, the significance of melanin in the cell bodies of neurons is not known.

Nerve Fibers

The Axon

The single axon of a neuron may be as short as 1 mm. or as long as several feet, depending on the kind of neuron. Its diameter is between 1 and 20 μm., and an axon with a large diameter conducts impulses more rap-idly than a narrower one. *Collateral* branches, where these exist, leave the axon virtually at right angles (Fig. 17-11) and then make another more or less right-angle turn to continue on in the same direction, or to run back

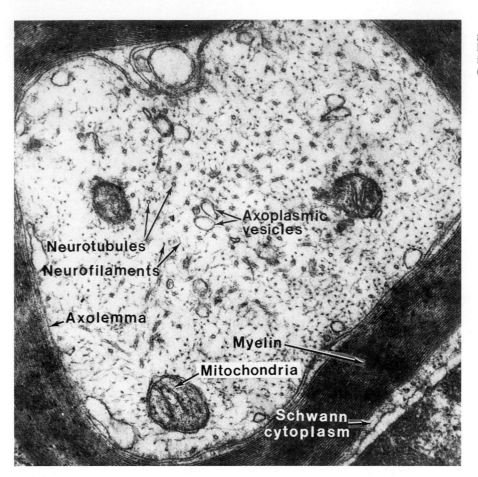

Fig. 17-16. Electron micrograph of a cross section of a myelinated nerve fiber (axon) showing its characteristic organelles. (Courtesy of B. Droz)

alongside the axon from which they branched as *recurrent collaterals* as in Figure 17-11. The region of the cell body from which the axon arises, which is called the *axon hillock* (labeled A in Fig. 17-15), is relatively free of rER but contains many filaments and microtubules.

Both efferent and afferent fibers situated in the white matter of the spinal cord and brain are myelinated. The proximal (initial) segment of the axon lying in the gray matter, however, remains devoid of myelin and instead is covered with cytoplasmic processes of oligodendrocytes and astrocytes. The proximal portion of the axon is also somewhat narrower than the more distal myelinated portion. However, as we shall see when we come to consider the autonomic nervous system, not all axons are myelinated.

Figure 17-16 illustrates the fine structure of a myelinated axon. Its cell membrane (commonly called the *axolemma*) lies just inside the myelin sheath surrounding the axon. Within its cytoplasm (similarly called *axoplasm*) there are numerous thread-shaped mitochondria arranged for the most part with their long axis along the axon. Small *axoplasmic vesicles* (Fig. 17-16) in the axon probably represent portions of the sER. There is an abundance of 10-nm. filaments (*intermediate filaments* or *neurofilaments*), especially at the nodes of Ranvier, and microtubules (*neurotubules*) are just as numerous (Figs. 17-16 and 17-19). The filaments and microtubules are mostly arranged longitudinally along the axon and hence may be seen in cross section in Fig. 17-16. Ribosomes are very seldom seen in the axoplasm and both rER and Golgi vesicles are altogether lacking. The axon is therefore virtually dependent on the cell body of the neuron for its supply of protein; hence, proteins and certain other macromolecular substances synthesized in the cell body are continuously transported toward the axon terminals by a process called *axoplasmic transport*, as follows.

Axoplasmic Transport. Due to the very great length of the axon, it is not unusual for it to have several hundred times the volume of the cell body of a neuron. Because there is little (if any) synthesis of proteins within the axon, required proteins, glycoproteins, and some other macromolecular substances, together with certain organelles such as mitochondria and vesicles, must be transported along the axon away from the cell body. Radioautography has shown that within a few minutes of being incorporated into proteins within the cell body, labeled amino acids move toward the axon hillock and migrate down the axon. Certain cytoplasmic proteins and organelles thus migrate in two main streams moving at different speeds along the axon.

First, there is a *slow stream* moving along the axon (away from the cell body) at a rate of 1 to 3 mm. per day. This slowly moving stream conveys vesicles, lysosomes, and some of the enzymes needed within axon terminals for the synthesis of neurotransmitter substances. An example of a protein transported by the slow stream is the enzyme tyrosine hydroxylase, which is involved in the synthesis of norepinephrine. This slow stream is thought to be necessary for axon growth and day-to-day maintenance of the axon.

Second, a *fast stream* also travels away from the cell body, but at a rate (5 to 10 mm. per hour) roughly 100 times faster than the slow stream. This fast-moving stream transports certain other components, mostly those necessary for synaptic function, including dopamine hydroxylase (another enzyme needed for synthesizing norepinephrine), glycoproteins, phospholipids, mitochondria, and neurosecretory granules. Other axon components seem to travel at speeds intermediate between those of the slow and fast streams. It is not known how axoplasmic flow is brought about, but it is widely held that microtubules may play some role.

Dendrites

These are commonly very much shorter than the axon and may extend in any direction from multipolar neurons (Fig. 17-2, *right*). Unlike the axon, dendrites branch dichotomously at acute angles, so that there are several orders of branching, with the final branches being small in diameter. There are commonly 5 to 15 major dendritic processes on a typical motor neuron in the spinal cord and it has been estimated that somewhere between 80 and 90 per cent of the surface of such a cell is represented by its dendrites, which present a considerable surface area for receiving impulses. Larger dendritic processes (labeled D in Fig. 17-15) differ from the axon in containing ribosomes and cisternae of rER (constituting the Nissl substance indicated by dark patches in these processes in Fig. 17-2, *right*) as well as abundant neurotubules, neurofilaments, and mitochondria (Fig. 17-15). Hence they contain the same kinds of organelles as the cell body.

Dendritic Transport. Certain proteins, for example acetylcholinesterase, the enzyme that destroys the neurotransmitter acetylcholine after it has been released at synapses, are transported toward the dendritic terminals

(away from the cell body) at a rate of about 3 mm. per hour, which is almost as rapid as the fast stream in axons.

Retrograde Flow. Not only do components migrate away from the cell body toward the axon or dendrite terminals, some migrate in the reverse direction (*retrograde flow*) away from either the presynaptic terminal of the axon or postsynaptic terminals of the dendrites and toward the cell body. These retrograde streams in the axon and dendrites are able to transport some of the cytoplasmic components toward the cell body almost as rapidly as the fast stream (described above) conveys others in the reverse direction. Retrograde flow, of course, returns many cytoplasmic components to the cell body so that they do not accumulate at the fiber terminals and it has even been suggested that it may also serve the purpose of allowing the neuron to monitor the welfare of its pre- and postsynaptic terminals in case anything is wrong with them.

NERVE IMPULSES

In order to properly appreciate the structural basis for function in nerve tissue at either the LM or EM level, it is essential to have some knowledge of the nature of the nerve impulse. This is a subject properly dealt with in depth in physiology courses and texts. However, since curricula differ, the study of histology may precede that of physiology, so for those who have not yet had the advantage of learning about nerve impulses in a physiology course, an introductory account is given here.

What Is Meant by the Term *Resting Potential*

Since the word *potential* or *potentiality* is so commonly used in histology with regard to the as yet unrealized capacities of cells for further differentiation, it should be pointed out that with regard to nerve cells the word *potential* is used as it is in electricity, where it refers to relative electrical charges between two points in a field or circuit. In other words, a potential refers to something that exists between two points. In the instance of a neuron it refers to the relative electrical charges present inside and outside the confines of its cell membrane. Thus it is sometimes referred to as the *transmembrane potential*. In a resting neuron the potential between the two sides of the membrane is called its *resting potential*, and it has been shown with electrodes, one inserted into the cell body or one of its processes and the other placed outside the plasmalemma, to be −70 mv.; hence the *inner side* of the plasmalemma of a neuron is *negatively charged* with respect to its outer side.

The Cause and Maintenance of the Resting Potential

The reason for there being a resting (transmembrane) potential when a neuron is not conducting is that the total concentrations of positively and negatively charged ions are unequal on either side of its cell membrane, with there being relatively more positively charged ions outside the membrane (the side in contact with the intercellular space) and more negatively charged ones on the inner aspect of the membrane (the side in contact with cytoplasm). The basis for this is as follows.

First, it will be recalled that the cell membrane is able to transport certain cations (by active transport) against their concentration gradients. Using ATP as a source of energy, the sodium-potassium pump (p. 111) of the cell membrane pumps sodium ions out of the cytoplasm and potassium ions into the cytoplasm from the intercellular fluid. Next, whether these ions stay where they are pumped depends on the selective permeability of the cell membrane, for it is this that determines which ions can or cannot diffuse back along their concentration gradients into the compartments from which they were pumped. Since the permeability of the nerve cell membrane for potassium ions is considerable, these ions rapidly leave the cytoplasm, in which their concentration by virtue of the sodium-potassium pump is higher than in the intercellular fluid. This tends to increase the number of positively charged ions outside the cell membrane. But the membrane is not as permeable to sodium ions, so that once pumped out into the intercellular fluid these do not re-enter the resting neuron. As a consequence of potassium ions (which are positively charged) constantly leaking out to join sodium ions (also positively charged) that are continuously being pumped out into the intercellular fluid, the total concentration of positively charged ions is greater in the intercellular fluid than in the cytoplasm; this is the primary reason for the inner aspect of the plasmalemma being negative with respect to its outer aspect in a resting axon.

Another factor of importance in maintaining negativity on the cytoplasmic side of the plasmalemma is that the cytoplasm contains relatively large numbers of negatively charged organic macromolecules. Due to their size these are unable to diffuse through the membrane, and because their numbers are not matched by similar large molecules in the tissue fluid outside the neuron, they also contribute to maintaining the negative charge on the inner aspect of the plasmalemma.

As a result of the factors described above, a resting potential of −70 mv. exists between the inner and outer sides of the nerve cell membrane, which is therefore said to be *polarized*.

The Nerve Impulse

A nerve impulse originates at the site of, and in response to, a stimulus. A *stimulus* may be one of a variety of kinds and can be, for example, of a mechanical, electrical, chemical, physical, or thermal nature. When applied to the plasmalemma at some site, a stimulus initiates an impulse in a neuron. Later we deal with impulses fired off at afferent nerve endings in response to certain stimuli and describe how they are transmitted across synapses from one neuron to another so that a second neuron, for example, can be stimulated by receiving impulses from another neuron. Here, since we intend to explain how nerve impulses are propagated along unmyelinated axons, we shall describe what would happen at the site of a stimulus applied to the plasmalemma of an unmyelinated axon at a given point along its length — with the realization, of course, that this would not be the usual part of a neuron to receive stimuli. When we have described how impulses are propagated along unmyelinated axons, we will then go on to explain the way they travel along myelinated ones. However, it should be borne in mind that in the following we are referring to axons of the *unmyelinated* type.

The first detectable effect of applying a so-called *effective stimulus* to an unmyelinated axon is the occurrence at the site of the stimulus of a sudden influx into the axoplasm of sodium ions from outside the axolemma. To understand why this could hap-

pen it should be remembered that up until now the sodium-potassium pump of the axolemma has maintained an excess of sodium ions outside the axolemma against a concentration gradient. The immediate influx of sodium ions into the axon at the site of the stimulus is explained by the axolemma at this site suddenly becoming permeable to sodium ions so they immediately move inward due to their concentration gradient.

Since sodium ions carry a positive charge, their sudden influx into the axoplasm reduces the total positive charge on the outer aspect of the axolemma and adds to the positive ions within the axoplasm to such an extent that the inner·side of the axolemma no longer remains negatively charged in relation to its outer surface. In other words, the *resting potential* of the axolemma rapidly *disappears*. Indeed, the influx is so great that the inner side of the axolemma very temporarily becomes slightly positively charged in relation to its exterior. Because of the movement of sodium ions inward being due to their moving along their concentration gradient, this movement is quickly stopped when their concentration in the axoplasm reaches that outside the axolemma. However, just as any further influx is thus arrested, a second event is occurring, which is that the axolemma suddenly becomes extremely permeable to potassium ions. Since these ions were previously in excess on the inner side of the axolemma due to the action of the sodium-potassium pump, and the axolemma now becomes readily permeable to them, they flow outwardly through the membrane to the exterior (because of their concentration gradient). This has two effects. First, it reduces the total positive charge in the axoplasm, and second, it increases the total positive charge outside the axolemma. The combined effect is, of course, to *restore the resting potential* of the axolemma. The membrane then regains its former ability to prevent free movement of sodium or potassium ions across it in accordance with their respective concentration gradients. The sodium-potassium pump again becomes effective and soon the site is once more operating under the conditions that pertained before the stimulus was applied.

The series of events outlined above can be described by saying that application of a stimulus to some site along an unmyelinated axon causes immediate *depolarization* of its membrane at that site and this is followed almost instantaneously by *repolarization*. However, what is very important is that when there is a depolarization (followed by repolarization) of any part of a neuron, the depolarization and then the repolarization spread in a wave-like manner along the cell membrane to the termination of the axon. Hence, the transmission of a nerve impulse amounts to a *wave of depolarization and repolarization* sweeping along the cell membrane.

The depolarization and repolarization of the cell membrane of a neuron (or muscle) cell are often described as an *action potential*. Semantically this is a puzzling term. It was probably devised to denote that an action potential was different from what is termed a *resting potential* (although the latter is really the potential of a *resting membrane*) and that the depolarization and repolarization of a stimulated cell membrane are transmitted along the cell membrane in a wave-like manner and hence the stimulus causes action.

Before describing the spread of an action potential, we should point out that for convenience in the foregoing, we have described what would happen if a stimulus were applied (artificially) to an unmyelinated nerve fiber at some point along its course. Actually, if this were done in the laboratory, a wave of depolarization and repolarization would spread from the site of stimulation toward both ends of the fiber. In life, however, afferent or efferent fibers are stimulated only at one end and hence the wave of depolarization (followed by one of repolarization) initiated at one end travels in only one direction to the other. Since a nerve fiber becomes repolarized immediately behind a wave of depolarization sweeping along it, the question arises as to why the wave of depolarization moving along it (in one direction) does not also spread backward to depolarize the repolarized site immediately behind it—which, of course, would initiate a retrograde wave of depolarization. The reason it does not spread backward is that the repolarized site immediately behind the wave of depolarization is temporarily refractive to stimulation. We shall now go on to explain how a wave of depolarization is propagated along a fiber.

As a result of the influx of positively charged sodium ions into the axolemma at the site of a stimulus, which is sufficient not only to destroy the negativity of the axoplasm at that site but also to make it transiently positive, an electrical current is set up between this axoplasm and the still negatively charged axoplasm farther along the axon so that positive charges (ions) flow forward toward the negatively charged axoplasm. Furthermore, the outer aspect of the axolemma at the site where it becomes depolarized attracts positive charges to it from the charged membrane farther ahead. As a result, the axoplasm just ahead of the site of the stimulus almost instantaneously becomes somewhat more positively charged and the outer aspect of the axolemma just ahead of the depolarized site becomes less positively charged. Accordingly, an electrical current flows outwardly through the axolemma from the axoplasm that has gained positive charges to the outside of the axolemma where positive charges were drawn away. The passage of current out through the membrane just ahead of the site where depolarization has occurred causes this region of the membrane in turn to become permeable to sodium ions, so that it then becomes depolarized just as the membrane did at the site of the stimulus. The depolarization occurring here then similarly brings about depolarization of the membrane slightly ahead of it, and so on, so that a wave of depolarization (followed by repolarization) sweeps progressively along the fiber.

Earlier in this account, we explained what would happen if an unmyelinated axon were stimulated at some point along its course, which does not happen under normal circumstances in the body, only under experimental conditions. Under such artificial conditions the wave of depolarization and repolarization (the action potential) would spread from the site of the stimulus in both directions. Within the body, however, the action potential is transmitted in only one direction along a nerve fiber. The nerve impulse does not travel in the reverse direction, restimulating the part of a nerve fiber over which it has just passed because when the axolemma has been depolarized and is becoming repolarized, it is refractory for a brief period to further excitation. Accordingly, a wave of depolarization that begins, for example, close to the cell body of an efferent neuron can only spread along its axon toward its termination because the part of the axon behind the wave of depolarization remains temporarily refractive to further stimulation. Furthermore, in chains of neurons, synapses, as we shall see, act as one-way gates and so permit impulses to pass from neuron to neuron in one direction only. These arrangements control the direction of flow of impulses in the nervous system.

The Function of Myelin—Saltatory Conduction. As already noted, the myelin of myelinated fibers is not continuous but interrupted at regular intervals by *nodes of Ranvier* (one is labeled n in Fig. 17-10). These nodes are present along myelinated fibers of both the CNS and PNS. The distance between consecutive nodes varies; it is at least 0.2 mm. but can be more than 1 mm. in large fibers. In myelinated fibers each region of the fiber between nodes is invested with a thick coat of myelin, which keeps tissue fluid away from the axon and acts as an electrical insulator. However, at the nodes there is no myelin so that here the axolemma is *exposed to tissue fluid.* Since the internodal regions of the axolemma are insulated, no current can flow from the axolemma to the exterior of the fiber in any of the internodal parts of the axolemma. At the nodes, however, the converse applies for here the axolemma lacks insulation by myelin so that at their nodes myelinated fibers behave like unmyelinated fibers. Hence depolarization (described above) can occur at the nodes.

When, for example, a motor neuron is stimulated, an action potential spreads into and along its axon. The very first (proximal) part of the axon is not myelinated and here the wave of depolarization spreads along the axon as it does in an unmyelinated fiber (as described above). But when the wave of depolarization enters the myelin sheath it cannot cause the axon immediately ahead of it to become depolarized, because the electrical current that would be set up between the interior and exterior of the axon (for the reasons described in the preceding text) cannot pass out through the myelin to the exterior at the site just ahead of the action potential. Since it is passage of this current through the axolemma that would make it permeable to sodium ions, the depolarization of the axolemma that would occur in an unmyelinated axon immediately ahead of the wave of depolarization does not occur in internodal portions of a myelinated one. However, the same difference in potential is nevertheless set up between the positively charged axoplasm and the outer surface of the membrane, but the current set up between them first has to flow through the axoplasm all the way to the next node of Ranvier before it can reach the exterior. When this occurs the passage of current out through the axolemma at this node makes it permeable to sodium ions so that the axon at this point becomes depolarized. This in turn sets up a current that, to reach the exterior, has to travel through the axoplasm to the next node, where it causes the axon at that node to become depolarized, and so on. So the passage of a nervous impulse along a myelinated fiber is not due to a continuous wave of depolarization sweeping along the fiber. It depends, instead, on local electrical currents being set up as each consecutive node becomes depolarized, with current passing to the next node and causing its depolarization and setting up a current that causes depolarization of the next node, and so on. Since an electric current travels much faster than a continuous wave of depolarization, transmission of impulses is much faster in myelinated fibers than in unmyelinated ones (up to 50 times faster). Because impulses thus "jump" along a myelinated fiber from one node to another, conduction along myelinated fibers is called *saltatory* (L. *saltare,* to jump) *conduction.*

The rate of conduction of nerve impulses in myelinated fibers is not only much faster than in unmyelinated fibers, it also increases in relation to the diameter of the myelinated fiber. Both findings are to be explained by the fact that conduction in myelinated fibers is primarily due to electrical currents. The reason for the speed of conduction being faster in larger fibers would seem to be explained by Ohm's Law, which postulates that the electrical resistance of a conductor varies inversely with its diameter.

HOW NERVE IMPULSES ARE TRANSMITTED AT AXON TERMINALS

Nerve impulses arriving at the termination of an axon on either another neuron or a muscle fiber are said to transmit impulses to them because a wave of depolarization is set up in the plasmalemma of the neuron or muscle cell. Nerve impulses arriving at the termination of an axon associated with gland cells or fat cells likewise bring about a response in these cells. How does the arrival of nerve impulses induce a response in another neuron, muscle fiber, gland cell, or fat cell?

Development of Knowledge. To explain this we should mention something here that is covered in more detail later in connection with the PNS. Among the efferent neurons of the PNS there is a division of labor between (*1*) those whose activities are under the control of the conscious mind and (*2*) those that function automatically outside its control. Collectively, the neurons of the latter group constitute the *autonomic nervous system,* which controls the contractile activity of muscle cells in the viscera and blood vessels, secretory activity of exocrine glands, and metabolic activities of certain other cells. There are two parts to the system, one called its *sympathetic division* and the other its *parasympathetic division.*

Further development of knowledge in this area depended on the discovery of a hormone called *epinephrine,* produced in the adrenal glands. It was noticed that giving an animal epinephrine produced most of the effects obtained by stimulating the *sympathetic* division of the autonomic nervous system. It was therefore thought that epinephrine might perhaps act by stimulating this division of the system. However, in 1904 Elliott found that administering epinephrine to an animal produced the effects obtained by stimulating sympathetic nerves in some parts of the body even after the sympathetic nerves to these parts had been severed. So in due course it was realized that epinephrine (actually it turned out to be the closely related hormone *norepinephrine*) brought about a response by directly affecting the cell membrane of the cells that responded. Meanwhile another substance, *acetylcholine,* was found to act the same way in connection with the *parasympathetic* division of the autonomic nervous system. These findings led to the concept that arrival of impulses at nerve endings caused them to *liberate a chemical substance,* such as norepinephrine or acetylcholine, that had a *direct effect on the cell membrane* of the cell that responded. This mechanism is referred to as *chemical mediation* of nerve impulses.

It was then found that chemical mediators were involved in transmitting nerve impulses not only at autonomic nerve endings but also at endings on muscles under voluntary control. Furthermore, it was discovered that chemical mediators were responsible for transmission of impulses from one neuron to another at most synapses, and that the arrival of a wave of depolarization along one neuron could cause a wave of depolarization to be initiated in a second by causing the release of a chemical mediator at the synapse.

The realization that impulses were mediated chemically, of course, helped to explain why synapses transmitted impulses only in one direction, a characteristic known long before chemical mediation was even discovered.

There are, however, some synapses at which transmission is electrical and these will be described later. Here we shall describe the type in which chemical mediators (*neurotransmitter substances*) are formed and liberated, and bring about transmission of impulses.

SYNAPSES INVOLVING CHEMICAL NEUROTRANSMITTERS

Some Terminology. The part of a neuron that delivers impulses at a synapse is referred to as a *presynaptic terminal* and the part receiving them is called a *postsynaptic terminal.* The presynaptic part of a synapse is commonly an axon terminal. Here the end of an axon branch is expanded into an *end bulb* (or *end foot*), the shape of which can be seen in Figure 17-18. The end bulb is, of course, bounded by axolemma, and the region of the axolemma that closely approaches the postsynaptic neuron at a synapse forms the *presynaptic membrane.* The region of cell membrane of the postsynaptic neuron closely associated with the presynaptic membrane is, as noted, referred to as the *postsynaptic membrane.* Between the pre- and postsynaptic membranes there is an intercellular space at most synapses, visible only with the EM, termed the *synaptic cleft* (labeled *cleft* in Fig. 17-20).

The Positions of Synapses on Neurons. Synapses can be classified on the basis of their position on the postsynaptic neuron. Only the common types will be mentioned here. Where axons terminate on dendrites, they form what are termed *axodendritic* synapses (Figs. 17-17A and 17-21B). In some of these the dendrite possesses little protrusions called *dendritic spines,* on or around which a terminal end bulb of the axon fits (Figs. 17-17B and 17-21C). Axon endings that terminate on the cell body of a neuron form what are termed *axosomatic* synapses (Figs. 17-17A and 17-21D). About half the total surface of the cell body of a neuron (Fig. 17-18) and almost all the surface of its dendrites may be involved in synaptic contact with other neurons. Axons that terminate on other axons form what are termed *axoaxonic* synapses (Fig. 17-17C). An axon can form a synapse with a second axon only at a region of the latter that is not myelinated. This situation is encountered in the *proximal segment* of an axon, for here the axon remains naked because myelination does not begin right at the axon hillock but at a short distance away from it. The *end bulb* regions of axons also lack myelin sheaths, so another way axoaxonic synapses can be formed is between terminal end bulbs of a presynaptic axon and those of a postsynaptic axon (Fig. 17-17C). There are other anatomical sites and arrangements of

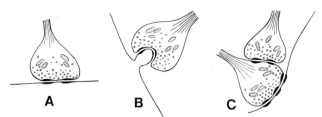

Fig. 17-17. Diagram illustrating some common kinds of synapses. (A) Axodendritic or axosomatic synapse. (B) Axodendritic synapse in which an end bulb synapses with a dendritic spine. (C) Axoaxonic synapse of the end bulb to end bulb type. (Barr, M. L.: The Human Nervous System. New York, Harper & Row, 1972)

synapses but these are more suitably described later in the chapter.

THE BASIC FINE STRUCTURE OF SYNAPSES

Since most synapses mediate impulses by means of chemical mediators, we shall here describe the basic electron microscopic structure of this type of synapse and its relation to function. In such a synapse there is a distinct space about 20 to 30 nm. wide, termed the *synaptic cleft*, between its parallel pre- and postsynaptic membranes (Fig. 17-20). The cytoplasm of the expanded end bulb region of the axon (which is called the *presynaptic terminal*) contains numerous mitochondria, indicating high metabolic activity, and abundant *synaptic vesicles* (Fig. 17-19), of which several kinds have been described. Those found at most synapses are spherical, with a diameter of 40 to 50 nm. At some synapses, however, the synaptic vesicles appear flattened when certain EM procedures are used, while at others the spherical vesicles show electron-dense cores. Each type of synaptic vesicle is believed to contain a particular kind of neurotransmitter substance.

Asymmetrical and Symmetrical Types of Synapses. As originally described by Gray, there is a type of synapse, often termed the *asymmetrical* type, that is found at axon terminals on small dendrites and dendritic spines. Within the synaptic cleft of such synapses, which is about 30 nm. wide, the EM discloses some slightly electron-dense material in a plaque-like arrangement. On the cytoplasmic side of the presynaptic membrane there are relatively small aggregations of moderately electron-dense material (Fig. 17-20, not labeled). However, on the cytoplasmic aspect of the postsynaptic terminal there is a considerable aggregation of relatively electron-dense material (Figs. 17-19 and 17-20, labeled postsynaptic density); hence the appearance of the postsynaptic terminal differs from that of the presynaptic one.

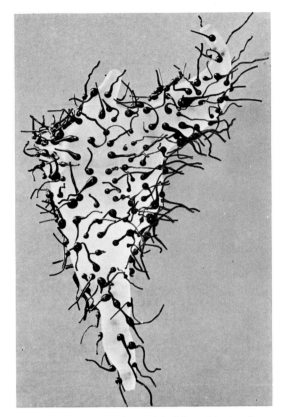

Fig. 17-18. Photograph of a model of the cell body of a neuron in the dorsal horn of the spinal cord (cat). The model shows the numerous fibers terminating as end bulbs (end feet) that synapse with the body of the cell. (Haggar, R. A., and Barr, M. L.: J. Comp. Neurol., *93*:17, 1950)

In the second type of synapse the synaptic cleft is slightly narrower (about 20 nm. wide) and the postsynaptic densities appear as more or less discrete patches somewhat similar to the patches seen in the presynaptic terminals. Since they thus appear like those on the presynaptic membrane, this type of synapse is sometimes called *symmetrical*. It is now conceded that besides these two slightly different kinds of chemical synapses recognized by Gray there are other synapses that are intermediate in structure.

The Presynaptic Membrane. Attached to its cytoplasmic face, this specialized region of the cell membrane has a hexagonal array of electron-dense particles, about 60 nm. in diameter, that project into the cytoplasm of the presynaptic terminal and are joined to one another by filaments. Further, there is an associated network of actin-like filaments ramifying throughout the cytoplasm of the presynaptic terminal. In between the particles attached to the presynaptic membrane there are spaces just wide enough to permit access of synaptic vesicles to the membrane.

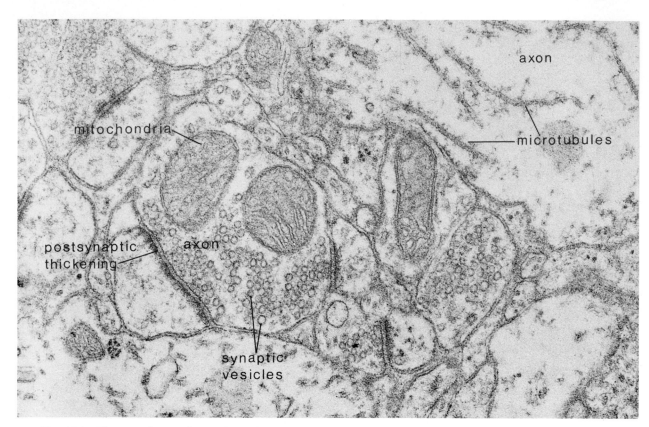

Fig. 17-19. Electron micrograph (×41,000) of asymmetrical synapses in occipital cortex (rat). (Courtesy of D. G. Jones)

The purpose of this elaborate arrangement, which is referred to as the *presynaptic vesicular grid,* has not yet been fully established, but it presumably delimits the sites at which synaptic vesicles can make contact with the presynaptic membrane.

The Synaptic Cleft. This cleft is filled with tissue fluid containing materials that after fixation for the EM can be seen in electron micrographs, where they are described as being somewhat more electron-dense in the asymmetrical than in the symmetrical kind of synapse. Certain EM methods disclose the material in the cleft as a double layer, separated by an electron-lucent gap of 2 nm. Furthermore, filamentous structures are sometimes seen traversing the cleft. This led Pfenninger to suggest that there are two layers of intercellular material in the synaptic cleft, each containing fine threads (perhaps macromolecules or molecular aggregates) that stick out from each synaptic membrane like bristles from a brush. This material appears to serve the purpose of holding the pre- and postsynaptic membranes together because presynaptic membranes tend to remain attached to their associated postsynaptic membranes when disrupted nerve tissue is submitted to cell fractionation. Both glycoproteins and glycolipids are found in the synaptic junctional fractions

of synaptosome preparations (the *synaptosome fraction* is the biochemical term for the pinched-off nerve endings obtained by fractionating disrupted nervous tissue) and there is histochemical evidence of carbohydrate-containing macromolecules in the synaptic cleft. Hence the intercellular material within the synaptic cleft is probably related to the cell coat material of the pre- and postsynaptic membranes. Moreover, markers such as horseradish peroxidase are able to penetrate the synaptic cleft, indicating that there is a true intercellular space in the synaptic cleft. No basal lamina is present between the pre- and postsynaptic membranes at neuronal synapses, but as we shall see there is one at motor nerve endings, which are commonly regarded as synapses between axons and muscle cells.

The Postsynaptic Membrane. As already noted, in asymmetrical synapses the densities on the cytoplasmic side of the postsynaptic membrane are far more prominent than those associated with the presynaptic membrane (Fig. 17-19). The densities seem to represent perforated plates of dense granular material. In symmetrical synapses they have the form of less noticeable, discrete patches on the cytoplasmic side of the postsynaptic membrane.

It has been pointed out that there are certain structural

and functional similarities between synaptic junctions and desmosomes. Thus, densities are associated with the cytoplasmic sides of both synaptic membranes and there are deposits of electron-dense intercellular material in the synaptic cleft. Moreover, as noted, synaptic membranes tend to remain associated with one another when disrupted nervous tissue is fractionated. Hence it appears that at chemical synapses there are junctions holding the pre- and postsynaptic membranes together and that these may serve the purpose that desmosomes do between other cell types.

Since Gray's first description of chemical synapses, several morphologically different kinds have been distinguished on the basis of the appearance of their synaptic vesicles, the width of their synaptic cleft, and the prominence of their postsynaptic densities. The functional role of each kind of synapse so distinguished is a matter of current investigation. We shall next consider the synaptic vesicles and their contents.

HOW NEUROTRANSMITTER SUBSTANCES ARE RELEASED AT SYNAPSES

The arrival of a nerve impulse at the termination of the presynaptic neuron at a synapse is manifested by a depo-larization of the presynaptic membrane. This makes the membrane more permeable to calcium ions so that an immediate influx of these occurs into the presynaptic terminal. Here they cause the synaptic vesicles containing the neurotransmitter to fuse with the presynaptic membrane. The fused membranes open up so that the contents of the vesicles are discharged into the synaptic cleft. The process here (exocytosis) is the same as that by which secretory vesicles from the Golgi empty their contents through the cell membrane of secretory cells (Figs. 5-21 and 5-32). The release of the transmitter substance into the synaptic cleft is what affects the postsynaptic neuron. This effect can be either of two kinds, as described shortly.

THE FORMATION OF SYNAPTIC VESICLES AND THE RECYCLING OF THE MEMBRANE OF THEIR WALLS

After synaptic activity involving the fusion of numerous synaptic vesicles with the presynaptic membrane, new vesicles must be formed to replace them. This entails new vesicles forming and budding off from the limiting membrane of the presynaptic terminal into the axoplasm close to the presynaptic membrane, by the same sort of mechanism as occurs in phagocytosis and pinocytosis

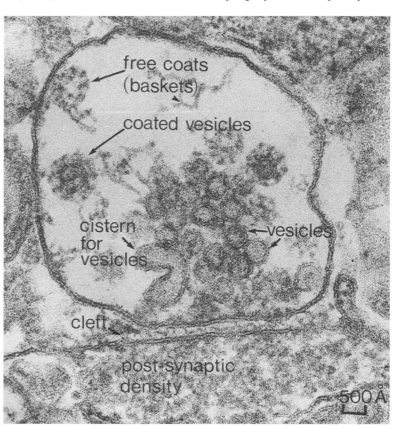

Fig. 17-20. Electron micrograph of a synapse in the cerebral cortex (rat). The synaptic vesicles fuse with the presynaptic membrane and release their contents of neurotransmitter. Coated vesicles subsequently arise from the membrane of the presynaptic terminal by endocytosis (the free coats may be contractile, initiating endocytosis). The free coats or baskets fall off, leaving smooth vesicles which fuse with the collecting cisterna. Vesicles later bud off from the cisterna and become reloaded with neurotransmitter. The postsynaptic region is a dendrite. (Courtesy of P. Seeman)

(shown in Fig. 5-39) or endocytosis (shown in Fig. 5-38). The vesicles thus forming from the limiting membrane of presynaptic terminals were found to be of the coated variety, the formation of which (in another site) was illustrated in Figure 5-43. The coats of these vesicles are termed *baskets* (Fig. 17-20). As the coated vesicles move inward they lose their baskets, so that their membranous walls become naked. In this state they fuse with a cisterna of smooth-surfaced membrane (Fig. 17-20), into which they presumably empty their contents. However, new vesicles bud off from the cisterna just as vesicles bud off from the Golgi (Fig. 5-32); these nascent synaptic vesicles accumulate and are therefore present and ready to fuse with the presynaptic membrane and empty their contents of neurotransmitter into the synaptic cleft the next time nerve impulses arrive at the end bulb. Thus the axolemma of the end foot is constantly recycled. The membrane "used up" in forming coated vesicles is added back to the axolemma when the vesicles fuse with the presynaptic membrane.

Since the neurotransmitter is present in the collecting cisterna, it is also present in the synaptic vesicles that bud off from it. Exactly where each of the various neurotransmitter substances are synthesized, and how they come to be contained in the cisterna from which the synaptic vesicles bud off, has not yet been clearly established. However, it appears likely that at least in the case of acetylcholine, synthesis occurs within the membranous cisterna in the presynaptic terminal.

EXCITATORY AND INHIBITORY SYNAPSES

Physiologically there are two types of synapses, excitatory and inhibitory, and these will be described below. But first we should realize that the concept of the function of synapses has changed over the years. The word *synapse* (Gr. *synapsis,* a conjunction or connection) was first used to denote the site of meeting of two neurons over which a nerve impulse could pass from the one to the other. This concept of synapses was essential for postulation of the neuron theory and for understanding how nerve impulses could travel over more than one neuron to pass, for example, from the brain to a toe. But while visualizing synapses as linking neurons in a chain was helpful, it was only part of the story because it was subsequently established that a neuron can synapse with hundreds of other neurons and indeed there can be so many synapses on the cell body of some neurons that they can scarcely be counted. Furthermore, it became apparent that synapses did not necessarily act by conducting nerve impulses from one neuron to another, but that some synapses act to *inhibit* the reactivity of the neuron with which they connect, while others on the same

neuron act to *excite* it. Accordingly, the net effect of both kinds of synapses on a neuron is the particular balance established at any given moment between these two opposite kinds of synaptic activity. We shall now consider the two physiological types of synapses, excitatory and inhibitory.

Relation to Morphological Types and Respective Modes of Action. In general, axodendritic synapses appear to be mostly of the excitatory kind, whereas axosomatic synapses are more commonly of the inhibitory type. However, before attempting to explain the difference between the two, we shall briefly review the ionic composition of the fluid in the synaptic cleft, which, of course, is comparable to the tissue fluid anywhere else in the body.

As was described earlier in this chapter (p. 498), the concentration of potassium ions is maintained at a higher concentration in the axoplasm than in the intercellular fluid by the action of the sodium-potassium pump. Sodium ions, however, are pumped out of the axon and hence are at a higher concentration in the intercellular fluid. Because the axon has an internal negative charge (its resting potential), chloride ions are repelled and hence leave the axon, so that like sodium ions they are present in excess in the tissue fluid of the cleft.

When a nerve impulse arrives at an excitatory type of synapse and causes release of neurotransmitter into its synaptic cleft, the neurotransmitter has the effect of making the postsynaptic membrane more permeable to sodium ions by opening up channels for them in it. This, of course, allows more and more positively charged sodium ions to pass from the synaptic cleft into the cytoplasm of the postsynaptic terminal so that its resting negative potential is reduced. If enough positive ions continue to enter, the point is reached at which a complete depolarization of the postsynaptic membrane occurs, with the result that a nerve impulse is generated in the postsynaptic neuron.

At inhibitory synapses, however, the situation is somewhat different. When impulses arrive at the presynaptic membrane of an inhibitory synapse, they cause the release of an inhibitory type of neurotransmitter substance into the synaptic cleft. This has the effect of opening up channels in the postsynaptic membrane for negatively charged (chloride) ions that, as they enter the postsynaptic terminal from the synaptic cleft due to their concentration gradient, act so as to *increase* its negative (resting) potential, an effect called *hyperpolarization*. Potassium ions also seem to be involved; they leave the postsynaptic terminal, thereby also increasing its internal negative potential.

From the foregoing it will be obvious that the arrival of impulses at excitatory synapses acts so as to *lower* the resting potential of the cell membrane of the postsynaptic neuron; hence excitatory impulses render the postsynaptic neuron more excitable. Impulses arriving at inhibitory synapses, however, have the opposite effect; they *raise* the potential difference across the cell membrane of the postsynaptic neuron and so render the postsynaptic neuron less excitable. When considerably more impulses have arrived at excitatory synapses than at inhibitory ones on a given neuron, the potential difference across the membrane of this postsynaptic neuron becomes reduced enough to trigger a depolarization, which, of course, initiates an impulse along the axon of the postsynaptic neuron.

How Particular Neurotransmitter Substances Can Be Detected in Nerve Fibers. There are two general ways in which this can be done. First, norepinephrine and the chemical family to which it belongs (referred to as the *catecholamines*) can be made to fluoresce by treating them under controlled conditions with formaldehyde vapor. Hence, the positions of tracts of those nerve fibers that transmit impulses by means of norepinephrine, which serves as the principal neurotransmitter at inhibitory synapses in the CNS and also as the chemical mediator at sympathetic endings on muscle and most gland cells, can be determined by suitably treating a section with formaldehyde vapor and observing it under the fluorescence microscope. A second approach that can be used is to prepare a specific antibody against an enzyme involved in the synthesis of the particular neurotransmitter being investigated, label it with a fluorescent dye, and utilize it for the same purpose. Alternatively, histochemical methods specific for the enzymes required for synthesis of the neurotransmitter may be employed.

ELECTRICAL SYNAPSES

Although impulses are mediated at most synapses by means of neurotransmitter substances (referred to as *neurochemical* transmission), there are some synapses where direct electrical transmission of impulses (*neuroelectrical* transmission) occurs. Such synapses, which are called *electrical synapses,* all have a symmetrical appearance and are characterized by having a much narrower synaptic cleft, only 2 to 4 nm. wide. Furthermore, since there is no delay in transmission due to chemical mediation, neuroelectrical transmission is virtually instantaneous. In the EM, electrical synapses (which have been demonstrated in certain regions of the brain) have all the characteristics of *gap junctions* and like them permit free movement of ions between the pre- and postsynaptic terminals.

Certain other synapses contain some regions similar to gap junctions and other regions where there are wider synaptic clefts, together with associated synaptic vesicles on the presynaptic side and postsynaptic densities on the

other. Such synapses are referred to as *mixed synapses* and apparently mediate impulses by both electrical and chemical means.

SYNAPTIC ARRANGEMENTS BETWEEN NEURONS

The presynaptic terminal in a synapse is commonly that of an axon, but this is not always the case. As noted earlier in this chapter, other kinds of synaptic arrangements also exist between neurons. Some of these are illustrated in Figure 17-21. *Dendrodendritic* synapses (between dendrites of separate neurons), for example, are found in cerebral cortex (Fig. 17-21F) and, in particular, in the olfactory bulbs (relay stations between the olfactory receptors and the olfactory area of the cerebral cortex), where they are involved in processing information about smells. At such synapses the presynaptic membrane possesses a feature unusual for a dendrite: it has synaptic vesicles associated with it. Moreover, in the olfactory bulbs dendrodendritic synapses with opposite polarities and functions are arranged in pairs, with an excitatory synapse between a dendrite of one neuron and a dendrite of another only a short distance away from an inhibitory one passing inhibitory impulses between the same two dendrites but in the reverse direction. Such complexities of synaptic transmission suggest that various levels of organization exist in the circuitry of the CNS, with one level consisting of microcircuits involving dendrodendritic synapses. Finally, Figure 17-21E shows synapses between dendritic spines and the cell body of another neuron, that is, *dendrosomatic* synapses. It therefore seems that any part of a neuron can synapse with any part of another neuron.

Postnatal Formation of Synapses. There is some indication that neurons retain their capacity for forming synapses, at least under certain conditions, into adult life. If, for example, a nerve of the PNS that has been severed is rejoined by means of sutures, new axon sprouts grow from the stump along the nerve toward the structure formerly innervated and there establish new synaptic contact with target cells. Both afferent and efferent fibers are able to do this, the process involving specificity. Regenerating fibers appear able to recognize appropriate target cells with which to establish synapses.

Within the confines of the CNS, regeneration of fibers in adult mammals is extremely limited and ineffective, though apparently not nonexistent. For example, one tract of the CNS that appears capable of regeneration, at least in the ferret, is the hypothalamo-hypophyseal tract (which connects the pituitary gland with the hypothalamus). Furthermore, axons grow for short distances across spinal cord transections in animals given certain

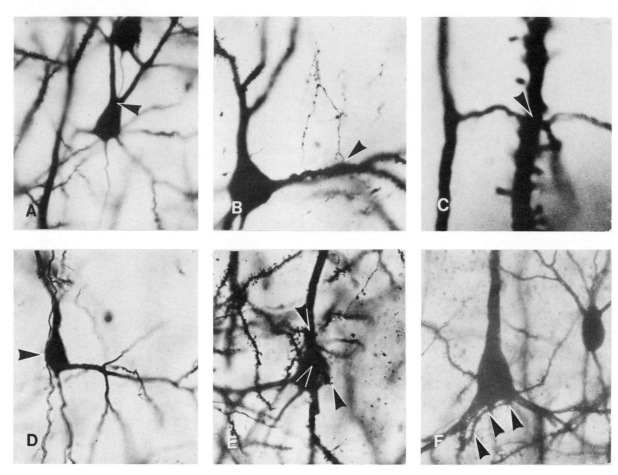

Fig. 17-21. Photomicrographs illustrating synaptic arrangements between pyramidal cells in the cerebral cortex of a cat (modified Golgi stain). The arrows indicate: (*A*) *axosomatic* synapse, between the *axon* of a neuron (cell body at *top center*) and the *cell body* of another neuron at *center;* (*B*) *axodendritic* synapse, between a terminal branch (*right of center*) of the *axon* of a neuron and a *dendrite* of another neuron whose cell body lies at *bottom left;* (*C*) *axodendritic* synapse, between a collateral branch (extending from *left* to *right* across middle of photomicrograph) of the axon (*left* border) of a neuron and a *dendritic spine* on a dendrite (*right of center*) of another neuron; (*D*) *axosomatic* synapse, between the *axon* (thin fiber running parallel to *left* border) of a neuron and the *cell body* of another neuron, with which it forms a *synapse en passant* (Fr., meaning in passing); (*E*) *dendrosomatic* synapses, between spines of a *dendrite* of a neuron whose cell body lies at *top left* and the *cell body* of the neuron at *center;* (*F*) *dendrodendritic* synapses between spines on a *dendrite* (which extends diagonally from *middle right* toward *bottom left*) and a major *dendritic* process that runs parallel to it and belongs to the neuron lying *left of center*. (Courtesy of E. G. Bertram)

drugs to reduce the amount of scar tissue formed in the lesion, although this very limited regeneration is not enough to restore lost functions. One difficulty in investigating whether new synapses form in the CNS is that the information about reconstituted or newly established neuronal pathways within the CNS comes chiefly from studies of recovery from induced lesions, since there are few other known ways of inducing continued formation of synapses. But interpretation of the findings is difficult because it is hard to determine whether recovery of function is due to regeneration of the cut fibers themselves, so as to re-establish their original synaptic connections, or due to collateral sprouting of adjacent intact fibers with the formation of new compensatory synapses. Moreover, it remains to be seen whether the synapse formed after inducing experimental lesions might not always represent synaptic replacement, that is, takeover of denervated former postsynaptic terminals, or whether some new synaptic sites are also formed. Accordingly, the extent to which new synapses form in the CNS in adult life and could contribute to learning and memory remains an unknown entity.

Fig. 17-22. Low- and high-power photomicrographs (*A* and *B*) of human cerebral cortex (H and E). Note the capillaries, separated from the neuropil (the gray background) by a shrinkage space. (*A*) The bodies of nerve cells and nuclei of neuroglia cells can be seen. (*B*) One nerve cell body at *middle right* has an oligodendrocyte as a satellite.

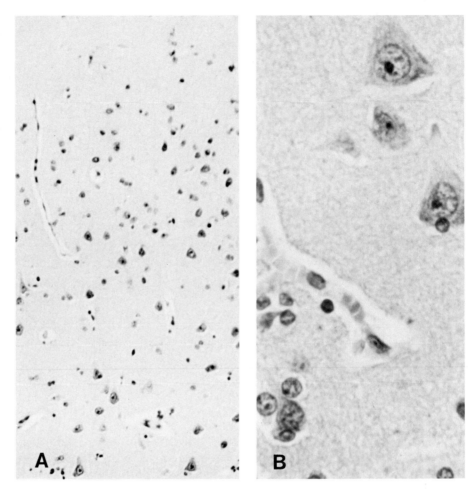

NERVE TERMINATIONS ON SECRETORY AND FAT CELLS

This topic will be considered later in this chapter in connection with the autonomic nervous system.

THE MICROSCOPIC STRUCTURE OF GRAY MATTER

We shall begin the study of the various cellular components of the CNS by commenting briefly on the general microscopic structure of gray matter and how this was determined. Before describing what has been learned about the microscopic structure of gray matter from the use of metallic impregnation methods, we should first comment on how little could have been learned about its complex structure from the study of routine sections and ordinary stains alone.

Figure 17-22A illustrates a low-power view of human cerebral cortex stained with H and E. Four components can be identified in it:

(*1*) The cell bodies of neurons. These are shown to better advantage in Figure 17-22B, at higher magnification.

(*2*) Nuclei, which are scattered about. There is insufficient cytoplasm for identification of the cells in which they reside. Some are nuclei of small neurons but most belong to supporting cells to be described shortly.

(*3*) Capillaries. These permeate the substance of gray matter (one can be identified in both parts of Fig. 17-22).

(*4*) The neuropil. This forms the pale blue-gray, seemingly structureless background seen in an H and E section, in which the three components mentioned above are contained. It constitutes the bulk of gray matter. What it consists of has been elucidated as a result of the development of metallic impregnation methods and more recently by electron microscopy, as will be described in the following pages.

Evolution of Silver Impregnation Methods. In 1872 the Italian anatomist Camillo Golgi was forced by economic

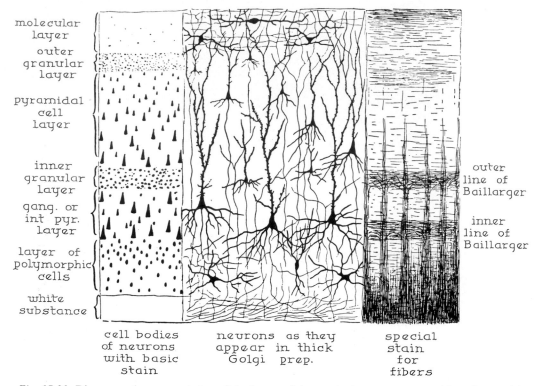

molecular
layer

outer
granular
layer

pyramidal
cell
layer

inner
granular
layer

gang. or
int. pyr.
layer

layer of
polymorphic
cells

white
substance

outer
line of
Baillarger

inner
line of
Baillarger

cell bodies
of neurons
with basic
stain

neurons as they
appear in thick
Golgi prep.

special
stain
for
fibers

Fig. 17-23. Diagrammatic representation of the layers of the cerebral cortex as seen with various staining methods. (Modified from Villiger, E.: Brain and Spinal Cord. Philadelphia, J. B. Lippincott, 1925)

circumstances to take a position as chief resident physician and surgeon in a hospital for incurable patients. Such was his zeal for anatomical research that he set up a rudimentary histological laboratory in his kitchen, equipped with little more than a microscope, where he worked at night and made a discovery that revolutionized the study of nervous tissue.

Golgi had fixed some tissue of the CNS in a solution of potassium bichromate and left it in this solution for a long time. He then soaked it in silver nitrate and, probably to his surprise, sections revealed that silver was deposited as a dark precipitate on only *some* of the cells in the tissue, but not most of them. Furthermore, the ones impregnated stood out against a clear background. By this means it is possible to demonstrate whole neurons (their cell bodies and their processes) in thick sections, where they appear as in Figure 17-23, *middle*. This method also shows supporting cells of the CNS with innumerable processes (Fig. 17-23).

Subsequently, a young man in Spain destined to become the greatest neurohistologist of his time, Santiago Ramon y Cajal, saw the possibilities of Golgi's method, made improvements in it, and systematically investigated the histology of nervous tissue.

With the development of metallic impregnation methods and the use of thick sections it was possible to demonstrate processes of neurons over considerable distances and show the different sizes and shapes of the nerve cell bodies from which they arose. It is now therefore possible to portray the arrangement in which they exist, for example, in the cerebral cortex, as shown in Figure 17-23, *middle*.

THE ORGANIZATION OF NEURONS IN THE CEREBRAL AND CEREBELLAR CORTEX

Cerebral Cortex. The gray matter constituting the cerebral cortex varies from about 1.5 to 4 mm. in thickness and covers the white matter of the cerebral hemispheres (Fig. 17-6). The convoluted surface of the hemispheres in man (Fig. 17-6) renders the gray matter much more extensive than in animals where it is smooth. Preparations made from different parts of the hemispheres show the same general plan of microscopic structure, but this is modified in different cortical areas where the cortex performs different functions. In general, the cortex exhibits 6 layers of cell bodies of neurons (Fig. 17-23, *left*). The extent to which each of these layers is developed differs in various areas, but the significance of this is more a matter for consideration in neuroanatomy textbooks. Here we shall describe only some of the characteristics of the 6 layers.

The most superficial is called the *molecular layer* (Fig. 17-23, *left*). It contains relatively few cell bodies and consists chiefly of fibers of underlying cells, the fibers of which run in many directions but generally parallel with the surface (Fig. 17-23, *right*). The second layer is called the *outer granular layer* because it contains the cell bodies of many small nerve cells, which gives it a granular appearance when examined under low power (Fig. 17-23, *left*). The third layer is called the *pyramidal cell layer* because of its content of pyramid-shaped cell bodies of neurons (Fig. 17-23, *left*). The fourth layer is termed the *inner granular layer* because it is "granulated" with small nerve cell bodies (Fig. 17-23, *left*). The fifth layer is termed the *internal pyramidal layer* because its most prominent feature is its content of pyramidal cell bodies. In one part of the cortex, the *motor area*, the pyramidal cells of this layer are huge; they are called *Betz cells*. The sixth and final layer is named the layer of *polymorphic cells* because the cells of this layer have many shapes. It will be noticed in Figure 17-22A that the size of the cell bodies of the neurons in the deeper parts of the cortex are larger than those in the more superficial parts, hence the existence of the layers described from impregnation methods can be correlated roughly with what is seen in an H and E section.

It has been estimated that there are close to 10 billion neurons in the cerebral cortex, and since one neuron may effect synaptic connection with as many as 10 thousand others, the possibilities with regard to the number of pathways that are available here are indeed overwhelming.

Cerebellar Cortex. The gray matter in the *cerebellar cortex* is arranged somewhat differently so as to form 3 layers. The superficial one is termed the *molecular layer* because it contains relatively few small neurons, together with numerous unmyelinated fibers. Deep to this there is a layer of huge flask-shaped cells named *Purkinje cells* after the Czech physiologist Johannes Purkinje who described them in 1837. The remainder of the gray matter of the cerebellar cortex consists of an inner *granular layer* containing abundant small neurons. The three layers are illustrated in Figure 17-24.

The several kinds of neurons and their fibers are arranged in a somewhat complex manner, with the Purkinje cells receiving both excitatory and inhibitory impulses. Their huge dendritic arborizations extend up into the molecular layer, as shown in Figure 17-25, to collect excitatory impulses arriving primarily from the motor area of the cerebral cortex. The cerebellum modulates and organizes the motor impulses so as to regulate and coordinate

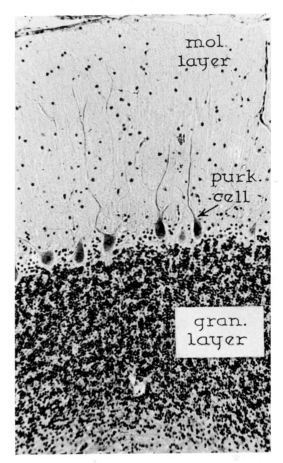

Fig. 17-24. Low-power photomicrograph showing the full thickness of the cortex of the cerebellum (H and E).

movements involving groups of muscles. Llinás has written a readable account of the neuronal and functional organization of the cerebellum that may be consulted for further details.

THE SUPPORTING CELLS OF THE CNS (NEUROGLIA)

In most body parts support is provided by various kinds of intercellular substance produced by connective tissue cells developing from the mesoderm. But gray and white matter of the brain and spinal cord develop from ectoderm and, except for endothelial cells of capillaries, do not contain connective tissue cells. Accordingly, the substance of the brain and cord is soft and delicate: indeed, a brain removed at autopsy cannot be cut into slices until it has been hardened in fixative. An important reason for the soft brain and cord not being damaged more commonly is that in life they are protected by being more or

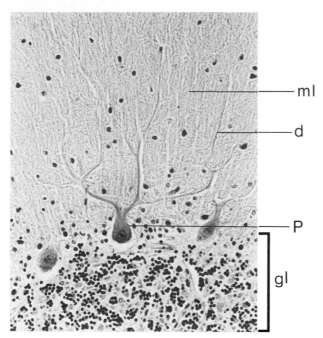

Fig. 17-25. Photomicrograph (×230) of cerebellar cortex, showing a Purkinje cell (P) with extensive dendritic tree (d) extending up into the molecular layer (ml). Part of the granular layer (gl) of the cortex is seen below. (Courtesy of C. P. Leblond)

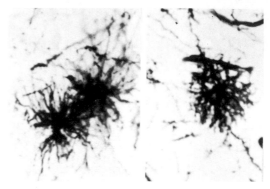

Fig. 17-26. Medium-power photomicrographs of two protoplasmic astrocytes in a Golgi preparation of the cerebral cortex (dog). The heavy black lines crossing the picture at *right* are blood vessels. Feet of processes of the astrocyte are attached to the lower one.

less suspended in a bath of fluid, the *cerebrospinal fluid,* as will be described shortly. Nevertheless, the neurons of the CNS are provided with an intimate type of support by *neuroglial cells;* these cells hold the cell bodies and processes of neurons in proper spatial arrangement with one another and also serve other purposes.

An understanding of the form and supporting functions of neuroglial cells in the CNS followed the development of metallic impregnation methods. Ordinary stains such as H and E give no intimation that these cells possess processes that permeate the substance of the CNS, binding it together and to the capillaries that course through it. Golgi preparations show that some glial cells, of which only the nucleus could be seen in an H and E section, possess innumerable processes connecting various parts of neurons to capillaries, as shown in Figure 17-26. Furthermore, refined impregnation methods and also studies with the EM show that the *neuropil* (the pale background of gray matter) is a vast conglomerate of cell bodies and processes of neuroglia and processes of neurons, which in the neuropil are mostly unmyelinated. But before considering the neuropil further, we shall describe the 3 types of neuroglial cells.

The use of silver and gold impregnation methods by Cajal and del Rio-Hortega (one of his pupils) permitted neuroglial cells to be classified into 3 groups as follows.

Oligodendrocytes (Fig. 17-7, *bottom right*) were so named because they were small, with tree-like processes. *Astrocytes* (Fig. 17-7, *bottom*) received their name to suggest their star-like processes. A third type of cell, which was given the name *microglial cell* because of its tiny size (Fig. 17-30), was also identified. However, as noted, microglial cells were since shown not to develop from neuroectoderm but instead from monocytes circulating in the bloodstream. They therefore represent small macrophages.

OLIGODENDROCYTES

Reliable methods of metallic impregnation exist for the identification of astrocytes and microglia but none is specific for oligodendrocytes. In order to study oligodendrocytes, Mori and Leblond used the reasonably specific metallic stains to mark astrocytes and microglia and assumed that the unstained cells were oligodendrocytes. These were studied with the EM and also in thin sections with the LM.

Whereas one type of oligodendrocyte was expected, three were found: large light cells, small dark ones, and cells of intermediate size and density. But the 3 types had certain features in common, such as an abundance of ribosomes and microtubules and fine nonbranching processes extending from their cell bodies. There are thus 3 classes of oligodendrocytes, referred to as *light, medium,* and *dark,* respectively. The cells of these 3 classes are equally numerous in the very young, but in the adult only the dark oligodendrocytes are common.

In the course of development neuroglia arise from a derivative of the ependyma of the neural tube, called the *subependymal layer.* The primitive cells, known as *spongioblasts (glioblasts),* proliferate actively and dif-

Fig. 17-27. (A) Electron micrograph (×15,000) of a *light oligodendrocyte* with a *dark oligodendrocyte* at *lower left* (from rat brain). The light oligodendrocyte has cytoplasm rich in ribosomes and microtubules. A Golgi stack (G) and a dense body (db) are indicated. The dark oligodendrocyte is small, shows densely staining cytoplasm, and has more condensed coarse chromatin in its nucleus. Golgi saccules are prominent in its cytoplasm.

(B and *C)* Photomicrographs (not electron micrographs). *(B)* A light oligodendrocyte (×3,000); and *(C)* a dark oligodendrocyte (×3,000) as seen in a thin section stained with toluidine blue. The light oligodendrocyte (LO) has a light nucleus with grainy chromatin and prominent nucleolus; its ample cytoplasm is less pale. The dark oligodendrocyte (DO) shows large dense chromatin patches in its nucleus and its cytoplasm stains very deeply. (Courtesy of E. Ling, J. Paterson, and C. P. Leblond)

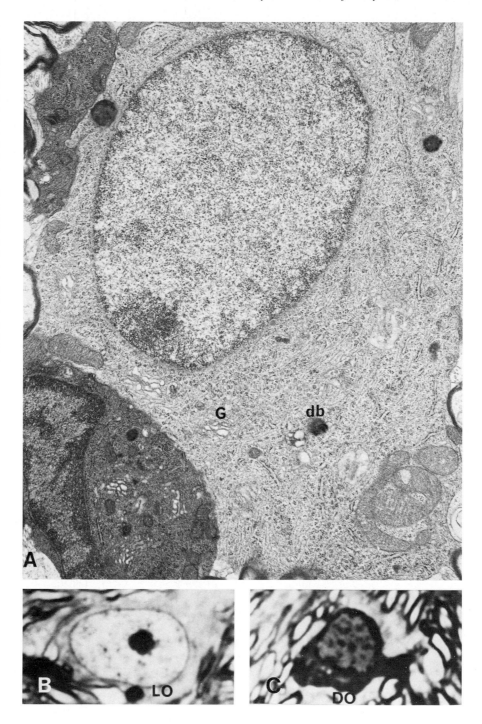

ferentiate into either *astroblasts* or *oligodendroblasts.* The last mitosis of astroblasts gives rise to *astrocytes* (*see* below), which under normal conditions do not have the ability to divide, whereas the last mitosis of oligodendroblasts gives rise to nondividing *light oligodendrocytes.*

The light oligodendrocyte (Fig. 17-27) has a relatively large, pale nucleus with a large nucleolus. Its cytoplasm is abundant and characteristically contains many evenly distributed free ribosomes and numerous cytoplasmic organelles. A light oligodendrocyte has a short life span (a few weeks at most), after which it gradually transforms into a medium oligodendrocyte, intermediate in size and electron density between a light and a dark oligodendrocyte. Then in a few weeks it transforms again into a dark oligodendrocyte; hence the dark oligodendrocyte is the last cell of the series. The volume of this cell is less than one quarter of that of the light cell. In the CNS tissue of the adult, dark oligodendrocytes appear as small cells with dark round nuclei; they are seen commonly in both gray and white matter.

Myelin-Forming Function. It has long been known that oligodendrocytes are often disposed in rows between myelinated fibers in white matter (*left* in Fig. 17-29). As already mentioned, they send off fine processes. These are extensions of their cell membrane with a minimal amount of cytoplasm containing mostly microtubules and an occasional mitochondrion. The extremity of each fine process spreads out into a thin sheet composed mainly of its two cell membranes, and this sheet wraps itself many times around a nerve fiber. Each process is able to wrap a different fiber, so that a single oligodendrocyte wraps several fibers (Fig. 17-10). Together, the many layers constitute an internodal segment of a *myelin sheath.* Thus, oligodendrocytes serve the same myelin-forming function as cells termed *Schwann cells,* which myelinate nerve fibers of the PNS, where the process is much easier to visualize and which will be described in detail in due course.

The light type of oligodendrocyte is abundant when myelination is active and therefore is believed to play a major role in producing myelin sheaths. Oligodendrocytes probably complete the job by the time they reach the medium stage. When they shrink to the dark final stage they remain connected to myelin sheaths through fine processes and probably play a role in maintaining the sheaths.

Turnover. Radioautography after tritiated thymidine labeling reveals that even after growth is completed there are occasional mitoses of glioblasts and oligodendroblasts. Even though these mitoses are few, they result in the production of new light oligodendrocytes that transform into the medium and dark cells just mentioned. Continuation of this process at a low rate throughout life suggests the possibility of some turnover of oligodendrocytes.

ASTROCYTES

Astrocytes are stained in a reasonably specific manner by Cajal's gold chloride-sublimate method. On a yellow background the astrocytes then appear as dark stars due to staining of processes that extend in various directions. Some astrocytes are also stained in Golgi preparations

(Fig. 17-26). The processes may go to blood vessels (Figs. 17-26 and 17-29); others go to the surface of neurons. In either case, as described in detail later, they widen at the end and spread out over the surface with which they are in contact—a capillary or neuron—to cover much of its surface, thus constituting what is known as an *astrocyte foot.* This foot spreads until it comes close to, and partly in contact with, another astrocyte foot. Hence, astrocytic feet make up an almost complete sheath around capillaries, interrupted only very occasionally with glial cells or processes of other kinds. They do the same around many neurons but with interruptions at synapses. Astrocyte feet also end on the basement membrane that separates brain tissue from the surrounding pia matter.

Examination of gold-stained astrocytes in the LM and EM reveals that two kinds of components are stained in their cytoplasm: *dense bodies* (referred to by Cajal as *gliosomes* and now presumed to be *lysosomes*), and bundles (fibrils) containing *filaments* (f in Fig. 17-28). These are the structures responsible for the dark staining of astrocytic processes shown in Figure 17-29. Each filament bundle arising in an astrocyte foot extends in a process to the perinuclear region of the cell and then continues on into another process to reach its end. The cytoplasm is thus arranged around straight or gently curving bundles of filaments. The filaments are described as being about 8 or 9 nm. in diameter and are of unknown composition, except that they contain a protein different from that characterizing the intermediate filaments of neurons. They are presumably responsible for providing rigidity or tensile strength for the astrocyte processes that extend from one capillary to the next, or from a capillary to a neuron or one of its processes, to provide a strong link between them (capillaries have some rigidity due to their basement membrane). Astrocytes are thus thought to play an important role in cohesion of nervous tissue of the CNS.

Astrocytes may be divided into two categories, referred to as *fibrous* and *protoplasmic.* Fibrous astrocytes are characterized in gold-stained preparations by long, straight processes that branch little or not at all (Fig. 17-29, *right*). These astrocytes are located in the white matter. Dense bodies (lysosomes) are found in the cytoplasm between the bundles of filaments in the processes and even the end feet. It was long held that fibrous astrocytes were the only ones to contain fibrils (that is, bundles of filaments), but the EM showed that the protoplasmic type also contains such bundles.

Protoplasmic astrocytes have branching cytoplasmic processes extending from all aspects of their cell bodies, so that after metallic staining they resemble bushy shrubs (Figs. 17-7, *bottom,* and 17-26). Their processes are

Fig. 17-28. (*A*) Electron micrograph (×13,800) of an astrocyte (from rat corpus callosum). Note the pale nucleus and cytoplasm. Bundles of filaments (f) may be seen in the cytoplasm. Two neighboring axons are indicated (ax). (*B*) Photomicrograph (×3,000) of two astrocytes (A) near a capillary lumen (L). Thin section, stained with toluidine blue. The ovoid astrocyte nucleus is pale, with a fine rim of chromatin along the nuclear envelope. A pale cytoplasmic process extends at *left,* between dark myelinated axons. (Courtesy of E. Ling, J. Paterson, and C. P. Leblond)

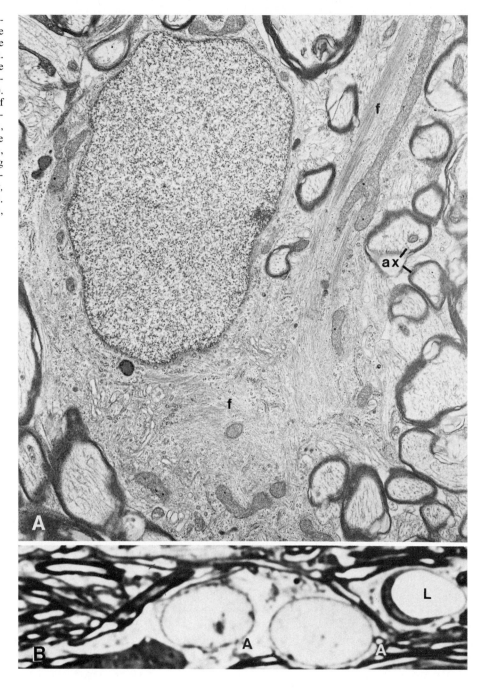

shorter and branch more extensively than those of fibrous astrocytes; as noted, the EM shows that these also are held rigid by bundles of filaments.

Examination of astrocytes of either type in the EM reveals a light, rather large nucleus (Fig. 17-28). Often the nucleus shows small indentations, due to pressure from bundles of filaments. The cytoplasm is also rather light because of its low content of ribosomes and rER. As shown in Figure 17-28, axons (which appear as dark rims) are often enveloped by astrocyte cytoplasm. Astrocytes

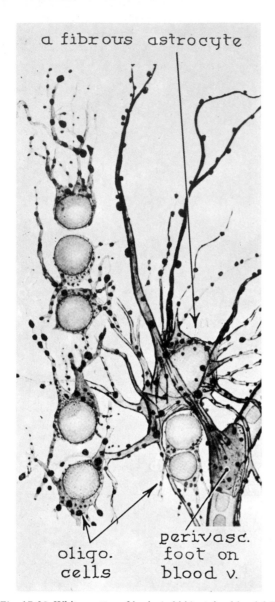

Fig. 17-29. White matter of brain (rabbit), stained by del Rio-Hortega's method for gliosomes (*see* text). It shows a row of oligodendroglial cells on the left and a fibrous astrocyte on the right. (Modified from Penfield, W.: Brain, *47:*430, 1924)

are fairly numerous; for instance, in the corpus callosum (the bundle of fibers joining the cerebral hemispheres) they make up one quarter of the glial cell population. Astrocytes arise from astroblasts, which contain only sparse filaments and are able to divide. Since an occasional degenerating astrocyte is encountered, degeneration may balance production of new astrocytes, suggesting a slow turnover of the astrocyte population.

EPENDYMAL CELLS

It is not unusual to classify these also as a type of neuroglial cell. The ependymal cells that line the lumen of the neural tube perform three more or less consecutive functions. At first their function is proliferative (Fig. 17-7). Their second function is supportive. As the wall of the neural tube thickens, the lining cells send out long processes that for a time reach the exterior of the tube and help to form the external limiting membrane that surrounds the tube. Still later they gradually relinquish their supporting role and function chiefly in forming a continuous epithelial lining, known as the *ependyma,* for the ventricles of the brain. They also persist in the central canal of the spinal cord. In certain sites in the ventricles, the ependyma is pushed inward by vascular tufts to form what are called *choroid plexuses,* as explained presently. The ependyma that comes to cover the capillaries of the choroid plexuses is thus termed *choroid plexus epithelium.*

MICROGLIA (BRAIN MACROPHAGES)

Microglia are small cells evenly scattered throughout white and gray matter, where they make up about 5 per cent of the glial cells in the white matter (in the corpus callosum). They are stained reasonably specifically by the so-called weak silver carbonate method of del Rio-Hortega, which stains both nucleus and cytoplasm as well as their long angular processes (Fig. 17-30). With the EM the cytoplasm of the cell body and processes is found to contain a little rER and a fair number of dense bodies. Microglia normally do not divide (nor do they take up tritiated thymidine) and show little indication of mobility and phagocytosis. However, whenever there is a local emergency, such as a stab wound or inflammation, dra-

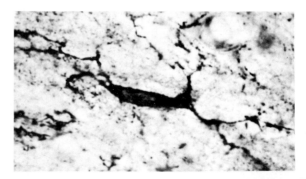

Fig. 17-30. Photomicrograph (×1,100) of a microglial cell (stained by del Rio-Hortega's weak silver carbonate method). The nucleus and cytoplasm are deeply stained. A number of long, dark, cytoplasmic processes extend out from the cell. (Courtesy of C. P. Leblond)

Fig. 17-31. Drawings illustrating nuclei of neuroglial cells as they appear in sections (stained with H and E under very favorable conditions). From *left* to *right*, the top row shows light, medium, and dark oligodendrocytes. The bottom row shows an astrocyte at *left* and a microglial cell at *right*. (Courtesy of C. P. Leblond)

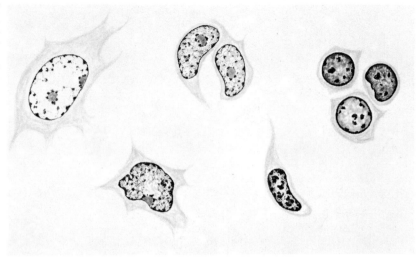

matic changes occur; both their nucleus and their cytoplasm enlarge, and they become mobile and fill up with phagocytosed material like other macrophages.

Origin. The origin of microglia has been a subject of speculation but the consensus of opinion is that they come from the blood, probably by transformation of monocytes. However, there may be some interference to their entry into brain substance because to do this they have to pass through the capillary basement membrane. What seems to happen is that after they have passed from the blood through the endothelium of a capillary they may become enclosed by an expansion of its basement membrane, thus becoming a so-called *perithelial cell.* Such cells stain like microglia by the del Rio-Hortega method, but their cytoplasm and processes are minimal. Eventually, however, they break out of this basement membrane enclosure, especially in emergencies, to enter the brain tissue.

It would have been less complicated if microglia had never been classed as neuroglia because they do not develop (as do the other cells of brain tissue) from neuro-epithelium, nor is their function to play a supporting role.

RECOGNITION OF DIFFERENT TYPES OF NEUROGLIA IN SECTIONS

Since the nucleus is all that can be recognized of glia in H and E sections, we should consider whether the different kinds can be recognized from the appearance of their nucleus alone. Certain differences do exist and typical nuclei are illustrated in Figure 17-31. However, identification by this means is *not* recommended for the inexperienced student and *thin* sections are essential if it is to be done with any degree of certainty.

THE NATURE OF THE NEUROPIL

As already described, between the capillaries and the cell bodies and processes of neurons, an H and E section reveals only a pale blue, finely mottled, seemingly structureless substance containing some nuclei, called the *neuropil* (Fig. 17-22). The EM, however, shows that this is a conglomerate of the cell bodies and processes of astrocytes, together with the processes of neurons, only a few of which are myelinated (Fig. 17-32). Between the cell bodies and processes of astrocytes there is a network of fine intercellular spaces. The total intercellular space is not inconsiderable; it is said to be 10 to 20 per cent of the brain volume. Glycosaminoglycans (hyaluronic acid and chondroitin and heparan sulfates), but not fibrous intercellular substances, are present between the cells, which are connected to one another at spots by desmosome-like junctions. The tissue fluid in the intercellular spaces would thus be held in place by a gel structure similar to that of the amorphous components of loose connective tissue, permitting diffusion to occur between capillaries and neurons. Neurons are, of course, very sensitive to a lack of oxygen or a low blood sugar level.

THE MENINGES

The spinal cord and brain are protected not only by a bony encasement (cranium and vertebral column) but also by 3 connective tissue wrappings called the *meninges* (Gr. pl. of *meninx,* membrane) (Fig. 17-33). Of these, the innermost is applied directly to the surface of the brain and cord; it is called the *pia mater* (Figs. 17-33 and 17-34).

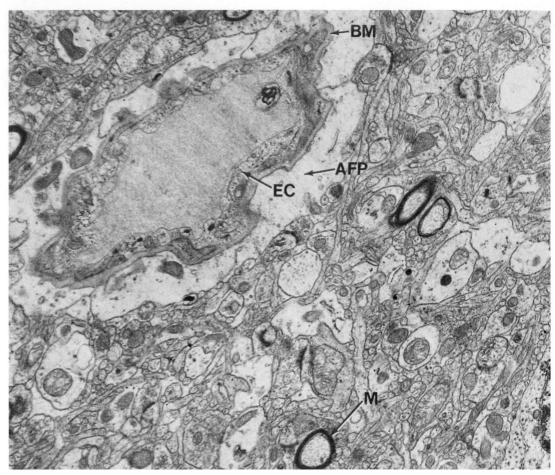

Fig. 17-32. Electron micrograph (×12,000) of a capillary (*upper left*) in the neuropil of cerebral cortex. An endothelial cell of the capillary is labeled EC and the basement membrane around the capillary, BM. Just outside the basement membrane there is a light zone around the capillary, AFP, representing expanded astrocyte feet attached to the basement membrane. The cell bodies of the astrocytes lie farther away from the capillary. Except for the capillary, most of the area seen is neuropil, which consists of a conglomerate of astrocyte processes intertwined with nerve fibers, most of which are unmyelinated; however, an occasional myelinated fiber (labeled M) is seen in the neuropil. (Courtesy of I. Robertson)

The middle one is called the *arachnoid* (Figs. 17-33 and 17-34), and the outermost one is called the *dura mater* (Figs. 17-33 and 17-34). The microscopic structure of each will now be considered.

THE PIA MATER

As indicated by its name (L. *pia*, tender; *mater*, mother), this membrane is delicate. It contains not only interlacing bundles of collagenic fibers but also fine elastic networks, and is covered with a continuous membrane of flattened squamous cells morphologically similar to mesothelial membranes of body cavities. The substance of the pia contains a few fibroblasts and macrophages and many blood vessels that are distributed by the pia over the surface of the brain (Fig. 17-33).

THE ARACHNOID

The middle layer of the meninges is called the *arachnoid* because it is separated from (but at the same time joined to) the pia by a cobweb-like (Gr. *arachnoeides*, like a cobweb) network of delicate connective tissue trabeculae (Fig. 17-33). The term *arachnoid* includes both the continuous roof over the pia and the network of trabeculae supporting this roof (like pillars) above the pia.

The pia and arachnoid are sometimes described as a combined membrane, the *pia-arachnoid* or *leptomeninges*.

The arachnoid membrane and its trabeculae are composed chiefly of delicate collagenic fibers, together with some elastic fibers. Both outer and inner surfaces of the membranous roof and trabeculae are covered with a continuous lining of thin, flat lining cells similar to those covering the pia. Between the membranous roof of the arachnoid and the pia mater below there is a space through which the arachnoid trabeculae extend like pillars to hold up the roof. This space is filled with *cerebrospinal fluid* and is termed the *subarachnoid space* (Figs. 17-33 and 17-34).

The surface of the brain, as noted, is extraordinarily convoluted (Fig. 17-6). Whereas the pia extends down into the sulci and fissures to cover the surface of the brain intimately, the membranous part of the arachnoid (except in some larger fissures) does not. Hence over grooves there is more accommodation for cerebrospinal fluid than at other sites. Indeed, there are sites termed *cisternae* where the brain surface lies at a considerable distance from the covering arachnoid so as to accommodate considerable amounts of cerebrospinal fluid.

THE DURA MATER

As its name suggests (L. *dura*, hard; *mater*, mother), this outermost membrane is of tough consistency and made up of dense connective tissue (Fig. 17-33). The collagenic fibers tend to run longitudinally in the spinal dura but more irregularly in the cranial dura. Some elastic fibers are mixed with the collagenic. There are certain differences between the dura of the vertebral canal and that of the cranium. In the vertebral canal the dura consists of a relatively free dense connective tissue sheath. The potential space between its inner surface and the outer surface of the arachnoid is called the *subdural space* (Fig. 17-34), and it normally contains a slight amount of fluid that is *not* cerebrospinal fluid. The outer surface of the spinal dura abuts on the *epidural (extradural) space* (Fig. 17-34), which is filled with loose areolar tissue containing a variable amount of fat and many veins. The internal periosteum of the vertebrae, which lines the vertebral canal, forms the outer limit of the epidural space. The space between the arachnoid roof and pia, as noted, is called the *subarachnoid space* (Fig. 17-34).

In the cranium there is no potential epidural space because here the dura is fused with the internal periosteum of the cranial bones.

Although the cranial dura is often described as having 2 layers, it is only the inner layer that forms the cranial dura that is continuous with the spinal dura in the vertebral canal. The so-called outer layer is not part of the dura but

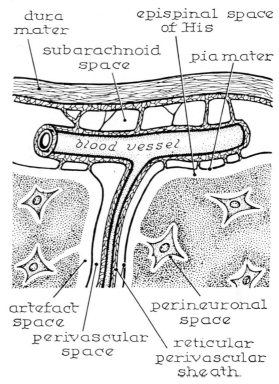

Fig. 17-33. Diagram illustrating the layers of the meninges and the perivascular space. Note that the "epispinal" and "perineuronal" spaces seen in routine LM sections are not true spaces but artifacts. (Redrawn from Woollam, D. H. M., and Millen, J. W.: J. Anat., *89:*193, 1955)

corresponds to the internal periosteum of the cranial bones. However, since these two layers adhere to one another, the cranial dura is also said to be adherent to the bones of the skull. The dura is much less vascular than the periosteum. Next, although the periosteum and the cranial dura are adherent to one another over most of the brain, they are separated in a few specific sites where the dura extends deep into the fissures of the brain to form large partitions or folds (Fig. 17-35). Along the line from which a partition extends into a fissure a cavity may exist between the folds of the dura. Such a cavity is roughly triangular in cross section (Fig. 17-35) and bordered above by periosteum (so-called outer layer of dura) and on the other 2 sides by the cranial dura, which sweeps from both sides of the fissure down into it to form a partition there (Fig. 17-35). These spaces between the folds of the dura, which are disposed along the lines from which partitions originate, are lined by endothelium and contain venous blood; they constitute the *sinuses of the dura mater* (Fig. 17-35) and the *venous lacunae*.

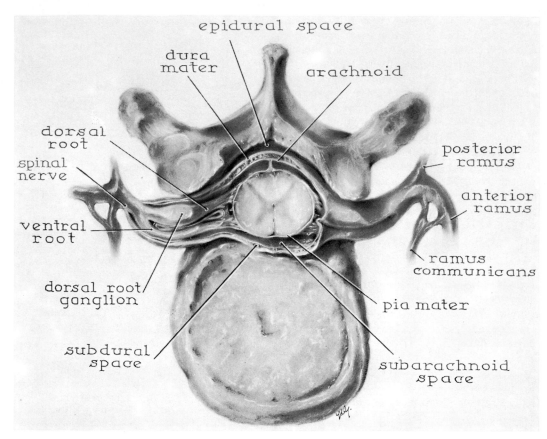

Fig. 17-34. Diagrammatic drawing of a cross section of the vertebral column at the level of intervertebral foramina. It shows the anatomical relation of the meninges to the spinal cord and the way the PNS is connected to the CNS. Note the spinal (posterior or dorsal root) ganglion containing the cell bodies of afferent neurons.

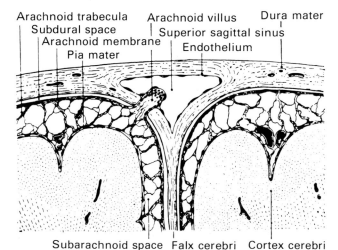

Fig. 17-35. Diagram illustrating the meninges, superior sagittal sinus, and an arachnoid villus. The potential subdural space is shown enlarged. The subarachnoid space over the convolutions also is increased so as to illustrate the subarachnoid mesh. (Weed, L. H.: Am. J. Anat., *31*:203, 1922)

HOW NUTRIENTS REACH THE CELL BODIES OF NEURONS OF GRAY MATTER

The capillaries that supply nutrients to cells within the substance of (*1*) the gray matter of the cortex of the cerebral and cerebellar hemispheres and (*2*) the gray matter of the cord are derived from arterial vessels close to the surface of the brain and cord. These vessels are conveyed in the deeper layers of the meninges. Small vessels from the pia mater penetrate the brain substance to terminate in capillaries supplying neurons and neuroglia as follows.

The Blood Vessels of the Pia Mater. The blood vessels penetrating the substance of the brain are covered proximally with a thin sheath of reticular connective tissue (Fig. 17-33). Furthermore, pia dips into the tunnels containing the vessels so as to line these tunnels (Fig. 17-33). Between the layer of connective tissue covering these vessels and that lining the tunnels (that is, the pia) there is a true *perivascular space* (labeled in Fig. 17-33). This is found only around the larger vessels and does not extend as far as the capillaries. Thus, the perivascular space communicates with the subarachnoid space and contains cerebrospinal fluid.

From the study of ordinary H and E sections of brain, two *false impressions* were gained over the years from *artifacts*. First, as a result of shrinkage a further space could be seen between (*1*) the pia that lines the tunnels and (*2*) the brain substance (labeled artefact space at *left* in Fig. 17-33). Second, another so-called "perineuronal space" was seen between the cell bodies of neurons and the neuropil (labeled in Fig. 17-33). Both of these spaces are artifacts. Furthermore, as noted above, the true perivascular space recognizable with the LM around larger vessels disappears as the capillaries are reached, so there are no continuous spaces around capillaries as there may appear to be in H and E sections, as for example at *lower middle* in Figure 17-22B. As noted, such spaces are also *artifacts*.

The Formation and Resorption of Tissue Fluid in Gray Matter

As described in connection with loose connective tissue, tissue fluid is formed from the arterial end of capillaries and resorbed at their venous end (Fig. 8-6). In most body sites, any excess is drained away by lymphatic capillaries (Fig. 8-6). The capillary endothelium normally permits escape of some blood protein but this does not accumulate because it is continuously drained away in the lymphatic capillaries.

The situation in gray matter, however, is very different. First, there are *no lymphatic capillaries in the CNS* to drain away tissue fluid, a situation that would result in edema elsewhere (refer to Fig. 8-7B). Next, the capillaries are of the continuous type and their endothelial cells are joined together by almost *continuous tight junctions* (described in Chap. 5). Little tissue fluid would therefore be produced by these capillaries. Furthermore, capillaries of gray matter are surrounded with a very substantial basement membrane (BM in Fig. 17-32); this is often split so as to accommodate a pericyte.

There has been difference of opinion as to whether the basement membrane of a capillary is completely surrounded by astrocyte feet or whether this covering is discontinuous. Robertson found that 88 per cent of the basement membrane is covered with astrocytic processes (Fig. 17-32). The cytoplasm of oligodendrocytes, moreover, accounted for covering 4 per cent of the basement membrane surface, and the remaining 8 per cent was covered by very small cell processes, either neuronal or neuroglial, the nature of which could not be determined precisely.

The Blood-Brain Barrier

Clinical and experimental findings suggested the existence of a *blood-brain barrier* before any studies were made with the EM to determine its basis. It was found, for example, that certain substances with therapeutic value if given intravenously did not enter the brain from the blood, as would occur in other body parts. Moreover, certain dyes that would gain entrance from the blood to other parts of the body were found not to pass into gray matter, so there is no doubt that there is some kind of a blood-brain barrier. From EM studies using electron-dense tracers this barrier seems to consist of (*1*) the continuous capillary endothelium with its *very extensive tight junctions* between contiguous cells that appear to form an almost complete seal between them, and (*2*) the very substantial basement membrane surrounding the capillaries. However, gases and small molecules essential for the nutrition of neurons and glial cells diffuse through this barrier relatively easily.

THE FORMATION, CIRCULATION, AND RESORPTION OF CEREBROSPINAL FLUID

The Distribution of Cerebrospinal Fluid. Protection is afforded the delicate tissue of the CNS by its being (*1*) contained in bony cavities and (*2*) more or less suspended in a fluid cushion. This fluid is contained in the pia-arachnoid, for all the interstices of its cobweb-like structure (Fig. 17-33) are filled with a modified tissue fluid called *cerebrospinal fluid* (CSF). The fluid-filled pia-arachnoid completely surrounds the brain and cord and functions as a hydraulic shock absorber.

The ventricles of the brain constitute a continuous passageway (Fig. 17-6) filled with CSF, which is in communication with CSF outside the brain in the pia-arachnoid through 3 openings in the roof of the fourth ventricle. Normally CSF flows through these openings from inside the brain to the outside.

Composition. Cerebrospinal fluid contains salts but very little protein and only a very few cells, mostly lymphocytes. The examination of CSF in suspected injuries or diseases of the CNS is valuable in diagnosis. For example, finding blood in CSF can confirm a skull fracture involving rupture of vessels. Or finding an increase in the number of cells in CSF may help in diagnosing certain inflammatory diseases of the nervous system or meninges. Even investigating the pressure of CSF may help in distinguishing certain pathologic conditions of the brain or cord.

The Sites of Formation of Cerebrospinal Fluid

Some CSF is formed on the exterior of the brain, but most is formed in the brain ventricles by the *choroid plex-*

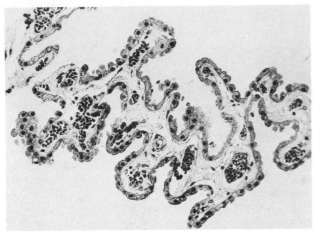

Fig. 17-36. Photomicrograph of a portion of a human choroid plexus. Note the cuboidal choroid plexus epithelium covering the villi and the congested tortuous capillaries of the plexus beneath. (Courtesy of E. Linell)

uses, which are little tufted structures rich in capillaries that project into the lumina of the ventricles (Fig. 17-36). These structures are specialized to produce tissue fluid. Their capillaries lie close to the free surface of the plexus, which is exposed to the fluid-filled lumen of a ventricle (Fig. 17-36). This free surface is covered with cuboidal epithelium (Fig. 17-36) through which tissue fluid must pass before it enters the lumen of a ventricle and becomes CSF; for this and other reasons it is more difficult for some substances, particularly macromolecular ones, to enter cerebrospinal fluid than to get into ordinary tissue fluid.

Development of Choroid Plexuses. The part of the neural tube forming the roof of the third and the fourth ventricles becomes very thin, consisting of no more than the single layer of cuboidal cells that comprises the ependyma plus the vascular pia-arachnoid covering it. In these sites the pia-arachnoid, pushing the ependyma ahead of it, invaginates into the ventricles to form choroid plexuses. A similar process results in development of choroid plexuses in the lateral ventricles. Thus 4 choroid plexuses are formed: one in the fourth, one in the third, and one in each of the lateral ventricles of the brain.

The Microscopic Structure of Choroid Plexuses. A choroid plexus comprises many leaf-like processes that hang, as it were, from a stem. Each process is supplied by a small artery or arteriole that opens into a capillary plexus. These capillaries are tortuous and produce elevations in the epithelium called *villi.* Figure 17-36 shows a process from which villi containing large capillaries project on either side.

The epithelium covering the choroid plexuses develops from the ependyma. It is of the cuboidal type (Fig. 17-36) and is termed *choroid plexus epithelium.* It rests on delicate connective tissue derived from pia-arachnoid pushed in behind it during development, ahead of its blood vessels. The EM discloses that the free surface of the epithelial cells is covered with microvilli with somewhat bulbous ends.

Degenerative changes occur in the plexuses of the lateral ventricles relatively early in life, manifested by calcium deposits or cysts.

The Circulation of Cerebrospinal Fluid

Cerebrospinal fluid produced in the lateral ventricles circulates through the interventricular foramina and, with that produced in the third ventricle, passes through the cerebral aqueduct of the midbrain to the fourth ventricle and out through its roof into the subarachnoid space. Most of the CSF in the pia-arachnoid spaces surrounding the brain and cord is formed inside the brain so that if outflow through the roof of the fourth ventricle is blocked, CSF accumulates in the ventricles and expands them, stretching the brain from within. This can occur as a result of disease or deformity, and the condition is called *internal hydrocephalus.*

A minor amount of CSF is formed by smaller blood vessels that penetrate the brain. These produce some tissue fluid that makes its way to the brain surface via the pia-arachnoid conveying the vessels. At the brain surface it mixes with, and becomes part of, the CSF.

Since CSF is formed continuously it must also be resorbed continuously, for otherwise increased intracranial pressure would result. The structures that resorb CSF back into the bloodstream at the same rate as it is produced are known as *arachnoid villi;* these are button-like projections of the arachnoid into certain venous sinuses of the dura mater (Fig. 17-35). The more or less hollow cores of arachnoid villi are filled with CSF, separated from the blood in the sinuses by only the thin covering of the villi (Fig. 17-35). CSF passes through the covering cells to enter the venous blood in the sinus.

The Relation of the Formation and Resorption of Cerebrospinal Fluid to the Formation and Resorption of Tissue Fluid Elsewhere

The arrangements for forming and resorbing CSF are not unlike those by which tissue fluid is formed and resorbed in most parts of the body. Presumably hydrostatic pressure in the capillaries of choroid plexuses is elevated (for capillaries); certainly they appear congested. Tissue fluid would thus be readily produced in choroid plexuses. On the other hand, the hydrostatic pressure in the venous sinuses into which the arachnoid

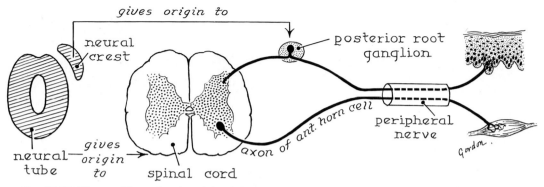

Fig. 17-37. Diagram illustrating the origin of the PNS. The neural crest gives rise to posterior root ganglion cells. Processes from each of these grow peripherally and centrally; hence the neural crests give rise to the afferent components of the PNS. The efferent components of the PNS develop from the neural tube by means of axons from anterior horn cells growing out from the developing spinal cord.

villi project is low. Furthermore, the greater osmotic pressure of blood (imparted by its protein content) would draw CSF, which is low in protein content, back into the blood through the cells of the arachnoid villi. However, this arrangement differs from that ordinarily concerned in resorption of tissue fluid because as noted, there are *no lymphatics in the CNS* to draw off excess fluid. But some CSF may be drained away by passing along spaces in nerves going to various parts of the body.

THE MICROSCOPIC STRUCTURE OF THE NERVOUS TISSUE OF THE PERIPHERAL NERVOUS SYSTEM

The PNS consists of the following 3 components:

(1) Ganglia. These are little nodules containing cell bodies of neurons. There are two general kinds of ganglia in the PNS: first, *cerebrospinal ganglia,* which contain cell bodies of afferent neurons of body segments (Figs. 17-5 and 17-34), and second, *autonomic ganglia,* which contain cell bodies of efferent neurons of the autonomic system.

(2) Nerves. These are branching, cord-like structures that extend out from the brain as cranial nerves, and from the spinal cord as spinal nerves, to reach almost every part of the body (Fig. 17-1). Nerves each contain many nerve fibers, commonly both afferent and efferent. Large nerves are sometimes termed *nerve trunks.*

(3) Nerve Endings and Organs of Special Sense. Detailed descriptions of the various kinds of endings of afferent (sensory) nerve endings and the organs of special sense are given in appropriate chapters later in this text, because they are studied to better advantage once the organs and structures in which they are distributed have

been described. All efferent fibers end in association with gland or muscle cells. Efferent nerve endings among secretory cells of exocrine glands will be described later in this chapter, while efferent (and also afferent) nerve endings in muscle will be dealt with in Chapter 18.

The following outline of the components of the PNS provides a basis for completing our classification of nervous tissue:

Nervous Tissue

The tissue of the CNS { Gray matter

White matter

The tissue of the PNS { Ganglia

Nerves

Nerve Endings

THE DEVELOPMENT OF THE PNS

The afferent and efferent components of the PNS develop from different sources. The afferent ones will be considered first.

Afferent Components. The neural plate gives rise to two neural crests (Fig. 6-3) as well as the neural tube. These neural crests breaks up into chains of nodules, the forerunners of the posterior (dorsal) root ganglia of the spinal cord and their cranial counterparts. Each segment of the cord has two such ganglia, one on each side in a posterolateral position (Figs. 17-34 and 17-37). The neuroectodermal cells of these ganglia differentiate along two main lines, as in the neural tube. Along one line they form neuroblasts. These are bipolar cells but, as noted, their two processes fuse so that the bipolar neurons forming from them take on a pseudo-unipolar shape (Fig. 17-2). However, their single process branches, with one branch

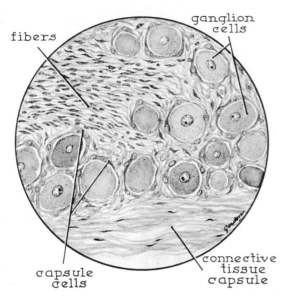

Fig. 17-38. Drawing of a portion of a spinal ganglion (high-power), showing the appearance of the ganglion cells and their capsule cells (amphicytes).

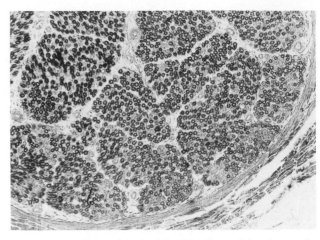

Fig. 17-39. Photomicrograph (×100) of a peripheral nerve in cross section, stained with osmic acid. Note the substantial perineurium at *bottom right* surrounding the fascicle (bundle) of myelinated nerve fibers, the myelin sheaths of which are stained black. The delicate loose connective tissue constituting the endoneurium may also be seen. (Courtesy of C. P. Leblond)

growing centrally toward the posterior root of the spinal cord; the other process grows peripherally, enclosed with other fibers in a nerve trunk, eventually to reach the tissue in which it is to provide a sensory ending (Fig. 17-37).

Some neuroectodermal cells in developing spinal ganglia differentiate along a second pathway to form supporting cells; these are not included with the neuroglia but represent their PNS counterparts. They are of two main types: *capsule cells,* which form capsules around the cell bodies of the ganglion cells (Fig. 17-38), and *Schwann cells (neurolemmal cells),* which form sheaths for the nerve fibers.

Efferent Components. These arise not from neural crests but from the middle layer of the neural tube (Fig. 17-37). Neuroblasts become efferent neurons and sprout axons that extend from the anterolateral surface of the spinal cord as efferent fibers of peripheral nerves. The efferent fibers of cranial nerves originate in the same way. The axons escape the confines of the CNS through foramina (Fig. 17-34), from there passing into nerve trunks, as shown in Figure 17-37, by which they are distributed to the structures they innervate.

When we deal with the autonomic nervous system, we shall find that it consists *only of efferent* neurons, and that the cell bodies of some of these lie in the brain and cord, but the cell bodies of others are scattered in *autonomic* (not posterior root) *ganglia* in various parts of the body. Therefore the cell bodies in these ganglia lie outside the confines of the CNS. They develop from neuroectodermal cells of the neural crests that migrate outward into the

body early in development. Where they go and what they do will be described shortly.

THE MICROSCOPIC STRUCTURE OF SPINAL GANGLIA

The bodies of nerve cells here are extremely rounded. Many of them are large, being as much as 120 μm. in diameter (Fig. 17-38), but some are small (15 μm.). Their central nucleus is large and pale-staining and commonly contains a single prominent nucleolus (Fig. 17-38). Their cytoplasm contains neurofibrils and basophilic material, the latter characteristically more dispersed than that in anterior horn cells. Accumulations of the yellow-brown pigment lipofuscin may be present in the cytoplasm (Fig. 5-62). The rounded cell bodies of ganglion cells are each separated from the connective tissue framework of a ganglion by a single layer of flattened *capsule cells* or *amphicytes* (Fig. 17-38), derived from neuroectoderm; as noted, these are the PNS counterparts of the neuroglia of the CNS.

The proximal process of each ganglion cell approaches the bundle of fibers in the posterior root, where it divides, as noted, into two branches. One passes into the spinal nerve, which conducts it out to a receptor ending (Fig. 17-37). The other passes inward via the posterior root to reach the posterior column of gray matter on that side of the cord (Fig. 17-37). Both branches have the appearance of axons and are commonly myelinated. The connective

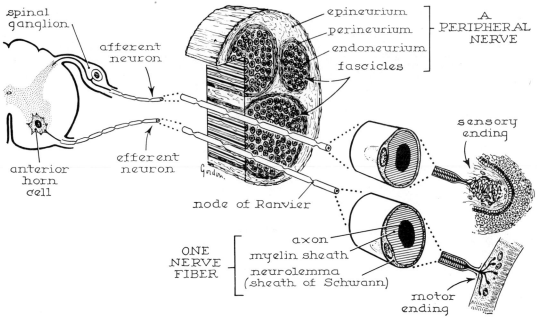

Fig. 17-40. Diagram showing the organization of the PNS and the various parts of a sizable peripheral nerve.

tissue in which the ganglion cells and their processes lie is the counterpart of the connective tissue sheath of nerves, as next described.

The same three orders of connective tissue wrappings (epi, peri-, and endoneurium) are found in the cerebrospinal ganglia.

THE MICROSCOPIC STRUCTURE OF PERIPHERAL NERVES

THE CONNECTIVE TISSUE COMPONENTS OF NERVES

In contrast to the nervous tissue of the CNS, the peripheral nerves encountered in gross dissection are cordlike and relatively strong. This is due to their fairly extensive connective tissue component, which is arranged to form tubular sheaths of three different orders. As may be seen in a cross section of a large peripheral nerve, a tube-like arrangement of connective tissue encases the whole nerve; this is called the *epineurium* (Fig. 17-40). Its wall is not as thick and strong, however, as that of the next size of connective tissue tube in its interior, which is called *perineurium* (Figs. 17-39 and 17-40). Each tube of perineurium encloses a *fascicle* (L. *fasciculus,* bundle) of nerve fibers, each fiber being enclosed in a tube of connective tissue termed *endoneurium* (Figs. 17-39 and 17-40). Smaller nerves, however, lack an epineurium. Hence small nerves such as the ones illustrated in Figures 17-39 and 17-48 consist of a tube of perineurium containing endoneurial tubes, each with a nerve fiber inside it.

THE NERVE FIBERS OF PERIPHERAL NERVES

The fine structure of nerve fibers (axons) was described in connection with Figure 17-16. Each nerve fiber in the PNS is covered with a thin, delicate cytoplasmic sheath termed the *neurolemma* (also spelled *neurilemma*) or *sheath of Schwann* (Fig. 17-41). The *Schwann cells* comprising this sheath are derived from neuroectodermal

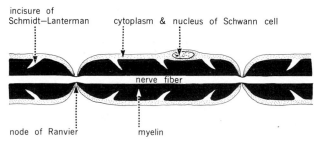

Fig. 17-41. Simplified diagram showing a portion of a myelinated nerve fiber of the PNS, its sheath of Schwann (neurolemma) consisting of Schwann cells, and two nodes of Ranvier. (Redrawn from Barr, M. L.: The Human Nervous System. New York, Harper & Row, 1972)

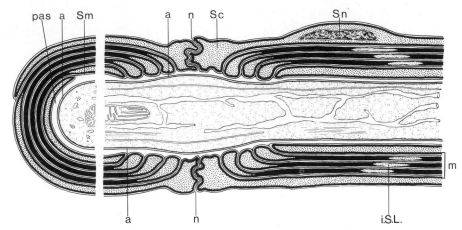

Fig. 17-42. Diagram illustrating the fine structure of the myelin sheath of a myelinated nerve fiber of a peripheral nerve in cross section (*left*) and longitudinal section (*right*). Surrounding the fiber is a sheath of Schwann, with a node of Ranvier (n). Between the axolemma (a) of the fiber and the Schwann cell membrane (Sm) there is a periaxonal space (pas). The myelin sheath (m) made of transformed Schwann cell membrane is interrupted where the Schwann cells join one another at the nodes. Here the processes of the neighboring Schwann cells interdigitate as shown but do not seal off the axolemma from intercellular space. Most of the Schwann cell cytoplasm (Sc) lies external to the myelin and contains the nucleus (Sn). An incisure of Schmidt-Lanterman (i.S.L.) is labeled at *bottom right;* it consists of pockets of Schwann cell cytoplasm trapped within the myelin. (Courtesy of C. P. Leblond)

cells of the neural crests and, to a lesser extent, the neural tube. In one kind of nerve fiber there is a substantial sheath of myelin between the nerve fiber and the Schwann cell cytoplasm (Figs. 17-41 and 17-44); such fibers are accordingly termed *myelinated fibers.* The other kind of fiber (and these tend to be smaller) is devoid of myelin, so fibers of this type are termed *unmyelinated* (*nonmyelinated*) *fibers.* Both myelinated and unmyelinated fibers are found in a given large nerve trunk. We next go on to describe myelinated fibers.

Schwann Cells and Nodes of Ranvier

The myelin of myelinated fibers is not continuous but interrupted at regular intervals, as noted, by constrictions called *nodes of Ranvier* (Figs. 17-40, 17-41, and 17-42). At nodes there is no myelin, so that processes of Schwann cells dip down toward the axolemma without completely covering it. In these sites a nerve fiber is therefore not covered by the sheath of Schwann. As shown in Figure 17-42, processes of neighboring Schwann cells interdigitate at the nodes and some lie apposed to the axolemma, embedded in amorphous intercellular material. A basal lamina that surrounds the sheath of Schwann extends in continuous fashion across each node from one Schwann cell to the next. There is one Schwann cell between every two nodes. The distance between consecutive nodes of a given fiber varies from 0.3 to 1.5 mm. Nodes of Ranvier, as noted, are also present in the CNS (n in Figure 17-10), but in the CNS the myelin is produced by oligodendrocytes. Where nerve fibers branch, they do so at nodes. The role of the nodes in saltatory conduction of nerve impulses along myelinated fibers was explained earlier in this chapter.

The Formation and Fine Structure of Myelin Sheaths in the PNS

A Schwann cell first enfolds an axon (Fig. 17-43, *left*) so that this comes to lie along a long trough in its cytoplasm. It is generally believed that the Schwann cell, or part of it, then begins to rotate around the axon (Fig. 17-43, *left, middle,* and *right*). The cell membrane of the Schwann cell is represented in this simple LM diagram (Fig. 17-43) as a single line; later its EM appearance is depicted as a double line. As the Schwann cell begins to wind around the axon, its cell membrane on one side of the groove (in which the axon lies) comes into contact with its cell membrane on the other side of the groove (Fig. 17-43, *middle* and *right*). These parts of its membrane approximate and stay together and thus are seen, as the cell continues to wind around the axon, as a spiral of rings each made of double lines; hence each single line in Fig. 17-43, *right,* represents one thickness of cell membrane. Between adjacent double rings there is at first a layer of cytoplasm (stippled in Fig. 17-43), but as the winding continues the cytoplasm is squeezed back into the cell body of the cell.

We next have to consider how a structure consisting of concentric rings, with each ring comprising two thicknesses of cell membrane, takes on the appearance of myelin. Under high magnification, with good resolution, a fully formed myelin sheath reveals concentric dark rings termed *major dense lines* (Fig. 17-44, *inset*), 2 to 3 nm. thick, separated from each other by a layer of a lighter material about 10 nm. thick (Fig. 17-44, *inset*). With special fixation and excellent resolution, a thinner dark line can be seen in the middle of each of the lighter layers; these fine lines halfway between the major dense lines are termed *intraperiod lines* (Fig. 17-44, *inset*).

As the body of the Schwann cell continues to rotate around the nerve fiber, *outer* aspects of its cell membrane keep coming in contact with one another and fusing (Fig. 17-45). The dark line so formed becomes compressed to form a fine *intraperiod line* (Fig. 17-45). Next, as the cytoplasm is squeezed away, the *inner* aspects of the same parts of the cell membrane (the side previously bordering on cytoplasm) come together and also fuse with one another so as to form the *major dense line* (Fig. 17-45). The material filling the spaces between the major dense lines

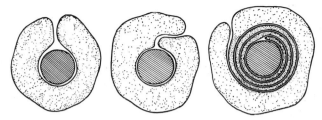

Fig. *17-43*. Diagram illustrating early stages of the formation of a myelin sheath by a Schwann cell of the PNS according to the jelly-roll hypothesis. (Based on Green, B. B., and Schmitt, F. O.: Symposium on the Fine Structure of Cells. Groningen, Holland, Noordhoff, 1955)

is derived chiefly from the lipid in the middle layers of the 2 regions of the cell membrane that fused together. But why fusion of the outer side of 2 parts of the cell membrane should give rise to only a thin, dark (intraperiod) line and fusion of 2 inner sides to a heavy (major dense) line is not clear. Both kinds of lines may be seen in Figure 17-44, *inset*.

The exact mechanism of myelination has not yet been clearly established, and winding of the body of the

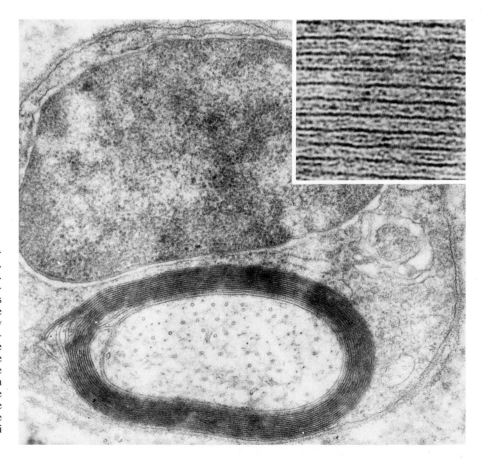

Fig. 17-44. Electron micrographs (×70,000; *inset*, ×360,000) of sciatic nerve (rat). This is a cross section of a myelinated nerve fiber surrounded by its sheath of Schwann. At *top* is the nucleus of a Schwann cell. Below the nucleus, lying in the cytoplasm of the Schwann cell, is the myelin sheath surrounding the nerve fiber. (*Inset*) This shows the major dense lines of the myelin sheath. Between the major dense lines, intraperiod lines can be seen; these are double in some places. (Courtesy of M. Nagai and A. Howatson)

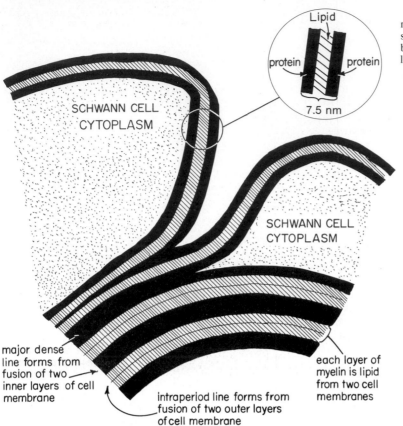

Fig. 17-45. Diagram illustrating how cell membranes of Schwann cells become myelin sheaths and which parts of the cell membrane become the dense major and the intraperiod lines of myelin sheaths. (After J. D. Robertson)

Lipid

protein   protein

7.5 nm

SCHWANN CELL
CYTOPLASM

SCHWANN CELL
CYTOPLASM

major dense
line forms from
fusion of two
inner layers of cell
membrane

intraperiod line forms from
fusion of two outer layers
of cell membrane

each layer of
myelin is lipid
from two cell
membranes

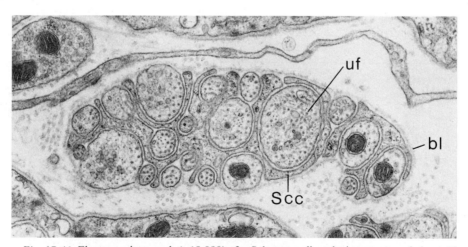

uf

bl

Scc

Fig. 17-46. Electron micrograph (×18,000) of a Schwann cell enclosing a group of about 20 unmyelinated fibers (uf), which are arranged so that each fiber lies in a groove in the cytoplasm of the Schwann cell. The fibers are cut here in cross section and appear as lighter rounded areas in contrast to the darker Schwann cell cytoplasm (Scc) enclosing them. Microtubules and occasional mitochondria may be seen in the nerve fibers. Each fiber is enclosed with its own cell membrane (axolemma) and surrounded by Schwann cell membrane. Between the two cell membranes there is an intercellular space of 10 to 15 nm. Surrounding the whole Schwann cell and covering over the grooves containing the nerve fibers there is a basal lamina (bl). These nerve fibers belong to the autonomic nervous sytem and are seen here in the heart of a hamster. (Courtesy of I. Taylor)

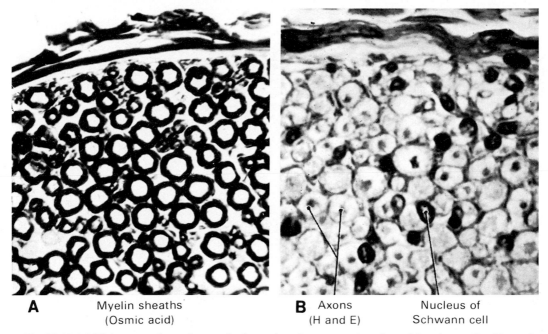

A   Myelin sheaths
         (Osmic acid)

B Axons   Nucleus of
       (H and E)   Schwann cell

Fig. 17-47. (A) High-power photomicrograph of a portion of a cross section of a peripheral nerve fixed in osmic acid. *(B)* A similar preparation stained with H and E. For details, *see* text.

Schwann cell together with the nucleus around the axon (like making a jelly roll) still appears to be the best explanation for myelination in the PNS. However, since an oligodendrocyte can myelinate segments of several different axons (Fig. 17-10), presumably all at the same time, it is difficult to believe that this could be the mechanism of myelination in the CNS.

In peripheral nerves there are little discontinuities termed *clefts (incisures) of Schmidt-Lanterman* (Figs. 17-41 and 17-42) in the internodal myelin sheath. These clefts represent places where the cytoplasm of Schwann cells was trapped during formation of myelin by rotation of the cells around the nerve fiber; hence they run spirally within the myelin.

Unmyelinated Fibers

Certain afferent and autonomic nerve fibers lack any myelin sheath. They are nevertheless protected by Schwann cells by bundles of them being so arranged that each extends in a groove through the cytoplasm of a Schwann cell. In this manner from 5 to 20 or so unmyelinated fibers lie protected by a Schwann cell at any given level (Fig. 17-46). The protective cellular sheath enclosing a group of unmyelinated fibers thus comprises a series of Schwann cells arranged end to end along the bundle, with the Schwann cells interdigitating to form a continuous column. Surrounding the external surface of

the Schwann cells in such a way as to cover over the grooves where they open to the exterior there is a basal lamina (Fig. 17-46, bl). Between the axolemma of each unmyelinated fiber and the Schwann cell membrane lining the groove housing it there is an intercellular space 10 to 15 nm. wide containing tissue fluid (which is involved in transmitting impulses) and probably also cell coat material.

THE LM APPEARANCE OF PERIPHERAL NERVES

In preparing an ordinary paraffin section the lipid in the myelin surrounding individual nerve fibers, unless specially treated, dissolves away in the dehydrating and clearing agents. This allows the nerve fiber to slip to one side of the tubular space left by the myelin dissolving away. Hence H and E cross sections of nerves show the site previously occupied by myelin as little rounded spaces, empty except for the nerve fiber, which may be situated toward one side of the space (Fig. 17-47B). Pale-staining Schwann cell cytoplasm is seen on the outer surface of the myelin space. The nuclei within a nerve bundle belong to Schwann cells, fibroblasts of the endoneurium, or endothelial cells of capillaries (also of the endoneurium). In an osmic acid-stained preparation, however, the myelin surrounding the nerve fiber is preserved and stains black so that the myelin sheaths appear as blackened rings (Figs. 17-39 and 17-47A).

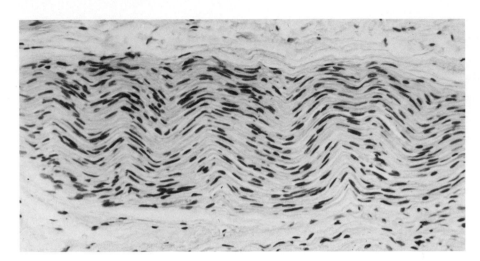

Fig. 17-48. High-power photomicrograph of a longitudinal section of a small peripheral nerve, showing the snake-like appearance typical of longitudinal sections of nerves in sections.

In routine H and E sections, nerves cut obliquely or in planes approaching the longitudinal may have a streaky appearance substantially different from what might be expected from their cross-sectional appearance. Moreover, the streaky appearance is accentuated by the long thin nuclei between fibers; these nuclei belong to Schwann cells and cells of the endoneurium (Fig. 17-48). The streaks run in a wavy snake-like manner along the nerve (Fig. 17-48).

In electron micrographs of myelinated nerve fibers cut in cross section a *periaxonal space* (pas in Fig. 17-42) 15 to 20 nm. wide is seen between the axolemma and the Schwann cell membrane. Just next to this part of the cell membrane of the Schwann cell (labeled Sm in Fig. 17-42) there is a thin layer of cytoplasm (stippled in Fig. 17-42) and encircling this are layers of transformed Schwann cell membrane constituting the myelin sheath (m in Fig. 17-42). External to the myelin lies the greater part of the Schwann cell cytoplasm (Sc in Fig. 17-42), bounded at its outer surface by the cell membrane and basal lamina of the Schwann cell. The periaxonal space is presumably sealed off from intercellular space to facilitate saltatory conduction of nerve impulses (described earlier in this chapter).

The Variability of Nerve Fascicles. Most peripheral nerves are said to be *mixed* in that they contain both afferent and efferent fibers (Fig. 17-40). However, these two types of fibers are not distinguishable from one another histologically. Toward the distal end of nerves the afferent and efferent fibers tend to segregate so that individual fascicles become predominantly motor or sensory.

A large nerve contains fascicles of fibers each surrounded with a dense sheath of perineurium (Fig. 17-40). Sunderland has shown that there is much communication between fascicles, in that nerve fibers pass from one to another. Consequently, the relative sizes and content of

fibers of the fascicles in a nerve changes continually along its course. Hence if a small section of a nerve is, for example, destroyed and an attempt is made to join the two stumps together the fascicles in the two stumps may not match each other.

In order to join the two stumps of a nerve, a portion of which has been destroyed, recourse may be taken to stretching the two parts of the nerve to be joined. Nerves can be stretched to some extent without damage to them. This is probably due at least in part to the fact that nerve fibers follow a zigzag course along a nerve (Fig. 17-48). Stretching a nerve (up to a point) merely straightens out the fibers and does not stretch them. The strong perineurial sheaths provide a limiting factor in stretching a nerve (for details *see* Sunderland).

Small nerves are composed of only a single fascicle surrounded by a perineurial sheath (Figs. 17-39 and 17-48).

The number of nerve fibers within a fascicle varies greatly, as does the diameter of the nerve fibers in the fascicle, and there are more fibers in the distal parts of some nerves than at more proximal levels. The increased number of fibers is attributable to the branching of fibers within nerves.

The Blood Supply of Nerves. In surgical procedures nerves must sometimes be freed of their attachments for certain distances and it is important to know whether this will cause serious damage within them. Fortunately, nerves are supplied by a profusion of vessels that anastomose freely. The vessels are of several orders. There are longitudinally disposed epineurial, interfascicular, perineurial, and intrafascicular arteries and arterioles. The endoneurium contains a capillary network. Nutrient arteries from vessels outside the nerve, and from longitudinally disposed vessels accompanying the nerve, penetrate the nerve frequently along its course to communicate with the neural vessels. The number of anastomoses between all these vessels is so great that nerves can be freed for considerable distances from their surrounding attachments. Sunderland stresses the importance of preserving the superficial vessels that run along nerves when the nerves are being freed from adjacent structures, for these superficial vessels are important links in the system that provides such efficient anastomoses.

The Regeneration of Peripheral Nerves

Nerve injuries are of different orders of severity, as follows.

First-Degree Injuries. These are common and generally caused by pressure being applied to a nerve at a particular site for a limited time; this can squeeze the blood vessels in the nerve sufficiently to cause local anoxia of axons and *interfere with their function.* Sensory fibers are more affected than motor ones, and different kinds of sensory fibers vary in susceptibility. After pressure is released, recovery of sensation or motor function may occur in a matter of minutes, hours or weeks, depending on the severity of the injury. If recovery does not occur in a few weeks, the injury must be regarded as more severe than a first-degree type, as will now be described.

Second-Degree Injuries. This kind is generally caused by prolonged and/or severe pressure on some part of the nerve—enough to destroy the axon where it is subjected to pressure. Nerves sometimes are injured purposefully in this fashion to bring about temporary paralysis of some muscle or muscles whose actions are interfering with others, or the recovery of some part of the body (for example, the nerves to one side of the diaphragm sometimes are squeezed hard enough to put the lung on that side to rest).

The severe pressure required to bring about second-degree injuries to nerves causes *death of axons* at the site where pressure is applied. In this respect the second-degree type of injury has fundamentally different consequences from the first-degree type. When even a small segment of an axon dies, the part of the axon distal to the injury also dies because it is separated from the cell body on which it depends for its existence. Accordingly, nerve function in a second-degree type of injury can be restored only by all parts of an axon distal to the injury being regenerated.

When the cell body recovers from the axon reaction (Fig. 17-14), it begins again to synthesize new cytoplasm. This results in new cytoplasm pushing into and through the site where the axon was crushed. To discuss the further fate of the axon we must consider certain other changes that result from the injury.

When myelinated axons distal to a site of injury die, their myelin sheaths also degenerate. Since degeneration of the axon and its myelin sheath was first described by Waller, the process often is termed *Wallerian degenera-*

tion. Macrophages from the endoneurium phagocytose the degenerating material. It has been suggested that Schwann cells may also become phagocytic and help rid the area of debris.

A second-degree type of injury, however, is believed not to interrupt the continuity of endoneurial tubes at the site of injury. Accordingly, when a cell body supplies cytoplasmic components to the damaged axon, it grows into the same endoneurial tube. The way the axon sprout becomes myelinated is similar to that in severed and reunited nerves, as will now be described.

Regeneration in Severed Nerves Rejoined Surgically

If a peripheral nerve is cut, the use of muscles in the part of the body it supplies and sensation from that part need not be lost forever. Provided the 2 cut ends of the nerve are brought together and fastened by sutures through their connective tissue wrappings (or held together by some other means), at least partial function may be restored to the part affected, but after a considerable period of time.

In the part of the nerve distal to the cut, the fibers of afferent and efferent neurons are, of course, severed from their cell bodies, so they die and become necrotic. Disintegration of axons takes a short time and in a few days only a little debris is left in the space the living axon formerly occupied (Fig. 17-49). The myelin sheaths of myelinated axons severed from their cell bodies also disintegrate (Fig. 17-49). The myelin breaks down rather more slowly than the material of the axon but soon becomes reduced to droplets (Fig. 17-49).

In axon regeneration the Schwann cells become proliferative and motile and are believed to form cords that lie in the endoneurial tubes (Fig. 17-49). Macrophages from the endoneurium phagocytose and digest droplets of broken-down myelin and remnants of dead axons and then move away. Fibroblasts close to the cut proliferate, but unless the site has become infected, not as rapidly as the Schwann cells. The latter bulge from the cut ends of endoneurial tubes of the distal and proximal stumps. The slit-like spaces between proliferating Schwann cells enable nerve fibers to push across the gap from the proximal to the distal stump (Fig. 17-49).

While all this is taking place distal to the cut, changes also occur in the proximal stump. Near the cut, axons at first degenerate. As already mentioned, Schwann cells proliferate and grow out into the gap to meet those from the distal stump. Thus continuity is established across the cut by Schwann cells with longitudinally disposed slits between them. Axons from the proximal portion now start to push forward a little each day and soon reach the space where union has occurred between the outgrowths of Schwann cells. Axons on growing into this maze-like arrangement often form many branches (Fig. 17-49),

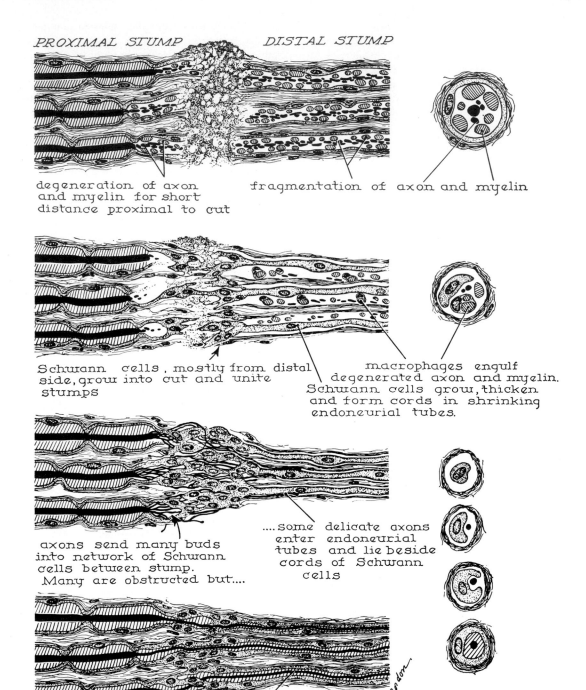

PROXIMAL STUMP   *DISTAL STUMP*

degeneration of axon
and myelin for short
distance proximal to cut

fragmentation of axon and myelin

Schwann cells, mostly from distal
side, grow into cut and unite
stumps

macrophages engulf
degenerated axon and myelin.
Schwann cells grow, thicken
and form cords in shrinking
endoneurial tubes.

axons send many buds
into network of Schwann
cells between stump.
Many are obstructed but....

....some delicate axons
enter endoneurial
tubes and lie beside
cords of Schwann
cells

axons continue to push along
endoneurial tubes of distal stump and are
enfolded by Schwann cells after which new myelin is formed

Fig. 17-49. Diagram showing the degenerative and regenerative changes that occur in a nerve when it is severed.

which push their way through any available slits and spaces. Many traverse the region of the cut and grow along the tiny passageways between Schwann cells into the open ends of endoneurial tubes of the distal stump; these are narrower but still open. Under good conditions fibers grow down these tubes at a rate estimated at from 1 to 4 mm. a day. As they near the termination of the nerve they grow somewhat more slowly.

No matter how carefully severed nerves are joined together, it could scarcely be expected that the majority of axons growing along it would ever find their proper paths. It seems incredible under the circumstances that efficient motor function and reasonably good sensation should return to a part of the body after the nerve supplying it has been severed. Nevertheless, good results are often obtained by joining cut nerves. Perhaps one thing that helps is that the axons form so many branches. More axons may try to grow down the severed nerve than were present in the first place and sometimes several enter one endoneurial tube.

In an endoneurial tube the axon sprout lies against a cord of Schwann cells (Fig. 17-49). The latter gradually enfold the axon, probably much as occurs in normal development (Fig. 17-49). New myelin may form and the cord-like Schwann cells then assume their mature appearance.

Unmyelinated fibers show a similar capacity for regeneration.

Nerve Transplantation. In certain types of injuries a whole segment of a nerve may be destroyed. Under these conditions the two cut ends cannot be approximated; hence recourse may be taken to what is called *nerve grafting.* In this procedure a piece of some superficial nerve that is not essential is removed, and placed and sutured so as to fill the gap. On transplantation, the Schwann cells in an autologous nerve graft appear to survive and proliferate. In this respect the graft acts very much like the distal stump as described above. However, even though Schwann cells proliferate at both of its cut ends to join with the distal and proximal stumps of the damaged nerve, it is obvious that the use of a graft necessitates axon branches finding their way through two mazes instead of one. So it is understandable why the results of nerve grafting are not nearly as satisfactory as those of joining cut ends of a nerve directly.

To complete our description of the 3 components of the tissue of the PNS (ganglia, nerves, and nerve endings), we next briefly consider afferent nerve endings.

AFFERENT NERVE ENDINGS

The Basis for Sensation. We are able to experience a variety of modalities of sensation, namely touch, pressure, heat, cold, pain, smell, sight, hearing, and position and movement of the parts of the body. In order for us to perceive a sensation, impulses initiated by stimuli at nerve endings of afferent neurons must be conducted via ascending tracts in white columns of the spinal cord to sensory areas of the cerebral cortex. All sensation is experienced in the brain, the kind perceived depending on the general sensory area of cortex stimulated by afferent impulses. Moreover, the particular region of cortical sensory area receiving impulses gives us an awareness of the location of the receptors that are stimulated. This is witnessed by the fact that, even when blindfolded, we know whether someone has touched us on a hand or a shoulder.

All afferent impulses begin by nerve terminals converting stimulus energy of some kind into nerve impulses. When an afferent nerve ending receives an effective stimulus, its cell membrane suddenly becomes freely permeable to sodium ions so that these enter the ending from the intercellular fluid. This influx of positive ions depolarizes the membrane, initiating a nerve impulse that is transmitted up the afferent fiber toward the CNS. Different kinds of sensory receptors seem to be designed to respond to particular kinds of energy and in some instances, such as receptors for touch and pressure, to different intensities of the same kind of energy. The receptors concerned with the senses of smell, taste, sight, hearing, and perception of movement and the position of the body in relation to gravity are assembled into what are termed the *organs of special sense.*

The microscopic structure of the various kinds of afferent nerve endings is much easier to understand if it is studied after that of the body parts they supply, so we describe them where we come to these parts in Part 3 of this textbook. Thus, many of the receptors detecting changes in our environment are associated with the skin and so will be described in Chapter 20. For convenience, however, references are provided at the end of this chapter, under Nerve Endings. Receptors in muscles and joints, which enable us to perceive limb movement and position, are appropriately dealt with in the next chapter. Olfactory receptors will be considered in Chapter 23 and taste receptors in Chapter 21. The photoreceptors in the eyes and the hair cells in the ears concerned with hearing and sensing position of the head will be described in Chapter 28.

EFFERENT NERVE ENDINGS

The endings of efferent nerve fibers on muscle cells are described in Chapter 18 and those in glands will be dealt with at the end of this chapter, after we have described the part of the PNS known as the autonomic nervous system.

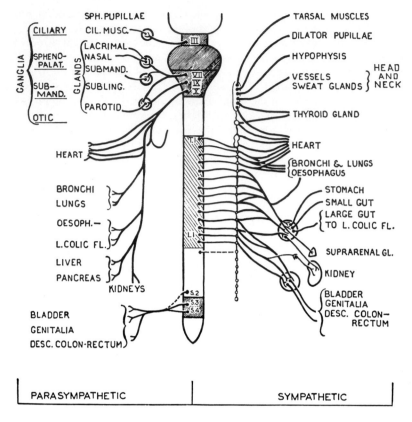

Fig. 17-50. Diagram illustrating the organization of the autonomic nervous system. The parasympathetic division is shown on the *left*, and the sympathetic division on the *right*. (After Stopford. *In* Grant, J. C., Boileau, and Basmajian, J. V.: Grant's Method of Anatomy. ed. 7. Baltimore, Williams & Wilkins, 1965)

THE AUTONOMIC NERVOUS SYSTEM

Nervous tissue is specialized so that it can be excited by different kinds of stimuli originating either within or without the body and so that it can conduct nerve impulses rapidly to (*1*) gland cells of the exocrine type and (*2*) muscle cells. These are the kinds of cells that account for *responses*.

Only some of these responses are under the control of the will, namely, those that occur in what we call our "muscles." The control of heart muscle and smooth muscle (the kind that controls the diameter of blood vessels and the intestine) and all exocrine glands is outside the direct influence of the conscious mind. However, these involuntary activities are controlled by reflex phenomena. Some of the afferent impulses concerned in these reflexes make their way into consciousness; for example, stimulation of the nerve endings in the taste buds of the mouth gives rise to the sensation of taste as well as initiating the response of salivation. But we are not even dimly aware of certain other afferent impulses, for example, those arising from the stimulation of nerve endings in the viscera. Hence the function of smooth and cardiac muscle and glands is said to be automatically controlled in the body.

The *efferent* innervation of the viscera, cardiovascular system, smooth muscle, and exocrine glands of the body is accordingly referred to as the *autonomic nervous system* (Gr. *autos,* self; *nomos,* law). The remainder of the PNS is sometimes referred to as the *somatic nervous system.* Cardiac muscle and most smooth muscle and glandular structures of the viscera are doubly innervated by the autonomic nervous system since it comprises *two divisions,* with each division sending efferent fibers to most parts of the muscle or gland the autonomic nervous system innervates (Fig. 17-50), so that each part has a double supply. Further, the efferent impulses arriving at muscle or gland cells from neurons of the two divisions tend to cause different physiological effects. For example, impulses arriving by way of one division may lead to the contraction of a certain region of smooth muscle, while those arriving at the same muscle from the other division cause it to relax. In the viscera the two divisions are thus functionally antagonistic to each other, with the responses of muscle and glands being the net result of the activities of the two divisions. These activities are integrated and coordinated in the hypothalamus. However, outside the viscera (for example in the skin) smooth muscle or secretory cells may be innervated by only one or the other of the two divisions. Hence, although the two

Fig. 17-51. Photomicrographs of ganglion cells as they appear in sections stained with cresyl blue. Note the larger size of the posterior root ganglion cell and the eccentric position of the nucleus in some of the sympathetic ganglion cells.

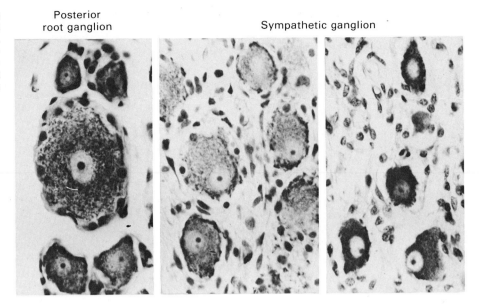

Posterior
root ganglion

Sympathetic ganglion

divisions of the system may be broadly said to be functionally antagonistic to one another, it does not mean that every structure innervated by the system receives innervation from both divisions.

The two divisions of the autonomic nervous system are termed the *sympathetic* (Gr. *syn*, with; *pathos*, suffering) and the *parasympathetic* (Gr. *para*, beside) *divisions.* Both arise in the CNS but from different parts of it (Fig. 17-50). The fibers of neurons innervating muscle and glands from the two systems therefore travel along different routes. Moreover, in both systems *two efferent neurons* are always required to join the CNS with each gland or muscle innervated (Fig. 17-50). In both systems the cell body of the first neuron in each efferent chain is situated in the CNS but that of the second neuron lies outside the CNS in a ganglion of the autonomic system. The two neurons involved in each instance are called *preganglionic* and *postganglionic*, respectively. We now consider briefly the microscopic structure of ganglia of the autonomic nervous system and then consider the two systems in more detail and describe where the ganglia are located.

AUTONOMIC GANGLIA

The ganglia of the autonomic nervous system are generally similar to cerebrospinal ganglia in that they have a connective tissue framework and contain ganglion and capsule cells. However, there are certain differences. The nerve cells of autonomic ganglia are *multipolar* and, since they possess many dendrites, have somewhat more irregular and less distinct contours than cerebrospinal ganglion cells (Fig. 17-51). Furthermore, their capsule cells constitute a less uniform layer due to the multipolar shape of the ganglion cells. In general, the nerve cells of autonomic ganglia are smaller than those of cerebrospinal ganglia and not all of them are surrounded by capsules. Moreover, their nucleus, which resembles that of cerebrospinal ganglion cells in having a single central nucleolus, is disposed more eccentrically than in cerebrospinal ganglion cells (Fig. 17-51). The terminal ganglia of the parasympathetic system may be very small and sometimes may consist of only a single ganglion cell.

We next give a short account of the anatomy of the sympathetic division of the autonomic nervous system. It is more complex than that of the parasympathetic division, a description of which follows.

THE SYMPATHETIC DIVISION

In the thoracic and upper lumbar portions of the spinal cord, intermediolateral as well as anterior and posterior columns of gray matter are present. The nerve cell bodies in these intermediolateral columns differ somewhat from those in the anterior columns; they are smaller and their mostly myelinated axons leave the cord by way of the anterior nerve roots (Figs. 17-52, 17-53, and 17-54). They extend into the anterior roots for only a short distance, whereupon they leave them by way of little nerve trunks (Fig. 17-52) called white *rami communicantes* (L. *ramus*, branch; *communicans*, communicating; and white because the axons are myelinated). Before considering the further course of these axons we shall describe the ganglia of the sympathetic

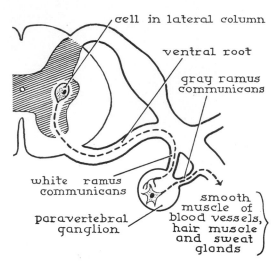

Fig. 17-52. Diagram showing one course taken by preganglionic and postganglionic fibers of the sympathetic division of the autonomic nervous system.

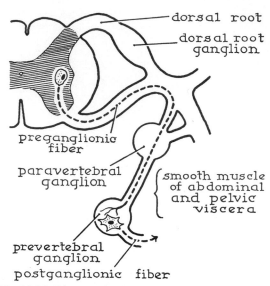

Fig. 17-54. Diagram showing a third course taken by preganglionic and postganglionic fibers of the sympathetic division of the autonomic nervous system.

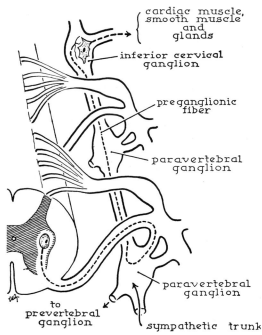

Fig. 17-53. Diagram showing a second course taken by preganglionic and postganglionic fibers of the sympathetic division of the autonomic nervous system.

The paravertebral ganglia are interconnected to form what are called *sympathetic chains* (*trunks*), one on each side of the vertebral column, from the sacral to the upper cervical level (Fig. 17-53). In the cervical region there are 3 ganglia in each chain: the superior, middle, and inferior cervical ganglia. The middle cervical ganglia are not always present. In the thoracic region 10 or 11 ganglia are distributed along each side of the vertebral column (Fig. 17-50). In some instances the first thoracic ganglion is fused with the inferior cervical to form the stellate ganglion. The lumbar region has 4 ganglia on either side of the vertebral column and so does the sacral region. Nerve fibers connect the ganglia of the left chain to those of the right in the lumbar and sacral regions.

The prevertebral ganglia constitute an abdominal plexus anterior to the vertebral column, in closer association with the viscera than the paravertebral ganglia. They comprise mainly the celiac, superior mesenteric, and inferior mesenteric ganglia. The terminal ganglia are situated peripherally, close to the organs they innervate.

Axons from bodies of nerve cells in the intermediolateral columns of the spinal cord extend through the white rami and then go on to synapse with neurons in paravertebral (Figs. 17-52 and 17-53), prevertebral (Fig. 17-54), or terminal ganglia. Therefore they are called *preganglionic* fibers.

Postganglionic fibers emerging from the ganglia of the sympathetic chains re-enter the spinal nerve by way of *gray rami communicantes*. The routes taken by pre- and postganglionic sympathetic fibers are illustrated in Figures 17-52, 17-53, and 17-54. The postganglionic fibers are unmyelinated.

division of the autonomic nervous system. According to their position in the body these are called *paravertebral, prevertebral,* or *terminal ganglia.* Since other courses deal with the positions and connections of autonomic ganglia in detail, a general understanding of them is all that is required here.

THE PARASYMPATHETIC DIVISION

Nerve fibers belonging to the parasympathetic division of the system innervate most glands and muscles innervated by the sympathetic division and, as noted, the two systems are to some extent antagonistic to each other. As in the sympathetic division, between each structure innervated by the parasympathetic division and the CNS (from which the parasympathetic division arises) a chain of *two efferent neurons* is always found.

The parasympathetic division takes origin from two widely separated parts of the CNS. The cell bodies of the nerve cells that give rise to some of its preganglionic fibers are situated in nuclei of gray matter in the medulla and the midbrain, and the preganglionic fibers arising from these cell bodies leave the CNS by way of the 3rd, 7th, 9th, and 10th cranial nerves (Fig. 17-50, *left*). The cell bodies from which the remainder of the preganglionic fibers arise are found in the lateral columns of the sacral portion of the spinal cord, and they make their way out of the CNS by way of the 2nd, 3rd, and 4th sacral spinal nerves, which they soon leave by way of the visceral rami of these nerves (Fig. 17-50, *bottom, left*).

Since the preganglionic fibers of the parasympathetic division of the autonomic system emerge by way of cranial and sacral nerves from the CNS, the parasympathetic division is also termed the *craniosacral division* of the autonomic system, in contrast to the *thoracolumbar division.*

The preganglionic fibers of the parasympathetic division are, in general, longer than those in the sympathetic division and with certain exceptions they proceed all the way to the muscle or gland with whose innervation they are concerned. Here they generally end in small *terminal ganglia* closely associated with the gland or muscle innervated. The postganglionic axons are generally short. However, in the head region the ganglia of the parasympathetic division are not closely associated with the glands or muscles innervated and the postganglionic fibers are correspondingly longer (Fig. 17-50, *top, left*).

AUTONOMIC NERVE ENDINGS

The endings of postganglionic fibers of the sympathetic and parasympathetic systems in smooth or cardiac muscle or glands cannot be seen in H and E sections, although the terminal ganglia of the parasympathetic system show to advantage. Nerve endings on muscle cells are described in the next chapter. However, the endings of efferent fibers of the autonomic system are essentially like the termination of a presynaptic neuron at a synapse and the stimulation of a muscle or gland cell is effected by nerve impulses causing a release of a chemical mediator that induces a response. Special technics are necessary for demonstrating endings of autonomic fibers in muscle or glands. Silver impregnation or staining of fresh tissue with methylene blue is commonly employed to reveal them. Even with special technics it is difficult to establish definitely how and where the fibers end. However, the EM disclosed that nerve endings on smooth muscle cells resemble very simple motor end plates on striated muscle fibers, as described in the next chapter. The effects of autonomic stimulation of smooth muscle cells will also be dealt with in that chapter. The nerve endings of the autonomic system at secretory cells will be described below.

THE EFFECT OF AUTONOMIC CHEMICAL MEDIATORS ON SECRETION BY CELLS OF EXOCRINE GLANDS

Chemical mediation of nerve impulses was described at some length in connection with synapses. In the development of knowledge about the autonomic system it was at first concluded that parasympathetic endings elaborated acetylcholine and endings of the sympathetic system elaborated norepinephrine. However, it was found later that some sympathetic fibers could elaborate acetylcholine, for it was shown that although the innervation of the sweat glands of the skin is provided by sympathetic fibers, the chemical transmitter liberated at their endings at sweat glands is acetylcholine. Accordingly, it became usual to class the fibers of the autonomic system, not necessarily as to whether they were parasympathetic or sympathetic fibers but as to whether they were *adrenergic* (which means the chemical mediator they elaborate is *norepinephrine*) or *cholinergic* (which means their endings elaborate *acetylcholine*). In the instance of sweat glands this means, for example, that cholinergic fibers are controlled by activities of the sympathetic division.

In general, the postganglionic fibers in the sympathetic division are adrenergic, but as noted those supplying the sweat glands are cholinergic. The preganglionic fibers of both the sympathetic and the parasympathetic divisions are cholinergic, as are postganglionic parasympathetic fibers.

Both adrenergic and cholinergic fibers innervate secretory cells of many glands—for example, the parotid glands of rats, as will be described shortly. (It should be pointed out, however, that there seems to be considerable variation with regard to innervation of the parotid and other salivary glands in different species.)

As Hand points out, the term *nerve ending* is rather inappropriate for describing innervation of secretory cells of glands. This is because the axon innervating them does not necessarily possess a single terminal bulb applied closely to the particular cells affected by the chemical mediator it liberates (as appears to be the case in Fig. 17-55). Instead, an axon may possess several swellings along its terminal part (Fig. 17-56), each of which can elaborate chemical mediator, and so the influence of a single axon is not limited to one particular site, as a single end bulb at an axon termination would be.

In order for nerve fibers to supply acinar cells of an exocrine gland they must be conducted in the connective tissue between acini. Here the fibers are covered by Schwann cells (Fig. 17-56) and sometimes more than one fiber is enclosed by the same Schwann cell. Usually the axon sheds its Schwann cell covering as or before it penetrates the basal lamina of an acinar cell, so that a bulb can come into close contact with the cell membrane of the

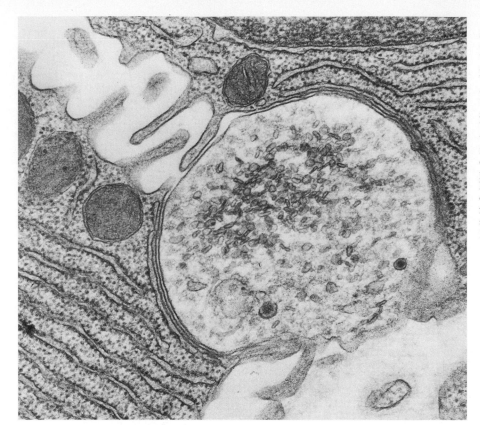

Fig. 17-55. Electron micrograph (×65,750) showing at *center* a bulb of an axon lying between the basal parts of two acinar cells of parotid gland (rat). Within the bulb there are vesicles containing neurotransmitter. The bulb is not separated from the acinar cells by basement membrane. The acinar cells in contact with the bulb have cytoplasm rich in free ribosomes and rER. The cisterna of ER that closely approaches the bulb and runs parallel with it has no ribosomes on its outer surface but its surface that faces the cytoplasm has ribosomes on it. (Hand, A. R.: J. Cell Biol., *47*:540, 1970)

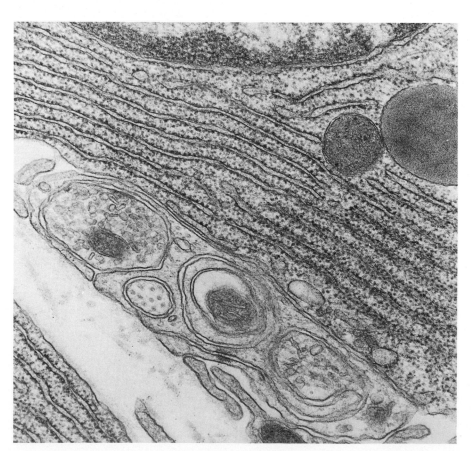

Fig. 17-56. Electron micrograph showing three axon bulbs (*lower left*) within the cytoplasm of a Schwann cell at the base of an acinar cell of rat parotid gland. There is a cisterna of ER lying close to, and parallel with, the area where it might be expected that chemical mediation would occur; note that this cisterna has no ribosomes on the surface near the axon bulbs. (Courtesy of A. Hand)

acinar cell (Fig. 17-55). However, sometimes only relatively close contact is achieved, without the bulbs along axons losing their Schwann cell covering, as in Figure 17-56.

Hand describes two types of bulbs that serve as the source of a chemical mediator in the rat parotid. About two thirds of them contain vesicles 30 to 70 nm. in diameter with electron-dense cores. The evidence indicates that these bulbs are adrenergic. The remaining one third of the bulbs are considered to be cholinergic.

The way the release of a chemical mediator affects the function of a secretory cell is not understood. Hand, however, notes that a cisterna of endoplasmic reticulum can often be seen close to, and parallel with, the cell membrane of the acinar cell at the site where an axon bulb is present; this occurs in both adrenergic and cholinergic types of bulbs. The side of the cisterna that faces the bulb is devoid of ribosomes but the other side has ribosomes attached to it (Figs. 17-55 and 17-56).

The number of bulbs associated with an acinus varies. Hand discusses the possibility that gap (nexus) type junctions between acinar cells participate in transmitting stimulation throughout a whole secretory unit.

REFERENCES AND OTHER READING

GENERAL

Bourne, G. H. (ed.): Structure and Function of Nervous Tissue. New York, Academic Press, vol. 1, 1968; vols. 2 and 3, 1969; vols. 4 and 5, 1972.
Koelle, G. B.: Neurohumoral transmission and the autonomic nervous system. *In* Goodman, L. S., and Gilman, A. (eds.): The Pharmacological Basis of Therapeutics. p. 404. New York, Macmillan, 1975.
Peters, A., Palay, S., and Webster, H.: The Fine Structure of the Nervous System: The Neurons and Supporting Cells. Philadelphia, W. B. Saunders, 1976.
Santini, M. (ed.): Golgi Centennial Symposium: Perspectives in Neurobiology. New York, Raven Press, 1975.

SPECIAL

Central Nervous System

Axelrod, J.: Neurotransmitters. Sci. Am., *230:*58, June, 1974.
Brightman, M. W.: The distribution within the brain of ferritin injected into cerebrospinal fluid compartments. II. Parenchymal distribution. Am. J. Anat., *117:*193, 1965.
Bunge, R. P.: Glial cells and the central myelin sheath. Physiol. Rev., *48:*197, 1968.
Bunge, R. P., Bunge, M. B., and Ris, H.: Ultrastructural study of remyelination in an experimental lesion in adult cat spinal cord. J. Biophys. Biochem. Cytol., *10:*67, 1961.
Caley, D. W., and Maxwell, D. S.: Development of the blood

vessels and extracellular spaces during postnatal maturation of rat cerebral cortex. J. Comp. Neurol., *138:*31, 1970.
————: An electron microscopic study of neurons during postnatal development of the rat cerebral cortex. J. Comp. Neurol., *133:*17, 1968.
Causey, G.: The Cell of Schwann. Edinburgh, E. & S. Livingstone, 1960.
Finean, J. B.: The nature and stability of nerve myelin. Int. Rev. Cytol., *12:*303, 1961.
Gabe, M.: Neurosecretion. Oxford, Pergamon Press, 1966.
Gray, E. G., and Guillery, R. W.: Synaptic morphology in the normal and degenerating nervous system. Int. Rev. Cytol., *19:*111, 1966.
Haggar, R. A., and Barr, M. L.: Quantitative data on the size of synaptic end-bulbs in the cat's spinal cord; with a note on the preparation of cell models. J. Comp. Neurol., *93:*17, 1950.
Hess, A., and Young, J. Z.: Nodes of Ranvier in the central nervous system. J. Physiol., *108:*52P, 1949.
Heuser, J. E., and Reese, T. S.: Evidence for recycling of synaptic vesicle membrane during transmitter release of the frog neuro-muscular junction. J. Cell Biol., *57:*315, 1973.
Hökfelt, T., Fuxe, K., Goldstein, M., Johansson, O., and Ljungdahl, A.: Transmitter histochemistry of the central nervous system. *In* Santini, M. (ed.): Golgi Centennial Symposium. Proceedings. p. 401. New York, Raven Press, 1975.
Hudson, A. J., and Smith, C. G.: The vascular pattern of the choroid plexus of the lateral ventricle. Anat. Rec., *112:*43, 1952.
Imamoto, K., and Leblond, C. P.: Presence of labeled monocytes, macrophages and microglia in a stab wound of the brain following an injection of bone marrow cells labeled with ³H-uridine into rats. J. Comp. Neurol., *174:*255, 1977.
Jones, D. G.: Some current concepts of synaptic organization. Advances in Anatomy, Embryology and Cell Biology. vol. 55, part 4. Berlin, Springer-Verlag, 1978.
King, J. S.: A light and electron microscopic study of perineuronal glial cells and processes in the rabbit neocortex. Anat. Rec., *161:*111, 1968.
Kruger, L., and Maxwell, D. S.: Electron microscopy of oligodendrocytes in normal rat cerebrum. Am. J. Anat., *118:*411, 1966.
Ling, E. A., Patterson, J. A., Privat, A., Mori, S., and Leblond, C. P.: Identification of glial cells in the brain of young rats. J. Comp. Neurol., *149:*43, 1973.
Llinás, R. R.: The cortex of the cerebellum. Sci. Am., *232:*56, Jan., 1975.
McEwen, B. S., and Graftsein, B.: Fast and slow components in axonal transport of protein. J. Cell Biol., *38:*494, 1968.
Maxwell, D. S., and Pease, D. C.: Electron microscopy of the choroid plexus. Anat. Rec., *123:*331, 1956.
Mori, S., and Leblond, C. P.: Identification of microglia in light and electron microscopy. J. Comp. Neurol., *155:*57, 1969.
————: Electron microscopic features and proliferation of astrocytes in the corpus callosum of the rat. J. Comp. Neurol., *157:*197, 1969.
————: Electron microscopic identification of three classes of oligodendrocytes and a study of their proliferative activity in the corpus callosum of young rats. J. Comp. Neurol., *139:*1, 1970.
Nathaniel, E. S. H., and Nathaniel, D.: The ultrastructural features of the synapses in the posterior horn of the spinal cord in the rat. J. Ultrastruct. Res., *14:*540, 1966.
Palay, S. L.: Synapses in the central nervous system. J. Biophys. Biochem. Cytol., (Suppl.) *2:*193, 1956.
————: The structural basis for neural action. *In* Brazier, M. A.

B. (ed.): Brain Function. vol. 2, p. 69. Berkeley, University of California Press, 1963.

Palay, S. L., and Palade, G. E.: The fine structure of neurons. J. Biophys. Biochem. Cytol., *1*:69, 1955.

Paterson, J. A., and Leblond, C. P.: Increased proliferation of neuroglia and endothelial cells in the supraoptic nucleus and hypophysial neural lobe of young rats drinking hypotonic sodium chloride solutions. J. Comp. Neurol., *175*:373, 1977.

Paterson, J. A., Privat, A., Ling, E. A., and Leblond, C. P.: Transformation of subependymal cells into glial cells as shown by radioautography after ³H thymidine injection into the lateral ventricles of the brain of young rats. J. Comp. Neurol., *149*:73, 1973.

Pfenninger, K. H., and Rees, R. P.: Properties of membranes in synapse formation. *In* Barondes, S. H. (ed.): Neuronal Recognition, Current Topics in Neurobiology. New York, Plenum Press, 1976.

Shepherd, G. M.: Microcircuits in the nervous system. Sci. Am., *238*:93, Feb., 1978.

Sotelo, C.: Morphological correlates of electronic coupling between neurons in mammalian nervous system. *In* Santini, M. (ed.): Golgi Centennial Symposium. Proceedings. p. 355. New York, Raven Press, 1975.

Weed, L. H.: The cerebrospinal fluid. Physiol. Rev., *2*:171, 1922.

———: Certain anatomical and physiological aspects of the meninges and cerebrospinal fluid. Brain, *58*:383, 1935.

———: Meninges and cerebrospinal fluid. J. Anat., *72*:181, 1938.

Woollam, D. H. M., and Millen, J. W.: The perivascular spaces of the mammalian central nervous system and their relation to the perineuronal and subarachnoid spaces. J. Anat., *89*:193, 1955.

Peripheral Nervous System

Droz, B., and Leblond, C. P.: Axonal migration of proteins in the central nervous system and peripheral nerves as shown by radioautography. J. Comp. Neurol., *121*:325, 1963.

Geren, B. B., and Raskind, J.: Development of the fine structure of the meylin sheath in sciatic nerves of chick embryos. Proc. Natl. Acad. Sci., *39*:880, 1953.

———: The formation from the Schwann cell surface of myelin in the peripheral nerves of chick embryos. Exp. Cell Res., *7*:558, 1954.

———: Structural studies on the formation of the myelin sheath in peripheral nerve fibers. *In* Cellular Mechanisms in Differentiation and Growth. Princeton, N.J., Princeton University Press, 1956.

Geren, B. B., and Schmitt, F. O.: Electron microscope studies of the Schwann cell and its constituents with particular reference to their relation to the axon. *In* Fine Structure of Cells. p. 251. Groningen, Holland, Noordhoff, 1955.

Hess, A.: The fine structure of young and old spinal ganglia. Anat. Rec., *123*:399, 1955.

Hess, A., and Lansing, A. I.: The fine structure of peripheral nerve fibers. Anat. Rec., *117*:175, 1953.

Landon, D. N. (ed.): The Peripheral Nerve. London, Chapman and Hall, 1976.

Robertson, J. D.: The unit membrane of cells and mechanism of myelin formation. *In* Ultrastructure and Metabolism of the Nervous System. p. 94. Proc. Assoc. Res. Nerv. Ment. Dis. Baltimore, Williams & Wilkins, 1962.

Schnapp, B., and Mugnaini, E.: The myelin sheath: electron microscopic studies with thin sections and freeze-fracture. *In*

Sanitini, M. (ed.): Golgi Centennial Symposium. Proceedings. p. 209. New York, Raven Press, 1975.

Shanklin, W. M., and Azzam, N. A.: Histological and histochemical studies on the incisures of Schmidt-Lanterman. J. Comp. Neurol., *123*:5, 1964.

Shanthaveerappa, T. R., and Bourne, G. H.: The "perineural epithelium," a metabolically active, continuous, protoplasmic cell barrier surrounding peripheral nerve fasciculi. J. Anat., *96*:527, 1962.

Smith, B. H., and Kreutzberg, G. W.: Neuron-target Cell Interactions. Neurosci. Res. Program Bull., *14*, No. 3:1, 1976.

Steer, J. C., and Horney, F. D.: Evidence for passage of cerebrospinal fluid along spinal nerves. Can. Med. Assoc. J., *98*:71, 1968.

Afferent Nerve Endings

For References on afferent endings in muscle, *see* lists at end of Chapter 18.

Cauna, N.: Structure of digital touch corpuscles. Acta Anat., *32*:1, 1958.

Cauna, N., and Mannan, G.: The structure of human digital Pacinian corpuscles and its functional significance. J. Anat., *92*:1, 1958.

———: Development and postnatal changes in digital Pacinian corpuscles in the human hand. J. Anat., *93*:271, 1959.

Chouchkov, C. V.: Cutaneous receptors. Advances in Anatomy, Embryology and Cell Biology. vol. 54, part 5. Berlin, Springer-Verlag, 1978.

Halata, Z.: The mechanoreceptors of the mammalian skin. Ultrastructure and morphological classification. Advances in Anatomy, Embryology and Cell Biology. vol. 50, Fasc. 5. Berlin, Springer-Verlag, 1975.

Iggo, A.: Cutaneous and subcutaneous sense organs. Br. Med. Bull., *33*:97, 1977.

Keller, J. H., and Moffett, B. C., Jr.: Nerve endings in the temporomandibular joint of the Rhesus macaque. Anat. Rec., *160*:587, 1968.

Lynn, B.: Somatosensory receptors and their CNS connections. Ann. Rev. Cytol., *37*:105, 1975.

Pease, D. C., and Quilliam, T. A.: Electron microscopy of the Pacinian corpuscle. J. Biophys. Biochem. Cytol., *3*:331, 1957.

Shanthaveerappa, T. R., and Bourne, G. H.: New observations on the structure of the Pacinian corpuscle and its relation to the perineural epithelium of peripheral nerves. Am. J. Anat., *112*:97, 1963.

Sinclair, D.: Cutaneous Sensation. London, Oxford University Press, 1967.

———: Normal anatomy of sensory nerves and receptors. *In* Jarrett, A. (ed.): The Physiology and Pathophysiology of the Skin. The Nerves and Blood Vessels. vol. 2, p. 371. London, Academic Press, 1973.

Straile, W. E.: Encapsulated nerve end-organs in the rabbit, mouse, sheep and man. J. Comp. Neurol., *136*:317, 1969.

Werner, J. K.: Trophic influence of nerves on the development and maintenance of sensory receptors. Am. J. Physical Medicine *53*:127, 1974.

Efferent Nerve Endings

For References on efferent endings in muscle, *see* lists at end of Chapter 18.

Hand, A. R.: Nerve-acinar relationships in the rat parotid gland. J. Cell Biol., *47*:540, 1970.

———: Adrenergic and cholinergic nerve terminals in the rat

parotid gland. Electron microscopic observations on permanganate-fixed glands. Anat. Rec., *173:*131, 1972.

Regeneration

Bueker, D., and Meyers, E.: The maturity of peripheral nerves at the time of injury as a factor in nerve regeneration. Anat. Rec., *109:*723, 1951.

Guth, L.: Regeneration in the mammalian peripheral nervous system. Physiol. Rev., *36:*441, 1956.

Gutmann, E., and Guttmann, L.: Factors affecting recovery of sensory function after nerve lesions. J. Neurol. Psychiat., *5:*117, 1942.

Gutmann, E., Guttmann, L., Medawar, P. B., and Young, J. Z.: The rate of regeneration of nerve. J. Exp. Biol., *19:*14, 1942.

Gutmann, E., and Sanders, F. K.: Functional recovery following nerve grafts and other types of nerve bridge. Brain, *65:*373, 1942.

————: Recovery of fiber numbers and diameters in the regeneration of peripheral nerves. J. Physiol., *101:*489, 1943.

Holmes, W., and Young, J. Z.: Nerve regeneration after immediate and delayed suture. J. Anat., *77:*63, 1942.

Horn, G., Rose, S. P. R., and Bateson, P. P. G.: Experience and plasticity in the central nervous system. Science, *181:*506, 1973.

Lund, R. D.: Development and Plasticity of the brain. An Introduction. New York, Oxford University Press, 1978.

Nesmeyanova, T. A.: Experimental Studies on Regeneration of Spinal Neurons. New York, Halsted Press, 1977.

Polezhaev, L. V.: Loss and Restoration of Regenerative Capacity in Tissues and Organs of Animals. Cambridge, Harvard University Press, 1972.

Ramon y Cajal, S.: Degeneration and Regeneration of the Nervous System. London, Oxford, 1928.

Sanders, F. K.: The repair of large gaps in the peripheral nerves. Brain, *65:*281, 1942.

Sanders, F. K., and Young, J. Z.: The degeneration and reinnervation of grafted nerves. J. Anat., *76:*143, 1941.

Seddon, H. J.: Three types of nerve injury. Brain, *66:*237, 1943.

————: War injuries of peripheral nerves. Br. J. Surg. (War Surg., Suppl. No. 2), p. 325, 1948.

Seddon, H. J., Medawar, P. B., and Smith, H.: Rate of regeneration of peripheral nerves in man. J. Physiol., *102:*191, 1943.

Sunderland, S.: The capacity of regenerating axons to bridge long gaps in nerves. J. Comp. Neurol., *99:*481, 1953.

————: A classification of peripheral nerve injuries producing loss of function. Brain, *74:*491, 1951.

————: Factors influencing the course of regeneration and the quality of the recovery after nerve suture. Brain, *75:*19, 1952.

Windle, W. F.: Regeneration of axons in the vertebrate central nervous system. Physiol. Rev., *36:*427, 1956.

Young, J. Z.: Factors influencing the regeneration of nerves. Adv. Surg., *1:*165, 1949.

————: Histology of peripheral nerve injuries. *In* Cope, Z. (ed.): Medical History of the Second World War: Surgery. p. 534. London, Her Majesty's Stat. Off., 1953.

————: Structure, degeneration and repair of nerve fibers. Nature, *156:*132, 1945.

Young, J. Z., Holmes, W., and Sanders, F. K.: Nerve regeneration—importance of the peripheral stump and the value of nerve grafts. Lancet, *2:*128, 1940.

Blood Supply of Nerves

Adams, W. E.: The blood supply of nerves. J. Anat., *76:*323, 1942.

Sunderland, S.: Blood supply of the nerves of the upper limb in man. Arch. Neurol. Psychiat., *53:*91, 1945.

————: Blood supply of peripheral nerves. Arch. Neurol. Psychiat., *54:*280, 1945.

————: Blood supply of the sciatic nerve and its popliteal divisions in man. Arch. Neurol. Psychiat., *54:*283, 1945.

18 Muscle Tissue

Muscle Tissue As a Composite. Epithelial glands, muscle tissue, and nervous tissue are all composites, meaning that although they consist primarily of the kinds of cells that give them their names (i.e., epithelial, muscle, and nerve cells), they also have a connective tissue component. Connective tissue is essential in muscle tissue for at least two reasons. First, muscle cells function vigorously and so require an abundant supply of oxygen and nutrients. These are brought by the capillaries that in most kinds of muscle lie between the muscle cells in delicate connective tissue. Second, muscle cells all have to pull together on something to do their work. The harness transmitting their pull consists of the fibrous intercellular substance of the connective tissue component of the muscle. Histological study of muscle tissue therefore involves both of these components.

Why Muscle Cells Are Called Muscle Fibers. Contractility, a fundamental property of all animal cells, attains its greatest expression in muscle cells. Indeed, almost all the cytoplasm of muscle cells consists of contractile machinery. For this to shorten a cell effectively, the cell, instead of being rounded, should be long and narrow and the contractile machinery should be arranged so as to pull the two ends of the cell closer together. Since muscle cells are thus long and narrow, they were long ago called muscle *fibers*. After studying lifeless collagen and elastic fibers it may seem strange to also designate living cells as fibers; the term *fiber,* however, denotes that a structure is thread-like but lacks connotation as to whether it is composed of living or nonliving substance.

The Three Kinds of Muscle Tissue. The needs of various parts of the body for particular kinds of contraction are somewhat different. For example, the kind of muscle required for a tennis player to run and hit a ball both hard and accurately is not the same kind he needs to move food along his intestinal tract to undergo digestion. For the various sorts of contraction needed in different parts of the body there are three kinds of muscle tissue, each with its own kind of muscle fibers. The first kind acquired four different names, as follows.

1. Skeletal (Also Called Voluntary, Striated, or Striped) Muscle Tissue. This kind comprises what people in general call their "muscles." Since most of these muscles are attached by at least one end to some part of the skeleton, this kind of muscle tissue was long ago called *skeletal muscle.* Then as physiological knowledge developed it was found that its function was controlled voluntarily — it could be contracted or relaxed at will — so skeletal muscle came to be known also as *voluntary muscle.* It should be appreciated, however, that skeletal muscle is capable of functioning without voluntary control, for example, when without conscious effort it maintains a state of partial contraction (termed *tonus*) as in holding one's head up. The same muscles that maintain tonus can be used voluntarily to move the head, for example in watching a tennis match from the side of the court.

Next, when it became possible to prepare good histological sections of skeletal (voluntary) muscle and examine them with the LM, fibers in longitudinal section were found to exhibit regular cross striations. Because this seemed due to the substance of a fiber being composed of alternate thin light and dark segments that crossed the fiber from one side to the other (look at Figs. 18-4 and 18-5), microscopists gave this kind of muscle yet another name, *striated muscle.* Moreover, having cross striations also led to its being termed *striped* muscle. The term now generally employed by histologists is *striated muscle,* but the student should remember that striated muscle is a synonym for voluntary or skeletal muscle, names that are still in common use.

2. Cardiac Muscle Tissue. This constitutes most of the substance of the heart, hence its name. However, it is not entirely confined to the heart because some is also normally present in the walls of the pulmonary vein and superior vena cava. Since its fibers possess cross striations, it might be thought that cardiac muscle would be classified as another type of striated muscle instead of having a special place in muscle classification. But cardiac muscle differs from striated (voluntary) muscle in not being under the control of the will, and so it was given a category of its own. It was fortunate that it was classed as a separate type of muscle, because the EM later showed that its fine structure differs in some respects from that of ordinary striated (skeletal) muscle, as will be described presently.

3. Smooth Muscle Tissue. Because its fibers lack any cross striations, this type was called *smooth* muscle (in the sense of not being striped). Since it is not under the control of the will, smooth muscle is also called *involuntary* muscle. It is of course controlled by the nervous system, but by its involuntary division, the autonomic nervous system.

The fibers of smooth muscles are commonly arranged in sheets and constitute one or more layers of the walls of tubes and certain hollow structures in the body, examples being blood vessels (except the tiniest), tubes conducting air into and out of the lungs, the urinary bladder and gallbladder, and all regions of the alimentary tube except its very beginning (where striated muscle is present). Accordingly, one can voluntarily initiate swallowing of food, but once the food reaches a certain point, its further passage along the tube cannot be controlled voluntarily. The chief role of smooth muscle in the walls of such tubular or bladder-like structures is to regulate the size of their lumina or cavities by its degree of contraction (tonus). In some cases it also propels their contents along with waves of contraction.

We shall now deal with each of the three types of muscle in detail.

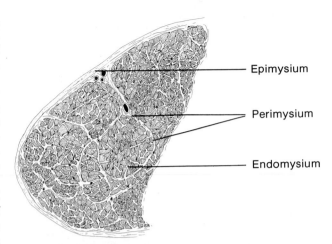

Fig. 18-1. Diagram of a small striated muscle in cross section under very low magnification, showing its connective tissue components and organization into bundles of muscle fibers. *Epimysium* encloses the entire muscle, *perimysium* surrounds each bundle of fibers, and *endomysium* lies in between the individual muscle fibers.

This contains extensive capillaries (Fig. 18-2) and nerve fibers supplying the muscle fibers. Hence striated muscle fibers are arranged longitudinally in the interstices of an endomysial network from which they are nourished and innervated.

At each end of a muscle the connective tissue elements continue on beyond the muscle fibers to blend with the strong connective tissue anchoring the muscle to the

STRIATED (VOLUNTARY) MUSCLE

MICROSCOPIC STRUCTURE AS SEEN IN H AND E SECTIONS

The Connective Tissue Component

This is most easily seen in a cross section of a muscle. As illustrated in Figure 18-1, the entire muscle is surrounded by a tough sheath of relatively dense connective tissue, called *epimysium* (Gr. *epi*, upon) because it encloses the muscle. From the epimysium, blood vessels enter or leave the interior of the muscle by way of fibrous partitions that extend into the muscle to surround fascicles (bundles) of muscle fibers; these partitions constitute the *perimysium* (Gr. *peri*, around) and serve also to conduct lymphatics and nerves into the muscle. From the perimysium, delicate sheets of connective tissue, comprising a few fibroblasts, some amorphous intercellular substance, and a few delicate collagenic fibers, provide a network extending between each and every muscle fiber and constituting the *endomysium* (Gr. *endon*, within).

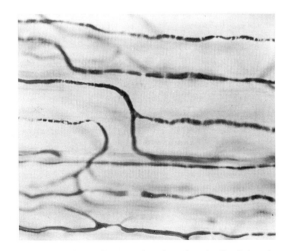

Fig. 18-2. Photomicrograph of a longitudinal section of striated muscle with its blood vessels injected with India ink. Note the capillaries in the endomysium running between and parallel to the muscle fibers. (Courtesy of W. Hartroft)

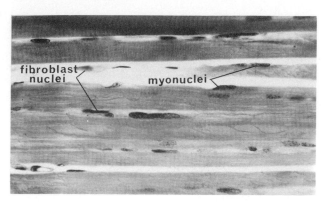

Fig. 18-3. Photomicrograph of striated muscle fibers in longitudinal section. Cross striations can be seen. Muscle nuclei (myonuclei) are located at the periphery of the fibers but sometimes appear to lie within them due to the plane of section. Some fibroblast nuclei can also be seen in the endomysium between the muscle fibers. (Courtesy of E. Schultz and C. P. Leblond)

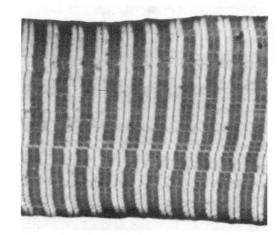

Fig. 18-4. Photomicrograph (×2,000) of a striated muscle fiber in longitudinal section (stained with toluidine blue). The thick dark vertical stripes are made up of the A bands of myofibrils; the light stripes contain the I bands, centered by Z lines. On close inspection, a paler region, the H zone, can be seen in the center of each A band. Note how the bands of the myofibrils all lie in register with one another, giving an impression of continuous striations across the fiber. Note also the pale fine lines running horizontally through the dark A bands; these are narrow regions of sarcoplasm lying between individual myofibrils. (Courtesy of E. Schultz)

structure on which it pulls. Thus a muscle may terminate in a tendon anchored by means of Sharpey's fibers into a bone (Fig. 16-8, p. 473) or into cartilage. However, certain muscles terminate in connective tissue anchorages that take the form of aponeuroses, raphes, periosteum, or even the dense connective tissue of the skin, without a definite tendon being required.

The Fibers of Striated Muscle

Compared with the cells of other tissues, fibers of striated muscle are extremely large and each contains, instead of a single nucleus, a relatively large number of nuclei that varies in relation to the mass of the fiber. These multinucleated fibers are of a cylindrical shape, tapered at each end. They are from 1 to 40 mm. long and may be up to 0.1 mm. in diameter. Fibers in any given muscle tend to be of more or less constant size, but some muscles have relatively large fibers and others have smaller ones.

Because striated muscle fibers are so long in relation to the field seen even with the low-power objective, the student should not expect to see fibers cut longitudinally from one end to the other. It is only possible to examine relatively short portions in longitudinal sections (Fig. 18-3), and even in excellent sections not every fiber will be cut exactly along its longitudinal axis. Fibers are nevertheless sufficiently narrow for several to be seen in *cross* sections (Fig. 18-6) even at higher magnifications.

Sarcolemma. Each striated muscle fiber is enclosed by its cell membrane, which is termed its *sarcolemma* (Gr. *sarkos,* flesh; *lemma,* husk). Although this is too thin for its cross-sectional appearance to be resolved with the LM, just external to it there is a basement membrane that

is sufficiently well stained by the PAS technic to be faintly visible with the LM. The sarcolemma plays a role in conducting contraction-eliciting impulses along and into the fiber, as will be described in detail in due course.

Nuclei. These have an elongated ovoid shape (Fig. 18-3). In human striated fibers they lie scattered in the peripheral cytoplasm just beneath, and with their long axes parallel to, the sarcolemma. In some other vertebrates, however, they lie deeper in the substance of the fiber. The nuclei of more or less flattened fibroblasts in the endomysium (labeled fibroblast nuclei in Fig. 18-3) may lie so close to the outer surface of muscle fibers that they can be confused with muscle nuclei (labeled myonuclei in Fig. 18-3), particularly in longitudinal sections. Nuclei of muscle fibers are, however, more easily distinguished from those of fibroblasts of endomysium in cross sections (Fig. 18-6) than in longitudinal sections.

Cross Striations. In perfectly cut longitudinal sections, alternating dark and light segments (called *bands*) run a straight course across fibers (Fig. 18-4). But in sections cut slightly obliquely these cross striations appear as crescents (Fig. 18-5), like coins in a stack seen at an angle from above.

When observed under polarized light, the dark-staining bands are birefringent (anisotropic), while the light-staining ones are isotropic. Accordingly, the dark bands are called *A bands* (A for anisotropic) and the light ones, *I*

Fig. 18-5. High-power photomicrograph of striated muscle fibers in slightly oblique longitudinal section. Note that the cross striations appear to be crescent-shaped. This is due to the section being somewhat oblique with respect to the longitudinal axis of the fibers. A bands (dark), I bands (light), and Z lines (bisecting the I bands) are all clearly visible in the lower fiber.

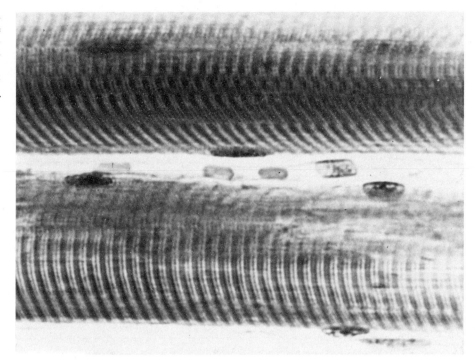

bands (I for isotropic). Thin, dark lines termed *Z lines* also cross the fiber, bisecting the I bands (Figs. 18-4 and 18-5). Sometimes a paler region, termed the *H zone,* can be observed crossing the fiber in the middle of the A band (Fig. 18-4). The cause and significance of these cross striations will become apparent when we deal with the fine structure of striated muscle fibers.

Myofibrils. Long ago it was observed that striated muscle fibers could be dissociated into component fibrils, called *myofibrils,* that were longitudinally oriented and had the same pattern of cross striations as the intact fiber. Hence the cross striations seeming in the LM to run right across the fiber are *not continuous* from one side of the fiber to the other. They appear so only because the myofibrils are packed together very closely, with all their cross striations in register, so that their borders are seldom resolved in longitudinal sections. However, it is easier to see the myofibrils in transverse sections (Fig. 18-6), where they appear as slightly darker staining dots separated by pale-staining cytoplasm, which in muscle fibers is called *sarcoplasm.* With this cross-sectional appearance in mind, a close scrutiny of a longitudinal section will occasionally disclose very fine longitudinal slits of sarcoplasm between myofibrils, as can be seen in Figure 18-4. However, such small traces of sarcoplasm usually pass unnoticed in routine LM sections.

Sarcomeres. This term (Gr. *meros,* part) denotes the portions of myofibrils, 2 to 3 μm. in length, lying along

their course between every two consecutive Z lines. Sarcomeres represent the ultimate contractile units of striated muscle, and muscles contract because sarcomeres shorten to as little as half their resting length; the mechanism involved will now be discussed.

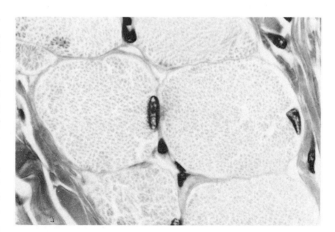

Fig. 18-6. Photomicrograph of striated muscle fibers cut in cross section (high-power). Their nuclei (*center* and *middle right*) lie peripherally in the fibers and are distinguishable by their position and appearance from nuclei of fibroblasts in the endomysium lying between the fibers (just below *center*). The myofibrils within the fibers are visible as gray dots in the pale-staining cytoplasm.

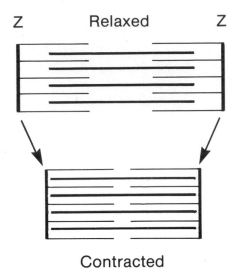

Z   **Relaxed**   Z

Contracted

Fig. 18-7. Diagram of a sarcomere of a striated muscle fiber in the relaxed (*top*) and contracted (*bottom*) state, showing the change in the relative positions of the thick and thin filaments and the Z lines. For details, *see* text.

DEVELOPMENT OF KNOWLEDGE ABOUT THE FINE STRUCTURE OF SARCOMERES AND THE MECHANISM OF CONTRACTION

As biochemical knowledge advanced in the first half of this century, it became known that the substance of muscle was composed largely of the two proteins *actin* and *myosin*. Furthermore, when these two proteins were extracted and then recombined in vitro they formed a complex called *actomyosin*. This complex could be precipitated in the form of threads, and in 1941 Szent-Györgyi discovered that threads of actomyosin shortened when ATP was added. Until the second half of this century, however, it was thought that individual protein molecules, attached to Z lines, would themselves have to shorten to draw the Z lines closer together in contraction.

When in the early 1950s it became practicable to study striated muscle with the EM, the internal structure of the sarcomere was found to be very different from what had been surmised from light microscopy. Instead of being composed of two different kinds or densities of homogeneous proteins, the A and I bands of myofibrils were found to contain characteristic but somewhat different arrangements of longitudinally oriented and rod-shaped structures, which were termed *filaments*. Two kinds of filaments were identified, thick ones and thin ones, each with its own special distribution, as shown in Figure 18-7. In the relaxed sarcomere, neither kind of filament extends all the way from one Z line to the next. As can be seen in the upper parts of Figures 18-7 and 18-9, the thick ones

occupy only the middle portion of the sarcomere—the part recognized in the LM as the A band. Both ends of the thick filaments are free. The thin filaments, however, have only one end free; the other is attached to a Z line. Thus the thin filaments extend from each Z line toward the middle of the sarcomere, where they project in between the thick filaments so as to interdigitate with them. However, in the relaxed sarcomere they extend only part way in between the thick filaments of the A band, without reaching the middle of the sarcomere (Fig. 18-7, *top*). It has since been established that the thick filaments contain myosin and the thin filaments contain actin. Thus the thin filaments correspond to the microfilaments seen in many others types of cells.

In contracting sarcomeres, the thin filaments move farther in between the thick filaments and in full contraction their free ends almost meet in the middle of the sarcomere (Fig. 18-7, *bottom*). Since their length remains unchanged, the only way the thin filaments can move farther in between the thick ones is by pulling on the Z lines to which they are attached, and this pulls the ends (the Z lines) of all the sarcomeres closer together, as shown in Figure 18-7, *bottom*.

The realization that thick filaments contained myosin and thin filaments contained actin suggested that some sort of increasing attraction between actin and myosin might be responsible for pulling the fine filaments farther in between the array of thick filaments. Such a mechanism would help explain why contraction in vitro also appeared to depend on some sort of interaction between actin and myosin. The concept of the two types of filaments moving with respect to one another is the basis of the *sliding filament model* of muscular contraction, proposed by H. E. Huxley and his coworkers in 1954 as the outcome of their EM and x-ray diffraction studies. This model revolutionized thinking about muscle contraction and almost immediately found wide acceptance. A more detailed consideration of the biochemical reactions involved will be given presently. But first we should correlate what is seen with the LM and EM in both relaxed and contracted striated muscle fibers.

HOW THE STRIATIONS SEEN WITH THE LM ARE RELATED TO THE FINE STRUCTURE OF SARCOMERES

The names of the cross striations of striated muscle fibers, as noted, were based on light microscopy. With the LM it was possible to discern A and I bands and Z lines, and sometimes in good preparations a lighter H zone could be seen in the middle of the A band (this is visible on close examination of Fig. 18-4). It was also noted with the LM that during contraction A bands remained con-

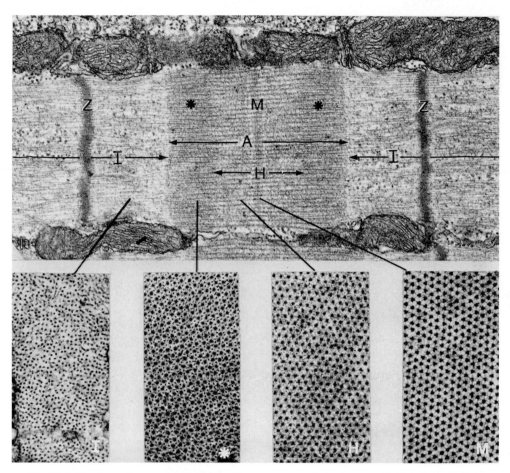

Fig. 18-8. Electron micrographs illustrating the appearance of a sarcomere of striated muscle in longitudinal and transverse sections. The *upper* micrograph shows a *longitudinal section* of a relaxed sarcomere. On either side of the Z lines are halves of lightly stained I bands containing only thin filaments; these filaments extend from the Z lines and interdigitate with thick filaments lying within the darker-staining A band. The regions of the A band that are marked (*) contain both thick and thin filaments and hence appear darker than the region where only thick filaments are present—the H zone (H). A darker M line (M) lies at the center of the A band.

   Cross sections taken at the levels indicated are shown in the *lower four* micrographs (×33,000). The *first* of these shows thin filaments in the I bands. The *second* shows thin filaments interdigitating with thick filaments in the A band, forming hexagonal patterns around them; this section is cut through the region marked *. The *third* shows thick filaments in the H zone. The *fourth* micrograph shows thick filaments at the level of the M line, where fine interconnections link them together. (Courtesy of E. Schultz and C. P. Leblond)

stant in length but I bands became increasingly shorter. The EM later disclosed why this was so.

   As can be seen from the upper part of Figure 18-8, the EM revealed that in relaxed fibers the greater density of the A band is due to the presence of thick filaments (about 1.5 μm. long and 10 nm. in diameter) and the lesser density of the I band is due to its having only thin filaments (about 1 μm. in length and 5 nm. in diameter). The thin filaments lying at each end of the relaxed sarcomere project

into the A band for about one quarter of its length and so leave a less dense middle section in the A band (Fig. 18-8, *top* micrograph) that corresponds to the lighter H zone seen with the LM (Fig. 18-4). As can be seen from the lower part of Figure 18-9, the H zone virtually disappears in a fully contracted sarcomere because in contraction the thin filaments move toward the middle of the A band and the latter thereupon becomes uniformly dense, revealing no H band because it now contains both thick and thin fil-

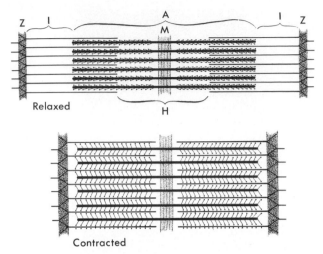

Fig. 18-9. Diagram of a sarcomere of striated muscle in the relaxed (*top*) and contracted (*bottom*) state, showing the detailed arrangements of its components. The thick filaments, which extend the full length of the A band, are about 1.5 μm. in length and approximately 10 nm. in diameter; the thin filaments interdigitating with them are about 1 μm. long and approximately 5 nm. in diameter. In the relaxed sarcomere, halves of I bands, containing only thin filaments, are evident on either side of the darker A band. In the middle of the A band there is a lighter region, the H zone, centered by the M line. Interdigitation is at a minimum in the relaxed state (*top*), so that the I bands and H zone are both relatively long, but these parts of the sarcomere shorten during contraction (*bottom*) due to the movement of the Z lines toward the free ends of the thick filaments. The change in position of the myosin heads (cross bridges) during contraction is also indicated. (Courtesy of E. Schultz and C. P. Leblond)

aments from one end to the other. The darker M line occasionally visible with the LM in the middle of the H band is seen in the EM to be due to fine threads that appear to interconnect the middle parts of the adjacent thick filaments (Fig. 18-9).

EM studies further show that thin filament attachments on one side of the Z line lie opposite spaces in between thin filament attachments on the other side; this is why the Z line has a characteristic zigzag appearance in electron micrographs (Figs. 18-8, *top*, and 18-10). The Z lines thus interconnect the thin filaments of adjacent sarcomeres. One interpretation of the arrangement is that the thin filaments are attached to a lattice of filaments of another type which are referred to as Z *filaments*. As can be seen in the electron micrograph in Figure 18-10, these Z filaments pursue a zigzag course across the myofibril. The *inset* in Fig. 18-10 represents a surface view of the Z line and shows diagrammatically how each thin filament (cross-hatched circles) in one sarcomere appears to be linked by Z filaments to the four nearest thin filaments (black circles) belonging to the adjacent sarcomere, at least in the simpler kinds of Z lines that have been studied. Finally, Z lines contain the protein α-actinin, but it is not yet clear which components of the Z line contain this protein.

CROSS-SECTIONAL APPEARANCE OF FIBERS SEEN WITH THE EM

The arrangements of filaments in various parts of sarcomeres can also be determined from cross sections of fibers. Thus in relaxed sarcomeres cross sections of I bands reveal only thin filaments (Fig. 18-8, *lower left*),

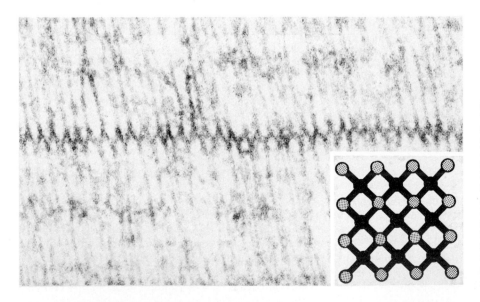

Fig. 18-10. Electron micrograph ($\times$150,000) of a Z line in a white striated muscle fiber of a species (a fish) in which a Z line is a comparatively simple structure. Its zig-zag appearance is due to darkly staining Z filaments, 4 nm. in diameter, to which the thin filaments are attached. (*Inset*) Diagram illustrating the structure of a Z line in surface view ($\times$700,000), showing the investigator's interpretation of how the thin filaments are connected to the Z filaments. For details, *see* text. (Franzini-Armstrong, C.: J. Cell Biol., *58*:630, 1973)

while cross sections through the ends of the A band show both thick and thin filaments (Fig. 18-8, *second* of the *lower* four micrographs). The thin filaments are arranged hexagonally with one thick filament in the center of each hexagon. Moreover, the thick filaments are arranged in a triangular pattern, each triangle with a thin filament in its center. Cross sections through the H zone show only thick filaments (Fig. 18-8, *third* of the *lower* four micrographs). Finally, cross sections through the M line show thick filaments with their fine interconnections (Fig. 18-8, *fourth* of the *lower* four micrographs).

THE FINE STRUCTURE OF THE OTHER COMPONENTS OF MUSCLE FIBERS

Now that we have described the fine structure of myofibrils and the way their thin filaments slide farther in between their thick ones during contraction, we shall next deal with the other components of muscle fibers before going on to discuss contraction at the molecular level. First we shall describe the component in which the myofibrils are embedded. This is called *sarcoplasm* (Gr. *sarkos*, flesh; *plasma*, something formed or molded) and is of significance in the metabolism of the muscle fibers. (Some authors include the myofibrils as part of the sarcoplasm.) Secondly we shall deal with the *sarcolemma* and the efferent nerve ending terminating on it, which is called a *motor end plate*. Further, we shall explain how impulses for contraction are conducted from the sarcolemma by means of invaginations termed *transverse tubules* into the substance of the fiber so that they reach each and every myofibril. Finally, we shall describe the counterpart of the sER which in striated muscle fibers takes the form of an elaborate system of interconnecting cisternae called the *sarcoplasmic reticulum:* this is very much involved in regulating contraction and relaxation. We now go on to discuss each of these in turn.

Sarcoplasm. Since muscle fibers have very substantial energy requirements, they have numerous capillaries close beside them (Fig. 18-2). Oxygen and nutrients from these capillaries diffuse through the sarcolemma into the sarcoplasm in which the myofibrils are embedded.

The elongated nuclei of striated muscle fibers in man, as noted, are characteristically distributed in the peripheral sarcoplasm close to the sarcolemma, with their long axis parallel to it. There are many mitochondria in this region. The peripheral sarcoplasm may also contain a few ribosomes and deposits of glycogen. Deeper within the fiber mitochondria are numerous in the sarcoplasm between adjacent myofibrils (Fig. 18-12B) and glycogen is also present (Fig. 18-12A). Hence the sarcoplasm has an abundance of mitochondria containing the respiratory enzymes so important for the active metabolism of muscle fibers. Moreover, the sarcoplasm also contains a supply

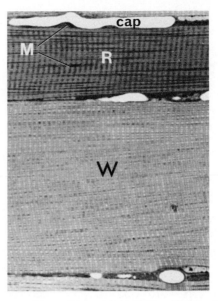

Fig. 18-11. Photomicrograph (×720) of striated muscle (stained with toluidine blue), showing two of its fiber types. The narrower red fibers (R) contain numerous mitochondria (groups of which are indicated by M) packed between their myofibrils, and also at their periphery, especially in association with capillaries (cap). The wider white fibers (W) contain fewer mitochondria. (Courtesy of E. Schultz)

of a free pigmented protein called *myoglobin*. Chemically this protein is closely related to the hemoglobin of erythrocytes and like hemoglobin it can take up, store, or give up oxygen as needed. Myoglobin is red to brown in color and muscle fibers with relatively large quantities of it are called *red fibers*. Meat containing large amounts of it—for example that of seals and whales and the dark meat of fowls—is brown in color and this is said to be due to the high content of myoglobin.

Because striated muscle fibers in different muscles vary in diameter and in their content of sarcoplasm (and hence myoglobin), they are classified as *red, white,* or *intermediate,* as will now be described. Most muscles of man contain all three types but their relative proportions vary with regard to the role of the muscle in the body.

Red fibers (labeled R in Figs. 18-11 and 18-12, *inset*) are characterized by their small diameter and abundance both of myoglobin in their sarcoplasm and of cytochromes (respiratory enzymes) in their numerous mitochondria. *White fibers* (labeled W in Figs. 18-11 and 18-12, *inset*) are somewhat wider and contain less myoglobin and fewer mitochondria. The characteristics of intermediate fibers (labeled I in Fig. 18-12, *inset*) lie between those of red and white fibers. Muscles made up predominantly of red fibers are capable of sustaining activity for longer periods of time than those with mostly white fibers be-

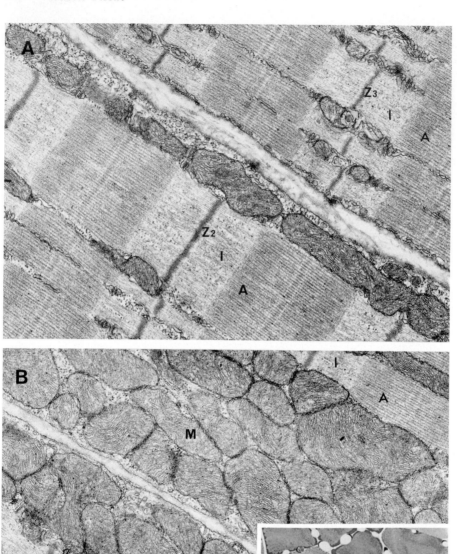

Fig. 18-12. Electron micrographs (×33,000) of striated muscle (longitudinal section) showing all three fiber types. (*A*) At *upper right* there is a white fiber (Z_3), characterized by relatively few mitochondria lying chiefly between myofibrils at the level of Z lines. At *lower left* there is a fiber of the intermediate type (Z_2). (*B*) Red fibers (Z_1) shown here contain an abundance of mitochondria (M) at their periphery as well as in between myofibrils. (*Inset*) Photomicrograph showing white (W), intermediate (I), and red (R) fibers in cross section. Note their relative diameters. The rounded pale areas between the muscle fibers are blood capillaries. (Courtesy of J. Dadoune)

cause their sarcoplasm is well adapted to supplying their energy requirements. White fibers, however, while able to undergo faster contractions than red fibers, are more suited for short bursts of activity. They fatigue relatively rapidly because their energy requirements cannot be met over prolonged periods. The difference between these two types of fibers becomes apparent when the muscles of domestic fowl are compared with those of wild fowl. In chickens, mostly red fibers (dark meat) are found in the much-used leg and thigh musculature while the little-used pectoral muscles, which would be used in flying, are white. Wild fowl capable of sustained flight, however, have red fibers in their pectoral muscles.

The Sarcolemma. This has the typical structure of a cell membrane, and external to it there is a well-developed basal lamina (BM in Fig. 18-23).

In order to understand how impulses for contraction reach the myofibrils it is important to appreciate that the sarcolemma of a striated muscle fiber has permeability characteristics essentially similar to those of the axolemma of an axon, so that it is *electrically polarized* during relaxation. The principal factors contributing to the resting potential of an electrically excitable membrane were discussed in Chapter 17 (p. 498). Thus, during relaxation the inside of the sarcolemma is maintained at a negative resting potential with respect to the outside. Impulses for contraction are, of course, propagated as waves of depolarization along a motor axon toward the terminals of its branches, each of which is apposed to the sarcolemma of a striated muscle fiber. On arriving at the terminal the almost immediate effect of these impulses is to initiate local depolarization of the sarcolemma, with the result that a wave of depolarization spreads out from the region under the terminal to sweep along the sarcolemma and down its tubular invaginations (transverse tubules), thereby passing from the surface of the muscle fiber deep into its sarcoplasm. Only then does the depolarization cause contraction. But before going into what happens inside the muscle fiber we must explain how nerve impulses become transmitted across the narrow gap between the axolemma of the nerve terminal and the sarcolemma apposed to it at what is termed a *motor end plate* (soon to be described). This in turn entails explaining how striated muscle fibers are arranged with respect to the efferent nerve fibers supplying them.

THE EFFERENT INNERVATION OF STRIATED MUSCLE

Motor Units

The efferent nerve supplying a given muscle contains the axons of numerous motor neurons. Each muscle fiber is supplied either by a single motor axon or by a branch of a motor axon. In some muscles, for example certain of the extrinsic eye muscles responsible for delicate eye movements, each muscle fiber is individually innervated by the axon of a single motor neuron. In most muscles, however, each motor axon branches so as to innervate many muscle fibers. This pattern of innervation is seen, for example, in trunk muscles responsible for maintaining posture, where each motor axon has abundant branches and supplies several hundred muscle fibers. In this type of arrangement, the muscle fibers supplied by any given motor axon (and hence any given motor neuron) are distributed widely throughout the muscle.

One motor neuron and its axon, together with the single or (more commonly) multiple muscle fibers it supplies, constitute what is termed a *motor unit*. The degree of contraction of muscle fibers belonging to any given motor unit is not subject to voluntary control: they either contract fully (though the force of their contraction can vary under differing circumstances), or else they do not contract at all. The strength of any given skeletal muscle contraction therefore depends on *how many* of its motor units fire off for the contraction. Because of the wide separation of the individual muscle fibers supplied by axon branches in any given motor unit, weak contractions that require the participation of relatively few motor units involve the muscle as a whole; if instead these fibers were all grouped together, such contractions would involve only localized regions of the muscle. Finally, it is of interest that within any one motor unit, all the muscle fibers can be either red or white, but not both.

Motor End Plates

Every striated muscle fiber is innervated by a terminal branch of a motor axon and thus belongs to some motor unit. A general term for a site at which an axon ends on a muscle fiber is a *neuromuscular (myoneural) junction*. The axon with its covering approaches the surface of a striated muscle fiber from the endomysium at an angle and generally makes contact with the muscle fiber midway between its ends. At the site of contact the axon and its covering form a little flattened mound on the surface of the muscle fiber, called a *motor end plate*. This may be stained for the LM by impregnation with gold or silver salts (Fig. 18-13) or methylene blue in fresh tissue. With the advent of the EM much has been learned about the motor end plate and how it functions.

The Fine Structure of the Motor End Plate—Relation to Function. The EM disclosed that the axon does not enter the substance of the muscle fiber. Instead, the little mound seen with the LM has the following structure. Where the axon branch reaches the mound its myelin sheath disappears but the Schwann cells investing it remain in the form of a continuous roof over the axon terminals (Figs. 18-14C and D and 18-15). Near its termination the axon again branches repeatedly to form a number of short *axon terminals* clustered together over the deep central part of the mound. These are seen most clearly in surface view (Figs. 18-13 and 18-14E) but can also be studied in sections cut perpendicular to the sarcolemma (Figs. 18-14A and B and 18-15). The appearance of a motor end plate as seen with the EM in a longitudinal section of a muscle fiber is illustrated diagrammatically in Figure 18-14C and D, which show that the axon terminals lie in troughs lined by sarcolemma. In these troughs the naked surface of the axon is separated from the sarcolemma by a gap about 20 to 60 nm. wide, termed the *synaptic cleft* (Fig. 18-14D). The surface area of the trough is greatly increased by being thrown into evenly

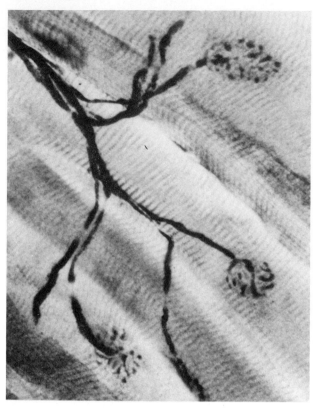

Fig. 18-13. Photomicrograph (×250) of a branch of a myelinated motor nerve fiber where it supplies several striated muscle fibers belonging to a motor unit (preparation stained with gold chloride). The smaller myelinated branches of the nerve fiber terminate at flattened end plates on the muscle fibers.

spaced folds invaginated into the sarcoplasm. These are called *junctional folds* (Fig. 18-14D and E and labeled JF in Fig. 18-15), and the spaces between them communicating with the synaptic cleft are termed *subneural clefts.* The synaptic cleft contains glycosaminoglycans and basal lamina components. Moreover, with regard to function it should be noted that it also contains the enzyme *acetylcholinesterase* necessary to inactivate the neurotransmitter substance acetylcholine liberated at the motor end plate (*see* below). The sarcoplasm associated with the motor end plate is relatively rich in mitochondria and nuclei.

How Impulses for Contraction Are Transmitted to Muscle Fibers From the Axon Terminals of Motor End Plates

With the EM the axon terminals lying in the troughs in the sarcolemma are seen to contain many mitochondria and accumulations of *synaptic vesicles* (V in Fig. 18-15).

These contain the neurotransmitter substance *acetylcholine.* When a wave of depolarization sweeps along the axolemma to reach the termination of a motor axon, the increased permeability leading to depolarization also permits calcium ions to enter the axon from the intercellular fluid. This causes synaptic vesicles to fuse with the axolemma and empty their contents of acetylcholine by exocytosis into the synaptic cleft, the number of vesicles discharged varying with the amount of motor stimulation received. The acetylcholine then becomes attached to acetylcholine receptor sites on the sarcolemma, located for the most part on the peaks of the junctional folds. When acetylcholine combines with these receptor sites it instantaneously increases the permeability of the sarcolemma in the end plate region. This permits sodium ions to pass into the sarcoplasm and potassium ions to move out in the reverse direction. As a result there is a substantial drop in the resting potential of the sarcolemma in this region and a wave of depolarization now moves away from the end plate and sweeps over the sarcolemma. Subsequent events will be described after the next section, which deals with the way membrane is conserved at the axon terminals.

Recycling of Synaptic Vesicle Membrane. Synaptic vesicles (V in Fig. 18-15) in axon terminals are about 40 to 50 nm. in diameter and are most numerous opposite the peaks of the junctional folds of the sarcolemma below. They cease to exist on liberating their acetylcholine in response to nerve impulses and so must be replaced continuously. Furthermore, so many synaptic vesicles fuse with the axolemma that axon terminals might be expected to grow due to accumulation of membrane. However, this does not happen because membrane contributed by the synaptic vesicles is retrieved by a recycling mechanism. As at other synapses (the motor end plate represents a synapse between an axon and a muscle fiber), *coated vesicles* are pinched off and hence removed from sites adjacent to the presynaptic membrane (refer to pp. 503 to 504) and these coated vesicles then move into the axoplasm. During the process of invagination the vesicles acquire the characteristic coating on their cytoplasmic surface; this surrounds the vesicle in the form of a basket. Once well within the cytoplasm of the terminal, coated vesicles lose their coating and coalesce so as to form a cisterna of smooth-surfaced membrane from which new synaptic vesicles proceed to bud off. The size of this membranous cisterna varies with the activity of the end plate. Since acetylcholine is synthesized in the cisterna (by the action of enzymes brought to the terminal by axoplasmic transport), it is already present within the synaptic vesicles at the time that they bud off from the cisterna.

Fate of Acetylcholine Released At Motor End Plates. After acetylcholine has been released into the synaptic cleft, it

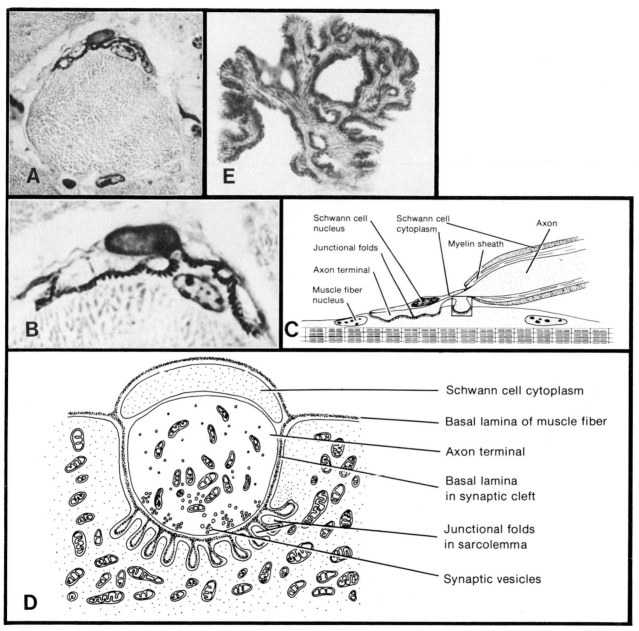

Fig. 18-14. Diagrams and photomicrographs illustrating the structure of a motor end plate. The photomicrographs are of motor end plates on intercostal muscle fibers (hedgehog), stained by the acetylthiocholine method for cholinesterase; nuclei are counterstained with hematoxylin. (A) Low-power photomicrograph (×1,000) showing a motor end plate (*top*) as it appears in a cross section through a muscle fiber (seen at *center*). Muscle fiber nuclei are present just beneath the end plate and at *bottom* (refer to diagram in C). (B) Photomicrograph showing the end plate at higher magnification (×2,500). The darkly stained nucleus just above *center* belongs to a Schwann cell; the paler one right of *center* belongs to the muscle fiber. Dark staining of the cholinesterase in the synaptic cleft clearly outlines the junctional folds in the sarcolemma (refer again to diagram in C). (C) Explanatory diagram showing, at the EM level, a motor end plate in a longitudinal section of a muscle fiber, and its continuity with a motor axon. Note how the terminal branches in the end plate are covered on their exposed side with Schwann cells. This diagram should be compared with Figure 18-15. (D) Details that would be seen with the EM in the area indicated at *lower right center* in (C). Note again the Schwann cell capping the axon terminal. For further details, *see* text. (E) Photomicrograph (×1,400) of a motor end plate in surface view (without counterstaining). In this plane of focus the junctional folds running along the synaptic troughs may be discerned. Note the way the terminal branches of the axon branch repeatedly so as to constitute the end plate. (Photomicrographs courtesy of, and diagrams modified after, R. Couteaux)

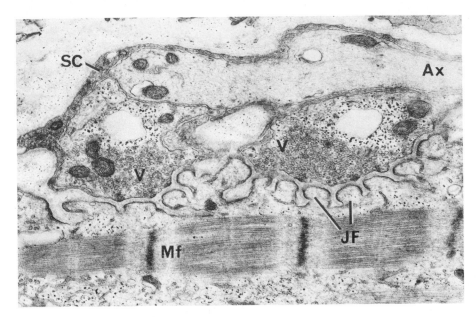

Fig. 18-15. Electron micrograph (×20,000) of a motor end plate (newt). The upper surface of the motor axon (Ax) is covered with a thin layer of Schwann cell cytoplasm (SC). The axon terminals contain abundant synaptic vesicles (V) and mitochondria. Note the junctional folds (JF) in the sarcolemma under the axon terminals. A myofibril (Mf) is visible in the sarcoplasm of the muscle fiber. This figure should be compared carefully with Figure 18-14C. (Courtesy of T. L. Lentz)

is promptly degraded into choline and acetate by *acetylcholinesterase.* This enzyme seems to be bound to the basal lamina component occupying the synaptic and subneural clefts. It is probably able to destroy some acetylcholine even before the neurotransmitter has had a chance to combine with the receptor sites on the sarcolemma, thereby reducing the risk of unwanted contractions as a result of spurious release of the neurotransmitter. Fast destruction of the transmitter substance is, of course, vital for rapid transmission of impulses to the muscle fiber because it permits the same receptor sites to be stimulated repeatedly.

It will be of interest to medical students that in a condition known as *myasthenia gravis* (Gr. *mys,* muscle; *astheneia,* weakness), characterized by muscular weakness, the sarcolemma has fewer acetylcholine receptor sites than normal. As a result, the arrival of motor nerve impulses frequently fails to elicit contraction of the required number of fibers in a muscle so that the muscle as a whole is capable of only feeble contractions. There is evidence that this condition is the result of autoimmune attack directed specifically against acetylcholine receptors (Drachman).

The Transverse Tubules (T Tubules). When a nerve impulse arrives at a motor end plate, a wave of depolarization, as noted, sweeps over the sarcolemma. Before the advent of the EM it was not known how depolarization was conducted into the fiber to the myofibrils, which, of course, are the contractile structures. However, the EM disclosed a system of narrow tubules (T tubules) extending from the sarcolemma into the fiber at fairly regular intervals along its length. Next, when ferritin, a marker

readily detectable in the EM, was injected in between muscle fibers, it passed deep into the fiber by way of the lumina of the T tubules; hence these lumina connect with intercellular space (Fig. 18-16, *inset*). Since T tubules are thus invaginations of the sarcolemma they readily conduct waves of depolarization into the substance of the fiber.

Within the fiber, T tubules branch extensively. In mammalian striated muscle fibers, branches of two T tubules encircle each sarcomere of every myofibril at positions close to the junctions of the A and I bands of relaxed fibers (Fig. 18-18). In amphibian striated muscle fibers, however (which were the first kind studied), the branching T tubules extend in at only *one* level per sarcomere, encircling the myofibrils at the level of each Z line (Fig. 18-16).

The system of T tubules would explain how a wave of depolarization could be conducted to the periphery of each and every sarcomere but not why this would bring about contraction. Contraction is not the result of a wave of depolarization directly affecting the contractile machinery inside the sarcomere, but is instead due to its setting in motion a further event in still another component of the sarcoplasm (again disclosed by the EM), termed the *sarcoplasmic reticulum.* The membranous walls of this reticulum are connected to those of T tubules in a manner that allows a wave of depolarization conveyed along the T tubules to elicit a change in permeability of the walls of the sarcoplasmic reticulum.

The Sarcoplasmic Reticulum. This organelle of a muscle fiber is the counterpart of the sER of other cell types. Since its form is complex, we first describe the sarcoplas-

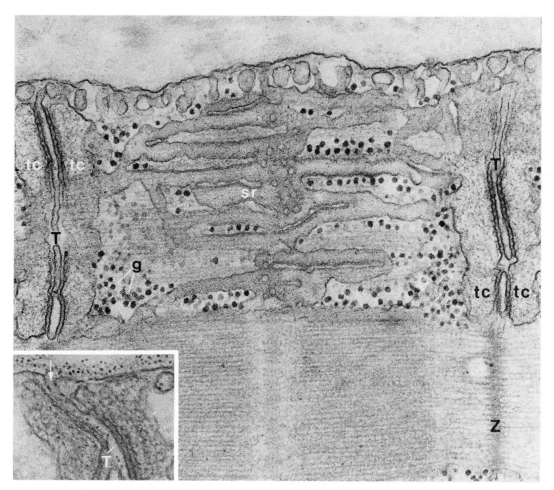

Fig. 18-16. Electron micrograph of a longitudinal section of a striated muscle fiber (frog), showing transverse (T) tubules and sarcoplasmic reticulum (sr). The top myofibril is not in the plane of section but has been cut tangentially, revealing in surface view the sarcoplasmic reticulum surrounding it. Two T tubules (T) enter the fiber at the level of Z lines (one Z line is labeled in the lower myofibril). These tubules are closely associated with the terminal cisternae (tc) of sarcoplasmic reticulum flanking them on either side to form triads. A unique kind of intracellular junction (*see* text) can be seen between the T tubules and terminal cisternae. The terminal cisternae at either end of the sarcomere are joined by longitudinal channels to a fenestrated region of the sarcoplasmic reticulum (sr) surrounding the middle of the sarcomere. Abundant β particles of glycogen (g) lie between the tubules of sarcoplasmic reticulum.

(*Inset*) Part of a striated muscle fiber that was immersed in a ferritin solution before fixation. Ferritin can be seen as black particles not only on the outer surface of the sarcolemma at *top* but also within the T tubule (T). This indicates the the ferritin marker in intercellular space has free access to T tubules through openings (indicated by arrow) onto the sarcolemma, and shows that lumina of T tubules are continuous with intercellular space. (Courtesy of R. Birks)

mic reticulum of amphibian striated muscle fibers, where it has been studied most extensively. Moreover, its arrangement in amphibian muscle fibers is relatively easy to understand since, as noted, sarcomeres are encircled by branches of T tubules at the level of Z lines, as shown in Figure 18-16.

The sarcoplasmic reticulum comprises a continuous system of components that range in shape from tubules to flattened cisternae. Around every sarcomere there is a collar-like complex of these components. Moreover, as Figure 18-17 illustrates, the collar is continuous with identical collars of sarcoplasmic reticulum surrounding sarcomeres at the same level in neighboring myofibrils. Accordingly, at any given level along the course of the

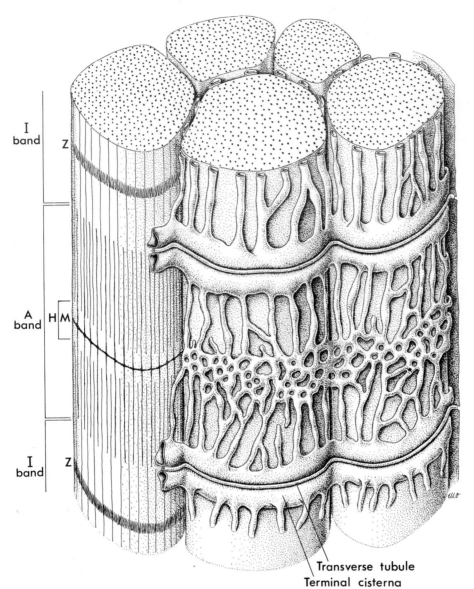

I
band

Z

A
band

H M

I
band

Z

Transverse tubule
Terminal cisterna

Fig. 18-17. Diagram of part of a mammalian striated muscle fiber, illustrating the layout of the sarcoplasmic reticulum surrounding its myofibrils. In the myofibril at *left* the A, I, and other bands and Z lines are indicated. The sarcoplasmic reticulum surrounding the myofibrils is illustrated at *middle* and *right*. Note that in mammalian striated muscle fibers two transverse (T) tubules supply a sarcomere. Each T tubule is located close to the junction between an A and an I band, where it is associated with two terminal cisternae of sarcoplasmic reticulum, one on each side of it. Each terminal cisterna connects with more or less longitudinal sarcotubules of the reticulum located around the A band and these in turn anastomose to form a network in the more central region of the band (extending across the H band). The triple structure seen in cross section where the two terminal cisternae (one from each adjacent sarcomere) flank a transverse tubule, one on either side of it, constitutes a triad; two triads are illustrated in front of the myofibril at *left*. (Courtesy of C. P. Leblond)

fiber all the sarcomeres (each belonging to a different myofibril) are surrounded by the same interconnecting and continuous complex of collars of sarcoplasmic reticulum. The components of the collar around each sarcomere are as follows.

At either end of the sarcomere there is a large and somewhat flattened cisterna, referred to as a *terminal cisterna* because of its position, that forms a hollow ring around the myofibril beside and parallel with the T tubule at that end of the sarcomere (as seen in Fig. 18-16). On the other side of this T tubule there is a corresponding terminal cisterna belonging to the adjacent sarcomere and this likewise forms a ring around the end of the adjoining

sarcomere. The lumina of these two terminal cisternae (which, as noted, belong to contiguous sarcomeres) are larger than that of the T tubule lying between them (refer to Fig. 18-16) and the three structures seen together in cross section are collectively referred to as a *triad*. No direct structural continuity has yet been detected between the lumen of the T tubule, which connects with intercellular space, and the lumen of the sarcoplasmic reticulum, which forms a distinct and separate intracellular compartment.

The remaining portion of the sarcoplasmic reticulum surrounding a sarcomere interconnects the terminal cisternae (tc in Fig. 18-16) lying at each end of the sar-

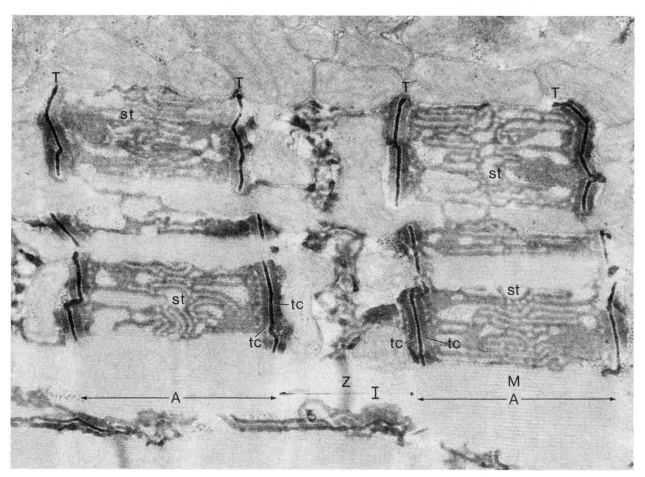

Fig. 18-18. Electron micrograph (×38,000) of part of a striated muscle fiber (mouse) postfixed in osmium-ferrocyanide, showing the layout of the sarcoplasmic reticulum around adjoining sarcomeres. Note that T tubules (T) are situated at the junctions of A and I bands in mammalian striated muscle. Terminal cisternae (tc) of the sarcoplasmic reticulum lie alongside the T tubules. The "torn sleeve" appearance of the sarcoplasmic reticulum is due to anastomosis of the sarcotubules (st) of the reticulum. Note also the fine filaments joining the thick filaments at the M lines of the sarcomeres. These are seen particularly well just above the label A at *bottom left.* (Forbes, M. S., Plantholt, B. A., and Sperelakis, N.: J. Ultrastruct. Res., *60:*306, 1977)

comere. It surrounds the more central region of the sarcomere like a lacy sleeve and consists of tubules called *sarcotubules* that are, for the most part, longitudinally arranged except in the midregion of the sarcomere (near the position indicated by sr in Fig. 18-16), where they anastomose freely to form a fenestrated collar. Figure 18-17 shows the parts of the reticulum in a mammalian fiber.

The sarcoplasmic reticulum of mammalian striated muscle fibers has not yet been described in such great detail. However, Forbes et al. recently demonstrated the general form of the sarcoplasmic reticulum very clearly by utilizing a selective cytochemical EM method. Furthermore, this procedure also demonstrates the way T tubules are associated with the reticulum. Fig. 18-18 shows the sarcoplasmic reticulum around contiguous sar-

comeres of myofibrils of mouse striated muscle. This tangential section was cut parallel to the surface of the myofibrils and shows not only sarcoplasmic reticulum but also the respective positions of T tubules (labeled T in Fig. 18-18) and triads in relation to A and I bands (also labeled in Fig. 18-18). The positions of the terminal cisternae (tc) and the complex of anastomosing sarcotubules (st) of the sarcoplasmic reticulum, the configuration of which resembles a torn sleeve, are also evident in this micrograph and, furthermore, the sarcotubules around A bands are clearly seen. Other planes of section also reveal sleeves of anastomosing sarcotubules around I bands and intervening Z lines, so that in mammalian fibers the terminal cisterna at either end of a sarcomere (and therefore not far from a Z line) is joined by sarcotubules to the

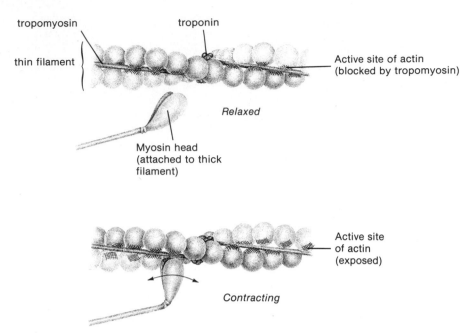

tropomyosin   troponin

thin filament {

Active site of actin
(blocked by tropomyosin)

Relaxed

Myosin head
(attached to thick
filament)

Active site
of actin
(exposed)

Contracting

Fig. 18-19. Diagrammatic representation of the structure of a thin filament of striated muscle at the molecular level, illustrating how in contraction the double head region of a myosin molecule of a thick filament (not shown) becomes able to interact with the actin molecules in the thin filament. As shown here, a thin filament comprises a double-stranded helix of G-actin molecules, with tropomyosin molecules (shown as rods) and units of troponin complex (shown in black) lying along the grooves between the strands. (*Top*) Note that the position of the tropomyosin molecules during relaxation is such that they block the active sites on the actin molecules so as to prevent myosin heads from interacting with them. (*Bottom*). The configuration of the troponin complex is altered by calcium ions during contraction. This in turn causes the tropomyosin molecules to move away from the active sites on the actin molecules so that these sites become exposed and able to interact with myosin heads of thick filaments.

neighboring terminal cisterna belonging to the adjoining sarcomere. Accordingly, in mammalian striated muscle fibers, collars of sarcoplasmic reticulum surrounding A bands alternate with collars surrounding I bands. The latter collars encircle the end regions of adjoining sarcomeres (Fig. 18-17).

It would be at triads that impulses for contraction would pass from T tubules to sarcoplasmic reticulum. It is interesting that at triads there are specialized junctions characterized by the presence of particulate structures between the membrane of the terminal cisterna and that of the T tubule (Franzini-Armstrong). However, the functional significance of these junctions (which can be seen in Fig. 18-16) is not clear. Their design, for instance, differs considerably from that of typical low-resistance pathways (gap junctions) and this raises the question of whether impulses are transmitted electrically from T tubules to the sarcoplasmic reticulum or by some other means.

How Contraction and Relaxation Are Controlled. The sarcoplasmic reticulum regulates muscular contraction by controlling the *concentration of calcium ions* within myofibrils and this in turn determines whether actin will interact with myosin. The principal integral membrane protein of the sarcoplasmic reticulum is the enzyme Ca^{++} $Mg^{++}ATPase$. During relaxation this enzyme, energized by ATP, pumps calcium ions out of myofibrils into the sarcoplasmic reticulum. Once within the sarcoplasmic reticulum, calcium ions are bound to certain proteins (one of which bears the appropriate name *calsequestrin,* from the L. *sequestrare,* to commit for sake keeping). These proteins are located on the inner surface of the membrane of the sarcoplasmic reticulum (MacLennan). When there is a low concentration of calcium ions in myofibrils, the active sites on actin molecules cannot interact with myosin because they are blocked by molecules of the regulatory protein tropomyosin (which is active in the absence of calcium ions). Since the concentration of calcium ions in myofibrils is low during relaxation, actin and myosin cannot interact with one another.

When a muscle fiber is stimulated to contract, however, calcium ions escape from the sarcoplasmic reticulum and immediately enter myofibrils, where they liberate actin molecules from their constraint in a manner to be described in a later section; this, of course, allows actin to interact with myosin. The link between conduction of a wave of depolarization into a muscle fiber and contraction of the fiber is sometimes referred to as *excitation-contraction coupling*.

THE MOLECULAR BASIS FOR MUSCLE CONTRACTION

The following section is intended as background information for those interested in the biochemical events in muscular contraction.

Thin Filaments. In addition to actin, thin filaments of striated muscle fibers contain two other proteins, *tropomyosin* and *troponin*. The manner in which molecules of these proteins fit together to form a thin filament is illustrated in Figure 18-19. Two rows of globular actin molecules are intertwined to form a double-stranded helix that constitutes the backbone of the thin filament (Fig. 18-19). There is thus a spiral groove along each side of the helix. Long, narrow tropomyosin molecules lie end to end in these grooves (Fig. 18-19), so that there are tropomyosin molecules lying along both sides of the helix. At regular intervals troponin molecules are bound to the tropomyosin molecules in the grooves. The name tropomyosin was coined because it was at first incorrectly believed that tropomyosin was a precursor of myosin. Later, however, it was discovered that tropomyosin had a different role — in conjunction with troponin, it plays a key role in *regulating interaction of actin with myosin* in a way that will be described later. Troponin was later found to be a complex of three subunits, each with its own role in regulating contraction.

Thick Filaments. These are composed of myosin molecules. A myosin molecule possesses a head and a long tail region and thus resembles a golf club in shape (Fig. 18-20). Its head region, which is actually a double structure, and the adjacent (proximal) portion of its tail, approximately 60 nm. in length, constitutes what is termed *heavy meromyosin* (Gr. *meros*, part) (Fig. 18-20). The remainder of the tail region (the handle and most of the shaft of the golf club), which totals about 90 nm. in length, constitutes its other part, called *light meromyosin*. As shown in Figure 18-20, a myosin molecule is flexible both at the junction of its heavy and light meromyosin portions and also at its neck region, allowing the double head and proximal tail portion to hinge on the rest of the molecule; the significance of this flexibility will become apparent in due course.

In a thick filament, myosin molecules are bundled together side by side as shown in Figure 18-21. Half of them have their heads toward one end of the filament and their tails toward the

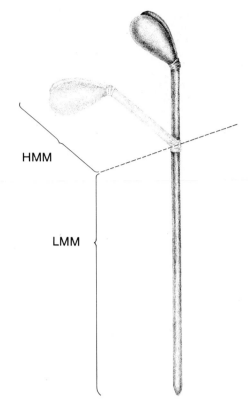

HMM

LMM

Fig. 18-20. Diagram illustrating how a myosin molecule changes in shape when it interacts with actin. The two subunits of a myosin molecule, heavy meromyosin (HMM) and light meromyosin (LMM), are also indicated. Bending at two hinge regions in the molecule permits movement of the double head region from its position during relaxation (indicated in solid lines) to another position (dotted) that allows it to interact with an actin molecule in an adjacent thin filament. The myosin head is believed to oscillate back and forth between these two positions with great rapidity, interacting with actin molecules one at a time and thereby helping to move the actin-containing filament along. Most of the tail region of the myosin molecule, corresponding more or less to light meromyosin, is embedded in a thick filament parallel with its longitudinal axis so as to support the oscillating head region.

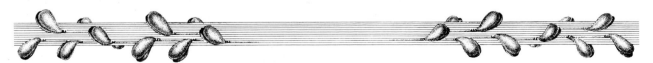

Fig. 18-21. Diagram of the middle of a thick filament of a striated muscle fiber, illustrating how its myosin molecules are arranged. The double head regions of the molecules are arranged in pairs, with each one of the pair on opposite sides of the filament. Note also the spiral arrangement of the heads (each pair being rotated in position with respect to the next) with the result that the heads come to lie in six longitudinal rows at intervals of 43 nm. along the filament. Due to the orientation of the myosin molecules, a bare region in the middle of the filament is devoid of myosin heads; it consists entirely of tail regions of the molecules.

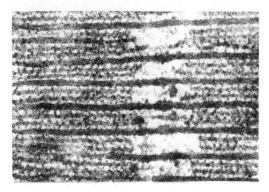

Fig. 18-22. Electron micrograph (×150,000) of part of a sarcomere of striated muscle (rabbit psoas), showing cross bridges on the thick filaments. (Courtesy of H. E. Huxley)

other; the other half have the reverse arrangement, with their heads toward the other end of the filament (and their tails pointing in the opposite direction). This arrangement of the myosin heads is important because it explains why the two sets of thin filaments in a sarcomere are pulled in *opposite directions.* Moreover, the myosin molecules are staggered so that their heads lie at regular intervals along thick filaments (Fig. 18-21) except in their middles (in the general region of the M line), where there are no heads. Hence the midsection of a thick filament consists entirely of tail regions of myosin molecules, the heads of which point toward the two ends of the filament (Fig. 18-21).

With the EM, heads of myosin molecules can just be seen on thick filaments as what have been termed *cross bridges* (Fig. 18-22) because, as we shall see, they repeatedly bridge the gaps between thick and thin filaments during contraction. The myosin heads are arranged helically so as to form six longitudinal rows along the filament (Fig. 18-21). Each rows of heads is thus perfectly aligned with one of the six thin filaments seen in cross sections to form a hexagon around each thick filament (Fig. 18-8, *second* of the *lower* four micrographs). Under conditions discussed below, the myosin heads associate with actin molecules in the adjacent thin filament during contraction.

The Intermolecular Reactions in Contraction

First, the role of troponin in thin filaments will be described. As noted, units of troponin complex are interposed between tropomyosin molecules at regular intervals (every 40 nm.) along the grooves between the double strands of actin, as shown in Figure 18-19. The troponin complex and tropomyosin molecules cooperate to form a molecular locking device that during relaxation *prevents* actin molecules from interacting with myosin heads on adjacent thick filaments. The actin in thin filaments can only be "unlocked" by *calcium ions,* which are liberated from the sarcoplasmic reticulum on arrival of an impulse (depolarization) along the T tubules. When the muscle fiber is not being stimulated to contract, calcium ions are quickly withdrawn from myofibrils into the sarcoplasmic reticulum so that their concentration falls below the minimum required to "unlock" actin; the contraction process therefore abruptly ceases. The mechanism

by which calcium ions "unlock" actin involves their binding to one kind of troponin. This causes a change in configuration of the troponin complex and in turn moves the tropomyosin molecules so as to expose the active sites on the actin molecules involved in interacting with myosin heads, as shown in Figure 18-19B. Cohen's paper may be consulted for further details about the troponin complex.

It is generally conceded that for contraction to occur myosin heads on the thick filaments must swivel on their tails and serially connect and then disconnect with actin molecules along the thin filaments, thereby moving the thin filaments along the thick ones. While there is evidence that myosin heads change their position during contraction, the precise way in which contractile force is generated by this occurring is still unknown.

The Role of ATP. The energy required to power muscular contraction is derived from ATP, the energy "currency" of the cell. This is hydrolyzed due to ATPase activity of the myosin heads. The manner in which energy released by hydrolysis from ATP is utilized in contraction is not well understood. It is presumably applied to bending myosin molecules at their hinge regions, so that the myosin heads change their position and move the thin filaments to which they attach along the thick ones.

Studies with soluble actin and myosin by Murray and Webber show that head regions of myosin molecules develop a high affinity for actin when they bind ATP. Furthermore, ATP is hydrolyzed extremely rapidly as soon as myosin heads bind to actin molecules. Since the complex of all three components (actin, myosin, and ATP) is not stable, it dissociates rapidly into (*1*) actin and (*2*) myosin-ATP; this is what may bring about *detachment of cross bridges* just at the moment when further molecules of ATP are bound to myosin heads. Hence initial binding of as yet unsplit ATP molecules to myosin heads may be the event that initiates each cycle of operation. This cycle would involve four further stages. First, a myosin head would disconnect from an actin molecule. Next, the head would shift to its new position at the other extreme of its range of movement (as shown in Fig. 18-20). Here it would attach to another actin molecule a little farther along the thin filament and then, using energy liberated from ATP, shift back to its original position, thereby moving the thin filament to which it was temporarily attached. It has been calculated that this whole cycle of operation would have to be repeated at the astonishing rate of 50 to 100 times per second.

An interesting corollary to the way ATP is used for contraction is that after death, when generation of ATP ceases, no ATP remains to dissociate myosin from actin in the muscles and so these proteins remain permanently complexed in the form of actomyosin. Accordingly, for several hours after death, the filaments of muscles are seized up and locked together in a fixed position. This state, called *rigor mortis* (L. meaning rigidity of death), persists until the muscles can be stretched passively after autolysis has set in.

When a muscle fiber is being stimulated it remains contracted as long as impulses keep arriving at the motor end plate. When the impulses cease or the energy reserves of the muscle fiber have become exhausted, the fiber relaxes. In the former case, relaxation is brought about by removal of calcium ions by the sarcoplasmic reticulum until they reach a low concentration in the myofibrils. The energy for pumping calcium ions out of the myofibrils into the sarcoplasmic reticulum is again provided by ATP. Hence ATP plays a role not only in contraction but also in relaxation.

The energy for *resynthesis* of ATP can be derived from the breakdown of glucose, glycogen, or free fatty acids. ATP can also be rapidly resynthesized during exercise by combination of ADP with phosphate groups from another high-energy com-

Fig. 18-23. Electron micrograph
(×22,000) of a satellite cell (*middle*), adjacent to a striated muscle fiber (*lower
right*) and enclosed by the same basal
lamina (BM). The myofibrils (A) of the
muscle fiber at *lower right* are cut in
cross section through an A band and
hence show both thick and thin filaments. A thin portion of fibroblast cytoplasm (F), a component of the endomysium, lies in the space between the
satellite cell and the other muscle fiber at
upper left. The nucleus of the satellite
cell is labeled N. (Courtesy of E.
Schultz)

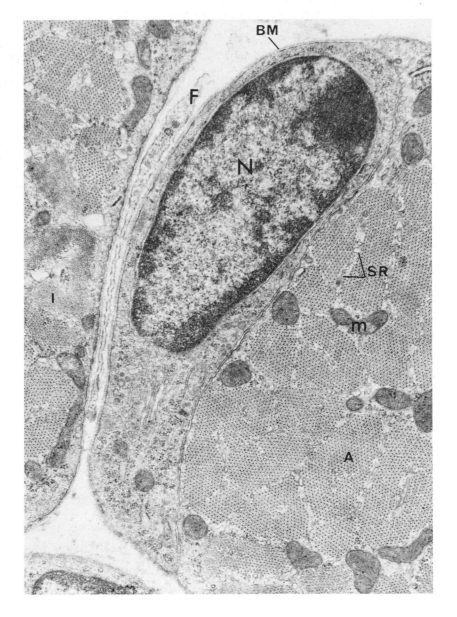

pound, *phosphocreatinine,* which in turn is reconstituted during
relaxation. This use of phosphocreatinine as an intermediary
may be likened to having additional currency of another denomi-
nation in the bank ready for a time of need. Whereas the efficient
way of producing ATP from glucose or glycogen is through oxidative phosphorylation, some energy can also be liberated in the
absence of oxygen, with the production of lactate and pyruvate
as metabolites. This latter pathway is an important alternative
during sustained exercise, when the oxygen supply may become
inadequate to permit continued oxidative phosphorylation.
Moreover, the various types of fibers differ with regard to which
pathway predominates. Thus oxidative phosphorylation is more
prevalent in red fibers, which have abundant mitochondria, and
anaerobic glycolysis is more important in white fibers.

THE DEVELOPMENT, GROWTH, REGENERATION, AND MAINTENANCE OF STRIATED MUSCLE FIBERS

The cells forming striated muscle fibers in the embryo
are called myoblasts. After repeated proliferation these
cells, which have a single nucleus and lack myofibrils,
commence to fuse with one another so as to form elongated multinucleated cylindrical structures known as
myotubes, which in due course develop myofibrils and
other organelles characteristic of striated muscle fibers.

Most striated muscle fibers develop before birth in hu-

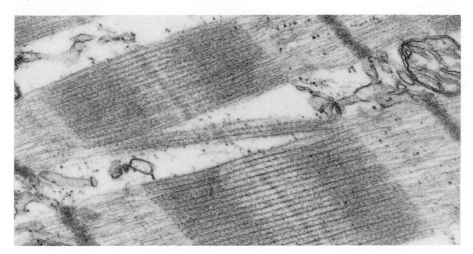

Fig. 18-24. Electron micrograph (×43,000) of part of a striated muscle fiber from a growing animal, close to a tendon. At *center* there is evidence that some filaments cross from one myofibril to another. This would be expected in regions where myofibrils had reached their maximal diameter and so were splitting longitudinally to form more myofibrils. (Courtesy of T. Harrop)

mans and virtually all are formed by the end of the first postnatal year, during which their numbers in a given muscle increase only slightly. In animals such as rats, however, the number of fibers can double in certain muscles during the postnatal growth period. The number of nuclei in each fiber also increases postnatally. The additional nuclei are derived by muscle fibers fusing with small uninucleated cells that seem to represent myoblasts left over from embryonic development. These are termed *satellite cells* and lie beside muscle fibers, enclosed within their basal lamina (Fig. 18-23). In studying satellite cells, Moss and Leblond found that tritiated thymidine became incorporated into their nucleus within 1 hour of injection into growing rats but none could be found at this time in nuclei of striated muscle fibers. A day later, however, the label was found in some myonuclei as well as in satellite cells, suggesting that labeled nuclei of former satellite cells had now become incorporated into these fibers.

The Growth of Skeletal Muscles

During the postnatal growth period, muscles have to increase in length and width in order to keep pace with growth of the skeleton. Their ultimate size depends on the amount of exercise obtained and much effort is often expended in achieving the desired results. All growth of striated muscles after the first year of life is due to *enlargement* of striated muscle fibers, which is termed *hypertrophy* (Gr. *hyper,* over; *trophe,* nourishment), and not due to *increase of numbers* of fibers, that is, *hyperplasia* (Gr. *plasis,* molding). We first describe how muscle fibers grow in width.

Growth in Width. Samples of skeletal muscles obtained at different times during postnatal growth show an increase in the number of myofibrils in each fiber. As the fibers grow, protein molecules for new filaments, synthesized on ribosomes in the sarcoplasm, become assembled onto the outer surface of existing myofibrils where there are in contact with the sarcoplasm. As growing myofibrils approach their maximum diameter, they appear to split longitudinally (Fig. 18-24) to create more myofibrils. Thus, striated muscle fibers grow in width by increasing the number of myofibrils (and other organelles) they contain.

Growth in Length. Fusion with satellite cells lengthens striated muscle fibers. Furthermore, the myofibrils of striated fibers can increase in length in post-natal life by having new sarcomeres built onto their ends at sites where the ends of the fibers attach to dense connective tissue. Thus, in growing animals the terminal sarcomeres of myofibrils show a relatively scanty content of filaments (Fig. 18-25) and numerous free ribosomes are seen in the sarcoplasm, indicating that it is at these sites that additional filament proteins are synthesized and newly synthesized filaments are assembled into new sarcomeres. The infoldings of the sarcolemma seen where connective tissue fibers attach to the ends of muscle fibers moreover appear to delimit the diameter of new sarcomeres being assembled at the ends of the fibers (Fig. 18-25).

Regeneration

In addition to providing a mechanism for striated muscle fibers to grow, satellite cells persist throughout adult life as a potential source of new myoblasts capable of fusing to form totally new muscle fibers. Thus satellite cells can divide to give rise to myoblasts following muscle trauma and in certain dystrophic conditions where there is an attempt at regenerating new fibers. This appears to be the only mechanism for regeneration of mammalian

Fig. 18-25. Electron micrograph (×25,900) showing a junction of a muscle with a tendon in a growing rat. Where the muscle fiber at *right* tapers toward the tendon at *left* the sarcolemma forms deep folds. In this region thin filaments are attached to the cytoplasmic surface of the sarcolemma and, outside the sarcolemma, collagen fibrils penetrate deeply into the invaginations and attach to the basal lamina. (Mackey, B., Harrop, T. J., and Muir, A. R.: Acta Anat., *73:*588, 1969)

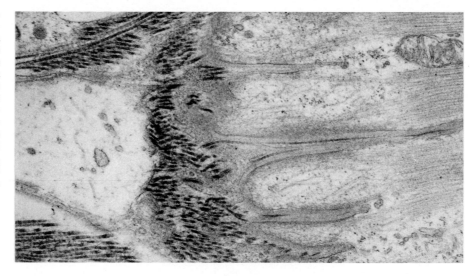

striated muscle fibers because myonuclei do not divide once incorporated into muscle fibers. Any large muscle defects due to severe trauma, however, become filled with fibrous scar tissue laid down by fibroblasts.

Maintenance

Striated muscle fibers require their motor nerve supply not only to elicit contraction but also for their general health and welfare. Loss of efferent innervation greatly increases their sensitivity to acetylcholine and can lead to their degeneration or atrophy.

Cross reinnervation experiments show that when white muscle fibers (faster contracting) are artificially supplied with motor nerves formerly supplying red fibers (slower to contract), they contract more slowly, like red fibers. Conversely, red fibers contract like white ones when supplied with motor fibers formerly supplying white fibers. This shows that the physiological characteristics of muscle fibers also are dependent on their efferent innervation.

Motor neurons are therefore said to exert a continuous *trophic influence* on the muscle fibers they innervate. Without this influence, which may turn out to be no more than the secretion of a steady supply of a neurotrophic factor from the terminals of motor axons, striated muscle fibers undergo degenerative changes. Some hold the view that at least some forms of *muscular dystrophy* (Gr. *dys,* bad or difficult), conditions characterized by atrophic changes in individual muscle fibers, may be the result of an inadequate supply of, or diminished responsiveness to, neurotrophic factors. However, this hypothesis is by no means the only one advanced to explain muscular dystrophy.

THE AFFERENT INNERVATION OF SKELETAL MUSCLES, TENDONS, AND SYNOVIAL JOINTS

Skeletal muscles have not only a motor (efferent) nerve supply but also an afferent one, by means of which they signal their degree of contraction to the CNS. This information is integrated in the CNS with afferent impulses from tendons, ligaments, and joint capsules, and gives an awareness of the positions and rates of movement of the various parts of the body that enables us to tell what positions our bodies and limbs are in, even when we cannot see, touch, or hear anything. The sensory receptors that send these afferent impulses are the *muscle spindles, tendon organs,* and *joint receptors.* Each of these will now be described in turn.

Muscle Spindles (Neuromuscular Spindles)

These are the length-registering receptors of muscles. They participate in several control mechanisms, the simplest of which are called *stretch reflexes* because they are responses to stretch in muscles. A familiar example is the *knee jerk* elicited by striking the patellar tendon so as to stretch the quadriceps femoris muscle. Reflex contraction of this muscle promptly makes the foot on the same side kick forward (Fig. 17-5, p. 486). However, before explaining how muscle spindles participate in this type of reflex, we must describe their structure and innervation.

The Structure of Muscle Spindles. A muscle spindle is fusiform in shape, 3 to 5 mm. long and about 0.2 mm. wide at its middle, and, as can be seen from Figures 18-26 and 18-27B, it is almost entirely enclosed by an extensible *capsule* of connective tissue (C in Fig. 18-27). Spindles lie longitudinally in muscles and are incorporated in

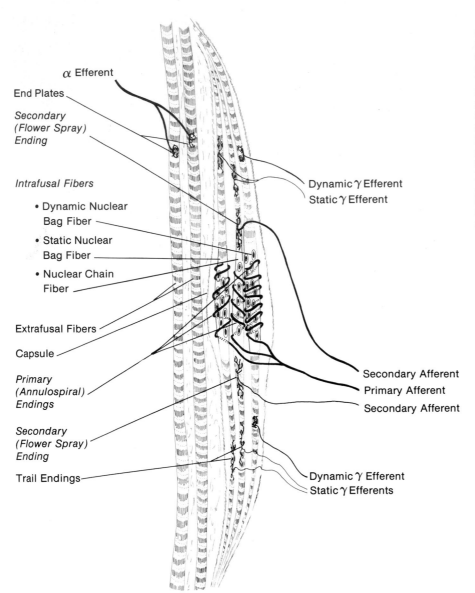

α Efferent

End Plates

*Secondary
(Flower Spray)
Ending*

Intrafusal Fibers

• Dynamic Nuclear
  Bag Fiber

• Static Nuclear
  Bag Fiber

• Nuclear Chain
  Fiber

Extrafusal Fibers

Capsule

*Primary
(Annulospiral)
Endings*

*Secondary
(Flower Spray)
Ending*

Trail Endings

Dynamic γ Efferent
Static γ Efferent

Secondary Afferent
Primary Afferent
Secondary Afferent

Dynamic γ Efferent
Static γ Efferents

Fig. 18-26. Schematic diagram of a muscle spindle, illustrating the innervation of the nuclear bag and nuclear chain fibers, as determined from muscles of the cat. There are up to 12 intrafusal fibers (with up to 10 of these being of the nuclear chain type); only two nuclear bag fibers and one nuclear chain fiber are shown here for clarity. The afferent fibers supplying the spindle are classified as follows: primary afferents, group IA; secondary afferents, group II. *See* text for further details. The β-innervation has been omitted and the diameter of the spindle was expanded in order to show details.

such a way as to be stretched when the muscle, as a whole, becomes stretched. They are scattered throughout the muscle and are most numerous in muscles requiring fine control. Each spindle contains from 2 to 12 muscle fibers that are narrower and different from ordinary striated muscle fibers, and accordingly are termed *intrafusal fibers* (L. *fusus,* spindle) to distinguish them from the *extrafusal fibers* outside the spindle. The intrafusal fibers are bathed in the tissue fluid occupying the expanded midsection of the spindle (Figs. 18-26 and 18-27B, labeled S).

There are two microscopically distinguishable types of

intrafusal fibers. The larger ones, for reasons that will soon be apparent, are called *nuclear bag fibers* and there are usually 1 to 4 such fibers in a spindle. The smaller *nuclear chain fibers* are more numerous; there are up to 10 of these in a spindle. Nuclear bag fibers are both wider and longer than nuclear chain fibers (Figs. 18-26 and 18-27; compare nb with nc in Fig. 18-27B). They are called *nuclear bag fibers* because their mid portions are expanded into noncontractile regions containing so many nuclei packed closely together that they literally look like bags of nuclei. Fibers of this type may be long enough to project beyond the ends of the capsule (Fig. 18-26).

Fig. 18-27. Photomicrographs illustrating the structure and innervation of a muscle spindle (cat). (*A*) Part of a spindle teased from a soleus muscle (stained with gold chloride), showing primary (annulospiral) afferent endings at *right* and secondary (flower spray) afferent endings at *left*. The primary endings are supplied by branches of a group IA afferent fiber (*top right*) and the secondary endings are supplied by a group II afferent fiber (*top center*). The top and bottom intrafusal fibers (nb) are of the nuclear bag type; closely packed nuclei (n) may be discerned beneath the primary ending in the top nuclear bag fiber. Between the two nuclear bag fibers lie four smaller nuclear chain fibers. (*B*) Transverse section of adductor digiti longus muscle (stained H and E) showing a muscle spindle sectioned through its midregion. Like the one above, this spindle contains two large nuclear bag fibers (nb) and four smaller nuclear chain fibers (nc). Note the smaller diameter of intrafusal compared with extrafusal fibers (ef). The connective tissue capsule (C) of the muscle spindle with its central fluid-filled space (S) is also evident. (Boyd, I. A.: Philos. Trans. R. Soc. Lond. [Biol. Sci], *245*:81, 1962)

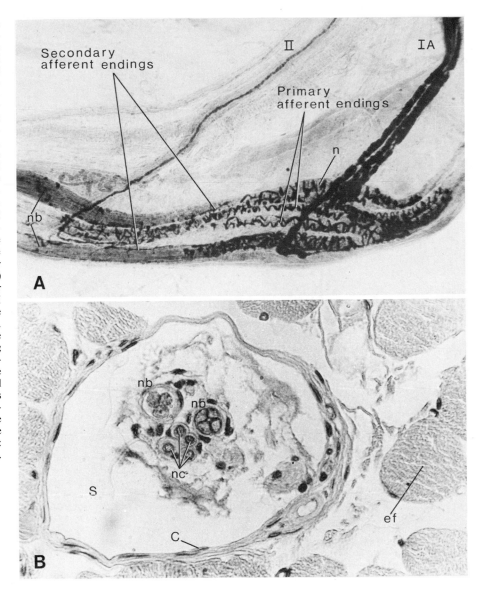

Nuclear chain fibers are narrower and shorter and do not have expansions in their middle regions, and their nuclei are all lined up in a single row resembling a chain (Figs. 18-26 and 18-27B, labeled nc).

For those interested in more details, the afferent and efferent innervation of the intrafusal fibers will now be described.

The Afferent Innervation of Nuclear Bag Fibers. Each nuclear bag fiber receives a terminal branch of a large myelinated sensory fiber (*primary afferent* in Fig. 18-26). As can be seen in Fig. 18-27A, the afferent ending of this group IA fiber winds around the nuclear bag more or less spirally and hence is sometimes called an *annulospiral ending*; however, in man it is not as spiral

as in other vertebrates and it is now more common to call it a *primary ending.*

The Afferent Innervation of Nuclear Chain Fibers. Unlike nuclear bag fibers, nuclear chain fibers receive afferent innervation from *two* sources. First, branches of the same large sensory fiber (*primary afferent* in Fig. 18-26) that terminates in primary endings in nuclear bag fibers form similar primary endings in the central regions of nuclear chain fibers. Second, branches of smaller and separate afferent fibers (*secondary afferent* in Fig. 18-26; II in Fig. 18-27) terminate in *secondary (flower-spray)* endings, one on each side of the primary ending. Thus, nuclear chain fibers are supplied with both primary and secondary afferent endings.

The primary ending responds to both degree and rate of stretch of a muscle, while the secondary endings respond only to

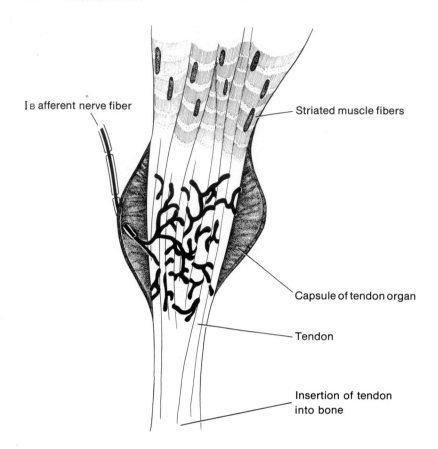

I B afferent nerve fiber

Striated muscle fibers

Capsule of tendon organ

Tendon

Insertion of tendon into bone

Fig. 18-28. Diagram of a tendon organ with its connective tissue capsule cut open and reflexed so as to reveal its innervation. The large myelinated afferent fiber (group IB) that supplies the organ terminates in numerous unmyelinated branches ramifying between the collagenic bundles of the tendon. These bundles are narrower and less closely packed in the region of the tendon organ than elsewhere in the tendon.

degree of stretch. The ways in which impulses from the two kinds of afferent endings participate in different reflexes are complex. Stretching afferent endings, for example by tapping a patellar tendon, initiates impulses that travel up afferent fibers to the spinal cord (as shown in Fig. 17-5), where afferent neurons synapse with large α motor neurons supplying numbers of ordinary (extrafusal) fibers in the muscle involved. The motor neurons thereupon elicit contraction of the extrafusal fibers they innervate so that the stretch reflex is completed. Stimulation of afferent endings ceases when tension in intrafusal fibers is unloaded by contraction of extrafusal fibers with which they are in parallel. The afferent neurons synapse in the spinal cord not only with efferent neurons of the same segment but also with intersegmental connector neurons that conduct impulses to parts of the brain concerned with muscular coordination.

The Efferent Innervation of Intrafusal Fibers. Intrafusal fibers, like extrafusal fibers, also have an *efferent* nerve supply. The purpose of this, however, is not to provide further contractile power for the muscle as a whole, but to cause the intrafusal fibers to contract and thereby increase their response at any given muscle length. Small motor fibers (*dynamic and static γ efferents* in Fig. 18-26) from γ motor neurons supply the contractile ends of intrafusal fibers. In cat muscle spindles studied by Boyd's group, nuclear bag fibers may receive either dynamic γ fibers or static γ fibers. There are thus two functionally different types of nuclear bag fibers. Nuclear chain fibers, however, all receive static γ fibers. As shown in Figure 18-26, γ fibers terminate in either multiple *en grappe* (Fr. *grappe,* cluster) *endings* or in more extensive *trail endings* on contractile portions of intrafusal

fibers. Efferent impulses from the γ motor neurons elicit contraction in these regions so as to stretch the afferent endings still further and this increases their response at any given muscle length. Some of the nuclear bag fibers also receive β efferent fibers (not shown in Fig. 18-26).

It will be appreciated from the foregoing that both degree and velocity of stretch of muscles are automatically monitored by muscle spindles, which operate by signalling to the CNS any temporary discrepancies that might exist between the length of intrafusal fibers and the length of the muscle as a whole. Misalignment signals are used to moderate contraction in the extrafusal fibers of the muscles concerned. This constitutes a servocontrol mechanism that has been likened to power-assisted steering of motor vehicles, in which misalignment between steering wheel and road wheel positions is measured and applied toward turning the road wheels in the desired direction. Muscle spindles, together with other afferent endings sensitive to tendon tension and joint position and motion, comprise a group of receptors called *proprioceptors* (L. *proprius,* own; *capio,* to take) that are involved in controlling motion and posture. The other types of proprioceptors will next be considered briefly.

Fig. 18-29. Low-power photomicrograph of cardiac muscle (sheep). Note how cardiac muscle fibers branch and anastomose with one another. The light-staining slit-like spaces between them are filled with endomysium conveying blood (and lymph) capillaries.

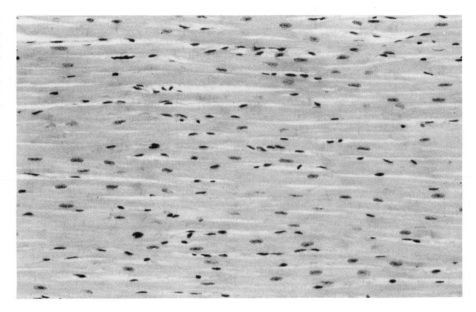

Tendon Organs

Also referred to as *Golgi tendon organs* or *neurotendinous organs,* these receptors are found at the junctions of muscles with their tendons and in aponeuroses (on which muscles pull). They are encapsulated structures about the same size as muscle spindles. As shown in Figure 18-28, the large myelinated afferent fiber supplying a tendon organ has small nonmyelinated branches that ramify within the tendon organ between the collagenic bundles of the tendon. Unlike muscle spindles, tendon organs lack efferent innervation. The afferent endings are probably stimulated by being compressed between the collagenic bundles when the tendon is under tension, since they respond to tension in muscles with which they are in series.

Joint Receptors

We have several types of sensory receptors in our joints. Internal and external joint ligaments, for example, possess receptors closely resembling tendon organs. The connective tissue capsules of joints contain numerous free nerve endings and Ruffini-type and paciniform corpuscles (described in Chap. 20, p. 642). Paciniform corpuscles (mechanoreceptors) present in synovial joints are positioned at sites compressed by joint movement. Together with muscle spindles and tendon organs they play an important role in *kinesthesia* (Gr. *kinesis,* motion; *aisthesis,* perception), that is, conscious perception of position and movement of the various parts of the body. It may be of interest to the medical student that kinesthetic sensation in the hip joint, for instance, is not lost after

total surgical replacement of the joint and remains virtually unimpaired even if the patient is given a ball-and-socket prosthesis. Since the majority of joint receptors would be totally incapacitated or removed by the surgical procedures employed, the importance of muscle spindles and tendon organs in maintaining awareness of limb position can be readily appreciated.

CARDIAC MUSCLE

Before the advent of the EM it was believed that cardiac muscle comprised a branching network of fibers that had no ends and hence represented a continuous multinucleated network of cytoplasm, which sort of arrangement is called a *syncytium* (Gr. *syn,* together). The LM appearance that gave this erroneous impression is seen in Figure 18-29, which shows that in cardiac muscle the structures called *fibers* branch and anastomose extensively so as to leave slit-like spaces between them. The EM, however, showed that cardiac muscle fibers were composed of individual cells joined end to end by cell junctions. The slit-like spaces between anastomosing fibers contain endomysium that carries capillaries and lymphatics close to the muscle fibers.

Microscopic Structure as Seen With the LM

With the LM it was found that cardiac muscle fibers possessed cross striations like those described in striated muscle and, furthermore, that they were crossed every so often by unique, darkly staining bands (marked with arrows in Fig. 18-30) wider than Z lines and called *in-*

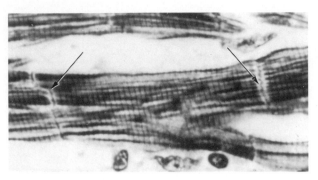

Fig. 18-30. Photomicrograph of a longitudinal section of a cardiac muscle fiber (stained with tannic and phosphomolybdic acids and amido black to demonstrate its cross striations). Cardiac muscle cell boundaries take the form of intercalated disks (indicated by arrows). These may pass straight across the fiber as on the *right,* or in a stepwise manner as on the *left.* Note the branching of the fiber. (Courtesy of Y. Clermont)

tercalated (L. *intercalatus,* to insert between) *disks.* While sometimes pursuing a straight course across a fiber (as at *right* in Fig. 18-30), these commonly cross it in a step-like fashion (as at *left* in Fig. 18-30 and in Fig. 18-31, *inset*). As explained in due course, the EM revealed that intercalated disks represent boundaries between individual cells in cardiac muscle. Thus it became clear that car-

diac muscle was not a syncytium but consisted, like the two other types of muscle, of discrete cells — with the difference, however, that the cells of cardiac muscle were joined end to end by cell junctions so as to form a network of cells. So the term *fiber* when used with regard to cardiac muscle refers not to a single cell but to what we now know represents a *chain of cells* joined together end to end. Whereas individual cardiac muscle cells are too short and thick to be considered thread-like, several such cells joined end to end would satisfy the definition of a fiber. However, since contiguous cells are commonly joined together in an irregular manner, as shown in Figure 18-30, cardiac muscle fibers appear to anastomose repeatedly with one another.

The individual cells in cardiac muscle fibers generally have a single nucleus but sometimes there are two. The nucleus is somewhat larger and paler than those of striated muscle fibers and generally it lies toward the middle of the fiber (Fig. 18-32). This helps in distinguishing cardiac from striated muscle, as does the fact that cardiac muscle fibers have the appearance of branching and anastomosing with one another.

Although cardiac muscle is striated, its rhythmic contraction is not under the control of the will; hence cardiac muscle is classed as *involuntary.* Cardiac muscle will contract spontaneously without any nerve supply whatsoever, but only at less than half its normal rate of contrac-

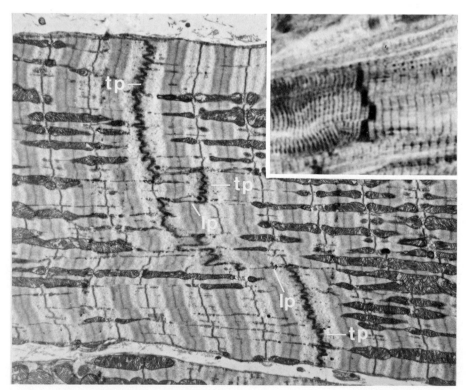

Fig. 18-31. Electron micrograph (×5,100) of an intercalated disk in ventricular heart muscle (dog). Note that this disk crosses the fiber in a stepwise fashion. Each transverse portion (tp) of the disk, which lies at the level of a Z line, is characterized by expanded desmosome-like junctions together with scattered small gap junctions. The longitudinal portions (lp) of the disk contain extensive gap junctions. (*Inset*) Photomicrograph (×1,000) of a comparable intercalated disk from the same source. Note the stepwise course this disk takes across the fiber. (Courtesy of A. Spiro)

tion. The heartbeat is regulated in a certain part of the heart, known as the *pacemaker,* composed of special cardiac muscle cells innervated by fibers of the autonomic nervous system. From the pacemaker, ordinary heart muscle fibers and a system of muscle fibers designed more for conduction than contraction function together to conduct impulses throughout the heart, with the result that the atria and (slightly later) the ventricles beat in a synchronized manner (as will be described in Chap. 19 in which we deal with the heart as an organ).

The Fine Structure of Cardiac Muscle Fibers

In many important respects the fine structure of cardiac muscle resembles that of skeletal muscle. The fibers of cardiac muscle are made up largely of myofibrils, between which there is sarcoplasm containing a great many mitochondria. However, as can be seen in Figures 18-33 and 18-34, myofibrils of cardiac muscle (m in Fig. 18-34) anastomose freely to form a continuous arrangement instead of being discrete cylindrical structures like those of striated muscle. Furthermore, as is evident in Figure 18-31, their cross striations are not always in perfect register with one another across the fiber. Mitochondria are abundant (as can be seen in Figs. 18-31, 18-33, and 18-34), reflecting the considerable energy requirements of cardiac muscle. Granules of glycogen are commonly present in the sarcoplasm in between the mitochondria. Moreover, mitochondria and glycogen are also present together with Golgi saccules and lipid droplets in the sarcoplasm at the poles of the nucleus (Fig. 18-33). In the atria (but not the ventricles) the sarcoplasm at the ends of the nucleus also contains secretory granules (300 to 400 nm. in diameter) that originate from the Golgi (Fig. 18-

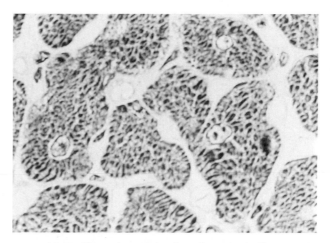

Fig. 18-32. Photomicrograph of cardiac muscle fibers cut in transverse section. The nuclei lie more or less centrally in the fibers and myofibrils are clearly visible due to the sarcoplasm between them being only very lightly stained.

33). The functional significance of these granules has not been established but there is some indication that they may contain catecholamines. Deposits of the lipochrome pigment *lipofuscin* are also common at the poles of the nucleus, particularly in older individuals.

The Fine Structure of Intercalated Disks

When intercalated disks were studied with the EM they were found to be sites where cell membranes at the ends of adjoining cardiac muscle cells interdigitated very extensively with one another and were joined by some sort

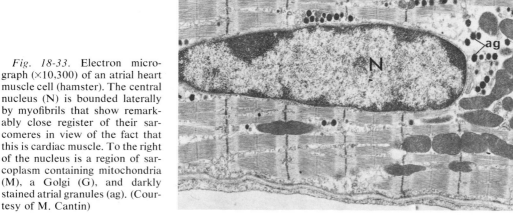

Fig. 18-33. Electron micrograph (×10,300) of an atrial heart muscle cell (hamster). The central nucleus (N) is bounded laterally by myofibrils that show remarkably close register of their sarcomeres in view of the fact that this is cardiac muscle. To the right of the nucleus is a region of sarcoplasm containing mitochondria (M), a Golgi (G), and darkly stained atrial granules (ag). (Courtesy of M. Cantin)

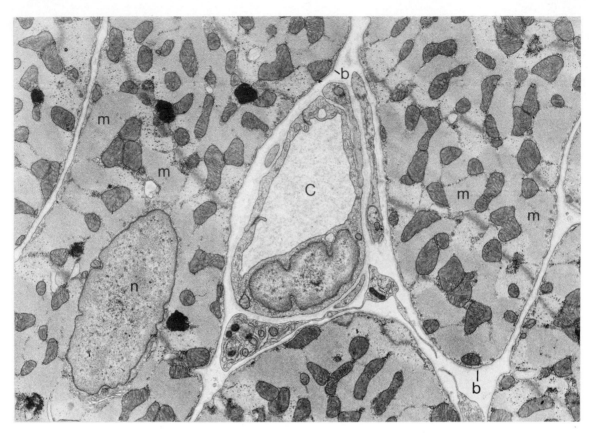

Fig. 18-34. Electron micrograph (low-power) of a transverse section of ventricular papillary muscle (cat) showing cardiac muscle fibers in cross section. The myofibrils (m) have irregular contours in cross section due to anastomosis of the myofibrils. Their filaments are just visible as closely packed dots. Note the abundant mitochondria between myofibrils, the central nucleus (n) in the fiber at *left,* and the basal lamina (b) surrounding the fibers. A blood capillary (C) lies in the endomysium at *center.* (Bloom, W., and Fawcett, D. W.: Textbook of Histology. Philadelphia, W. B. Saunders, 1975)

of junctional complex. At intercalated disks that cross fibers in a stepwise manner, relatively large projections on the end of one cell fit into equally large depressions in the adjoining cell (as shown at *left* in Fig. 18-35A). In addition, smaller papilla-like projections (with the corresponding smaller depressions into which they fit) are associated with all intercalated disks, whether they cross the fiber in a stepwise fashion or not; these smaller projections are shown in Figure 18-35B. Both large and small interdigitations are presumably necessary to ensure satisfactory adhesion between the ends of the adjoining cells (otherwise repeated contractions might eventually pull the cells apart). To further aid this adhesion, the membranes at the ends of adjacent cells are joined by a special sort of junctional complex, which we shall now describe.

As can be seen from Figures 18-31 and 18-35, intercalated disks that run a stepwise course across a fiber consist of *transverse portions* (crossing the fiber at right angles to its longitudinal axis at the level of Z lines) and *longitudinal portions* (lying parallel to the long axis of the fiber). Two different types of cell junctions have been observed in the transverse portions of such intercalated disks. First, there are abundant cell junctions of the *fascia adherens* type; these are of the nature of expanded desmosomes. This type of junction is associated with dense material on the inner surface of the cell membrane, thought to provide anchorage for the thin filaments and at the same time provide a site of particularly strong adhesion to help prevent separation of adjoining muscle cells when they contract. Second, there are scattered small *gap junctions* believed to permit rapid conduction of impulses for contraction from each cell to the next. However, larger gap junctions (Fig. 18-36) are common in the longitudinal portions of step-shaped intercalated disks and these are believed to play the principal role in conducting impulses through ordinary heart muscle. Unlike the adherens type of junction, gap junctions are not attached to

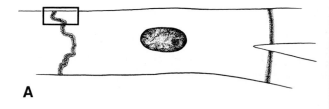

A

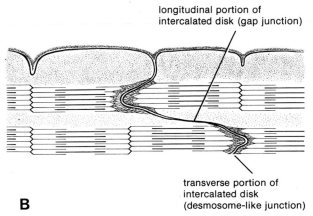

longitudinal portion of
intercalated disk (gap junction)

transverse portion of
intercalated disk
(desmosome-like junction)

B

Fig. 18-35. (*A*) Diagram of a component cell of a cardiac muscle fiber. This cell interdigitates with the one on its left, so the intercalated disk between the two crosses the fiber in a stepwise manner. (*B*) Diagram showing the area indicated above in the detail that would be seen with the EM. The transverse portions of the intercalated disks consist predominantly of expanded desmosome-like junctions but also contain a few small gap junctions. The longitudinal portions of the disks have extensive gap junctions. Note that the transverse portions of the disks are situated at the level of Z lines and that the thin filaments of the I bands insert into a filamentous network associated with the desmosome-like junctions.

any filaments. Thus, the fine structure of the intercalated disk indicates that it serves a mechanical function in holding cardiac muscle cells together and transmitting their pull and yet permits electrical communication from one cell to another by allowing direct exchange of ions through gap junctions.

The Sarcoplasmic Reticulum and T Tubules

The sarcoplasmic reticulum is less well developed in cardiac muscle cells than in striated muscle cells and lacks large terminal cisternae. It consists of an irregular system of narrow tubular cisternae (Sr in Fig. 18-37) that, as in striated muscle, surround each myofibril (Fig. 18-37).

In mammalian cardiac muscle cells the T tubules enter at the level of Z lines, so that, as in amphibian striated

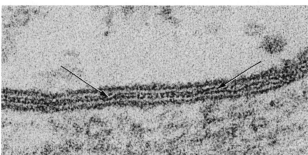

Fig. 18-36. Electron micrograph (×200,000) of a gap junction (located between the arrows) in an intercalated disk between cardiac muscle cells (mouse). (Courtesy of N. McNutt)

muscle, the number of levels at which T tubules enter corresponds to the number of sarcomeres in a myofibril. The T tubules are more than twice as wide as those of striated fibers and also differ in being lined with basal lamina continuous with the basal lamina external to the sarcolemma. Triads are not evident because the cisternae of sarcoplasmic reticulum that make contact with T tubules of cardiac muscle cells are small and do not form continuous rings around myofibrils. The T tubules of cardiac muscle are thought to conduct impulses for contraction into the cell interior (as described on p. 552) so as to facilitate stimulation of contraction in the myofibrils.

The Growth and Regenerative Capacity of Cardiac Muscle

Heart muscle responds to increased demands by increase of the size of its existing fibers, that is, by compensatory *hypertrophy*. It is generally believed that cardiac muscle cells have no capacity for mitosis in postnatal life. Moreover, they lack the satellite cells responsible for regeneration in striated muscle. Nevertheless there are reports that a few poorly differentiated cardiac muscle cells may form in experimentally traumatized hearts of animals (Polezhaev). This new potential muscle tissue, however, quickly becomes replaced by connective tissue scars. Due to the obvious difficulty in studying regeneration of human heart muscle, it is not known whether a similar (though ineffective) attempt at regeneration might occur in humans. All that can be found at autopsies in regions where heart muscle was damaged is fibrous scar tissue.

SMOOTH MUSCLE

In smooth muscle, the term *fiber* is used in much the same sort of way as in skeletal muscle, that is, to denote a single cell. Each smooth muscle fiber, however, has only one nucleus and as in cardiac muscle it is located near the

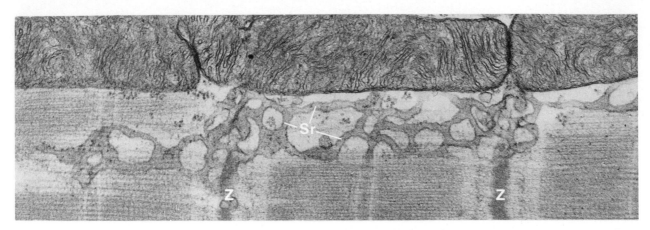

Fig. 18-37. Electron micrograph (×47,000) of part of a cardiac muscle fiber (ventricular papillary muscle of cat), showing sarcoplasmic reticulum surrounding a myofibril. In this longitudinal section part of the reticulum has been cut tangentially and so is seen here in glancing section. Narrow tubules of the reticulum (Sr) lie between the myofibril extending across the bottom of the micrograph and the row of mitochondria (between myofibrils) extending across the top. In cardiac muscle the sarcoplasmic reticulum consists of an irregular arrangement of narrow tubules. It has no special distribution over A bands or Z lines and lacks the large terminal cisternae seen in skeletal muscle fibers. (Fawcett, D. W., and McNutt, N. S.: J. Cell Biol., *42:*1, 1969)

center of the cell. As implied by its name, a smooth muscle cell lacks any cross striations.

The Arrangement and Characteristics of Smooth Muscle Fibers

As noted, most of the smooth muscle of the body lies in the walls of hollow viscera and blood vessels. It is com-

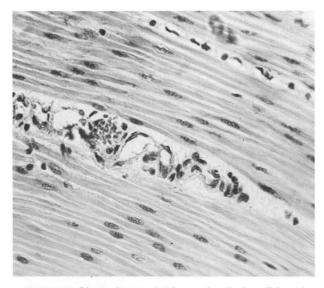

Fig. 18-38. Photomicrograph of part of wall of small intestine (dog), showing bundles of smooth muscle fibers cut longitudinally. Loose connective tissue (*center* and *upper right*) invests each bundle, supplying it with capillaries and nerve fibers.

monly arranged in two *layers* in the walls of viscera, in most places with the inner layer arranged in a circular manner and the outer one running longitudinally, but we shall find that there are exceptions to this general rule in certain of the viscera. Smooth muscle fibers are arranged spirally in parts of the gastrointestinal and respiratory tracts and in arterial blood vessels, where the angle the spiral makes to the long axis of the vessel increases with distance along the arterial tree. Thus, while lying obliquely in the walls of the larger arterial vessels, smooth muscle cells become less oblique in smaller ones and eventually form a truly circular layer in the smallest arterioles.

Layers of smooth muscle are commonly subdivided into *bundles* of fibers, each of which is invested with connective tissue supplying it with capillaries and nerve fibers (Fig. 18-38). These bundles commonly anastomose with one another. The ends of muscle fibers in a bundle interdigitate with those of other bundles so as to form a tightly knit group of fibers that functions more or less as a single unit.

Smooth muscle, which like cardiac muscle is innervated by the autonomic nervous sytem and is thus *involuntary*, is able to stay partly contracted (that is, maintain *tonus*) for prolonged periods and so is of great importance in regulating the size of the lumen of tubular structures. When, for example, the degree of tonus in a circular layer of smooth muscle increases, the diameter of the lumen becomes smaller. Excessive tonus, however, can have pathological repercussions. In the condition called *asthma*, for example, increased tonus in the smooth muscle of the walls of certain tubes conducting air in and out of the lungs so narrows their lumina that it becomes difficult to expel air. Again, increased tonus in circular smooth muscle in the walls of arterioles can so restrict the outflow of blood from arteries that blood backs up to raise the blood pressure.

As well as maintaining tonus, smooth muscle fibers in the walls of blood vessels have the important role of producing elastin, the significance of which will be discussed in Chapter 19. In the walls of the gastrointestinal tract, and to a lesser extent the oviducts and ureters, smooth muscle fibers undergo rhythmic contractions and give rise to *peristaltic waves* that sweep down these tubes and propel their contents along. The contraction of smooth muscle is usually sluggish compared with that of striated muscle, but the smooth muscle fibers of the *sphincter pupillae* (the circular fibers of the iris that constrict a pupil) contract relatively quickly.

Microscopic Structure as Seen in the LM

As seen in Figure 18-38, smooth muscle fibers have an elongated, tapered form. Their size varies considerably with their location. The smallest are about 30 μm. long and lie in the walls of small blood vessels. The largest are about 0.5 mm. long and are found in the walls of the uterus during pregnancy. However, most are about 0.2 mm. long and up to 8 μm. wide. The nucleus, which lies in the widest part of the fiber (usually toward its middle), can become pleated passively when the fiber contracts (Fig. 18-39). In routine H and E sections the cytoplasm appears uniform, but improved methods have revealed the existence of tiny dark patches (labeled db in Fig. 18-40) along the cell membrane and within the cytoplasm. These were subsequently called *dense bodies* from their

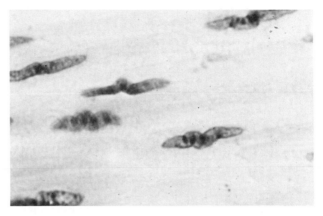
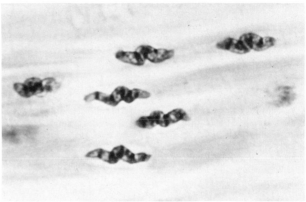

Fig. 18-39. High-power photomicrographs of partly contracted smooth muscle fibers. Note the way their nuclei become progressively pleated as the fibers contract.

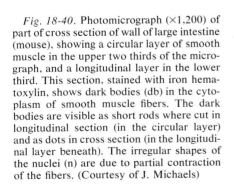
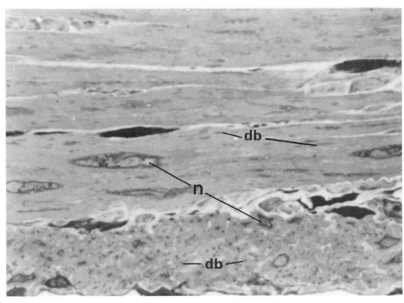

Fig. 18-40. Photomicrograph (×1,200) of part of cross section of wall of large intestine (mouse), showing a circular layer of smooth muscle in the upper two thirds of the micrograph, and a longitudinal layer in the lower third. This section, stained with iron hematoxylin, shows dark bodies (db) in the cytoplasm of smooth muscle fibers. The dark bodies are visible as short rods where cut in longitudinal section (in the circular layer) and as dots in cross section (in the longitudinal layer beneath). The irregular shapes of the nuclei (n) are due to partial contraction of the fibers. (Courtesy of J. Michaels)

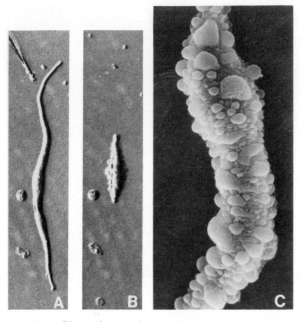

Fig. 18-41. Photomicrographs (*A* and *B*) and scanning electron micrograph (*C*) illustrating how the contours of a smooth muscle fiber change during contraction. The two photomicrographs (×310) are frames from a film, showing a living smooth muscle fiber (*A*) before stimulation and (*B*) undergoing maximal contraction. The scanning electron micrograph (×1,800) shows an isolated smooth muscle cell (C) contracted to about one third of its resting length. Note that in (*B*) and (*C*) the cell membrane of the fiber balloons out during contraction. (Fay, F. S., and Delise, C. M.: Proc. Natl. Acad. Sci. U.S.A., *70*:641, 1973)

appearance in the EM and their significance will be discussed shortly.

When relaxed, smooth muscle fibers are spindle-shaped and have a smooth outline. But when undergoing contraction, they assume a more ellipsoid shape and the cell membrane and cytoplasm bulge out into bubble-like expansions (Fig. 18-41C). The reason for this will be apparent when we describe how smooth muscle fibers contract.

The intercellular space between smooth muscle fibers is occupied by the basal lamina surrounding each fiber, collagen, elastin, and an amorphous component. All these materials (or their precursors) appear to be synthesized by the muscle cells themselves. The collagen in the intercellular spaces merges with that laid down by fibroblasts in the connective tissue surrounding fiber bundles and thus participates in harnessing the pull of the muscle fibers.

It is often difficult for a student to distinguish between the appearance of a layer of smooth muscle and that of connective tissue in which fibrocyte nuclei lie between, and are compressed by, parallel fibers of collagen. In H and E sections the student usually has to rely on being able to distinguish nuclei of smooth muscle cells from those of fibroblasts. It is sometimes desirable to use other staining methods to make the distinction clearer and those in common use include Mallory's and Van Gieson's stains.

Two other types of cells resembling smooth muscle cells should also be mentioned. First, there are certain cells around the secretory alveoli of exocrine glands such as mammary, sweat, lacrimal, and salivary glands (Fig. 7-25) that have prominent filaments in their processes. In the breast, these cells contract in response to the hormone oxytocin (p. 872) in much the same way as smooth

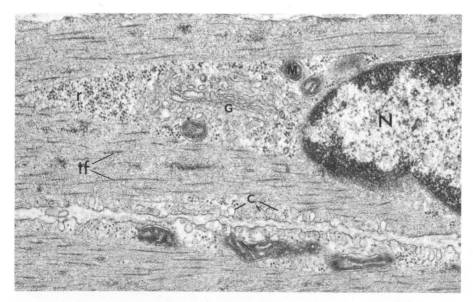

Fig. 18-42. Electron micrograph (×38,000) of part of a smooth muscle cell in longitudinal section. Numerous thick filaments (tf) are visible in the cytoplasm, with thin filaments between them. The sarcoplasm at one end of the central nucleus (N) contains ribosomes (r), mitochondria (M), and Golgi saccules (G). Note also the caveolae (c) in the cytoplasm beneath the cell membrane. (Somlyo, A. P., Devine, C. E., Somlyo, A. V., and Rice, R. V.: Philos. Trans. R. Soc. Lond. [Biol. Sci.], *265*:223, 1973)

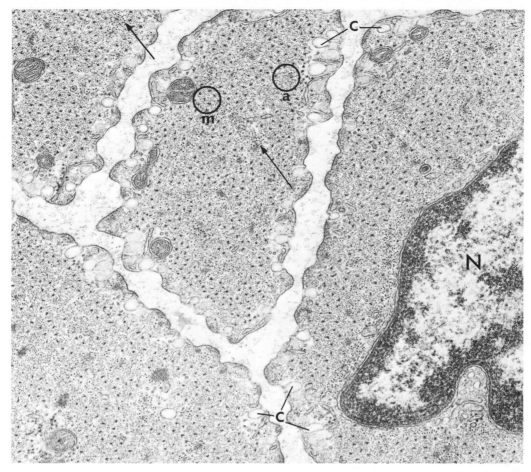

Fig. 18-43. Electron micrograph (×34,000) of smooth muscle fibers in transverse section, showing thick filaments (m) and a relatively large number of thin filaments (a). Bundles of intermediate (10-nm.) filaments are also present (indicated by arrows). The large fiber at *right* shows a central nucleus (N). Note also the caveolae (c) lying beneath the cell membrane. (Somlyo, A. P., Devine, C. E., Somlyo, A. V., and Rice, R. V.: Philos. Trans. R. Soc. Lond. [Biol. Sci.], *265:*223, 1973)

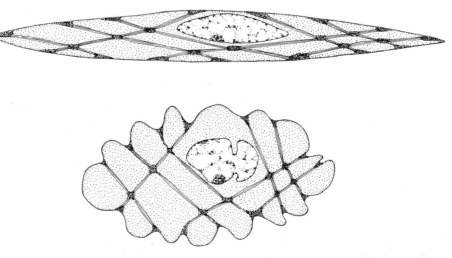

Fig. 18-44. Diagram illustrating how contraction is brought about in a smooth muscle fiber. Bundles of intermediate (10-nm.) filaments are shown here attached to dense bodies distributed in the cytoplasm and attached to the cell membrane. Contractile forces are believed to be transmitted through this system of bundles of intermediate filaments to the cell membrane, which in full contraction changes from the shape shown at *top* to that depicted at *bottom*. (Courtesy of C. P. Leblond and E. Schultz)

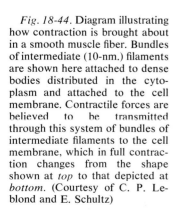

573

muscle cells in the walls of the uterus. However, because these cells are derived from ectoderm instead of mesoderm they are called *myoepithelial cells.* Second, in the testis Clermont has described flattened contractile cells called *myoid cells* in the walls of the seminiferous tubules.

The Fine Structure of Smooth Muscle Fibers

With the EM, mitochondria, ribosomes, glycogen, and Golgi saccules, together with a small amount of rER, can all be seen in the cytoplasm of smooth muscle fibers. However, these organelles and inclusions are mostly confined to the perinuclear cytoplasm at the poles of the nucleus (Fig. 18-42). Until comparatively recently, little could be recognized in the more peripheral regions of the cytoplasm except for *dense bodies* corresponding to the dark patches seen with the LM. However, with improved methods of fixation thin and thick filaments containing *actin* and *myosin,* respectively, similar to those of striated muscle but arranged in a less orderly way, were demonstrated in the cytoplasm. Intermediate (10-nm.) filaments were also demonstrated and these together with the thin and thick filaments are believed to act in a manner soon to be described to shorten the cell and produce contraction.

The first filaments to be discovered in smooth muscle fibers were *thin filaments* (microfilaments) with a diameter of 7 nm., since no special conditions were needed to preserve them (Figs. 18-42 and 18-43). Later, with improved fixation, *thick filaments* with a diameter of 17 nm. were also observed (Figs. 18-42 and 18-43). Both types of filaments have a predominantly longitudinal orientation in relaxed fibers but are more randomly arranged in contraction. Smooth muscle fibers lack cross striations because their thin and thick filaments overlap each other in no definite pattern and they do not lie in discrete sarcomeres between Z lines, which also are absent. The proportion of actin (relative to myosin) is higher in smooth than in striated fibers, and the regulatory proteins tropomyosin and troponin are also present.

More recently, intermediate filaments with a diameter of 10 nm. have been demonstrated in the cytoplasm of smooth muscle fibers. These filaments are indicated by arrows in Figure 18-43. They are made up of a protein of molecular weight 55,000 (Cooke) and are believed to constitute a more or less continuous system that pulls on dense bodies scattered throughout the cytoplasm and attached to the cell membrane (Fig. 18-44). These dense bodies contain α-actinin, a protein associated with the Z lines of striated muscle, and hence dense bodies may represent the counterparts of Z lines but arranged in a much more haphazard way. However, it is not yet known how 10-nm. filaments or dense bodies might be connected to actin or myosin filaments. The force of contraction is nevertheless believed to be generated by a sliding filament

mechanism like that of striated muscle, and it is probably transmitted by the 10-nm. (intermediate) filaments to the dense bodies attached to the cell membrane so that the longitudinal axis of the fiber is shortened in the manner depicted in Figure 18-44. As a consequence the parts of the cell lying between these dense bodies balloon out during contraction, as shown by Fay and Delise (Fig. 18-41) and illustrated in Figure 18-44, *bottom.*

The *sarcoplasmic reticulum* is less well developed in smooth muscle than in striated muscle. As can be seen in Figure 18-45, narrow tubules of the reticulum are associated with longitudinal rows of subsurface vesicles termed *caveolae* (L. for small vesicle) invaginated from the cell membrane. Since these caveolae open onto the surface of the muscle fiber it is possible that they may play a role like that of T tubules of striated fibers, namely carry impulses for contraction into the cell. It has been further suggested that they may participate with the sarcoplasmic reticulum in regulating the calcium ion concentration reaching the filaments.

The Efferent Innervation of Smooth Muscle

As noted, there are really two different types of smooth muscles. First, there are layers of smooth muscle fibers in walls of tubes and hollow viscera that undergo sustained partial contraction or participate in peristaltic waves of contraction. Then there are others like the sphincter pupillae that undergo relatively fast, precisely graded contractions. Those of the former type are called *visceral smooth muscles* and they have a different pattern of innervation from those of the latter type, which for reasons given below are called *multi-unit smooth muscles.*

In *visceral smooth muscle* (found for instance in the walls of the intestine and uterus), few of the muscle fibers of a bundle are supplied with neuromuscular junctions. Instead, impulses for contraction pass from one muscle cell to the next through *gap junctions* (these are common between the fibers of this type of smooth muscle) in the same sort of way as in cardiac muscle. Here efferent nerve impulses *regulate* contraction instead of initiating it. Furthermore, smooth muscle fibers of this type also contract in response to a variety of non-neural stimuli, including histamine, the hormone oxytocin, and even physical stretch.

In *multi-unit smooth muscle* (such as that of the iris and the wall of the vas deferens) every muscle fiber is *individually innervated.* Gap junctions may be present between the fibers but the extent to which they might participate in conducting impulses from one muscle fiber to another has not been established. The pattern of innervation of multi-unit smooth muscles is similar to that found in motor units of striated muscles except that the muscle fibers in the unit are *localized* instead of being distributed throughout

Fig. 18-45. Electron micrograph (×53,000) of smooth muscle fiber, cut tangentially along its longitudinal axis, and disclosing numerous caveolae in the cytoplasm immediately under its cell membrane. These caveolae are intimately associated with tubules of sarcoplasmic reticulum (SR). Note also the cell membrane-associated dark body (db) at *lower left* and the bundle of filaments extending from it toward the interior of the cell. (Devine, C. E., Somlyo, A. V., and Somlyo, A. P.: J. Cell Biol., *52*:690, 1972)

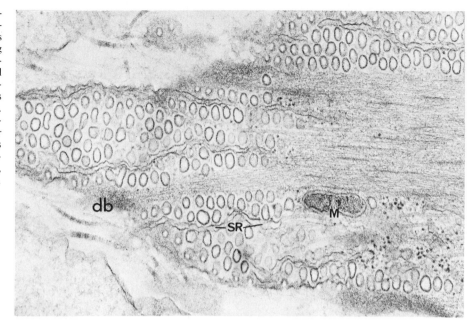

the muscle. This arrangement allows impulses for contraction to be delivered simultaneously to all the smooth muscle fibers in a given local region so that they all participate in a relatively fast local contraction.

In some parts of the body the smooth muscle is of an *intermediate* type in which about 20 to 50 per cent of the muscle fibers are individually innervated.

Neuromuscular Junctions on Smooth Muscle Fibers

The structure of neuromuscular junctions between autonomic nerve fibers and smooth muscle fibers is less complex than that between motor nerves and striated muscle fibers. Efferent autonomic nerve fibers branch repeatedly and each branch crosses and supplies a number of smooth muscle fibers, making synapses *en passant*. These branches are commonly swollen to form series of *axon varicosities* that lie like strings of beads in grooves in the surface of the muscle fibers. There is a synaptic cleft of 20 to 100 nm. between the axolemma and the sarcolemma. Within the axon varicosities there are numerous mitochondria and synaptic vesicles containing either *acetylcholine* (parasympathetic fibers) or *norepinephrine* (sympathetic fibers). On stimulation the neurotransmitter is released in the usual manner by exocytosis from the varicosities into the synaptic cleft and combines with receptor sites in the sarcolemma. As well as having receptor sites for acetylcholine, smooth muscle fibers have two different types of receptor sites for norepinephrine and other adrenergic neurotransmitter substances, referred to as α- and *β-adrenergic receptors*.

Much will be learned in pharmacology about the relative effects of various adrenergic drugs on smooth muscle cells with one or the other kind of receptor in different parts of the body. For example, certain of these drugs used to alleviate attacks of asthma by relaxing smooth muscle cells in the walls of the airways are specific enough to act on pulmonary smooth muscle cells (which have β-adrenergic receptors) with little effect on the heart rate or blood pressure, unwanted effects that would negate their usefulness.

The Growth and Regeneration of Smooth Muscle

Like the other two types of muscle, smooth muscle responds to increased demands by undergoing compensatory hypertrophy, but this is not its only response. During pregnancy, for example, the smooth muscle cells in the wall of the uterus increase not only in size (hypertrophy) but also in number (hyperplasia). Smooth muscle cells also increase in number in certain pathological conditions. Thus focal proliferation of smooth muscle cells can be demonstrated in atherosclerosis, a disease affecting arteries, as will be described in the next chapter (p. 597).

In hormone-treated or pregnant animals mitotic figures are frequently observed amongst smooth muscle cells of the uterus, so it is generally accepted that smooth muscle cells themselves retain the capacity for mitosis. McGeachy has studied reconstitution of smooth muscle bundles in the wall of the large intestine of guinea pigs following a crush injury. In the damaged region small, spindle-shaped cells (which he considered to be myoblasts) went on to proliferate and differentiate into smooth muscle cells. The spindle-shaped cells (myoblasts) appeared to be progeny of smooth muscle cells that had divided close to the injury. In the next chapter we discuss how smooth muscle cells in the walls of new blood vessels differentiate from the pericytes associated with existing small vessels.

REFERENCES AND OTHER READING

GENERAL

Comprehensive General Reference

Goldman, R., Pollard, T., and Rosenbaum, J. (eds.): Cell Motility. Book A, Motility, Muscle and Non-Muscle Cells; and Book B, Actin. Myosin and Associated Proteins. Cold Spring Harbor Conferences on Cell Proliferation, vol. 3, Cold Spring Harbor Laboratory, 1976.

STRIATED MUSCLE

Betz, E. H., Firket, H., and Reznik, M.: Some aspects of muscle regeneration. Int. Rev. Cytol., *19*:203, 1966.

Bourne, G. H. (ed.): The Structure and Function of Muscle. vols. 1 to 3. New York, Academic Press, 1960.

Cohen. C.: The protein switch of muscle contraction. Sci. Am., *233* (No. 5):36, May, 1975.

Ebashi, S., Endo, M., and Ohtsuki, I.: Control of muscle contraction. Quart. Rev. Biophys., *2*:351, 1969.

Forbes, M. S., Plantholt, B. A., and Sperelakis, N.: Cytochemical staining procedures selective for sarcotubular systems of muscle: modifications and applications. J. Ultrastruct. Res., *60*:306, 1977.

Forssmann, W. G., and Girardier, L.: A study of the T-system in rat heart. J. Cell. Biol., *44*:1, 1970.

Franzini-Armstrong, C.: Studies of the triad. I. Structure of the junction in frog twitch fibers. J. Cell Biol., *47*:488, 1970

———: The structure of a simple Z line. J. Cell Biol., *58*:630, 1973.

Granger, B. L., and Lazarides, E.: The existence of an insoluble Z disc scaffold in chicken skeletal muscle. Cell, *15*:1253, 1978.

Hanson, J., and Huxley, H. E.: The structural basis of contraction in striated muscle. Symp. Soc. Exp. Biol., *9*:228, 1955.

———: Structural basis of the cross-striations in muscle. Nature, *172*:530, 1953.

Huddart, H.: The Comparative Structure and Function of Muscle. Oxford, Pergamon Press, 1975.

Huxley, H. E.: The double array of filaments in cross-striated muscle. J. Biophys. Biochem. Cytol., *3*:361, 1957.

———: The contraction of muscle. Sci. Am., *199*:66, Nov., 1958.

———: The mechanism of muscular contraction. Science, *164*:1356, 1969.

———: The structural basis of muscular contraction. Proc. R. Soc. Lond. [Biol.], *178*:131, 1971.

———: Introductory remarks: the relevance of studies on muscle to problems of cell motility. *In* Goldman, R., Pollard, T., and Rosenbaum, J. (eds.): Cell Motility. Book A, Motility,

Muscle and Non-Muscle Cells. p. 115. Cold Spring Harbor Conference on Cell Proliferation, Cold Spring Harbor Laboratory, 1976.

MacConnachie, H. F., Enesco, M., and Leblond, C. P.: The mode of increase in the number of skeletal muscle nuclei in the postnatal rat. Am. J. Anat., *114*:245, 1964.

MacKay, B., Harrop, T. J., and Muir, A. R.: An experimental study of the longitudinal growth of skeletal muscle in the rat. Acta Anat., *73*:588, 1969.

MacLennan, D. H.: Resolution of the calcium transport system of sarcoplasmic reticulum. Can. J. Biochem., *53*:251, 1975.

Mauro, A.: Satellite cell of skeletal cell fibers. J. Biophys. Biochem. Cytol., *3*:193, 1961.

Moss, F. P., and Leblond, C. P.: Satellite cells as the source of nuclei in muscles of growing rats. Anat. Rec., *170*:471, 1971.

Murray, J. M., and Webber, A.: The cooperative action of muscle proteins. Sci. Am., *230* (No. 2):59, Feb., 1974.

Sandow, A.: Skeletal muscle. Annu. Rev. Physiol., *32*:87, 1970.

Szent-Györgyi, A.: Chemistry of Muscular Contraction. ed. 2. New York, Academic Press, 1951.

Efferent Nerve Endings in Striated Muscle

Andersson-Cedergren, E.: Ultrastructure of motor end plate and sarcoplasmic components of mouse skeletal fiber as revealed by three-dimensional reconstructions from serial sections. J. Ultrastruct. Res., Suppl. *1*, 1959.

Couteaux, R.: Motor end plate structure. *In* Bourne, G. H. (ed.): The Structure and Function of Muscle. vol. 1, p. 337. New York, Academic Press, 1960.

Drachman, D. B.: Myasthenia gravis. N. Engl. J. Med., *298*:136 and *298*:186, 1978.

Kelly, A. M., and Zacks, S. I.: The fine structure of motor endplate morphogenesis. J. Cell Biol., *42*:154, 1969.

Lester, H. A.: The response to acetylcholine. Sci. Am., *236*(No. 2):106, Feb., 1977.

Reger, J. F.: Electron microscopy of the motor end-plate in rat intercostal muscle. Anat. Rec., *112*:1, 1965.

Smith, B. H., and Kreutzberg, G. W.: Neuron-target cell interactions. Neurosci. Res. Program Bull., *14* (No. 3): 1, 1976.

Zacks, S. I.: The Motor End Plate. Philadelphia, W. B. Saunders, 1964.

Afferent Nerve Endings in Striated Muscle

For Afferent Endings in Synovial Joints, *see* References on Nerve Endings in Chapter 17.

Boyd, I. A.: The response of fast and slow nuclear bag fibers and nuclear chain fibers in isolated cat muscle spindles to fusimotor stimulation, and the effect of intrafusal contraction on the sensory endings. Q. J. Exp. Physiol., *61*:203, 1976.

Boyd, I. A., and Ward, J.: Motor control of nuclear bag and nuclear chain intrafusal fibers in isolated living muscle spindles from the cat. J. Physiol., *244*:83, 1975.

Bridgman, C. F.: Comparisons in structure of tendon organs in the rat, cat and man. J. Comp. Neurol., *138*:369, 1970.

Cooper, S., and Daniel, P. M.: Muscle spindles in man; their morphology in the lumbricals and the deep muscles of the neck. Brain, *85*:563, 1963.

Kennedy, W. R.: Innervation of normal human muscle spindles. Neurology, *20*:463, 1970.

Matthews, P. B. C.: Mammalian Muscle Receptors and Their Central Actions. London, Edward Arnold, 1972.

Merton, P. A.: How we control the contraction of our muscles. Sci. Am., *226*(No. 5):30, May, 1972.

Moore, J. C.: The Golgi tendon organ and the muscle spindle. Am. J. Occup. Ther., *28:*415, 1974.

CARDIAC MUSCLE

Cantin, M., Veilleux, R., and Huet, M.: Electron and fluorescence microscopy of hamster atrium after administration of 6-hydroxydopamine. Experientia, *29:*882, 1973.

Challice, C. E., and Virágh, S. (eds.): Ultrastructure of the Mammalian Heart. Ultrastructure in Biological Systems. vol. 6. New York, Academic Press, 1973.

Fawcett, D. W., and McNutt, N. S.: The ultrastructure of the cat myocardium. I. Ventricular papillary muscle. J. Cell Biol., *42:*1, 1969.

McNutt, N. S., and Fawcett, D. W.: The ultrastructure of the cat myocardium. II. Atrial Muscle. J. Cell Biol., *42:*46, 1969.

Rumyantsev, P. P.: Interrelations of the proliferation and differentiation processes during cardiac myogenesis and regeneration. Int. Rev. Cytol., *51:*188, 1977.

Sjostrand, F. S., Andersson-Cedergren, E., and Dewey, M. M.: The ultrastructure of the intercalated discs of frog, mouse and guinea pig cardiac muscle. J. Ultrastruct. Res., *1:*271, 1958.

SMOOTH MUSCLE

Becker, C. G., and Nachman, R. L.: Contractile proteins of endothelial cells, platelets and smooth muscle. Am. J. Pathol., *71:*1, 1973.

Bulbring, E., Brading, A., Jones, A., and Tomita, T. (eds.) Smooth Muscle. London: Edward Arnold, 1970.

Cooke, P.: A filamentous cytoskeleton in vertebrate smooth muscle fibers. J. Cell Biol., *68:*539, 1976.

Cooke, P. H., and Fay, F. S.: Correlation between fiber length, ultrastructure and the length-tension relationships of mammalian smooth muscle. J. Cell Biol., *52:*105, 1972.

Devine, C. E.: Vascular smooth muscle, morphology and ultrastructure. *In* Kaley, G., and Altura, B. M. (eds.): Microcirculation. vol. 2. Baltimore, University Park Press, 1978.

Devine, C. E., and Somlyo, A. P.: Thick filaments in vascular smooth muscle. J. Cell Biol., *49:*636, 1971.

Devine, C. E., Somlyo, A. V., and Somlyo, A. P.: Sarcoplasmic reticulum and mitochondria as cation accumulation sites in smooth muscle. Philos. Trans. R. Soc. Lond. [Biol. Sci.], *265:*17, 1973.

Fay, F. S.: Structural and functional features of isolated smooth muscle cells. *In* Goldman, R., Pollard, T., and Rosenbaum, J. (eds.): Cell Motility. Book A, Motility, Muscle and Non-Muscle Cells. p. 185. Cold Spring Harbor Conference on Cell Proliferation, Cold Spring Harbor Laboratory, 1976.

Fay, F. S., and Delise, C. M.: Contraction of isolated smooth muscle cells—structural changes. Proc. Natl. Acad. Sci. U.S.A., *70:*641, 1973.

Gabella, G.: Fine structure of smooth muscle. Proc. Trans. R. Soc. Lond. [Biol.], *265:*7, 1973.

Kelly, R. E., and Rice, R. V.: Ultrastructural studies on the contractile mechanism of smooth muscle. J. Cell Biol., *42:*683, 1969.

Lowey, J., and Small, J. V.: Organization of myosin and actin in vertebrate smooth muscle. Nature, *227:*46, 1970.

McGeachie, J. K.: Smooth muscle regeneration. Monographs in Developmental Biology 9. Basel, S. Karger, 1975.

Polezhaev, L. V.: Organ Regeneration in Animals. Chap. 6, p. 100. Springfield, Charles C Thomas, 1972.

Rice, R. V., Moses, J. A., McManus, G. M., Brady, A. C., and Blasik, L. M.: The organization of contractile filaments in a mammalian smooth muscle. J. Cell Biol., *47:*183, 1970.

Richardson, K. C.: The fine structure of autonomic nerve endings in smooth muscle of the rat vas deferens. J. Anat., *96:*427, 1962.

Somlyo, A. P., Devine, C. E., Somlyo, A. V., and Rice, R. V.: Filament organization in vertebrate smooth muscle. Philos. Trans. R. Soc. Lond. [Biol. Sci.], *265:*223, 1973.

Somlyo, A. P., Somlyo, A. V., Ashton, F. T., and Vallières, J.: Vertebrate smooth muscle: ultrastructure and function. *In* Goldman, R., Pollard, T., and Rosenbaum, J. (eds.): Cell Motility. Book A, Motility, Muscle and Non-Muscle Cells. p. 165. Cold Spring Harbor Conference on Cell Proliferation, Cold Spring Harbor Laboratory, 1976.

(Further references on smooth muscle are given in connection with arteries in Chap. 22.)

PART FOUR

THE SYSTEMS OF THE BODY

The remaining chapters of this textbook will each deal with the histology of one of the systems. The term *system* is used in histology, physiology, and other subjects to designate a group of organs and/or structures that collaborate to carry out some important function for the body. For example, the circulatory system consists of the heart and all the vessels concerned with circulating blood and lymph throughout the body. After we finish with the circulatory system, we shall take up the other systems of the body one by one, a chapter at a time. It should be noted, however, that our presentation of nervous tissue in Chapter 17 also dealt with the nervous system (brain, spinal cord, and peripheral nervous system), so there will be no separate chapter on the nervous system.

19 The Circulatory System

General Structure, Functions, and Terminology. In any society of individuals in which there is division of labor, there must be an efficient transportation system so that goods can be exchanged between its specialized workers. Whereas railways, trucks, planes, ships, and pipelines serve this function in modern societies of people, the system used in the community of cells comprising the human body is equivalent to a pipeline and is called the circulatory system.

Two fluids, blood and lymph, circulate in the body. The circulation of lymph was dealt with to some extent in Chapter 13, and more will be said at the end of this chapter. Here we shall consider the blood circulatory system.

THE PARTS OF THE CIRCULATORY SYSTEM AND THEIR PARTICULAR FUNCTIONS

Pumps are required to move fluid through pipelines. Since there are *two circuits* involved in the circulatory system, each requires a pump; this is provided by the heart, which consists of two pumps side by side. These two sides of the heart, each a separate pump, are often referred to as the *left* and *right hearts*, and each is connected to a different circuit. The right heart pumps blood through what is termed the *pulmonary* circuit (L. *pulmo,* lung), so this maintains the *pulmonary circulation.* The left heart pumps blood through the remainder of the body, and since the body is well organized it can be said to constitute a system, so this circulation is called the *systemic circulation.*

In each circuit the pump delivers blood under pressure into thick-walled strong tubes called *arteries* that branch repeatedly and finally terminate in strong tubes with narrow lumina called *arterioles*. These act as pressure reduction valves and deliver blood into the thin-walled *capillaries* under relatively low pressure. The capillary beds of the lungs permit carbon dioxide of the blood to be released into inspired air and oxygen to be absorbed into the erythrocytes. In the systemic circulation the capillaries permit oxygen and nutrients to pass through their walls and so provide these essentials to body cells. The blood from capillary beds in both circuits is delivered first into *venules* and then into *veins*. The veins are so arranged that the blood received from the *lungs* is delivered to the *left heart,* which can then pump it through the systemic circulation, whereas the blood returned from the *systemic* circuit is delivered to the *right heart* which pumps it through the lungs, where it is again oxygenated and cleared of carbon dioxide.

Next, the right and left hearts each have two main parts, an upper *atrium* (Gr. *atrion,* hall) in which the blood being returned to that side of the heart collects (right and left atria are labeled in Fig. 19-1) and a *ventricle* (L. for a small belly or cavity; right and left ventricles are also labeled in Fig. 19-1). Both the atria and the ventricles are sac-like structures, the walls of which consist of cardiac muscle. The walls of the ventricles are much thicker and stronger than those of the corresponding atria (both are stippled in Fig. 19-1). The chief function of the atria is to act as reservoirs between contractions of the heart. However, most of the blood that between heartbeats enters an atrium passes on through the valve that guards the passageway into the ventricle below it. The valve between the right atrium and the right ventricle is termed the *tricuspid valve* (labeled in Fig. 19-1) and the one between the left atrium and ventricle is called the *mitral valve* (also labeled in Fig. 19-1). (Reasons for these names will be given later.) Both of these valves are open when the heart fills between beats and they remain open as the atria contract. But when the ventricles contract both valves are forced closed by pressure being built up in the contracting ventricles. This pressure, however, forces the pulmonary valve (labeled in Fig. 19-1) to open so that the right ventricle can pump its contents through the pulmonary circulation, and it forces open the aortic valve (labeled in Fig. 19-1) so the blood in the left ventricle can be pumped all through the body.

When the ventricles finish their contraction and begin to relax, the pressure within them drops below that in the arteries into which they have pumped most of their contents. So the pulmonary and aortic valves (Fig. 19-1) are both forced, by the pressure in the arteries above them,

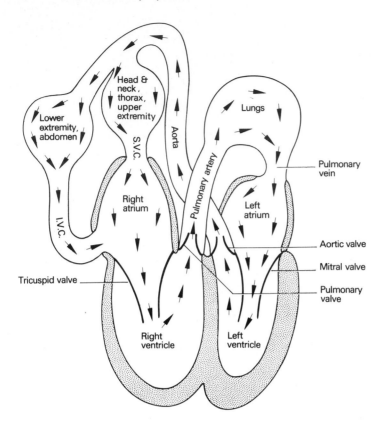

Fig. 19-1. Schematic diagram illustrating important parts of the heart in relation to other components of the circulatory system. (Thompson, J. S.: Core Textbook of Anatomy. Philadelphia, J. B. Lippincott, 1977)

into the closed position, in which they remain until the ventricles are refilled and contract again. While the relaxing ventricles are being refilled, the tricuspid and mitral valves open because the pressure of the venous blood emptying into them is then greater than that existing in the relaxing ventricles.

The tubes into which blood is pumped by ventricular contractions are called *arteries* for the curious reason that they were once believed to contain air (L. *aer,* air). In arteries blood is under pressure, the pressure being higher in the systemic circulation than in the pulmonary. Since artery walls have elastin and smooth muscle as their chief components, they accommodate the pressure inside them. The elastin, moreover, is stretched by ventricular contractions, and in returning to a less stretched state it maintains pressure in the arteries between heartbeats as will be described presently.

The different parts of the circulatory system will be described in more detail under the following main headings:

1. The Heart
2. Arteries and Arterioles
3. The Peripheral Circulation
4. Veins and Venules
5. The Lymphatic Division of the Circulatory System

THE HEART

THE MYOCARDIUM

The muscular walls of the atria and ventricles comprise the *myocardium.* This consists of anastomosing cardiac muscle fibers, with the interstices of the network being filled with the cardiac equivalent of the endomysium found in skeletal muscle (Fig. 18-29). In cardiac muscle this contains a very rich supply of capillaries, required for the extensive energy requirements of the heart. Cardiac muscle was described in detail in Chapter 18.

In understanding features of the myocardium to be described here it should be recalled that, as described in the previous chapter, cardiac muscle cells are connected end to end by intercalated disks (Fig. 18-31) and these have two components. At sites where individual cardiac muscle cells are joined end to end (transverse portions of intercalated disks) extensive desmosome-like junctions are much in evidence. But scattered between these, and constituting the chief type of cell junction in the longitudinal parts of intercalated disks (Fig. 18-31), there are gap junctions (Fig. 18-36). These, of course, permit rapid transmission of waves of depolarization from one cardiac muscle cell to another. With this in mind it will be easier

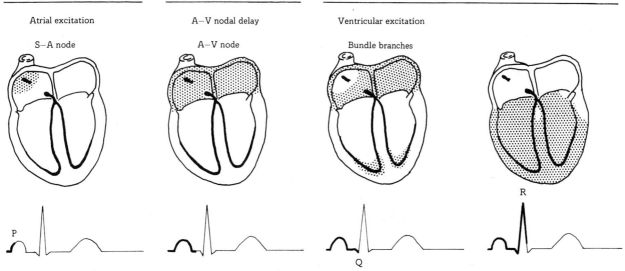

Fig. 19-2. Schematic diagram illustrating the sequence of contraction in the heart in relation to the cardiac cycle. Below each stage, in which the contracting region is shown stippled, the corresponding wave that appears at this time on an electrocardiogram is indicated by a heavy line. For further details, *see* text. The waves in an electrocardiogram are also illustrated in Figure 19-8. (Shepard, R. S.: Human Physiology. Philadelphia, J. B. Lippincott, 1971)

to understand how the heart contracts and relaxes as it does with each cardiac cycle.

The Cardiac Cycle. What is termed a *cardiac cycle* comprises the succession of events that occurs in a heart from the beginning of one beat to the beginning of the next. In one phase of the cycle the heart is relaxing. In this phase blood is flowing from the venae cavae into the relaxing right atrium and from there through the open tricuspid valve into the relaxing right ventricle. Simultaneously, blood from the pulmonary vein is flowing into the relaxing left atrium and on through the open mitral valve into the relaxing left ventricle. In the next phase of the cycle the two atria contract, with the process of contraction beginning in the right atrium near the entrance of the superior vena cava (stippled area in the left diagram in Fig. 19-2). The contraction spreads over both atria so that most of the blood they contain is forced into their respective ventricles. The wave of contraction that sweeps over the atria *is not, however, immediately transmitted to the ventricles.* There is a brief enough delay for the atria to finish their contraction. Furthermore, when contraction occurs in the ventricles it does not begin, as might be thought, next to the atria but near the apex of the heart (stippled area in third from left diagram in Fig. 19-2). From here it spreads rapidly throughout the myocardium of both ventricles, thereby causing them to deliver their contents into the pulmonary artery and aorta, respectively. We shall now describe the system in which the impulse for contraction originates and by means of which it is transmitted in the heart.

THE IMPULSE-CONDUCTING SYSTEM OF THE HEART

The Histological Basis for Two Hearts Beating as One, and for Other Synchronized Events Occurring in the Heart

The efficiency of the heart as a dual pump depends on contractions in the left and right hearts being simultaneous and on the different events in the cardiac cycle described above following each other in orderly sequence. The synchronization of these events and their occurring in an orderly sequence depend on the impulse for contraction sweeping through the heart down what is termed its *impulse-conducting system* (Fig. 19-3). This system is composed of a special type of cardiac muscle cell that is variously specialized for either initiating an impulse for contraction or for conducting the impulse through parts of the heart, as next described. It should be mentioned that passage of the impulse through the heart and the contraction it incites can be traced by means of what are termed *electrocardiograms,* as will be described presently. This is of enormous value in establishing accurate diagnosis of various disorders of the heart originating either from failure of conduction in some part of the conducting system or from lesions (from the L. *laedere,* to hurt, meaning damaged tissue) of the heart muscle itself, in particular lesions caused by thrombosis (p. 270) having occurred in some part of the coronary circulation.

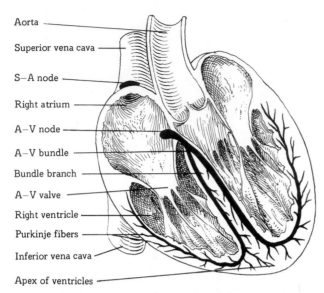

Aorta

Superior vena cava

S—A node

Right atrium

A—V node

A—V bundle

Bundle branch

A—V valve

Right ventricle

Purkinje fibers

Inferior vena cava

Apex of ventricles

Fig. 19-3. Diagram of the impulse-conducting system of the heart. The heart has been cut open in the coronal plane to expose its interior and the main parts of its impulse-conducting system (indicated in black). For details, *see* text. (Shepard, R. S.: Human Physiology. Philadelphia, J. B. Lippincott, 1971)

The Initiation of the Impulse for Contraction — the Sinoatrial (S-A) Node. What is termed the S-A node is a little mass of specialized cardiac muscle fibers contained in substantial amounts of fibroelastic connective tissue richly supplied with capillaries. It is located in the right-hand wall of the superior vena cava at its junction with the right atrium (Figs. 19-3 and 19-4A). Its capillaries are supplied by a *nodal artery* (Fig. 19-4), and numerous nerve fibers belonging to both divisions of the autonomic nervous system enter the node. The cells responsible for its specialized function are cardiac muscle cells but they (Fig. 19-4B) are narrower, and like the cells of other parts of the system (to be illustrated shortly) they contain fewer myofibrils than ordinary cardiac muscle cells.

The S-A node is termed the *pacemaker* of the heart. This is because in most people at rest it "fires off" an impulse approximately 70 times a minute and this is transmitted throughout the heart so as to cause its parts to contract in proper sequence.

Some Background on How Pacemaker Cells Function. As was described in the chapters on nervous and muscle tissue, the cell membrane of a resting nerve cell or striated muscle fiber is electrically *polarized,* with its outer aspect being positively charged with respect to its cytoplasmic side, so that it exhibits a resting potential. When, however, a nerve cell receives an effective stimulus at some site, the cell membrane becomes permeable at that site to sodium ions which, of course, are positively charged. These ions are maintained by the sodium-potassium pump of the cell membrane in greater concentration outside the cell; but when a stimulus is received they immediately diffuse into the cytoplasm through the membrane and as a result the outside of the cell membrane is suddenly no longer positive in relation to the inner side. So at this site the resting potential between the two sides of the membrane suddenly disappears; in other words, the membrane becomes *depolarized.* A further phenomenon also occurs, namely, the depolarization spreads along the membrane in a wave-like manner with great speed. It is the arrival of such waves of depolarization (nerve impulses) at a motor end plate that, through the action of a neurotransmitter, initiates a wave of depolarization that sweeps over the sarcolemma of a striated muscle fiber, to be conducted into the fiber by transverse tubules so as to cause it to contract.

The important point to make here is that striated muscle fibers, being under voluntary control, remain polarized until arriving nerve impulses act so as to depolarize them. In this respect cardiac muscle fibers are fundamentally different from voluntary muscle fibers in a way that accounts for at least some cardiac muscle fibers being able to act as pacemakers, as will now be explained.

Pacemaker Cells. Unlike voluntary skeletal muscle fibers, which remain polarized until their contraction is initiated by the arrival of nerve impulses at an end plate, there are certain cardiac muscle cells, termed *pacemaker cells,* that have an unstable resting membrane potential: this is due to their cell membrane losing its permeability to potassium ions so that with the passage of time (a small fraction of a second) their resting potential becomes diminished to the point where the membrane ceases to act as a barrier. This permits such an influx of sodium ions into the cell that the cell membrane is immediately and completely depolarized. Such cells are connected, presumably by gap junctions, to adjacent cardiac muscle cells that have a more stable (or even entirely stable) resting potential. Cardiac muscle cells that connect with pacemaker cells are called *follower cells,* and when a wave of depolarization generated in a pacemaker cell is transmitted through a gap junction to a follower cell the latter also is immediately depolarized. Since the follower cell is in turn connected to further follower cells with stable resting potentials, a whole succession of cells becomes depolarized. Thus, pacemaker cells in the S-A node initiate regular waves of depolarization that are conducted through the heart to cause the contraction of its different parts in proper sequence, as will next be described. But first we should mention that whereas the rate at which pacemaker cells in the S-A node become depolarized is in a resting person around 70 times per minute, under conditions of physical exercise the pulse rate quickens. It also sometimes becomes accelerated under conditions of emotion that lead to increased activity of the sympathetic division of the autonomic nervous system. This can happen because, as noted, the S-A node is richly supplied with fibers from both divisions of the autonomic nervous system. These, however, are *not* responsible for *initiating* depolarization of pacemaker cells, they can only *modify* the rate at which they become depolarized. The sympathetic system tends to stimulate the rate at which pacemaker cells depolarize, whereas parasympathetic fibers tend to slow the rate. Certain hormones can also affect the rate at which they depolarize.

The Pathway of the Wave of Depolarization Through the Heart

From the S-A node the wave of depolarization is conducted to the cardiac muscle cells of the right atrium and

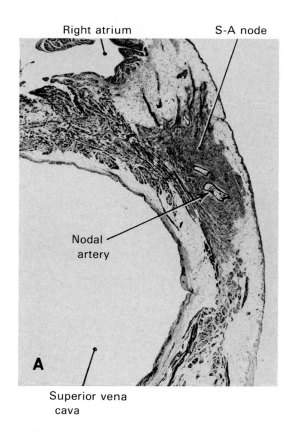

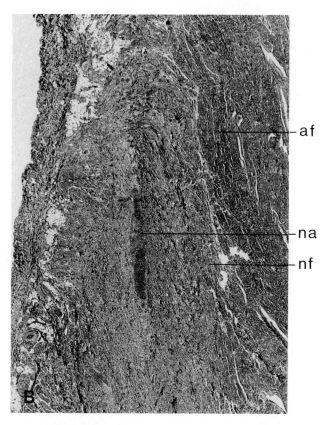

Fig. 19-4. (A) Very low power photomicrograph of a cross section of the right-hand wall of the superior vena cava at its junction with the right atrium. This shows the sinoatrial (S-A) node, the pacemaker of the heart. *(B)* Low-power photomicrograph showing the S-A node in longitudinal section. A part of the lumen of the superior vena cava is seen as a white space at *upper left,* and atrial muscle is the darker tissue at *right.* Note that the nodal fibers (nf) of the node, which occupies the middle part of the picture, are narrower than the darker-staining atrial fibers (af) at *right.* The nodal fibers are embedded in abundant collagenic fibers. Part of the wall of the nodal artery (na), which pursues a curving course through the middle of the node, is also seen near *center.* (Courtesy of J. Duckworth)

from there it spreads over all the cardiac muscle cells of both atria to more or less converge on another node of specialized cells called the *atrioventricular (A-V) node* (Fig. 19-3, A-V node) that lies in the lower part of the interatrial septum immediately above the attachment of the septal cusp of the tricuspid valve (labeled A-V valve in Fig. 19-3). Anteriorly, the A-V node is continuous with the *A-V bundle* (Figs. 19-3 and 19-5), described below. The conduction of the wave of depolarization over the atria is, of course, associated with contraction of its cardiac muscle cells, and so by the time the wave of depolarization reaches the A-V node most of the atrial muscle is contracting.

The A-V Bundle. For a long time it was believed that there was a continuous fibrous partition between the atria and the ventricles in the human heart. But in 1893 His showed that the partition was pierced by a *bundle* of cardiac muscle fibers. In the same year, Kent noted that the

partition in the monkey heart was pierced by a bundle of muscle fibers but these were somewhat different from ordinary cardiac muscle fibers. It was then established that this *atrioventricular (A-V) bundle* of muscle fibers (Figs. 19-3 and 19-5, avb), or, as it is often called, the *bundle of His,* provides the means whereby each wave of depolarization that sweeps over the atria can be conducted to the ventricles to institute their contraction at precisely the time when they have been completely filled with blood due to contraction of the atria. The cardiac muscle fibers in the A-V bundle are specialized to *conduct* rather than contract, and, as we shall see presently, they have a different microscopic appearance from fibers of ordinary cardiac muscle.

After entering the interventricular septum, the A-V bundle forms two main branches (Fig. 19-3), and about half way down the septum the fibers of the two branches of the bundle become of a type called *Purkinje fibers* (Fig.

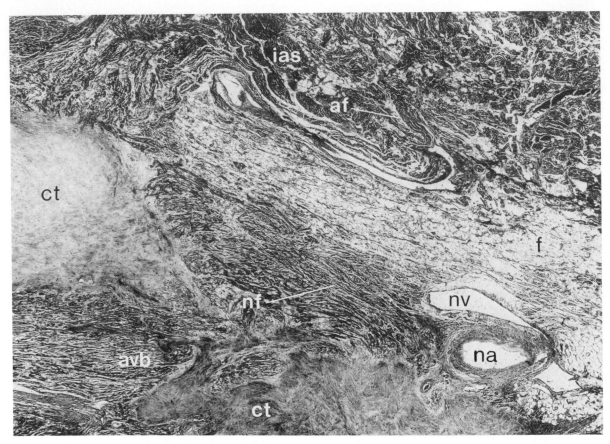

Fig. 19-5. Low-power photomicrograph of a sagittal section of the atrioventricular (A-V) node of the heart. For orientation purposes note that the left-hand side of the picture is anterior, the right posterior. Atrial muscle of the interatrial septum (ias) extends along the top margin. The grayish areas at *left* and *bottom* are fibrous connective tissue (ct) of the so-called skeleton of the heart. Pale areas containing fat cells (f) are present at *middle* and *lower right*. Both the nodal artery (na) and the nodal vein (nv) are included in the section at *lower right,* posterior to the node. The darkly staining A-V node lies anterior to these vessels, in between them and the fibrous tissue at *bottom* and *left* and the fatty connective tissue above. Note that the nodal fibers (nf) are narrower than the atrial fibers (af) of the interatrial septum above the node. Nodal fibers extend anteriorly at *lower left* to join the A-V bundle (avb), which runs anteriorly from the node. The fibers of the A-V bundle are also narrower than ordinary cardiac muscle fibers. (Courtesy of J. Duckworth)

19-3). But before discussing these further, we should comment briefly on the microscopic structure of the cells of the conducting system thus far considered.

The Microscopic Structure of the S-A and A-V Nodes and the Bundle of His. The S-A node is a small mass of specialized cardiac muscle fibers that lie in substantial amounts of fibroelastic tissue (Fig. 19-4). It is supplied by a *nodal artery*. As may be seen in Figure 19-4B, the nodal fibers are of a finer caliber than ordinary cardiac muscle fibers outside the node, with which fibers the nodal fibers connect, presumably by gap junctions. The nodal fibers can be seen, even with the LM, to contain fewer myofibrils than ordinary atrial fibers.

The A-V node (Fig. 19-5) is similar to the S-A node in many respects. It too is supplied by a special nodal artery

(na in Fig. 19-5) and consists of fine cardiac muscle fibers that branch and anastomose very extensively. These nodal fibers connect on the atrial side with ordinary atrial muscle fibers and near the A-V septum with the specialized cardiac muscle cells of the A-V bundle (labeled avb, *bottom left* in Fig. 19-5).

The Fine Structure of Pacemaker and Specialized Conducting Cells. The EM appearance of some of the types of cardiac muscle cells seen in the lower part of the A-V node is illustrated in Figure 19-6. Like cells of the conducting system of the heart in general, they contain relatively few, poorly organized myofibrils. The cells along the bottom of the micrograph are more representative of those seen further along in the A-V bundle in that they possess somewhat more myofibrils, but in fewer numbers

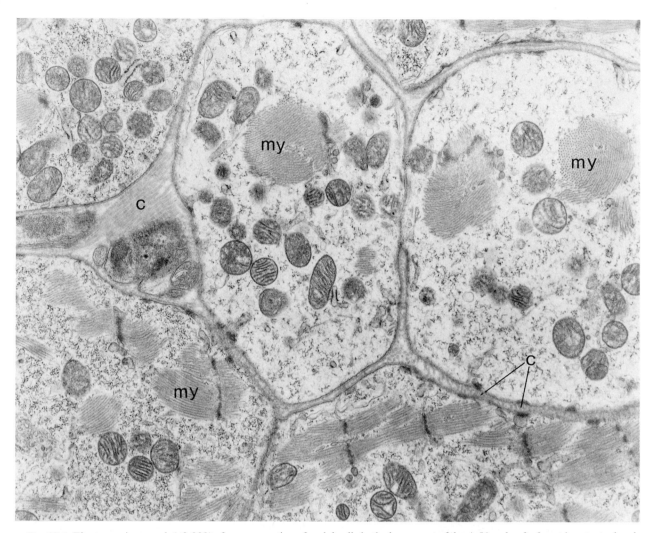

Fig. 19-6. Electron micrograph (×9,000) of a cross section of nodal cells in the lower part of the A-V node of a ferret heart, at a level where conducting cardiac muscle fibers leave the node anteriorly to enter the A-V bundle. These are all cells of nodal fibers. Both types illustrated contain numerous ribosomes and mitochondria but have a variable small number of myofibrils (my). Very few myofibrils are present in the pale type of cell seen at *middle* and *right*. The cells at *top left, bottom left,* and *bottom right* more closely resemble ordinary cardiac muscle cells but they have fewer myofibrils (though slightly more than pale fibers). The irregular orientation of the myofibrils in both kinds of nodal cells accounts for the myofibrils being seen cut in oblique section. Some collagenic fibrils (c) are visible in the endomysium (together with some small nerve fibers) at *middle left,* and at *lower right* between the fibers. (Courtesy of I. Taylor)

and more variable arrangements than are seen in ordinary cardiac muscle cells. Although normally the cells of the A-V node do not function as pacemaker cells, but instead as specialized conducting cells that slightly delay transmission of impulses from the atria to the ventricles, they can under certain circumstances take on pacemaker function, and so it would seem that the fine structure of the two cells illustrated at *upper right* in Figure 19-6 would be representative of pacemaker cells in general.

Purkinje Fibers. These begin in the A-V bundle about halfway down each of its two branches. They were first seen by Purkinje in 1845. Seen with the LM, they resemble ordinary cardiac muscle fibers in that they have centrally located nuclei and cross striations (Fig. 19-7A). However, they differ from ordinary cardiac muscle fibers in that they are generally wider, and also because the myofibrils in each fiber tend to be disposed around its periphery; this leaves the central core relatively empty of myofibrils, their place being taken by considerable amounts of glycogen. In H and E sections the glycogen is

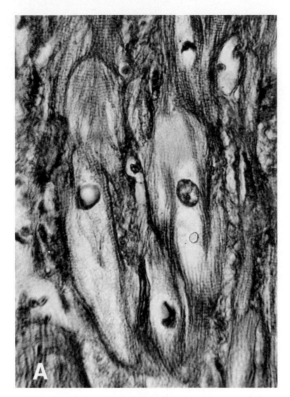
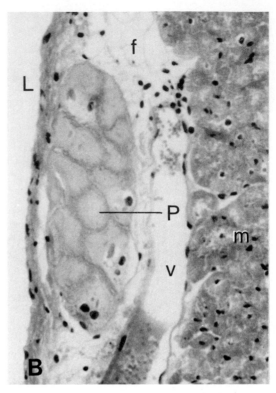

Fig. 19-7. Photomicrographs of Purkinje fibers from the wall of the right ventricle. (*A*) Purkinje fibers from human heart in longitudinal section. Note their large size and the way myofibrils occupy the periphery of the fibers. (Courtesy of J. Duckworth) (*B*) Purkinje fibers from sheep heart in transverse section. A bundle of Purkinje fibers (P) is seen here embedded in loose connective tissue of the endocardium. To the left of the bundle lies the lumen (L) of the ventricle. To the right of the bundle there is an endocardial blood vessel (its lumen labeled v) and, farther to the right, cardiac muscle (m) of the myocardium is seen. Some fat cells (f) are present in the endocardium.

not seen; hence the central part of each Purkinje fiber appears to be empty except where nuclei are present (Fig. 19-7). Bundles of Purkinje fibers can also be seen deep in the endocardium (Fig. 19-7B).

It is important to realize that Purkinje fibers supply the papillary muscles before they supply the lateral walls of the ventricles, up which they spread as a subendocardial network. Since these fibers conduct the impulse for contraction much more rapidly than the ordinary heart muscle, this arrangement ensures that the *papillary muscles* will *take up the strain* on the leaflets of the mitral and the tricuspid valves before the full force of ventricular contraction is thrown against them. It should also be noted by referring to Figures 19-2 and 19-3 that the distribution of the branches of the rapidly conducting Purkinje system is such that the relatively thick exterior walls of the ventricles near the apex of the heart are depolarized before the impulse reaches the ventricular walls at the base of the heart. Hence, in general the apical parts of the ven-

tricles contract before their basal parts (*see* third diagram from *left* in Fig. 19-2 and compare it with the diagram on its right).

The fine structure of Purkinje fibers is to a great extent what would be anticipated from their LM appearance in that they contain relatively few myofibrils (which demonstrate cross striations similar to those seen in ordinary cardiac muscle and are peripherally disposed), many mitochondria, and much glycogen. The sarcoplasmic reticulum is not as well developed as in ordinary cardiac fibers, and Purkinje fibers are relatively, if not completely, deficient in transverse tubules.

There would seem to be no reason to believe that the type of junctions connecting the cells in Purkinje fibers to one another and to cells of ordinary cardiac muscle fibers would be any different from those that connect ordinary cardiac muscle cells together, and hence there would be sufficient gap junctions to readily transmit waves of depolarization from one cell to another.

The Basis of Electrocardiograms. The progressive passage of a wave of depolarization over the heart from the S-A node to the terminations of the Purkinje system, with the resulting depolarization and contraction of the cardiac muscle that occurs in sequence in different parts of the heart, can be followed by viewing (from *left* to *right*) the diagrams in Figure 19-2. Next, if one could place two electrodes on the heart at given sites between which a portion of cardiac muscle became depolarized (and hence contracted), the depolarization would set up an electrical current between the electrodes and this could be detected by a galvanometer. If an instrument serving this function were designed to record on a moving strip of paper temporary currents set up by depolarizations and repolarizations of heart muscle occurring between the two electrodes, these currents could be recorded in relation to the times at which they occurred in the cardiac cycle. This is achieved by the instrument known as an electrocardiograph and the record it produces is called an *electrocardiogram* (ECG or EKG). Next, because body tissues are good conductors, it is not necessary to implant electrodes on the heart itself to obtain an electrocardiogram. Instead, the electrodes can be connected externally to body parts representing projections of different parts of the heart, for example, the right and left arms and the left leg. Other combinations of leads can be used for special purposes. Depolarizations of muscle that occur between points in different planes can thus be measured.

In a normal electrocardiogram, currents detected in the heart in a cardiac cycle show as deflections (deviations) from what would otherwise be a straight line. The major component waves of a normal electrocardiogram are shown in Figure 19-8; they are known as P, Q, R, S, and T, respectively.

Electrocardiograms are of such interest to those who will go on into clinical medicine that a short introduction is warranted here. First, the P wave (Figs. 19-2 and 19-8) is due to depolarization of the atria. Subsequent repolarization of the atria is not registered because it is masked by the following waves. The next obvious wave is the R wave (Fig. 19-8), but just before it and also immediately after it there are little dips called Q and S waves, respectively (Fig. 19-8). So the Q, R, and S waves are commonly referred to as the QRS complex. The R wave results from depolarization of the bulk of the ventricular muscle, whereas the Q and S waves are due to depolarization of the first and last parts of it, respectively. The T wave is caused by repolarization of the ventricular muscle. Figure 19-2 correlates the waves seen in an electrocardiogram with what is happening in the heart at any given moment in the cardiac cycle. The region stippled in the diagram on the *left* in Figure 19-2, for example, shows where depolarization is occurring at the beginning of the P wave, which is indicated in the electrocardiogram in Figure 19-8. Figure 19-2 from Shepard is a particularly helpful one to study in order to understand the cardiac cycle.

Relation to Medicine. Most heart ailments seen by physicians involve abnormal functioning of the impulse-conducting system of the heart. The list of abnormalities is long and electrocardiograms are of paramount importance in detecting sites of heart muscle damage or altered function in the conducting system. One type of malfunction in particular should be mentioned because it demonstrates that potential pacemaker cells exist in parts of the heart other than the S-A node, and furthermore that the reason for them not normally functioning as pacemakers (and so upsetting the normal cardiac cycle) is that they do not spontaneously depolarize at as rapid a rate as the cells of the S-A node. Accordingly, under normal conditions such cells become depolarized by the wave of depolarization that sweeps over the atria and down through the impulse-conducting system of the heart, after which they become repolarized. However, before they have

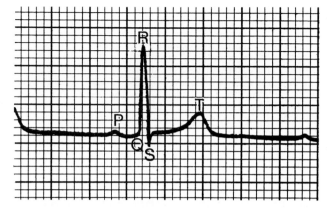

Fig. 19-8. An electrocardiogram obtained from a normal human heart. For details, *see* text.

time to spontaneously depolarize, they become depolarized again by the next wave of depolarization that sweeps down over the atria and on through the conducting system.

Other potential pacemaker cells make their presence felt if, for example, conduction is blocked in the A-V bundle, which is far from being a rare event and can be permanent or intermittent. Under such conditions of bundle block, the wave of depolarization originating about 70 times per minute in the S-A node does not reach the ventricles. This would lead to immediate death if it were not for the fact that there are potential pacemaker cells among the ordinary cardiac muscle cells of the ventricles. These, however, spontaneously depolarize at a much slower rate (28 to 40 times per minute) than those of the S-A node, so the contractions they spontaneously institute in the ventricle are out of synchrony with those of the atria (which continue to contract at their normal rate). So an individual suddenly incapacitated by a bundle block collapses but, because there are potential pacemaker cells in the ventricles, produces just enough ventricular contractions to stay alive, at least in a prone position. Thanks to modern science, such a patient can now be restored to normal health by providing him with an artificial pacemaker connected to the ventricles. This takes over pacemaker function from the slowly depolarizing pacemaker cells of the ventricles, inducing the ventricles to contract regularly at the normal 70 or so beats per minute. With most artificial pacemakers (described below), ventricular contractions are not synchronized with atrial contractions so it might be thought that the ventricles would not fill properly before ventricular contraction occurred. However, atrial contractions do not play as important a role in filling the relaxed ventricles as was once thought. Their main function is to serve as reservoirs, and when the ventricles relax after contraction enough blood flows into them to provide for subsequent effective contraction. For those who might be interested in further details about artificial pacemakers, an introductory account follows.

Artificial Pacemakers. These are battery-powered electronic devices about the size of a pocket watch. A pacemaker can be implanted under local anesthesia into subcutaneous tissue at a site where a wire from the pacemaker can be inserted into, and slipped down, a vein into the right heart so that, while being viewed with a fluoroscope, its terminal can be passed through the tricuspid valve to enter the right ventricle, where it lodges firmly in the trabeculae so as to make good electrical contact with the endocardium at that site. Pacemakers, however, can be lodged in other sites and connected to a ventricle by other routes.

The usual kind of artificial pacemaker is designed to send an electrical impulse sufficient to set off a wave of depolarization in the ventricles, and hence ventricular contraction, at some regular rate such as 72 times a minute. However, in patients with only intermittent bundle block their own pacemaker (S-A node) would sometimes also transmit impulses to the ventricles. So impulses from either their own pacemaker or from the artificial pacemaker could arrive at times when the ventricular muscle was already depolarized and hence not reactive; furthermore, such a situation could result in irregularly spaced ventricular contractions, many of which could be relatively ineffective. This is avoided by using what are termed *standby* pacemakers. In these, the same lead to the heart that conducts impulses to depolarize the ventricles is used in between beats as a sensor for detecting whether a normal R wave appears in the ventricles during those periods when the patient's A-V bundle is functioning normally. In a pacemaker of this type, sensing a normal R wave prevents it from sending its signal, just in time to stop it firing off an R wave itself. Thus, when a patient with a standby pacemaker and intermittent bundle block takes exercise, his pulse rate will go up if his bundle is conducting, and his artificial pacemaker will be continuously inhibited; but if his bundle is not conducting, his pulse rate will remain steady at the pacer rate. There are now artificial pacemakers designed to send ventricular signals at the proper times in response to atrial depolarizations, and in this sense they reproduce the normal physiological control of ventricular contractions.

THE COVERINGS AND LININGS OF THE HEART

The Pericardial Cavity. The myocardium is covered with a fibroelastic connective tissue membrane, which, in turn, is covered with a single layer of mesothelium. This mesothelially covered, fibroelastic membrane which is bound to, and hence continuous with, the endomysium of the myocardium is termed the *epicardium* (Gr. *epi,* upon). Outside this layer there is, however, another fibroelastic membrane, the *pericardium,* which is lined with mesothelium. Between the mesothelium lining the pericardium and that covering the epicardium there is a potential space, the *pericardial cavity,* which in health contains up to 50 ml. of fluid distributed as a thin film between the apposed mesothelial surfaces. The epicardium becomes continuous with the pericardium at the roots of the great vessels entering or leaving the heart. The mesothelial covering of the epicardium thus also becomes continuous with the mesothelial lining of the pericardium, so the former can also be referred to as the *visceral layer of serous pericardium* and the latter as the *parietal layer of serous pericardium,* with the outer, fibroelastic part of the pericardium being called *fibrous pericardium.* The lubricating film of fluid between the mesothelial lining of the pericardium and the mesothelial covering of the epicardium provides a slippery surface that permits the heart to move freely during contraction and relaxation. In certain

diseases the amount of fluid in the pericardial cavity becomes greatly increased; in others the epicardium becomes united by fibrous connective tissue adhesions to the pericardium. Both conditions impede the action of the heart.

Epicardium. The histological features of the epicardium vary over different parts of the heart. Its superficial (mesothelial) layer is a pavement of thin flattened cells typical of simple squamous epithelium (Fig. 7-4). This layer rests on a layer of ordinary connective tissue containing small blood vessels, lymphatics, and nerve fibers. Deeper in this layer there are larger blood vessels and varying amounts of fat. The deepest part of the connective tissue layer blends with the endomysium of the underlying cardiac muscle.

Endocardium. This membrane forms a complete lining for the atria and ventricles and covers all the structures projecting into them, such as valves, chordae tendineae, and papillary muscles, soon to be described. In general, the thickness of the endocardium varies inversely with the thickness of the myocardium it lines. The endocardium consists of three layers. The innermost comprises an endothelium supported by delicate connective tissue; this layer is continuous with the lining of the blood vessels opening into the heart. The next (middle) layer is the thickest. It consists of dense connective tissue in which many elastic fibers are present, particularly in its inner part. These commonly are disposed parallel with the surface, and in some sites where they are abundant they alternate with layers of collagenic fibers. In the outer part of this layer some smooth muscle fibers may also be present. The third (deepest) layer of the endocardium consists of more irregularly arranged connective tissue. Fat may be present here (f in Fig. 19-7B). This layer contains blood vessels and in certain sites it also contains branches of the impulse-conducting system (Purkinje fibers, Fig. 19-7) described in the foregoing. The connective tissue of this layer is continuous with the endomysium of the myocardium.

SKELETON OF THE HEART

The aorta and the pulmonary artery arise from the left and the right ventricles, respectively. At its point of origin each is surrounded by a fibrous ring. The dense connective tissue (Fig. 19-9) of these rings is continuous, either directly or indirectly, through the medium of a triangular mass of dense connective tissue that may show some tendency toward cartilage formation, the trigonum fibrosum, with the connective tissue of fibrous rings that surround the atrioventricular orifices. The fibrous rings surrounding the outlets of the atria and ventricles prevent the valve-containing outlets from becoming dilated when the muscular walls of the chambers contract and force their contents through them. These fibrous structures, together with the fibrous (membranous) part of the interventricular septum, (Fig. 19-5, ct) also provide a means for insertion of the free ends of the fibers of the cardiac musculature. For this reason, these various fibrous structures sometimes are said to constitute the *skeleton* of the heart.

VALVES OF THE HEART

Each ventricle has an intake and an exhaust valve of the leaflet (flap) type (Figs. 19-9 and 19-10). The leaflets of these valves consist essentially of folds of endocardium (Fig. 19-9). But, since 2 layers of endocardium alone would not be strong enough to withstand the pressures generated, the middle of each leaflet is reinforced with a flat sheet of dense connective tissue.

The intake valve of the right ventricle consists of 3 leaflets and so is called the *tricuspid valve.* Although the Latin *cuspis* means a point, it has become common to speak of the leaflets themselves as cusps. The intake valve of the left ventricle consists of only 2 leaflets; hence it is occasionally called the *bicuspid valve.* More commonly it is known as the *mitral valve* because of its resemblance to a bishop's miter (tall cap). The leaflets of both atrioventricular valves have a similar histological structure. They are covered on both sides with endocardium and have a middle supporting layer of dense connective tissue containing numerous elastic fibers.

At the base of the leaflet the middle collagenic plate becomes continuous with the dense connective tissue of the rings surrounding the orifices. Smooth muscle fibers have been described at this site and sphincter-like action attributed to them. Capillaries may be present at the base of the leaflet (where smooth muscle fibers are present) but they do not extend up into the valves in man. Such cells as are distributed throughout the dense connective tissue of the valves live in tissue fluid derived from the plasma of the blood within the heart that bathes the valves.

Tendinous cords of dense collagenic connective tissue (chordae tendineae), which are covered with thin endocardium, extend from the papillary muscles to connect with the ventricular surface of the middle (collagenic) supporting layer of each leaflet. It should be realized that the exhaust valves of the ventricles (the aortic and the pulmonary valves) open on ventricular contraction and that only the closed intake (the tricuspid and mitral) valves have to withstand the full pressure of ventricular contraction. There is a danger, then, that unless they were specially protected, they might during strong ventricular contraction behave like umbrellas on windy days and be blown inside out. The chordae tendineae and the papillary muscles from which they arise limit the extent to which

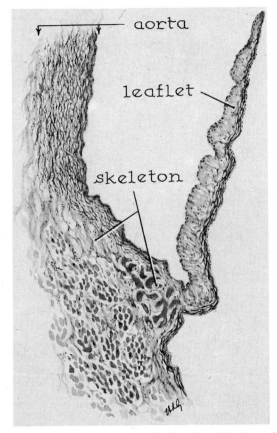

Fig. 19-9. Drawing of a longitudinal section of the heart (low-power) cut through the site where the wall of the ventricle (*bottom left*) is continuous with an aortic valve leaflet. The tissue of the base of the leaflet merges into the skeleton of the heart. Part of the wall of the aorta is labeled; the aortic wall on the opposite side of the lumen of the vessel would lie to the right of the general area illustrated.

the portions of the valves near their free margins can be "blown" toward the atria. (See Fig. 19-3.)

The exhaust valve of the right ventricle is termed the *pulmonary semilunar* (L. *semi,* half; *luna,* moon) *valve* because its leaflets are crescent-shaped. The exhaust valve of the left ventricle is termed the *aortic semilunar valve,* and it, too, has 3 leaflets (Fig. 19-10). The leaflets of these valves are thinner than those of the atrioventricular valves. However, they are of the same general construction, being composed essentially of folds of endocardium reinforced with a middle layer of dense connective tissue; the folds of endocardium at their bases become continuous with the skeleton of the heart (Fig. 19-9). They have no chordae tendineae. The leaflets contain a considerable amount of elastic tissue on their ventricular sides (Fig. 19-9).

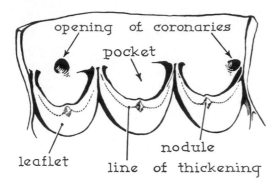

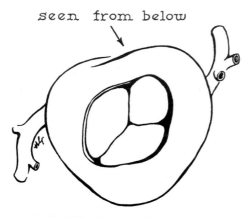

Fig. 19-10. (*Top*) The 3 leaflets of the aortic valve as they appear when the aorta is cut open and spread out flat. Note that the openings of the coronary arteries are located just above this valve. (*Bottom*) The appearance of the aortic valve in its closed position, as seen from below.

In a semilunar valve leaflet the dense middle layer becomes somewhat thickened along a line close to, and parallel with, its free margin, particularly near the middle of the leaflet. This thickened line, not the free margin, is the line along which the leaflets touch one another when the valves close; hence the tissue here must be strong. Between this line of thickened tissue and their free margins, the leaflets are more flimsy and film-like. These very pliable free margins permit a more perfect seal than could be obtained by stiffer tissue unless it were perfectly "machined."

For the free edges of 3 pocket valves bulging inward from the lining of a vessel to make a perfect seal requires that each leaflet, when the valve is closed, have a triangular appearance with its apex reaching the center of the vessel (Fig. 19-10). At the apex of each leaflet, the thickening along the line close to the free margin is accentuated to form a nodule (Fig. 19-10). The free margin of a closed valve curves upward to peak at this point so that

this pointed portion constitutes a true cusp (Fig. 19-10), but the whole leaflet is often called a cusp.

Diseases affecting the valves of the heart may cause serious problems. In particular, in children suffering from rheumatic fever, the leaflets may become the seat of an inflammatory process that can deform their line of closure. The healing of the leaflets is often associated with considerable increase in their collagenic component; as a result, they become stiffer and shorter or deformed in other ways. Leaflets can even adhere to one another. In any event, the end result is likely to be a valve that does not open or close properly. In his clinical years, the student will see many examples of valves so affected. It is now possible to replace diseased valves of certain types with artificial ones or transplants.

ARTERIES AND ARTERIOLES

There are 3 main kinds of arteries. Although all conduct blood, the 3 kinds perform somewhat different and important functions, to which their structure is particularly adapted. They are: (*1*) elastic arteries, (*2*) muscular (distributing) arteries, and (*3*) arterioles. These types are not sharply divided, for type 1 merges with type 2 and type 2 with type 3. Each kind will be described in turn.

Elastic Arteries. To simplify the following account, we shall deal only with the systemic circulation. The left ventricle delivers blood into the aorta in spurts, ordinarily slightly more than 70 spurts per minute. During contraction of the ventricle, the pressure generated is relatively high. But between contractions the pressure in the arterial system would fall to zero if the walls of the arterial system were rigid, like the walls of metal pipes. However, a reduced pressure in the arterial system between contractions of a ventricle is maintained because the walls of the arteries that lead directly from each ventricle are constructed chiefly of many layers of elastic laminae. Such arteries are termed *elastic* arteries. Blood delivered into them by the contracting heart stretches the elastin in their walls. Then, after a ventricle has finished contracting, its exhaust valve closes, and the walls of the elastic arteries (stretched when the ventricle contracted) passively contract to maintain pressure within the system for the short interval elapsing before the ventricle fills and contracts again.

Systolic and Diastolic Blood Pressure. The pressure within the arterial system generated during the contraction of the ventricles is called the *systolic* (Gr. *systole,* a contracting) blood pressure, and it is slightly more than half as much again as the pressure that is maintained by the stretched elastic tissue of the arterial walls between contractions of the heart; the latter is called the *diastolic* (Gr. *diastole,* dilation) pressure.

The function of maintaining pressure within the arterial system during diastole is performed chiefly by the largest arteries of the body because their walls consist chiefly of elastin. The branches that arise from the largest arteries to deliver blood to the different parts of the body have a different function and they have walls of a somewhat different character, as will now be described.

Muscular (Distributing) Arteries. Since the parts of the body under varied conditions of activity require different amounts of blood, the arteries supplying them must be capable of having the size of their lumina regulated so that appropriate amounts of blood can be delivered at any given time. For example, the muscles in the right arm of a right-handed tennis player require more blood during a match than those of his left arm. Regulation of the size of the lumina of these *distributing* arteries is under the control of the sympathetic division of the autonomic nervous system, through its innervating smooth muscle. The walls of distributing arteries consist chiefly of so-called circularly disposed smooth muscle fibers (which are actually arranged in a spiral) and these fibers respond to nerve impulses and other stimuli by regulating the size of the lumen of the artery they surround. If the walls of these arteries were made of elastin, which can only recoil passively, nervous control would not be possible. Because the important component of their walls is smooth muscle, distributing arteries are also called *muscular* arteries. They variously regulate the flow of blood to different parts of the body according to the needs of these parts.

Arterioles. In order for man to stand erect, a substantial pressure must be maintained within the arterial system; otherwise, blood would not be delivered in sufficient quantities to the various capillary beds such as those of the brain, for this requires that the force of gravity be overcome. However, pressure must be maintained within the arterial system in such a way that blood is delivered into capillary beds under reduced pressure because the walls of capillaries must be thin (and therefore weak) to permit ready diffusion through them. Delivery of arterial blood into capillary beds under relatively low pressure is achieved by *arterioles*. These, as their name implies, are essentially very small arteries, but they have a relatively narrow lumen and thick muscular walls. Since blood is of a certain viscosity, their narrow lumen offers considerable resistance to its flow, and this permits relatively high pressures to be built up behind them. The degree of pressure within the arterial system as a whole is regulated mainly by the *degree of tonus of the smooth muscle cells in the walls of arterioles* and this in turn is controlled by the autonomic system, and by hormones as will be described in a later chapter. If the tonus of the smooth muscle cells becomes increased above the normal range, *hypertension* (high blood pressure) results.

THE MICROSCOPIC STRUCTURE OF ARTERIES

The walls of arteries consist of 3 coats or tunics that are by no means always as clear-cut as the following description may suggest. They are (*1*) the tunica intima (the innermost coat), (*2*) the tunica media (the middle coat), and (*3*) the tunica adventitia (the outermost coat). The relative thickness of each coat and the type of tissue it contains depend on whether the vessel is an elastic artery, muscular artery or arteriole.

BOUNDARIES AND COMPOSITION OF THE THREE COATS AS SEEN IN H AND E SECTIONS

The 3 coats are most easily distinguished in muscular arteries, so we begin with them.

Muscular Arteries. The *intima* is bounded on its inner surface by *endothelium* (which is included as part of the intima) and at its outer surface by a substantial lamina of elastin termed the *internal elastic lamina;* this lamina too is regarded as part of the intima. This lamina is most easily seen in muscular arteries where it appears in an artery that has contracted after death (because there was no blood pressure to keep its wall stretched) as a wavy, bright pink line. This is seen as a dark wavy line just beneath the endothelium in Figure 19-11A. In many muscular arteries the endothelium lining the artery seems to lie directly on the internal elastic lamina. Sometimes the internal elastic lamina is duplicated; this is described as a *split internal elastic lamina* (Fig. 19-12).

The *media* of a muscular artery is composed essentially of more or less spirally disposed smooth muscle cells (Figs. 19-11A and 19-12). The intercellular substance holding the smooth muscle cells together is made by the smooth muscle cells themselves and is chiefly *elastin*. There is relatively more elastin in the media of a large muscular artery than in a small one. The outer border of the media of a muscular artery is marked by a substantial lamina of elastin, called the *external elastic lamina*.

The *adventitia* of a muscular artery varies but is commonly one half to two thirds the thickness of the media (Fig. 19-11A). It consists chiefly of elastic fibers (darkly stained in Fig. 19-11A) but it also contains collagenic ones. So most of the elastin in the wall of a muscular artery lies in the tunica adventitia. Tiny blood vessels called *vasa vasorum* (vessels of vessels) supply the adventitia, particularly in larger arteries. Lymphatics are also present in the adventitia.

Coronary Arteries. Because thrombosis here is an important cause of disability and death, the coronary arteries, which supply the musculature of the heart, deserve special attention. They are of the muscular type. They differ somewhat, however, from the usual type of muscu-

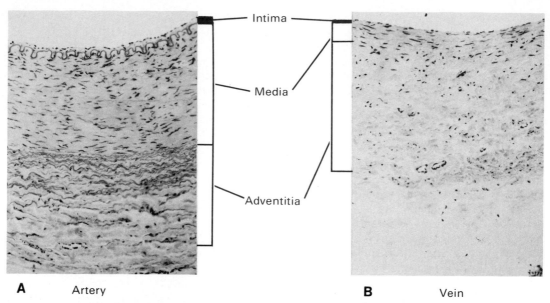

Intima

Media

Adventitia

A   Artery   **B**   Vein

Fig. 19-11. (*A*) Medium-power photomicrograph of a cross section of part of the wall of a distributing artery. (*B*) Photomicrograph (same magnification) of a cross section of part of the wall of one of its companion veins. Note the great disparity in the thickness of the media between the artery and the vein.

lar artery. Usually the endothelium of a small muscular artery lies directly on the internal elastic lamina as in Figure 19-12. However, it is not true for some parts of the coronary arteries of newborn children as will now be explained.

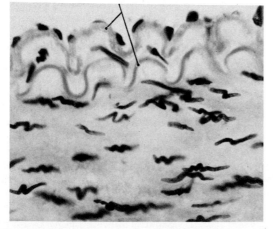

Split internal elastic lamina

Fig. 19-12. High-power photomicrograph of a cross section of the wall of a distributing artery, showing a split internal elastic lamina in the intima and smooth muscle cell nuclei (in the contracted configuration) in the media below.

Jaffé, Hartroft, Manning, and Eleta described intimal thickenings, termed musculo-elastic cushions, at the sites of branching of coronary arteries in newborn babies (Fig. 19-13). It is thought that the tissue in these sites has its origin from undifferentiated smooth muscle cells of the media, which migrate from the media through fenestrae in the internal elastic lamina (Fig. 19-13) to take up a subendothelial position. Here they produce elastin in the form of fibers or incomplete laminae. In addition, they probably produce other types of intercellular substance (mostly ground substance but sometimes a little collagen as well) in these cushions.

Cells other than undifferentiated smooth muscle cells may also make their appearance in these thickenings very early in life. Monocytes, for instance, gain entrance so that it seems likely that the macrophages seen later in thickened intimas could originate from cells coming to the intima via the blood.

The musculo-elastic cushions, as may be seen at *lower left* in Figure 19-13, tend to have 2 layers. The superficial layer contains more amorphous intercellular substance and fewer fibers than the deeper layer.

Next, as Jaffé, Hartroft, Manning, and Eleta show, and what could be very important with regard to the development of atherosclerosis (soon to be discussed) in coronary arteries is that intimal thickening tends to become general along the coronary arteries in the early decades of life. The thickening is of the same nature as that seen in

Fig. 19-13. Diagram of the wall structure of the coronary arteries, based on a study of coronary arteries of newborn babies. The thickenings of the intima vary in thickness. (Based on Jaffé, D., Manning, M., and Hartroft, W. S.: Coronary arteries in the earlier decades of man. Fed. Proc., *27*:575, 1968)

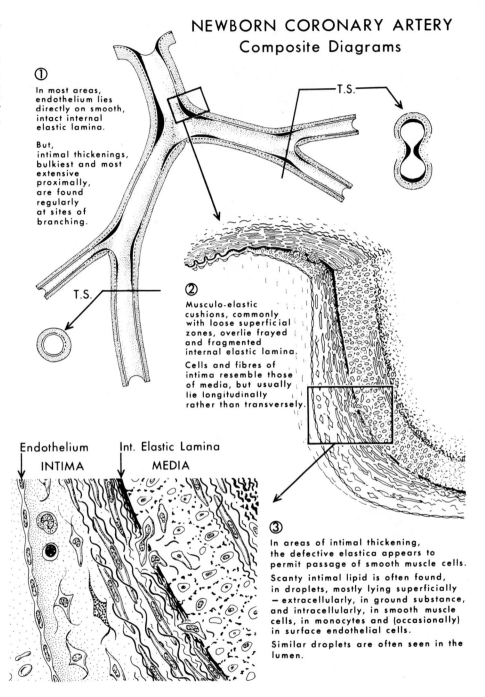

NEWBORN CORONARY ARTERY
Composite Diagrams

① In most areas, endothelium lies directly on smooth, intact internal elastic lamina.

But, intimal thickenings, bulkiest and most extensive proximally, are found regularly at sites of branching.

T.S.

T.S.

② Musculo-elastic cushions, commonly with loose superficial zones, overlie frayed and fragmented internal elastic lamina.

Cells and fibres of intima resemble those of media, but usually lie longitudinally rather than transversely.

Endothelium   Int. Elastic Lamina
INTIMA   MEDIA

③ In areas of intimal thickening, the defective elastica appears to permit passage of smooth muscle cells.

Scanty intimal lipid is often found, in droplets, mostly lying superficially — extracellularly, in ground substance, and intracellularly, in smooth muscle cells, in monocytes and (occasionally) in surface endothelial cells.

Similar droplets are often seen in the lumen.

newborns at bifurcations, but not so pronounced. As a result of the thickening there are often elastic fibers rather than an internal elastic lamina directly beneath the endothelium, and there may also be little deposits of collagen in the intima in these sites. The cells in this subendothelial layer are mostly cells of the undifferentiated smooth muscle type already described. In the intima, however, they are disposed longitudinally, whereas in the media they are arranged circularly (though somewhat spirally) (Fig. 19-14).

Elastic Arteries. In these the *intima* is very much *thicker* than that of a muscular artery (Fig. 19-15). For example,

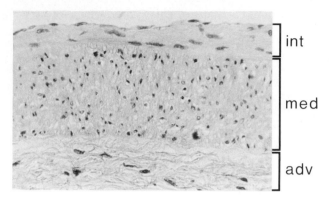

Fig. 19-14. Photomicrograph of part of the wall of a coronary artery (cut in *longitudinal* section) from a 5-year-old child. Note that the intima (int) has become thickened by smooth muscle cells, mostly of the undifferentiated type; these are disposed longitudinally under the endothelium. Deep to this, smooth muscle cells of the media (med) form a circular layer and so have been cut in cross section. Collagenic fibers and fibroblasts are visible in the adventitia (adv). (Courtesy of D. Jaffé)

the intima of the aorta makes up about 20 per cent of the total thickness of its wall. In the H and E section on the left of Figure 19-15, it appears paler than the media, and in the section stained for elastin on the right, it can be seen that the intima contains less elastin than the media.

The elastic component of that part of the intima between the endothelium and the internal elastic lamina is in the form of fibers and incomplete laminae embedded along with cells in amorphous intercellular substance. It seems most probable that the main cell type in a normal intima is the same as that already described for coronary arteries, namely, a relatively undifferentiated type of smooth muscle cell that can produce the various types of intercellular substance seen in the intima. However, other types of cells are commonly described as being present in the intima of elastic arteries—for example, fibroblasts and macrophages.

The external border of the intima is marked by an internal elastic lamina; this is considered to be part of the intima, but it is similar to the other laminae that are such a prominent feature of the media and that will be described shortly. However, it is not always easy to distinguish the

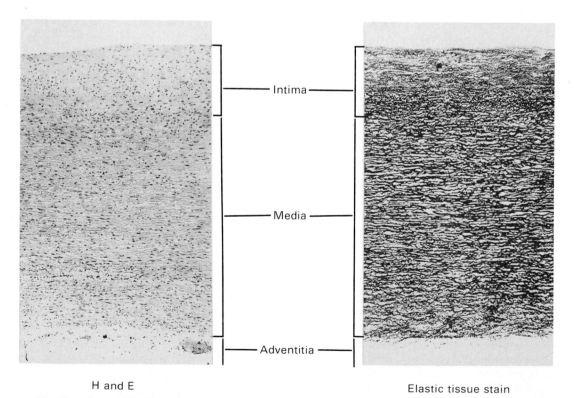

H and E   Elastic tissue stain

Fig. 19-15. Low-power photomicrographs of serial sections of the wall of the aorta, with the elastic fibers and laminae stained specifically in the section on the right.

internal elastic lamina as such because there is so much elastin in the intima.

The media of an elastic artery constitutes the bulk of its wall and consists chiefly of concentrically arranged fenestrated laminae of elastin similar to the internal elastic lamina of the intima. They appear as dark lines in Figure 19-15 (*right*), and as lighter ones in Figure 19-15 (*left*). The number of these varies with age. There are about 40 in the newborn and up to 70 in the adult. The laminae also become thicker in adults than they are in childhood.

The smooth muscle cells between adjacent laminae are of the type already described that produce, in addition to the elastin of the laminae and also fine elastic and collagenic fibers in the interstices between laminae, the considerable amount of amorphous intercellular substance also present between adjacent laminae in which the cells of the tunica media are embedded. The intercellular substance here is commonly more basophilic than the ground substance of ordinary connective tissue, suggesting that it contains a greater proportion of sulfated glycosaminoglycans. Furthermore, there is additional evidence that the amorphous intercellular substance here is the product of a cell type that, in some species at least, has some of the attributes (or at least potentialities) of chondrocytes. In unreported experiments Ham found that the administration of a very large dose of vitamin D to rabbits, a dose that caused calcification of the media, was followed afterward by the development of rings of cartilage in the aortic wall. Curiously enough, the rings were so regularly disposed as to mimic the distribution of rings of cartilage in the trachea. Hartroft (personal communication) has also found rings of cartilage forming in the aortic wall in animals in which arterial disease was produced by dietary means. As already noted, the undifferentiated smooth muscle cells of arteries seem to have a broad potentiality.

The outermost limit of the media is marked by the external elastic lamina.

The adventitia of an elastic artery is thin (Fig. 19-15). It consists of irregularly arranged connective tissue containing both collagenic and elastic fibers. Small blood vessels are present in it and supply also the outer one third of the tunica media; these constitute the *vasa vasorum*. Lymphatic capillaries are also present in the adventitia. The reason capillaries and lymphatics are not present in the inner part of the wall of an artery will soon be described. The collagen in the adventitia of elastic arteries may serve as a sheath to restrain overexpansion of the artery.

The Changes in Arterial Walls Associated With Atherosclerosis. Since this type of arterial disease is a major cause of death, we shall here discuss some histological features of elastic and muscular arteries that may have a bearing on it. Atherosclerosis, so prevalent in our society, involves degeneration of portions of the *intima* and also sometimes even deeper layers of important arter-

ies. The lesions themselves suggest that lipid metabolism is involved in their formation, since lipids—for example, cholesterol —often accumulate in them. Lesions of this type are commonly called *atheromata* because the contents, at least sometimes, have a gruel-like (Gr. *athere*, gruel) appearance.

Atherosclerosis (Gr. *athere* + *sclerosis*, hardening) would not be such a serious matter if it were not for the fact that platelets may begin to adhere to the rough inner surface of a vessel at the site of atherosclerotic lesions and there, particularly if they come into contact with collagen (p. 273), institute the formation of a thrombus. So, from the standpoint of preventative medicine, there are really 2 interrelated problems: (*1*) preventing the development of atherosclerosis, and (*2*) preventing the formation of thrombi on atherosclerotic lesions. It is the latter phenomenon—the formation of a thrombus—that causes the coronary thrombosis or cerebral stroke that may cause death, because the part of the heart or brain supplied by the affected artery dies.

So we might ask if there are any peculiarities about the histology of the walls of elastic and certain muscular arteries (for example, coronary arteries) that might give some clue as to why they should so commonly be sites of degenerative lesions and thrombus formation. In pursuing this thought, we shall consider briefly the mechanism by which artery walls must be nourished; this is different from most other body parts.

Some Problems Associated With Supplying Oxygen and Nutrients to the Arterial Wall and Removing Waste Products From It. The wall of an artery is stretched by pressure from within the artery and this presents unique problems for its nutrition.

The usual arrangement for supplying any considerable mass of tissue with oxygen and nutrients is for it to be permeated with capillaries. Ordinarily, capillaries are supplied with blood under very low pressure. But if low-pressure capillary beds were present in the inner parts of the walls of arteries, they would collapse because the relatively high pressure of the blood within the lumen would be transmitted to at least the inner layers of the artery walls and this is a much greater pressure than exists in capillaries. Low-pressure capillaries are not present in the walls of arteries except as vasa vasorum in their outer layers; here they can remain open because the force of the pressure of the blood in the lumen is taken up by the inner and the middle layers of the artery walls and hence does not reach them. Lacking capillaries, cells in the intima and inner two thirds of the media of the walls of arteries must be nourished by diffusion of substances from the blood in the lumen through the intercellular substances of the intima and most of the media. This is a long distance for a diffusion mechanism to operate effectively. The situation is not unlike that in hyaline cartilage, where diffusion must also occur over relatively long distances. It will be recalled that precipitation of mineral in cartilage matrix can interfere with diffusion and hence nutrition of its cells. Slow deposition or accumulation of substances in artery walls might likewise interfere with the diffusion mechanism on which their cells are dependent.

The removal of products of metabolism, or in particular macromolecular products of degeneration, from the cells in the inner layers of arterial walls would seem to be an even greater problem because there are no lymphatic capillaries in the inner parts of the wall to help remove waste products and, in particular, macromolecules. Even if they were present here, because the pressure within lymphatic capillaries is so low in lymphatic capillaries, they would collapse due to the arterial pressure in the lumen.

From the foregoing it might be expected that degeneration would be more likely to occur in arterial walls than in most other sites in the body, and further, that arterial walls would be more likely to become sites of accumulation of macromolecular mate-

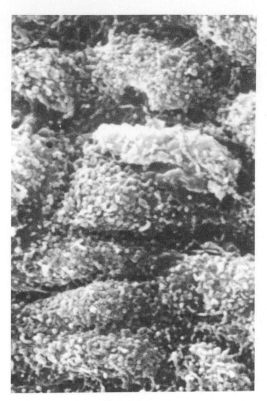

Fig. 19-16. Low-power scanning electron micrograph of the endothelial surface of the lining of the pulmonary artery. The surface presented to the lumen is studded with innumerable microvillus-like projections. (Smith, V., Ryan, J. W., Michie, D. D., and Smith, D. S.: Science, *173*:925, 1971)

rials than tissues where lymphatic capillaries drain away macromolecules. It seems to the authors that in the study of atherosclerosis the mechanism of nutrition in artery walls deserves more attention than it has received.

Another histological feature of artery walls of significance in atherosclerosis is the undifferentiated type of smooth muscle cell already mentioned. This kind of cell, which inhabits the intima, has broad potentiality and there is much evidence that its proliferation is involved in the atherosclerotic process. The experimental approach described on page 303 whereby the enzyme G-6-PD can be used in heterozygous females as a tracer to show that in certain blood disorders certain types of blood cells are all members of the same clone has also been used in connection with tracing (again in heterozygous females) the origin of the aggregations of undifferentiated smooth muscle cells seen in atherosclerotic lesions. These experiments have shown that the muscle cells all have the same form of the enzyme and hence are clones (Benditt and Benditt). For those who have read about control of cell populations in Chapter 6, it might be of interest to know that a hypothesis has been advanced by Martin and Sprague that as an individual becomes older, the well-differentiated smooth muscle cells of his arteries may not be able to produce enough chalone-like inhibitor to restrain the prolifer-

ative activity of the less-differentiated smooth muscle cells in the intima, so that these would multiply to form tumor-like aggregates that incite, or are otherwise involved in, the atherosclerotic process.

A further histological point of interest relates to the presence of collagen in the intima; for the more there is, the greater is the danger of abrasions or other defects in the endothelium permitting platelets to come into contact with it to bring about their aggregation as was described in Chapter 10.

Finally, scanning electron microscopy has revealed that the endothelial lining of an artery can be studded with microvillus-like projections (Fig. 19-16) and these could exert hemodynamic effects.

The regenerative capacity of endothelial cells seems to be considerable and, as a result, defects made in normal endothelial linings are repaired very quickly. Moreover, there is some experimental evidence to suggest that cells in the blood may be able to settle out and form new endothelium where there was none. This could be due to endothelial cells becoming detached from other sites and circulating and becoming implanted at sites where endothelium is needed.

Elastin Formation in Developing Arteries. In the formation of arteries, mesenchymal cells loosely encircle developing endothelial tubes and differentiate into a type of cell that eventually assumes all the characteristics of a smooth muscle cell. This type of cell is believed to produce the elastin and other intercellular substances of the intima and media of a developing artery. A small portion of such a cell is labeled Sm at *bottom left* in Figure 19-17, which is an electron micrograph of the intima of the developing aorta of a fetus. The micrograph shows the elastin of the internal elastic lamina (labeled iel) of the intima forming in close association with differentiating smooth muscle cells. The way the homogeneous elastin (e in Fig. 19-17) comes to lie within a scaffolding of microfibrils (m in Fig. 19-17) was described in Chapter 9 (p. 235).

The processes of synthesis and secretion of proelastin are probably very similar to those of procollagen, which were described in Chapter 9 and illustrated in Figures 9-7 and 9-8.

The Growth of Elastic Laminae of Arteries. During the postnatal growth period these have to cover a wider area in order to encompass the lumen of growing arteries. This requires that more elastin somehow make its appearance *within the substance* of a lamina. Yet elastin is formed by an appositional growth mechanism. In this connection, however, it should be observed that elastic laminae are fenestrated. It is usually and correctly assumed that the function of fenestrae is to serve as holes through which dissolved substances can diffuse to nourish cells deep to the lamina concerned. However, fenestrae would also permit growth of the laminae, as follows.

During growth, the aorta (for example) increases both in length and width. Hence the elastic laminae in its wall would have to stretch in two directions. But if a lamina

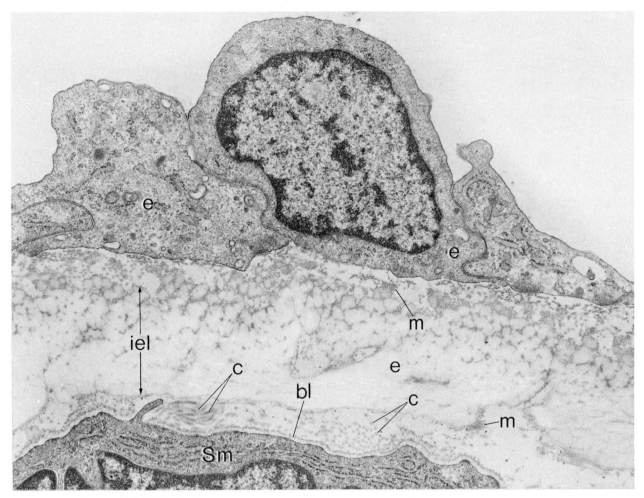

Fig. 19-17. Electron micrograph (×16,000) of the intima of the developing aorta of a human fetus, showing the internal elastic lamina (iel) beneath the endothelial cells (e). At *bottom left* part of a differentiating smooth muscle cell (Sm) is present; this cell is probably producing elastin and other intercellular substances of the wall. It is enclosed in a basal lamina (bl) and also has collagenic fibrils (c) associated with it. Note also the microfibrils (m) forming a scaffolding for the amorphous elastin (e) of the internal elastic lamina. (Courtesy of M. D. Haust)

were to be stretched in both directions, its fenestrae would become increasingly larger. The inner surfaces of these holes would then provide sites where elastin could continually be added to a surface to increase the total amount in the lamina. So fenestrae may also serve as sites where the appositional deposition of elastin can occur during growth.

The Possibility of Regeneration of Elastic Laminae. There has been some question as to whether new elastic laminae can form in arteriosclerotic arteries. Ham's studies on arteriosclerosis (a general term for hardening of the arterial wall) in rats given very large doses of vitamin D, by which

method the greater part of the media of a coronary artery becomes almost immediately calcified, indicated that as time went on new elastin formed on each side of the calcified ring.

ARTERIOLES

Arterial vessels with overall diameters of less than 100 μm. are called *arterioles.* As can be seen from Fig. 19-18, the thickness of the wall of an arteriole, seen in a section of fixed tissue, is generally only slightly less than the diameter of its lumen. The walls of larger arterioles have the usual

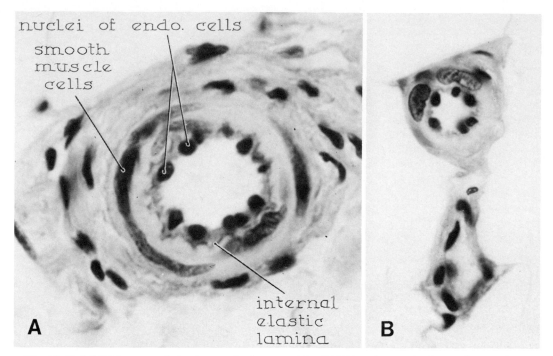

Fig. 19-18. (*A*) High-power photomicrograph of an arteriole. (*B*) Photomicrograph of a small arteriole (*top*) and its companion venule (*bottom*).

3 coats. The intima consists of endothelium, the basal lamina of which is applied to an internal elastic lamina in larger arterioles. The media contains up to about 3 so-called circular layers of smooth muscle cells that are actually arranged in the form of a spiral, and an external elastic lamina is also present in larger arterioles. The adventitia may be as thick as the media; it contains a mixture of collagenic and elastic fibers.

As arterioles branch and become smaller, their walls become thinner and their lumina smaller. The ratio between the wall thickness and the diameter of the lumen, however, remains about the same (compare Fig. 19-18A and 19-18B, *top*), and this together with a rough estimate of the number of layers of smooth muscle cells in the media are criteria that are often used for recognizing arterioles. The internal and external elastic laminae become very thin in smaller arterioles (Fig. 19-18B), and in the smallest (those less than 35 μm. in diameter) they are absent. The smooth muscle cells of the media of small arterioles are correspondingly small (compare those in part A and part B, *top*, of Fig. 19-18). In the smallest arterioles only one or two layers of smooth muscle cells can be seen in a cross section (Fig. 19-18B). The adventitia of small arterioles is very thin and consists chiefly of collagenic fibers.

THE PERIPHERAL CIRCULATION

CAPILLARIES AND CAPILLARY BEDS

Capillaries are commonly arranged in the form of anastomosing networks called *capillary beds;* it is from these beds that tissue fluid is formed and hence oxygen and nutrients are provided for cells in their vicinity. The blood flowing through a capillary bed arrives through arterioles and is carried away by venules, with the volume flowing through a given bed at any given time being under the control of the autonomic nervous system. This control is mediated by smooth muscle cells that are arranged so as to encircle blood vessels of different calibers. For example, if the smooth muscle cells of arterioles are contracted so as to restrict the arteriolar lumen, less blood is delivered to the capillary beds they supply. If dilated, arterioles supply more blood to the beds. But they are not the only vessels involved in controlling circulation in capillary beds, as will now be described.

Perhaps the first point to emphasize is that it would be impossible to elucidate how blood circulated through what is generally termed the *terminal vascular bed* by studying sections of fixed tissue. It can only be done by examining living preparations with the LM. Much of our present-day knowledge on this matter comes from the detailed studies of Zweifach, who provided Figure 19-23, which we describe in detail later. But first we shall describe capillaries.

The Appearance of Capillaries in H and E Sections. Since capillaries are disposed in so many different planes in most tissues, and since most of them pursue irregular courses, it is seldom that they are seen cut longitudinally in sections. Striated muscle is an exception, for here they run parallel to the muscle fibers. Because of this they are relatively straight and hence the cross-sectional appearance of capillaries may be studied to advantage in cross sections of striated muscle (Fig. 19-19). Such sections cut through most capillaries without passing through nuclei of any of their endothelial cells; hence these capillaries appear as simple tubes (Fig. 19-19, *bottom*). However, in some instances the nucleus of one of the endothelial cells of a capillary wall will be cut and, if so, appears as a dark crescent partly encircling the lumen (Fig. 19-19, *upper left*). In cross sections some capillaries are seen to contain red blood cells (Fig. 19-19, *right of center*) and sometimes leukocytes (Fig. 19-19, *upper right*).

As noted in Chapter 9, the EM disclosed that there are 2 main types, respectively termed *continuous* and *fenestrated*. We shall deal with these in turn.

The Fine Structure of Continuous Capillaries. In life the lumen of a continuous capillary is around 8 to 10 μm. in diameter, that is, slightly wider than an erythrocyte. Erythrocytes are not circulating through every capillary at any given time and so many will not be fully open. The capillary shown in Figure 19-20, for instance, is partly collapsed. In some cross sections of capillaries one endothelial cell may seem to encircle the lumen. However, in others parts of two or more endothelial cells may be seen. The capillary shown in Figure 19-20 reveals parts of two endothelial cells. Since these are fitted together in an irregular fashion, a thin *cross section* would still cut through parts of two endothelial cells even if each of the two endothelial cells completely surrounded the capillary.

As can be seen in Figure 19-20, the nucleus of an endothelial cell creates a bulge in the capillary wall; nevertheless, it is covered on all sides with cytoplasm. The cytoplasm contains all the usual organelles and in most capillaries is replete with pinocytotic vesicles (some are indicated by arrows in Fig. 19-20). These vesicles seem to form on both the inner and outer surfaces of a capillary endothelial cell, so that a mixture is seen of vesicles traversing the cytoplasm in either direction. They are thought to be a way for macromolecular substances to be brought back into, or transported out of, capillaries.

The edges of endothelial cells are somewhat irregular in outline so that contiguous cells interdigitate and form serrated joints with one another. In most capillaries the

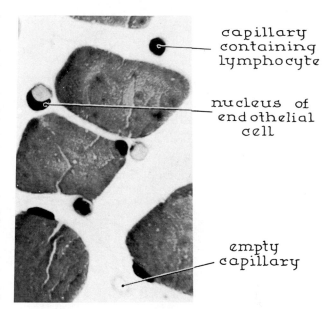

Fig. 19-19. Oil-immersion photomicrograph of striated muscle, showing various appearances presented by capillaries in cross section. The section can pass through a capillary where a nucleus of an endothelial cell is present; if so, the nucleus appears as a blue crescent (*upper left*). If a capillary is cut where no nucleus is present, it appears as a thin cytoplasmic ring (right of center, and *bottom*). Either red blood cells or leukocytes may be present in capillaries where they are sectioned (*top right*).

parallel edges of contiguous cells over most of their courses are separated by a space that is normally about 20 nm. wide; this space is filled with material of low electron density (Fig. 19-20).

In most parts of the body, the edges of contiguous endothelial cells of capillaries of both the continuous and the fenestrated kind seem to be joined by *tight junctions* of the fascia occludens type, so that these junctions do not occupy the entire margin of the contiguous cells. Between these junctions there are slit-like clefts through which tissue fluid can pass out of the capillary. In the brain, however, as noted in Chapter 17, the tight junctions between contiguous endothelial cells are continuous in that they extend right around the margins of the cells and hence they are of the zonula occludens type; furthermore, the capillaries are also completely surrounded by a very substantial basement membrane, so there is an effective blood-brain barrier. At points of contact between contiguous endothelial cells of capillaries, one cell generally overlaps another slightly and commonly forms a flap or fold called a *marginal fold* that projects a little into the lumen of the capillary, as can be seen at *lower left* in Figure 19-20. The capillary as a whole is enclosed by a basement membrane (Fig. 9-4).

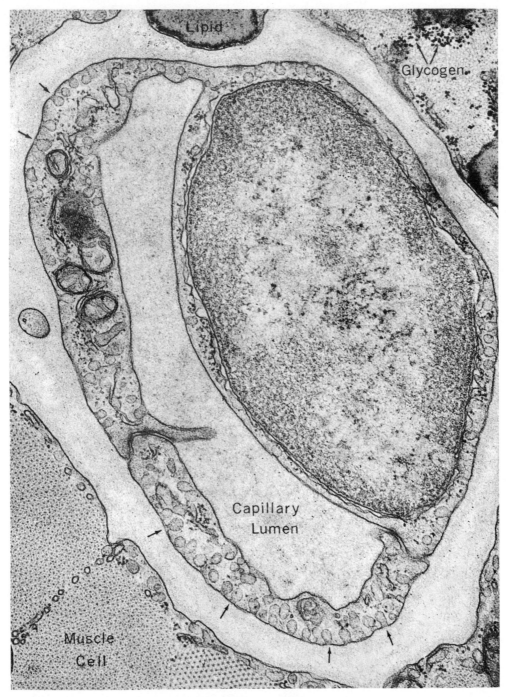

Fig. 19-20. Electron micrograph of a continuous capillary, seen in cardiac muscle. The section passes through the nucleus of an endothelial cell. Parts of two endothelial cells are present; junctions between them are seen at *lower left* and *lower right*. A marginal fold projects into the lumen just above the one on the left. Note the numerous pinocytotic vesicles; several sites where they are originating are indicated by arrows. (Fawcett, D. W.: J. Histochem. Cytochem., *13:*75, 1965)

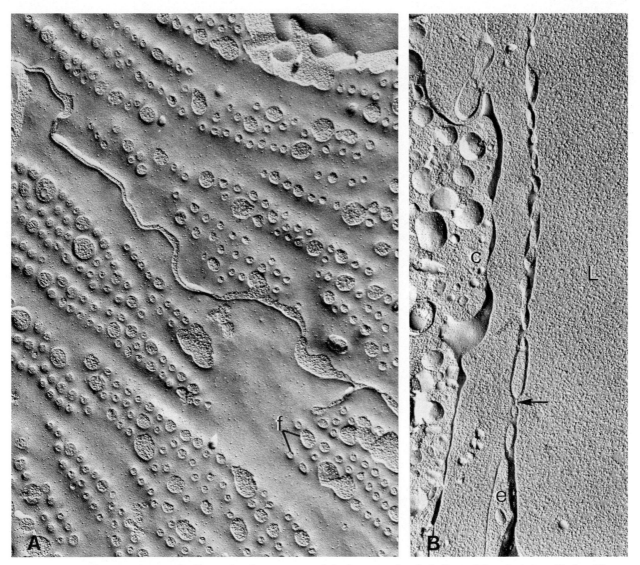

Fig. 19-21. Electron micrographs illustrating the structure of the fenestrated endothelium of fenestrated capillaries. These depict freeze-fracture replicas of capillary endothelial cells of the adrenal gland (hamster). (*A*) Endothelial cells in surface view (×152,000), showing the disposition of the fenestrae (f) in well-defined tracts. The biggest fenestrae here (in the adrenal cortex) are 166 nm. in diameter, which is uncommonly large for fenestrated capillaries in general. (*B*) Endothelial cells fractured transversely (×107,000). The endothelium (e) is seen lying at a short distance to the right of the cytoplasm (c) of an adrenal cell (at *left*) that borders on the capillary; the lumen (L) of this capillary is seen at *right*. Note the diaphragms closing over the fenestrae (a diaphragm is indicated by the arrow). (Ryan, U. S., Ryan, J. W., Smith, D. S., and Winkler, H.: Tissue and Cell, *7*:181, 1975)

The Fine Structure of Fenestrated Capillaries. These are not unlike capillaries of the continuous type, as described above, except that some of the attenuated regions of cytoplasm of their endothelial cells are riddled with circular perforations, commonly around 60 to 80 nm. in diameter but somewhat larger than this in certain sites (as, for example, illustrated in Fig. 19-21). These perforations are of a permanent nature and are called *fenestrae* (L. for windows). They are not open, but are closed by a thin *diaphragm* in all but the fenestrated capillaries of kidney glomeruli, where it is generally agreed that most, if not all, of the fenestrae lack diaphragms. Although little is known about the permeability properties of these fenestrae, it is widely believed that their presence facilitates exchange across the endothelial membrane.

The diaphragm closing over a fenestra appears in the

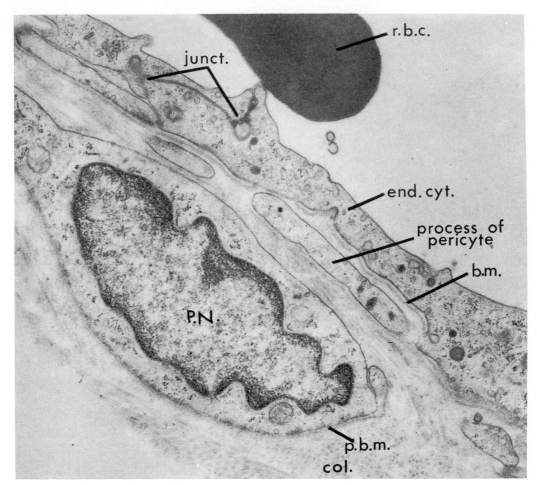

Fig. 19-22. Electron micrograph of the wall of a small blood vessel with a pericyte. A red blood cell (r.b.c.) is seen at *top,* within its lumen. Below this, two endothelial lining cells (end. cyt.) are attached to each other by tight junctions (fascia occludens); two of these are labeled junct. A basal lamina (b.m.) can be seen underlying the endothelium. Deep to this is the process of a pericyte (labeled) and farther out from the lumen is its cell body and nucleus (P.N.). A basal lamina (p.b.m.) also surrounds the cell body of the pericyte. Some collagen fibrils (col.) are present at *bottom.* (Courtesy of N. Taichman and H. Movat)

EM as a single structure that is described as being somewhat thinner than a single cell membrane and possessing a central thickening about 10 to 15 nm. across. Rather than a circumscribed region of ordinary cell membrane, it is more likely to be a special kind of structure that is inserted, as it were, into the attenuated cytoplasm. Hence all around the periphery of the fenestra, cell membrane on the luminal side of the endothelial cell would be in direct continuity with cell membrane on the surface facing the surrounding tissue. If it were otherwise, with the cell membranes extending across the fenestra instead of meeting around it, the diaphragm might be expected to be more of the thickness of 2 cell membranes and perhaps even to appear as a double structure.

The disposition of fenestrae in this type of capillary is

often studied by means of freeze-fracture replicas (this technic was described on p. 111), and an example of a fenestrated capillary seen in this way is shown in Figure 19-21. Such replicas show that in some places in the body the fenestrae are aligned in tracts along the endothelial cells (Fig. 19-21A). Figure 19-21B also clearly shows that the fenestrae in capillaries of the adrenal gland, for example, are closed over by diaphragms and not patent.

Pericytes. Many years ago occasional contractile cells (called Rouget cells) were observed lying along the sides of the capillaries in the eyes of frogs. So when occasional cells were also found beside capillaries in mammals it was at first incorrectly thought that they were the counterparts of Rouget cells and hence were contractile. It took a long time to establish that these cells have no contractile role and that capillaries are only passive tubes, so that the control of blood flow in capillary beds has to be looked for elsewhere.

These cells scattered along the sides of capillaries and certain other small blood vessels in mammals, and which are referred to as *perivascular cells* or *pericytes,* were, however, shown to be of great importance for other reasons, which were described on page 228. Although in the growth of new blood vessels pericytes can develop into smooth muscle cells, in their normal relatively undifferentiated state they are seen to differ from smooth muscle cells in several respects. Their organelles, for instance, are distributed more diffusely and their cytoplasm lacks filaments and dense bodies. They also have long cytoplasmic processes extending from their cell body (Fig. 19-22, process of pericyte) whereas smooth muscle cells have the elongated shape of fibers.

Since the perivascular cells of capillaries play no contractile role, we must look to other vessels in the microvasculature for those responsible for controlling blood flow through capillary networks.

THE VESSELS THAT CONTROL BLOOD FLOW THROUGH THE TERMINAL VASCULAR BED

Only vessels with smooth muscle in their walls are able to regulate the distribution and rate of flow of blood through the capillary beds. This regulation is effected by narrowing (*vasoconstriction*) or widening (*vasodilation*) of the lumen of these vessels. Continuous adjustment of the caliber of their lumina, which is referred to as *vasomotor activity,* is mediated by autonomic nervous impulses and also locally by certain chemical mediators and metabolites.

There are several levels in the terminal vascular tree at which blood flow is regulated. The first is the level of the *terminal arterioles* delivering blood into the capillary networks. These vessels are small in diameter (30 to 50 μm.) but still have a single continuous layer of smooth muscle cells in the tunica media of their walls, and it is the degree of tonus in these cells that determines the diameter of their lumina at any given moment.

Next, as may be seen in the diagram of the terminal vascular bed (Fig. 19-23), a terminal arteriole opens into 2 types of vessels. At *top left* and also at *top right* in Figure 19-23 it opens into true *capillaries.* Although we have said that there are no smooth muscle cells associated with true capillaries, there are smooth muscle cells encircling each of these capillaries at their respective sites of origin from the arteriole and these smooth muscle cells constitute what are termed *precapillary sphincters* (Gr. *sphink-*

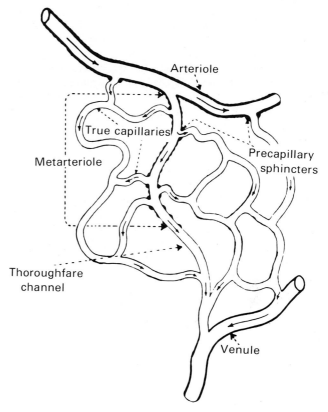

Fig. 19-23. Schematic diagram of the types of vessels constituting the terminal vascular bed and regulating microcirculation through it. For details, *see* text. (Courtesy of B. Zweifach)

ter, band), labeled in Figure 19-23. By changing their degree of tonus and hence constricting the opening into the capillary to a greater or lesser extent, the tiny sphincters control the flow of blood entering these true capillaries. The second type of vessel, arising from the midpart of the terminal arteriole shown in Figure 19-23, is a larger kind of vessel termed a *metarteriole* (labeled in Fig. 19-23). This vessel pursues a course that traverses the whole capillary bed, eventually to drain into a venule, as shown at the bottom of Figure 19-23. Many true capillaries of the bed arise from its proximal portion, so there are precapillary sphincters here also. Moreover, many true capillaries drain into its distal part (the portion known, for reasons soon to be explained, as a *thoroughfare channel,* labeled in Fig. 19-23). A metarteriole is wider than a true capillary and moreover it is encircled by smooth muscle cells at many, but somewhat scattered, sites along approximately the first half of its course (these smooth muscle cells are indicated by black semicircles in Fig. 19-23). Hence the volume of blood entering a capillary bed is controlled by precapillary sphincters at sites where true capillaries open directly from a terminal arteriole or from a metarteriole. Furthermore, the volume of blood flowing along a metarteriole itself is controlled by the tonus in the encircling smooth muscle cells scattered along its course. In some tissues, however, vasomotor activity in terminal arterioles is the main factor controlling local blood flow in capillary beds. Moreover, vasomotor activity of precapillary sphincters can be independent of that of the terminal arterioles and metarterioles from which the capillaries originate.

The metarterioles in some sites can serve another purpose, that of acting as low-resistance channels for an increased blood flow. This occurs especially in mesenteries and body sites where thermoregulation is important, such as in the skin and ear. As can be seen in Figure 19-23, these low-resistance pathways, which are called *preferential (thoroughfare) channels,* represent continuations of the distal ends of metarterioles and empty into venules. Preferential channels (which are not present to the same extent in all tissues) open when constriction of precapillary sphincters reduces blood flow through the local capillary network; the channels thus bypass the capillary bed and sustain blood flow through the region when the capillaries are not being utilized. In sections, these channels would be indistinguishable from large capillaries or postcapillary venules (*see* below).

Most of the knowledge we have gained about the terminal vascular bed comes from studies on flattened tissues such as mesenteries. However, microvascular beds extend in 3 dimensions in most parts of the body and hence are a good deal more complex. For details about microcirculation in other kinds of terminal vascular beds, *see* Sobin and Tremer and also Baez.

ARTERIOVENOUS ANASTOMOSES
(AV SHUNTS)

It should be realized that not all the blood has to pass through the terminal vascular bed. In certain regions of the body there are alternative channels called *arteriovenous anastomoses (AV shunts)* that permit blood to pass directly from the arterial to the venous side of the circulation, without having to go through capillaries, metarterioles, or preferential channels.

In the liver, for instance, short unbranched vessels (up to 45 μm. in diameter) connect some of the arteries directly to veins. Elsewhere, anastomoses may be longer and narrower (5 to 18 μm. in diameter) and connect arterioles to venules. The proximal half or two thirds of such vessels has a well-developed smooth muscle layer in its walls, and the distal segment has a somewhat wider lumen.

Arteriovenous anastomoses exhibit vasomotor activity and are extremely responsive to thermal, mechanical, and chemical stimuli. They are fairly numerous in the skin, where they are considered to be of importance in bypassing the capillary beds of the dermis in order to conserve heat.

VEINS AND VENULES

VENULES

Capillaries and thoroughfare channels open at their venous end into *postcapillary venules* (8 to 30 μm. in diameter in life), which have increasing numbers of pericytes associated with them as their diameter increases. These in turn open into *collecting venules* (30 to 50 μm. in diameter) that as well as having pericytes also possess an adventitia consisting of fibroblasts and collagen fibers. The *muscular venules* (50 to 100 μm. in diameter) into which the collecting venules empty have 1 or 2 layers of smooth muscle cells in their media. A very thin internal elastic lamina is present in the media and the adventitia is relatively well developed. In routine sections, however, all venules tend to look alike except for the size of their lumina. The venules empty the venous blood they collect from the microcirculation into small *collecting veins* (100 to 300 μm. in diameter) that have several layers of smooth muscle cells in their media.

The Fine Structure of Venules. Venules are probably the most significant of all vessels of the terminal vascular bed with regard to the study of inflammation. It is known that migration of leukocytes can occur through the walls of venules, and venules have been shown to be sites where blood plasma passes out into the tissue in the inflammatory process.

As shown in Figure 19-24, venules, like all blood vessels, are lined by *endothelial cells.* Except at sites where there are tight junctions there is a space of about 10 to 20 nm. between the cell membranes of contiguous cells. As was shown in Figure 11-5, leukocytes migrate through the walls of venules, and to do so they effect separation between the borders of contiguous cells to leave the vessels through the openings so formed; this in itself suggests that the tight junctions must be of the fascia (or even macula) type and not in the form of zonulae. Furthermore, endothelial cells are rich in actin-containing microfilaments, suggesting that they are able to alter their shape, and such movements under inflammatory conditions may be of assistance in permitting fluid and leukocytes to leave these vessels.

Just outside the endothelium is a *basement membrane* (Fig. 19-22, b.m.). The basement membrane surrounding the endothelium of capillaries and venules is about 50 nm. in thickness and is thought to become thicker with age.

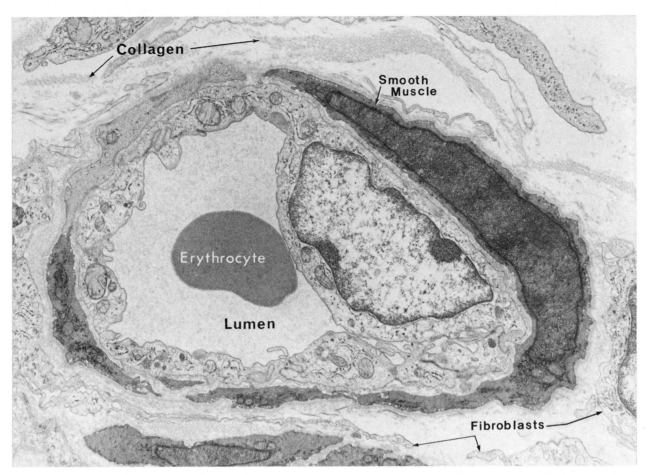

Fig. 19-24. Electron micrograph of a venule or small vein. Note that smooth muscle cells (dark) do not completely surround the lumen as in arterioles. To the right of the erythrocyte the nucleus of an endothelial lining cell is seen. A basal lamina is present between the endothelium and the smooth muscle cell, and also surrounding the smooth muscle cell. (Courtesy of M. Weinstock)

The large nucleus at *lower left* in Figure 19-22 (labeled P.N.) is the nucleus of a *pericyte*. The processes of pericytes are often cut in oblique or cross section as they extend along or around the endothelial tube of the venule. Pericytes and their processes are also enclosed with basement membrane, which is continuous with the basement membrane that surrounds the tube of endothelium. In this sense the basement membrane of the endothelial tube splits so as to envelop the pericyte and its processes as well as the endothelial tube. Basement membrane can be seen on the pericyte at the site marked p.b.m. in Figure 19-22. One process of the pericyte is labeled.

Some *collagen* can be seen surrounding the endothelial tube and pericyte external to the basement membrane. This is in the form of fibrils that here are mostly cut in cross section (Fig. 19-22, col.).

As venules merge into small veins, the character of the cells described as pericytes changes in that they become replaced by fully differentiated smooth muscle cells (Fig. 19-24).

VEINS

Veins of Small and Medium Size. The structure of these varies greatly. In general their walls, like those of the corresponding arteries, consist of 3 tunics (Fig. 19-11B). The *intima* consists of endothelium, which either rests directly on a poorly defined internal elastic membrane or is separated from it by only a slight amount of subendothelial connective tissue. The *media* is generally much thinner than that in the companion artery (Fig. 19-11). It consists chiefly of circularly disposed smooth muscle fibers. Smooth muscle cells, where present in the walls of venules, may not completely encircle the lumen (Fig. 19-24)

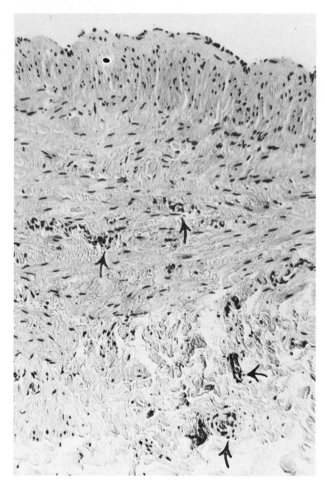

Fig. *19-25*. Medium-power photomicrograph of the wall of a saphenous vein as it appears in cross section. All the smooth muscle seen in the wall of this vein lies in the media. Note the inner layer of longitudinal muscle and observe that vasa vasorum (indicated by arrows) penetrate deeply into the media from the adventitia, which extends across the bottom third of the micrograph.

as they do in arterioles. More collagenic fibers and fewer elastic fibers are mixed with them than in arteries. In some veins the innermost smooth muscle fibers of the media have a longitudinal course. In general, the media is much less muscular, and hence thinner, in veins that are protected, for example, by muscles or by pressure of abdominal contents, than in veins that are more exposed. The cerebral and the meningeal veins have almost no muscle in their walls. The *adventitia* of veins of medium size is often their thickest coat (Fig. 19-11B). It commonly consists chiefly of collagenic connective tissue.

The muscular media is well developed in the veins of the limbs, particularly in those of the lower ones. This is

particularly true of the saphenous veins (Fig. 19-25). Being superficial, these are not supported by the pressure of surrounding structures to the same extent as deeper veins. Furthermore, when a person stands erect, their walls must withstand the hydrostatic pressure generated by a long column of blood. For these reasons their walls must be thicker than those of most veins. This is accomplished chiefly by a very substantial media. The innermost part of this consists chiefly of longitudinally disposed smooth muscle fibers associated with elastic fibers (Fig. 19-25), and the outermost and thicker part, of circularly disposed smooth muscle fibers (Fig. 19-25).

Large Veins. The structure of different large veins varies considerably. In general, the tunica intima resembles that of veins of medium size, but the subendothelial layer of connective tissue is thicker. In most of the largest veins there is little smooth muscle in the media and the *adventitia is by far the thickest* of the 3 coats (Fig. 19-26);

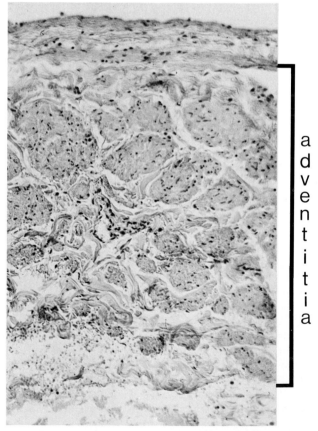

a
d
v
e
n
t
i
t
i
a

Fig. *19-26*. Medium-power photomicrograph of the wall of the inferior vena cava in cross section. Note the longitudinal muscle bundles in the adventitia.

it contains both collagenic and elastic fibers. In many instances — for example, the inferior vena cava — the innermost part of the tunica adventitia contains bundles of longitudinally disposed smooth muscle fibers (Fig. 19-26).

The Vasa Vasorum of Veins. Veins are *supplied much more abundantly* with vasa vasorum than are arteries. Since veins contain poorly oxygenated blood, the cells in the walls of veins would probably need more oxygen on occasion than could be obtained by diffusion from the lumen of the vessel. Vasa vasorum carrying arterial blood into the substance of the walls of veins would supply this need. Furthermore, since the blood in veins is under low pressure, vasa vasorum can approach the intima of the walls of veins without collapsing due to the pressure within the vein. Hence, the vasa vasorum of veins penetrate much closer to the intima than do those of arteries. They are seen to advantage in the thick walls of the saphenous vein (Fig. 19-25).

The Lymphatics of Veins. Since the walls of veins do not have to withstand great pressures, as do the walls of arteries, lymphatics, as well as vasa vasorum, can be present in a patent state within the substance of their walls. The walls of veins are *supplied much more abundantly* with lymphatic capillaries than walls of arteries. Indeed, this probably explains why tumors that spread by way of lymphatics invade the walls of veins but not the walls of arteries. Lymphatic capillaries may approach the inner surface of veins so closely that the tissue fluid that enters them to become lymph is probably a filtrate or dialysate of the blood plasma in the lumen of the vein itself.

The Valves of Veins. Veins are provided with valves arranged so as to permit blood to flow toward the heart but not in the opposite direction. The valves of veins are of the flap (leaflet) type. Most have two leaflets, but some have only one. The leaflets are folds of intima with central reinforcements of connective tissue. Elastic fibers are disposed on the side of the leaflet that faces the lumen of the vessel.

Valves are especially abundant in the veins of the extremities, but they are generally absent from the veins of the thorax and the abdomen. Valves are commonly located immediately distal to sites where tributaries enter veins. Immediately proximal to the attachment of a valve a vein is always dilated slightly to form a pouch or sinus. Hence, in distended superficial veins, localized swellings indicate the sites of valves.

The roles of valves in veins are several. First, they help overcome the force of gravity by preventing backflow. But they may also act in other ways. For example, valves in veins that are squeezed when surrounding muscles contract would enable the surrounding muscles to serve as pumps. Moreover, valves in such veins would prevent muscular contractions from creating back pressure on the capillary beds drained by the veins.

Varicose Veins. Superficial veins, as noted, are relatively unsupported, and the weight of the blood within those below the heart is a factor tending to cause their dilatation. Under conditions in which there is some resistance or obstruction to the return of blood from a part, or in which the walls of the veins are not as strong as usual (because of heredity or disease), superficial veins gradually dilate. As dilation proceeds, the valves become incompetent and, as a result, gravity exerts a still greater dilating force on their walls. Superficial veins that under these conditions become tortuous, irregular, and wider than usual are called *varicose veins.*

THE TRANSPLANTATION OF BLOOD VESSELS

The use of autologous transplants of blood vessels is limited because there is no source of autologous transplants for replacing any of the larger vessels of the body (except under certain circumstances where anastomoses are abundant). Some types of arterial defects can be repaired with autologous venous grafts, but the use of these is also limited. Transplants of homologous blood vessels were used to some extent but they have now been superseded by transplants of synthetic materials formed into the tubular shape of blood vessels. These materials do not stir up a tissue reaction and have led to tremendous development in the field of blood vessel surgery.

SENSORY RECEPTORS IN THE BLOOD CIRCULATORY SYSTEM

The Carotid Sinus and the Carotid Body. These are examples of two kinds of sensory receptors that are involved in reflex control of the blood circulation. The *carotid sinus* is a slight dilatation of one of the carotid arteries near the bifurcation of the common carotid artery. Usually, the site of the dilatation is the internal carotid artery immediately above its point of origin (Fig. 19-27). In the dilated part the media of the vessel is relatively thin, and the adventitia is relatively thick. Many nerve endings of afferent fibers from the carotid branch of the glossopharyngeal nerve are present in the adventitia. Since the media is thin at this site, the adventitia must bear more of the brunt of withstanding the pressure within the vessel than is usual in arteries; hence the nerve endings within it are readily stimulated by pressure changes. Nerve impulses set up by pressure changes within the sinus are conducted to the centers in the brain that control motor activity of the heart and arteries.

In addition to the carotid sinus, there are other areas along the common carotid artery of the cat that have *baroceptor* (Gr. *baros,* weight) activity. Boss and Green

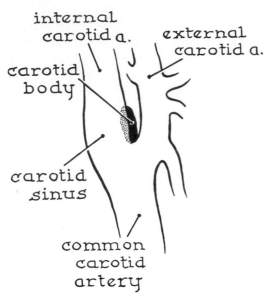

Fig. 19-27. Diagram of carotid sinus and carotid body.

studied the histology of these baroceptor areas and found it similar to that of the carotid sinus. In each area, myelinated fibers ramify in the adventitia of the vessel. Furthermore, at these sites there is generally less muscle and sometimes less elastin in the media, and the collagenic fibers of the adventitia are in the form of finer fibers that are intricately interwoven.

The *carotid body* is a small condensation of tissue on the wall of the internal carotid artery (Fig. 19-27). It consists of cords and clumps of ovoid cells and is abundantly provided with wide (sinusoid-like) capillaries. Its cells are richly supplied with nerve endings. These seem to be stimulated by changes in the concentrations of carbon dioxide and oxygen and pH changes in the blood. Nerve impulses arising from these *chemoreceptor* endings are also conducted to the centers in the brain that control the activities of the heart and the arteries.

Small structures similar to the carotid body are also present in the arch of the aorta, in the pulmonary artery, and at the origin of the right subclavian artery. Delicate pressure receptors are also present in the walls of the great veins close to the heart.

THE LYMPHATIC DIVISION OF THE CIRCULATORY SYSTEM

Lymphatic Vessels. The vessels in the body that conduct lymph are called *lymphatics*. The walls of the smallest of these—the kind into which the lymphatic capillaries

empty—consist of a thin layer of connective tissue and an endothelial lining. When lymphatics become larger (0.2 to 0.5 mm. in diameter) their walls show indications of being composed of the usual 3 layers: *intima, media,* and *adventitia.* These 3 layers, however, are not well defined in the walls of smaller lymphatics (Fig. 19-28). The *intima* commonly contains elastic fibers. The *media* of larger lymphatics consists chiefly of circularly and obliquely disposed smooth muscle fibers. The muscle fibers are supported by some connective tissue that contains elastic fibers. The *adventitia* is relatively well developed, particularly in the smaller vessels, and contains smooth muscle fibers; these run both longitudinally and obliquely. Small blood vessels are present in the outer coats of lymphatics of medium and large size.

The lymphatics, which collect lymph from lymphatic capillaries and carry it to the larger lymphatic vessels that finally deliver it into the blood circulatory system, commonly pass through tissue along with a vein and its companion artery. However, lymphatic vessels do not show as much tendency to converge on one another to form a single large vessel as do small veins; hence it is common for several lymphatics to be associated with a vein and its companion artery. Furthermore, lymphatics, as they pass through tissues, may unite with one another but they also branch again and so remain numerous.

Lymphatic vessels, except for the smallest ones, commonly (but not always) possess valves. These are more numerous and hence closer together than valves of veins. Indeed, valves in lymphatics may be so close together that a distended lymphatic appears to be beaded, because of the dilated sections between the numerous valves. Lymphatic valves commonly have 2 leaflets; these consist of folds of intima with delicate connective tissue in

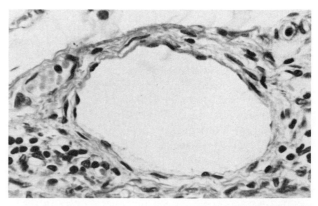

Fig. 19-28. High-power photomicrograph of a small lymphatic vessel. The nuclei of a few smooth muscle fibers may be seen in its wall, but the various layers of the wall are not clearly defined in lymphatics.

their middle, and endothelial coverings (Fig. 19-29). The endothelial cells on the leaflets of valves in both lymphatics and veins are said to be oriented differently on the 2 surfaces of a leaflet, with their long diameters being parallel with the stream on the side of the leaflet that faces the stream and at right angles to the stream on its sheltered side.

It is easy to understand how each segment of a lymphatic situated between 2 valves could act as a pump if (*1*) the wall of the lymphatic in that segment contracted, or (*2*) that segment were squeezed because of compression from outside the lymphatic. In frogs there are lymph hearts to propel lymph, but it seems doubtful that lymph is propelled along the lymphatics of mammals by contractions of the smooth muscle in their walls. The compression of lymphatics occasioned by pulsating blood vessels in their vicinity, or by active or passive movements of the parts in which they are contained, may cause lymphatic vessels to serve as pumps to some extent and so aid in propelling lymph along them. This explains why massage may be employed to improve lymphatic drainage of a body part. However, it seems doubtful if there is very much lymph flow from normal tissues that are at rest. As we shall see when the intestine is studied, the lymphatics draining it participate in absorbing fat. After a fatty meal the lymph from the intestine is milky in color and is termed *chyle*.

The lymph collected in the body is returned to the bloodstream by means of 2 main vessels; the *thoracic duct* and the *right lymphatic duct* (the latter may be represented by several vessels). At its beginning in the abdomen, the thoracic duct is somewhat dilated to form what is termed the *cisterna chyli,* and from here it extends to open into the left innominate vein in the angle of its junction with the internal jugular and left subclavian veins. Sometimes it is represented by several smaller vessels which open separately into the great veins. The right lymphatic duct or, more commonly, several representatives of the right lymphatic duct enter the great veins on the right side at sites comparable with those at which the thoracic duct enters the great vessels on the left side. The thoracic duct receives all the lymph that forms in the abdomen; hence, it is much the larger vessel of the two.

Lymphatic Capillaries. Although these resemble blood capillaries in general, there are certain differences. First, lymphatic capillaries are not surrounded with a well-developed basement membrane; if one is present, it is only very poorly developed and in itself probably presents virtually no barrier to the entry of macromolecular substances. Second, lymphatic capillaries can end blindly whereas blood capillaries always have an arterial and a venous end. Third, lymphatic capillaries do not have pericytes associated with them. The last and important difference is that lymphatic capillaries have, attached

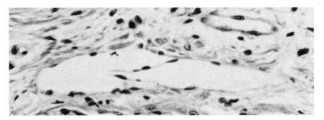

Fig. 19-29. Photomicrograph of an oblique section of a lymphatic, showing one of its valves. (Courtesy of Y. Clermont)

to the surface of their endothelial cells that faces the surrounding tissue, bundles of filaments (of unknown composition) that extend out into the connective tissue all around the capillary (*see* Leak). These are known as *anchoring filaments* and their role seems to be that of holding lymphatic capillaries open under conditions of edema, where pressure in the surrounding tissue might otherwise cause them to collapse.

REFERENCES AND OTHER READING

THE HEART AND THE IMPULSE-CONDUCTING SYSTEM OF THE HEART

Herman, L., Stuckey, J. W., and Hoffman, B. F.: Electron microscopy of Purkinje fibers and ventricular muscle of dog heart. Circulation, *24:*954, 1961.

Keith, A., and Flack, M.: The auriculoventricular bundle of the human heart. Lancet, *2:*359, 1906.

Kent, S.: Researches on the structure of function of the mammalian heart. J. Physiol., *14:*233, 1893.

Muir, A. R.: Observations on the fine structure of the Purkinje fibers in the ventricles of the sheep's heart. J. Anat., *91:*251, 1957.

Rhodin, J. A. G., Delmissier, P., and Reid, L. C.: The structure of the specialized conducting system of the steer heart. Circulation, *24:*349, 1961.

Virágh, S., and Challice, C. E.: The impulse generation and conduction system of the heart. *In* Challice, C. E., and Virágh, S. (eds.): Ultrastructure of the Human Heart. New York, Academic Press, 1973.

Wellens, H. J. J., Lie, K. I., and Janse, M. J. (eds.): The Conduction System of the Heart. Structure, Function and Clinical Implications. Leiden, Stenfert Kroese, 1976.

(For fine structure of cardiac muscle, *see* References for Chap. 18.)

ARTERIES, VEINS, AND LYMPHATICS

Abramson, D. I. (ed.): Blood Vessels and Lymphatics. New York, Academic Press, 1962.

Boss, J., and Green, J. H.: The histology of the common carotid baroceptor areas of the cat. Circ. Res., *4:*12, 1956.

Boyd, J. D.: Observations on the human carotid sinus and the nerve supply. Anat. Anz., *84:*386, 1937.

Burton, A. C.: Relation of structure to function of the tissues of the wall of blood vessels. Physiol. Rev., *34:*619, 1954.

Cervós-Navarro, J., and Matakas, F. (eds.): The Cerebral Vessel Wall. New York, Raven Press, 1975.

Clark, E. R.: Arterio-venous anastomoses. Physiol. Rev., *18:*229, 1938.

Jaffé, D., Hartroft, W. S., Manning, M., and Eleta, G.: Coronary arteries in newborn children. Acta Paediatr. Scand. [Suppl.], *219:*1, 1971.

Keech, M. K.: Electron microscope study of the normal rat aorta. J. Biophys. Biochem. Cytol., *7:*533, 1960.

Kjærgaard, J.: Anatomy of the Carotid Glomus and Carotid Glomus-like Bodies (Non-chromaffin Paraganglia). Copenhagen, F. A. D. L.'s Forlag, 1973.

Lansing, A. I.: The Arterial Wall. Baltimore, Williams & Wilkins, 1959.

Leak, L. V.: Electron microscopic observations on lymphatic capillaries and the structural components of the connective tissue-lymph interface. Microvasc. Res., *2:*391, 1970.

Luft, J. H.: The fine structure of the vascular wall. *In* Jones, R. J. (ed.): Evolution of the Arteriosclerotic Plaque. p. 3. Chicago, University of Chicago Press, 1963.

Parker, F.: An electron microscope study of coronary arteries. Am. J. Anat., *103:*247, 1958.

Pease, D. C., and Molinari, S.: Electron microscopy of muscular arteries: Pial vessels of the cat and monkey. J. Ultrastruct. Res., *3:*447, 1960.

Pease, D. C., and Paule, W. J.: Electron microscopy of elastic arteries: The thoracic aorta of the rat. J. Ultrastruct. Res., *3:*469, 1960.

Pritchard, M. M. L., and Daniel, P. M.: Arterio-venous anastomoses in the human external ear. J. Anat., *90:*309, 1956.

———: Arterio-venous anastomoses in the tongue of the sheep and the goat. Am. J. Anat., *95:*203, 1954.

Rhodin, J. A. G.: Fine structure of the vascular wall in mammals. Physiol. Rev., *42* (Suppl. 5):48, 1962.

Ryan, T. J.: Structure and shape of blood vessels of skin. *In* Jarrett, A. (ed.): The Physiology and Pathophysiology of the Skin. The Nerves and Blood Vessels. vol. 2. London, Academic Press, 1973.

Simionescu, M., Simionescu, N., and Palade, G. E.: Segmental differentiations of cell junctions in the vascular endothelium. Arteries and Veins. J. Cell Biol., *68:*705, 1976.

Smith, V., Ryan, J. W., Michie, D. D., and Smith, D.: Endothelial projections, as revealed by scanning electron microscopy. Science, *173:*925, 1971.

Wollard, H. H.: The innervation of blood vessels. Heart, *13:*319, 1926.

Wollard, H. H., and Weddell, G.: The composition and distribution of vascular nerves in the extremities. J. Anat., *69:*165, 1935.

ELASTOGENESIS IN ARTERIES

Bierring, F., and Kobayasi, T.: Electron microscopy of the normal rabbit aorta. Acta Pathol. Microbiol. Scand., *57:*154, 1963.

Haust, M. D., More, R. H., Bencosme, S. A., and Balis, J. U.: Elastogenesis in human aorta: an electron microscope study. Exp. Mol. Pathol., *4:*508, 1965.

Paule, W. J.: Electron microscopy of the newborn rat aorta. J. Ultrastruct. Res., *8:*219, 1965.

Rhodin, J. A. G.: Fine structure of vascular walls in mammals with special reference to smooth muscle component. Physiol. Rev., *42*(5):447, 1962.

Ross, R., and Bornstein, P.: Elastic fibers in the body. Sci. Am., *224:*44, June, 1971.

ARTERIAL WALL IN RELATION TO ATHEROSCLEROSIS

Benditt, E. P.: The origin of atherosclerosis. Sci. Am., *236:*74, Feb., 1977.

Benditt, E. P., and Benditt, J. M.: Evidence for a monoclonal origin of human atherosclerotic plaques. Proc. Natl. Acad. Sci. U.S.A., *70:*1753, 1973.

Martin, G. M., and Sprague, C. A.: Symposium on in vitro studies related to atherogenesis: life histories of hyperplastoid cell lines from aorta and skin. Exp. Mol. Pathol., *18:*125, 1973.

Paoletti, R., and Gotto, A. M., Jr. (eds.): Atherosclerosis Reviews. vol. 1. New York, Raven Press, 1976.

Ross, R., and Glomset, J. A.: The pathogenesis of atherosclerosis. N. Engl. J. Med., *295:*369 (Part I), 420 (Part II), 1976.

THE TERMINAL VASCULAR BED

Comprehensive General Reference

Kaley, G., and Altura, B. M. (eds.): Microcirculation. vols. 1, 2, and 3. Baltimore, University Park Press, 1977 to 1978.

Special References

Baez, S.: Skeletal muscle and gastrointestinal microvascular morphology. *In* Kaley, G., and Altura, B. M. (eds.): Microcirculation. Vol. 1, p. 69. Baltimore, University Park Press, 1977.

Beacham, W. S., Konishi, A., and Hunt, C. C.: Observations on the microcirculatory bed in rat mesocecum using differential interference contrast microscopy in vivo and electron microscopy. Am. J. Anat., *146:*385, 1976.

Bruns, R. R., and Palade, G. E.: Studies on blood capillaries. I. General organization of blood capillaries in muscle. J. Cell Biol., *37:*244, 1968.

Farquhar, M.: Fine structure and function in capillaries of the anterior pituitary gland. Angiology, *12:*270, 1961.

Fawcett, D. W.: Comparative observations on the fine structure of blood capillaries. *In* The Peripheral Vessels, Internat. Acad. Pathol. Monograph No. 4. p. 17. Baltimore, Williams & Wilkins, 1963.

Fernando, N. V. P., and Movat, H. Z.: The smallest arterial vessels: Terminal arterioles and metarterioles. Exp. Mol. Pathol., *3:*1, 1964.

———: The capillaries. Exp. Mol. Pathol., *3:*87, 1964.

Karnovsky, M. J., and Cotran, R. S.: The intercellular passage of exogenous peroxidase across endothelium and mesothelium. Anat. Rec., *154:*365, 1966.

Majno, G., Palade, G. E., and Schoefl, G. I.: Studies on inflammation. II. The site of action of histamine and serotonin along the vascular tree: a topographic study. J. Biophys. Biochem. Cytol., *11:*607, 1961.

Minot, C. S.: On a hitherto unrecognized form of blood circulation without capillaries in the organs of Vertebrata. Proc. Boston Soc. Nat. Hist., *29:*185, 1901.

Movat, H. Z., and Fernando, N. V. P.: Small arteries with an internal elastic lamina. Exp. Mol. Pathol., *2:*549, 1963.

————: The venules and their perivascular cells. Exp. Mol. Pathol., *3:*98, 1964.

Nelemans, F. A.: Innervation of the smallest blood vessels. Am. J. Anat., *83:*43, 1948.

Palade, G. E.: Blood capillaries of the heart and other organs. Circulation, *24:*368, 1961.

Ryan, U. S., Ryan, J. W., Smith, D. S., and Winkler, H.: Fenestrated endothelium of the adrenal gland: freeze-fracture studies. Tissue and Cell, *7:*181, 1975.

Simionescu, M., Simionescu, N., and Palade, G. E.: Segmental differentiations of cell junctions in the vascular endothelium. The microvasculature. J. Cell Biol., *67:*863, 1975.

Sobin, S. S., and Tremer, H. M.: Three-dimensional organizational organization of microvascular beds as related to function. *In* Kaley, G., and Altura, B. M. (eds.): Microcirculation. vol. 1, p. 43. Baltimore, University Park Press, 1977.

Zweifach, B. W.: Introduction: perspectives in microcirculation. *In* Kaley, G., and Altura, B. M. (eds.): Microcirculation. vol. 1. Baltimore, University Park Press, 1977.

Zweifach, B. W., Grant, L., and McCluskey, R. T. (eds.): The Inflammatory Process. ed. 2, vols. 1 to 3. New York, Academic Press, 1974.

20 The Integumentary System (The Skin and Its Appendages)

The skin is the largest organ of the body. It consists of 2 layers, of different origins, that are firmly attached to one another. The outer is stratified squamous keratinizing *epithelium* (described in Chap. 7) derived from ectoderm. It has no blood vessels and so has to be nourished by tissue fluid from the second and deeper layer of the skin, which consists of irregularly arranged *connective tissue* of mesenchymal origin and hence contains blood vessels (*see* Fig. 7-1, p. 188).

Terminology. The word *dermis* (Gr. for skin) is sometimes used to refer to the skin as a whole—that is, to describe a membrane that consists of 2 layers. This, for example, is the way it is used in the term *dermatology,* which refers to the branch of medical science concerned with diseases of the skin, in which both layers may be involved. However, when a dermatologist, histologist, or histopathologist studies skin with the microscope he will call its outer (epithelial) layer the *epidermis* (Gr. *epi,* upon) and the deeper (connective tissue) layer of the skin the *dermis,* thus using the latter term to mean the same as the Latin word *corium,* which means hide. Hides, in the form of leather, have had the epidermis removed.

The deeper part of the epidermis consists of living epithelial cells. The cells in the deepest layer next to the dermis proliferate throughout life. As a result, epithelial cells are always being pushed toward the surface, and as they are pushed progressively farther away from their source of nutrients (the dermis) they die and become transformed into a horny material called *keratin.* The thickness of the keratin is different in the 2 types of skin we shall now briefly describe.

Skin is commonly classified into two types, *thick* and *thin.* Actually, these terms refer to the thickness of the epidermis and not to the thickness of the whole skin, as will become apparent in the following.

The Structure and Distribution of So-Called Thick and Thin Skin. Thick skin covers the palms of the hands and the soles of the feet; thin skin covers the rest of the body. Thick skin is characterized by a *thick epidermis,* which has a particularly thick layer of keratin on its outer surface (Fig. 20-1A). The skin covering the remainder of the body, although it has a thick *dermis* in some sites, as on the back, has a relatively *thin epidermis,* and the outer keratinized layer of this is relatively thin (Fig. 20-11, *top*). Note also the connective tissue dermis in Figure 20-1. The structure of thick and thin skin will be described in detail shortly.

The Relation of Skin to Subcutaneous Tissue (Hypodermis). The 2 layers of the skin are firmly joined together to form a cohesive membrane that varies in thickness from less than 0.5 mm. to 3 or 4 mm. (or even more) in different parts of the body. The skin rests on subcutaneous tissue, which varies from being of the loose or adipose to the dense variety in various sites on different people. The subcutaneous connective tissue (Fig. 20-1) corresponds to the *superficial fascia* of gross anatomy. It is sometimes also called the *hypodermis,* but it is not part of the skin. Irregularly spaced bundles of collagenic fibers extend from the dermis into the subcutaneous tissue to provide anchorage (Fig. 20-1A), and the subcutaneous tissue permits skin over most parts of the body considerable latitude of movement.

The Appendages of the Skin. During embryonic development, cells of the ectoderm-derived epidermis grow down into the dermis to give rise to epithelial glands and glandlike structures that include sweat glands, hair follicles (which form hairs), and sebaceous glands. The way glands develop was described in Chapter 6 (review Fig. 6-2). Epidermal invasion of the connective tissue is also responsible for the grooves of epidermis that produce fingernails and toenails.

So a consideration of the skin includes study of the epidermis and dermis and also the epidermal appendages. The latter constitute the sweat glands, hair follicles, sebaceous glands, nail grooves, and nails.

Some Functions of Skin. The epidermis, particularly its layer of keratin, is a barrier to disease organisms. Keratin is nearly waterproof; this permits an internally fluid body to exist in what is often a very dry atmosphere. The keratin makes it possible to have a bath in fresh water without the body becoming swollen with water, or in salt water without the body becoming shrunken. Furthermore, this keratin acts as a barrier against water loss from the surface of the body.

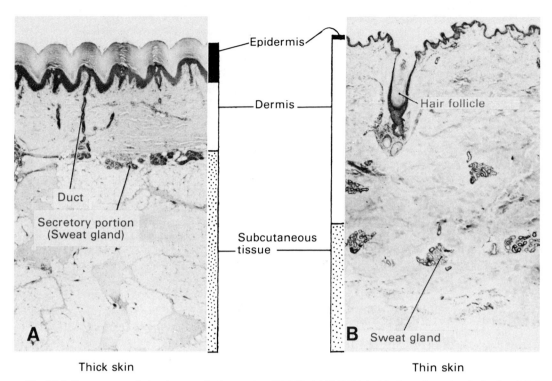

Fig. 20-1. Low-power photomicrographs (same magnification) of (*A*) thick skin from the sole of a foot and (*B*) thin skin from the abdomen. Note that thick skin has a thick epidermis, consisting mostly of keratin, whereas thin skin has a thin epidermis but a thick dermis. Note also the parts of eccrine sweat glands in (*A*) and the positions of these glands in each kind of skin.

The epidermis, however, is not impervious to everything; for example, certain chemicals can be absorbed through it into the capillaries and lymphatics of the underlying dermis. Accordingly, care has to be taken in many instances that poisonous chemicals do not come into direct contact with the epidermis.

The epidermis, because it contains certain cells that can produce the dark pigment melanin, can protect the body from the harmful effects of too much ultraviolet light.

The skin (epidermis and dermis) has many other useful functions. It is of the greatest importance in relation to regulating the temperature of the body; how it does this will be described later. Furthermore, by sweating the skin functions as an excretory organ. Vitamin D, the antirachitic vitamin, is made in skin exposed to ultraviolet light. Without vitamin D from other sources, children kept out of the sun develop rickets (Fig. 15-61). The skin contains nerve endings responsible for picking up stimuli that evoke various types of sensation in consciousness (touch, pressure, heat, cold, and pain). Hence the skin is of the greatest importance in permitting man to adjust in relation to his environment.

Medical students will learn to appreciate the particular importance of the skin in a physical examination. No exploratory operations are necessary to see it; of all the important structures of the body, it alone is exposed so that it may be examined with the unaided eye. Yet its appearance may reflect, just as truly as the appearance of deep-seated organs, the existence of a general disease. Moreover, its appearance often gives the physician a useful check on a patient's statement about his or her age. The presence and amount of hair in certain sites give information about how much of certain sex hormones is being secreted. The color of the skin may indicate a variety of conditions: it becomes yellow in jaundice, bronzed in certain glandular deficiencies, dry and hard in others, and warm and moist in still others. Cyanosis may give the skin a blue-gray appearance and so reflect generalized impairment of circulatory or respiratory functions. In vitamin A deficiencies, the skin of extensor surfaces may lose its hair and become rough, like sandpaper. In certain other vitamin deficiencies the skin around the corners of the mouth may become cracked and scaly. Many infectious diseases that affect the whole body produce characteristic rashes or other kinds of lesions on the skin (for example, scarlet fever, measles, chickenpox, syphilis, and others). The skin very commonly is affected when individuals are allergic (hypersensitive) to certain proteins and other substances; for example, some women develop rashes from certain kinds of makeup. In addition to involvement of the skin in conditions and diseases of fairly general character, there is a whole host of skin diseases proper.

Since the skin is the most exposed part of the body, it is very susceptible to various kinds of injuries. The treatment of cuts, abrasions, burns, and frostbites is part of routine medical or paramedical practice. Much skin is often destroyed by accidents and it is fortunate that it can be grafted so readily from one part of the body to another; indeed, as will be described presently, one type of skin graft can be cut so that the skin at the site from which it is taken is renewed at the same time as the graft is providing skin for the site from which it has been lost. In this way areas of skin on the body can, in a sense, be multiplied.

THE MICROSCOPIC STRUCTURE OF THICK SKIN

The First Thief Identified by Fingerprints. In 1880 Henry Faulds, a Scottish medical missionary, published a note in *Nature* entitled "On the Skin Furrows of the Hand." He described these as "forever unchangeable" and pointed out that "finger marks" might be used for scientific detection of criminals. Indeed, he reported some experience in this matter and described how greasy finger marks on a bottle had led to the identification of the individual who had been drinking the rectified spirits from the dispensary. From this beginning, fingerprinting developed into a most useful tool in crime detection.

Significance and Development of Surface Ridges and Grooves. If the palms of the hands (including the fingers) and the soles of the feet (including the toes) are examined with the naked eye or, better, with a magnifying glass, they are seen to be covered with ridges and grooves in a fashion reminiscent of a field plowed by the contour method. On the hands and feet of dark-skinned races the ridged area is clearly marked off by its lighter color.

The ridges and furrows develop during the 3rd and the 4th fetal months. The pattern that then forms never changes afterward except to enlarge. Patterns are determined chiefly by hereditary factors, as is shown by the close similarity of pattern in monozygotic twins and by the resemblances in fingerprints between members of a given family. Racial differences are reflected in the patterns.

The patterns can be greatly modified by growth disturbances in the fetus during the 3rd and/or 4th months. This is strikingly shown in children that are born with Down's syndrome (due to a chromosomal anomaly described in Chapter 3, p. 78). Some 70 per cent of such children

show combinations of patterns not seen in normal babies; hence an analysis of the skin patterns of a newborn baby may give very important information on whether it has been born with this anomaly.

The *epidermal ridges,* which are the ones that can be seen with the naked eye, are caused by the epidermis following the contours of underlying *dermal ridges.* The latter may be studied in sections of skin cut perpendicular to its surface. Sections so cut would be easier to interpret if they were to appear as illustrated in the upper drawing in Figure 20-2, which shows clear-cut *primary dermal ridges* underlying the epidermal ridges. However, actual sections of skin do not appear this way, but as shown in the lower picture in Figure 20-2. This (real) appearance is due to the fact that epidermis grows down into the peak of each primary dermal ridge so that each primary dermal ridge is split into 2 ridges. Each half of the split ridge, from the appearance it presented in a single section, was termed a *papilla,* and, as a consequence, the epidermal downgrowth that lies between each half of the ridge was termed an *interpapillary peg.* However, the structures termed *papillae* and *interpapillary pegs* are not actually cone-shaped papillae or pegs, because they appear consistently in sections (*see* Fig. 20-1A). If they were true papillae and pegs, they would be seen only in occasional sections where the plane of section happened to pass through one of them. Because they appear consistently, they are actually *ridges;* however, they are deficient occasionally along their courses. As we shall see, one kind of sweat gland in the skin opens through the tops of the so-called interpapillary pegs.

THE EPIDERMIS

The following account deals in particular with the epidermis of thick skin but much of it applies equally to that of thin skin.

Basement Membrane. A well-developed basement membrane is present between the epidermis and the dermis. It is variable in thickness in various body sites and in different species. In the skin of the pig it is sufficiently well developed to be resolved with the LM, particularly after thermal burns, which do enough damage to cause exudation of plasma from the abundant capillaries in the interpapillary pegs of dermis and lift the epidermis from the dermis so as to form blisters. It can be seen readily just below the middle in illustration B in Figure 20-23, which should be inspected briefly at this time. The fine structure of basement membranes was described in Chapter 8 (p. 222).

The Cells of Epidermis. Four cell types have been described, with their relative proportions varying with regard to species and body site. Mouse skin has been investigated extensively and here about 85 per cent of the cells are derived from ectoderm and are termed *keratinocytes*. They are the kind we shall first deal with in the following. The other types of cells of the epidermis will be described later; they are (*1*) *melanocytes*, the pigment-forming cells of epidermis and which are derived from migratory cells from the neural crests; (*2*) *Langerhans' cells*, which are probably macrophages that have invaded epidermis; and (*3*) *Merkel cells*, which are sensory receptors (described at the end of this chapter).

Keratinocytes and Keratinization

In approaching a study of the epidermis it is important to appreciate that the keratin that constitutes the outer layer of the epidermis is not a secretion of cells but instead is the end result of *transformation* of epithelial cells into scales. Hence, when keratin scales are worn away or desquamate from the surface, they can only be replaced by underlying living cells becoming keratinized and this means that there must be as much cell multiplication in the deep layer of the epidermis as there is loss of keratinized cells from its surface. Indeed, it has been shown that the cells of the plantar epidermis of a rat are completely replaced every 19 days and in humans it takes up to 1 month, depending on the body site. Several processes, then, are more or less constantly taking place in the epidermis: (*1*) cell division in the deep layer; (*2*) cells being pushed toward the surface as a result; (*3*) cells farthest away from the dermis being transformed into keratin; and (*4*) keratin desquamating from the surface.

Next, the fact that the cells are constantly changing in appearance as they move from the bottom to the top of the epidermis is reflected by the epidermis seemingly being composed of different *layers* that can be distinguished from one another in the LM by their appearance. Hence it is a time-honored custom to name and describe the histology of the different layers of the epidermis as seen with the LM. We shall do this in the following and amplify what gives rise to these appearances by describing what is seen with the EM.

The Layers of the Epidermis

Stratum Germinativum. The deepest layer, which abuts on the basement membrane, is termed the *stratum germinativum* (Fig. 20-3) or *stratum basale* (Fig. 20-5). The surface of cells of the stratum germinativum that abuts on the basement membrane is irregular (Fig. 20-5) and on the cytoplasmic aspect of the cell membrane abutting on the basement membrane there are *hemidesmosomes* (Figs. 7-18 and 20-5). The cells of the stratum germinativum are more or less columnar in shape (Fig. 20-5, *bottom*). The borders of these cells are not distinct in the usual H and E

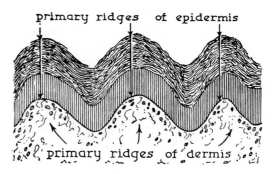

primary ridges   of epidermis

primary ridges of dermis

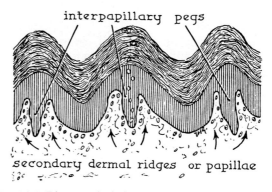

interpapillary pegs

secondary dermal ridges or papillae

Fig. 20-2. Diagrams depicting the relation between epidermal and dermal ridges. (*Top*) This diagram is not factual but illustrates the concept of a primary dermal ridge below each epidermal ridge. (*Bottom*) Actually, each primary dermal ridge is split into two secondary ridges as a result of growth of epidermis down into the primary ridge along its crest.

section, and the inexperienced student must avoid thinking of their nuclei, which are distinct, as being the cells themselves. The deepest layer is called the *stratum germinativum* because it generates new cells; this accounts for cells being pushed from this layer into the next one above.

The cells in this germinal layer (Fig. 20-5) have a large content of free ribosomes and polyribosomes that are probably concerned in synthesis for growth (cell proliferation) and synthesis of the considerable content of intermediate (10 nm.) filaments (tonofilaments) that form in the cells of this layer and eventually become part of the keratin. By the time the cells pass into the next layer above, bundles of 10-nm. filaments have become wide enough to be seen with the LM. These bundles represent what were called *tonofibrils* and, as will now be explained, account for this second layer of the epidermis being called the *prickle cell layer* or the *stratum spinosum*.

Stratum Spinosum. The cells of this second layer are not columnar like those of the basal layer, but are more or

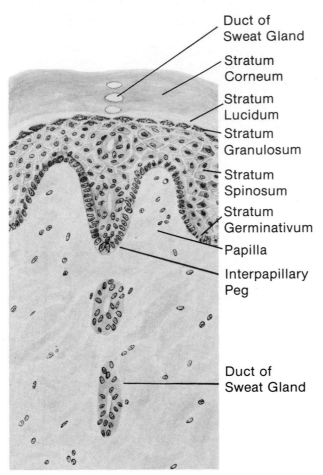

Fig. 20-3. Drawing of a section of thick skin, illustrating the various layers of the epidermis and the way in which the duct of a sweat gland enters an interpapillary peg. Note how the wall of the duct thereafter is constituted by cells of the different layers of epidermis through which it passes.

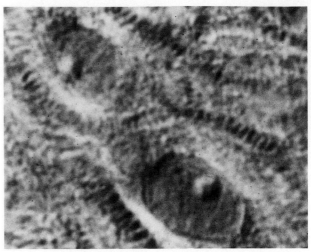

Fig. 20-4. Photomicrograph (interference contrast) of cells of stratum spinosum of human thick skin, unstained section. Note the spinous processes joining adjacent cells and giving them a prickly appearance. They are sites where the cell membranes of contiguous cells are held together by desmosomes. (For illustrations of the fine structure of desmosomes, *see* Figs. 7-17 and 7-18). The nucleus and nucleolus of a prickle cell are evident at *lower right* (the three-dimensional appearance is due to their respective interference properties).

less polyhedral in shape. Furthermore, as shown in Figure 20-4, with the LM their borders appear separated from one another by small spaces traversed by fine spine-like processes; this gives the cells of this layer a prickly appearance and accounts for the name of the layer.

It was once incorrectly thought that fibrils called tonofibrils actually crossed from the interior of one cell to the interior of another. However, the EM showed that what is actually seen is strands of cytoplasm extending out from adjacent cells to meet and come into very firm contact by means of a *desmosome* (Fig. 7-17). Most of the substance of the spinous processes seen with the LM is cytoplasm with a considerable content of 10-nm. filaments; this is what constitutes the dense masses of filaments seen closely associated with desmosomes in Figure 7-17 (where they are labeled T). These wide bundles of

filaments are what were termed *tonofibrils*, but they do not, of course, pass from one cell into another and they are always contained in cytoplasm.

The intercellular spaces seen in Figure 20-4 are in large part due to shrinkage artifact. If cells are separated slightly, for this or any other reason, the sites where cytoplasm is drawn out into processes are sites where their membranes are attached by desmosomes. Moreover, there is reason to believe that in life the cell membranes of contiguous cells of this layer at least would not, except at the sites of desmosomes, be everywhere in intimate contact with one another because in a thick epithelial membrane there is need for at least a little tissue fluid in between cells to ensure efficient diffusion of nutrients and waste products between the more superficial living cells and the capillaries of the dermis.

Stratum Granulosum. This layer of thick skin (the third layer of the epidermis) is from 2 to 4 cells thick and lies immediately superficial to the stratum spinosum (Fig. 20-3). In cross sections of skin its cells are roughly diamond-shaped (Figs. 20-3 and 20-5) and they are fitted together with the long axis of each parallel to the contour of the overlying ridge or groove. The cytoplasm of the cells of this layer is characterized by its containing granules that stain deeply with hematoxylin; these are called *keratohyalin* granules.

Fig. 20-5. Drawing of the layers of the epidermis, based on electron micrographs of stratified squamous keratinizing epithelium. Shown are a representative cell of each layer and the keratin of the stratum corneum. Note the desmosomes and tonofibrils (bundles of tonofilaments). Hemidesmosomes are present on the cytoplasmic side of the basal cell membrane of the cell of the stratum basale where it abuts on the basement membrane. (Courtesy of A. Weinstock)

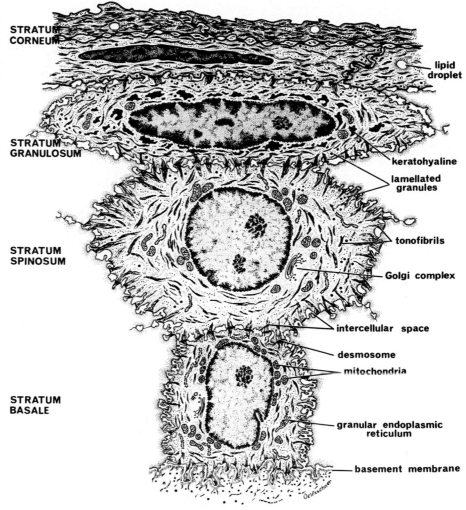

Stratum Lucidum. The next and fourth layer is not always seen to advantage. When visible, it is thin and appears as a clear, bright, homogeneous line. For this reason it is called the *stratum lucidum* (Fig. 20-3). It is said to consist of a substance called *eleidin,* which is presumed to be a transformation product of the keratohyalin observed in the stratum granulosum.

Stratum Corneum. As cells are pushed more superficially into the fifth and final layer, the *stratum corneum* (which is the name for the layer of keratin), their nuclei and all cytoplasmic organelles seemingly disappear. Even their keratohyalin granules fade away, all of which suggests intracellular activity of lysosome-derived enzymes. Nevertheless, desmosomes connecting the drawn-out squames (formerly living cells) can still be distinguished in the EM. There are different hypotheses as to what happens. One view is that the keratohyalin granules become converted into a homogeneous matrix in which all the previously formed filamentous material of the cell becomes embedded and that also infiltrates nuclei and other organelles. In this manner, each cell is transformed into one of the squames of keratin that constitute the keratin layer (stratum corneum). Not everything in the cells becomes keratin, because there is still some other protein and certain other materials that can be recovered from the keratinized layer.

It should perhaps be noted that keratohyalin granules are not essential for keratinization. Some species have keratinized skin in which keratohyalin granules are not visible.

Finally, keratin is a tough fibrous protein, highly resistant to chemical change. From what has been said in previous chapters about the syntheses of proteins that either remain within a cell or are exported from it, it might

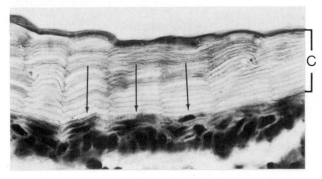

Fig. 20-6. Photomicrograph (×650) of thin skin, from an ear of a mouse. This is a frozen cross section stained with methylene blue after alkali treatment to swell the cells. Note the stacking of the cells, particularly evident in the stratum corneum (c). The arrows indicate the most superficial nucleated cell in each vertical column (these cells are in the stratum granulosum). Note how the cells in each column interlock with those in adjacent columns. (Menton, D. N.: Am. J. Anat., *145:*1, 1976)

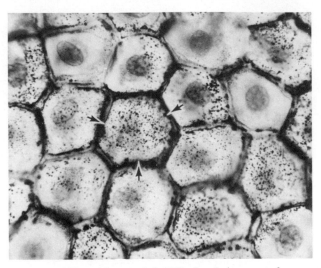

Fig. 20-8. Photomicrograph (×730) of a whole mount of mouse ear epidermis (with its cells outlined with silver nitrate and nuclei counterstained by the Feulgen reaction) seen by transillumination. Most of the cells at this level belong to the stratum granulosum, hence the granules in their cytoplasm. These are the most superficial nucleated cells. Note their hexagonal outline and the way they interlock with the cells in surrounding columns (one column is indicated by arrows). The double line at the periphery of each column indicates the dimensions of the overlap between adjacent columns. (Menton, D. N.: Am. J. Anat., *145:*1, 1976)

be thought that keratin also would be synthesized in cells as keratin either in association with free polyribosomes or even rough-surfaced endoplasmic reticulum. However, the production of keratin seems to be more complex than this, for part of it at least does not seem to be synthesized as keratin itself but, as described above, to result from transformation of other cell constituents.

It is of interest in connection with the synthesis of keratin that certain other types of epithelium in the body that ordinarily do not keratinize do so under conditions of prolonged vitamin A deficiency.

How the Squames of Stratum Corneum Are Fitted Together. Anyone who has tried to crowd more cartons, bottles, and jugs into a refrigerator than its shelf can hold will be aware of how much space can be wasted in fitting objects together. The same problem arises in connection with cells, but for the most part it would seem to be solved because of their being soft enough to be molded into shapes that fit their local environment. However, there is more of a problem in connection with the stratum corneum because in this layer the cells, as they become keratinized, become more rigid. Moreover they must adhere to one another firmly with no spaces between them if the stratum corneum is to be impervious, for instance, to water.

According to Menton, only recently has it been established that squames of the stratum corneum are stacked, one upon another, in neat contiguous vertical columns and that the edges of every squame in a stack interlock with those in the surrounding stacks in the best possible way for avoiding waste space (Fig. 20-6). This requires that the squames be of a special geometric form, and to describe this further we should mention Lord Kelvin, one of the most eminent physicists of the last century. (Students might be interested in knowing that besides being responsible for impressive advances in knowledge in physics, this great scientist was not only known for behaving toward his most elementary students with the greatest of modesty and kindliness, but also found great pleasure in acknowledging the work of even his humblest assistants.) What concerns us here is that, according to Menton, Kelvin showed from studies on liquid films that 14-sided polygons (which are known as orthic tetrakaidecahedrons) are more economical than any other kind of polygon for being fitted one to another so as to fill space without there being any interstices between them. Menton notes that the tetrakaidecahe-

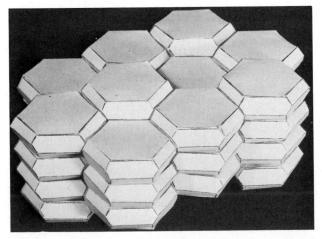

Fig. 20-7. Photograph of model illustrating how the cells of stratum corneum are packed together in interlocking columns, with each cell having the shape of a flattened tetrakaidecahedron (shown here as they appear in an alkali-swollen preparation; *see* Fig. 20-6). (Menton, D. N.: J. Invest. Dermatol., *57:*925, 1971)

dron is the only geometric form that can be stacked into regular columns and have all its units interdigitate with adjacent units in 6 surrounding columns. As matters turned out it seems that the squames of the stratum corneum are flattened tetrakaidecahedrons. One of the models constructed by Menton is shown in Figure 20-7. It is to be noted that in surface view each squame is hexagonal. Furthermore, its 6 edges are beveled into a V-shape. A V-shaped edge would, of course, fit perfectly into a reverse V formed at the edge of one hexagonal cell placed on another, but this would require that the 6 stacks surrounding any given stack be composed of flattened hexagonal cells (squames) disposed in planes half the thickness of a squame above and below it as shown in Figure 20-7. It is by this means that a perfect fit is obtained between adjacent stacks.

How the cells of the stratum corneum could become arranged in this distinctive manner is difficult to understand. One factor is that since the outer part of the stratum corneum is fairly rigid and cells are being pushed continually toward it from the stratum germinativum, cells in the stratum granulosum and the lower part of the stratum corneum would be under some pressure. This would seem to be enough to cause them to become flattened and assume hexagonal outlines when viewed from above (Fig. 20-8). One idea is that the pressure might lead to at least a few cells nearer the surface becoming stacked in the form of flattened tetrakaidecahedrons quite by chance, but once this pattern was established it could become general and would be followed automatically by other cells being pushed upward from below, providing they were still soft enough to be molded into that shape.

Aspiring dermatologists would doubtless find Menton's discussion of disruption of the normal stacking arrangement of epidermal cells, a feature associated with certain skin diseases characterized by increased turnover of the epidermal cell population (and also certain other conditions), most instructive.

Chalones and the Control of Cell Multiplication in Epidermis

This was discussed in Chapter 6 and further references on the topic are given at the end of this chapter.

THE DERMIS

The thickness of the dermis varies greatly in relation to different body sites. It consists of 2 layers of connective tissue that merge into one another. The outer is by far the thinner and is composed of loose connective tissue. It is called the *papillary layer* because the connective tissue papillae that extend up into the epidermis constitute most of it (Figs. 20-1 and 20-2, *bottom*). This layer extends only slightly below the bases of the papillae, where it merges and blends with the thicker *reticular layer,* which consists of dense irregularly arranged connective tissue. It comprises the remainder of the dermis (the bulk of what is labeled dermis in Figure 20-1A). It is called the *reticular layer* of dermis because the bundles of collagenic fibers of which it is composed interlace with each other in a net-like manner.

Elastic fibers are arranged as a network of very fine fibers in the papillary layer and coarser fibers lie randomly distributed in the reticular layer. The elastin content of the dermis is, however, not very great.

The Capillary Content of the Two Layers of the Dermis. A very important difference between the papillary and reticular layers of the dermis is their respective content of capillaries. As will be described in detail shortly, the capillary blood supply of the papillary layer is extensive. One group of capillaries extends in loops up into the so-called papillae (ridges) projecting into the epidermis; these provide nourishment for the epidermis and also act in heat regulation. Another group of so-called capillaries (really more of the nature of venules) forms a flat bed below the bases of the papillae. The papillary layer thus has a rich blood supply. Capillaries are scarce in the reticular layer, being numerous only in association with epidermal appendages that project down into the reticular layer.

The cells of the dermis of thick skin are mostly fibroblasts, and these are scattered about sparingly. A few macrophages are also present. Fat cells may be present, singly or more commonly in groups.

SWEAT GLANDS

Sweat glands are commonly classed as being of the *apocrine* or *eccrine* type, which words are given special meanings in relation to skin, as will be explained in a later section.

Apocrine Sweat Glands

This type probably evolved first, since apocrine sweat glands are of considerably more practical use and much more numerous in other mammals than they are in man. Their chief function seems to be the production of relatively small amounts of secretions which, on reaching the skin surface, give rise to distinctive *odors* (body odor in man) that enable animals to recognize the presence of others. In man, however, their distribution is very limited, for they are mostly confined to the thin skin of the axilla, pubic region, and areolae of the breasts. They develop from the same downgrowths of epithelium that give rise to hair follicles and their ducts open, not onto the skin surface, as do the ducts of the infinitely more numerous eccrine sweat glands, but into hair follicles, above the openings of the sebaceous glands soon to be described.

A sweat gland of the apocrine type has a large secretory portion and a duct. Both are coiled, and hence different coils of the same gland are often seen in a given section, where they appear as a group of secretory units. The secretory units have a wide lumen bounded by a layer of cuboidal or columnar secretory cells. It is believed that they secrete more or less continuously but the secretion is not abundant. The secretory units are sur-

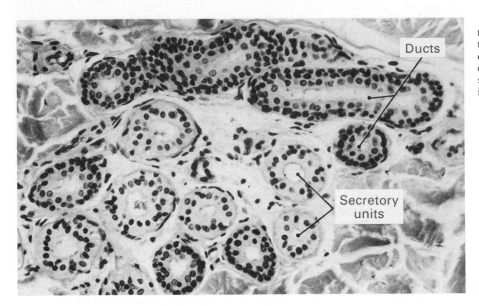

Fig. 20-9. High-power photomicrograph of dermis, showing the pale-staining secretory units of eccrine sweat glands cut in cross section and the darker-staining ducts of these glands cut in cross and oblique sections.

rounded by *myoepithelial cells* innervated by the autonomic nervous system. Their contraction can express secretion from the secretory units under conditions of excitement or aroused emotions. The ducts are similar to those of ordinary (eccrine) sweat glands, to be described next. However, as noted, the ducts of apocrine sweat glands *empty into hair follicles*.

The secretion of human apocrine sweat glands has no odor, but it contains substances readily degraded by bacteria into odoriferous (sometimes offensive) breakdown products.

Eccrine Sweat Glands

These are the common type of sweat glands in man. They are simple tubular glands distributed all over the body except in a very few sites (lips and certain parts of external genitalia of both males and females). It has been estimated that there are around 3 million of them in the skin. They are particularly numerous in thick skin (it has been estimated that there are 3 thousand per square inch in the palm of the hand). Each consists of a secretory part and an excretory duct. The secretory part of most eccrine sweat glands is situated immediately below the dermis *in the subcutaneous tissue* (Fig. 20-1). The secretory part of the tubule is coiled on itself; hence in sections it appears as a little cluster of tubes in cross and oblique section (Figs. 20-1 and 20-9). The secretory cells are of two types. Most are cuboidal or columnar in shape and have pale cytoplasm containing some glycogen. These cells are wider at their bases than at their luminal surface. Canalic-

uli between adjacent cells of this type are believed to conduct sweat to the lumen. The other and less common type of cell is narrower at its base than at its luminal surface. Its cytoplasm can be shown to contain granules that stain well enough for these cells to be known as *dark cells*.

The lumen of the *secretory part* of a sweat gland is about as wide as its wall is thick. Cells that may be spindle-shaped or have branching processes, and that resemble smooth muscle cells but are derived from ectoderm, are disposed around the secretory portions of the tubules on the inner aspect of the basement membrane. These are called *myoepithelial cells,* and it is believed that their contractions assist in expelling sweat. Immediately outside these flattened cells and the basement membrane of the tubule, connective tissue is condensed as a sheath around the secretory portions of the glands.

After pursuing a tortuous course in a limited area, the secretory portion of the gland becomes continuous with a *duct* that extends to the surface. The epithelial walls of ducts of sweat glands stain more deeply, on the whole, than the secretory cells. This is because the lining cells of these ducts form *2 layers* and are smaller than those of the secretory units; hence they contain relatively more nuclei (to take up stain) than do walls of secretory units. Ducts, therefore, can be distinguished readily in sections (Fig. 20-9) because they appear *darker.* Furthermore, the lumen of the duct is *narrower* than that of the secretory part of the gland; this is unusual, for in most glands the lumina of ducts are much wider than the lumina of secretory units. The ducts, which follow a tortuous, somewhat spiral course through the dermis, enter the tips of the interpapillary pegs of epidermis that project down between the double rows of so-called papillae (Fig. 20-3). The epithelium of the ducts at this site merges with that of the interpapillary pegs, and, from this point on, the cells of the epidermis become the cells of the walls of the ducts. Ducts so constituted pursue a spiral course through the epidermis, and when the stratum corneum is reached, the spiral nature of their course becomes accentuated (Fig. 20-3). The ducts of eccrine sweat glands finally *open on the surfaces of the ridges;* their openings are obvious in a good fingerprint.

Among other things, sweat contains sodium and chloride ions, water, and certain metabolites and nitrogeneous waste substances. Some of the sodium (but not water) is resorbed as the secretion passes through the duct.

The nervous control of sweat glands and the way sweating acts to help control body temperature will be described after we consider the blood supply of the skin.

Terminology

To clear up any confusion that may have arisen in the mind of the reader with regard to the terminology used for sweat glands, we should emphasize that *apocrine* (Gr. *apokrinesthai,* to be secreted) sweat glands received their name before the EM showed that, with the exception of holocrine glands, in which entire cells go to make up the secretion, cytoplasm is generally not lost during the release of secretion from a cell. Hence, while this type of sweat gland still retains the name *apocrine,* it is now rightly classified as merocrine with regard to mechanism of release of its secretion. To make matters worse, the way the secretion is released in *eccrine* (Gr. *ek,* out; *krinein,* to separate) sweat glands is no different, so that these too are rightly classed as merocrine. So the names *apocrine* and *eccrine* used in connection with sweat glands can suggest inappropriate connotations about the ways their secretions are released that are better forgotten.

THE MICROSCOPIC STRUCTURE OF THIN SKIN

Thin skin covers all of the body except for the palms of the hands and the soles of the feet. As noted before, it should be understood that "thick" and "thin" apply to the epidermis only and not to the skin as a whole. Actually, thin skin varies greatly in thickness in different parts of the body. These variations are due almost entirely to variation in the thickness of the dermis. The skin covering extensor surfaces is usually thicker than that covering flexor surfaces. The skin covering the eyelid is the thinnest in the body (0.5 mm. or less), and that covering the shoul-

ders and the back the thickest (up to 5 mm.) of the thin type. Figure 20-10 illustrates samples of thin skin from different regions of the body.

Thin skin contains sweat glands (Fig. 20-1B), but they are not as numerous as in thick skin. Thin skin differs from thick in that it contains *hair follicles.* These are highly developed in the scalp and in certain other regions, but are also present in the thin skin over the whole body, with a few minor exceptions (e.g., glans penis). Moreover, the surface of thin skin, unlike that of thick skin, is not thrown into ridges and grooves.

Epidermis. This has fewer layers than in thick skin (Fig. 20-11). The stratum germinativum is similar to that of thick skin, but the stratum spinosum is thinner. The stratum granulosum may form a distinct continuous layer, but if not, numerous cells containing keratohyalin granules will be seen scattered along the line where this layer might be expected. No stratum lucidum is present, and the stratum corneum is relatively thin (Fig. 20-11).

Dermis. The surface presented by the dermis to the epidermis of thin skin is considerably different from that presented in thick skin. Instead of being arranged in ridges, the dermis of thin skin projects here and there into the epidermis in the form of true papillae. However, their presence is not reflected by any unevenness of the epidermal surface above them. The pattern seen on the epidermal surface of thin skin is not due to underlying dermal papillae but is caused chiefly by lines that tend to connect the slightly depressed openings of hair follicles.

THE PIGMENTATION OF THE SKIN

The important pigment of the skin is *melanin* (Gr. *melas,* black). Melanins are widely distributed in the animal kingdom and range from yellow through brown to black in color. In man, melanin occurs chiefly in the epidermis, in white races in the cells of the basal layers, where it tends to be disposed, as a student once wrote in a histology examination, on the sunny side of the nucleus (Fig. 20-12B). Melanin occurs in the form of fine brown to black granules, but these commonly clump together if the pigment is abundant. The relative content of melanin in the epidermis is responsible for the different color of skin in differences races (black, brown, yellow, and white). All, however, have *some* melanin in their skins. An inherent *inability* in an individual of any race to produce melanin results in his being what is called an *albino* (L. *albus,* white).

Increased amounts of melanin normally appear in the epidermis of white skin when it is exposed to ultraviolet light. It is the ultraviolet light in sunlight that causes a

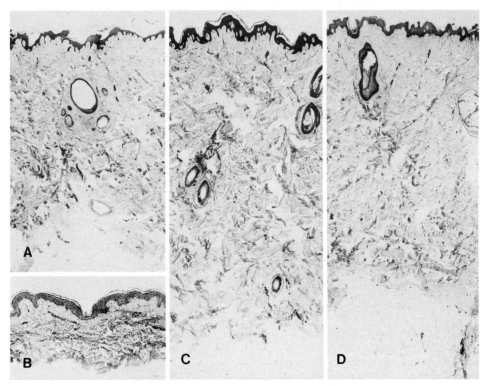

Fig. 20-10. The three large photomicrographs (taken at the same magnification) show thin skin from different parts of the body. (*A*) Skin from inside of leg. (*B*) Relatively thick split skin graft. Note that it contains a substantial content of dermis. (*C*) Skin from abdomen grafted to wrist, where it had been in position for some time. (*D*) Skin from lateral side of thigh.

Keratin

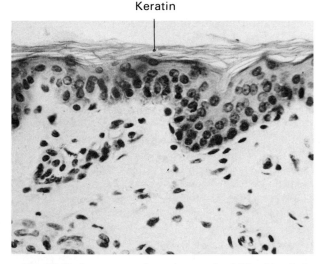

Fig. 20-11. Low-power photomicrograph of thin skin of abdomen. Here the stratified squamous epithelium is only a few cells thick. At the surface the epithelial cells undergo transformation into scales (squames) of keratin. The pale tissue beneath the epithelium is loose connective tissue of the papillary layer of dermis.

suntan to develop. Brunettes usually tan more readily than blondes. In some individuals, however, epidermal melanin tends to form in little patches (freckles).

Melanocytes

As was mentioned at the beginning of the section on epidermis, four kinds of cells are found in it. Next to keratinocytes, *melanocytes* are the most numerous. These are the cells that *produce melanin*. In the older literature the cells that produced melanin were called *melanoblasts*. However, this latter term is now used only for cells that in embryonic life develop in the neural crest and migrate to the epidermal-dermal junction, where they remain. Until melanoblasts take up a position at or in the basal layer of the epidermis, where they differentiate into *melanocytes*, they do *not* make melanin.

The cell bodies of melanocytes are disposed either just beneath or in between the cells of the basal layer of the epidermis. Before they make melanin, they may appear in the basal layer as so-called *clear cells* (Fig. 20-12A). The cell bodies of melanocytes in either position send out long

Fig. 20-12. (*A*) High-power photomicrograph of skin, showing a "clear cell" (indicated by arrow) in the stratum germinativum. (*B*) Oil-immersion photomicrograph of pigmented skin, showing melanin granules in the cytoplasm of the cells of the stratum germinativum.

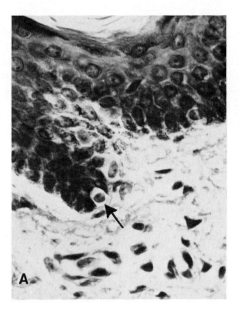

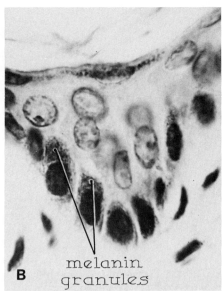

Fig. 20-12. (*A*) High-power photomicrograph of skin, showing a "clear cell" (indicated by arrow) in the stratum germinativum. (*B*) Oil-immersion photomicrograph of pigmented skin, showing melanin granules in the cytoplasm of the cells of the stratum germinativum.

processes between or under epidermal cells (Fig. 20-13), mostly those of the basal layer. Melanin granules made by melanocytes and apparently released from the tips of their processes are somehow taken into the cytoplasm of epithelial cells. If, as has been suggested, this is done by phagocytosis, it would require that the granules enter the intercellular space during transfer. By this or some other means the ordinary epithelial cells of the basal layer also come to contain melanin pigment. It follows, therefore, that melanocytes cannot be distinguished from true epidermal cells by their containing pigment. Although it has been suggested that before they become functioning melanocytes they appear as *clear cells* (Fig. 20-12A), functioning melanocytes can only be distinguished from ordinary epidermal cells by a histochemical test that demonstrates cells with the metabolic equipment required to make this pigment. This test, known as the "dopa reaction," will now be described.

Recognizing Melanocytes by the Dopa Reaction. The ability of melanocytes to produce melanin depends on their ability to synthesize the enzyme *tyrosinase*. If they possess this enzyme in active form, and are provided with the correct substrate, the tyrosinase will react with the substrate to form melanin. In man, however, the addition of tyrosine to samples of epidermis does not lead (at least not immediately) to the melanocytes forming melanin. (The reactions involved are complicated.) However, if dihydroxyphenylalanine, which is referred to as *dopa*, is added to a suitable preparation of epidermis, the tyrosinase within the melanocytes converts the dopa into melanin, which then is seen in the cytoplasm as dark pigment. This test, termed the *dopa reaction*, can be used to distinguish cells that have the ability to *make* melanin from cells that merely *take up* this pigment.

The dopa reaction has shown that melanocytes are very numerous in epidermis. According to Montagna, 10

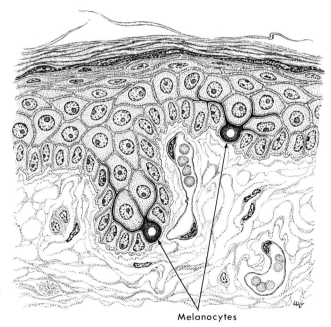

Fig. 20-13. Diagram illustrating the position of melanocytes in the skin. Note the way their branching processes (indicated in black) extend between the epidermal cells to supply them with melanin.

to 25 per cent of the cells in the basal layer of the epidermis of man are melanocytes. The dopa reaction has also been helpful in demonstrating the complicated arrangements of processes that extend from the cell bodies of melanocytes to intertwine with epidermal cells and supply them with pigment (Fig. 20-13).

Melanin Synthesis in Melanocytes. Synthesis of tyrosinase starts in the rER, from which the protein is transferred to the Golgi. Here the product is packaged in smooth-surfaced membranous vesicles, the content of which is now termed *protyrosinase.* As these vesicles change further they become known as *premelanosomes.* Active tyrosinase now appears in the contents of the vesicles and this results in melanin being synthesized in, or in association with, these vesicles. As this happens, the vesicles finally become known as *melanosomes,* which are oval, membrane-enclosed granules a little over 0.5 μm. in length. Before being obscured by melanin the granules reveal an internal arrangement of concentrically arranged lamellae. Each melanosome eventually becomes converted into a *melanin granule,* and when this has happened, the structure no longer contains demonstrable tyrosinase. The process is similar to the formation of secretory granules (described in Chap. 5) except that the enzymes in the secretory granules do their work while the vesicles are still within the cytoplasm.

Melanin-Containing Cells of the Dermis. Such melanin-containing cells as are seen in the dermis, with one exception, are cells that have not made melanin but have phagocytosed it. The one exception is infants of the Mongol race, for in these babies there may be true melanocytes deep in the dermis of the sacral region. Seen through the tissue that covers them, the pigment in these cells appears blue (this is the color of melanin seen through overlying tissue). The blue spot thus apparent is called a Mongol spot. Melanocytes are seldom seen in this site in children of the white race.

The Role of Melanin. While melanin serves to camouflage and protect certain animals from their predators, in man its primary function is to protect the deepest layers of the epidermis and the underlying dermis from the harmful effect of excessive ultraviolet light by scattering it. The fact that a person becomes tanned is evidence of an increased amount of melanin being produced by melanocytes for this purpose. Ultraviolet light on the skin is, of course, helpful to a point, because it irradiates ergosterol (a derivative of cholesterol), and irradiated ergosterol is one form of vitamin D; this vitamin, which is absorbed from the skin, is an essential factor in proper mineral metabolism. Indeed, a lack of vitamin D can cause rickets in children. Nowadays, however, in order to prevent rickets, infants are given vitamin D preparations by mouth.

LANGERHANS CELLS

These comprise the third kind of cell found in epidermis. That there were certain cells in the epidermis with shapes and properties different from those previously described was noted in the last century by Langerhans. These cells can be demonstrated to advantage by certain metallic impregnation methods, which disclose that they have branching processes that extend (like those of melanocytes) from their cell bodies between adjacent epidermal cells. The most widely accepted view about them was once that they were old melanocytes, but studies with the EM showed that they are healthy active cells (Fig. 20-14).

Under conditions of vitamin A deficiency, various kinds of membranes not ordinarily of the stratified squamous type become stratified squamous (this can happen for example in the trachea, which is normally lined by pseudostratified columnar ciliated epithelium). Langerhans cells are not present in the normal type of epithelium in these locations but they do appear in the stratified squamous epithelium that replaces the normal type and furthermore they make an appearance in the loose connective tissue underlying it. From these studies, Wong and Buck consider that the origin of Langerhans cells is more likely to be from mesenchyme than from epidermis. There is other evidence that supports this view.

Langerhans cells are not connected by desmosomes to the epidermal cells with which they are in contact. They have a very irregular shape and their nucleus is greatly indented. With the EM the rER is not very prominent but the Golgi is well developed. The cytoplasm contains some microtubules. Furthermore, it contains characteristic granules not seen in melanocytes; these are elongated structures showing longitudinal striations and some granules have a racquet shape. The function of Langerhans cells, and why they should have an association with stratified squamous epithelium, present problems. They are probably macrophages.

HAIR FOLLICLES

Development. Early in the 3rd month of fetal life the epidermis begins to send downgrowths into the underlying dermis (Fig. 20-15). They develop first in the region of the eyebrows, the chin, and the upper lip, and, soon after, they develop in all parts of the body that later will be covered with thin skin. These epidermal downgrowths become hair follicles, and give rise to hairs (Fig. 20-15, IV). By this means the fetus, at about the 5th or 6th month, has become covered with very delicate hairs.

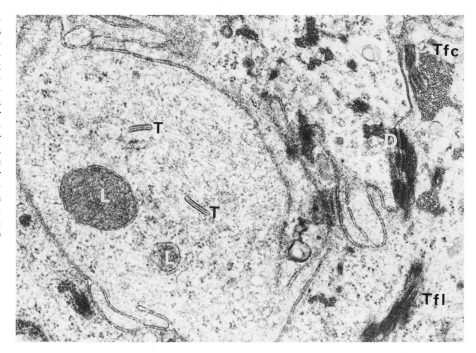

Fig. 20-14. Electron micrograph (×37,000) of a Langerhans cell in epidermis. The large pale-staining oval at *left* is the cytoplasm of a Langerhans cell. It contains lysosomes (L), and vermiform tubules (T), which are invaginations of the plasmalemma (note the line running along their axis). Possibly because of confinement in the intercellular spaces of stratified epithelia, Langerhans cells do not show the irregular outline typical of other macrophages. The adjacent stratified epithelial cells show bundles of tonofilaments cut in cross section (Tfc) and longitudinal section (Tfl), as well as desmosomes (D) along the intercellular spaces. (Courtesy of C. P. Leblond)

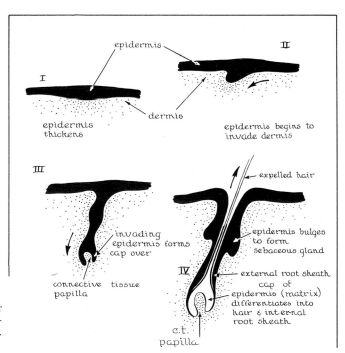

Fig. 20-15. Diagrams illustrating the development of a hair follicle and sebaceous gland in the fetus. (Redrawn from Addison, W. H. F. (ed.): Piersol's Normal Histology. ed. 15. Philadelphia, J. B. Lippincott, 1932)

627

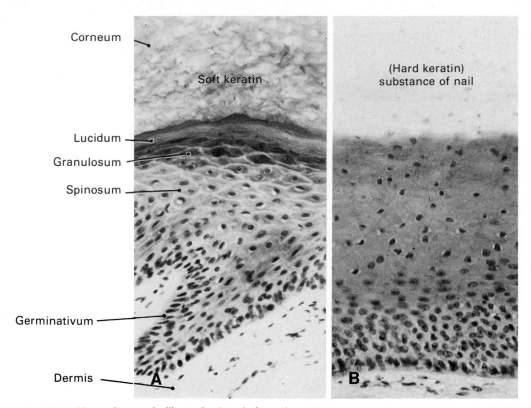

Fig. 20-16. Photomicrographs illustrating keratin formation. (*A*) The process by which soft keratin of thick skin is formed. Note keratohyalin granules in the stratum granulosum, and that a stratum lucidum is present. (*B*) The process by which hard keratin of the nail is formed. Note the gradual transition of cells into nail substance, with no stratum granulosum or lucidum being present, and note that hard keratin is more homogeneous than soft keratin.

They constitute the *lanugo* (L. *lana,* wool) of the fetus. This coat of hair is shed before birth except in the region of the eyebrows, the eyelids, and the scalp, where the hairs persist and become somewhat stronger. A few months after birth these hairs are shed and replaced by still coarser ones, while over the remainder of the body a new growth of hair occurs, and the body of the infant becomes covered with a downy coat called the *vellus* (L. for fleece). No hair follicles are formed after birth. At puberty, coarse hairs develop under the influence of male sex hormones in the axilla and pubic regions and, in males, also on the face and (to a variable extent) other parts of the body. The coarse hairs of the scalp and the eyebrows and those that develop at puberty are termed *terminal hairs* to distinguish them from those of the lanugo and vellus.

The human species, of course, is not very hairy. Most of the body is generally not covered with anything more than down-like vellus. Hair, then, is not a very important factor in keeping the body warm. It is, nevertheless, of

the greatest importance that the skin of the human species should contain hair follicles. They are, as we shall see, instrumental in repairing epidermis injured by burns and abrasions, and they make split-skin grafting possible. We shall explain the reason for this presently.

The Two Kinds of Keratin in Hair Follicles and Hairs. There are two kinds of keratin. These, the *soft* and the *hard* types, can be distinguished by histological means, and they have different physical and chemical properties. Both types are encountered in hair follicles.

Soft keratin covers the skin as a whole; hard keratin is found only in certain of the skin appendages, namely the fingernails and toenails, cuticle and cortex of hairs of man, and feathers, claws, and hooves of animals. Its formation is *not* manifested histologically by epidermal cells developing granules of keratohyalin in their cytoplasm; instead, the formation of hard keratin involves a gradual transition from living epidermal cells into keratin (Fig. 20-16B). Hard keratin is solid and does not desquamate; hence, it is a more permanent material than soft keratin (nails and hair must be cut if they are not to grow too long). Chemically, hard keratin is relatively unreactive and contains cystine and disulfide bonds than the soft variety.

THE STRUCTURE OF A HAIR FOLLICLE

A hair follicle develops by downgrowth of cells of the epidermis into the dermis and subcutaneous tissue.

The deepest part of the epithelial downgrowth becomes a cluster of cells called the *germinal matrix* of the hair follicle (Figs. 20-15 and 20-17) because it germinates the hair. It becomes fitted over a *papilla* of connective tissue (Figs. 20-15, III and 20-17) that provides capillaries and hence a source of tissue fluid into its central part.

The External Root Sheath. The part of the epidermal downgrowth that connects the germinal matrix with the surface becomes canalized and thereafter is called the *external root sheath* of the hair follicle (Figs. 20-15 and 20-18). Near the surface of the skin, the external root sheath exhibits all the layers of epidermis of thin skin (Fig. 20-17, *top*). This, of course, is to be expected since the external sheath represents a downward continuation of the epidermis. Therefore the external sheath near the surface of the skin is lined with soft keratin that is continuous at the mouth of the follicle with the soft keratin of the epidermis of the skin (Fig. 20-17). But deep down in the follicle, the external root sheath becomes thinner and does not exhibit some of the more superficial layers of the epidermis. At the bottom of the follicle, where the external root sheath surrounds and becomes continuous with the germinal matrix, the external root sheath consists of only the *stratum germinativum* of the epidermis (Fig. 20-17).

Formation and Growth of a Hair. For hair to grow in a follicle, the cells of the germinal matrix must proliferate. This forces the uppermost cells of the germinal matrix up the lumen of the external root sheath. As the cells are pushed up, they get farther and farther away from the papilla, which is their source of nourishment, and they turn into keratin. Those cells that become the cuticle and the cortex of the hair, which is hard keratin, do so without developing keratohyalin granules. The cellular area where the transition from cells into hard keratin occurs is called a *keratogenous zone* (Fig. 20-17). Hairs grow because of continued proliferation of the epidermal cells of the germinal matrix and successive conversion of these cells into keratin as they are forced up the follicle.

The Internal Root Sheath. The proliferating cells of the matrix form another structure in addition to a hair. This takes the form of a cellular tubular sheath which is pushed up around the hair to separate it from the external root sheath. This is called the *internal root sheath* (Figs. 20-17 and 20-18). It extends only partway up the follicle (Fig.

20-17). It is formed of *soft* keratin (Fig. 20-17); hence granules of keratohyalin can be seen in its cells as they become keratinized. In this region the granules are generally called *trichohyalin* (Gr. *thrix*, hair; *hyalos*, glass) *granules*, and instead of being basophilic they stain a bright red (Fig. 20-18).

THE PIGMENTATION OF HAIR

The pigment of hair, like that of the epidermis, is primarily *melanin*. The melanin of hair is also formed by *melanocytes;* these are distributed in the matrix of a hair follicle close to the papilla. The melanocytes in this region, like those of the epidermis, send out cytoplasmic processes that reach and provide melanin for the epithelial cells that will, by undergoing keratinization, become the cortex and the medulla of the hair. As the cells that form by means of cell division in the matrix move upward, they take up melanin in the upper part of the bulbous base of the hair, and then move up farther and become keratinized to become the cortex and the medulla of the hair. The melanin they contain becomes incorporated into the keratin of the hair, primarily that of the cortex, and gives it color.

There is evidence to indicate that the melanocytes of the bulb of the follicle divide by mitosis and so perpetuate themselves.

As people become older, their hair turns "gray." The lack of pigment in the hair of older people is ascribed to an increasing inability of the melanocytes of the bulbs of their hair follicles to make tyrosinase.

Although hair has many different colors, hair *pigments* of only 3 colors can be seen with the microscope; these are black, brown, and yellow. The yellow pigment is termed *pheomelanin,* and its formation seems to be under the control of genes other than those that control the formation of black and brown *melanin.* The metabolic pathways concerned in its formation are different from those producing black and brown melanin.

THE STRUCTURE OF HAIR

The cross-sectional shape and other features of terminal hairs vary in relation to race. Three chief types of hair are recognized; straight, wavy, and woolly. Straight hair is found in the Mongol races, Chinese, Eskimos, and the Indians of America; it is characteristically coarse and lank and rounded in cross section. Wavy hair is found in a number of ethnic groups, including Europeans, and woolly hair is characteristic of nearly all black races. A cross section of a wavy hair is oval and of woolly hair, elliptical or kidney-shaped.

A terminal hair consists of a central *medulla* of soft keratin (Figs. 20-17 and 20-18) and a *cuticle* and a *cortex*

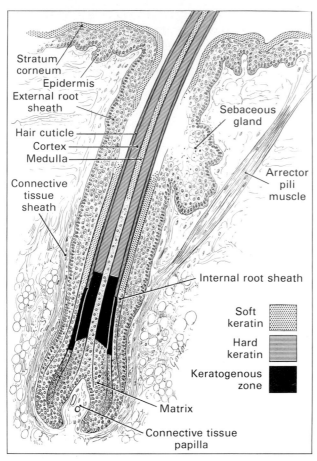

Stratum
corneum
Epidermis
External root
sheath

Hair cuticle
Cortex
Medulla

Connective
tissue
sheath

Sebaceous
gland

Arrector
pili
muscle

Internal root sheath

Soft
keratin

Hard
keratin

Keratogenous
zone

Matrix

Connective tissue
papilla

Fig. 20-17. Diagram of a hair in a hair follicle, showing the distribution of soft and hard keratin and the keratogenous zone in which the hard keratin of the hair is produced. (Based on Leblond, C. P.: Ann. N.Y. Acad. Sci., *53:*464, 1951)

of hard keratin (Figs. 20-17 and 20-18). Some hairs contain virtually no medulla; hence they show only a cuticle and a cortex of hard keratin. It is the pigment in the cells of the cortex that gives color to hair.

The cuticle consists of very thin, flat, scale-like cells arranged on the surface of a hair like shingles on the side of a house, except that their free edges point upward instead of downward (Fig. 20-19). The free edges of these cells interlock with the free edges of similar cells that line the internal root sheath and whose free edges point downward. This arrangement makes it difficult to pull out a hair without at least part of the internal root sheath coming with it. This can be of medicolegal interest.

The medulla consists of soft keratin. In it cornified cells are commonly separated from one another. Air or liquid may be present between the cells of the medulla.

THE CYCLIC ACTIVITY OF HAIR FOLLICLES

Hair coming out on a brush or comb is not an omen of imminent baldness. Reassurance for worried patients is gained by their learning that hair growth is cyclic. Animals that live in the far north, for example, commonly grow a new coat for each winter and lose it for each summer. The hair follicles of man also alternate between *growing* and *resting phases.* During the former the cells of the germinal matrix continue to proliferate and differentiate, and the hair elongates. However, the growing phase merges into a resting phase as the germinal matrix becomes inactive and atrophies. The root of the hair then becomes detached from its matrix and gradually moves up the follicle, gaining for a time a more or less secondary attachment to the external root sheath as the lower end of the hair approaches the neck of the follicle. Meanwhile, in the deeper part of the follicle, the epidermal external root sheath has retracted upward toward the surface. Finally, the hair comes right out of the follicle. Either before or after this event, the deeper parts of the external root sheath grow downward again to cover either the old papilla, which becomes rejuvenated, or a new one. A new germinal matrix develops, and this leads to a new hair beginning to grow up the follicle again.

The cyclic activity of the hair follicles of man differs in two ways from that of those animals forming and shedding a new coat each year. First, the cycles of activity are longer in the scalp hair of man. The hairs of the scalp last about 2 to 3 years before entering their short resting phase of 3 to 4 months. In other parts of the body, however, the growing phase is shorter than this and the resting phase is relatively long. The hairs of the eyebrows, for example, grow for 1 to 2 months and then their follicles rest for 3 to 4 months. The second difference is that adjacent follicles in man are commonly in different phases of activity at any given time. Trotter found, for example, that at one particular time 45 per cent of the follicles of the leg were in growing phase while the remainder were resting. In the scalp, however, 80 to 90 per cent of the follicles are in the growing phase at any given time. It is easy to see why the replacement of hair in man usually goes unnoticed.

Common Baldness. This is not common in women, which in itself suggests that male sex hormone may have something to do with baldness developing. Hamilton found that castration, and hence a lack of male sex hormone (testosterone) holds in check the hereditary tendency to develop baldness, and that administration of male sex hormone to individuals deficient in the hormone permits a hereditary tendency toward baldness to become operative, with baldness resulting. In other words, the genetic factors which tend to cause baldness are fully effective only if male sex hormone is present in the individ-

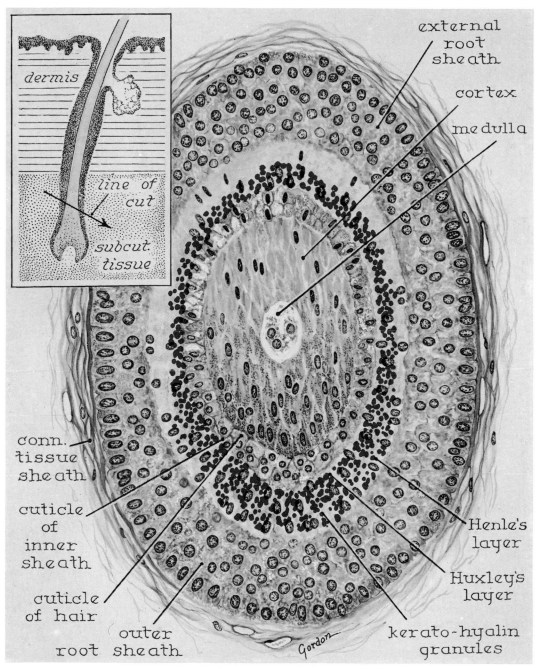

Labels on figure:
- external root sheath
- cortex
- medulla
- Henle's layer
- Huxley's layer
- kerato-hyalin granules
- conn. tissue sheath
- cuticle of inner sheath
- cuticle of hair
- outer root sheath

Inset labels:
- dermis
- line of cut
- subcut. tissue

Gordon

Fig. 20-18. High-power drawing of an oblique section through the keratogenous zone of a hair in its follicle. The plane of section is shown in the *inset.* (Hair follicles extend down into the subcutaneous tissue but not always as far as shown in the *inset.*) Nuclei in both the internal root sheath and the hair are becoming pyknotic, and red granules of trichohyalin (labeled kerato-hyalin) are present in the cells of the internal root sheath, indicating that it is forming soft keratin. No similar granules are seen in the cortex or cuticle of the hair. The inner root sheath comprises a cuticle, Huxley's and Henle's layers.

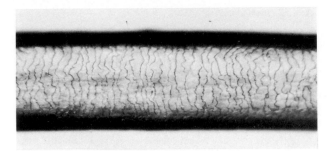

Fig. 20-19. Oil-immersion photomicrograph of the surface of a hair, showing its shingle-like cuticular scales.

ual concerned. Although baldness is an obvious sign of male sex hormone activity, the corollary should not be assumed by balding men that they are necessarily more virile than those with good heads of hair. Male sex hormone does not cause baldness unless the hereditary disposition to develop baldness is present.

The Effect of Cutting on the Growth of Hair. Another question often asked about hair is whether shaving or cutting hair encourages its growth. This has been the subject of much careful enquiry and long and painstaking experimentation (see Trotter). The general conclusion from these experiments is that cutting or shaving hair has no effect on its growth (which is about 0.4 mm. per day in scalp hair).

THE CONNECTIVE TISSUE SHEATH

Although the hair follicle is an epithelial structure, it is surrounded by a condensation of connective tissue that forms a *connective tissue sheath* about it (Figs. 20-17 and 20-18).

SEBACEOUS GLANDS

Development. As a hair follicle develops, cells from what would become the external root sheath of the upper third of the follicle grow out into the adjacent dermis and differentiate so as to form sebaceous glands (Fig. 20-15IV). When these are formed, their ducts open into the follicle at the site from which the outgrowth occurred; hence the sebaceous glands empty into the upper third of the follicle, below its mouth (Fig. 20-17). This part of the follicle is often called the *neck*.

Structure and Function. Most hair follicles slant somewhat from the perpendicular so that the hair points in a particular direction. Sebaceous glands are commonly disposed on the side of the follicle toward which the hair slants (Figs. 20-17 and 20-18, *inset*).

It is usual for several sebaceous glands to form from each follicle. Sebaceous glands secrete a fatty material called *sebum* that oils the hair and lubricates the surface of the skin. Sebum is said to possess some bactericidal and fungicidal properties but this has been disputed. Its chief function is probably that of acting as a natural "cold cream." It prevents undue evaporation from the stratum corneum in cold weather and so helps to conserve body heat. In keeping the stratum corneum oiled, it helps to keep it from becoming cracked and chapped, which can happen if it becomes too dry.

Sebaceous glands are holocrine glands; the mechanism of secretion in this type of gland was described in Chapter 7.

For a sebaceous gland (Fig. 20-20) to secrete sebum, many processes occur more or less simultaneously. These are: (*1*) proliferation of cells of the basal layer of the gland; (*2*) pushing of the extra cells formed as a result of proliferation toward the middle of the gland; (*3*) synthesis and accumulation of fatty material in the cytoplasm of these cells as they move away from the basal layer; and (*4*) necrosis of these cells as they are pushed still farther toward the middle of the gland because they are so far removed from their source of nourishment.

That sebaceous glands develop from hair follicles explains why no sebaceous glands are found in the skin that covers the soles of the feet or the palms of the hands. However, sebaceous glands develop in a few sites in the body without hair follicles (eyelids, papillae of breasts, labia minora, and corners of lips near the red margins in some people). And in some sites, in particular the skin covering the nose, the sebaceous glands that develop from hair follicles become much more prominent than the hair follicles themselves; the hair follicle in these sites is, as it were, a means to an end.

The Hormonal Control of the Activity of Sebaceous Glands and Its Relation to Acne. As will be described in Chapter 25, sex hormones begin to be secreted into the bloodstream in significant amounts at puberty (which they cause). Although secretion of male hormones is predominant in males and female sex hormones in females, the chemistry of sex hormones is inter-related and their metabolism complicated, and for one reason or another there is some female sex hormone activity in males and some male sex hormone activity in females. There is a substantial increase in the secretion of sebum at the time of puberty and experiments have shown that this is a result of male hormone. It has been shown moreover that this increased output in sebaceous glands is the result of a great increase in mitosis, bringing about more rapid turnover of the cell population of the glands. Unfortunately, the structural arrangements for delivering this greatly increased sebum to the skin surface do not seem adequate, with the result that sebum, instead of being freely ex-

Fig. 20-20. Medium-power photomicrograph of sebaceous glands opening into a hair follicle in thin skin.

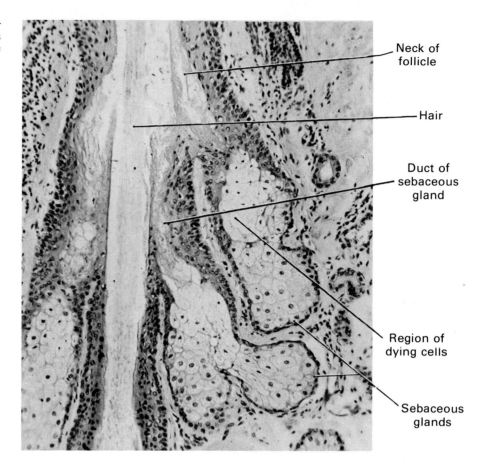

Neck of follicle

Hair

Duct of sebaceous gland

Region of dying cells

Sebaceous glands

pressed from the hair follicle, sometimes bulges into the skin so as to cause a condition called *acne* (pimples). Since this predisposes to further problems such as local infection, it is a condition that requires medical attention. Although female sex hormone acts to depress synthesis of sebum in sebaceous glands it apparently does not suppress mitosis, and it seems that at the time of puberty girls as well as boys begin to secrete either enough male sex hormone or some female hormone that at this time acts similarly on sebaceous glands to stimulate mitosis, because girls too are prone to acne at puberty. Experimental work has shown that male sex hormone needs help from certain pituitary hormones to achieve its effect, since male hormone in animals from which the pituitary gland has been removed is inactive as far as sebaceous glands are concerned.

ARRECTOR PILI MUSCLES

In the hairs of all but the beard and pubic regions, a small fan-shaped bundle of smooth muscle fibers called the *arrector pili* muscle (erector of the hair) is attached to the connective tissue sheath at a point about halfway down the follicle, or deeper. It passes obliquely upward to reach the papillary layer of the dermis a short distance away from the mouth of the hair follicle (Figs. 20-17 and 20-21). This muscle, like the sebaceous glands, is on the side of the follicle toward which the hair slants. In a section this bundle of muscle thus makes a third side to a triangle, the other two sides of which are the follicle and the surface of the skin. The sebaceous glands are situated within this triangle (Fig. 20-17). Hence, when the arrector pili muscle contracts, it not only pulls the whole hair follicle outward but also, by pulling from one side, makes the follicle more perpendicular (the hair "stands up"). Moreover, contraction of the muscle tends to "dimple in" the skin over the site of its attachment to the papillary layer of the dermis. The net result is to produce "goose pimples." The contraction furthermore squeezes the sebaceous glands contained in the triangle previously described (Fig. 20-17), and this causes their oily secretion to be expressed into the neck of the follicle and onto the skin.

The arrector pili muscles, being smooth muscle, are in-

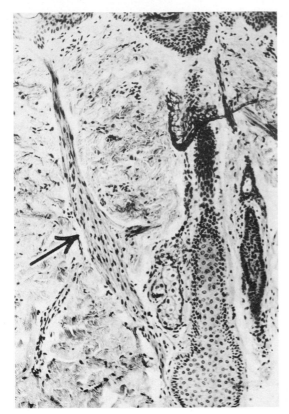

Fig. 20-21. Low-power photomicrograph of part of a hair follicle in thin skin at the site of its arrector pili muscle (indicated by arrow). The lumen and upper part of the hair follicle do not show in this plane of section. (Courtesy of E. Linell)

nervated by the sympathetic nervous system. Cold is an important stimulus for the reflex that leads to their contraction. The purpose of this reflex may be to express more oil onto the surface of the body from the sebaceous glands so that less evaporation, and hence less heat loss, occurs from the skin. Intense emotional states energize the body through the sympathetic nervous system and the release of epinephrine, so these, too, cause these muscles to contract. Fear can make one's hair "stand on end." This response is useful in the porcupine, and other animals are also said to "bristle with rage."

THE BLOOD SUPPLY OF THE SKIN

Arteries. The largest arteries supplying the skin are arranged in the form of a flat network in the subcutaneous tissue immediately below the dermis, called the *rete cutaneum.* From these vessels, branches pass both more deeply and also toward the surface. Those that pass more

deeply supply the adipose tissue of the more superficial parts of the subcutaneous tissue and the parts of hair follicles disposed therein. Those that pass superficially supply the skin. As these arteries penetrate the reticular layer of the dermis, they generally pursue a curved course and give off side branches to the adjacent hair follicles and sweat and sebaceous glands. On reaching the junction of the reticular layer and the papillary layer, they form a second flat network, composed of smaller arterial vessels, called the *rete subpapillare.*

Capillary Beds. Knowing the sites of the capillary beds in skin is of great importance in understanding how the temperature of the body is controlled and where fluid loss occurs from burns of different degrees.

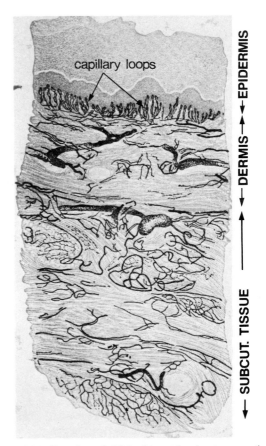

Fig. 20-22. Drawing of thick skin and subcutaneous tissue, showing the blood vessels (injected with opaque material) supplying the skin. Note the general disposition of the larger vessels in the dermis and subcutaneous tissue, and also that there are very few capillaries in the dermis. The numerous capillary loops in the connective tissue papillae that project into the lower border of the epidermis are shown to advantage. (Addison, W. H. F. (ed.): Piersol's Normal Histology. ed. 15. Philadelphia, J. B. Lippincott, 1932)

Since dermis consists chiefly of the relatively inert intercellular substance collagen, it does not require a very extensive capillary blood supply. Indeed, most of it is very sparingly supplied with capillaries. The capillary beds of the skin are extensive only in the region of the dermis that is in close association with epithelial cells requiring abundant nourishment for their function and growth, so they are confined to the connective tissue that (*1*) immediately underlies the epidermis, (*2*) surrounds the matrix of hair follicles, and (*3*) surrounds sweat and sebaceous glands.

The first capillary bed mentioned requires some further comment. Arterioles from the rete subpapillare pass toward the epidermis and give rise to capillaries that extend as loops up into the so-called connective tissue papillae (Figs. 20-22 and 20-23A). These capillaries supply tissue fluid to the basal cells of the epidermis. However, the capillary loops in the papillae are not the cause of the pink color of the skin, for they do not contain sufficient blood. The pink (bluish under certain conditions) color is due to the blood in flat networks of small thin-walled vessels (venules) in the deeper part of the papillary and in the superficial part of the reticular layers of the dermis. These flat networks of what are best regarded as venules constitute the *subpapillary plexuses* of the skin. The small venules drain into large ones, which, in turn, drain into small veins. In general, the veins leave the skin with the arteries.

Function of the Superficial Capillaries and Venules in Temperature Regulation. In man, body heat is lost directly through the skin. If the temperature of the air is lower than that of the body, the rate of heat loss can be increased or decreased by varying the extent to which the capillaries and venules in the papillary and subpapillary layers of the skin are open to the circulation. This is controlled both by the luminal size of metarterioles and the other vessels of the terminal vascular bed controlling the patterns of blood flow in these layers, and also by the luminal size of arteriovenous anastomoses that are relatively numerous in skin and enable blood to bypass the terminal vascular bed entirely so as to conserve heat when this is required.

If the temperature of the air is close to or higher than that of the body, the *effect* of a lower outside temperature can be achieved by the sweat glands pouring sweat onto the surface of the body, where it evaporates and so cools the skin. Hence, blood circulating through the papillary and subpapillary regions of skin from which sweat is evaporating loses heat. To keep down the temperature of an individual who performs violent muscular exercise on a very hot day and so generates a great deal of heat, both profuse sweating and dilation of the superficial blood vessels are needed. Some unfortunate individuals are born with very few or no sweat glands. When the temperature rises sufficiently, such individuals while at work can keep their body temperature down to the correct level only by frequently changing into fresh wet clothing.

Nervous Control of Sweating. The secretory cells of sweat glands are innervated by the sympathetic division of the autonomic nervous system. The postganglionic sympathetic fibers that innervate sweat glands produce *acetylcholine* at their endings, not norepinephrine as do most postganglionic sympathetic fibers. The activity of the nerves and hence of the sweat glands is controlled by a heat-regulating center in the hypothalamus.

It should be pointed out that many animals cannot lose heat in hot weather by sweating. The hairy coats of animals serve primarily as insulation. There is, then, no need for these animals to have sweat glands and extensive nets of capillaries and venules in the papillary and the subpapillary parts of the skin. (Dogs, for example, lose heat by evaporation as a result of panting.) Indeed, the blood supply of the skin of most laboratory animals is very different from that in man, so that deductions made from experiments on the skin of animals are not necessarily applicable to man. For example, a light burn on the shaved skin of a rat does not turn red as it does in man. The common pig is an exception. Its skin has an excellent supply of capillaries (Fig. 20-23), and its blood supply is similar to that in man. It is one of the few animals that can become sunburned. Its skin is so similar to that of man that it lends itself to experimental studies on skin grafting, burns, and healing of incisions.

THE RELATION OF THE CAPILLARY BLOOD SUPPLY OF SKIN TO BURNS AND PLASMA LOSS

A light sunburn, such as is commonly obtained on the first visit of the year to a beach, produces enough ultraviolet injury to cause capillaries and venules in the papillary and subpapillary layers of the skin to become widely open to the circulation (Fig. 20-23A). This makes the skin red.

The Nature of a Blister. In a slightly more severe burn, capillaries and venules of the papillary and subpapillary regions, in addition to dilating, allow plasma to leak from them (Fig. 20-23B). This causes an edema of the outer part of the dermis and often results in blisters. In thin skin, the common site of burns, blisters are the result of accumulations of plasma between the dermis and epidermis (Fig. 20-23C). In thick skin, blisters sometimes may be due to intraepidermal accumulations of plasma.

The Regeneration of Epidermis After a Burn. If thin skin has been burned severely enough for blisters to have formed, the burn would be severe enough to have destroyed the epidermis. Under these circumstances, a new epidermis is regenerated over the blister from the living

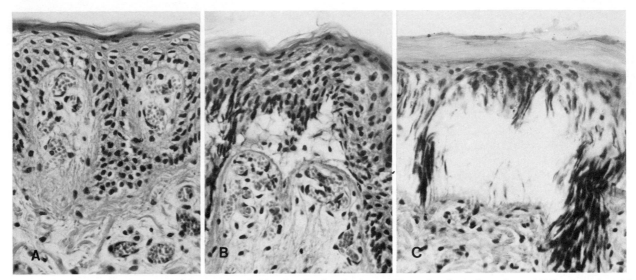

Fig. 20-23. Medium-power photomicrographs of skin of a pig, showing how a blister develops after a burn. (*A*) Section taken 15 minutes after a light burn. Note that the capillaries at *upper left* and *upper right* in the dermal papillae (close to the epidermis) are dilated and congested with blood. (*B*) Section taken 1 hour after the skin was burned lightly. The capillaries of the papillae (just below *center*) are still dilated and congested, and plasma has leaked from them and is accumulating between the dermis and the epidermis. Separation has occurred above the basement membrane, which is seen as a gray line covering the two papillae at *middle.* (*C*) Section taken 4 hours after the skin was burned slightly. The epidermis has been lifted a considerable distance from the dermis by plasma that has leaked from damaged capillaries of the dermis. (Ham, A. W.: Ann. Surg., *120:*692, 1944)

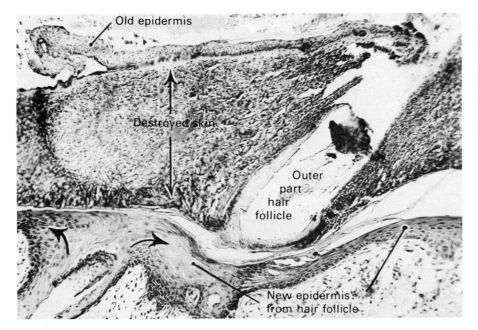

Fig. 20-24. Low-power photomicrograph of skin of a pig, some days after it was burned sufficiently to destroy the epidermis and outer part of the dermis. The former epidermis, now dead, may be seen at *top.* Below it, a considerable layer of dead dermis, containing the destroyed outer part of a hair follicle, may be seen. Below the layer of dead dermis, a new thin line of epidermis is growing out from the deeper part of the hair follicle. The newly formed epithelial cells are migrating along the line between the living and the destroyed skin. The destroyed skin eventually will be sloughed off as a scab when the new epidermis forms a continuous covering for the living skin below. Subsequently, the epidermis becomes thick, and so does the dermis beneath it, so that the skin is restored to its former thickness.

epithelium that persists deeper down in the hair follicles —just as it does when split skin grafts are cut from skin, as will be described later. Epidermis grows out from the external root sheaths of hair follicles to cover the denuded dermis (Fig. 20-24). Even if a burn is severe enough to destroy the more superficial part of the dermis (as well as the epidermis), the epithelial cells from the deeper parts of the hair follicles will survive and still grow out along the line between the living and the dead dermis (Fig. 20-24) to form new epidermis at this level.

Fig. 20-25. Drawings illustrating how a split skin graft is taken. The drawing at *left* depicts a split skin graft being cut at a level about halfway down the dermis. Such a graft (the part above the cut) can be transplanted to another site on the same individual and live. As illustrated at *right*, the site from which the graft is removed becomes covered in due course with new epidermis that grows up from hair follicles, and in man also from sweat glands, as is shown on the *right*. The dermis later becomes thickened.

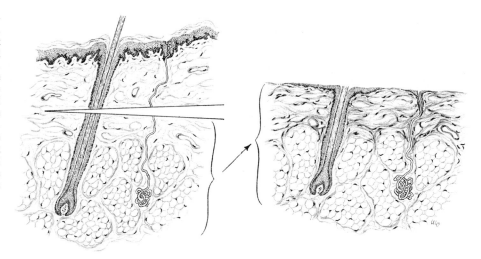

If, however, a burn is severe enough to destroy the epithelium deep in the hair follicles, a burned area can become re-covered naturally only by epithelium growing in from the edges of the injured area. This is a slow process, and if the burned area is large it takes months or years to heal, and indeed might never heal. In the meantime exposed dermis would become the seat of an inflammatory process that, in all probability, would cause huge scars to form. Nowadays, such burns are treated promptly by skin grafting, to be described shortly.

Sites of Plasma Loss in Burns of Different Depths. In superficial burns, plasma leakage occurs chiefly from dilated and injured capillaries and venules of the papillary and subpapillary layers of the dermis. Such burns appear red because these superficial vessels become dilated by the injury (Fig. 20-23A). In more severe burns these superficial vessels become coagulated by heat; hence, more severe burns may at first be *white in color*. In these, plasma leaks from deeper capillary beds associated with the hair follicles and sweat glands. In still more severe burns, plasma leaks from the capillary beds that supply the fat cells in the subcutaneous tissue. If a large area of skin is burned, even if the burn is not deep, enough plasma may leak from injured capillaries and venules to cause death of the patient. In modern treatment of burns, every effort is made to prevent hemoconcentration by administering blood plasma intravenously to the patient. Plasma leakage can be controlled by applying pressure bandages, since plasma cannot leak out into tissues unless it can expand the tissues.

SKIN GRAFTING

Skin can be successfully grafted from one part of an individual's body to another by two general methods.

By the first method (much used for example in reconstruction of part of the face) skin is moved from one part of the body to an adjacent part (for example, skin of the arm is brought close to the face and kept there for some time) without the skin ever being severed completely from its blood supply. While one edge of the graft is left connected with its original blood supply, the other is attached to a new bed. When the graft (after several days) has sufficient blood supply from the new site to which it has been attached, it can be severed from its original site and fixed in place in its new site. However, under most conditions where skin grafting is required—for example, the covering of a large area where the skin has been completely destroyed by a burn—*free* skin grafts, that is, grafts completely severed from their blood supply, are made as follows.

FREE SKIN GRAFTS

Autologous skin grafts are of two general types: split and full-thickness. Since in many kinds of accidents—in particular, thermal burns—large areas of skin may be destroyed, and since homografts do not take, it is fortunate that in the skin of man there is provision for the surgeon to multiply its extent; this is done by means of split skin grafts. By the use of these it is possible for a patient eventually to have much more skin than he possessed before grafting.

How Skin Is Multiplied by Split Grafts

A split skin graft is a shaving cut from the skin. A relatively thick one (thicker than now used) is shown in part B of Figure 20-10. The left diagram in Figure 20-25 shows about half the thickness of the skin being taken as a shaving. The piece taken can be placed on an area denuded of epidermis, and if kept in place its cells will be nourished by tissue fluid from the raw surface on which it has been placed. In due course, connective tissue cells from its bed will grow and form new intercellular substance to attach it firmly in place, and so it will provide a new epidermis for the skin. It will also become revascularized.

The reason why the site from which the split graft was taken becomes re-covered with epidermis is that the hair follicles and sweat glands of the skin extend all the way through the skin. When the superficial part of the skin is removed (to serve as a split graft) the external root sheaths of the hair follicles and the ducts of sweat glands, as is shown in the diagram on the right in Figure 20-25, serve as sources of new epidermal cells that grow out from these structures to re-cover the surface with new epidermis. Ham's studies in this connection were made on pigs, animals with excellent skin for skin-grafting experiments. In pigs

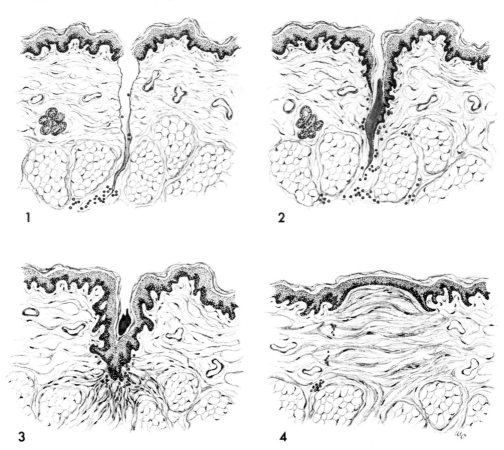

Fig. 20-26. Drawings showing the sequence of events in the healing of an incision made in skin under conditions where the edges of the wound are approximated by sutures, (*1*) A few hours after the incision was made; (*2*) after about 1 week; (*3*) about 2 weeks afterward; and (*4*) after about 1 month. For details, *see* text. (Based on Lindsay, W. K., and Birch, J. R.: Can. J. Surg., *7:*297, 1964)

the growth of new epidermis is chiefly, if not entirely, from the external root sheaths of hair follicles. It is said, however, that in man there is considerable growth of epidermis from sweat glands.

Full-Thickness Grafts

In certain cases, particularly where good cosmetic effects are desirable, full-thickness autologous free grafts are used. Here, however, there is no skin-multiplying effect because the skin appendages as well as epidermis and dermis are taken for the graft. So the edges of the site from which the full-thickness graft is cut must be sewn together, or the area covered with a split graft.

How Free Grafts Become Vascularized. It might be thought that a full-thickness graft would be too thick for its cells to be nourished by diffusion from tissue fluid from the bed in which the graft was placed. But full-thickness grafts do survive and soon develop a proper blood supply without the necessity of their blood vessels having to be connected to those of the bed. Cloutier and Ham showed by injection experiments in pigs (Fig. 13-4) that the capillaries of the graft and capillaries in its bed soon become joined, and that by 7 days blood would be flowing

again in the larger vessels of the graft, which must have remained alive by diffusion during the interim. The old vessels of the graft are used again, but it seems probable that new vessels grow into such a graft to supplement the original ones that become connected by new capillaries.

HEALING OF SKIN AFTER A SURGICAL INCISION OR ACCIDENTAL CUT

The old, widely held view was that following a surgical incision closed with sutures, fibrin formed between the edges of the incision and served as a weak bonding agent to help keep the cut edges together. It was assumed that fibroblasts from the dermis on each side of the cut, together with capillaries, grew into the fibrin and joined the edges together with new collagen. Meanwhile, the epidermis was thought to grow across the top, covering the new connective tissue forming below it.

Gillman reexamined the older concepts in the light of modern knowledge about the repair of tissue, and from experimental studies found them wanting in several respects. More recently, Lindsay and Birch made a study of the subject in young children, and their results, like those of Gillman, indicate that there has been much misunderstanding about what actually happens. The diagrams used here to illustrate the healing of a skin incision as we now understand it (Fig. 20-26) are redrawn from those of Lindsay and Birch, and the sequence of events they illustrate is in general similar to that postulated by Gillman.

First, the role of fibrin in the repair process was overestimated. Second, the dermis is a poor source of fibroblasts because fibroblasts are scarce in the reticular layer of the dermis (it consists mostly of collagen). Third, the dermis is a poor source of new capillaries because the reticular layer of the dermis is relatively nonvascular.

Next, the concept of epidermis growing over glued-together edges of dermis is also not in accord with fact. Indeed, the edges of the dermis are *not* glued firmly together, and as a result a V-shaped slit extends down from the surface to the subcutaneous tissue (Fig. 20-26, diagrams 1 and 2). A little fibrin soon forms near the bottom of the slit (dark in diagrams 2 and 3, Fig. 20-26). The epidermis on each side of the slit begins to bend downward (diagram 1 in Fig. 20-26).

A feature noticed about a week afterward is that the epidermis has extended down the sides of the slit, adhering to tissue on either side (diagram 2 in Fig. 20-26). If fibrin is present, the epidermis remains attached to healthy dermis. The epidermis that grows down the sides would be in the way if fibroblasts from the dermis on either side tried to grow across the gap. After about 2 weeks the epidermis that has grown down one side meets that on the other side so that epidermal continuity is restored deep in the cleft (diagram 3 in Fig. 20-26).

Meanwhile, fibroblasts and capillaries repair the connective tissue of the skin. However, the chief source of fibroblasts and capillaries is not dermis but subcutaneous tissue. This is because the subcutaneous tissue has a much more abundant supply of capillaries and hence many more pericytes than the relatively nonvascular and noncellular dermis. At the junction between dermis and subcutaneous tissue an abundant growth of fibroblasts, probably derived from pericytes (diagram 3 in Fig. 20-26), and capillaries forms a ridge of new tissue. As it grows, this bulges up at the bottom of the epithelially lined cleft, pushing the bottom of the cleft toward the surface until the surface is level again (diagram 4 in Fig. 20-26). This action requires, of course, that the area newly covered by epidermis (that formerly lined the cleft) be enlarged, just as the surface of cloth is enlarged if it is pulled on each side to straighten out a depressed wrinkle. So in due course the area previously occupied by the epidermally

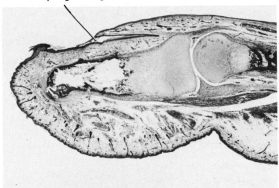

Developing nail groove

Fig. 20-27. Photomicrograph of a longitudinal section of a terminal phalanx of a fetus, showing how the epidermis invades the dermis proximally to form a nail groove.

lined cleft becomes occupied by new connective tissue derived chiefly from subcutaneous tissue, and this is covered with thin epidermis (Fig. 20-26, diagram 4)—thin because it is stretched as the connective tissue growth from below wells upward and expands the surface.

For a long time the epidermis here remains thin and lacks the usual uneven undersurface created by connective tissue papillae that normally project into the epidermis of thin skin (Fig. 20-26, diagram 4).

Lindsay and Birch also give helpful advice on how to suture skin so as to minimize scarring.

NAILS

Development. Toward the end of the first trimester of fetal life, epidermis covering the dorsal surface of the terminal phalanx of each finger and toe invades the underlying dermis along a transverse curved line. The invading epidermis has the form of a curved plate that slants proximally; later, the invading plate splits so that it forms the nail groove (Fig. 20-27). The epidermal cells making up the deeper wall of this groove proliferate to become the *matrix* of the nail (Fig. 20-28). The cells in the matrix proliferate, and the upper ones differentiate into *nail* substance, which is *hard* keratin (Fig. 20-16B). With continuing proliferation and differentiation of cells in the lower part of the matrix, the forming nail is pushed out of the groove and slowly slides along the dorsal surface of the digit toward its distal part, remaining firmly attached to it all the while. The epidermis over which it slides is called the *nail bed* (Fig. 20-28). It consists of only the deeper layers of the epidermis; the nail, as it were, serves as its stratum corneum. The skin of the dorsal surface of the digit is formed into a *lateral nail groove* along each side of

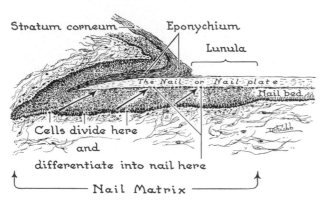

Fig. 20-28. Diagram of a longitudinal section of a nail groove with the root of its growing nail.

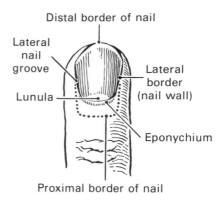

Fig. 20-29. Diagram of the end of a finger showing its fingernail.

the nail (Fig. 20-29). With sufficient growth, the *free margin* of the nail projects beyond the distal end of the digit (Fig. 20-29).

Microscopic Structure. The *body* of the nail is the part that shows; the part hidden in the nail groove is called the *root*. A crescent-shaped white area appears on the part of the body nearest the root. This is called the *lunula* (Fig. 20-29); it is seen to advantage on the thumb and is usually absent from the little finger. The nail is usually pink because the blood in the capillaries of the dermis under the nail bed shows through; the lunula is white because the capillaries under it do not show through. Some think the lunula indicates the extent of the underlying matrix (Fig. 20-28). Since the matrix is thicker than the epidermis of the nail bed, capillaries beneath it would not show through it as readily as through the epidermis of the nail bed. However, the lunula is not always correlated with the site of the matrix in sections. Hence some think its whiteness is due to the first formed nail substance being more opaque than the more mature nail substance found over the bed.

The dermis beneath the nail bed is arranged in longitudinal grooves and ridges; in cross sections these ridges appear as papillae. The dermis in this site is very vascular. The ridges and the grooves do not continue proximally under the matrix, but there are some papillae in this region.

At the proximal border of the nail, the stratum corneum of the epidermis projects over and is adherent to the nail. This, together with the stratum corneum of the epidermis that makes up the proximal superficial wall of the nail fold and is adherent to the proximal and outer surface of the nail root, constitutes the *eponychium* (Gr. *epi*, upon; *onyx*, nail) (Fig. 20-28); it consists of *soft* keratin.

Some Characteristics and Problems. On the average, nails grow about 0.5 mm. a week. Fingernails grow more rapidly than toenails and both grow faster in summer than in winter. The rate of growth of nails is different at different ages. Nail growth may be disturbed when the body suffers from certain diseases. Even psychological upsets are said to be reflected sometimes by the pitting of nails. Certain hormone deficiencies and excesses affect the growth of nails; hence the condition of the nails sometimes may help to indicate an endocrine gland disturbance.

Infections in the region of the eponychium or along the lateral borders of the nail (Fig. 20-29) are not uncommon. Sometimes, in order to permit these regions to heal, it is necessary to remove the root of a nail. When it is pulled out, the nail root is seen to be shaped like a curved chisel (it does not extend into the nail groove as far as might be thought). Provided the matrix is not destroyed, a new nail will grow out of the nail fold; however, if the matrix is destroyed, a new nail will not form.

Sometimes, from wearing improper shoes, the curvature of toenails becomes accentuated, and they pierce the dermis along one of their lateral grooves. The condition is called an *ingrown toenail*. Sometimes it is necessary to cut away some matrix at one side of the nail groove to cure this condition, since new nail will not grow from the region from which matrix is removed. Hence, cutting away matrix at one side results in formation of a narrower nail that does not impinge on the skin at the bottom of the lateral groove, and so the pierced skin at this point can heal.

THE SENSORY ROLE OF THE SKIN

Many different types of sensations experienced by the brain are due to nerve impulses being received by it from the skin. For example, the sensation experienced because of some part of one's body being touched depends on there being specialized nerve endings in the skin that have a low threshold for initiating nerve impulses when they are contacted even lightly, say with a feather. Impulses thus instituted travel to the brain to a site where they give rise not only to the sensation of touch, but also to perception of the site where the impulses originated.

The Role of Sensory Receptors in Sensation. It is important to emphasize that sensory receptors are merely tissue arrangements designed to have low thresholds that allow different kinds of stimuli to initiate nerve impulses from them. Only nerve impulses, and not different kinds of stimuli, pass to the brain. The experiencing of a sensation is a function of the brain resulting from impulses arriving in the sensory area of the cortex. If the nerve fiber from a receptor responding to a particular kind of stimulus is stimulated, for example, somewhere along its course, the sensation perceived is the one that would have ordinarily been experienced had impulses been initiated at the receptor itself. Moreover, the sensation is felt at the site from which the impulses would ordinarily have been derived. For example, a person with part of his leg amputated may, because of cut nerve fibers that formerly served the foot attempting to regenerate, and hence becoming stimulated at their ends, complain of feeling pain in the foot he no longer possesses.

The Functional Types of Sensory Receptors in Skin. The various types of sensory receptors in muscle and tendon have already been described (p. 561). Those in skin are of 3 main functional types: (*1*) those with a low threshold for temperature changes, and hence termed *thermoreceptors;* (*2*) those with low thresholds for stimuli resulting from touch, skin distortion, or pressure (in other words, mechanical stimulation), and hence called *mechanoreceptors* (Gr. *mechane,* contrivance); and (*3*) those with low thresholds for injuries leading to the sensation of pain; these are termed *nociceptors* (L. *nocere,* to injure).

The Afferent Nerve Supply of the Skin. Afferent nerve fibers, both myelinated and unmyelinated, extend from the cell bodies of afferent neurons in posterior root ganglia, to constitute a *subpapillary dermal plexus* that lies below but close to the epidermis, in the dermis. This supplies the fibers that lead to the sensory receptors of the skin, details of which are provided below for those interested.

THE MORPHOLOGICAL TYPES OF CUTANEOUS SENSORY RECEPTORS

There are two broad types: (*1*) free nerve endings and (*2*) encapsulated endings (often termed *corpuscular* receptors). We shall consider the free endings first; these are mostly derived from nonmyelinated fibers of the plexus.

FREE NERVE ENDINGS

As nonmyelinated fibers enter the epidermis, some become free of their investment of Schwann cells (Fig. 20-30A). The basal lamina of the most distal Schwann cells fuses with that of the stratum germinativum so that the afferent fibers continue on

as so-called *free endings* into the epidermis where they lie between the cell membranes of contiguous epithelial cells, extending as far as the stratum granulosum (Fig. 20-30A).

Similar free endings in the papillary layer of the dermis lie parallel with the dermal-epidermal border instead of perpendicular to the skin surface. They are also more bulbous and run a more tortuous course than free endings in the epidermis. The function of free endings in skin is not entirely clear. However, it is probable that they serve as *thermoreceptors* and *nociceptors.*

Basket-like arrangements of free nerve endings surround hair follicles and free endings enter the external root sheath, particularly in tactile hairs such as cat whiskers and other long coarse hairs on the snouts of animals. Since these respond to displacement of the hairs they are *mechanoreceptors.*

Merkel Endings. These are present in the deep layers of the epidermis of the palmar surface of the hands and the plantar surface of the feet. Here free nerve endings are attached to modified epidermal cells called *Merkel cells* found in the stratum germinativum. Merkel cells interdigitate with, and are larger than, the ordinary epidermal cells to which they are anchored by desmosomes. As shown in Figure 20-30B, nonmyelinated terminal branches of myelinated afferent nerve fibers each penetrate the basal layer of the epidermis, lose their investment of Schwann cells, and become expanded into a terminal disk attached to the base of a Merkel cell. The Merkel endings are also regarded as mechanoreceptors.

ENCAPSULATED NERVE ENDINGS

Pacinian Corpuscles (Corpuscles of Vater-Pacini). These are mechanoreceptors distributed throughout the dermis and subcutaneous tissue, particularly in the fingers, external genitalia, and breasts. They are also present in other sites that may be deformed by pressure, for example, joint capsules, mesenteries, and the wall of the urinary bladder.

A pacinian corpuscle is an ovoid structure, 1 to 4 mm. long and 0.5 to 1 mm. in diameter. It is supplied by a long myelinated nerve fiber that enters at one pole and loses its myelin sheath at a node of Ranvier just inside the corpuscle (Fig. 20-30C). The fiber then runs axially through the corpuscle to become expanded terminally into several club-like processes. Within the corpuscle, the nerve fiber is covered by numerous concentric layers of flattened cells, and hence in longitudinal section a pacinian corpuscle has the appearance of a longitudinally sliced onion (Fig. 20-30C).

The region immediately surrounding the nerve fiber is described as a *core* with an inner and outer part. The *capsule* surrounds this core. The flattened cells forming the core probably correspond to modified Schwann cells. In the inner part of the core (which contains up to 80 lamellae), the cells alternate with one another on opposite sides of the nerve fiber so as to form a series of concentric semicircles when seen in cross section. The cells in the inner part of the core are extremely flattened and packed together closely so that the intercellular spaces between them are narrow. However, the cells in the outer part of the core entirely surround the nerve fiber, forming about 60 complete concentric layers. The peripheral cells in the outer part of the core are somewhat thicker and more widely separated than the deeper ones. Desmosome-like junctions join all the cells forming the core, and there are sparsely distributed collagen fibers and tissue fluid, as well as basal laminae, in the intercellular spaces between them.

External to the core of the corpuscle lies the connective tissue capsule, which is continuous with the endoneural sheath of the afferent fiber supplying the corpuscle. The thickness of the cap-

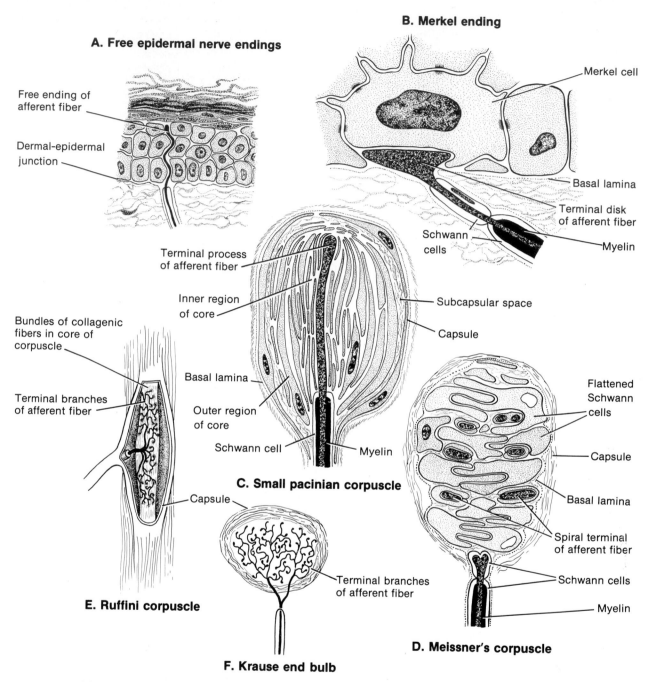

A. Free epidermal nerve endings

Free ending of
afferent fiber

Dermal-epidermal
junction

B. Merkel ending

Merkel cell

Basal lamina

Terminal disk
of afferent fiber

Schwann
cells

Myelin

Terminal process
of afferent fiber

Inner region
of core

Bundles of collagenic
fibers in core of
corpuscle

Terminal branches
of afferent fiber

Basal lamina

Outer region
of core

Schwann cell

Subcapsular space

Capsule

Myelin

C. Small pacinian corpuscle

Flattened
Schwann
cells

Capsule

Basal lamina

Spiral terminal
of afferent fiber

Schwann cells

Myelin

Capsule

E. Ruffini corpuscle

Terminal branches
of afferent fiber

D. Meissner's corpuscle

F. Krause end bulb

Fig. 20-30. Diagram of the sensory receptors in the skin. (*A*) Free nerve ending in epidermis. (*B*) Merkel ending in epidermis. (*C*) Small pacinian corpuscle in dermis. (*D*) Meissner's corpuscle in dermis. (*E*) Ruffini corpuscle in dermis. (*F*) Krause end bulb (mucocutaneous corpuscle) in dermis. For details, *see* text.

sule is variable; in large corpuscles it may contain as many as 30 concentric layers of flattened cells but in small ones, such as that depicted in Figure 20-30C, it consists of only 1 or 2 layers. These cells also are joined to one another by desmosomes. The intercellular spaces between them contain bundles of collagenic

fibers, tissue fluid, and basal lamina components. The deeper the position of the pacinian corpuscle in the skin, the greater the number of layers in the corpuscle. Between the core and the capsule of the corpuscle there is a narrow *subcapsular space* containing collagenic fibers and some fibroblasts.

Why the structural arrangements described above facilitate response of pacinian corpuscles to mechanical displacement of the skin due to pressure is not clear. They also detect vibrations.

Meissner's Corpuscles. These receptors are most numerous on the palmar surface of the fingers, the plantar surface of the feet, the lips, eyelids, external genitalia, and nipples. They lie just below the epidermal-dermal border in the papillary layer of the dermis. They are almost certainly mechanoreceptors, responding to skin displacement due to touch.

Each corpuscle is an ovoid structure about 100 μm. long and 50 μm. in diameter, lying with its long axis perpendicular to the skin surface. It consists of flattened cells that for the most part lie transversely in the corpuscle (Fig. 20-30D) and interleave with one another. These flattened cells are probably modified Schwann cells. The expanded nerve endings are so arranged that they lie parallel with the skin surface. As shown in Figure 20-30D, the myelinated afferent nerve fiber supplying the corpuscle loses its myelin sheath where it branches. From 2 to 9 branches enter at the base of the corpuscle and then branch repeatedly. The terminal branches may pursue a tortuous course through the corpuscle but are commonly arranged more or less in the form of a spiral. There are collagen fibers in the intercellular spaces between the nerve endings and flattened Schwann cells.

Surrounding the core of flattened cells with expanded nerve endings interleaved with them, there is a well-developed connective tissue *capsule*. This is continuous with the endoneurial sheath of the afferent fiber and is anchored to the epidermal-dermal border by bundles of collagen fibers.

It is significant that Meissner's corpuscles are situated in regions of tactile sensitivity.

Ruffini Corpuscles. These receptors lie deep in the dermis and subcutaneous tissue and are particularly numerous on the plantar surface of the feet. Each is a small elongated structure about 1 mm. long and 0.1 mm. in diameter. The large myelinated afferent nerve fiber that supplies the corpuscle branches repeatedly to form a diffuse arborization of nonmyelinated terminal branches. These end in flattened terminals ramifying extensively between bundles of collagenic fibers in the core of the corpuscle (Fig. 20-30E). Modified Schwann cells such as those seen in pacinian and Meissner's corpuscles are lacking. The nerve endings in Ruffini corpuscles appear to be stimulated by displacement of the collagen fibers with which they are intertwined. These collagen fibers run axially through the corpuscle and constitute its *core*. They pass right through both ends of the corpuscle (Fig. 20-30E) to merge with the collagen in the surrounding regions of the dermis. The *capsule* is relatively thin and is continuous with the endoneurial sheath of the afferent fiber.

There is a striking resemblance between Ruffini corpuscles and Golgi tendon organs (Fig. 18-28), so they are thought to be mechanoreceptors that respond to displacement of collagenic fibers in the surrounding connective tissue, much as tendon organs respond to pull in tendons.

Krause End Bulbs (Mucocutaneous Corpuscles). These are situated in the dermis of the conjunctiva (the covering of the whites of the eyes and the lining of the eyelids), tongue, and external genitalia. Two structurally different sub-types have been described; both are very lightly encapsulated compared with the other types of encapsulated receptors.

The afferent myelinated fiber of the simpler type ends in a single nonmyelinated bulbous expansion near the distal end of a poorly formed capsule. The afferent myelinated fiber of the more complex type branches repeatedly within an ill-defined capsule, forming a network of nonmyelinated endings (Fig. 20-30F).

The function of the end bulb receptors has not been established but it appears likely that they are mechanoreceptors.

REFERENCES AND OTHER READING ON SKIN AND SKIN APPENDAGES

GENERAL

Champion, R. H., Gillman, T., Rook, A. J., and Sims, R. T. (eds.): An Introduction to the Biology of the Skin. Oxford and Edinburgh, Blackwell, 1970.

Della Porta, G., and Muhlbock, O. (eds.): Structure and Control of the Melanocyte. New York, Springer, 1966.

Elgjo, K.: Epidermal Cell Population Kinetics in Chemically Induced Hyperplasia. p. 116. Scandinavian University Books. Oslo, University Press, 1966.

Jarrett, A. (ed.): The Physiology and Pathophysiology of the Skin. vol. 2. The Nerves and Blood Vessels. vol. 4. The Hair Follicle. London, Academic Press, 1973 and 1977.

Montagna, W.: The Structure and Function of Skin. ed. 2. New York, Academic Press, 1962.

Montagna, W., and Ellis, R. A. (eds.): The Biology of Hair Growth. New York, Academic Press, 1958.

———: Advances in the Biology of the Skin. vol. 6. New York, Pergamon Press, 1965.

Montagna, W., and Lobitz, W., Jr. (eds.): The Epidermis. New York, Academic Press, 1964.

Riley, V., and Fortner, J. G. (eds.): Pigment cell. Ann. N.Y. Acad. Sci., *100:*1, 1963.

Zelickson, A. S. (ed.): Ultrastructure of Normal and Abnormal Skin. Philadelphia, Lea & Febiger, 1967.

SPECIAL

Skin and Skin Appendages

Allen, T. D., and Potter, C. S.: Desmosomal form, fate and function in mammalian epidermis. J. Ultrastruct. Res., *51:*94, 1975.

Billingham, R. E., and Silvers, W. K.: The melanocytes of mammals. Q. Rev. Biol., *35:*1, 1960.

Breathnach, A. S.: The cell of Langerhans. Int. Rev. Cytol., *18:*1, 1965.

Brody, T.: The keratinization of epidermal cells of normal guinea pig skin as revealed by electron microscopy. J. Ultrastruct. Res., *2:*482, 1959.

Chacko, L. W., and Vaidya, M. C.: The dermal papillae and ridge patterns in human volar skin. Acta. Anat., *70:*99, 1968.

Chase, H. B.: Growth of the hair, Physiol. Rev., *34:*113, 1954.

Ellis, R. A.: Vascular patterns of the skin. *In* Montagna, W., and Ellis, R. A. (eds.): Advances in Biology of the Skin. vol. 2, p. 20. New York, Pergamon Press, 1961.

Fitzpatrick, T. B., and Szabo, G.: The melanocyte, cytology and cytochemistry. J. Invest. Dermatol., *32:*197, 1959.

Fowler, J., and Denekamp, J.: Regulation of epidermal stem cells. *In* Cairnie, A. B., Lala, P. K., and Osmond, D. G. (eds.): Stem Cells of Renewing Cell Populations. New York, Academic Press, 1976.

Hamilton, J. B.: Patterned loss of hair in man: types and incidence. Ann. N.Y. Acad. Sci., *53:*395, 1968.

Laurence, E. B., and Thornley, A. L.: The influence of epidermal chalone on cell proliferation. *In* Cairnie, A. B., Lala, P. K., and Osmond, D. G. (eds.): Stem Cells of Renewing Cell Populations. New York, Academic Press, 1976.

Menton, D. N.: A minimum-surface mechanism to account for the organization of cells into columns in the mammalian epidermis. Am. J. Anat., *145:*1, 1976.

Potten, C. S.: Identification of clonogenic cells in the epidermis and the structural arrangement of the epidermal proliferative unit (EPU). *In* Cairnie, A. B., Lala, P. K., and Osmond, D. G. (eds.): Stem Cells of Renewing Cell Populations. New York, Academic Press, 1976.

Ryan, T. J.: Structure and shape of blood vessels of skin. *In* Jarrett, A. (ed.): The Physiology and Pathophysiology of the Skin. vol. 2. The Nerves and Blood Vessels. London, Academic Press, 1973.

Seiji, M., and Bernstein, I. A.: Biochemistry of Cutaneous Epidermal Differentiation. Baltimore, University Park Press, 1977.

Seiji, M., Shimao, K., Birbeck, M. S. C., and Fitzpatrick, T. B.: Subcellular localization of melanin biosynthesis. Ann. N.Y., Acad. Sci., *100:*497, 1963.

Thodin, J. A. G., and Reith, E. J.: Ultrastructure of keratin in oral mucosa, skin, esophagus, claw and hair. *In* Fundamentals of Keratinization. p. 61. Washington, D. C., Am. Assoc. Adv. Sci., 1962.

Wolff, K., and Konrad, K.: Melanin pigmentation: an in vivo model for studies of melanosome kinetics within keratinocytes. Science, *174:*1034, 1971.

Wong, Yong-Chuan, and Buck, R. C.: Langerhans cells in epidermoid hyperplasia. J. Invest. Dermatol., *56:*10, 1971.

For References about tonofilaments and desmosomes, *see* Chapter 5.

Skin Healing

Croft, C. B., and Tarin, D.: Ultrastructural studies of wound healing in mouse skin. I. Epithelial behaviour. J. Anat., *106:*63, 1970.

Gillman, T., et al.: A re-examination of certain aspects of the histogenesis of the healing of cutaneous wounds; a preliminary report. Br. J. Surg., *43:*141, 1955.

Ham, A. W.: Experimental study of histopathology of burns, with particular reference to sites of fluid loss in burns of different depths. Ann. Surg., *120:*689, 1944.

Lindsay, W. K., and Birch, J. R.: Thin skin healing. Can. J. Surg., *7:*297, 1964.

Tarin, D., and Croft, C. B.: Ultrastructural studies of wound healing in mouse skin. II. Dermo-epidermal interrelationships. J. Anat., *106:*79, 1970.

Cutaneous Sensory Receptors

See under Afferent Nerve Endings at end of Chapter 17.

21 The Digestive System

The digestive system (Fig. 21-1) consists of: (*1*) a long muscular tube that begins at the lips and ends at the anus, at which two sites its epithelial lining becomes continuous with the epidermis of the skin; starting from the mouth, the tube is composed of the pharynx, esophagus, stomach, small and large intestine; and (*2*) certain large glands situated outside the tube proper (salivary glands, liver, gallbladder, and pancreas) that empty their secretions into it.

Digestion Occurs Outside the Body Proper. The semifluid material in the lumen of the digestive tube is as much outside the body as the water in which an ameba lives is outside the ameba. Food must be absorbed through the epithelial lining of the tube before it can be said to have gained entrance to the body proper. But most food taken in at the mouth is not in a form that can be used by cells. The carbohydrate of bread and potatoes, for example, is in the form of starch and must be broken down to glucose before it can be absorbed. The proteins of meat must be broken down to amino acids, and ingested fat must be likewise split into monoglycerides, fatty acids, and glycerol. The process by which foods taken in at the mouth are converted into substances that are absorbed is known as *digestion*. Digestion occurs in the lumen of the digestive tube and is brought about by food being acted upon by digestive juices secreted by glands in the wall of the tube and by other glands situated outside the tube but emptying into it. The products of fully digested food are absorbed through the epithelial cells lining the tube.

Definition and Description of a Mucous Membrane. The wet epithelial lining of the digestive tube and (as we shall see) other internal passageways that open to its surface constitutes, like the epidermis of skin, a barrier between the cells of the body and the outside world. The problem of providing protection along the vast wet epithelial surface of the digestive tube is considerably greater than that it is in the skin because a large part of the epithelial membrane of the intestinal tract must be thin enough to be absorptive. One of the chief safeguards ensuring integrity of the epithelium of a mucous membrane is its lubrication with *mucus*. From one end to the other, the digestive tube is richly provided either with individual cells or with glands that produce mucus. Wet epithelial membranes thus equipped, which line the various tubular and bladder-like structures in the body, are termed *mucous membranes*. But the term *mucous membrane* usually refers to something more than an epithelial membrane

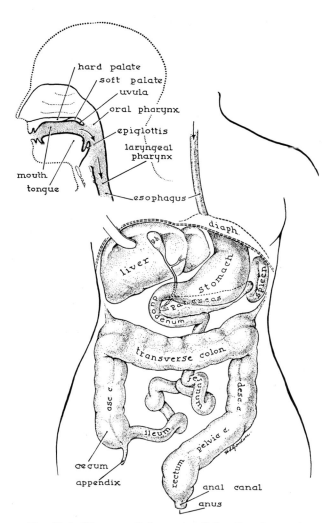

Fig. 21-1. Diagram of the parts of the digestive system. (Redrawn and modified from Grant, J. C. B.: A Method of Anatomy. ed. 4. Baltimore, Williams & Wilkins, 1948)

645

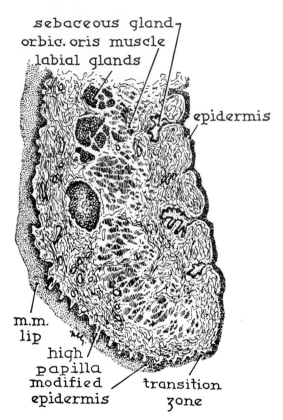

sebaceous gland
orbic. oris muscle
labial glands

epidermis

m.m.
lip

high
papilla
modified
epidermis

transition
zone

Fig. 21-2. Diagram of a sagittal section of a lip (low-power). (After Addison, W. H. F. (ed.): Piersol's Normal Histology. ed. 15. Philadelphia, J. B. Lippincott, 1932)

alone; it also includes the underlying connective tissue that supports the epithelial membrane. This connective tissue layer is termed the *lamina propria (tunica propria)* of the mucous membrane. In some instances mucous membranes are limited on the tissue side by a thin sheath of smooth muscle known as *muscularis mucosae* (muscle of the mucosa). The 3 main layers of a mucous membrane are shown in Figure 21-21.

THE ORAL CAVITY

THE LIPS

The substance of the lips consists of striated muscle fibers and fibroelastic connective tissue. The muscle tissue consists chiefly of the fibers of the orbicularis oris muscle and is distributed in the more central part of the lip (Fig. 21-2).

The outer surface of each lip (*right* in Fig. 21-2) is covered with skin that contains hair follicles, sebaceous

glands (Fig. 21-2, *top right*), and sweat glands. The red free margin of the lip is covered with a modified skin that represents a transition zone (*bottom* in Fig. 21-2) from skin to mucous membrane and is relatively transparent. The connective tissue papillae of the dermis beneath it are numerous, high, and vascular (Fig. 21-2, *bottom*), and, as a result, the blood in their capillaries readily shows through the transparent epidermis to make the lips appear red. No sweat or sebaceous glands or hair follicles are present in the skin of the red free margin of the lip. Since the epithelium is not heavily keratinized and is not provided with sebum, it must be occasionally wetted with saliva by the tongue to avoid "chapped" and "cracked" lips.

As the skin of the red free margin passes onto the inner surface of the lip (*left* in Fig. 21-2), it becomes transformed into mucous membrane. The epithelium of this surface is thicker than the epidermis covering the outer surface of the lip and is of the stratified squamous nonkeratinizing type. However, some granules of keratohyalin may be found in the cells of the more superficial layers. High papillae of connective tissue of the lamina propria (which, in mucous membranes, replaces the dermis of skin) extend into it. Small clusters of mucous glands, the labial glands (*top center* in Fig. 21-2), are embedded in the lamina propria and connect with the surface by means of little ducts.

THE CHEEKS

The mucous membrane lining the cheeks has, like that of the lips, a fairly thick stratified squamous nonkeratinizing epithelium. This is the kind of epithelium characteristically found on wet epithelial surfaces where there is considerable wear and tear and from which no absorption occurs. The superficial cells are rubbed off the surface and replaced from below. This, of course, requires that the cells in the deeper layers of the epithelium divide as rapidly as cells are worn away. Thus, if a finger or spatula is drawn across the inside of the cheek, many of the flat surface cells will be removed. If these are smeared on a slide and stained with methylene blue, their relatively small, central nucleus can be seen readily. As shown in Figure 4-10, Barr bodies can be seen and counted in such stained smears of oral mucosal cells.

The lamina propria of the cheeks consists of fairly dense fibroelastic tissue and extends into the epithelium in the form of high papillae. The deeper part of it merges into what is termed the *submucosa* of the lining of the cheek. This layer contains flat elastic fibers and many blood vessels. Strands of fibroelastic tissue from the lamina propria penetrate through the fatty elastic submucosa to join with the fibroelastic tissue associated with the muscle that underlies the submucosa and forms the chief substance of the wall of the cheek. These strands fasten the mucous membrane to underlying muscle at intervals, with the result that when the jaws are closed the relaxed mucous membrane bulges inward in many small folds instead of in one large fold (which would project inward so far that it would be an inconvenience and might even be bitten inadvertently).

There are small mucous glands, some of which have a few serous secretory demilunes, in the inner part of the cheek.

THE TONGUE

The tongue is composed chiefly of striated muscle, the fibers of which are grouped into bundles that interlace with one another and are disposed in 3 planes. Hence, in a longitudinal section of the tongue cut perpendicular to its dorsal surface (that is, a sagittal section), longitudinal and vertical muscle fibers are cut longitudinally and horizontal fibers are cut in cross section. The mucous membrane covering the undersurface of the tongue is uniformly thin and smooth, whereas that covering the dorsal surface shows a variety of features (Fig. 21-3). Moreover, certain diseases—for example, scarlet fever and pernicious anemia—may cause specific alterations of the dorsal surface which are of importance in diagnosis.

The mucous membrane covering the dorsal surface of the tongue is divided into 2 parts: (*1*) the anterior two thirds, or *oral part* (corresponding to the *body* of the tongue); and (*2*) the posterior one third, or *pharyngeal part* (corresponding to the *root* of the tongue). A V-shaped groove, the *sulcus terminalis,* extending across the dorsal surface, marks the border between these 2 parts. It lies directly anterior to the row of vallate papillae shown in Figure 21-3, *center.*

THE ORAL PART OF THE TONGUE

The mucous membrane covering the oral part of the tongue is covered by little projections of the mucous membrane called *papillae.* There are 3 kinds of these in man—*filiform, fungiform,* and *vallate.*

Filiform papillae (L. *filum,* thread) are relatively high, narrow, conical structures composed both of lamina propria and epithelium (Fig. 21-3, *top left*). Each has a *primary papilla* of lamina propria from which much smaller *secondary papillae* of lamina propria may extend toward the surface. The primary papilla is covered by a cap of epithelium that also forms caps over each secondary papilla. Sometimes the epithelial caps over the secondary papillae are thread-like, justifying the term *filiform,* and their consistency is horny, but there is some

question whether the surface cells become converted into true keratin in man. In some animals the filiform papillae are hard enough to make the dorsal surface of the tongue distinctly rasp-like, and it is said that a friendly lick from such an animal may draw blood.

Filiform papillae are very numerous and distributed in parallel rows across the tongue. Near the root these rows follow the V-shaped sulcus demarcating the body from the root of the tongue (Fig. 21-3, *center*).

Fungiform papillae are so called because they project from the dorsal surface of the oral part of the tongue like little fungi, narrower at their bases and with expanded smooth rounded tops (Fig. 21-3, *top center*). They are not nearly as numerous as filiform papillae, among which they are scattered; they are somewhat more numerous at the tip of the tongue than elsewhere. Each has a central core of lamina propria termed the *primary papilla,* and from this, *secondary papillae* of lamina propria project into the covering epithelium. The epithelial surface does not follow the contours of the secondary papillae of lamina propria as it does in filiform papillae; hence the secondary papillae of lamina propria bring capillaries very close to the surface of the epithelium. Since the covering epithelium is not keratinized, it is relatively translucent; this permits the blood vessels in the high secondary papillae to show through, and as a result the fungiform papillae in life are red.

Vallate Papillae. From 7 to 12 *vallate* (also called *circumvallate*) *papillae* are distributed along the V-shaped sulcus between the body of the tongue and the root (Fig. 21-3). The name (L. *vallum,* a rampart) suggests that each, like an ancient city, is surrounded by a rampart. Actually, each is like a turreted castle surrounded by a moat (Fig. 21-3, *bottom left*). The moat is kept flooded and cleansed of debris by glands disposed deep to the papilla, which empty by means of ducts into the bottom of the moat.

Each vallate papilla has a central *primary papilla* of lamina propria (Fig. 21-3, *bottom left*). *Secondary papillae* of lamine propria extend from this into the stratified nonkeratinizing epithelium that covers the whole papilla. Vallate papillae are narrower at their points of attachment than at their free surfaces; hence their shape is not unlike that of fungiform papillae.

Functions of Papillae. Animals in which filiform papillae are highly developed are capable of licking layers off solid and semisolid material with sandpaper-like efficiency. Even though filiform papillae are not very highly developed in man, they permit children to lick ice cream satisfactorily. Such papillae contain nerve endings specialized for touch. Most fungiform and all vallate papillae contain taste buds in which there are specialized nerve endings which, on being stimulated by contact with food, give rise to the nerve impulses that result in sensations of taste.

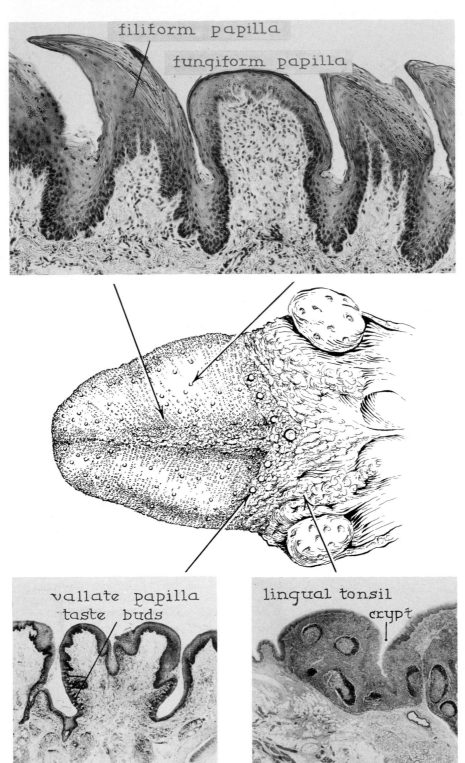

Fig. 21-3. Diagram and photomicrographs illustrating the structure of the dorsal surface of the tongue. The photomicrographs show sections cut from representative regions of its mucous membrane. *See* text for details. The sulcus terminalis is a V-shaped groove that can be discerned immediately anterior to the row of vallate papillae shown in the middle diagram. (*Top* illustration courtesy of C. P. Leblond)

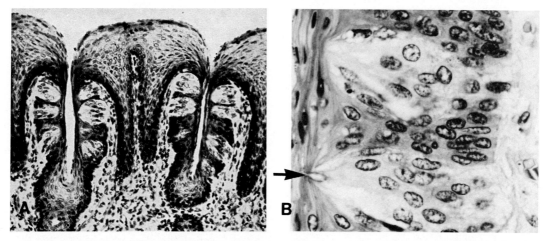

Fig. 21-4. (*A*) Low-power photomicrograph of a portion of the upper surface of the tongue of a rabbit, showing a foliate papilla. This kind of papilla (well developed only in certain animals) provides a good opportunity for seeing taste buds, which are seen as white bud-shaped structures in this illustration. (*B*) High-power photomicrograph of two taste buds in the tongue of a monkey. Pale-staining lamina propria is seen at *right*. The position of a taste pore is indicated by the arrow. (Courtesy of C. P. Leblond)

Taste Buds and Taste Receptors. Gustatory receptors lie protected in little bud- or barrel-shaped structures known as *taste buds*. These are arranged perpendicular to the surface in the epithelial covering of the tongue and the lining of the mouth and throat. Taste buds are most numerous on the dorsal surface of the tongue, particularly along the sides of vallate papillae (Fig. 21-3, *bottom left*). As noted, they are also present in most fungiform papillae. In certain animals they are particularly common in papillae of a type known as foliate (Fig. 21-4A).

From LM studies it was established that taste buds contain supporting (*sustentacular*) cells and *taste receptor* cells. In sections the sustentacular cells look like segments of orange (Fig. 21-4B) in that they follow a slightly curved course through the taste bud. They are arranged around a small cavity that communicates with the surface through a *taste pore,* the position of which is indicated with an arrow in Figure 21-4B. With the EM, long microvilli have been observed on the apical surface of both the so-called receptor cells and the cells supporting them.

The studies of Beidler and Smallman indicate that both types of cells differentiate from a third kind found in a basal position in the taste bud. They demonstrated a turnover of cells in the taste bud, the average life span of each cell being as short as 10 days or so, and also movement of cells from the periphery of the bud, where they are formed, to its middle.

Murray et al. described yet another kind of cell in taste buds of rabbits. This is characterized by its basal cell membrane possessing presynaptic densities and there

being synaptic vesicles associated with this membrane. The nerve terminals with which these cells synapse are not all bulbous and some are relatively narrow. There is thus the possibility that this is the type of cell that represents the true gustatory chemoreceptor.

In order to be tasted, substances must exist in solution and pass through taste pores into taste buds. Here they stimulate the chemoreceptors to generate impulses in the afferent nerve fibers with which they synapse. There are only 4 basic tastes (sweet, sour, salty, and bitter), so the great variety of subtle flavors we can appreciate is due to combinations of these basic tastes. Certain parts of the tongue discern some tastes more readily than others and certain flavors are also smelled at the time they are being tasted. The mechanism of flavor discrimination is not known. Individual taste receptors seem capable of responding to several flavors, so taste discrimination is thought to be based on recognition of patterns of responses from large numbers of receptors.

Taste receptors are as vulnerable to hazards as the epithelium in which they are located, so it is fortunate that new receptors are formed continuously by differentiation of the basal cells of the taste buds (Beidler and Smallman).

Taste impulses from the anterior two thirds of the tongue are carried by the chorda tympani division of the facial nerve, and from the posterior third by the glossopharyngeal nerve. Nonmyelinated afferent fibers of these nerves enter the proximal end of taste buds and synapse with at least one type of taste cell, as described above.

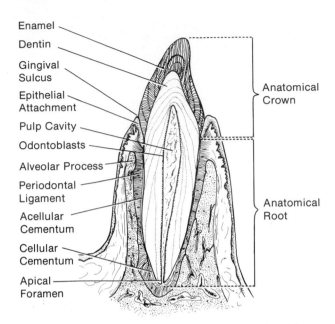

Enamel
Dentin
Gingival
Sulcus
Epithelial
Attachment
Pulp Cavity
Odontoblasts
Alveolar Process
Periodontal
Ligament
Acellular
Cementum
Cellular
Cementum
Apical
Foramen

Anatomical
Crown

Anatomical
Root

Fig. 21-5. Diagram of a lower central incisor tooth and its attachments, in sagittal section.

THE ROOT OF THE TONGUE

Lingual Tonsil. No true papillae are present on the mucous membrane covering the root of the tongue. The small humps seen over this part of the tongue are due to discrete aggregations of lymphatic nodules in the lamina propria beneath the epithelium (Fig. 21-3, *bottom right*). Such an arrangement, namely aggregations of lymphatic nodules in close association with a wet (in this instance, stratified squamous) epithelium, is generally called *tonsillar tissue*. That over the root of the tongue constitutes the *lingual tonsil*. Many of the lymphatic nodules in the lingual tonsil have germinal centers and diffuse lymphatic tissue fills the spaces between them. Along with lymphocytes there are many plasma cells. The stratified squamous nonkeratinizing epithelium overlying the lymphatic tissue extends down into it in many sites to form *crypts* (Gr. *kryptos*, concealed) (Fig. 21-3, *bottom right*). Lymphocytes migrate through the epithelium covering these patches of lymphatic tissue, especially through the walls of the crypts, to gain entrance to their lumina. The superficial cells lining the crypts desquamate, with the result that lymphocytes and desquamated epithelial cells both enter the crypts. However, ducts from underlying mucous glands open into the bottoms of many crypts and this arrangement, where present, serves to keep the lumina of the crypts washed out and free from debris. For this reason, infected crypts are not as common in the

lingual tonsil as in tonsillar tissue where no underlying glands open into the crypts.

THE TEETH

THE GENERAL PARTS OF AN ADULT TOOTH AND ITS ATTACHMENTS

Each curved row of teeth, located in the upper and lower jaws respectively, constitutes a *dental arch*. The upper arch is slightly larger than the lower; hence, the upper teeth normally slightly overlap the lower ones.

The bulk of each tooth consists of a special type of calcified connective tissue called *dentin*. Dentin is covered with a layer of one or another of 2 calcified tissues. The dentin of that portion of the tooth that projects through the gums into the mouth is covered with a cap of very hard, calcified, epithelially derived tissue called *enamel* (Fig. 21-5). The part of the tooth covered with enamel constitutes its *anatomical crown*. The remainder of the tooth, the *anatomical root* (Fig. 21-5), is covered with a special calcified connective tissue called *cementum*.

The junction between the crown and the root of the tooth is termed the *neck* or *cervix*, and the visible line of junction between enamel and cementum is termed the *cervical line*.

Within each tooth is a space that conforms to the general shape of the tooth; this is called the *pulp cavity* (Fig. 21-5). Its more expanded portion in the coronal part of the tooth is called the *pulp chamber*, and the narrowed part that extends through the root is called the *pulp* or *root canal*. The pulp consists of loose connective tissue, which is well supplied with nerve fibers and small blood vessels. The dentin that surrounds the pulp cavity is lined with a layer of special cells called *odontoblasts* (Fig. 21-5) whose function, as their name implies, is related to the production of dentin. Odontoblasts bear the same relation to dentin as osteoblasts do to bone and indeed are like osteoblasts in several respects. The nerve and the blood supply of a tooth enters the pulp through a small hole (or holes) through the apex of the root called the *apical foramen* (Fig. 21-5).

How the Roots of Teeth Are Attached to Bone. The roots of the lower teeth are set into a bony ridge that projects upward from the body of the mandible, and the roots of the upper teeth are set into a bony ridge that projects downward from the body of the maxilla; these bony ridges are termed *alveolar processes*. In these processes there are *sockets (alveoli)*, one for the root of each tooth. The teeth are held firmly in their alveoli by bundles of connective tissue fibers known collectively as *periodontal ligaments* (Fig. 21-5). This ligament consists of dense bundles of collagenic fibers extending in various directions from the bone of the socket wall to the cementum that covers the root. The collagenic fibers are embedded at one end in the calcified intercellular substance of the bone of the socket and at the other in the cementum of the tooth. The embedded regions are sometimes referred to as *Sharpey's fibers* (labeled SF in Fig. 21-15). The fibers not only hold the tooth in place but also are arranged so that when pressure is exerted on its biting surface the tooth is not pushed down into its socket.

The mucous membrane of the mouth forms an external covering for the bone of the alveolar process known as the *gum*. That part of the gum extending beyond the crest of the alveolar process in contact with the tooth is termed the *gingiva*.

The part of the tooth that extends into the mouth beyond the gingiva is called the *clinical crown* (as distinguished from the anatomical crown described above). The clinical crown may or may not be identical with the anatomical crown of a tooth (in Fig. 21-5 it is not). When the tooth erupts, the gingiva is attached to the enamel somewhere along the anatomical crown. As the tooth ages, however, the gingiva recedes; there is a time when the gingiva is attached to the tooth at the cervical line and at this stage the clinical and the anatomical crowns are identical. In older people, the gingiva recedes still farther and becomes attached to cementum, so that the clinical crown is now longer than the anatomical crown.

THE DENTITIONS IN MAN

Two separate sets of teeth, or *dentitions*, develop during life. The first or *primary* dentition serves during childhood. The teeth comprising this dentition are called *deciduous* (L. *decidere*, to fall down), *baby*, or *milk* teeth. These teeth are shed progressively and replaced by permanent teeth that should serve the individual for the rest of his life.

There are 20 teeth in the primary dentition – 10 in the upper and 10 in the lower jaw. The shape of all these teeth is not the same; each is modified for a particular function related to mastication. The first 2 teeth on each side of the midline in the upper and the lower jaws are called *central* and *lateral incisors* respectively (L. *incidere*, to cut into). They appear in a baby at about the age of 6 months. The next tooth lateral to the incisors is the *canine* or *cuspid* tooth, the free-biting surface of which has a single *cusp* (conical projection). Next in line, in the posterior part of a child's mouth, are 2 *molar* teeth on each side. Each molar tooth is modified for grinding food; hence its biting surfaces are wider and flatter than those of the other teeth and have 3 or more cusps projecting from them. They erupt at approximately 2 years. This set of teeth serves the child for the next 4 years or so, at which time the primary teeth begin to be shed and replaced by the permanent ones. This period of replacement of primary teeth extends over approximately 6 years, from about 6 through 12 years of age.

The permanent dentition consists of 32 teeth – 16 upper and 16 lower. Their shape is similar to that of the primary teeth, but they are somewhat larger. The anterior or front teeth, as in the primary set, are the *central* and *lateral incisors* and the *cuspid*. Immediately lateral to the cuspid are the 1st and the 2nd *bicuspids* or *premolars*, which are the teeth that occupy the spaces formerly occupied by the primary molars. Behind the bicuspids in each side of each jaw are 3 *molar* teeth. These are named the 1st, 2nd, and 3rd *molars;* they have no predecessors in the primary dentition but erupt behind the last of the primary teeth, in order. The 1st molar, or "6-year molar," erupts at about the age of 6 years. The 2nd molar erupts at about the age of 12 and is called the 12-year molar. The 3rd molar, or "wisdom tooth," erupts considerably later, if at all. This tooth is subject to much variation in size and shape and all too frequently remains suppressed or impacted within the jaw.

THE DEVELOPMENT AND ERUPTION OF A TOOTH

Two Germ Layers Participate in Forming a Tooth. The enamel of a tooth is derived from *ectoderm*. The dentin, cementum and pulp are all derived from *mesenchyme*.

The formation of a tooth – and to facilitate description we shall here consider a lower primary incisor so that we can speak of things growing up or down – depends *initially* on epithelium growing down into mesenchyme and assuming the form of the bowl of an inverted cup. Mesenchyme grows up into the bowl of this cup. Here inductive phenomena occur. The cells of the epithelium that lines the cup become *ameloblasts* and produce enamel. The mesenchymal cells in the bowl of the cup that are adjacent to the developing ameloblasts differentiate into *odontoblasts* and form successive layers of dentin to support the enamel that covers them. Thus the crown of a tooth develops from *2 different germ layers*.

Early Development

In the 6th week of embryonic life, a section through a developing jaw cuts across a line of thickening of the oral ectoderm. Teeth will develop along and beneath this line. From this line of thickening an epithelial shelf called a *dental lamina* (Fig. 21-6A) grows into the mesenchyme. From the lamina little epithelial buds, termed *tooth buds*, develop and from each of these a deciduous tooth will form (Fig. 21-6A).

As the dental lamina grows, each tooth bud increases in size and penetrates deeper into mesenchyme, where it assumes the form of an inverted cup (Fig. 21-6B). This structure forms what is called the *enamel organ* while, beneath it, the mesenchyme (which fills the bowl) is called the *dental papilla* (Fig. 21-6B).

The enamel organ then increases in size, its shape changes somewhat, and the alveolar process of the jaw grows up to partly enclose it (Fig. 21-6C). The line of contact between the enamel organ and dental papilla now assumes the shape and the size of the future line of contact between the enamel and dentin of the adult tooth. By the 5th month (Fig. 21-6D), the enamel organ loses direct connection with the oral epithelium, although remnants of the dental lamina may persist (sometimes giving rise to cysts in later life).

Just before this, the cells of the dental lamina produce a second bud of epithelial cells from which the permanent tooth will develop (Fig. 21-6C and D).

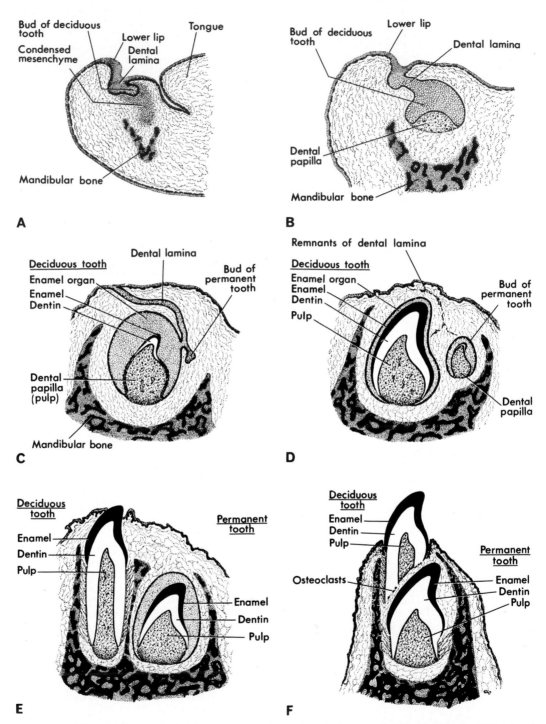

Fig. 21-6. Diagrams illustrating the development and eruption of a lower incisor tooth of the deciduous dentition, and how a tooth of the permanent dentition develops and erupts to replace the deciduous tooth.

Fig. 21-7. High-power photomicrograph of the dentino-
enamel junction of a developing
tooth, shortly after dentin formation has begun. Note the light
predentin between the odontoblasts and the dentin.

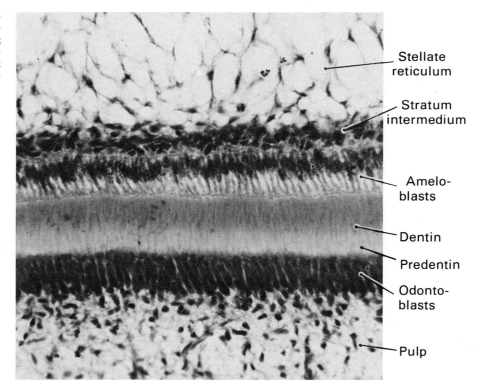

Stellate
reticulum

Stratum
intermedium

Amelo-
blasts

Dentin

Predentin

Odonto-
blasts

Pulp

The dental papilla, which will later become the pulp of the
tooth, consists of a network of mesenchymal cells embedded in
amorphous intercellular substance. This tissue becomes increasingly vascular as development proceeds.

Differentiation Within the Enamel Organ and the
Beginning of Hard Tissue Formation

At the stage depicted in Figure 21-6C, the cells of the enamel
organ adjacent to the tip of the dental papilla become tall and
columnar. These cells are *ameloblasts* (Fig. 21-7) and start
producing tooth enamel. Next to these cells is a layer (1 to 3 cells
thick) called the *stratum intermedium,* whose cells are connected
to ameloblasts and to each other by desmosomes; the rest of the
enamel organ is called the *stellate reticulum* because the cells are
star-shaped with long extensions (Fig. 21-7). The basement
membrane of the enamel organ separates the stellate reticulum
from the mesenchyme.

Ameloblasts first appear next to the tip of the dental papilla
and then down the sides toward the base of the crown. Meanwhile, mesenchymal cells of the dental papilla immediately adjacent to them become tall columnar *odontoblasts* (Figs. 21-7
and 21-8) that start forming dentin before the ameloblasts form
enamel. Dentin is first produced at the tip of the papilla, as
shown in white in Figure 21-6C. After a thin layer of dentin is deposited, the ameloblasts start producing enamel matrix, shown in
black in Figure 21-6C. The formation of dentin and enamel differs from bone formation in that the formative cells are not
trapped within the matrix they produce. Instead, as the cells
produce the hard tissue matrix they retreat away from it, the
ameloblasts outward and the odontoblasts inward.

The Formation of the Root and Its Role in Eruption

As dentin and enamel are deposited, the shape of the future
crown appears (Fig. 21-6D). Enamel forms down to what will be
the future line of junction of the anatomical crown and the root

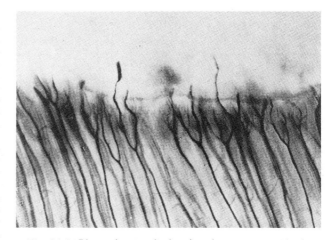

Fig. 21-8. Photomicrograph showing the processes of odontoblasts lying in canals known as dentinal tubules in the dentin.
(Churchill, H. R.: Meyer's Histology and Histogenesis of the
Human Teeth and Associated Parts. Philadelphia, J. B. Lippincott, 1935)

(Fig. 21-6D); meanwhile cells of the dental papilla differentiate into odontoblasts. Immature ameloblasts at the line of junction proliferate and migrate down into the underlying mesenchyme in the form of a tube (Hertwig's epithelial root sheath). As this sheath grows, it induces mesenchymal cells on the inside to differentiate into odontoblasts and sets the pattern for the shape of the root. However, there is little space for the root to develop; hence, space has to be created by the crown being pushed out through the oral mucous membrane (Fig. 21-6E). The formation of the root is, therefore, important in causing the tooth to erupt.

As the root sheath grows downward its older part (toward the crown), once it has served its purpose, detaches from the dentin making up the root and becomes disorganized. This allows mesenchymal cells to deposit *cementum* on the outer surface of the dentin and elaborate the fibers of the periodontal ligament. As cementum is laid down, it traps the ends of these fibers.

These processes continue downward until the root of the tooth is completed. Thus, the fibers of the periodontal ligament are firmly anchored in calcified cementum, which itself is firmly bound to the dentin of the root. The epithelial cells of the disorganized root sheath remain scattered within the periodontal ligament. They are called the *epithelial rests of Malassez,* and may later give rise to dental cysts.

The Permanent Tooth

By the time the deciduous tooth erupts into the dental arch, the tooth bud of the corresponding permanent tooth has been building up enamel and dentin in exactly the same manner as the deciduous tooth (Fig. 21-6E). When the crown is complete and the root partly formed, the permanent tooth prepares to erupt. However, in accordance with one of Wolff's laws, which states that pressure causes resorption of hard tissues, growth of the permanent tooth and the pressure of its enamel against the root of the deciduous tooth causes the softer of the two tissues, the dentin of the deciduous tooth, to be resorbed by osteoclasts (Fig. 21-6F). By the time the permanent tooth is ready to erupt into the dental arch, the root of the deciduous tooth above has been completely resorbed. The deciduous tooth is then shed and replaced by its permanent successor.

THE MICROSCOPIC STRUCTURE AND FUNCTIONS OF THE PARTS OF THE TOOTH

DENTIN

Odontoblasts begin to form dentin matrix soon after they assume their typical form. Initially they are separated from ameloblasts by an extension of the basement membrane of the enamel organ. However, this extension disappears as the odontoblasts mature and secrete the small collagen fibrils that constitute the bulk of dentin matrix. In addition, long and thick collagen fibrils, known as *Korff's fibers,* extend between odontoblasts in the direction of what was the basement membrane, but fan out before they reach its location.

It will be recalled that bone becomes larger by addition of new layers to one or more of its surfaces (Fig. 15-8). This is also true of dentin, except that growth is more limited because odontoblasts are present only along the inner (pulpal) side of dentin. Hence, new layers of dentin can be added only on its pulpal surface and these layers necessarily encroach on the pulp.

Furthermore, osteoblasts possess cytoplasmic processes around which the organic intercellular component of bone matrix is laid down. These are found within canaliculi (Fig. 15-5). Similarly, each odontoblast is also provided with a cytoplasmic process (Figs. 21-8, 21-9, and 21-10) extending outward from the apex of the cell to the dentino-enamel junction. When dentin matrix is deposited around these cytoplasmic processes, they also become enclosed in tiny canals called *dentinal tubules* and the processes within them are called *odontoblastic processes* (labeled in Fig. 21-10). With the addition of more dentin, odontoblasts are displaced progressively farther away from the dentino-enamel junction, with the odontoblastic processes becoming increasingly elongated along with the dentinal tubules containing them.

Two separate steps occur as bone tissue is developing: (*1*) synthesis of the organic component of bone matrix, and (*2*) its calcification. Similarly, dentin matrix is first formed and then calcifies, usually about 1 day later. Uncalcified dentin matrix is called *predentin* and a layer of it is located between the apex of odontoblasts and recently calcified dentin (Figs. 21-9 and 21-10).

It is well known that teeth are extremely sensitive to stimuli arising on a dentin surface. The sensitivity of dentin is attributed to the cytoplasmic processes of odontoblasts in the dentinal tubules, which would pass impulses to nerve fibers located at the pulp border. The sensitivity of dentin generally decreases with age, as a result of calcification within dentinal tubules.

The Fine Structure of Odontoblasts

In contradistinction to ameloblasts, which are tightly apposed to one another, odontoblasts may be separated from each other by intercellular clefts that may contain Korff's collagenic fibers and capillaries (Fig. 21-9). They are, however, held together by junctional complexes, visible in Figure 21-10 at each end of the terminal web. When viewed in the EM (Fig. 21-10), odontoblasts consist of a long cell body (at the periphery of the pulp) and a long odontoblastic process located within dentin. The cell body contains abundant rER and a prominent Golgi near the center of the cell. The odontoblastic process lies above the terminal web and contains no rER; however, it does contain secretory granules, a few vesicles, microtubules, and filaments.

Predentin and Dentin Matrix

The intercellular space surrounding the base of the odontoblastic processes contains predentin matrix. This is at first an amorphous ground substance with few or no

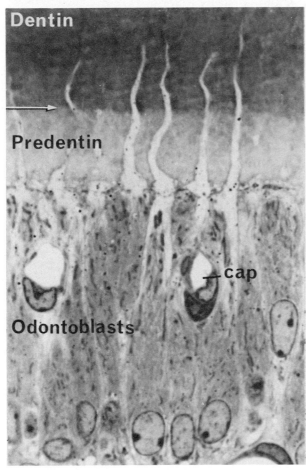

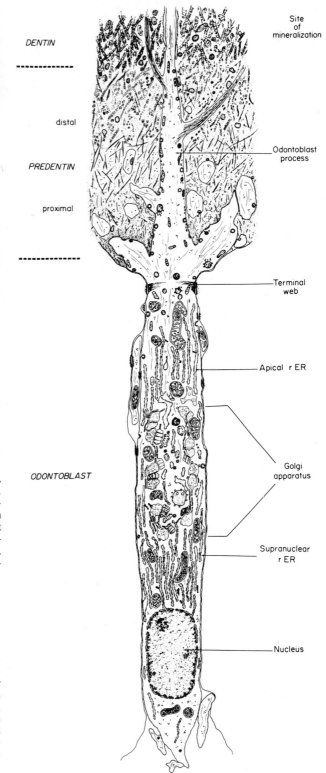

DENTIN

- - - - - - - - -

distal

PREDENTIN

proximal

- - - - - - - - -

ODONTOBLAST

Site of mineralization

Odontoblast process

Terminal web

Apical r ER

Golgi apparatus

Supranuclear r ER

Nucleus

Fig. 21-9. Photomicrograph (×1,000) showing odontoblasts, predentin, and dentin from the growing end of a rat incisor tooth. The cells are tall and polarized and arranged parallel to one another, each with a basal nucleus. Extending into the predentin from the apical pole of each cell is a light-staining odontoblast process. Predentin extends from between the bases of the processes to a sharply defined predentin-dentin junction (arrow). The dentin located beyond stains darker than predentin. (Courtesy of M. Weinstock)

Fig. 21-10. Diagram of an odontoblast, showing the arrangement of its organelles and the adjacent predentin and dentin matrix. An elaborate Golgi apparatus lies between the supranuclear and apical rER-rich regions; rER cisternae and Golgi saccules are absent from the odontoblastic process, which extends from the apical pole into the predentin and dentin. Branches of the process also project into the matrix. Within the process and its branches are secretory granules originating in the Golgi apparatus. The secretory product is released into predentin by exocytosis.

The collagenic fibrils of dentin possess finely granular material on their surface. Dentin matrix also contains crystals of apatite. (Weinstock, M., and Leblond, C. P.: J. Cell Biol., *60*:92, 1974)

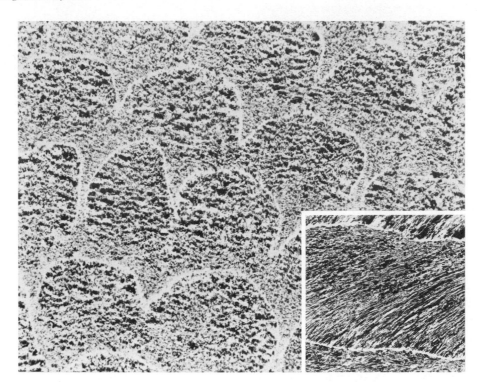

Fig. 21-11. Electron micrographs illustrating the orientation of the crystals of apatite in an un-decalcified section of dental enamel, showing the way this orientation accounts for what is called its rod (or prism) structure. In the large micrograph the enamel is cut in cross section; in the *inset* it is cut in longitudinal section. Apatite crystals contain calcium phosphate and so are electron-dense (and appear black). The upper, rounded part of each fan-shaped area seen, for example, at *upper left*, corresponds to the so-called rod component of enamel substance; here the crystals have a predominantly longitudinal arrangement (*see inset*). Along its lower (cervical) side, a rod extends into a relatively deep V-shaped ridge of what is termed the inter-rod component of enamel substance; this is the handle of each fan-shaped area. In the inter-rod component, the crystals lie progressively more obliquely the farther they are situated from the rod substance (*see inset*). The white line delimiting the fan-shaped areas is referred to as the rod sheath; it has a higher organic content than the rod and inter-rod matrix. (*Inset*) One rod cut in longitudinal section through its middle. Note the inter-rod matrix extending along its lower border but not delimited from the substance of the rod. It should be understood that because the inter-rod substance is continuous with rod substance, it can be recognized only by the gradual change in orientation of its apatite crystals, which lie progressively more obliquely the farther they are away from the rod substance. Rod sheath (white) is seen near upper and lower margins. (Courtesy of A. R. Ten Cate)

collagenic fibrils. Above and adjacent to this, the matrix contains progressively denser arrangements of fibrils, well packed at the predentin-dentin junction (Fig. 21-10). As noted, predentin matrix is not calcified, but dentin matrix is; the line of demarcation represents the calcification front. Once dentin is calcified its fine structure becomes obscured by apatite crystals, but decalcified sections show granular material on the collagenic fibrils (Fig. 21-10, *top*).

The process of procollagen synthesis and secretion in odontoblasts was described in detail in Chapter 9 (p. 231) and illustrated in Figure 9-7. Collagen accounts for al-most 90 per cent of dentin matrix; about 10 per cent is phosphoprotein and there are also small amounts of glycoprotein and glycosaminoglycan present. Phospho-protein is synthesized by odontoblasts and released to predentin, but it diffuses to the dentinal side of the junction with predentin, where it forms the granular material seen on the surface of the collagenic fibrils (Weinstock and Leblond).

This junction is the site of calcification of dentin. Immediately after injection of isotope-labeled phosphate or calcium salts, label is found in this region, with no radioautographic reaction on the predentinal side of the junction and a strong one on the dentinal side. Precipitation of calcium phosphate seems to occur just beyond the predentin-dentin junction (Munhoz and Leblond).

Although there may be some minor differences, the factors concerned in the calcification of bone described on pages 399 to 401 would seem to apply also to the calcification of dentin.

DENTAL ENAMEL

After the odontoblasts have produced the first thin layer of dentin, ameloblasts (Fig. 21-7) begin to make enamel. Enamel soon covers the dentin over the anatomical crown of the tooth (Fig. 21-6C). It forms first as a poorly calcified matrix that later calcifies almost completely. The material of the mineralized matrix is described as being in the form of rods. To some extent these enamel rods retain the shape of the ameloblasts that made them (Fig. 21-11). The elongated ends of ameloblasts where rods are formed are termed *Tomes' processes* (Fig. 21-12).

The Fine Structure of Ameloblasts

Individual ameloblasts are tall, columnar cells (Fig. 21-12). Their mitochondria lie close to the base of the cell. Narrow cisternae of rER extend above the nucleus to just below the terminal web (Fig. 21-12). An elongated Golgi lies along the axis of the cell above the nucleus (Figs. 21-13 and 21-14). Its cross section is circular (Fig. 21-13A) because it is roughly tubular in shape; it is surrounded by a peripheral network of cisternae of rER (Fig. 21-14). Secretory granules originate from Golgi saccules (Fig. 21-14) and mainly gather in the Tomes' process (Fig. 21-12). A few granules are also seen in small extensions of cytoplasm, from nearby ameloblasts, that lie at the base of the Tomes' process (Fig. 21-12). Extending through the middle of the Golgi, along its long axis, is a thick bundle of densely packed filaments called an *axial fibril* (Fig. 21-13A, labeled F). On reaching the nucleus, this bundle divides into several branches that continue downward along the sides of the nucleus (Fig. 21-13B, labeled f) to join a basal cell web (Kallenbach *et al.*).

Fig. 21-12. Diagram of the fine structure of an ameloblast. The nucleus is close to the base. Mitochondria are located beneath, and rER above, the nucleus. The supranuclear region also contains a Golgi apparatus comprising flattened saccules arranged so as to form the wall of a tubule. Small numbers of secretory granules lie inside the tubular Golgi region. The apical projection, called a Tomes' process, extends into the newly formed enamel matrix and contains large numbers of secretory granules. On either side of the Tomes' process are cytoplasmic extensions contaning a few secretory granules. The cell contains a basal web beneath the mitochondria as well as an apical terminal web beneath the Tomes' process. (Courtesy of H. Warshawsky)

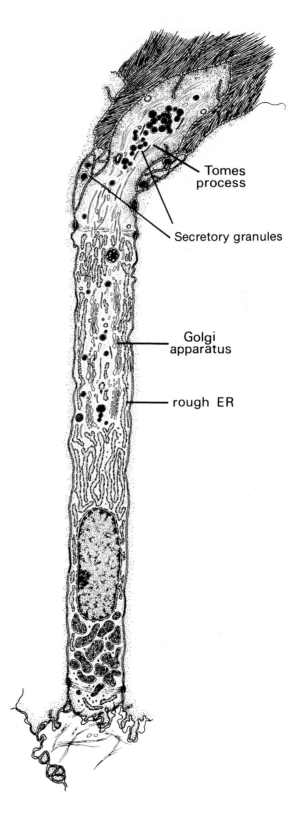

Tomes process

Secretory granules

Golgi apparatus

rough ER

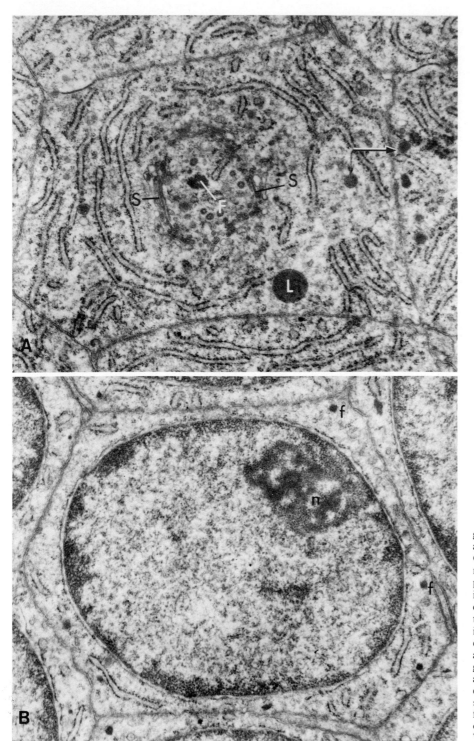

Fig. 21-13. (*A*) Electron micrograph of a cross section of an ameloblast at the level of the Golgi region. Its cell walls and rER are distinct. The Golgi appears nearly circular because of its tubular arrangement of saccules (S). An axial fibril (F) lies in the middle of the Golgi region. L is a dense body (lysosome). Secretory granules are indicated by an arrow. (*B*) Electron micrograph of a cross section of an ameloblast at the level of its nucleus and nucleolus (n). Little is seen in the cytoplasm except for a few cisternae of rER and longitudinal fibrils (f). (Courtesy of H. Warshawsky)

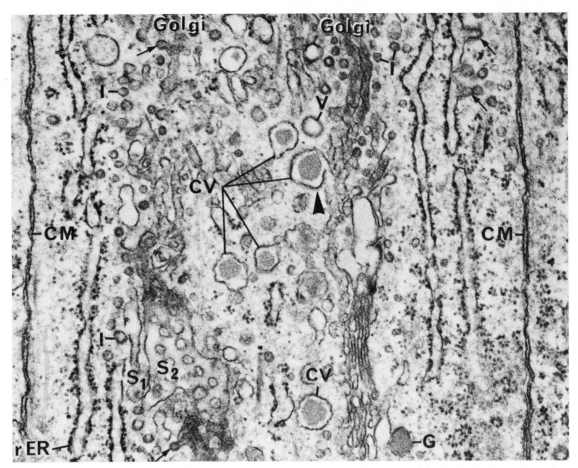

Fig. 21-14. Electron micrograph of the Golgi region of an ameloblast as seen in longitudinal section. The membrane of the cell (CM) may be seen extending down the left and right margins. Parallel to them are rows of rER cisternae studded with ribosomes. At *upper right*, coated vesicles (*oblique arrows*) are budding from a cisterna of rER. These will become transfer vesicles (I).

More centrally, two incomplete rows of Golgi saccules lie parallel to the lateral cell membranes; they are sections of the roughly tubular Golgi apparatus.

In the *middle*, prosecretory granules (condensing vacuoles) may be seen (CV). Bristle-coated patches (arrowhead) are giving rise to bristle-coated vesicles (V); as a result the content of prosecretory granules condenses. They become secretory granules that migrate in the direction of the Tomes' process. One of these granules may be seen at *lower right* (G). (Courtesy of A. Weinstock and C. P. Leblond)

Enamel Matrix

This consists of an organic matrix containing protein and carbohydrate, with calcium phosphate in the form of *apatite:* $Ca_{10}(PO_4)_6(OH)_2$. Each cell produces one enamel rod, the structural unit of enamel (Fig. 21-11). In decalcified sections examined in the EM, the matrix of the rod is seen to be composed of tiny tubular subunits with an oval diameter of about 25 nm. These are closely packed and run parallel to the axis of the rods. The tubules probably have a glycoprotein component since glycoprotein appears to be the secretory product that is

packaged into secretory granules (G at *bottom right* in Fig. 21-14) in the Golgi apparatus of ameloblasts. The content of these granules is released into the intercellular space by exocytosis and becomes part of the enamel matrix. However, whereas each Tomes' process forms the matrix of a rod, the cytoplasmic extensions at its base give rise to inter-rod matrix.

Calcification begins in relation to the tubules constituting the rods of enamel matrix. Enamel crystals initially appear as very thin ribbons of apatite (Warshawsky). There seems to be one crystal per tubule. As the rods lengthen, each crystal also lengthens indefinitely. The far-

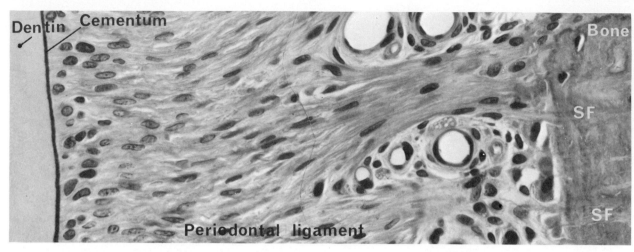

Fig. 21-15. High-power photomicrograph of a portion of a decalcified tooth and its associated alveolar bone (rat), showing the collagenic fibers of the periodontal ligament. From *left* to *right,* note the periphery of dentin, cementum (acellular), periodontal ligament, and the edge of alveolar bone. The fibers of the ligament abut on the cementum at *left* and extend between blood vessels to reach the alveolar bone into which they are inserted. The fibers seen within bone are known as Sharpey's fibers (SF at *lower right*). (Courtesy of H. Warshawsky)

ther from a Tomes' process the crystal is, the more intensely calcified it becomes. Hence, the mineral content of the crystal, and also of the whole matrix, increases as the dentino-enamel junction is approached. Along with the increase in mineral content, there is loss of water and decrease in organic content. When the mineral content reaches 95 per cent or so, calcification stops and the enamel is said to be mature.

Besides secreting a rod from its Tomes' process, each ameloblast, as noted, has apical extensions at the base of the Tomes' process (Fig. 21-12) that secrete inter-rod matrix of dental enamel. Although identical in composition, rod and inter-rod matrix characteristically differ in the arrangement of their tubular subunits and apatite crystals. The unique disposition of apatite crystals in these 2 components is illustrated in Figure 21-11, the legend of which should be consulted for details.

Fully formed enamel is relatively inert; no cells are associated with it because ameloblasts degenerate after they have formed enamel and the tooth erupts. Thus enamel is incapable of repair if it is damaged by decay, fracture, or other means. However, there is some exchange of mineral ions between enamel and saliva and this can effect minimal recalcification at the surface, but the effect is negligible deeper in the enamel.

Relation to Dental Caries (Tooth Decay). Tooth minerals are readily dissolved by acids, so that the acids in food and certain drinks in particular may produce tiny pits and crevices on the surface of enamel. Food debris commonly becomes trapped in such areas and acts as a substrate for acid-producing bacteria. Furthermore, sugar in sweet foods, candy, and beverages also acts as a substrate for these bacteria. Progressive loss of enamel (which is not replaced with new enamel) due to decalcification by the acids produced leads to the formation of *cavities.* Unless such cavities are filled, sooner or later they reach the dentin and extend into the dentinal tubules to reach the pulp of the tooth. When they near the pulp, they are prone to cause inflammation in it and, as will be explained below, this can cause its death.

A developing cavity causes no pain when confined to the enamel. When it reaches the dentin, it may or may not cause increased sensitivity of the tooth; increased sensitivity may be related to certain stimuli, for example, sweet materials. The presence of cavities should be determined by regular dental inspection. To treat them, all of the affected enamel and dentin must be drilled away and the cavity shaped so that it will retain a filling. Fillings must be used because there are no cells on the outer aspects of the tooth to make new enamel or surface dentin.

CEMENTUM

Some cells of the mesenchyme outside the developing root differentiate to become *cementoblasts.* These are similar to osteoblasts, but lay down another calcified connective tissue that is nonvascular and called *cementum.* The role of cementum is to anchor the fibers of the periodontal ligament and so attach them to the tooth (Fig. 21-15, *left*).

Cementum on the upper part of the root is acellular (Figs. 21-5 and 21-15); on the lower part there are cells within its matrix. The latter are called *cementocytes* and they, like osteocytes, reside in small spaces (*lacunae*) within the calcified matrix and communicate with their source of nutrition through canaliculi. Cementum, like bone, can only grow by the appositional mechanism.

PERIODONTAL LIGAMENT

As the root forms and cementum is deposited on its surface, the periodontal ligament arises from the surrounding mesenchyme. It consists of wide bundles of collagenic fibers arranged in the form of a suspensory ligament between the cementum covering the root of the tooth and the bony wall of its socket (Fig. 21-15). At both ends the fibers are embedded in hard tissue, suggesting that the matrix of alveolar bone on the one hand and that of cementum on the other are laid down around preexisting collagenic fibers. Nevertheless, the turnover rate of collagen in the periodontal ligament is exceptionally high, so that a good deal of remodeling of at least the nonembedded region of the ligament occurs throughout life. The collagen fibers in the ligament pursue a slightly wavy course (Figs. 21-5 and 21-15) and this arrangement permits very slight movement of the tooth within its socket.

The periodontal ligament is richly supplied with nerve endings sensitive to pressure so that inappropriate hard particles in soft foods, for example, can be readily detected.

EPITHELIAL ATTACHMENT

The gingiva surrounds each tooth like a collar and if the gums are healthy the inner surface of this collar is attached tightly to the tooth. In longitudinal section the gingiva extends a little way up the periphery of the tooth in the form of a narrow triangle (Fig. 21-5). Its epithelium on the side adjacent to the tooth becomes separated from the tooth at the apex of the triangle to form a narrow *gingival sulcus* encircling the tooth (Fig. 21-5). The epithelium at the bottom of this sulcus adheres to the tooth by virtue of its basal lamina and its hemidesmosomes over a collar-shaped zone; this is labeled *epithelial attachment* in Figure 21-5. Moreover, in recently erupted teeth the epithelium extending from the bottom of the sulcus to the base of the anatomical crown is attached not only to enamel but also extends down as far as the cementum.

Relation to Periodontal Disease. From the ions normally present in the saliva a calcified material termed *calculus* (L. for pebble) may form and accumulate in the gingival sulcus, and this tends to separate the epithelial attachment from the tooth. Once the epithelial seal around the tooth is broken, bacteria can gain entrance to the connective tissue of the gingiva, so the gingival sulcus is a danger zone. Eventually *pockets* may develop down the sides of a tooth and these can become infected, as a result of which the tooth is loosened. This process, known as *periodontal disease,* causes more loss of teeth than any other condition. Nutritional factors—for example, vitamin C deficiency—and metabolic factors can also be involved in periodontal disease.

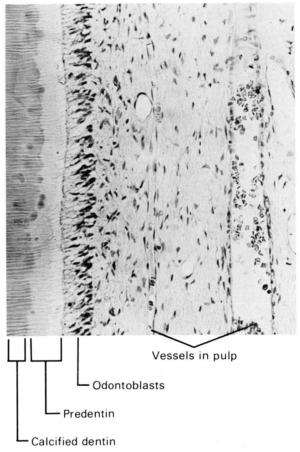

Vessels in pulp

Odontoblasts

Predentin

Calcified dentin

Fig. 21-16. High-power photomicrograph of a child's tooth showing its pulp. Dentin is still forming at this stage. (Courtesy of K. Paynter)

DENTAL PULP

Dental pulp is connective tissue derived from the mesenchyme of the dental papilla (Fig. 21-6C); it occupies the pulp chamber and root canals of teeth (Fig. 21-5). It is a soft tissue that retains its mesenchymal appearance throughout life (Fig. 21-16). The bulk of its cells appear stellate, being connected to one another by long cytoplasmic processes. Pulp is very vascular; the main vessels enter and leave it through the apical foramina. However, the pulpal vessels, even the large ones, have very thin walls (Fig. 21-16). This, of course, renders this tissue very susceptible to changes in pressure because the walls of the pulp chamber cannot expand. Even fairly mild inflammatory edema can lead to compression of the blood vessels and hence to necrosis and death of the pulp. Following pulp death, sometimes the pulp can be removed surgically and the space it occupied filled with

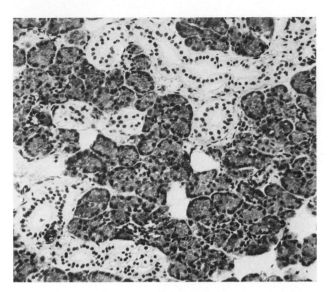

Fig. 21-17. Medium-power photomicrograph of parotid gland. The cytoplasm of the cells of the many intralobular ducts is light, and that of the cells of the serous secretory units, dark. A few fat cells are present near *center* and at *lower right*.

inert sealing material. Such a tooth is what is commonly called a "dead" tooth.

The pulp is richly supplied with nerves, and nerve endings have been observed in close association with the odontoblast layer between the pulp and the dentin. There are some reports of nerve fibers entering dentinal tubules, but there is no indication that they proceed more than a short distance within the tubules.

Any new dentin added to the walls of the tooth must be deposited on the surface abutting on the pulp, because this is the only place where odontoblasts exist. Dentin is produced throughout life and compensates for attrition of biting surfaces. Under certain conditions it may form rapidly (for example, under a cavity), but then appears more irregular and is designated *secondary dentin*. Dentin deposition gradually reduces the size of the pulp chamber and canals; hence, in older people the pulp is much reduced in size. The character of the pulp also changes in that it becomes more fibrous and less cellular.

THE SALIVARY GLANDS

There are a great many glands that deliver their secretion into the oral cavity, so they are all salivary glands. However, most are small, and so the term *salivary glands* is commonly used to indicate the 3 largest paired glands: (*1*) the parotid, (*2*) the submandibular (also called submaxillary), and (*3*) the sublingual glands.

Saliva and Its Functions

The mixed secretion of all the salivary glands is called *saliva*. It contains salts, gases, and organic components and usually also some cellular and bacterial debris and leukocytes. Two enzymes (*ptyalin* or *salivary amylase*, and *maltase*) and mucus are present in saliva.

Saliva has several functions. (*1*) It lubricates and moistens the buccal mucosa and lips, thus aiding articulation. The moistening must be carried on continuously because of evaporation and the swallowing of saliva. (*2*) It washes the mouth clear of cellular and food debris. (*3*) It moistens food and transforms it to a semisolid mass that may be swallowed easily (animals such as the cow, which live on a fairly dry diet, may secrete up to 60 liters of saliva daily). Moreover, moistening food allows it to be tasted. Taste buds are stimulated chemically, and substances that stimulate them must be in solution. (*4*) It buffers acidity in the oral cavity. (*5*) The role of salivary enzymes in the digestion of food is questionable. Amylase breaks down starch to maltose, but food is not retained in the mouth long enough for significant digestion to occur there.

The Parotid Glands

These are the largest of the 3 pairs of salivary glands proper. Each gland lies packed in the space between the mastoid process and the ramus of the mandible and extends below the zygomatic arch. From this part of the gland, its duct (Stensen's duct), running parallel with and immediately below the arch, plunges through the buccinator muscle to open into the vestibule of the mouth opposite the second upper molar tooth.

The gland is enclosed in a well-defined fibrous connective tissue capsule and is a compound tubulo-alveolar gland of the *serous* type. The microscopic details of the secretory units of such glands were described on page 203, and the mechanism of secretion in cells that secrete zymogen granules, on page 125. In addition to the usual features to be seen in a gland of this type, it is specially characterized by *many and prominent intralobular ducts* (Fig. 21-17). Accumulations of fat cells in the connective tissue septa are also characteristic of this gland.

The Submandibular (Submaxillary) Glands

These lie in contact with the inner surface of the body of the mandible, and their main ducts (Wharton's) open onto the floor of the oral cavity beside each other, anterior to the tongue and behind the lower incisor tooth. They also are compound alveolar or tubulo-alveolar glands. Although of the mixed type, the majority of their secretory units are of the *serous* variety. Mucous units are usually capped by serous demilunes (Fig. 7-24). Like the parotid glands, the submandibular glands have well-defined capsules and fairly prominent duct systems.

The Sublingual Glands

Unlike the other salivary glands, the sublingual glands are not so definitely encapsulated. They lie well forward, near the midline, below the mucous membrane of the floor of the mouth, and their secretions empty by several ducts (of Rivinus) that open along a line behind the openings of Wharton's ducts. They are compound tubulo-alveolar glands of the mixed type, but differ from the submandibular gland in that the majority of their alveoli are of the *mucous* type. Their microscopic appearance is different in different parts of the gland. In some areas only mucus-secreting units and mucous units with serous demilunes may be found. The connective tissue septa are usually more prominent than they are in the parotid or the submandibular glands.

The Control of Salivary Secretion

Ordinarily, salivary secretion is controlled by reflexes. Briefly, the efferent (secretory) fibers to the salivary glands are derived from the cranial outflow of the parasympathetic system and the thoracic outflow of the sympathetic system. There are many afferent pathways that may be concerned in salivary reflexes. The stimulus that evokes secretion reflexly may be mechanical or chemical. For example, the presence of food (or even pebbles or dry powders in the mouth) stimulates ordinary sensory nerve endings and causes salivary secretion. The taste buds, as noted, are receptive to chemical stimulation. Stimulation of sensory nerves other than those of the oral cavity may initiate a salivary reflex if that reflex has been conditioned (*see* p. 487). The amount (1 to 1.5 liters per day in man) and composition of saliva depend on the nature of the stimulus that initiates the reflex, and on whether sympathetic or parasympathetic fibers are predominantly involved in the efferent path. Stimulation of sympathetic fibers causes a thick, viscous secretion to be formed, whereas parasympathetic stimulation causes copious watery secretion. Nerve endings in the parotid are shown in Figures 17-55 and 17-56.

It was mentioned in Chapter 7 that acini of salivary glands include a cell flattened between the acinar cells and their basement membrane (Fig. 7-25), the cytoplasm of which contains well-developed contractile filaments; this cell is accordingly called a *myoepithelial cell.* Myoepithelial cells are particularly well developed in serous acini. Both acinar cells and myoepithelial cells are under autonomic control.

There is evidence in mice that sex hormones, ap-

parently in conjunction with thyroid hormone, are important in maintaining function in the secretory and duct cells of salivary glands.

THE PALATE AND PHARYNX

THE HARD PALATE

The mouth needs a strong roof so that the anterior part of the tongue, the part of the tongue that moves most freely, can bring force to bear against it in the process of mixing and swallowing food. Furthermore, the mucous membrane lining the roof of the mouth in this site has to be firmly fixed to the strong roof so that forceful movements of the tongue do not dislodge it, and its epithelium must be capable of withstanding wear and tear. These requirements are met by there being a bony roof over the mouth lined on its undersurface by a mucous membrane, the lamina propria of which is continuous with the periosteum of the bone above, and the epithelium of which is of the stratified squamous keratinizing variety. This constitutes the hard palate (Fig. 21-1).

Laterally, the mucous membrane is not so evenly adherent to the bony roof and is connected to it by strong bundles of connective tissue. Fat cells are disposed between these anteriorly, and glands, posteriorly.

In the median line is a ridge of bone to which the epithelium is attached by a very thin lamina propria. This ridge is called the *raphe.* Rugae with connective tissue cores radiate out from this laterally. They are more prominent in early than in later life.

THE SOFT PALATE

The soft palate continues posteriorly from the hard palate (Fig. 21-1). Its functions are different from those of the hard palate. It does not have to bear the thrust of the tongue and it must be movable so that in the act of swallowing it can be drawn upward and thus close off the nasopharynx to prevent food from being forced up into the nose. This requires that it contain muscle. It must also be reasonably strong, and this requires that it contain connective tissue which is disposed in it as an aponeurosis.

The soft palate projects backward into the pharynx from the hard palate (Fig. 21-1). Hence, the mucous membrane on its upper surface forms part of the lining of the nasopharynx, and the mucous membrane on its lower surface forms part of the lining of the oral pharynx. From its upper surface downward it exhibits the following layers (Fig. 21-18): (*1*) stratified squamous or pseudostratified ciliated columnar epithelium: (*2*) a lamina propria which contains a few glands and, near the hard

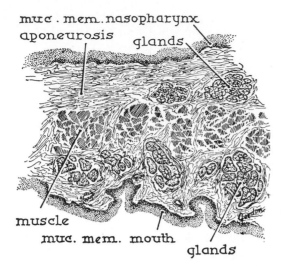

muc. mem. nasopharynx
aponeurosis   glands

muscle
muc. mem. mouth
          glands

Fig. 21-18. Drawing of a very low power section of the soft palate. (After Addison, W. H. F. (ed.): Piersol's Normal Histology. ed. 15. Philadelphia, J. B. Lippincott, 1932)

palate, has the form of a strong aponeurosis; (*3*) a muscular layer (posteriorly); (*4*) a thick lamina propria containing many glands; and (*5*) stratified squamous nonkeratinizing epithelium.

THE PHARYNX

The pharynx is a somewhat conically shaped chamber that serves as a passageway for both the respiratory and the digestive systems. Under conditions of nose breathing it conducts air between the nasal cavities and the larynx, and also to the eustachian (pharyngotympanic) tubes (Fig. 23-1). It also conducts food from the mouth to the esophagus, with which its apex is continuous (Fig. 21-1). But, since the pharynx is common to both systems, it permits an individual whose nasal passages are obstructed to breathe through his mouth or, when his mouth is immobilized for surgical reasons, to be fed with a tube through his nose.

The pharynx is divided into 3 parts. The *nasopharynx,* which lies above the level of the soft palate, is lined by a

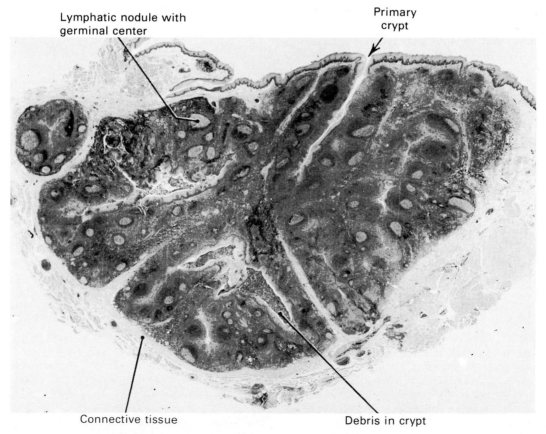

Lymphatic nodule with germinal center

Primary crypt

Connective tissue

Debris in crypt

Fig. 21-19. Very low power photomicrograph of a section of palatine tonsil.

pseudostratified columnar ciliated epithelium, as are the nasal cavities (Fig. 21-1). The posterior limit of the mouth is indicated by the glossopalatine arches, and the part of the pharynx behind these is the *oral pharynx* (Fig. 21-1). The *laryngeal pharynx* is the part that continues from the oral pharynx, from below the level of the hyoid bone, into the esophagus (Fig. 21-1). Both the oral and the laryngeal pharynx are lined with stratified squamous nonkeratinizing epithelium, as is the oral cavity.

The epithelial lining rests on a fairly dense connective tissue layer that contains many elastic as well as collagenic fibers. At the side of this layer farthest from the epithelium there is usually a stout layer of elastic fibers. Outside this again is striated muscle—the longitudinal and constrictor muscles of the pharynx.

Glands are present deep to the epithelium of some parts of the pharynx, particularly near the openings of the eustachian tubes. In some instances, the glands extend into the muscle coat. A slight rise along the midline of the nasopharynx indicates the location of the single *pharyngeal tonsil* (sometimes called the *adenoid,* especially when hypertrophied). This comprises a group of lymphatic nodules, separated by loose lymphatic tissue, lying under the pseudostratified columnar epithelial lining of the nasopharynx.

THE PALATINE TONSILS

So far mention has been made of the two *lingual* tonsils, located within the root of the tongue, and of the single *pharyngeal* tonsil in the nasopharynx. Far more prominent are the two *palatine* tonsils. These ovoid masses of lymphatic tissue thicken the lamina propria of the mucous membrane that extends between the glossopalatine and the pharyngopalatine arches. The epithelium here is of the stratified squamous nonkeratinizing type and dips into the underlying lymphatic tissue to form 10 to 20 little pits (*primary crypts*) in each palatine tonsil (Fig. 21-19). The stratified squamous epithelium lining the primary crypts may extend out into the adjacent lymphatic tissue to form secondary crypts. Either primary or secondary crypts may extend deeply enough to reach the outer limits of the tonsil.

The lymphatic tissue in the tonsil mostly lies directly below the epithelium and extends down along the sides of the crypts. It consists of lymphatic nodules, with or without germinal centers, that may be so close together that they fuse, or they may be separated by looser lymphatic tissue. In addition to small lymphocytes there are generally many plasma cells in this tissue.

Tonsillar tissue is strategically located near the entrances of the digestive tube and respiratory tree to serve as a sentinel on guard for infective agents against which antibodies are to be made as soon as possible. However,

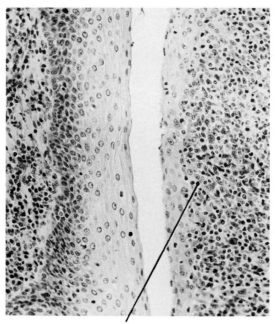

Lymphocytes invading
epithelium of crypt

Fig. 21-20. High-power photomicrograph of palatine tonsil, showing lymphocytes migrating through the epithelial lining of a crypt.

this is a hazardous occupation, and the infective agents may conquer the sentinel tissue and become so well established in the tonsils that the latter must be removed (*tonsillectomy*).

Many small lymphocytes formed in the tonsil leave it by migrating through the crypt epithelium (Fig. 21-20). Lymphocytes may so infiltrate the epithelium that it becomes difficult to establish its deep border. The lymphocytes that escape into the pharynx degenerate in the saliva and are called *salivary corpuscles.*

Glands are associated with the palatine tonsils, but their ducts open beside it and not into its crypts; hence, the crypts are not flushed out as they are in the lingual tonsil, and debris can accumulate in them and predispose them to infection.

THE GENERAL PLAN OF THE GASTROINTESTINAL TRACT

The wall of the gastrointestinal tube consists of 4 main layers (*see* Fig. 21-21, *lower right*): the *mucous membrane, submucosa, muscularis externa,* and *serosa.* The relation of the structure to the function of these 4 layers will now be described.

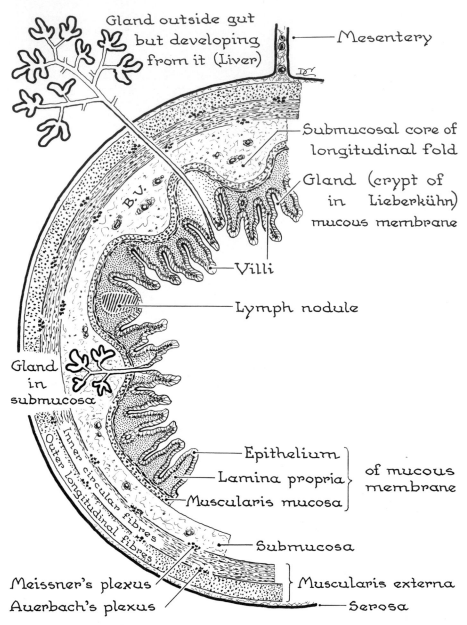

Fig. 21-21. General plan of the gastrointestinal tract.

Gland outside gut but developing from it (Liver)

Mesentery

Submucosal core of longitudinal fold

Gland (crypt of in Lieberkühn) mucous membrane

B.V.

Villi

Lymph nodule

Gland in submucosa

Inner circular fibres

Outer longitudinal fibres

Epithelium

Lamina propria

Muscularis mucosa

of mucous membrane

Submucosa

Meissner's plexus

Auerbach's plexus

Muscularis externa

Serosa

MUCOUS MEMBRANE

This comprises 3 layers: an *epithelial lining,* a supporting *lamina propria,* and a thin, usually double layer of smooth muscle, the *muscularis mucosae* (Fig. 21-21).

Epithelium. The type varies in relation to the function of the part of the tube it lines. In some sites it is primarily protective, for instance the stratified squamous epithelium of esophagus and anus; in others it is mostly secre-

tory, as in the mucous epithelium of the stomach; and in still others, it is primarily absorptive, as in the columnar epithelium of small and large intestine.

In addition to the secretory epithelium lining the stomach, individual secretory cells may lie scattered in the epithelial lining—for example, mucus-secreting goblet cells in the lining of the intestine. There are also definite glands extending to the submucosa, as in esophagus and duodenum. Finally, glands arising from the lining of the gastrointestinal tract may come to be located outside the tract altogether. The salivary glands, liver, and pancreas are all glands of this sort (Fig. 21-21, *upper left*). Nevertheless, since they all arise from the lining of the alimentary tract, they all drain into it by ducts, the sites of which indicate their respective sites of origin.

Lamina Propria. This layer consists of connective tissue that is best described as loose connective tissue with a tendency to form lymphatic nodules.

The functions of the lamina propria are numerous. In order to support the epithelium and to connect it with the muscularis mucosae, it contains collagenic, reticular, and, in some sites, elastic fibers. The lymphatic tissue so characteristic of this layer is of the nonencapsulated type and hence typical of lymphatic tissue commonly disposed under wet epithelial surfaces. Another common cell type is the plasma cell. Lymphocytes and plasma cells constitute a further line of defense against bacteria or other antigenic substances that gain entrance to the tissues across the epithelial membrane. After entry of a given antigen, the plasma cells produce a kind of immunoglobulin called *IgA* directed against it. This is known as *secretory immunoglobulin* since it has the ability to enter epithelial cells and be secreted by them into the lumen, where it can neutralize the antigen if it reappears in the digestive tube.

The lamina propria carries both blood and lymphatic capillaries close to the epithelial surface, particularly in the finger-like *villi* that project into the lumen from the small intestine (Fig. 21-21). Consequently, the products resulting from digestion of carbohydrates, proteins, and fats do not have to diffuse any great distance through tissue fluid of the lamina propria in order to gain entrance to one or the other type of capillary.

Muscularis Mucosae. This, the third and outermost layer of the mucous membrane, consists generally of 2 thin layers of smooth muscle, together with varying amounts of elastic tissue. In the inner layer the muscle fibers are circularly disposed, and in the outer, longitudinally (Fig. 21-21). The muscularis mucosae probably permits localized movement of the mucous membrane. Increased local tonus of the circular fibers would tend to throw the mucous membrane into transverse (circular) folds.

The muscularis mucosae sends off small bundles of smooth muscle fibers in the direction of the epithelium. In the small intestine, where the mucosa forms villi (Fig. 21-21), one smooth muscle bundle from the muscularis mucosae goes to the tip of each villus, where it ends on the basement membrane of its epithelium. These bundles contain the longest smooth muscle cells in the body. In the large intestine, where the free surface is rather flat, the bundles end on the basement membrane of the epithelial cells on that surface.

Submucosa. This coat connects the mucous membrane to the muscularis externa. It consists of loose connective tissue and houses plexuses of larger blood vessels (Fig. 21-21). The elastic fibers of these impart an elastic quality to the coat as a whole. This is augmented, particularly in the upper part of the gastrointestinal tract, by a considerable number of elastic fibers distributed throughout its substance. The elastic quality of the submucosa permits it to form the cores of such folds of mucous membrane as are present in different parts of the tract (Fig. 21-21, *top*).

A plexus of nerve fibers with which some ganglion cells are associated is present in the submucosa. This is called *Meissner's plexus* or the *submucosal plexus* (Fig. 21-21, *bottom left*). The fibers in it are mostly nonmyelinated, derived chiefly from the superior mesenteric plexus (a prevertebral plexus); hence they are postganglionic fibers from the *sympathetic* division of the autonomic nervous system. The relatively few ganglion cells in the submucosal plexus are terminal ganglion cells of the *parasympathetic* division; the preganglionic fibers that synapse there are derived from the vagus nerve (cranial outflow).

Muscularis Externa. This coat consists characteristically of 2 fairly substantial layers of smooth muscle. The inner layer has circularly disposed fibers and is somewhat thicker than the outer layer, which has longitudinally disposed fibers (Fig. 21-21). However, it is probable that these layers are not truly transverse or longitudinal and that the fibers of both layers pursue a somewhat spiral course. By seeing whether the fibers in the inner and the outer coats are cut in cross or longitudinal section a student can tell whether he is examining a cross or a longitudinal section of any part of the tract. Hence, if in a given section the fibers of the inner layer are cut in cross section, and the ones in the outer layer in longitudinal section, the section is a longitudinal one.

Functions. The muscularis externa is the primary means of propelling the contents of the tube downward from pharynx to anus. The orderly functioning of the muscularis externa is unquestionably an important requisite for health and happiness. The various kinds of actions it performs and their control are complex, so only introductory comment will be made here.

(*1*) The smooth muscle of the muscularis externa constitutes a surrounding sheath for the tract. Smooth muscle, it will be recalled, is adapted to maintaining different degrees of tonus (sustained contraction). The tonus of the muscularis externa is of prime importance in regulating the overall size of the lumen of the bowel.

(*2*) Smooth muscle has the inherent property of undergoing spontaneous and rhythmic contractions. The way impulses are conducted between smooth muscle cells by gap junctions was explained in Chapter 18.

(*3*) The muscularis externa is responsible for *peristaltic movements*. These are the primary cause of food being moved along the bowel. They are waves of constriction that sweep downward, pushing the contents of the bowel ahead of them. There are two kinds: slow gentle ones and vigorous rapid ones, called *peristaltic rushes.*

For effective waves of peristaltic contraction to sweep down the bowel, coordination is provided by a plexus of nerve fibers (associated with numerous ganglia) situated chiefly between the circular and longitudinal layers of muscle in the muscularis externa. This plexus is called *Auerbach's plexus* or the *myenteric plexus* (Fig. 21-21, *bottom left*). It contains preganglionic fibers of the *parasympathetic* division of the autonomic nervous system, which fibers (except in the distal part of the large intestine) are derived from the vagus nerve, and hence from the cranial outflow of the system. These fibers synapse with the cells of the terminal ganglia in the plexus which therefore correspond to parasympathetic ganglion cells. The postganglionic fibers given off by these ganglion cells terminate, for the most part, on muscle cells, which they stimulate. Postganglionic fibers of the *sympathetic* division of the autonomic nervous system, most of which arise from ganglion cells of the prevertebral ganglia, also contribute to Auerbach's plexus, though they have no cell stations there; they reach the muscle cells directly. Whether there are any afferent fibers in the myenteric plexus is a question that has been much discussed. Reflex actions seem to occur in the bowel, but there is little anatomical evidence to indicate that afferent neurons are involved. Perhaps something of the nature of an axon reflex (that will be learned about in physiology) operates in this situation.

Impulses traveling down the vagus nerve (parasympathetic division) tend to augment the tone and peristaltic movement of the muscularis externa. Impulses traveling down the sympathetic fibers from the prevertebral ganglia tend to inhibit both tone and peristaltic movements. A vast amount of gastrointestinal malfunction seems to be due to emotional disturbance affecting smooth muscle function in the bowel. Therefore many frustrated individuals suffer not only the unhappiness of not having what they want in life but also gastrointestinal difficulties due to their sustained emotional state.

Serosa or Adventitia. This, the fourth and outermost coat of the wall of the alimentary tube, is of a serous character; that is, it consists of loose connective tissue, covered with a single layer of squamous mesothelial cells and known as a *serosa.* In portions of the tract that are connected to adjacent tissues, the loose connective tissue is not covered by mesothelial cells, but merges with the connective tissue associated with the surrounding structures. In this case it is known as an *adventitia.*

Sheets of mesentery (Fig. 21-21, *top*) are covered on both sides by mesothelium and have a core of loose connective tissue containing a variable number of fat cells,

together with the blood and lymphatic vessels and the nerves that it conducts to the intestine.

THE ESOPHAGUS

The *esophagus* is a fairly straight tube extending from the pharynx to the stomach (Fig. 21-1). Its wall consists of the usual 4 layers described above in connection with the general plan of the gastrointestinal tract. Such variations from the general plan as are found in these layers are adaptations to its special function.

The Epithelium and Its Renewal. For protection against the rough material often swallowed, the esophagus is lined by stratified squamous epithelium. In man and primates this epithelium is of the nonkeratinizing type (Figs. 21-22 and 21-23), but in animals that swallow rough material, the keratinized type is present.

The stratified squamous epithelium of the esophagus needs to undergo continuous renewal. Mitosis occurs in the deeper layers, while superficial cells desquamate into the lumen. In the rat esophagus mitosis occurs only in the basal layer, but in other species cells of the 2 or 3 deepest layers may undergo mitosis. In all cases the deep layers where mitosis occurs are composed of small, deeply basophilic cells. As cells are displaced toward the lumen, they lose their ability to divide; this is associated with loss of cytoplasmic basophilia and the appearance of tonofilaments, together with overall enlargement of the cells. Differentiation of the cells is eventually followed by their desquamation.

The progeny cells of a mitotic division in a deep layer may take either of 2 courses. Some remain in the deeper layers to divide again; others differentiate as described, eventually to be shed from the surface. Marques-Pereira and Leblond showed that it is a matter of chance whether a cell divides again or undergoes differentiation.

Glands. There are only a few mucous glands scattered in the submucosa; these are called *esophageal glands* (Fig. 21-22). There are also some glands in the lamina propria near the stomach, and since these resemble the glands in the cardiac portion of the stomach, they are called *cardiac glands.*

Muscularis Externa. The muscle associated with the pharynx is striated, and muscle of this type continues into the upper third of the esophagus, where it forms its muscularis externa. In the middle third of the esophagus, smooth muscle makes its appearance in the muscularis externa and begins to take the place of the striated type, and in the lower third smooth muscle generally comprises all the muscle present. The section illustrated in Figure 21-22 was taken from the middle third and so shows muscle of both types in the muscularis externa, smooth to the inside and striated in the external, longitudinal layer.

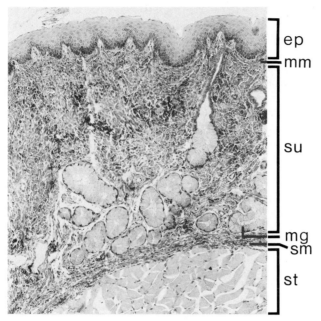

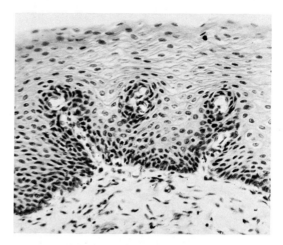

Fig. 21-23. High-power photomicrograph of the lining of the esophagus, showing its stratified squamous nonkeratinizing epithelium and the connective tissue of the lamina propria below. Papillae of lamina propria extend up into the epithelium and are seen as light areas (*center*) where they extend into it at an angle.

Fig. 21-22. Low-power photomicrograph (×70) of a portion of the wall of the middle third of the esophagus of a monkey. Stratified squamous nonkeratinizing epithelium (ep) lines the mucous membrane; it is supported on a lamina propria between it and the muscularis mucosae, the position of which is indicated by mm. Esophageal (mucous) glands (mg), a duct of which is seen at *upper right*, are evident in the submucosa (su). The inner, circular layer of the muscularis externa at *bottom* consists of smooth muscle (sm); the outer, longitudinal layer is composed of striated muscle (st). (Courtesy of C. P. Leblond)

The striated muscle of the pharynx and upper part of the esophagus is an exception to the general rule that striated muscle is voluntary, that is, under the control of the will. The muscle in the muscularis externa of the esophagus is innervated chiefly by parasympathetic fibers from the vagi. Hence, swallowing is in part an involuntary act, a reflex action set in motion by stimulation of afferent endings distributed chiefly in the posterior wall of the pharynx. Because the striated muscles of the mouth are under voluntary control, swallowing can be initiated, but continuation of swallowing from the pharynx onward is involuntary and due to operation of the autonomic reflex.

In man the muscularis externa of the esophagus is not thickened sufficiently at its point of entrance into the stomach (the cardia) to justify its being called a cardiac sphincter.

Adventitia. Since the esophagus is not covered with peritoneum, it has an adventitia rather than a serosa. This consists of loose connective tissue that connects the esophagus to the surrounding structures.

THE STOMACH

The stomach is the considerably expanded portion of the alimentary tube lying between the esophagus and the small intestine (Fig. 21-1). It acts as a reservoir, a function facilitated by the elasticity of its walls, which can stretch to give it a capacity of from 1 to 1½ quarts; its contents are retained in the stomach by the well-developed pyloric sphincter at its outlet. The stomach has a digestive role due to the action of the gastric juice secreted by the cells in the glands of its mucous membrane. Gastric juice contains 3 enzymes as well as hydrochloric acid and mucus. Of the 3 enzymes, *pepsin* is the most important. This enzyme is secreted in the form of its precursor, *pepsinogen.* In the acid environment it forms pepsin and begins the digestion of proteins. The other 2 enzymes are *rennin*, which curdles milk, and *lipase*, which splits fats. However, this last action is not extensive in the stomach.

The hydrochloric acid in the gastric secretion is present in sufficient concentration to kill the living cells present in uncooked food (fruit, oysters, etc.) and yet it does not destroy the cells that line the stomach, except under certain pathological conditions (such as excessive stress, when ulcers are produced). Obviously, there must normally be protection mechanisms operating to prevent this. It is believed that the coating of mucus, mainly secreted by the surface epithelial cells, is protective in this respect. Indeed, the mucus is produced so as to form a series of dis-

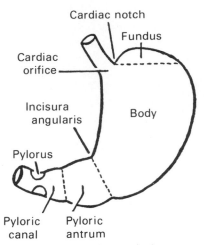

Cardiac notch

Fundus

Cardiac orifice

Incisura angularis

Body

Pylorus

Pyloric canal

Pyloric antrum

Fig. 21-24. Diagram of the parts of the stomach. (Grant, J. C. B.: A Method of Anatomy, ed. 4 Baltimore, Williams & Wilkins, 1948)

tinct layers; if one layer is damaged, the next one protects, and so forth. Finally, as will be described shortly, another form of protection is due to the epithelial cells lining the stomach being replaced every 3 days or so.

The stomach acts as an efficient mixer by virtue of its muscular movements. With the help of the enzymes, the stirring of the stomach converts its contents, diluted with gastric juice, into a semifluid of even consistency; this is called *chyme*. The stomach is also concerned in producing the factor necessary for absorption of vitamin B_{12} and it serves to some extent as an absorptive organ, but its function in this respect is limited to the absorption of water, salts, alcohol, and certain drugs.

Gross Characteristics. The shape of the stomach and its component parts is illustrated in Figure 21-24. Anatomically, the fundus is that part lying above a horizontal line drawn through the lower end of the esophagus. About two thirds of the remainder is called the *body of the stomach*. The distal part of the organ comprises the *pyloric antrum, pyloric canal,* and *pylorus.* Together, these last 3 portions are often collectively referred to as the *pylorus* or *pyloric region.* Histologically, 3 regions are described: (*1*) the *cardiac* region, which surrounds the cardiac orifice; (*2*) the body or *fundic* region, which includes the anatomical body and fundus; and (*3*) the *pyloric* region comprised of antrum, canal, and pylorus.

If an empty (contracted) stomach is opened, its mucous membrane shows branching folds, most of which are disposed longitudinally; these folds are termed *rugae.* Their cores consist of submucosa (Fig. 21-25, *top*). When the stomach is full, however, the rugae are almost completely "ironed out."

GENERAL MICROSCOPIC FEATURES

The wall of the stomach is composed of the 4 usual layers already described. The mucous membrane is relatively thick and contains numerous simple tubular glands, described below. In some sites the muscularis mucosae has 3 layers instead of the usual 2 described in the general plan. The small bundles of smooth muscle fibers going from the muscularis mucosae to the surface travel in between the glands. There are no glands in the submucosa except in the pyloric part adjacent to the duodenum. The muscularis externa also consists of 3 instead of 2 layers. The fibers of the innermost layer are disposed obliquely, those of the middle coat, circularly, and those of the outermost coat, longitudinally. A serosa is present on the outside surface of the stomach.

Pits and Glands of the Mucosa. If the gastric mucosa of the 3 histological regions is examined with the scanning electron microscope, for example, it is seen to be studded with tiny little openings through which the gastric juice wells up when the stomach is actively secreting. These are the openings of what are termed *gastric pits* or *foveolae.* The pits descend into the mucous membrane to become continuous with the upper ends of the gastric glands opening into them. Two or three glands deliver secretion into each pit, from which their secretion reaches the stomach lumen.

The gastric *pits* are relatively uniform in appearance throughout the stomach, differing only in length. Each is lined with mucus-secreting epithelial cells similar to the cells lining the entire stomach surface. The gastric *glands,* on the other hand, differ somewhat in the cardiac, fundic, and pyloric regions, so the glands of these areas are termed *cardiac, fundic,* and *pyloric glands,* respectively.

The lamina propria, which occupies the narrow space between adjacent glands, contains muscle fibers, blood vessels, lymphatics, and the usual connective tissue components.

The Surface Epithelium (Which Also Extends Down the Sides of the Pits to Line Them). The surface epithelium of the stomach is composed of only one kind of cell— *mucous columnar cells*—which are all alike, whereas in the small and the large intestine goblet cells alternate with absorptive columnar cells that do not produce mucus. The apical cytoplasm of these surface epithelial cells is filled with secretory vesicles containing mucus. When damage is done to the mucus sheets and underlying cells by certain types of food and drink (particularly straight liquor), some of the surface epithelial cells are shed into the lumen of the stomach. The mortality of surface cells is compensated for by migration of new cells arising in the isthmus region of gastric glands, as described below. When more extensive damage is done to the stomach, for

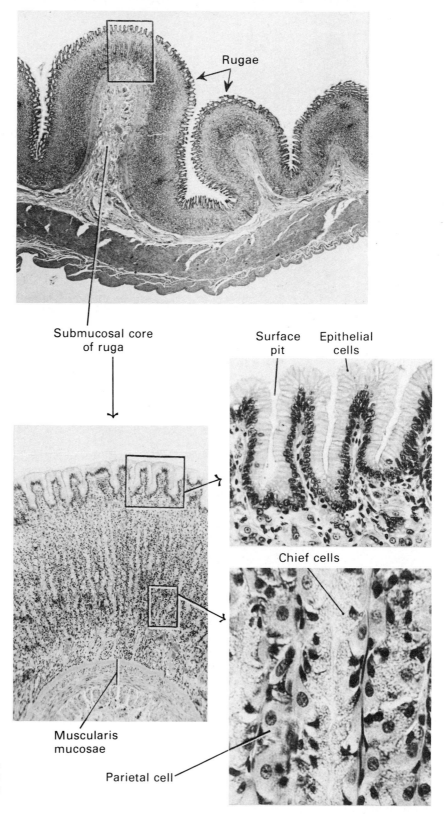

Rugae

Submucosal core
of ruga

Surface
pit

Epithelial
cells

Chief cells

Muscularis
mucosae

Parietal cell

Fig. 21-25. Photomicrographs of the
body of the stomach of a cat, illustrating
the structure of its rugae and fundic pits
and glands.

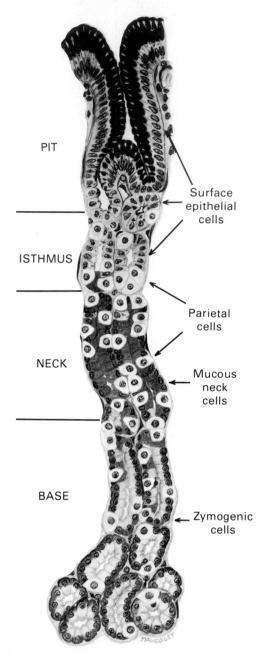

PIT

Surface
epithelial
cells

ISTHMUS

Parietal
cells

NECK

Mucous
neck
cells

BASE

Zymogenic
cells

Fig. 21-26. Drawing of a fundic pit and gland in the stomach of a monkey, stained with PAS and hematoxylin. (Courtesy of C. P. Leblond)

instance in surgical operations, the surface epithelium heals rapidly, again presumably because of entry of new cells.

Glands of the Cardiac Region. In the region immediately

surrounding the opening of the esophagus into the stomach, the glands at the bottoms of the pits are small and composed of mucous cells with a pale cytoplasm, suggesting low secretory activity. In places, a few parietal cells (to be described below) are scattered among the gland cells.

Glands of the Fundic Region. These produce nearly all the enzymes and hydrochloric acid secreted in the stomach; they also produce some of the mucus. In the body of the stomach the pits extend into the mucous membrane for only one quarter to one third of its thickness (Fig. 21-25, *lower left*). Therefore the glands that extend from the bottoms of the pits to the muscularis mucosae are 2 to 3 times as long as the pits are deep. The glands here are fairly straight except near the muscularis mucosae, where they may be bent (Fig. 21-26).

According to Stevens and Leblond, the glands may be divided into 3 segments. The deepest part is the *base* (Fig. 21-26), the middle part, the *neck,* and the upper part, the *isthmus* (Fig. 21-26). The isthmus is continuous with a pit. It should be understood that *pits* are not parts of glands; they are merely little wells sunk from the surface and lined with surface epithelial cells. Several glands may open into a pit.

The gastric juice is secreted by the glands, which contain 4 main kinds of secretory cells, demonstrated to advantage in sections stained by the PA-Schiff method and counterstained with hematoxylin.

The *isthmus* contains 2 types of cells, *surface epithelial cells* and *parietal cells.* The surface epithelial cells along the sides of pits have a considerable apical content of mucus (represented in black in Fig. 21-26). Deep down in the pits the content of mucus in the apical region of the cells is considerably less (Fig. 21-26), and in the isthmus the surface epithelial cells demonstrate only a few apical vesicles of mucus. Scattered between the surface epithelial cells in the isthmus are large *parietal cells;* these have relatively clear, pale cytoplasm when stained by the PA-Schiff method and hematoxylin. In good H and E preparations the cytoplasm of these cells is pink. The parietal cells seen in a section vary from being rounded to triangular in shape (Figs. 21-25 and 21-26). Their nucleus is spherical and generally central; their fine structure and function will be described presently.

The *neck* of a gastric gland is made up of *mucous neck cells* interspersed with *parietal cells* (Fig. 21-26). With PA-Schiff staining the cytoplasm of the mucous neck cells appears stuffed with pink mucus (dark in Fig. 21-26) and has a foamy appearance, but this is not readily seen in H and E sections. The nucleus is generally pressed against the base of the cell and often has a more or less triangular shape.

The *base* of a gastric gland contains mostly *zymogenic*

Fig. 21-27. Electron micrograph (×9,500) of a parietal cell in a gastric gland of a bat. Note the C-shaped intracellular canaliculus, filled with numerous long microvilli, and also the microvilli projecting from the surface of the cell. The dark, rounded structures in the cytoplasm are mitochondria. The other cells lining the lumen of the gland, seen at *upper right*, are mucous neck cells, characterized by having mucus globules in their apical cytoplasm and short microvilli on their apical surface. (Courtesy of S. Ito, R. Winchester, and D. Fawcett)

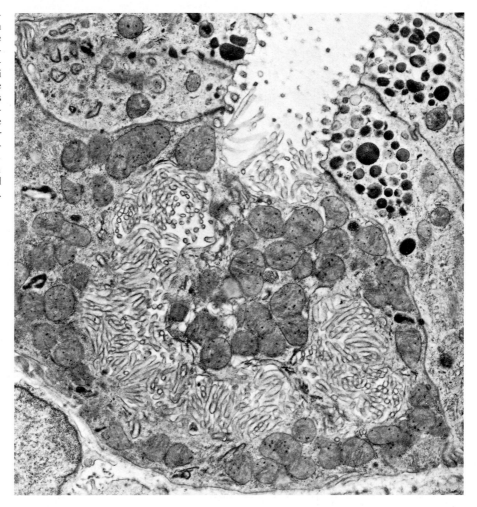

(chief) cells. These have accumulations of basophilic material in their cytoplasm, near their base (Fig. 21-26). The cytoplasm between the nucleus and the free surface appears granular if well fixed. *Parietal cells* are sprinkled here among the zymogenic cells. Not uncommonly a triangular parietal cell will be seen that is arranged so that one of its 3 sides lies along the basement membrane of the gland, and the other 2 border the bases of adjacent chief cells. The secretion from such a parietal cell must then pass between the two chief cells (that almost cover it) to reach the lumen. With good fixation, secretory canaliculi (described below) may be seen in their cytoplasm. These open on the side of the cell nearest to the lumen of the gland.

The zymogenic (chief) cells produce the enzymes of the gastric secretion, and the parietal cells produce the hydrochloric acid. The other types of cells produce only mucus.

THE FINE STRUCTURE OF THE CELLS OF THE GLANDS OF THE FUNDIC REGION

Parietal Cells. In the EM the parietal cell is characterized by a branching *canaliculus* extending into it from its apex, by which it delivers its secretion into the lumen of a gastric gland (Fig. 21-27). In addition to intracellular canaliculi, there may be intercellular canaliculi between adjacent parietal cells. An outstanding feature of the intracellular canaliculus is the innumerable microvilli projecting into it (Fig. 21-27). There are also finger-like invaginations between the bases of the microvilli. Some believe these invaginations can be inverted to become microvilli and vice versa, and that this phenomenon is related to acid secretion. The intracellular canaliculus occupies a considerable amount of space in a parietal cell and so encroaches on the cytoplasm that the cytoplasm that remains is literally stuffed with mitochondria. There

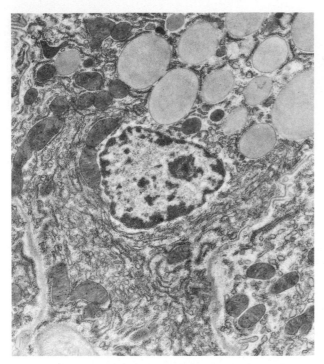

Fig. 21-28. Electron micrograph (×14,000) of a portion of a chief (zymogenic) cell in a gastric gland of a bat. Its nucleus is seen at *center*, large secretory vesicles at *upper right,* and well-developed cisternae of rER below *center.* The dark ovoid or elongate organelles toward the periphery of the micrograph (but not seen at *top right*) are mitochondria. (Courtesy of S. Ito, R. Winchester, and D. Fawcett)

are a few ribosomes, a little rER, and no secretory granules. A small Golgi apparatus can be seen.

The use of indicators on suitable sections shows that the cytoplasm of a parietal cell, as a whole, has a normal pH. However, the canaliculi have an extremely acid pH. The enzyme carbonic anhydrase is abundant in parietal cells and may be responsible for catalyzing the formation of carbonic acid. One theory is that hydrogen ions from this carbonic acid are transported, by an active transport mechanism, through the membrane that lines the finger-like invaginations and covers the microvilli, where they combine with chloride ions.

Besides producing hydrochloric acid, parietal cells are believed to secrete the so-called *intrinsic factor* necessary for absorbing vitamin B_{12} in the small intestine.

Chief (Zymogenic) Cells. These cells are characterized by an abundance of cisternae of rER and secretory vesicles (Fig. 21-28). The way the rER is concerned in forming secretory proteins such as the precursors of the enzymes made by these cells was described in detail in Chapter 5.

Mucous Neck Cells and Surface Epithelial Cells. Both cell types show numerous mucus droplets, particularly near the apex of the cell through which their secretion is delivered. Mucus-secreting cells were dealt with in detail in Chapters 5 and 7.

Less Common Cell Types. It has long been known that the cytoplasm of certain cells of both the gastric and the intestinal epithelium contains granules capable of reducing silver nitrate. They were called *argentaffin cells,* and also *enterochromaffin* cells because they are strongly stained also by bichromate salts. Certain slightly different cells can reduce silver nitrate only in the presence of a reducing agent; these were called *argyrophil* cells. Argentaffin and argyrophil cells are now classified as *endocrine cells* of the gastrointestinal tract. By analogy with the endocrine elements of the nervous system called *neuroendocrine cells,* it is appropriate to call these *enteroendocrine cells.* In the stomach several types are found. A strongly argentaffin kind, the *EC cell,* produces *serotonin* and also, according to recent work, *endorphin,* a morphine-like substance first identified in the brain. This cell, like most other enteroendocrine cells, is characterized by the presence in its base of dense secretory granules (Fig. 21-41), which release their content into the lamina propria for passage into the circulation.

THE RENEWAL OF CELLS IN THE GASTRIC MUCOSA

Stevens and Leblond found mitotic division only in the isthmus and neck regions of the glands, in the 2 mucus-containing types of cells. The surface epithelial cells are maintained by division of immature and partly mature cells in the isthmus. Daughter cells migrate into the pits, where they stop dividing, and then back up to the free surface, where they are eventually lost to the lumen. The mucous neck cells divide about half as often and cell production is balanced by loss into the gland lumen. The surface epithelium in the stomach is renewed (every 3 days in the rat) by cells in the isthmus dividing and daughter cells pushing up along the sides of the crypts and over the surface to replace those constantly lost through desquamation.

A more recent proposal is that around the junction of the isthmus and neck regions, a few cells with features characteristic of immaturity (abundant free ribosomes, few organelles, etc.) would give rise not only to surface epithelial and mucous neck cells, but also (at a much slower rate) to the other sorts of cells in the glands (namely, parietal, chief, and enteroendocrine cells). However, the situation is less clear here than in the small intestine, where cell production will be explained in more detail.

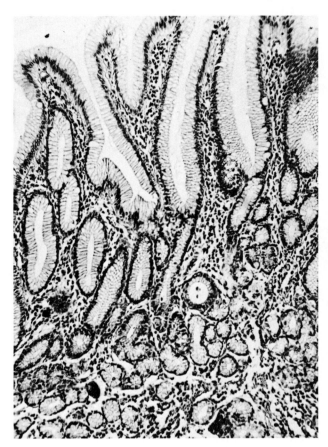

Fig. 21-29. Low-power photomicrograph of the mucous membrane of the pyloric region of the human stomach, showing pyloric pits and glands.

THE FINE STRUCTURE AND THE RENEWAL OF THE CELLS OF THE GLANDS OF THE PYLORIC REGION

The pits of the pyloric region are considerably longer than those of the fundic region. Furthermore, the accompanying glands are much shorter than those observed in the fundic region (compare Figs. 21-25, *lower left,* and 21-29). This difference should enable the student to distinguish sections of pylorus from those of the body of the stomach.

The pyloric glands contain *mucus-secreting* cells similar to mucous neck cells of the fundic region. The mucus globules in these cells, however, have a protein core (Fig. 21-30) and histochemical methods indicate that this contains pepsinogen (Zeitoun et al.). Hence their secretory activity results in release of the precursor of pepsin along with mucus.

In addition to mucus-secreting cells, *enteroendocrine*

cells are also observed in pyloric glands and, less commonly, in the lining of the pits into which they empty. These enteroendocrine cells include *EC cells* (as in the fundus) and 2 other cell types. One type secretes *somatostatin,* a hormone inhibiting the release of growth hormone by the somatotroph cells of the anterior lobe of the pituitary. Another type produces *gastrin,* a peptide that stimulates secretion of hydrochloric acid by parietal cells. Gastrin cells (Fig. 21-31) differ from other enteroendocrine cells by their secretory granules being distributed

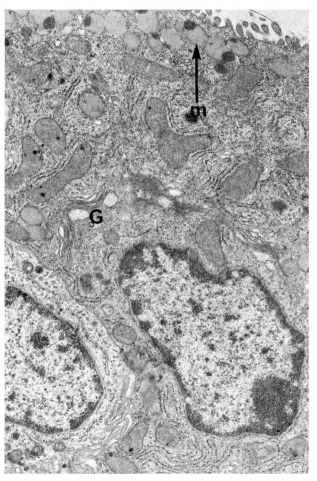

Fig. 21-30. Electron micrograph of a mucus-secreting cell of a pyloric gland of the stomach. Note the mucus globules (m) at top in the apical cytoplasm of the cell. Their contents are light-staining except for a dark-staining core that contains pepsinogen. Note also the abundant mitochondria and prominent Golgi apparatus (G) between the nucleus and the apical surface, and the well-developed rER. A portion of the lumen of the gland is seen at *top right,* with microvilli projecting into it. (Courtesy of C. P. Leblond and E. Lee)

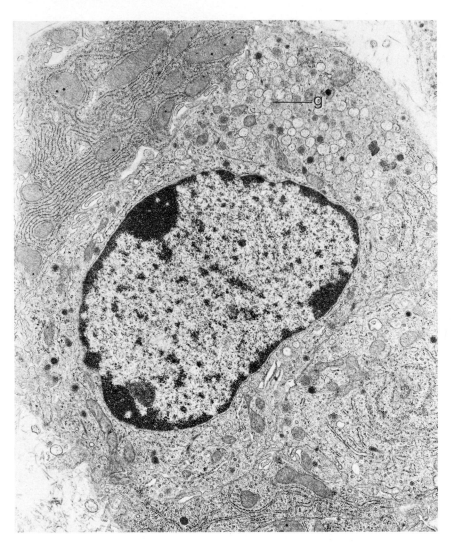

Fig. 21-31. Electron micrograph of a gastrin cell in a pyloric gland of the stomach. The secretory granules (g) of this type of enteroendocrine cell contain gastrin and appear pale. Some cisternae of rER and free polysomes are visible at *middle right*. Part of a chief (zymogenic) cell with extensive well-developed rER and numerous mitochondria is seen at *upper left*. (Courtesy of C. P. Leblond and E. Lee)

throughout the cytoplasm instead of accumulating in the base. Because of this feature, some think that gastrin cells release their secretion to the lumen rather than to the lamina propria. It may also be seen in Figure 21-31 that the granules are pale instead of electron-dense as in other enteroendocrine cells.

Some parietal cells are also observed in human pyloric glands, especially next to the duodenum. In other mammals, however, the parietal cells are not a usual component of the glands in the pyloric region; thus in the mouse, parietal cells are observed only in the transitional area between pyloric and fundic glands. As for chief (zymogenic) cells, they are absent in pyloric glands.

The turnover of cells in the pyloric *pit* is comparable with that in the fundic area, their life span being about 3 days. Turnover in the *gland*, however, is not nearly as

rapid; in animals the cells of pyloric glands are renewed in about 3 weeks. The enteroendocrine cells are renewed at an even slower race.

As in the fundus of the stomach, most pit and gland cells originate from the isthmus region located between a pit and a gland. Again there are indications that immature cells give rise to both pit and gland cells. As the pit cells mature, they migrate up along the walls of the pit, reaching the surface, from which they are later lost. The events in the maturation of the gland cells, however, are not as clear.

At the pylorus, the circular layer of smooth muscle in the middle coat of the muscularis externa is very well developed and forms a thick band encircling the exit of the stomach. This band is called the *pyloric sphincter*. It causes the submucosa and mucous membrane to bulge inward so that they are thrown into a transverse (circular) fold. The chief component of the core of this particular fold, it should be noted, is the thickened middle coat of the muscularis externa. This differs from most other folds in the alimentary tract, which have cores of submucosa.

In the stomach peristaltic movements begin near the middle and spread down to the pylorus. The pyloric sphincter automatically opens to permit food that is sufficiently fluid and acidified to enter the small intestine. At the same time it holds back solid undigested food.

The Control of Secretion of Gastric Juices

In dogs the surface of the resting stomach is coated with mucus; gastric juice wells up from the glands to flood the surface only when a meal is in prospect or actually being consumed. However, Carlson showed that in man there is more or less continuous secretion of modest amounts of gastric juice (10 to 60 ml. per hour). This is augmented when food is about to be eaten or is eaten. Several factors are concerned in augmenting the secretion. Psychic factors, as shown by Pavlov, play an important part and so justify the efforts of the imaginative cook. Psychic factors operate through nervous control of secretion via the vagus nerve. Certain foods, when they reach the stomach, have the ability to stimulate secretion directly, since they do so even if the nerves to the stomach are cut. Hence, if they stimulate secretion by a reflex initiated in the mucosa of the stomach, the reflex concerned must be a local one. Then, in addition to certain foods stimulating secretion, breakdown products of a wide variety of foods also have this property, particularly when they reach the small intestine, where they act on its mucosa possibly to make a substance that circulates by the bloodstream to reach the gastric glands. Accordingly, the gastric glands are said to secrete through 3 phases: (*1*) the cephalic (psychic factors), (*2*) the gastric, where consumed food either directly or indirectly stimulates the mucosa to induce secretion, and (*3*) the intestinal, where the breakdown products of digestion, and the gastric juice itself, reach and affect the intestinal mucosa to make it produce something that circulates by the bloodstream to stimulate further the gastric glands.

THE SMALL INTESTINE

Relation of General Structure to Functions

The small intestine is about 20 feet long. Its first foot or so constitutes the *duodenum* (Fig. 21-1). Almost all of this is relatively fixed in position, not being suspended by a mesentery. It pursues a horseshoe-shaped course around the head of the pancreas to become continuous with the *jejunum,* which constitutes the next part of the small intestine (Fig. 21-1). The last portion is termed the *ileum* (Fig. 21-1).

The small intestine has 2 chief functions: (*1*) completing digestion of food delivered into it from the stomach, and (*2*) selectively absorbing the products of digestion

into its blood and lymph vessels. In addition, it also makes some hormones.

The structure of the small intestine is specialized for both its digestive and its absorptive functions. It will be more convenient to describe how its structure is specialized for absorption before describing how it is specialized for digestion.

Features Relating to Absorption — Folds, Villi, and Microvilli

To perform its absorptive function efficiently, the small intestine requires a vast surface of epithelial cells of the absorptive type. The great length of the small intestine helps considerably in providing such a surface, but provision is made for increasing the absorptive surface in 3 other ways, as follows.

(*1*) Beginning about an inch beyond the pylorus, the mucous membrane is thrown into circularly or spirally disposed folds called the *plicae circulares* or *valves of Kerckring* (Fig. 21-32). These folds are generally crescentic and extend from one half to two thirds of the way around the lumen. However, single folds may extend all the way around the intestine or even form a spiral of 2 or 3 turns; the highest ones project into the lumen for about 1 cm. They all have cores of *submucosa,* are not "ironed out" if the intestine is full, and at the proximal end of the small intestine are large and close together (Fig. 21-32). In the upper part of the jejunum they become smaller and farther apart. In the middle or lower end of the ileum they disappear.

(*2*) The surface of the mucous membrane over and between the folds is studded with tiny leaf-, tongue-, or finger-like projections that range from 0.5 to 1 mm. or more in height. These are called the *intestinal villi* (Fig. 21-33). Since they are projections of mucous membrane, they have cores of *lamina propria.* The muscularis mucosae and the submucosa do not extend into them as they do into the plicae circulares.

The villi of the duodenum are broader than those elsewhere, and many examples of leaf-like ones can be found in this region. In the upper part of the jejunum, the villi, in general, are said to be tongue-shaped. Farther down, they become finger-shaped. However, these shapes are variable for different individuals. More important are the length and surface area of villi. In general, length and surface area are maximal at the beginning of the small intestine (that is, immediately after the pylorus) and they decrease gradually to reach a minimum in the ileum just before the ileocecal junction (Fig. 21-34). At first, it would appear that the size of villi varies with the extent of absorption taking place. However, the large villus size in the duodenum seems to be maintained by factors arising locally as well as coming from stomach and pancreas,

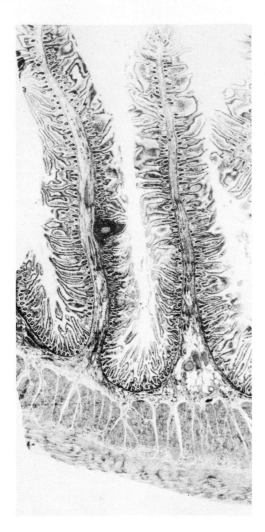

Fig. 21-32. Low-power photomicrograph of a *longitudinal* section of the wall of the jejunum of a dog, showing 2 plicae circulares (valves of Kerckring) cut in *cross* section. These plicae are covered with irregularly shaped villi.

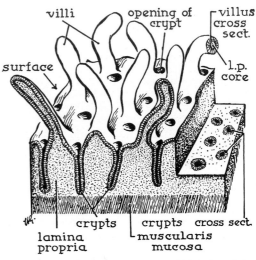

Fig. 21-33. Three-dimensional schematic drawing of the lining of the small intestine. Observe that villi are finger-like processes, with cores of lamina propria, that extend into the lumen. Note also that crypts of Lieberkühn are glands that dip down into the lamina propria. Observe particularly the difference in cross-sectional appearance between villi and crypts.

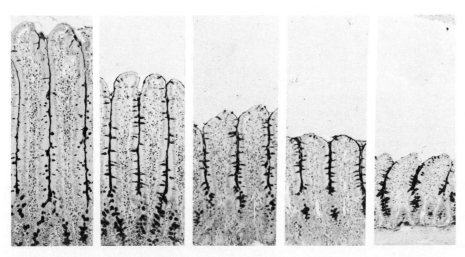

Fig. 21-34. Photomicrographs of villi in different regions of rat small intestine. From *left* to *right* are: beginning of duodenum; jejunum; junction of jejunum and ileum; mid ileum; and terminal ileum. Note the gradual decrease in villus size from pylorus to ileocecal valve, and that villi lie fairly close to one another (much more so than is depicted in Fig. 21-33). (Courtesy of G. Altmann and C. P. Leblond)

because when duodenum is connected to terminal ileum in such a way that secretions are shared, ileal villi become taller and duodenal villi smaller than normal (Altmann and Leblond).

(*3*) The absorptive surface is made still greater by the microvilli present on the free surfaces of the epithelial cells; these were described in Chapter 5 and are illustrated in Figures 5-7 and 21-37.

Features Relating to Digestion — Glands and Their Enzymes

In order to perform its other chief function (completing the digestion of food received from the stomach), the small intestine requires large supplies of digestive enzymes and mucus. The digestive enzymes are provided by glands; mucus is provided both by definite glands and by innumerable goblet cells that are intermingled with absorptive cells along the mucous membrane. The glands that provide the digestive juices and the mucus necessary for the function of the small intestine are distributed in 3 general sites: (*1*) outside the intestine, but connected with it by ducts, (2) in the submucosa, and (*3*) in the lamina propria.

The microscopic structure of the pancreas and liver, 2 glands that are situated outside the small intestine and deliver their secretions into it, will be considered in Chapter 22. Here we are concerned only with effects of their secretions on the digestive process. Their ducts, usually conjoined, open into the duodenum about 3 inches from the pylorus (Fig. 21-1). The exocrine secretion of the pancreas, delivered into the duodenum at this site, is alkaline (and helps neutralize the acid stomach contents), and it contains enzymes concerned in the digestion of proteins, carbohydrates, and fats. Several enzymes that effect different steps in protein digestion are probably elaborated. The enzymes are not active until they reach the intestine, where they are rendered potent. Together they can break down proteins to amino acids; it is in this form that proteins are absorbed. The pancreatic juice also contains enzymes that break down starches to sugars. Some sugars, for example, maltose, must be acted on further by enzymes produced by villous epithelial cells, and converted to monosaccharides before they are absorbed. The pancreatic juice also contains lipolytic enzymes that emulsify fat and break it down to free fatty acids or monoglycerides. The effect of these enzymes is facilitated by the presence of bile, the secretion of the liver.

The second group of glands to consider are those situated in the submucosa. Glands are found in this position only in the *duodenum*. These are compound tubular in type and are called *glands of Brunner* (Fig. 21-35). Generally, they are most numerous in the proximal part of the

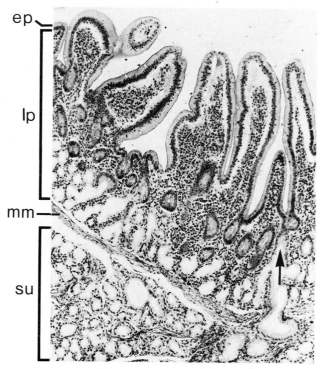

Fig. 21-35. Low-power photomicrograph (×100) of part of the wall of human duodenum. Note the pale-staining Brunner's glands (mucus-secreting) in the submucosa (su). They extend up through the muscularis mucosae (mm) into the lamina propria (lp) underlying the simple striated columnar epithelium (ep), which also contains goblet cells. The arrow indicates a site where the duct of a gland of Brunner empties into a crypt of Lieberkühn. The broad, leaf-like shape of the villus seen at *upper left* is characteristic of this part of the small intestine. (Courtesy of C. P. Leblond)

duodenum and less numerous (finally disappearing) in its more distal parts.

The secretory portions of Brunner's glands have the characteristic acinar appearance of mucous glands (Fig. 21-35) and lie mainly in the submucosa. Their ducts extend through the muscularis mucosae (Fig. 21-35) and empty their mucous secretion into the crypts of Lieberkühn, to be described shortly.

The third set of glands are the *crypts of Lieberkühn;* these dip down from the surface between villi to reach almost to the muscularis mucosae (Fig. 21-21 and 21-36A). Their openings on the surface of the intestine are shown diagrammatically in Figure 21-33, but these openings are difficult to see in life because they are kept tightly closed. Of the various enzymes secreted by the small intestine, one is exclusively produced within the crypts; it is *lysozyme*, a bactericidal enzyme elaborated by Paneth cells (described below). Most of the enzymes produced

Villus
oblique section

Villus
longitudinal section

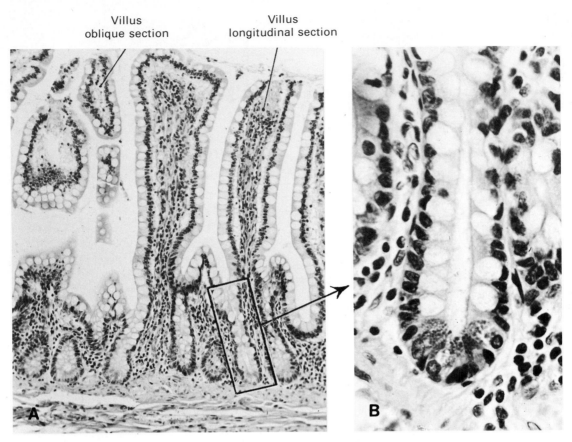

Fig. 21-36. (A) Low-power photomicrograph of part of the wall of the small intestine of a child, showing villi in longitudinal and oblique section and crypts of Lieberkühn. Lymphocytes are numerous in the cores of the villi. The muscularis mucosae extends along the lower margin of the picture. *(B)* High-power photomicrograph of a crypt of Lieberkühn, showing pale-staining goblet cells along its sides and Paneth cells with granules at its base.

by the small intestine, however, arise from the microvilli of columnar cells and remain associated with its striated (brush) border, as explained below.

SOME DETAILS OF THE STRUCTURE OF THE MUCOUS MEMBRANE

General Features of the Epithelium of Villi

Whereas the surface epithelial cells of the stomach secrete mucus and are all of the same type, the cells of the villi are of *2 main types*. About 90 per cent of them are tall, cylindrical cells with a thick "striated border" as described in Chapter 7 and illustrated (as it appears with the LM) in Figure 7-8. The EM shows that the border is composed of packed microvilli (Fig. 21-37, *top*); these cells are called *absorptive*, or more commonly *columnar*,

cells. The rest of the villous epithelium consists of mucus-secreting *goblet cells* (except for less than 0.5 per cent, which are enteroendocrine cells).

Columnar cells have much cytoplasm and highly convoluted lateral cell membranes; mitochondria are abundant (Fig. 21-37). Free ribosomes, however, are scarce. Cisternae of rER and Golgi saccules are well developed in columnar cells at the base of villi, but less prominent toward the tips of villi (Altmann). Furthermore, cell coat production is also more intense in cells at the base of villi and decreases toward their tips (Bennett and Leblond).

There is turnover of the cell coat of villous columnar cells. Some of the glycoproteins in their thick cell coat are hydrolytic enzymes; one is alkaline phosphatase; others convert disaccharides into monosaccharides. Thus lactase is important in the digestion of milk lactose by babies; the complex of sucrase and isomaltase plays a role in older children and adults. These enzymes turn over, with their rate of production and appearance on the microvillar surface balancing their rate of loss by shedding into the lumen.

Goblet cells (Fig. 21-38) are of 2 types. Those of the common type have been described previously. Their Golgi apparatus is prominent and their apical cytoplasm is usually distended with mucus globules (Fig. 21-38A). The cells of the other type show small dense granules within the mucus globules (Fig. 21-38B); they are not numerous in villi.

Cell Types in the Epithelium of Crypts

The cells in the epithelium lining the glands that dip down into the mucous membrane (the crypts of Lieberkühn) vary in relation to depth. The base of the crypt contains about equal numbers of Paneth cells, with characteristic large secretion granules, and small columnar cells in between them (Fig. 21-39). In electron micrographs the small columnar cells of the crypt base are seen to have little cytoplasm; they appear squeezed between Paneth cells (Fig. 21-40). Unlike villous columnar cells (Fig. 21-37), they have smooth lateral membranes. Their cytoplasm contains only few mitochondria and cisternae of rER and a small Golgi apparatus, but it is packed with free ribosomes. These features are characteristic of a relatively undifferentiated type of cell that, as might be expected, undergoes extensive proliferation. These cells were shown by Cheng and Leblond to be the stem cells giving rise to all the cell types found in the epithelium, as will be described in further detail in due course.

Paneth cells, in contrast, are highly differentiated and possess abundant rER and a prominent Golgi. Their zymogen granules (which are surrounded by a halo in the mouse, as seen in Fig. 21-40, but are not in man) are released to the lumen by exocytosis. Paneth cells contain zinc, but the significance of this in obscure. Nor is the nature of the enzymes they secrete known with certainty, except for the fact that they elaborate lysozyme (Erlandsen and Taylor).

The cells located above the crypt base are mostly columnar in shape. They show a gradual transition between crypt base columnar cells and villous columnar cells; their size increases progressively and their content of free ribosomes decreases, whereas the number of cisternae of rER increases. Furthermore, the columnar cells in the crypts divide, but those on the villi do not. Hence, in certain respects these two types of columnar cells are somewhat different. However, study of their embryonic development reveals that the epithelia of both the crypts and the villi have the same origin, and furthermore, they transform into one another, as described below.

Next to the Paneth cell region, cells with few mucus

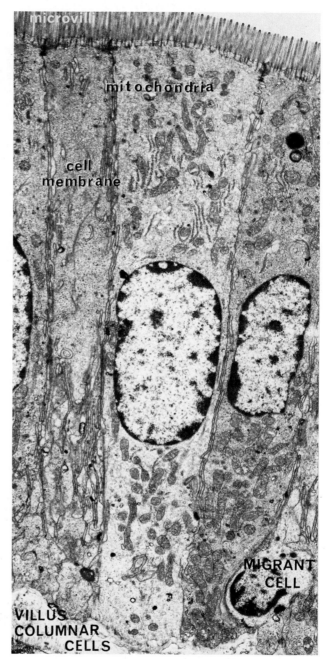

Fig. 21-37. Electron micrograph showing at *middle* a villous columnar cell of small intestine (mouse). This is a tall cylindrical cell with ample cytoplasm, numerous tall microvilli at the free surface. complex convolutions of the lateral membranes (well seen at *left,* particularly in the columnar cell showing no nucleus), numerous mitochondria, and very few free ribosomes. A few cisternae of rER are seen between mitochondria in the supranuclear region of the cell. (Courtesy of H. Cheng and C. P. Leblond)

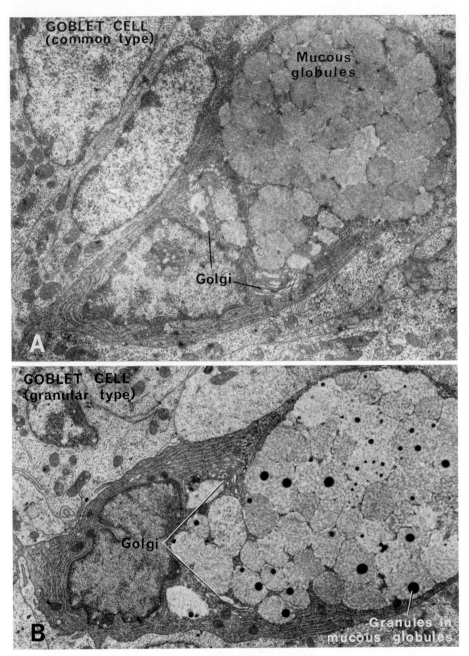

GOBLET CELL
(common type)

Mucous
globules

Golgi

A

GOBLET CELL
(granular type)

Golgi

Granules in
mucous globules

B

Fig. 21-38. Electron micrographs of goblet cells in the upper part of intestinal crypts (mouse small intestine). Their apex is distended by mucus globules to form a goblet shape. The Golgi apparatus is prominent. In about 25 per cent of the mucous cells of the crypts, dense granules are present within the globules, as shown (*B*). As these granular mucous cells migrate out of the crypts and along the villus walls, they secrete the granule-containing globules and elaborate new mucus globules that are free of granules. (Courtesy of H. Cheng)

globules may also be encountered. These cells, known as *oligomucous cells,* arise by differentiation of certain crypt base columnar cells (the type shown in Figs. 21-39 and 21-40). Furthermore, they retain their ability to divide, but only temporarily, for as soon as they start to become distended by mucus globules this capacity is lost. In the lower half of the crypt, most mucous cells contain only few mucus globules, while in the upper half they have the typical appearance of goblet cells (Fig. 21-38). Furthermore, in the crypts, one quarter of the goblet cells contain dense granules within their mucus globules, as illustrated in Figure 21-38B.

In this region, *enteroendocrine* cells constitute about 1 per cent of the cells present. They are characterized by a narrow apex and wide basal region packed with dense granules (Fig. 21-41), which, as in the stomach, may be argentaffin or argyrophil. Some of these cells produce *serotonin.* Others produce intestinal hormones, namely, *secretin, cholecystokinin,* and a substance similar to *glucagon.* Recent evidence indicates that in the small intestine, as in the stomach, some of the enteroendocrine cells produce *somatostatin* and *endorphin.*

Even less common is another cell type, the *caveolated cell,* a strange-looking cell (Fig. 21-42) characterized by invaginations of its cell membrane extending into its cytoplasm as irregular tubules, called *caveolae* (one is indicated by an arrow at *upper left* in Fig. 21-42). Polyplike structures arise from the walls of the caveolae and become free in their lumen in the form of small spheres, which eventually come out between the microvilli to join the chyme. Other noteworthy features of these cells are microvilli twice the length of those of the nearby cells, long bundles of straight filaments extending from the core of microvilli deep into the cytoplasm (so that some authors call it a *brush cell*), and filaments encircling the apical region. Caveolated cells, although rare, are found not only in the crypts and villi of the small intestine, but also in the stomach and large intestine (Nabeyama and Leblond). Their role remains undetermined.

Mention should be made of migrating cells found within the epithelium. These include not only lymphocytes and other kinds of leukocytes, but also an interesting cell type known as the *globule leukocyte.* This kind of cell is present in the epithelium of normal and, more commonly, parasite-infested individuals. The globule leukocyte (Fig. 21-43) is characterized by having large inclusions with properties similar to those of mast cell granules. Cells similar to globule leukocytes are also occasionally seen in the lamina propria (Fig. 21-43).

Cell Renewal in the Epithelium of the Mucous Membrane

Radioautographic studies have shown that columnar cells dividing in the crypts appear on the surface of villi within 1 day. By about 3 days they reach the tips of the villi (Fig. 21-44) and become extruded into the intestinal lumen. Hence in experimental animals the intestinal epithelium is entirely renewed every third day. In man the turnover time is believed to be every 5 or 6 days.

Migration within the crypts is largely attributable to population pressure, since continuous procreation there squeezes cells up the walls of the crypts and out of their openings. However, if cell division is interrupted artificially cells continue to come out of the mouths of the crypts and ascend the villi. Hence migration up the villi seems to be due to ameboid movement of columnar cells.

The functions of the cells change somewhat during their journey to the tips of the villi. As noted, the production of surface glycoprotein declines as the tips are

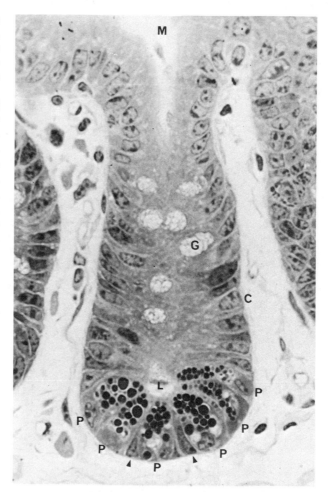

Fig. 21-39. Photomicrograph of a crypt of small intestine (mouse). From its base crowded with Paneth cells (P) to its mouth (M), cells surround its narrow lumen, part of which is seen at the base (L). The Paneth cells of the crypt base are recognizable by their granules. Those Paneth cells that have small granules (the two cells labeled P at *right*) are younger than those with large granules. Along the crypt walls, there are columnar cells (C) and mucous cells with light-staining mucus globules (G). The narrow cells indicated by small arrowheads between Paneth cells are crypt base columnar cells. (Courtesy of H. Cheng, J. Merzel, and C. P. Leblond)

reached. When Altmann measured protein synthesis from villus base to tip, a gradual decrease was noted. Thus it seemed that it might be a gradual decrease in the production of glycosylated protein that permitted cells to be liberated from the tips of villi. Then Altmann went on to show that an inhibitor of protein synthesis (cycloheximide) enhanced extrusion of cells from the villus tip. So it seems that a glycoprotein secreted by villus cells and deposited on their surface causes them to adhere to the

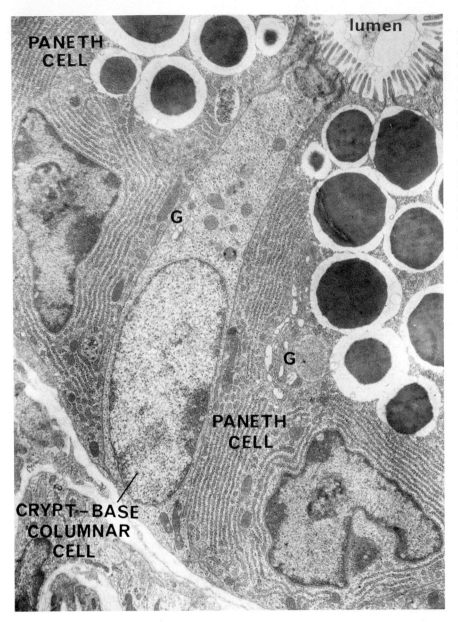

lumen

PANETH CELL

G

G

PANETH CELL

CRYPT–BASE COLUMNAR CELL

Fig. 21-40. Electron micrograph of a crypt base region of mouse intestine, showing a small columnar cell in between Paneth cells. This crypt base columnar cell (*middle*) has smooth lateral cell membranes. The cytoplasm is packed with free ribosomes; it also contains a poorly developed Golgi (G) and a few other organelles. This type of cell may be considered immature.

The cells on either side are Paneth cells characterized by their large zymogen granules, which have clear halos in the mouse. The Paneth cell at *right* shows the irregular nucleus characterizing mature Paneth cells. The Golgi apparatus is extensive (G). To its right, a pale ovoid prosecretory granule lies between the Golgi region and the dark secretory granules. (Courtesy of H. Cheng and C. P. Leblond)

basement membrane and to each other; as elaboration of this substance is gradually reduced, adhesion weakens to a point where the cells are extruded.

Goblet cells (Figs. 21-36 and 21-38), like columnar cells, arise from mitosis in the crypts. Typical goblet cells, however, do not divide. Mitosis occurs only in the oligomucous cells mentioned above and these later transform into typical goblet cells. There is evidence that the oligomucous cells come from the undifferentiated columnar cells at the base of the crypts. Later, goblet cells migrate

from crypt to villus in the same manner and at the same speed as the columnar cells to which they are bound by junctional complexes.

The least numerous of the cells of the crypts and villi are the enteroendocrine cells. These are of the various types described above. They all renew at about the same rate as the other cells (Ferreira and Leblond), to which they are also attached by junctional complexes. Incidentally, curious little tumors (carcinoids), not uncommon in the appendix, have been traced to enteroendocrine cells.

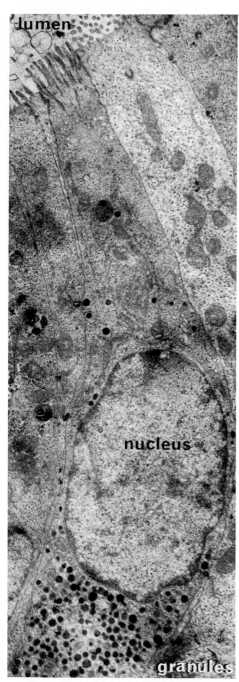

Fig. 21-41. Electron micrograph of an enteroendocrine cell of mouse small intestine, characterized by dense secretory granules in its basal region and a narrow apex reaching the lumen.

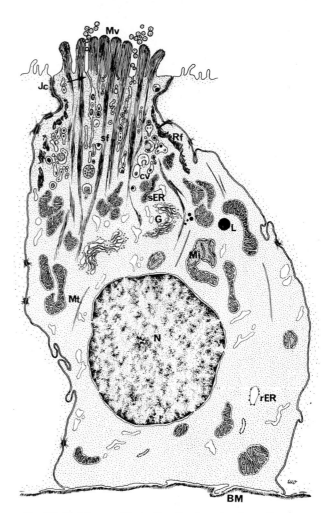

Fig. 21-42. Diagram illustrating the fine structure of a caveolated cell. It is characterized by its having caveolae, which are long irregular invaginations of the apical cell membrane that open between bases of microvilli (Mv), as indicated by the arrow at *top left.* Most caveolae are seen in cross section as vesicular profiles. Their lumina contain small spheres that are released from the caveolae. Microvilli, the cores of which consist of straight filaments that extends deep into the supranuclear region, are present on the apical surface. A ring of filaments (Rf) surrounds the apical region. (Courtesy of A. Nabeyama and C. P. Leblond)

Summary. The types of epithelial cells found in the lining of the small intestine and their relations and origins are shown in Figure 21-45. Here the various types of mature cells in the small intestine are shown above the cells that are intermediate between them and their common stem cell, the crypt base columnar cell.

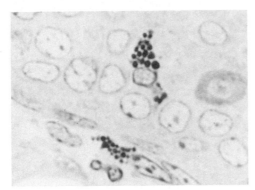

Fig. 21-43. Photomicrograph of intestinal epithelium, showing a globule leukocyte, recognized by large dense granules and a nucleus smaller than the nuclei of columnar cells nearby. At *bottom center* the lamina propria contains a similar cell. (Courtesy of R. Alexander)

Lamina Propria

The cores of villi are composed of lamina propria. In this particular site it consists of loose connective tissue with many of the attributes of lymphatic tissue. Its chief supporting element is a network of reticular fibers that extends throughout its substance and, at the sides and the tip of the villus, unites with the basement membrane under the surface epithelium. Branching cells with the pale cytoplasm are irregularly scattered throughout the

network and lymphocytes are common (Fig. 21-36). Plasma cells are fairly abundant and eosinophils are also sometimes seen. Furthermore, smooth muscle fibers extending from the muscularis mucosae are disposed along the axis of each villus, usually around a single large lymphatic capillary that ends blindly near its tip; this lymphatic capillary is usually termed the *lacteal* of the villus.

A single arterial twig from the submucosa usually penetrates the muscularis mucosae below each villus and ascends into it for some distance before breaking up into a capillary network. The capillaries approach the epithelial cells very closely. Separate arterial twigs break up into capillary nets surrounding the crypts of Lieberkühn. Nerve fibers from Meissner's plexus in the submucosa likewise penetrate the muscularis mucosae to ascend into each villus. Nodules of lymphatic tissue are not uncommon in the lamina propria of any part of the digestive tract, but they are particularly numerous in the small intestine, especially the ileum. They appear either singly, as solitary nodules, or in such close association with others that confluent masses are formed. The role of lymphatic tissue in the lamina propria was discussed in considering the general plan.

Solitary lymphatic nodules may be present almost anywhere in the lamina propria in the small intestine. They range from 0.5 to 3 mm. in diameter. Smaller ones are entirely confined to the lamina propria, but the larger ones may bulge through the muscularis mucosae into the submucosa. The epithelium over them and the other tissues

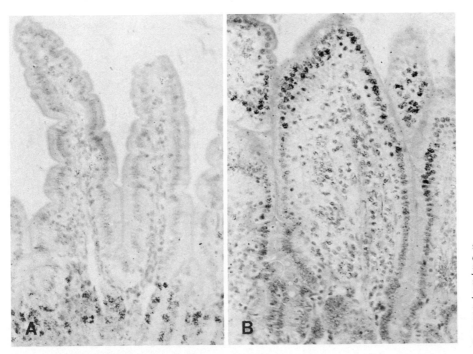

Fig. 21-44. Radioautographs showing how labeled epithelial cells migrate up the villi of mouse jejunum. (*A*) Labeled cells are seen in the crypts 8 hours after injecting tritiated thymidine. (*B*) After 3 days, the labeled cells have migrated to the tips of the villi. (Courtesy of C. P. Leblond and B. Messier)

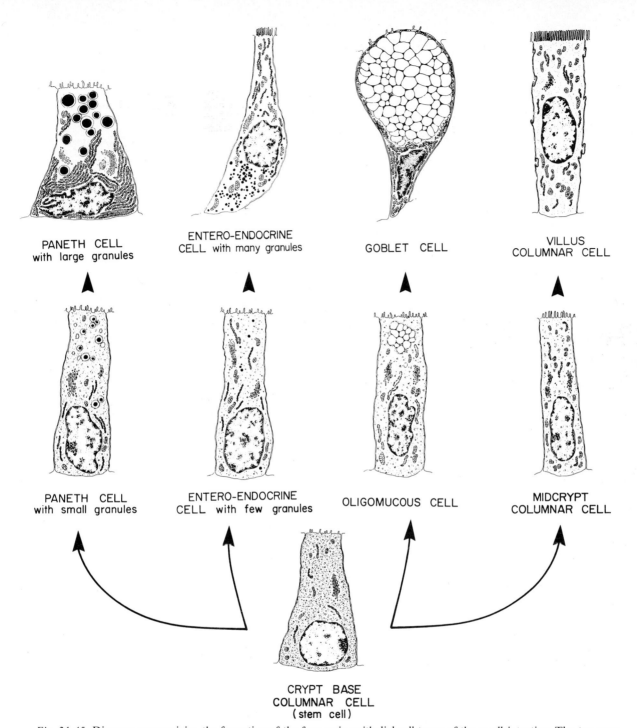

PANETH CELL
with large granules

ENTERO-ENDOCRINE
CELL with many granules

GOBLET CELL

VILLUS
COLUMNAR CELL

PANETH CELL
with small granules

ENTERO-ENDOCRINE
CELL with few granules

OLIGOMUCOUS CELL

MIDCRYPT
COLUMNAR CELL

CRYPT BASE
COLUMNAR CELL
(stem cell)

Fig. 21-45. Diagram summarizing the formation of the four main epithelial cell types of the small intestine. The top row shows mature cells; the second, intermediate cell types; the bottom row shows the crypt base columnar cell believed to be the stem cell of all these cell types.

The crypt base columnar cell divides actively. At *left*, a small proportion of cycling cells acquire a few granules characteristic of either Paneth or enteroendocrine cells, and later a full granule complement to become the corresponding mature cell. Some crypt base columnar cells acquire mucus globules (oligomucous cells in the third column); they remain able to divide and give rise to other mucous cells that accumulate more and more mucus. When the globules distend the cell apex into a goblet, the ability to divide is lost. The majority of crypt base columnar cells give rise to taller columnar cells found in the midcrypt region, as shown at *right*. These divide actively, giving rise to more columnar cells. Paneth cells degenerate in about 3 weeks but do not leave the crypt base. The three other cell types are bound together by junctional complexes and desmosomes; they migrate together toward the villus tips where they are lost to the lumen. (Courtesy of H. Cheng and C. P. Leblond)

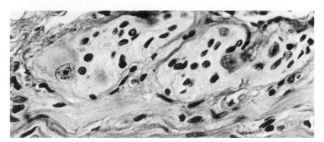

Fig. 21-46. High-power photomicrograph of part of the wall of the small intestine of a child, showing a portion of Auerbach's plexus between the two layers of the muscularis externa. Note the large ganglion cell at *left*. Its cytoplasm lies mostly above and to the left of its nucleus. Pale-staining unmyelinated nerve fibers and their Schwann cells (with dark nuclei) lie to the *right*. Smooth muscle cells are seen extending across the field at *bottom*.

about them are usually infiltrated with lymphocytes derived from these nodules. The larger confluent masses have an elongated oval shape and are confined to the side of the intestine opposite the mesenteric attachment. They vary from 1 to 12 cm. in length and from 1 to 2.5 cm. in width, and are called *Peyer's patches* after their discoverer. There are usually 20 to 30 of them, but more have been observed in young individuals. They are present mostly in the *lower part of the ileum,* where they are largest, but they are also found in the upper part of the ileum and lower part of the jejunum and have even been observed in the lower part of the duodenum. Villi are usually absent over them. They were of particular interest when typhoid fever was a prevalent disease, for in this condition they exhibit a profound inflammatory reaction and are common sites of ulceration, hemorrhage, and even perforation. Like lymphatic tissue as a whole, both solitary and confluent nodules become less prominent as an individual ages. In old age, Peyer's patches disappear almost completely.

The *muscularis mucosae* and the *submucosa* of the small intestine require no further description other than that given in the general plan.

The *muscularis externa* of the small intestine exhibits no special features, but sections of the small intestine provide a good opportunity for the student to see and examine the ganglion cells and nerve fibers of Auerbach's plexus, which coordinates peristaltic contractions. This is situated between the 2 muscle layers (Fig. 21-46).

Absorption From the Small Intestine

Sugars. Polysaccharide molecules are hydrolyzed only as far as disaccharides by pancreatic amylase. The final stage of their degradation into monosaccharides requires the participation of disaccharidases situated on the outer surface of microvilli of the villous columnar cells responsible for absorption, as described on page 680 (such enzymes are therefore sometimes referred to as "brush border enzymes"). Monosaccharides are readily absorbed by these columnar cells and pass into the blood capillaries coursing in the underlying lamina propria.

Proteins. These are broken down by several proteolytic enzymes into amino acids, in which form they are readily absorbed.

Fats. The digestion of fat in the intestine was described in Chapter 9 in connective with adipose tissue. The role of columnar absorptive cells of the small intestine in absorbing the products of digestion of fat and the formation of chylomicrons and their entrance into lymphatics were considered on page 240. Triglycerides are not taken up into columnar cells, but their breakdown products (fatty acids, monoglycerides, and possibly glycerol itself) are. In the gut lumen, these substances are combined into particles called *micelles,* 5nm. in diameter, that are produced under the influence of bile acids. There is difference of opinion as to whether micelles are absorbed as such by columnar cells or release their component fatty acids, monoglycerides and glycerol at the cell surface for absorption, but the latter seems more likely. In their free or micellar state, these substances enter columnar cells readily by a diffusion process that does not require energy.

Once within the cells, fatty acids, monoglycerides and possibly glycerol find their way into the endoplasmic reticulum (both smooth and rough ER seem to be involved), where they are recombined into fats by a process that does require energy. The rebuilt fat is readily visible in the EM within cisternae of sER.

Some authors believe the newly synthesized fat migrates from sER to the Golgi and comes out of the Golgi in fat-containing vesicles that open by exocytosis at the *lateral* cell membrane and thus release their fat content to the intercellular spaces. Other authors deny the passage of fat through the Golgi apparatus, but all agree that the newly synthesized fat does find its way into the intercellular spaces.

The fat appearing outside the cell is readily seen in the EM, for instance 1 hour after a fatty meal. It is in the form of globules enclosed by a very delicate protein-containing layer. These globules are known as *chylomicrons* and contain triglycerides, which make up 86 per cent of their weight, and also 8.5 per cent phospholipid, and 3 per cent cholesterol, as well as 2 per cent protein (probably associated with their outside layer).

The chylomicrons then pass into the small lymphatic vessels of the lamina propria and, from there, mostly into the thoracic duct, which delivers them to the main circulation. Their fate was discussed in connection with mast cells in Chapter 9 on page 247 and will be discussed further in connection with the liver in the next chapter (p. 716).

The lymphatics that drain the intestine contain considerable amounts of emulsified fat after a fatty meal; this creamy lymph is termed *chyle.*

Fig. 21-47. Medium-power photomicrographs of part of the wall of the large intestine, showing its mucous membrane. (*A*) Crypts of Lieberkühn cut in oblique section. (*B*) Crypts cut in longitudinal section. They extend down to the muscularis mucosae, which lies near the bottom margin in both pictures. Note the abundant goblet cells (pale-staining); the other epithelial cells are absorptive.

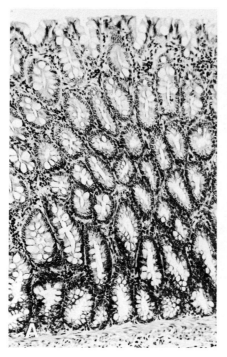
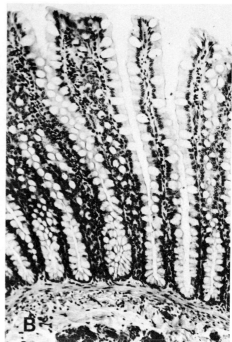

THE LARGE INTESTINE

Parts. The large intestine consists of the *cecum, (vermiform) appendix, ascending, transverse, descending* and *pelvic colons,* and *rectum* (including the *anal canal*). It terminates at the *anus* ((Fig. 21-1).

Function. The unabsorbed residue from the small intestine is emptied into the cecum in a fluid state. By the time the contents reach the descending colon, however, they have acquired the consistency of feces. Absorption of water by the mucous membrane is thus an important function of the large intestine.

Although a great deal of mucus is present in the alkaline secretion of the large intestine, no enzymes of importance are secreted with it. Nevertheless, some digestion occurs in its lumen. Part of this is due to enzymes derived from the small intestine remaining active in the material delivered into the large intestine, and part is to be explained by the putrefactive action of bacteria that thrive in its lumen breaking down cellulose which, if consumed in the diet, survives to reach the large intestine because the intestine of man secretes no enzymes capable of degrading it.

Feces consist of bacteria, products of bacterial putrefaction, such undigested material as survives passage through the large intestine, cellular debris from the lining of the intestine, mucus, and a few other substances.

MICROSCOPIC STRUCTURE

The mucous membrane of the large intestine differs from that of the small intestine in several respects. It has *no villi* in postnatal life. It is thicker; hence the crypts of Lieberkühn are deeper (Fig. 21-47). The crypts, which are distributed all over the lining surface of the large intestine, contain *no Paneth cells* (except in the young), but they usually have more *goblet cells* than are present in the small intestine (Fig. 21-47) and the proportion of goblet cells increases from the beginning of the colon to the rectum. The ordinary surface epithelial cells have striated borders like those of the small intestine. Finally, enteroendocrine cells of the various types already described are present.

Cell migration occurs in the large intestine, with epithelial cells dividing in the lower half of the crypts and migrating to the surface, where they are eventually extruded to the lumen.

At the base of the crypts in the colon and rectum, there are immature-looking cells believed to function as stem cells for the epithelium. However, whereas the presumptive stem cells in the ascending colon appear to be small columnar cells, those of descending colon and rectum contain secretory vacuoles in their apex and are, in fact, often called *vacuolated cells* (V in Fig. 21-48). As these cells migrate toward the crypt mouth, they at first become

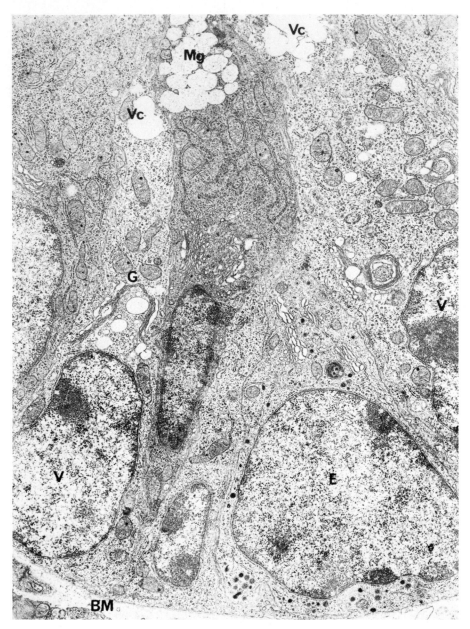

Fig. 21-48. Electron micrograph of a crypt base of descending colon. The columnar cells contain pale secretory vacuoles (Vc) and are often referred to as vacuolated cells (V). The Golgi apparatus (G) shows developing secretory vacuoles. The cytoplasm of these cells is lighter than that of the oligomucous cell seen at *middle,* in which a group of mucus globules (Mg) may be distinguished. At *lower right,* a young enteroendocrine cell (E) contains only a few dense granules.

As vacuolated cells migrate toward the crypt mouth, they become typical columnar cells with microvilli packed into a striated border. (Courtesy of A. Nabeyama)

filled with secretory vacuoles but, before approaching the surface, they lose all their vacuoles and become typical columnar cells with microvilli packed into a striated border (Chang and Leblond).

Crypts of Lieberkühn are not found in the anorectal canal at the junction of rectal and anal epithelium. The stratified squamous anal epithelium is not keratinized and extends over about 2 cm. At its outer border it becomes continuous with the stratified keratinized epidermis of the skin and on its inner border with the simple columnar epithelium that lines the remainder of the rectum. At the junction between anal and columnar epithelium, circumanal glands are present. These glands have a stratified columnar epithelium and are of the branched tubular type but do not seem to be actively functioning. They probably constitute an atrophic organ corresponding to functioning glands of certain mammals.

In the anorectal canal, the mucous membrane is thrown into a series of longitudinal folds known as the *rectal columns* or *columns of Morgagni.* Below, adjacent columns are connected by folds. This arrangement produces a series of so-called *anal valves.* The concavities of the pockets so formed are called *rectal sinuses.*

The muscularis mucosae continues only to the region of the longitudinal folds, and in them it breaks up into bundles and finally disappears. Hence there is not the same demarcation between lamina propria and submucosa in this region as in other parts of the tract. The merging lamina propria and submucosa contain many convolutions of small veins. A very common condition, *internal hemorrhoids,* is the result of the dilatation of these veins so that they bulge the mucous membrane inward and encroach on the lumen of the anal canal. *External hemorrhoids* result from the dilatation of veins at, and close to, the anus.

Muscularis Externa. In the large intestine this layer differs somewhat from its arrangement in other parts of the tract. Beginning in the cecum, the longitudinally disposed fibers of the outer coat, though present to a certain extent over the whole circumference of the bowel, are for the most part collected into 3 flat bands, the *teniae coli.* These are not as long as the intestine along which they are disposed; hence, they are responsible for gathering the wall of this part of the bowel into sacculations (*haustra*). Thus if the teniae are cut or stripped away, the bowel immediately enlongates, and the sacculations disappear. The 3 teniae extend from the cecum to the rectum, where they spread out and fuse to some extent so as to form a muscle coat that is thicker on the anterior and posterior aspects of the rectum than on its sides. The anterior and

the posterior aggregates of longitudinal smooth muscle are somewhat shorter than the rectum itself, and this results in a type of sacculation in this region also. It causes the underlying wall of the rectum to bulge inward to form two transverse shelves, one from the right and a smaller one from the left, called the *plicae transversales* of the rectum. These help to support the weight of the rectal contents and so make the work of the anal sphincter less arduous.

The circularly disposed smooth muscle fibers of the inner coat of the muscularis externa form a thicker coat between sacculations than they do over sacculations. In the anal canal they are increased to form a sphincter muscle, the *internal sphincter of the anus.*

Serosa. Along the colon and upper part of the rectum, the serous coat leaves the outer surface of the intestine at regular intervals to form little peritoneal sacs that enclose fat. These peritoneal redundancies hang from the external surface of the bowel and are termed *appendices epiploicae.* In some sites they contain only loose connective tissue.

THE VERMIFORM APPENDIX

This worm-like appendage of the cecum (Fig. 21-1) is the seat of so much disease that it merits separate description. Developmentally, it is the lower, blind end of the cecum that has failed to enlarge as rapidly as the remainder, and as a result it appears as a diverticulum arising

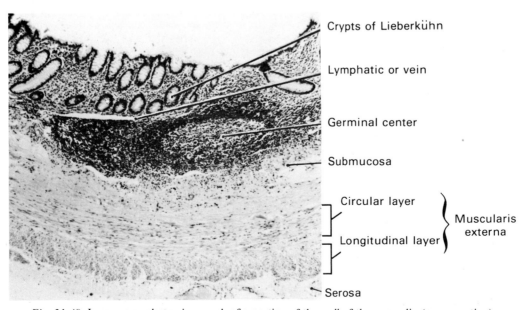

Fig. 21-49. Low-power photomicrograph of a portion of the wall of the appendix (cross section).

from the cecum, 1 inch or less below the entrance of the ileum. In many animals it is larger than in man and so provides a good-sized pouch off the main track of the intestine where cellulose can be subjected to prolonged digestion. In man it is too short and has too narrow a lumen to serve a similar function. Indeed, its form is commonly so bent and twisted that the lumen is often blocked, thus enhancing the danger of bacterial activity destroying not only the contents of the lumen but also the lining of the organ itself. As a result, organisms sometimes gain entrance to the tissues of its wall and lead to its infection. For this reason, surgical removal of the infected organ (*appendectomy*) is one of the commonest abdominal operations.

The appendix usually is studied microscopically by means of cross sections (Fig. 21-49). In preparations of this sort, the lumen of the appendix of a young person often appears somewhat 3-cornered instead of circular. In adults it is usually rounder, and in advancing years it may have become obliterated by connective tissue replacing its mucous membrane as well as filling its lumen.

The epithelium of the mucous membrane is similar to that of the large intestine (Fig. 21-49). However, the lamina propria contains *much more lymphatic tissue;* indeed, confluent lymphatic nodules may completely surround the lumen, though the amount diminishes with age. The muscularis mucosae is not well developed and may be missing in some areas. A few eosinophils are normally present in the lamina propria but, if present in the submucosa, are considered as being of significance in indicating a chronic inflammatory condition of the organ. Neutrophils in any numbers in the lamina propria or any other layer of the appendix wall indicate an acute inflammatory lesion (*acute appendicitis*). The muscularis externa conforms to the general plan in the intestine, and the longitudinal fibers form a complete coat. The appendix has a rudimentary mesentery.

REFERENCES AND OTHER READING

ORAL CAVITY AND SALIVARY GLANDS

Dewey, M. M.: A histochemical and biochemical study of the parotid gland in normal and hypophysectomized rats. Am. J. Anat., *102:*243, 1958.

Garrett, J. R., Harrison, J. D., and Stoward, P. J.: Histochemistry of Secretory Process. London, Chapman Hall, 1977.

Parks, H. F.: Morphological study of the extrusion of secretory materials by the parotid glands of mouse and rat. J. Ultrastruct. Res., *6:*449, 1962.

Travill, A.: The effect of pregnancy on the submandibular glands of mice. Anat. Rec., *155:*217, 1966.

Travill, A. A., and Hill, M. F.: Histochemical demonstration of myoepithelial cell activity. Q. J. Exp. Physiol., *48:*423, 1963.

TASTE BUDS

Beidler, L. N., and Smallman, R. L. S.: Renewal of cells within taste buds. J. Cell Biol., *27:*263, 1965.

Murray, R. G., Murray, A., and Fujimoto, S.: Fine structure of gustatory cells. J. Ultrastruct. Res., *27:*444, 1969.

TEETH

GENERAL REFERENCES

Books and Symposia

Anderson, D. J., Estoe, J. E., Melcher, A. H., and Picton, D. C. A. (eds.): The Mechanism of Tooth Support — A Symposium. Bristol, John Wright, 1967.

Gaunt, W. A., Osborne, J. W., and Ten Cate, A. R.: Advances in Dental Histology. Bristol, John Wright, 1967.

Stack, M. V., and Fernhead, R. W. (ed.): Tooth Enamel. Its Composition, Properties and Fundamental Structure. Bristol, John Wright, 1965.

Symons, N. B. B. (ed.): Dentine and Pulp: Their Structure and Reactions. Edinburgh, Livingstone, 1967.

Ten Cate, A. R.: Oral Histology. Chicago, Science Research Associates, 1979.

Termine, J., and Nylen, M.: Proceedings of the third international symposium on tooth enamel. J. Dent. Res., *in press.*

SPECIAL REFERENCES

Garant, P. R., and Nalbandian, J.: Observations on the ultrastructure of ameloblasts with special reference to the Golgi complex and related components. J. Ultrastruct. Res., *23:*427, 1968.

Garant, P., Szabo, G., and Nalbandian, J.: The fine structure of the mouse odontoblast. Arch. Oral Biol., *13:*857, 1968.

Kallenbach, E.: The cell web in the ameloblasts of the rat incisor. Anat. Rec., *153:*55, 1963.

Leblond, C. P., and Weinstock, M.: A comparative study of dentin and bone formation. *In* Bourne, G. H. (ed.): Biochemistry and Physiology of Bone. vol. 4, p. 517. New York, Academic Press, 1976.

Reith, E. J.: The ultrastructure of ameloblasts during early stages of maturation of enamel. J. Cell Biol., *18:*691, 1963.

Slaven, H. C., and Bavetta, L. A. (eds.): Developmental Aspects of Oral Biology. New York, Academic Press, 1972.

Warshawsky, H.: The fine structure of secretory ameloblasts in rat incisors. Anat. Rec., *161:*211, 1968.

———: A light and electron microscope study of the nearly mature enamel of rat incisors. Anat. Rec., *169:*559, 1971.

Weinstock, M., and Leblond, C. P.: Radioautographic visualization of the deposition of a phosphoprotein at the mineralization front in the dentin of the rat incisor. J. Cell Biol., *56:*838, 1973.

———: Synthesis, migration and release of precursor collagen by odontoblasts as visualized by radioautography after ^{3}H-proline administration. J. Cell Biol., *60:*92, 1974.

ESOPHAGUS AND STOMACH

Comprehensive General References on Stomach and Intestine

Crane, R. K. (ed.): Gastrointestinal Physiology II. International Review of Physiology. vol. 12. Baltimore, University Park Press, 1977.

Friedman, M. H. F. (ed.): Functions of the Stomach and Intestine. Baltimore, University Park Press, 1975.

Johnson, L. R. (ed.): Gastrointestinal Physiology. St. Louis, C. V. Mosby, 1977.

Special References

Bertalanffy, F. D.: Cell renewal in the gastrointestinal tract of man. Gastroenterology, *43:*472, 1962.

Ito, S.: The fine structure of the gastric mucosa. *In* Proc. Symp. Gastric Secretion; Mechanisms and Control. p. 3. Oxford, Pergamon, 1967.

————: Anatomic structure of the gastric mucosa. *In* American Physiological Society: Handbook of Physiology. Section 6 (Cole, C. F., ed.): Alimentary Canal. vol. 2, p. 705. Baltimore, Williams & Wilkins, 1967.

Ito, S., and Winchester, R. J. The fine structure of the gastric mucosa in the bat. J. Cell Biol., *16:*541, 1963.

Marques-Pereira, J. P., and Leblond, C. P.: Mitosis and differentiation in the stratified squamous epithelium of the rat esophagus. Am. J. Anat., *117:*73, 1965.

Sedar, A. W.: The fine structure of the oxyntic cell in relation to functional activity of the stomach. Ann. N.Y. Acad. Sci., *99:*9, 1962.

————: Stomach and intestinal mucosa. *In* Electron Microscope Anatomy. p. 123. New York, Academic Press, 1964.

Zeitoun, P., Duclert, N., Liautaud, F., Potet, F., and Zylberberg, L.: Intracellular localization of pepsinogen in guinea pig pyloric mucosa by immunohistochemistry. Histochemical and electron microscopic correlated structures. Lab. Invest., *27:*218, 1972.

SMALL AND LARGE INTESTINE

Altmann, G. G.: Factors involved in the differentiation of the epithelial cells in the adult rat small intestine. *In* Cairnie, A. B., Lala, P. K., and Osmond, D. G. (eds.): Stem Cells of Renewing Cell Populations. New York, Academic Press, 1976.

Bertalanffy, F. D., and Nagy, K. P.: Mitotic activity and renewal rate of the epithelial cells of human duodenum. Acta Anat., *45:*362, 1961.

Bloom, S. R. (ed.): Gut Hormones. Edinburgh, Churchill, 1978.

Cardell, R. R., Jr., Badenhausen, S., and Porter, K. R.: Intestinal triglyceride absorption in the rat. J. Cell Biol., *34:*123, 1967.

Chang, W. W. L., and Leblond. C. P.: Renewal of the epithelium in the descending colon of the mouse. I. Presence of three cell populations: vacuolated-columnar, mucous, and argentaffin. Am. J. Anat., *131:*73, 1971.

Cheng, H., and Leblond, C. P.: Origin, differentiation and renewal of the four main epithelial cell types in the mouse small intestine. I. Columnar cells. Am. J. Anat., *141:*461, 1974 (and the 4 next articles).

Ferreira, M. N., and Leblond, C. P.: Argentaffin and other "endocrine" cells of the small intestine in the adult mouse. II. Renewal. Am. J. Anat., *131:*331, 1971.

Irwin, D. A.: The anatomy of Auerbach's plexus. Am. J. Anat., *49:*141, 1931.

Leblond, C. P., and Cheng, H.: Identification of stem cells in the small intestine of the mouse. *In* Cairnie, A. B., Lala, P. K., and Osmond, G. G. (eds.): Stem Cells of Renewing Cell Populations. New York, Academic Press, 1976.

Leblond, C. P., and Walker, B. E.: Renewal of cell populations. Physiol. Rev., *36:*255, 1956.

Lesher, S., Fry, R. J. M., and Cohn, H. I.: Age and degeneration time of the mouse duodenal epithelial cell. Exp. Cell Res., *24:*334, 1961.

Lipkin, M., Sherlock, P., and Bell, B.: Cell proliferation kinetics in the gastrointestinal tract of man. II. Cell renewal in stomach, ileum, colon, and rectum. Gastroenterology, *45:*721, 1963.

Merzel, J., and Leblond, C. P.: Origin and renewal of goblet cells in the epithelium of the mouse small intestine. Am. J. Anat., *124:*281, 1969.

Moe, H.: The goblet cells, Paneth cells and basal granular cells of the epithelium of the intestine. Int. Rev. Gen. Exp. Zool., *3:*241, 1968.

Mooseker, M. S.: Brush border motility. Microvillar contraction in Triton-treated brush borders isolated from intestinal epithelium. J. Cell Biol., *71:*417, 1976.

Neutra, M., and Leblond, C. P.: Synthesis of the carbohydrate of mucus in the Golgi complex, as shown by electron microscope radioautography of goblet cells from rats injected with ^{3}H-glucose. J. Cell Biol., *30:*119, 1966.

Palay, S. L., and Revel, J. P.: The morphology of fat absorption. *In* Meng, H. C.: Lipid transport. pp. 1–11. Springfield, Ill., Charles C Thomas, 1964.

Richardson, K. C.: Electron microscopic observations on Auerbach's plexus in the rabbit, with special reference to the problem of smooth muscle innervation. Am. J. Anat., *103:*99, 1958.

Spencer, R. P.: The Intestinal Tract; Structure, Function and Pathology in Terms of the Basic Sciences. Springfield, Ill., Charles C Thomas, 1960.

Strauss, E. W.: Morphological Aspects of Triglyceride Absorption. *In* Codel, C. F., and Heidel, W. (eds.): Handbook of Physiology. vol. 3, sec. 6, chap. 71. American Physiological Society, Washington, 1968.

Trier, J. S.: Studies on small intestinal crypt epithelium of the proximal small intestine of fasting humans. J. Cell Biol., *18:*599, 1963.

Weirnik, G., Shroter, R. G., and Creamer, B.: The arrest of intestinal epithelial "turnover" by the use of x-irradiation. Gut, *3:*26, 1962.

22 The Pancreas, Liver, and Gallbladder

THE PANCREAS

General Features. The pancreas lies in the abdomen with its head resting in the concavity of the duodenum and its body extending toward the spleen, which its tail touches. A fresh pancreas is white with a pink tinge. Its surface appears lobulated because its capsule is thin enough not to obscure the structure beneath it.

The pancreas is *both an exocrine and an endocrine gland.* The bulk of its cells are arranged in acini (Fig. 5-19); these produce its exocrine secretion. This is collected and delivered by a duct system into the duodenum. The functions of the exocrine secretion in digestion were described on page 679. The endocrine secretion is made by little clumps of cells, richly supplied with capillaries and scattered throughout its substance (Fig. 22-1, islet). These little endocrine units are termed *islets* and named after Langerhans, who described them. The first hormone shown to be produced by the *islets of Langerhans* was called *insulin* (L. *insula,* island). Insufficient production of this hormone leads to *diabetes mellitus,* a disease that will be described when the islets of Langerhans are described in Chapter 25. The production of a second hormone, *glucagon* (*see* Chap. 25), was subsequently also attributed to the islets.

Development. The pancreas develops from 2 outgrowths from the epithelial (endodermal) lining of the developing duodenum. The developing duct system gives rise to acini whose exocrine secretion drains into the duct system, and to little islands of cells that will be endocrine units and empty their secretion into the bloodstream.

The clumps of cells destined to become islets fail to develop a lumen. In many instances (though by no means always) these clumps of cells become completely detached from the duct system to become truly isolated islets of Langerhans. The developing duct system gives rise to an ill-defined network of cords or tubules of cells disposed irregularly through the substance of the pancreas between acini. The cells of this network are relatively undifferentiated, and under certain circumstances they appear to give rise to new endocrine cells. This is the probable origin of those islet cells that sometimes seem to be scattered singly among the acini.

THE MICROSCOPIC STRUCTURE OF THE PANCREAS

Capsule

The connective tissue *capsule* that separates the pancreatic tissue from adjacent structures is remarkably *thin;* indeed it scarcely merits being called a capsule. The capsule is covered with peritoneum.

Septa

Partitions (*septa*) of connective tissue extend in from the capsule to divide the pancreas into *lobules.* These septa, like the capsule, are very *thin* (Fig. 22-1, interlobular septum). Furthermore, separation commonly occurs along them when pancreatic tissue is fixed, and in sections lobules are often clearly indicated because they are separated by artifacts.

Although the septa are thin, considerable condensations of dense connective tissue are often present around the main duct of the organ and its more immediate branches (Fig. 22-1, interlobular duct). These provide some internal support.

Acini

These comprise most of the substance of lobules. The way to find individual acini was described in Chapter 5 in connection with Figure 5-19 (*see* p. 123).

Within lobules acini are packed together in a most irregular way, with little loose connective tissue containing capillaries between them, so that a section cuts across acini in every conceivable plane. Most are cut in oblique section. In many sections of pancreas acini do not stand out clearly as individual structures. It may be helpful to realize that under the high-power objective an acinus is approximately one tenth of the field in width. Since the nuclei of the secretory cells that make up the acinus lie toward their bases, the nuclei in a single acinus tend to be arranged so as to form a rough ring of nuclei in its outer part (Fig. 22-2). The sides of the more or less pyramidal cells fitted together to form acini are so close together that cell boundaries between individual cells are not always

Fig. 22-1. Very low power photomicrograph of the pancreas, showing islets (*top left* and *bottom right*), a large interlobular duct (just below *center*), intralobular ducts, acini, and an interlobular septum (extending along *bottom*).

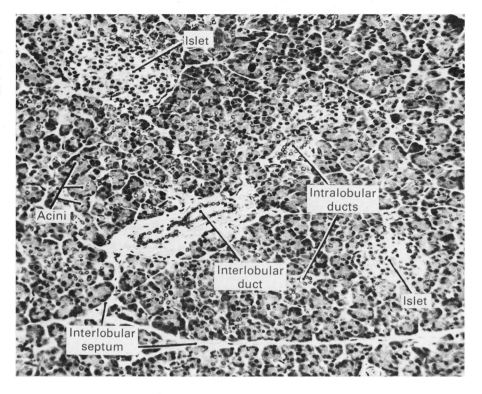

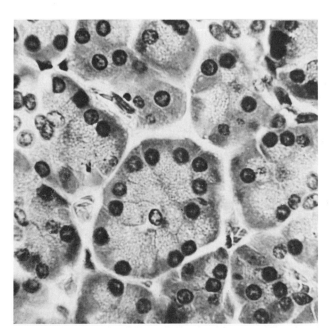

Fig. 22-2. High-power photomicrograph of a pancreatic acinus with the nucleus of a centro-acinar cell at its center.

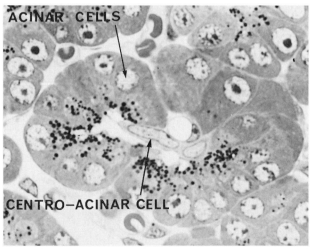

Fig. 22-3. Photomicrograph of a pancreatic acinus, stained with toluidine blue. The acinus is cut in such a way as to show a centro-acinar cell and the beginning of an intercalated duct. Zymogen granules are prominent in the acinar cells. (Courtesy of Y. Clermont)

distinct (Fig. 22-2). The apices of the cells of an acinus do not quite meet in the middle of each acinus; hence, a very small lumen is present in this site (Figs. 5-19 and 22-3). The cytoplasm between the nucleus and apex of each secretory cell contains acidophilic zymogen granules

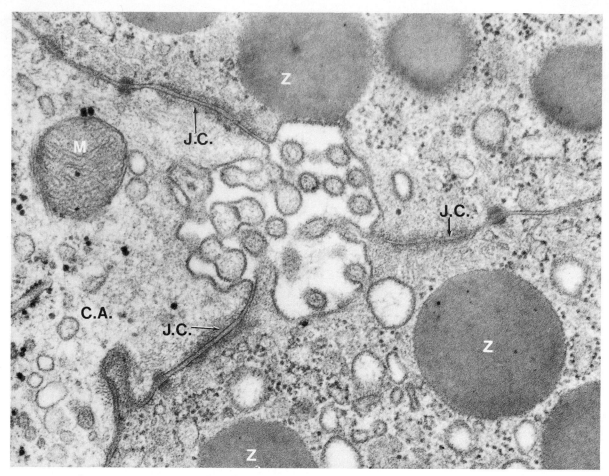

Fig. 22-4. Electron micrograph (×50,000) of a section through the lumen of a pancreatic acinus (guinea pig). At *center,* microvilli project into the lumen. The cell at *left* is a centro-acinar cell (C.A.). It is distinguished readily by an absence of zymogen granules; it does, however, contain a mitochondrion (M). At *top* a zymogen granule (Z) is about to be secreted from an acinar cell. Another acinar cell is seen at *lower right.* Junctional complexes (J.C.) are present at each site where the membranes of adjacent cells come into contact close to the lumen. (Farquhar, M. G., and Palade, G. E.: J. Cell Biol., *17:*375, 1963)

(Figs. 7-22 and 22-3). The nuclei are rounded and lie toward but not against the bases of the cells; they exhibit prominent nucleoli. The cytoplasm between the nuclei and the bases of the cells, and on each side of the nuclei, is basophilic because of its content of rRNA (Fig. 22-2), as expected in a cell synthesizing a great deal of protein.

Centro-acinar Cells

Nuclei can often be seen in the central part of an acinus (Fig. 22-2). These are the nuclei of what are appropriately termed *centro-acinar cells.* If an acinus is cut centrally (which happens once in a while), these cells can be seen to be cells of the little so-called *intercalated duct* that drains the acinus (Fig. 22-3). These ducts will be de-

scribed in due course. The proximal duct cells, lying on what would seem to be one side of the little duct, are more or less *invaginated into the lumen* of the acinus on one side, as is shown in Figure 22-3. Since the duct cells thus begin in the *center* of an acinus, they are termed *centro-acinar cells.*

The Fine Structure of Acinar Cells

This, together with the mechanism of secretion, was dealt with in detail in Chapter 5 and illustrated in Figure 5-21.

The junctional complexes between the borders of adjacent acinar cells close to the lumen of an acinus are illustrated in Figure 22-4. They are of the same type as those between the lining cells of the intestine. There are *zonulae occludentes* (continuous tight junctions) between their lateral borders close to the lumen. Below these there are *zonulae adherentes* (belt desmosomes), and also spot *desmosomes* deeper down toward the bases of the cells. Figure 22-4 also shows zymogen granules about to be secreted in the apices of acinar cells and that the centro-acinar cell at *left* (seen in the illustration) contains no zymogen granules because it is a duct type of cell. Both centro-acinar and acinar cells have short microvilli on their free borders (Fig. 22-4).

A delicate reticular connective tissue fills the space between individual acini and brings capillaries close to the bases of the secretory cells. The bases are covered with a thin basement membrane enclosing the whole acinus. Some of the capillaries have fenestrated endothelium. Nerve fibers of the autonomic system are also conveyed in this connective tissue.

Finding Islets of Langerhans

If in H and E sections enough lobules are inspected with the low-power objective, pale areas considerably larger than cross or oblique sections of acini will be seen (Fig. 22-1, islet). These areas are *islets of Langerhans* and contain cords and irregular clumps of cells and capillaries. However, it takes practice to identify islets readily with the low-power objective; a beginner may confuse an islet with a duct or a little patch of connective tissue. With the high-power objective, its characteristic structure of cords and clumps of cells separated by capillaries can be seen clearly. Islets are *not* encapsulated and so are separated from acinar tissue by only a trace of reticular tissue. Internal support in islets is provided by reticular fibers that are associated with capillaries. But there is not much connective tissue in islets; otherwise, the secretion of the cells might have difficulty gaining entrance to the capillaries.

How the Amount of Islet Tissue in a Pancreas Is Determined

Any estimate of the relative amount of islet tissue made from a single section has little value. The total amount of islet tissue could, of course, be determined by cutting a pancreas into serial sections and measuring the area of islets seen in each and every section. Bensley, however, described a simpler method in which he perfused the blood vessels of the fresh organ with neutral red or Janus green. As reduction occurs on standing, the dye fades from the acinar tissue, so that the islets stand out as either red or blue areas, depending on the dye used (Fig. 22-5). If pancreas so prepared is cut into little pieces it can be mounted on slides and observers can count the number of

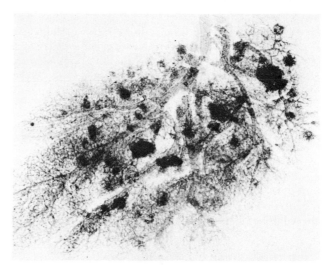

Fig. 22-5. Very low power photomicrograph of a piece of pancreas (from guinea pig) perfused with Janus green. The blood vessels subsequently were injected with opaque material. The islets appear as dark patches, and the network in which they lie corresponds to the injected blood vessels. (Courtesy of S. Bensley)

islets in the pieces and so determine the total number of islets in the pancreas. Other technics based on the same staining principles permit not only the number of islets but also the total volume of islet tissue to be estimated.

The different types of cells in islets and their appearance in different physiological states will be described in Chapter 25.

Ducts

Before describing the microscopic appearance of ducts, their general arrangement should be explained. The main duct of the pancreas (duct of Wirsung) is enveloped by connective tissue and serves as a backbone. From it, side branches emerge regularly at an angle, so that the duct system resembles a herring bone. The side branches run between lobules and hence are *interlobular* ducts. These branch to give rise to *intralobular* ducts, which enter the substance of lobules. Intralobular ducts are not nearly so prominent in the pancreas as they are in salivary glands. A relative *paucity of intralobular ducts* is, then, a useful criterion by which a student can quickly distinguish a section of pancreas from parotid gland (which it closely resembles in many respects). The presence of islets of Langerhans in the lobules is, of course, another, but in some preparations more than a glance is needed before islets are noticed and identified with certainty.

The larger of the relatively few intralobular ducts are ensheathed by dense connective tissue derived from the septa from which they emerge (Fig. 22-1). The intralobular ducts give rise to very small ducts lined with flattened epithelium. These lead to acini and are called *intercalated* (L. *intercalare,* to insert) *ducts* because they are inserted, as it were, between the secretory units and intralobular ducts proper. As noted, the intercalated ducts extend into the central part of acini and are seen as centro-acinar cells (Figs. 22-2, 22-3, and 22-4).

The lumen of the main duct is lined by columnar epithelium and goblet cells may be interspersed between ordinary columnar cells. Near the duodenum, small mucous glands may be associated with the main duct. The interlobular ducts are lined by low columnar epithelium. In the intralobular ducts, the epithelium is low columnar to cuboidal, and in the intercalated ducts, flattened cuboidal.

THE CONTROL OF EXOCRINE SECRETION OF THE PANCREAS

Pancreatic juice contains many important enzymes (including trypsin, chymotrypsin, lipase, DNAase, RNAase, phospholipase A, amylase, carboxypeptidases A and B, and elastase) that are needed to carry on further digestion of food that has passed through the stomach. There is a need for a mechanism to regulate pancreatic secretion in accordance with deliveries of stomach contents into the duodenum. Such a mechanism exists in the form of 2 hormones made by the mucosa of the duodenum when the acid contents of the stomach are delivered into it. The hormones circulate to the capillaries of the pancreas and stimulate exocrine secretion. *Secretin* stimulates secretion of the nonenzymatic ingredients of pancreatic juice, so its action may be primarily on cells of the small ducts. The second hormone, *pancreozymin,* however, is much more effective than secretin in stimulating secretion of enzyme-rich pancreatic juice, so it is believed to act on acinar cells. Stimulation of the vagus nerve induces some secretion, but the control of secretion seems to be primarily hormonal.

MAINTENANCE OF THE ACINAR CELL POPULATION

It might be thought that acinar cells would be so highly specialized that they would have lost their ability to divide. However, in studies on diabetes induced with anterior pituitary extracts, Ham and Haist found numerous mitotic figures in acinar cells as well as duct cells. This effect was probably due to growth hormone in the extracts used. It therefore seems that under ordinary conditions mitosis can occur in acinar cells to replenish their numbers as they wear out.

THE LIVER

LIVER STRUCTURE, FROM GROSS TO MICROSCOPIC

The liver is a huge gland, the largest in the body, weighing about 3 pounds in the adult. It is reddish brown and covered with a thin strong connective tissue *capsule* often termed *Glisson's capsule.* Most of the liver lies on the right side of the body, with its smooth upper convex surface fitting the undersurface of the dome-shaped diaphragm (Fig. 21-1). It has two main lobes, with the right being much larger than the left (Fig. 21-1). Its inferior surface is exposed in Figure 21-1, showing the impressions of the several organs it normally contacts (parts of the alimentary tract and the right kidney, which are separated from it in Figure 21-1), so its inferior surface is often called its *visceral* surface. This surface exhibits a short deep transverse fissure called the *porta* (L. for door) of the liver (not shown in Fig. 21-1). The porta is of particular interest with regard to the microscopic structure of the organ as follows.

The liver, like other glands, consists of parenchyma and stroma. The parenchyma consists of epithelial cells of endodermal origin termed liver cells, or more commonly, *hepatocytes.* The stroma is derived from mesoderm and consists of ordinary connective tissue. The liver is both an exocrine and an endocrine gland. Its endocrine secretions are delivered into the bloodstream as will be described persently. Its exocrine secretion is termed *bile* and is delivered into a duct system that eventually empties it into the duodenum.

The liver has a unique blood supply because it is supplied both with venous and arterial blood. The former is blood that as arterial blood supplied a major part of the intestinal tract, where the capillaries through which it circulated absorbed, for example, glucose and amino acids resulting from digestion of starch and proteins within the tract and other substances besides. This blood, more or less laden with products of digestion, drains into the *portal vein,* which enters the liver at its porta. However, the liver also requires arterial blood and this is delivered to it by the hepatic artery, which also enters the liver at its porta. Moreover, since the liver is both an exocrine and an endocrine gland, in serving the first role it must have a duct system. Its exocrine secretion, *bile,* is collected in the liver as will be described presently. The terminal duct into which it is collected is termed the *hepatic duct* and this *leaves* the liver at its porta. Furthermore, some lymph is formed in the liver and this is drained away from the liver by lymphatics that converge near the porta and leave it at that site. (The venous drainage of the liver is accomplished by hepatic veins; these, however, make

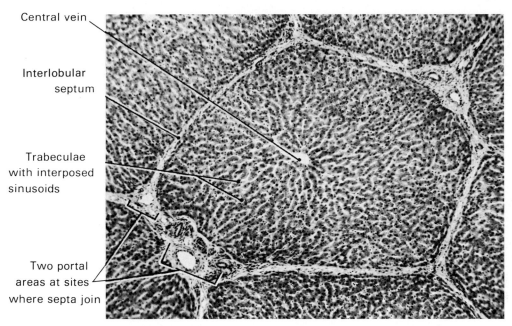

Central vein

Interlobular
septum

Trabeculae
with interposed
sinusoids

Two portal
areas at sites
where septa join

Fig. 22-6. Low-power photomicrograph of liver of pig, illustrating a classic hexagonal lobule as it appears in this species.

their way from the liver by another route). So there are four main tubes that enter or leave the porta; the two that *enter* its substance at this point are the portal vein and the hepatic artery and the two that *leave* are the hepatic (bile) duct and lymphatic.

THE MICROSCOPIC STRUCTURE OF THE LIVER AS SEEN WITH THE LM

Perhaps the most important thing to keep in mind in learning the histology of the liver is that not only is it both an exocrine and an endocrine gland, it is unique in that there is *no division of labor* between those cells that produce the exocrine secretion and those that elaborate the endocrine ones. All its parenchymal cells (hepatocytes) produce both kinds of secretions. The parenchyma of the liver must therefore be arranged so that every hepatocyte on one or more of its surfaces (*1*) abuts on a passageway that connects with a duct system to carry away its exocrine secretion (bile) and (*2*) abuts on a blood vessel into which it delivers its endocrine secretions. Before we can explain in detail how this is accomplished, it is necessary to describe what is termed the *classic lobule* of the liver because it is within such lobules that the arrangement exists that provides for production and delivery of both exocrine and endocrine secretions.

THE CLASSIC LOBULE OF THE LIVER

As will be explained later, two kinds of liver lobules have been visualized. At this point we shall describe only the *classic lobule,* for this was the first kind to be described and it is still what is implied when the term *liver lobule* is used without qualification.

As was described in Chapter 7, the lobules of a gland are generally separated from one another by thin partitions of ordinary connective tissue termed *interlobular septa.* Hence, lobules are identified as the segments of a gland that are enclosed by interlobular septa. This was the criterion adopted when liver lobules were first described. However, a difficulty arose because in human liver no interlobular septa could be found. (How this problem is overcome in histology will be described presently.) Septa were found, however, in arrangements that could demarcate lobules perfectly in pigs (Fig. 22-6) and certain other animals. It was noticed, moreover, that seen in cross section, the lobules of pig liver were polyhedral in form, often being hexagons. These can be fitted together side by side so that at each corner of each hexagon the partitions between 3 lobules meet (Fig. 22-6). Moreover, at each corner of a lobule (where the 3 interlobular partitions meet) the connective tissue is more abundant and on close inspection reveals a cross section of a branch of the portal vein, hepatic artery, and bile duct, together with a lymphatic. This grouping together of branches of the four

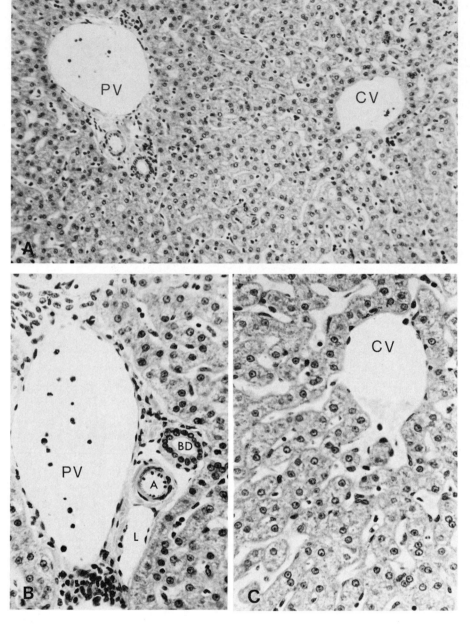

Fig. 22-7. (A) Low-power photomicrograph of liver showing at *left* a portal tract with a branch of the portal vein (PV) and, at *right,* a central vein (CV). Between these there are trabeculae of liver cells with sinusoids situated between them. *(B)* Portal tract at higher magnification. A branch of the portal vein is labeled PV; that of the hepatic artery. A: that of the bile duct, BD; and what is probably a lymphatic, L. Note that the vein, artery, bile duct, and lymphatic are enclosed in a connective tissue stroma. *(C)* Central vein at higher magnification. Note the sinusoids emptying into the central vein (CV) just below *center,* and that the endothelium lining it is associated with very little connective tissue. (Courtesy of H. Whittaker)

tubes, together with the connective tissue that contains them, constitutes what is termed a *portal area* or *portal tract.* Two can be seen (but not very clearly) at lower left in Figure 22-6. As we shall see, these portal tracts are also present in human liver (Fig. 22-7) but they *are not connected with each other by connective tissue partitions.* Nevertheless, they serve as landmarks that if connected by imaginary lines permit the outline of lobules to be visualized.

Finally, before finishing our discussion of liver lobules

of the pig we should note another landmark, which indicates the axis of a polyhedral lobule: it is the *central vein* (Fig. 22-6), through which blood drains away from the lobule.

The Classic Lobule in Man

In man, classic lobules are more difficult to identify because they are not separated from one another by partitions. Hence to visualize a classic lobule the observer has to be able to recognize the 2 kinds of landmarks, portal tracts and central veins. These will now be described in more detail.

Portal Tracts and Their Origin. As already noted, the liver of man is covered with a thin connective tissue *capsule* (of Glisson), which contains regularly arranged collagenic fibers and scattered fibroblasts; this in turn is covered with a layer of mesothelial cells. Second, at the porta of the liver the connective tissue of the capsule extends like the trunk of a tree into the substance of the liver. Within the liver this tree of connective tissue branches very extensively, with branches extending in so many different directions that no part of the liver parenchyma is ever farther than a millimeter away from one or more of its branches. Since these branches pursue somewhat irregular courses, thin slices cut for microscopic study commonly cut them in cross or oblique section and so they appear under the low or high power of the LM as little more or less triangular patches of connective tissue that commonly contain what appear to be four holes (Fig. 22-7B). These holes, of course, are the lumina of branches of the four kinds of tubes reaching all parts of the liver. The nature of these tubes will now be described.

The Tubes in Portal Tracts. The largest tube seen in every branch of the connective tissue tree is a branch of the *portal vein*. This is labeled PV in Figure 22-7A and B. The complementary blood supply of the liver is arterial; the arterial blood is conveyed into the substance of the liver by the branches of the *hepatic artery* that also travel in the portal tracts. These, of course, have a much smaller lumen than the branches of the portal vein, as can be seen clearly in Figure 22-7B, where the branch of the hepatic artery is labeled A. It is therefore via the branches of the connective tissue tree that blood from the portal vein and hepatic artery is conveyed to all parts of the liver from the porta.

The other two tubes seen in branches of the connective tissue tree permit certain fluids to *leave* the liver. One of these tubes in each branch of the connective tissue tree is a *bile duct* made of epithelial cells (BD in Fig. 22-7B) and it drains the exocrine secretion of the parenchymal cells (bile) out of the liver. The little ducts in the various branches on their way out of the liver all eventually join in the trunk of the tree and eventually empty into the hepatic duct. The fourth type of tube seen in every branch of the tree has a very thin wall and is a *lymphatic*. The lymphatics in the various branches also join up in the trunk of the tree and drain lymph from the liver. What is probably a lymphatic is labeled L in part B of Figure 22-7 (the only other possibility is that it might be a tiny branch of the relatively large portal vein).

It should next be noted that when the student looks over a section of human liver the size of a portal tract varies in relation to the size of the branch of the tree that happens to be cut. For example, a stout branch near the trunk would be large and would contain large tubes while a section through a small branch near its termination would be small and have small tubes within it. Sometimes portal tracts are seen that represent cuts through sites where one or more of the tubes are branching, and where this happens the portal tract reveals more than four tubes.

Central Veins and Where They Drain. As just described, blood is brought into the liver by the portal vein and the hepatic artery in portal tracts and from these it is delivered into branching *sinusoids* that pass through the parenchyma of the lobule from its periphery to empty into its central vein. Sinusoids will be described in more detail presently. A central vein is shown in Figure 22-6 and at the right side of the illustration in part A of Figure 22-7, where it is labeled CV. Another is shown in greater detail in part C in the same figure. In the latter illustration the sinusoids (seemingly empty passageways) can clearly be seen emptying into it. Central veins drain into larger veins, often called *sublobular veins,* and these in turn drain into the hepatic veins which leave the liver posteriorly, emptying their blood into the vena cava. The system of veins that drains blood from the liver does not travel in any substantial tree of connective tissue as do the portal vein and hepatic artery that supply blood to the liver, and, furthermore, throughout the liver the two systems of blood vessels remain apart from one another. The central veins of the liver, because they are not associated with any other vessels, constitute a useful landmark that can be used to locate centers of lobules, as will be described in the following.

Outlining Cross Sections of Classic Lobules in Sections of Human Liver

Classic lobules are somewhat longer than they are wide. They are packed together in a haphazard way so that in any given section of liver, lobules are sliced in every conceivable plane. Hence it is usually rather difficult to find a lobule that has been cut approximately in cross section. The first landmark to look for is a central vein that appears as a circle because it has been cut in cross section. The next thing to do is to determine whether or not there are portal tracts around it that could be connected up with imaginary lines to form the outline of what could be the periphery of that lobule. The student should not expect the imaginary lines connecting portal tracts to form a perfect hexagon, but by performing this exercise with enough central veins he will generally find a central vein around which there are several portal tracts (which can be discerned in Fig. 22-8) at more or less the same distance from the central vein. Such areas if connected by imaginary lines would delineate lobules, the contents of which we shall now describe.

The Parenchyma. Under the low magnification necessarily used to study or photograph a complete cross sec-

Portal area

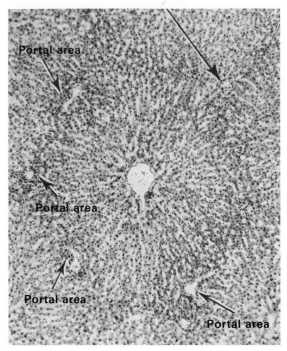

Fig. 22-8. Low-power photomicrograph of a classic lobule of human liver. Five portal areas are included; these indicate the periphery of the lobule. Note that the connective tissue septa seen in pig liver in Figure 22-6 are not present in human liver.

tion of a lobule of pig liver (Fig. 22-6) or lobule of human liver (Fig. 22-8), the parenchymal cells of the lobule, the hepatocytes (dark in Figs. 22-6 and 22-8), appear to be arranged in irregular rows that branch and converge as they pass from the periphery of the lobule to the central vein. Between these irregular rows of hepatocytes are light slit-like spaces representing the liver *sinusoids*.

The Three-Dimensional Arrangement of Hepatocytes

Attempting to visualize in 3 dimensions how hepatocytes and sinusoids are arranged from observing sections (which for all practical purposes reveal only two dimensions) is probably the hardest exercise that exists in histology. The 3-dimensional structure to be visualized must permit every hepatocyte to abut on a passageway that can conduct its exocrine secretion (bile) to the bile duct in a portal tract, and at the same time that same hepatocyte must also abut on at least one sinusoid in order to deliver its internal secretion into the bloodstream. We next consider how the latter is achieved.

Figure 22-9 is a high-power photomicrograph of part of a section of human liver in which the sinusoids (some of which are labeled S) are somewhat more distended than usual and hence easily seen. It would seem to be clear in this illustration that the cell membrane of almost every hepatocyte is, at some site around its circumference, in contact with a sinusoid and, in many instances, with two. In view of this we can be assured that if any hepatocyte does not *seem* to be in contact with a sinusoid in a given section, a section taken above or below the plane examined or photographed would show that it was.

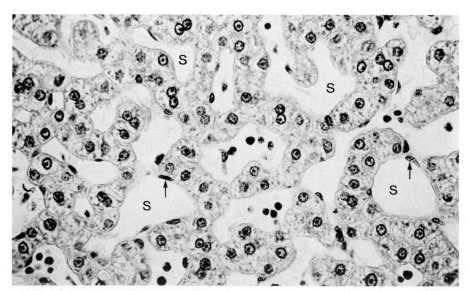

Fig. 22-9. Photomicrograph of human liver. The sinusoids are somewhat distended and hence the trabeculae are spread farther apart than usual. Note that the trabeculae are continuous with one another and always surround a sinusoid, some of which are labeled S. Nuclei of endothelial or Kupffer cells are indicated by arrows. Note that most trabeculae appear 1 or 2 cells wide in this section. (Courtesy of H. Whittaker)

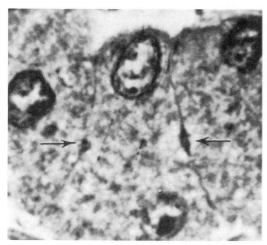

Fig. 22-10. Oil-immersion phase contrast photomicrograph of an H and E section of liver, showing 2 bile canaliculi (indicated by arrows). The clear space at *top right* is a sinusoid.

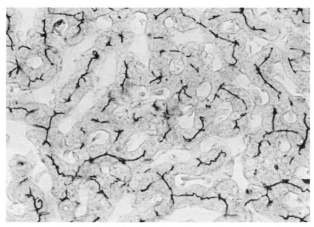

Fig. 22-11. Photomicrograph of liver trabeculae, showing their bile canaliculi, which are demonstrated here by a histochemical reaction for alkaline phosphatase. The cells of the trabeculae are gray (their nuclei do not show) and the sinusoidal spaces are pale. (Courtesy of M. Phillips and J. Steiner)

Next, how could every hepatocyte seen in Figure 22-9 abut on a passageway into which it could secrete its exocrine secretion with the passageway leading to a bile duct in a portal tract? Perhaps it should first be explained that the passageway into which a hepatocyte secretes its exocrine secretion is termed a *bile canaliculus,* which is no more than an intercellular cleft between the cell membranes of two or more contiguous hepatocytes. Two canaliculi, indicated by arrows, are shown between hepatocytes in a cross section of a 3-cell row of hepatocytes in Figure 22-10. Hence canaliculi cannot exist unless they are between at least 2 hepatocytes and they cannot be continuous unless a row of at least 2 hepatocytes is continuous. So for canaliculi to exist and be continuous so as to drain bile from hepatocytes to the bile ducts in portal areas, hepatocytes must always be arranged in what are probably best called *trabeculae,* each of which must be at least 2 cells thick or wide so there can always be a canaliculus running along it between two cells. A trabecula can be either more than 2 cells wide or more than 2 cells thick, but it cannot be both because if it were, for example, 3 cells wide and 3 cells thick its innermost cells, while they could have access to bile canaliculi, would not have access to blood in a sinusoid. Furthermore, trabeculae of hepatocytes must anastomose throughout the lobule in such a way as to permit the bile in their canaliculi to drain into a bile duct in a portal area. Likewise the sinusoids in the meshes of the trabecular network must all connect with one another to empty the blood that passes along them into the central vein of the lobule. The continuity of the bile canaliculi in trabeculae of hepatocytes can be shown by taking advantage of the histochemical method demonstrating the enzyme alkaline phosphatase, which delineates bile canaliculi as shown in Figure 22-11. Here it is evident that the bile canaliculi run between the hepatocytes of the trabeculae in which they are present and that these are all at least 2 cells wide or thick. Since the trabeculae of hepatocytes anastomose with one another, canaliculi can be continuous from any given site within a liver lobule to a portal tract, where they empty their contents into a bile duct as will be described presently.

In conclusion, it would seem from the foregoing that the easiest way to visualize a 3-dimensional structure for the parenchyma of the liver lobule, that would fit the requirements of having every hepatocyte abut on both a canaliculus and a sinusoid, is to conceive of it as consisting of a 3-dimensional network of irregular trabeculae of hepatocytes that are always at least 2 hepatocytes wide or thick and that branch and anastomose with one another so as to enclose branching sinusoids in the interstices of the 3-dimensional trabecular network. The above-described concept would readily explain in particular what is seen in Figures 22-9 and 22-11 (which should be compared with each other) as well as what is seen in Figures 22-6 and 22-7. One more point should be mentioned here, which is that the general direction in which the branching and anastomosing trabeculae of hepatocytes are disposed is from the periphery of a lobule radially toward its central vein, as is shown to advantage in Figure 22-6.

Another Concept of the Arrangement of Hepatocytes. What appear to be single rows of hepatocytes are often seen in sections of liver. But from all the foregoing it is

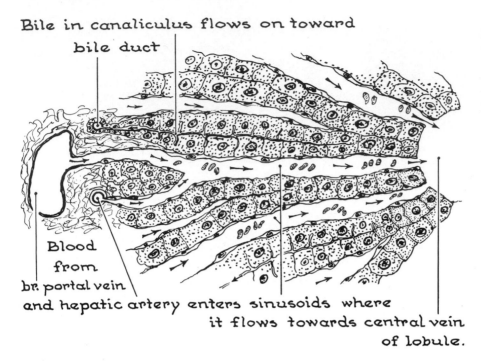

Bile in canaliculus flows on toward
bile duct

Blood
from
br. portal vein
and hepatic artery enters sinusoids where
it flows towards central vein
of lobule.

Fig. 22-12. Diagram illustrating how blood from branches of the portal vein and hepatic artery (*left*) flows into sinusoids that lie between trabeculae and empty into a central vein (*right*). The way bile travels in the opposite direction in canaliculi to empty into bile ducts in portal areas is also shown.

obvious that if there were single rows of hepatocytes in the liver there could not be such a thing as a continuous canaliculus along their lengths. Accordingly, when single rows are seen in sections (and these are still unfortunately often termed liver cords), there must always have been at least another row above or below them so that there could have been a continuous canaliculus present between 2 rows. However, there is a question as to how many rows of hepatocytes might have been present above or below a given single row seen in a section.

As was shown in Figure 1-15, a slice cut from a plate of cells one cell thick but many cells "deep" would appear in a section as a single row of cells. Hence a single row of hepatocytes, seen in any section, could be either a slice through a trabecula that was a few cells deep or so many cells deep that it could be termed a "plate" of cells. And indeed the concept of the liver parenchyma being composed of "plates" of hepatocytes has received a good deal of attention. However, in our opinion, if what might be regarded as "plates" of cells were present in the liver parenchyma, they would, in random sections, sometimes be cut parallel to their broad surfaces and hence appear here and there as large patches of contiguous hepatocytes, and it might be expected that such patches would be seen fairly commonly. However, if the term "plate" is used not to depict flat arrangements of hepatocytes that are one cell thick, but with reference to curving arrangements of hepatocytes that are freely perforated by sinusoids, it becomes questionable as to whether the groups

of hepatocytes between the sinusoids would not be better termed anastomosing *trabeculae*. We think it is stretching the concept of what constitutes a "plate" rather too far to attempt to interpret what is seen, for example, in Figures 22-6, 22-7, and 22-11 as constituting sections through "plates" and hence it seems more logical to interpret sections of the substance of liver lobules as being composed of anastomosing trabeculae of hepatocytes with sinusoids in their interstices. For references to the plate hypothesis, *see* Elias.

Blood and Bile Flow in Opposite Directions. Within lobules, as shown in Figure 22-12, blood from both the portal vein and the hepatic artery of the portal tract enters (but not as directly as is shown in this simple diagram) the sinusoids between the trabeculae of hepatocytes and in these sinusoids it is mixed and flows along so as to enter central veins. The bile secreted by hepatocytes into the canaliculi of trabeculae flows along these canaliculi to enter a bile duct in a portal tract. Hence in the tissue between portal tracts and central veins blood and bile flow *in opposite directions*.

FURTHER COMMENT ON LIVER LOBULES

A *lobule* means a "little lobe" and the term *lobe* seems to have been first used to describe any projecting rounded part of a structure (for example, the lobe of the ear). In connection with glandular organs it was employed to designate any part that projected from the main mass of an organ or was separated from other parts of the organ by fissures, connective tissue septa, or indentations. The term *lobule* was first used to designate small parts of lobes separated from each other by a smaller order of fissures, septa or indentations. However, with the LM, lobules of *exocrine* glands were generally found to be not only parts separated from one another by partitions but also parts in which the secretory units all drained into a common intralobular duct or set of intralobular ducts. So, a second definition for lobules came into being—that lobules are small subdivisions of an organ that are constituted of groups of closely adjacent secretory units draining into a common duct or set of ducts. This second definition proved useful; for example, it enables lobules to be identified in the kidney even though they are not separated from one another by fissures, septa, or indentations. However, the fact that there are 2 ways to define lobules causes complications with regard to the liver because the area defined in the one way is not the same as that defined in the other. Both kinds of lobules will now be described.

The classic liver lobules in man are relatively soft, and where stacked side by side, they may not be stacked evenly (one may overlap the next). Furthermore, they are not necessarily stacked side by side, but instead in such a way that one lobule may point one way and the next in a somewhat different direction. A second difficulty is that it is easy to think of there being 6 portal tracts that *belong* to each lobule; but even in an ideal arrangement each portal tract serves and so "belongs" to the 3 lobules between which it lies. Portal tracts therefore do not "belong" to any particular lobule; they merely *run between* lobules, and so if lobules are not stacked evenly, a portal tract that runs parallel with 1 lobule would probably not run parallel with the long axis of the lobules between which it lies. There is only a remote chance of the 6 portal tracts that run between such haphazardly stacked lobules ever running in the same direction, so that they would all be cut in cross section in the same plane at 6 points around the lobule. More likely, portal tracts would be "missing" in any given section at several points around the periphery of a lobule cut in cross section, because at these points—where they are "missing"—they are running in some other direction, parallel with some other lobule, and so would lie beneath or above the section being examined.

The reason why it is important to indulge in this difficult exercise in 3-dimensional thinking is that the liver can be affected, for example, by nutritional deficiencies, toxins, and impaired circulation, and it is very important in interpreting the cause of liver damage to know which parts of the lobules seen in a section have the best and the poorest blood supply. We shall explain later why attempting to interpret lesions seen in liver lobules according to the concept of the classic lobule is not altogether satisfactory and why a different unit of structure, proposed by

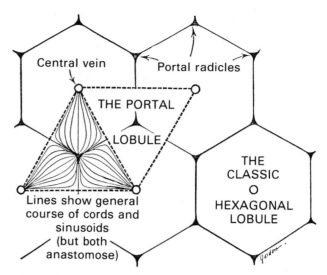

Fig. 22-13. Diagram illustrating the concepts of liver substance being composed of (*1*) classic lobules, or (*2*) portal lobules (as seen in a cross section).

Rappaport and called the *liver acinus,* has proved to be helpful in this and other respects. But before describing the liver acinus we shall, in order to round out our account of lobules, comment on the second type of lobule, termed the *portal lobule,* that has been described.

The Portal Lobule

As already noted, another way of defining a lobule of an exocrine gland is to consider that any group of secretory units emptying their secretion into small ducts, that in turn connect with one another so as to empty the secretion from a given region into a main duct, constitutes a *lobule.* In many exocrine glands such regions are separated from one another by connective tissue septa, so that the region implied by the term *lobule* is the same if either definition of a lobule is used. But the little portions of liver whose secretory units (liver trabeculae) empty into a common main duct (a bile duct in a portal area) are not the same portions of liver tissue that are surrounded by connective tissue partitions in the liver of a pig or are considered to constitute classic liver lobules in man. In the *classic lobule,* the parenchyma of the lobule is the tissue (trabeculae of hepatocytes) that surrounds a *central vein* (Fig. 22-13). But in the *portal lobule* the parenchyma is the tissue that surrounds a portal area because it is this area that contains the *bile duct* into which the surrounding liver trabeculae empty their exocrine secretion (Fig. 22-13). As shown in Figure 22-13, portal lobules are roughly triangular in cross section and there are twice as many of them as classic lobules (in those species that have hexagonal classic lobules). As shown at the left side of Figure 22-13, the liver trabeculae (represented by lines) that lead from a central vein diverge and then converge again to empty their bile (via ductules, to be described later) into the bile duct of a portal area.

It may seem (at least superficially) that, for anyone studying any aspect of the flow of bile through a lobule, the portal lobule would be the more suitable concept to employ. But if one were studying blood flow through the sinusoids of a lobule, the classic lobule would have certain advantages. However, in thinking of classic lobules it has often been more or less assumed that, at any given site seen in a section, blood derived from the hepatic artery and portal vein in the portal tract, at the level seen in that section, flows directly into the sinusoids seen around the portal area in that particular section. This oversimplified view proved to be a misconception and the elucidation of how blood from portal tracts is really delivered into sinusoids led in due course to the concept of the units of structure called *acini* instead of that of lobules; this will soon be described. But first we should explain why differences in the quality of the blood that passes along different segments of sinusoids in the liver is so important. This is done in the following section.

Introductory Comment on the Metabolic Role of Hepatocytes

To explain why the blood supply of hepatocytes is so important, we should first admit that it is very much of an understatement to describe, as we have done, the liver as if it were only an exocrine and endocrine gland. This is only excusable because it facilitates its histological description. It is now time to point out that hepatocytes perform, in addition to their purely secretory functions, a vast number of *metabolic* functions (estimated at well over 500) of the greatest importance in maintaining viability and health of the body. It is in connection with these functions and their possible impairment due to the quality and quantity of blood passing along sinusoids that knowledge of the course of blood flow through the liver parenchyma is of such great importance.

The manifold metabolic functions performed by the liver are facilitated by hepatocytes being the first parenchymal cells with which the many kinds of nutrients absorbed from the intestine into the blood of the portal system have direct contact. Hepatocytes are concerned with the processing and distribution of these nutrients. For example, it is in hepatocytes that absorbed monosaccharides are converted into glycogen and stored so as to keep the blood sugar level from rising unduly after meals. Hepatocytes can subsequently convert the glycogen back to glucose and release it to maintain a proper glucose level in the blood. They are also profoundly concerned in protein and fat metabolism and with the metabolism of hormones and vitamins. In addition they are called upon to detoxify drugs and certain compounds that otherwise could cause damage. In other words, hepatocytes constitute an enormous bank of cells specialized to perform a vast number of metabolic duties. Their fine structure and the ways in which this is adapted to performing some of these duties will soon be described. The sites in the liver at which these various duties are performed are in part related to the concentrations of the various substances in blood plasma as this passes from one end of a sinusoid to the other. So, in relating various liver functions to the microscopic structure of hepatocytes, we should know as far as possible where both portal and arterial blood enters and leaves the sinusoids. This requires that we now describe the liver acinus.

The Liver Acinus

The subdivision of liver tissue known as an *acinus* is neither easy to explain nor easy to understand. It may help first to explain what it is *not*.

In studying the pancreas, we learned that *acini* are small exocrine secretory units housed in lobules. There are hundreds or thousands of acini within a lobule of the pancreas; hence in the pancreas acini are much smaller subdivisions of structure than lobules. The *liver acinus*, on the contrary, is *not* an exocrine secretory unit. Furthermore, it is *not* a subdivision of a classic lobule because, even though in a cross section of a classic lobule an acinus is only one third the size of the classic lobule, it is made up of *parts of two adjacent classic lobules*. So it is easiest to think of liver acini as subdivisions of liver structure in their own right, so that, instead of thinking of the liver as being made up of lobules, one can think of the liver as being made up of acini. But in order to describe how to distinguish liver acini, everyone assumes the reader knows all about portal lobules. Furthermore, to distinguish acini we have to use the same guideposts that are used to locate either kind of lobule that we have described. The guideposts are *portal tracts* and *central veins*. We shall go on to describe how to locate acini after the following discussion.

Why It Is Advantageous to Think of the Liver as Being Composed of Acini Instead of Portal Lobules. It is obvious that the parts of liver trabeculae that are closest to central veins are exposed to blood of the poorest quality, because to reach a central vein blood must have passed along a sinusoid that was at least as long as the distance from a portal area to a central vein. Along a sinusoid blood would continue to lose oxygen and accumulate carbon dioxide. Parenchymal cells immediately adjacent to central veins are thus supplied by blood with the lowest oxygen and nutrient content as compared with the parenchymal cells situated closer to portal areas. Furthermore, blood here would have the greatest content of carbon dioxide and other waste products of metabolism.

Next, in days past before the concept of acini was developed, it was often assumed that sinusoids of the parenchyma that immediately surrounds a portal area would receive the freshest blood; this concept was based on the idea that at any given site along a portal tract blood was emptied almost directly from the hepatic artery and portal vein of that portal tract into the sinusoids that radiated from that portal tract. However, this view disregarded the fact that there would be smaller vessels leading off from the larger vessels in the portal tracts to deliver blood into the sinusoids of the parenchyma. It would be an exception if, in any vascular tree, blood did not flow through progressively smaller vessels until the peripheral circulation was reached, in which blood is emptied into either capillaries or sinusoids. The concept of acini takes into account the fact that in order for blood to be delivered from the hepatic artery and portal vein into sinusoids, there have to be branches of the hepatic artery and portal vein that extend off at intervals, more or less at right angles, from the hepatic artery and portal vein in a portal tract and into the parenchyma, where they branch into small vessels that empty into sinusoids.

These side branches of the hepatic artery and portal vein of portal tracts constitute the backbones of the liver acini (Fig. 22-14), and it is from these branches that twigs empty blood into sinusoids (Fig. 22-14), providing blood that is the freshest in any part of the parenchyma. So to know where the best quality blood is to be found in liver, we must ascertain where these tiny branches of vessels in portal areas are located.

How to Find an Acinus. Finding 6 portal areas in any given section that can be connected by imaginary lines to form a hexagon, with a central vein in the center, is seldom possible in human liver for reasons already given. Rappaport suggests that the observer is much more likely to find only 2, 3, or 4 well-defined portal tracts around the periphery of any hexagon visualized around a central vein. In other words, if one thinks of hexagons around central veins, about half of the portal areas that should be around the hexagon are missing.

What could be considered to be a classic lobule showing only 3 portal areas in its periphery is illustrated in Figure 22-14, at *right;* this figure also indicates by an "M" where portal tracts are "missing." Rappaport believes that distributing terminal branches of the portal vein and hepatic artery in any portal tract extend out from these vessels more or less at right angles (as shown just above *center* in Fig. 22-14), toward angular points around the hexagon where well-defined portal areas are "missing" ("M" in Fig. 22-14). Since these smaller terminal vessels extend roughly at right angles from the main vessels, they

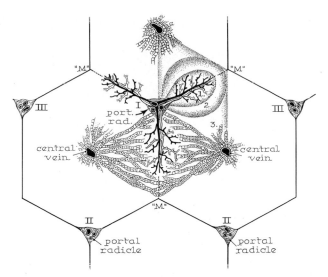

Fig. 22-14. Diagram illustrating the concept of liver substance being composed of acini. So that the relation of acini to classic lobules can be visualized, classic lobules are also outlined. Only two acini are shown. In the one to the *upper right of center,* the three zones are indicated in stippling. The shape of the one just *below center* is indicated by the layout of the trabeculae that have been drawn in. Note that acini are diamond-shaped in cross section. (For further details, *see* text.)

are not cut transversely in cross sections of lobules. However, they are occasionally cut obliquely because they pursue irregular courses. On their arched and irregular course toward the points of the lobule where triangular portal tracts are "missing" (Fig. 22-14, "M"), they may be cut repeatedly or not at all in any given section. These terminal portal and arterial branches, in association with the terminal bile ductules, form the backbones of masses of hepatic parenchyma that are roughly diamond-shaped in cross section and which constitute *acini* as described below.

At the *top center* in Figure 22-14 there is a central vein. A short distance below this there is a typical triangular-shaped portal tract. We shall concentrate first on the two small blood vessels that branch at right angles from the hepatic artery and the portal vein, respectively, of the tract to descend *vertically* in this illustration (that is, away from the central vein at *top center*), toward an "M" (a site where a portal tract is "missing") to form the backbone of one acinus. The extent of this acinus (in 2 dimensions) is indicated in the illustration because the area occupied by its parenchyma is shown complete with liver trabeculae that extend out from its backbone to the left and to the right, and on each side the trabeculae in this acinus converge on central veins. The acinus is therefore roughly diamond-shaped in cross section and it includes liver

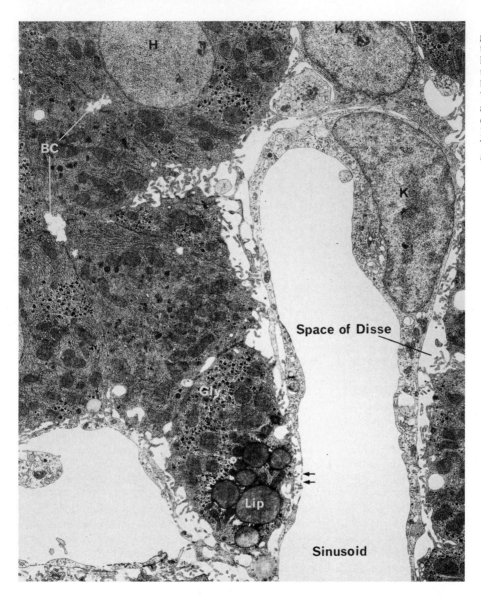

Fig. 22-15. Electron micrograph (×5,100) of liver (rat). Note the space of Disse between the lining cells of sinusoids and hepatocytes (H). Between hepatocytes bile canaliculi (BC) can be seen. Within the hepatocytes glycogen areas (Gly) alternate with regions containing rER and mitochondria. Lipid droplets are labeled Lip. Two Kupffer cells (K) are seen at *top right*. Courtesy of E. Rau)

parenchyma that is situated in parts of 2 different classic lobules, as shown in Figure 22-14.

The parenchymal cells closest to the vascular backbone of the acinus have the *best blood supply* of any of its parts. This part, which Rappaport terms *Zone 1* of an acinus, is more or less oval-shaped in cross section; it is labeled 1 in another diamond-shaped acinus present at *upper right* in Figure 22-14. The liver parenchyma that surrounds Zone 1 is roughly circular in cross section and is indicated in the same acinus as *Zone 2*. This zone has the second best blood supply in this acinus. The irregularly shaped outer part of an acinus that reaches to the central veins is termed *Zone 3*, and it has the *poorest blood supply* of any part of an acinus.

Summary. In cross section, acini are more or less diamond-shaped, with each end converging on a central vein. A cross section, if cut through its middle, would show its backbone of vessels. But an acinus has thickness and if it were too thick it would not be efficient with regard to its vessels supplying blood to parenchyma relatively far away from them. Acini are therefore not as thick as classic lobules are long. So when we say there are 3 times as many acini as portal lobules, we are only speaking of what is seen in a cross section. If they are not as thick as lobules are long there would, of course, be many more than 3 times as many acini along the length of a portal area extending along the side of a classic lobule.

By thinking in 3 dimensions it can be appreciated that since the vascular backbones of acini run more or less at right angles to the vessels in portal tracts, the parenchyma

Fig. 22-16. Electron micrograph (×11,000) of a rat liver sinusoid (S), showing an endothelial lining cell (E), surrounded on all sides by hepatocytes (H). The numerous microvilli on the sinusoidal surface of each hepatocyte extend right across the space of Disse (D) to reach the endothelial cell. Note that there is no basal lamina surrounding the endothelial cell along its border with the space of Disse. The arrow indicates an extension of a supporting cell (fat-storing cell or lipocyte, illustrated in Fig. 22-20). (Courtesy of A. Blouin)

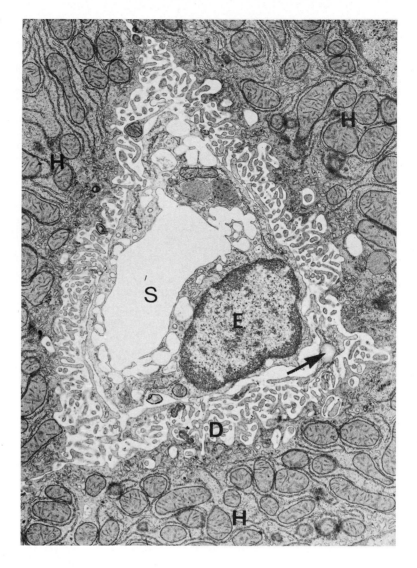

seen in the periphery of a lobule in a given section could be part of Zone 1, 2, or 3 of an acinus whose vascular backbone ran parallel to the plane of the section but might have been considerably below or above the plane of the section. For this reason, what appears as a peripheral part of a lobule in any given section, even a part adjacent to a portal tract, may not have the best blood supply because it may lie relatively far from the vascular backbone of an acinus.

The Acinus as a Metabolic Unit. There is now evidence indicating that the kinds of metabolic processes that occur in the 3 zones of an acinus are somewhat different; this explains why certain toxic agents or nutritional deficiencies affect different zones to different extents. For details, Rappaport's articles should be consulted.

The concept of the acinus helps in understanding why certain regions of liver lobules are more damaged than others under different conditions, and why the extent of damage within the periphery of lobules may seem to vary from section to section.

THE HEPATIC SINUSOIDS AND THE SPACE OF DISSE

Studies with the LM suggested the existence of a space between the walls of sinusoids and the hepatocytes bordering on them. That this space, called the *space of Disse,* was not a shrinkage artifact was established by EM studies (Figs. 22-15 and 22-16). This true space contains blood plasma, but blood cells are normally not seen in it in postnatal life. It contains vast numbers of microvilli that project from the free surfaces of the hepatocytes bordering it (Figs. 22-16 and 22-17).

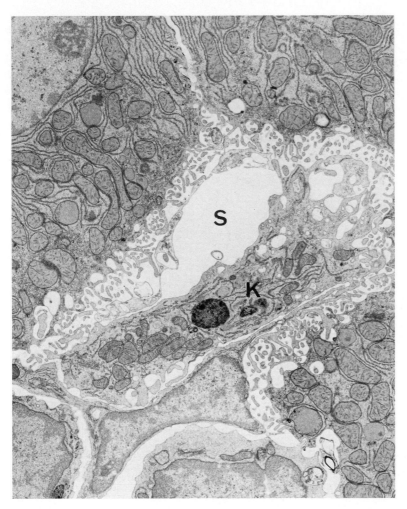

Fig. 22-17. Electron micrograph (×9,700) of a Kupffer cell (K) in the lumen of a sinusoid (S) of rat liver. Dense bodies (probably secondary lysosomes) are evident near the middle of the cell; one is particularly large and rounded. Note the numerous pseudopodia on this type of macrophage; they are readily seen *right of center.* Some mitochondria are also present, especially in the left half of the Kupffer cell. (Courtesy of A. Blouin)

THE CELLS OF THE WALLS OF SINUSOIDS

Development of Knowledge. Long ago it was observed with the LM that the lining of the liver sinusoids differed from the lining of ordinary capillaries in that 2 different types of cells were involved. Cells of the one type were relatively thin and flat, resembling the endothelial cells of ordinary capillaries but those of the other kind were much larger. In sections they often appeared to be stellate (shaped like a star) and they became known as the stellate cells of von Kupffer who, in the last century, was the first investigator to describe them. They are now known as *Kupffer cells* (Fig. 22-15K). They have a different origin from endothelial cells in that they are derived from monocytes and so for all practical purposes are to be regarded as *macrophages.*

It was noted in describing sinusoids of bone marrow and lymph nodes that sinusoids in these tissues are lined with ordinary endothelial cells. EM studies suggest that phagocytic cells are only associated with these sinusoids. They may, however, give the appearance of being parts of their lining because although they lie against the outer surfaces of the sinusoidal walls they commonly, by means of pseudopodia, protrude between endothelial cells into the lumina of sinusoids. However, in the liver the Kupffer cells actually *form part of the lining,* being interposed between endothelial cells.

Fine Structure of Kupffer Cells. As may be seen in Figure 22-17, Kupffer cells have an irregular outline; their cytoplasm projects in the form of pseudopodia and microvilli and clefts extend into the cytoplasm between projections. A feature of Kupffer cells is that they contain worm-like tubules in their cytoplasm that probably represent reservoirs of cell membrane available for a rapid phagocytic response to particulate matter. The nucleus of Kupffer cells resembles that of macrophages.

Fig. 22-18. Electron micrograph (×14,300) of a rat liver sinusoid (S) in cross section, showing an endothelial lining cell (E). Intercellular gaps or cytoplasmic fenestrae (C) could provide communication between the lumen of the sinusoid and the space of Disse (D). Note that a basal lamina is absent in the space of Disse. The arrows indicate cytoplasmic extensions of supporting cells (fat-storing cells, as illustrated in Fig. 22-20). Note the numerous microvilli on the sinusoidal surface of the surrounding hepatocytes (H). (Courtesy of A. Blouin)

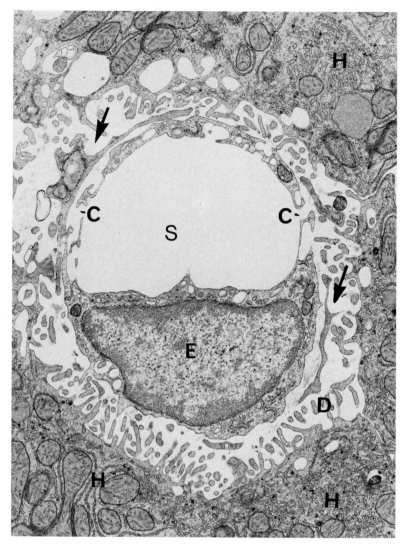

Within the cytoplasm there are membrane-enclosed spaces that could represent either pinocytotic or phagocytic vesicles. Phagocytosed material may be present—for example, iron in the form of hemosiderin, resulting from phagocytosis and destruction of old erythrocytes. Mitochondria are also present (Fig. 22-17). There is some rER (as seen in Fig. 22-17), but the Golgi apparatus is not prominent. Dense bodies (secondary lysosomes) are fairly common; some can be seen in Figure 22-17. Wisse found that the cytoplasm of Kupffer cells, unlike that of endothelial cells, is peroxidase-positive. This provides another means of distinguishing between Kupffer and endothelial cells and, of course, it also seems to suggest an origin from monocytes (which possess peroxidase-positive granules).

Fine Structure of the Endothelial Cells Lining the Sinusoids. After the EM established that there was a space of Disse, it became of interest to ascertain how a sinusoidal wall permitted plasma and chylomicrons to pass out through it and yet excluded platelets and blood cells. Many EM studies disclosed tiny openings through the lining (Fig. 22-18C) which could be taken to represent either gaps between contiguous endothelial cells or fenestrae through their cytoplasm. However, it could be argued that such minute deficiencies in the lining might be the result of fixation artifacts.

Wisse in his studies of liver perfused with fixative came to somewhat different conclusions about the lining of the sinusoids in that he found no gaps between the contiguous endothelial cells, and so conceived of the sinusoids as

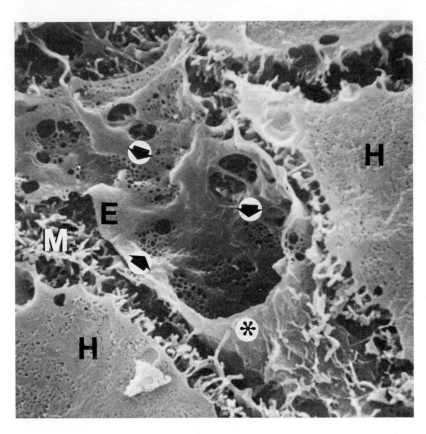

Fig. 22-19. Scanning electron micrograph illustrating the endothelial lining of a sinusoid and the space of Disse in rat liver. The freeze-fractured surface shown extends across a sinusoid at *middle* and includes parts of two hepatocytes (H) on opposite sides of the sinusoid. Microvilli extending from the surfaces of these into the space of Disse are seen to advantage; one site where they are abundant is labeled M. The inner surface of the endothelial wall of the sinusoid (fractured obliquely) is labeled E. The outer surface of the sinusoid is indicated by an asterisk. Some reticular fibers are seen on the outer surface of the sinusoid. Fenestrated areas of the endothelium (sieve plates) are indicated by arrows. (Brooks, S. E. H., and Haggis, G. H.: Lab. Invest.. *29*:60. 1973).

having *continuous* walls. Furthermore, he observed that the fenestrae are confined to very attenuated regions of the cytoplasm at sites that he termed *sieve plates,* which are illustrated in Figure 22-19. According to his view the fenestrae of the sieve plates would be the only passageways by which the sinusoidal lumen communicates with the space of Disse. The fenestrae in the sieve plates are oval in shape and not closed over by diaphragms as they are in the common type of fenestrated capillary; their average diameter is about 100 nm. With no other gaps in sinusoidal walls, the sieve plates could serve a filtering role so that chylomicrons, for instance (which are roughly the same size as the fenestrae), would gain access to the space of Disse, whereas larger (particulate) matter could not. Furthermore, there is no basal lamina associated with the endothelial cells that might interfere with their passage (as is evident in Figs. 22-16 and 22-18).

How the Walls of Sinusoids Are Supported. In view of the fact that the endothelium that lines sinusoids is unsupported by a basal lamina, we have to consider what it is that prevents this lining layer from being flattened against the sinusoidal surfaces of hepatocytes, obliterating the space of Disse. First, it should be appreciated that the fenestrae in the sieve plates do not impede free passage of plasma into the space. Hence the hydrostatic pressure in

the space of Disse would be no different from that in the sinusoid, and there would be no great force to cause flattening.

The space itself contains a variety of supporting structures. First, as may be seen in Figures 22-16 and 22-18, it is permeated by the innumerable microvilli on the sinusoidal surfaces of hepatocytes. Second, as demonstrated by Wisse, the endothelial layer is supported in places by cytoplasmic extensions of fat-storing cells, sometimes referred to as *lipocytes.* These storage cells are situated between hepatocytes in association with the space of Disse of sinusoids, so they may be regarded as an interstitial cell type of the parenchyma. A lipocyte, containing lipid storage droplets, is labeled F in Figure 22-20; one of its processes is also indicated (arrow). Two lipocyte processes supporting the endothelial lining of another sinusoid are illustrated in Figure 22-18 (*see* arrows).

A further factor to be considered is that the endothelial cell cytoplasm is probably not as fragile as it looks, since it contains microtubules and filaments. Furthermore, endothelial cells are joined together by cell junctions, probably of the fascia occludens type.

Finally, there are *reticular fibers* in the space of Disse. Some may be seen at *bottom right* in Figure 22-19. These delicate intercellular fibers are regarded by many as being

Fig. 22-20. Electron micrograph (×11,500) showing a fat-storing cell (lipocyte) labeled F lying in between two hepatocytes (H) of rat liver. It also lies in association with a Kupffer cell (K) in a sinusoid (the lumen of which is seen as a clear space at *bottom right*). The lumen of another sinusoid, with an endothelial lining cell (E), is seen at *top right*. The fat-storage globules (G) of the lipocyte are partly extracted by fixative. The arrow indicates a cytoplasmic process extending from the lipocyte; such processes are considered to provide support for the endothelial lining cells (E) of sinusoids, as seen at *top right*, and also for Kupffer cells in the walls of sinusoids. (Courtesy of A. Blouin)

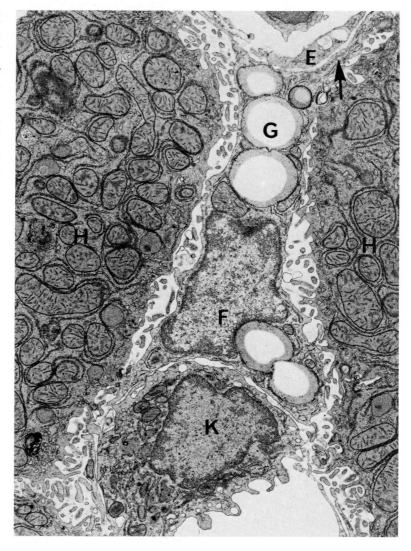

the principal supporting structures not only in the walls of hepatic sinusoids but also for the soft tissue of the liver lobule as a whole.

THE MICROSCOPIC STRUCTURE OF HEPATOCYTES

Hepatocytes illustrate many features of general interest to those studying cell biology and were used for this purpose in the early chapters of this textbook, so it is unnecessary to repeat everything dealt with earlier. However, for convenience we review here some main points of interest.

Hepatocytes storing glycogen (stained for glycogen and not so stained) were illustrated in Figure 1-19 and hepa-

tocytes containing excessive amounts of fat, in Figure 1-20. Figures 3-17 and 3-18 show polyploid hepatocytes.

Fine Structure. A hepatocyte nucleus is illustrated in Figure 4-3; nuclear envelope and pores may be seen in more detail in Figure 4-4.

The cytoplasm of hepatocytes literally abounds in all sorts of organelles and inclusions. Mitochondria are particularly numerous (Figs. 22-17 and 22-20); it is estimated that each hepatocyte contains 1,000 or more. Mitochondria are of particular importance to hepatocytes because of the many and varied types of metabolic activity carried out by these cells. Free and membrane-bound polyribosomes are abundant in hepatocytes. Both rER and sER are prominent; the significance of this will be apparent when we describe the endocrine functions of hepatocytes. Many Golgi stacks, probably interconnected by

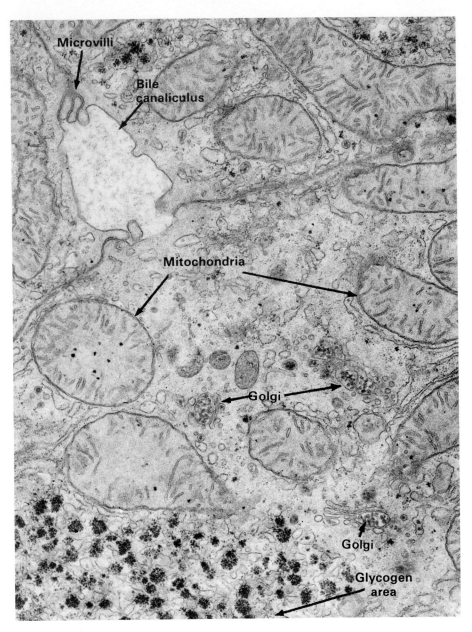

Fig. 22-21. Electron micrograph (×30,000) of hepatocytes of mouse liver. A bile canaliculus is seen at *upper left*, with microvilli projecting into its lumen. The abundant large mitochondria have numerous cristae. Within the Golgi saccules present below *center*, note the electron-dense lipoprotein particles which are the precursors of the lipoproteins released to the plasma. Glycogen granules, arranged in rosettes (α-particles), are seen at *bottom left*, with tubules of sER between the rosettes. (Courtesy of A. Jézéquel)

tubules as explained in Chapter 5, are scattered about in the cytoplasm. Some lie close to the nucleus, others near the bile canaliculi, as seen in Figure 22-21. The Golgi saccules also are concerned in the endocrine functions of hepatocytes (*see* below). Lysosomes of all kinds are present, particularly close to the bile canaliculi (Fig. 22-22). Some of the lysosomes contain lipofuscin, the wear-and-tear pigment, because the lipofuscin in hepatocytes is taken up by lysosomes (which are thereupon called *lipofuscin bodies*). Hepatocytes also contain a number of vesicular organelles called *microbodies* (labeled in Fig.

22-22). In most species (but not man) these have a dense body in their centers that seems to be crystalline. Microbodies have a surrounding membrane and contain several enzymes. The crystalline structure in the center of those of many species is uricase. This enzyme is concerned with metabolizing uric acid further in order for it to be eliminated from the body. Humans, however, seem to lack this enzyme and so have to excrete uric acid as such in their urine. An inability to metabolize or eliminate all the uric acid produced, as well as that absorbed from food, leads to the condition *gout*. It has recently been ob-

Fig. 22-22. Electron micrograph (×13,000) of three hepatocytes bordering in a bile canaliculus in the liver of a ground hog. The cells are joined at this site by junctional complexes. The component of the complex closest to the lumen is a continuous tight junction (zonula occludens). At some distance away there is a desmosome. In the hepatocyte at *upper right* some rER can be seen (*right of center*). Note also a lysosome and two microbodies with characteristic crystalline internal structure. Some sER is also present. (Courtesy of J. Steiner)

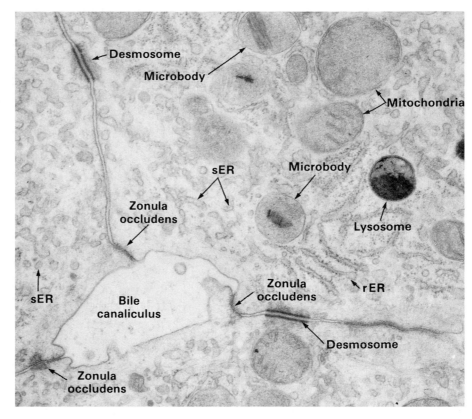

served that microbodies contain enzymes important in metabolizing fatty acids by β-oxidation and that their numbers increase when certain drugs are given to reduce serum lipid levels.

Following this general account of the organelles of hepatocytes we shall soon attempt to relate the presence of some of them more particularly to the functions of hepatocytes. But first we must mention the various kinds of surfaces of hepatocytes.

The Three Kinds of Surfaces of Hepatocytes

(*1*) The surface bordering on the space of Disse has numerous microvilli projecting from it into the space (Fig. 22-16), which, of course, provides each hepatocyte with an enormous surface for *absorption* of substances from the bloodstream. Between microvilli there is space for hepatocytes to *secrete* substances into plasma. (2) Sides of hepatocytes in most species have projections and indentations to fit complementary ones on the hepatocytes beside it, but these are not prominent in man; they help hold hepatocytes together. (*3*) At some site on the surface of a hepatocyte there is a bile canaliculus between it and one or two other hepatocytes (Figs. 22-21 and 22-22). The surface bordering on the canaliculus is secretory.

Bile canaliculi will be described further in connection with the exocrine function of the liver.

THE FUNCTIONS OF HEPATOCYTES

Without going into the functions of the liver in depth we shall comment briefly on some of the kinds of functions it performs and relate these to the organelles concerned. We begin with the endocrine functions of the liver.

SOME ENDOCRINE FUNCTIONS OF HEPATOCYTES IN RELATION TO THE ORGANELLES CONCERNED

As already noted, the liver is an *exocrine* gland because hepatocytes secrete bile into canaliculi and this is carried away by a duct system to the intestine. But decades ago it was also described as an *endocrine* gland. At that time a gland was considered to be endocrine if it secreted any useful substance into the bloodstream. So when it was found that the liver secreted sugar into the blood it was considered an endocrine gland as well as an exocrine gland. It is now known that it secretes several useful substances into the bloodstream, as next described. It is noteworthy that its exocrine and endocrine functions are both performed by the same specialized secretory cells—

the hepatocytes. It should also be mentioned that although it is convenient here to discuss the liver as an endocrine gland, the latter term is now generally used in a more restricted way for those glands that secrete hormones.

The Synthesis of Glycogen and Secretion of Glucose

After a substantial carbohydrate-containing meal, the blood glucose level would escalate uncontrolled were it not for the hepatocytes, removing excess glucose from the blood and, in the presence of *insulin,* storing it as glycogen. Conversely, when the blood sugar level begins to fall, they convert glycogen back into glucose and release it into the blood. Seen with the EM, glycogen deposits formed from glucose take the form of electron-dense particles a little larger than free ribosomes and arranged together to form rosettes (Fig. 5-60). These are closely associated with tubules of sER (Figs. 5-60 and 22-21). This characteristic association between glycogen deposits and tubules of sER is probably due to the enzyme glucose-6-phosphatase, an enzyme important in glycogen metabolism, being located in the sER.

The hormone *hydrocortisone,* which is produced by the adrenal cortex, also can cause glycogen to form in hepatocytes; but this is due to glycogen being formed from proteins or their precursors, and such glycogen formation results in liberation of glucose into the blood and not subtraction of glucose from it. (This will be discussed more fully in Chapter 25.)

The Secretion of Blood Proteins

Hepatocytes synthesize the albumins, fibrinogen, and most of the globulins of blood plasma as well as other proteins concerned in blood coagulation, and secrete these into the sinusoids. Hepatocytes do not, of course, produce immunoglobulins; these are produced by plasma cells.

The proteins secreted by hepatocytes into the blood are synthesized in cisternae of rER, seen here and there in the cytoplasm (as shown *right of center* in Fig. 22-22). After their synthesis the blood proteins are delivered via the Golgi to the free surface of the cell, which is bathed by plasma, and released by exocytosis.

The Secretion of Lipoproteins

Hepatocytes are also concerned in controlling the level of lipids in the blood. Although some lipid in the blood is in the form of a loose complex of fatty acids and albumin, most is in the form of little particles in which lipid is combined in some fashion with protein. These particles are referred to as the *lipoproteins* of the blood. Lipid particles

themselves would be hydrophobic and so would not remain in suspension in plasma. But the protein with which they are associated acts so as to make the particles sufficiently hydrophilic to remain in suspension in plasma.

There are 4 kinds of lipoprotein particles in blood. (*1*) The *chylomicrons,* which are described in Chapter 9 in connection with adipose tissue (p. 240), are the largest of these particles and, as already described, they are formed in the intestinal absorptive cells. Hepatocytes participate with other cells in the body in removing these from the blood after a fatty meal. Since chylomicrons are suspended in blood plasma they readily enter the space of Disse and are probably absorbed as such by liver cells, where they are broken down, with their constituents being utilized by the hepatocytes. The other lipoproteins are called (*2*) *pre-beta lipoprotein,* (*3*) *beta lipoprotein,* and (*4*) *alpha lipoprotein* respectively. Particles of pre-beta lipoprotein are somewhat smaller than chylomicrons and relatively richer in protein. They are believed to be made in hepatocytes. The particles of beta lipoprotein are smaller still and denser and have less lipid. These, too, are synthesized by hepatocytes and they are the chief medium by which cholesterol is transported throughout the body. They are probably secreted along with, or as part of, the pre-beta lipoprotein. The alpha lipoprotein forms the smallest of all lipoprotein particles and its lipid is chiefly in the form of phospholipid, an essential component of cell membranes.

The lipoproteins made by hepatocytes seem to be assembled in a step-by-step manner. Their protein content is synthesized in the rER, which is continuous with the sER. The sER is concerned with the synthesis of lipids. So it appears that the protein and lipid of the particles are synthesized in the same tubule, with the protein being formed where it is rough and the lipid where it is smooth. Of course, the Golgi is also involved and vesicles containing lipoprotein particles bud off from its saccules (Fig. 22-21) to move to the sinusoidal surface, where the contained particles are released to the blood. Within the cytoplasm the membrane-surrounded particles appear as dark granules.

METABOLIC AND DETOXIFYING ROLE OF HEPATOCYTES IN RELATION TO THE ORGANELLES CONCERNED

Another function of hepatocytes (over and above their endocrine function just described and exocrine function next to be described) will only be touched on here; it involves transformations and conjugations that detoxify dangerous substances that when absorbed from the gut or formed in the body might have a deleterious effect. For example, ammonia formed in connection with the metabolism of amino acids is toxic once it reaches a certain concentration. Hepatocytes prevent such concentrations being attained by using ammonia to form either useful substances or urea; the latter is nontoxic (unless concentrations are excessive) and eliminated from the body by the kidneys.

Many substances, ranging from prescribed drugs to chemicals absorbed from various sources, are metabolized and detoxified by hepatocytes. In some instances the breakdown products of these substances are more damaging than the substances themselves.

Steroid hormones and alcohol are also metabolized in hepatocytes. In connection with their continued detoxification there is marked increase of sER in hepatocytes.

THE EXOCRINE SECRETION OF THE LIVER

The exocrine secretion of the liver is *bile*. About 0.5 to 1 liter is emptied into the intestine daily. Bile contains bile pigments (bilirubin), bile salts, protein, cholesterol, and crystalloids of tissue fluid. *Bilirubin* pigment is primarily a waste product, formed not in hepatocytes but from the breakdown of hemoglobin in macrophages of the spleen and bone marrow, and to a lesser extent by Kupffer cells of hepatic sinusoids. This non-iron-containing breakdown product of hemoglobin passes into the blood and is absorbed from the plasma in the space of Disse by hepatocytes. These render it water-soluble by conjugating it with *glucuronic acid,* and then they secrete it as one component of bile. Bile salts, in contrast to bile pigments, are useful substances that once they reach the intestine facilitate greatly the digestion of fats. Like cholesterol, the third component of bile, bile salts are produced in hepatocytes.

There is yet another component of bile. The hormones produced by the adrenal cortex and sex glands are constantly absorbed from the blood by hepatocytes and metabolized to different extents. The products so formed, or even active unchanged steroid hormones, are partly secreted into the bile. From the bile in the intestine some hormone may be resorbed into the bloodstream. Hence, there is said to be an enterohepatic circulation of steroid hormones.

There is also an enterohepatic circulation of bile pigment, for when bilirubin reaches the intestine, it is changed into urobilinogen and stercobilinogen by the action of bacteria that live in the intestine. Part of the urobilinogen is subsequently reabsorbed into the capillaries of the intestine. These, of course, drain into the portal system, and as the blood containing reabsorbed urobilinogen passes along the sinusoids of the liver, the urobilinogen is taken up by hepatocytes and changed into bilirubin again, after which it is again secreted into the bile.

Although bile is secreted by the liver at a fairly regular rate, it is delivered into the intestine irregularly, generally when it will do most good; this requires that it be temporarily stored and concentrated in the gallbladder between meals, as described later in connection with the gallbladder.

Bile Canaliculi. The cell membranes of adjacent cells bordering on the lumen of a bile canaliculus are tightly bound together by a junctional complex (Fig. 22-22). Close to the lumen there is a zonula occludens. Farther away from the lumen, the junctional complex only occasionally shows a zonula adherens. Farther out there are desmosomes (Fig. 22-22) as well as gap junctions.

The cell membranes that form the wall of a bile canaliculus project irregularly into the lumen of the canaliculus as short microvilli (see Figs. 22-21 and 22-22). Histochemical studies indicate that there is a substantial amount of ATP-ase at the border of the cytoplasm that abuts on the bile canaliculus and this enzyme is perhaps involved in the secretion of bile. There is also some condensation of filaments in this location.

The Connections Between Canaliculi and Bile Ducts. Bile canaliculi can be demonstrated in the LM by different methods. Sometimes they can even be seen in H and E sections, but their demonstration without special treatment probably depends on their being somewhat distended as in Figure 22-10. Gomori showed that histochemical methods for alkaline phosphatase revealed them; alkaline phosphatase is known to be present in bile (Fig. 22-11). Bile canaliculi can also be injected with opaque materials through the bile ducts and studied in cleared sections.

The EM showed that bile canaliculi are sequestered spaces between the membranes of contiguous hepatic cells. In some species (but not much in man), there is condensation of cytoplasmic filaments beneath the cell membranes that border canaliculi. This, together with the junctional complexes on each side of the canaliculi (Fig. 22-22), permits canaliculi to withstand some pressure without rupturing.

Bile canaliculi begin from blind endings within hepatic trabeculae in the regions around central veins of lobules. As they pass along the trabeculae toward the periphery of lobules, they anastomose freely (Fig. 22-11). The bile that flows along them drains finally into *bile ductules,* which are the smallest branches of the bile ducts surrounded by connective tissue in portal tracts. The connections between the bile canaliculi of the trabeculae and bile ducts of portal tracts have been studied vigorously over the years, and a certain confusion about terminology has resulted. However, the EM has clarified many of the points previously unsettled, as follows.

First, the bile canaliculi in trabeculae of human liver are bounded usually by 2, but in some places by 3, hepatocytes (Figs. 22-10 and 22-22). At sites where trabeculae approach and abut on portal tracts, the canaliculi empty into what are called *canals of Hering.* Canals of Hering along their short courses (Fig. 22-23) are bordered in part by hepatocytes and in part by a *duct type* of cell. There are no types of cells in the walls of the canals

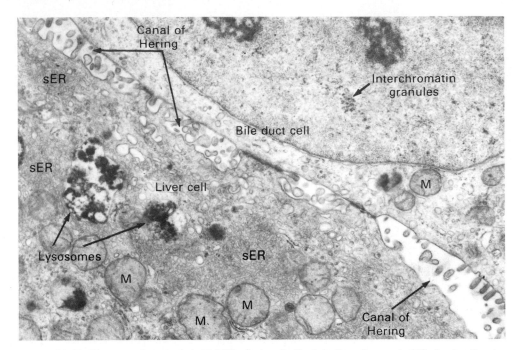

Fig. 22-23. Electron micrograph (×13,300) of a longitudinal section of a canal of Hering (rat liver). (These passages are difficult to find in normal liver; this is from an animal given large doses of alpha-naphthyl-isothiocyanate, which makes them easier to find.) At *lower left* is a hepatocyte, and at *upper right* a bile duct cell. The channel between them, into which microvilli of both types of cells project, is a canal of Hering. The mitochondria (M) of the duct cell are somewhat smaller than those of the hepatocyte. The sER and lysosomes of the hepatocyte have undergone marked hypertrophy in response to the chemical. (Courtesy of J. Steiner)

of Hering that represent transitions between hepatocytes and duct cells. There is instead a mixture of hepatocytes and duct cells along the course of the canals (Fig. 22-23). The canals of Hering are very short and connect with *bile ductules* (the finest branches of the bile duct system). These are present in the connective tissue of portal tracts. However, the canals of Hering are not the *only* channels by which bile from canaliculi reaches the bile ductules in the portal radicles, because leading off at angles from the canals of Hering there are little bypasses termed *preductules* (*cholangioles*) and these, too, drain into the bile ductules in the portal tracts. Preductules differ from canals of Hering in having no hepatocytes along their course; their walls are made entirely of cells of the duct type (Fig. 22-24). The walls of preductules are seen in cross sections to consist of no more than 2 or 3 cells of the duct type (Fig. 22-24). The bile ductules (small bile ducts) in the portal tracts, into which both canals of Hering and preductules drain, where seen in cross section, always have more than 3 cells around their walls (Fig. 22-25). The bile ductules, as noted, are the smallest branches of the branching bile ducts contained in the connective tissue tree that sends its branches to the periphery of all liver lobules.

Cells of the *duct type* along canals of Hering and in the walls of preductules differ from hepatocytes in several ways. They are smaller and have much less cytoplasm than hepatic cells (Figs. 22-23 and 22-24). Their cytoplasm contains only a little rER but does contain a moderate number of ribosomes. The Golgi apparatus is not well developed and is commonly disposed between the nucleus and the lumen. They contain no glycogen, and their mitochondria are smaller than those of hepatocytes. Basement membrane is present at the base of cells of the duct type but not in association with hepatocytes. Junctional complexes hold the cell membranes of contiguous cells firmly together at the sites of canaliculi. Elsewhere contiguous membranes interdigitate to help keep adjacent cells together. Microvilli project into the lumina of bile ductules. All these features are illustrated in Figures 22-23 and 22-24.

Bile Ducts. The bile ductules, the smallest branches of the bile duct system, have walls of low cuboidal epithelium (Fig. 22-25). The slightly larger ducts seen in portal areas have walls of cuboidal epithelium (Fig. 22-7B). Still larger bile ducts have columnar epithelium, so in general the height of the epithelium varies in relation to the size of the duct, a usual feature of ducts of glands. The 2 main

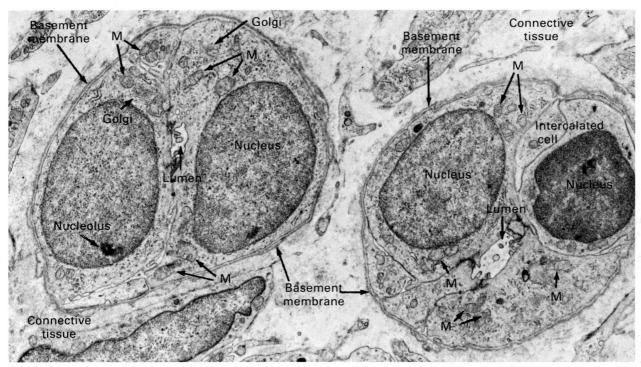

Fig. 22-24. Electron micrograph (×8,500) of two bile preductules (cholangioles) in the connective tissue of a portal tract of the liver. Each is surrounded by a basal lamina. The one on the *left* is lined by two bile ductule cells, the one on the *right* by three. The one at *right* also shows a cell which in this plane of section is not in contact with the lumen; such cells are designated intercalated cells. Note the simple fine structure of the duct cells, with small, inconspicuous mitochondria, sparse Golgi saccules, and virtually no endoplasmic reticulum. These cells are not very active metabolically. (Courtesy of J. Steiner)

hepatic ducts, which leave the liver at the site of the porta (transverse fissure), unite to form the *hepatic duct.* The extrahepatic ducts require more support than the intrahepatic ones embedded in the connective tissue of the portal tracts. This is provided by dense connective tissue and smooth muscle arranged so as to surround the epithelially lined lumen of the tube.

In bile ducts large enough to be lined by columnar epithelium, fat droplets are not uncommon within the cytoplasm of their lining cells. In the larger intrahepatic bile ducts, and in the extrahepatic ones, tubuloalveolar glands are present in the much-folded mucous membrane.

LYMPHATICS AND THE FORMATION OF LIVER LYMPH

There is nothing special about the appearance of the lymphatics in portal tracts; their size and number vary with the size of the tract in which they are seen. There is, however, a problem in ascertaining the source of the lymph they contain.

The liver produces a great deal of lymph relatively rich in protein. There has been controversy about where it is

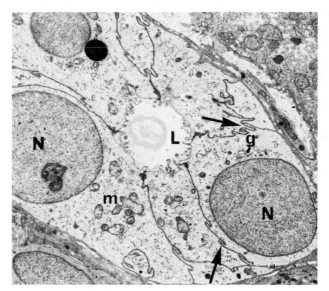

Fig. 22-25. Electron micrograph of a cross section of a bile ductule in a portal tract of human liver. Note the interlocking folds (indicated by arrows) along the cell membranes of the bile ductule cells. Mitochondria are few. (Courtesy of H. Sasaki and F. Schuffner. *In* Steiner, J. W., Phillips, M. J., and Miyai, K.: Ultrastructural and subcellular pathology of the liver. Int. Rev. Exp. Pathol., *3*:65, 1964)

formed. Lymphatics have not been demonstrated with certainty in or around liver trabeculae or sinusoids, but only in the connective tissue components of the liver, that is, in (*1*) the connective tissue of the capsule, (*2*) the tree of connective tissue that carries the branches of the portal vein, hepatic artery, and bile duct to the sides of each lobule, and (*3*) the sparse connective tissue associated with hepatic veins.

JAUNDICE

Jaundice means yellow. Under normal conditions the amount of yellow bile pigment in blood is not enough to color the skin. But under certain conditions blood can contain enough to cause the skin, mucous membranes, and whites of the eyes to take on a yellow color. A person so affected is said to have *jaundice*.

Jaundice can occur in 3 different ways, as will now be described.

(*1*) Normally, hepatocytes remove bilirubin from the blood at the same rate at which it is produced by macrophages. But under conditions in which erythrocyte destruction becomes greatly increased, the uptake of bilirubin by hepatocytes may lag behind its rate of production by macrophages, with the result that the concentration of bilirubin increases in the blood sufficiently to cause jaundice. This type is generally termed *hemolytic jaundice* because it is caused by increased hemolysis of red blood cells. (This is also the mechanism responsible for physiological jaundice of the newborn, due to the nucleated red blood cells persisting from prenatal life being rapidly destroyed by macrophages.)

(*2*) The ability of the liver to absorb bilirubin, process it metabolically, and secrete it into canaliculi may become impaired in various ways. First, in a rare condition there is a block at the cell membrane of the hepatocytes, which becomes altered in such a way that bilirubin is prevented from entering them from the bloodstream as readily as it should. Next, hepatocytes may have hereditary enzyme defects that prevent them handling bilirubin properly, or hepatocytes may be damaged through various causes so that there are not enough healthy cells to handle the bilirubin coming to them from blood. Finally, they may be so damaged that the bilirubin they absorb is not properly secreted and leaks back into the sinusoids.

(*3*) The production of bilirubin and its uptake and secretion by hepatocytes can be normal, but the bile secreted into the duct system can be prevented from flowing properly to the intestine because of some obstruction to the duct system. The common obstruction is a stone in one of the main drainage ducts. Another cause of obstruction can be a malignant growth of cells in the head of pancreas, which obstructs the duct opening into the duodenum. Under these conditions bile is dammed back through the hepatocytes into sinusoids.

THE REGENERATIVE CAPACITY OF THE LIVER AND THE PROBLEM OF CIRRHOSIS

Over 60 per cent of the cells in the liver are hepatocytes. If a portion of the liver is excised from an experimental animal, the hepatocytes soon undergo mitosis and restore the liver to its normal size in a few days. The factors that operate to cause this rapid regeneration are not thoroughly understood. The concept that the control of the cell population in the liver is mediated by a

chalone was described in Chapter 6. According to this concept, when part of the liver is excised not enough chalone is produced to restrain cell proliferation. If, however, hepatocytes are damaged by nutritional deficiencies, or toxic substances in the circulation (or for other reasons), the problem of regeneration becomes much more complicated. This is due primarily to the fact that not all the structures essential for regeneration of functional hepatic tissue may be able to regenerate in a harmonious way so as to restore the normal complicated architecture of the organ; there are just too many tubes and passageways, within and without lobules, to re-form and become connected together again properly.

In the healing of a fracture, osteogenic cells may fail to effect a cartilaginous and bony type of union. Fibroblasts from adjacent connective tissue may grow between the fragments at the fracture site and fill the gap with ordinary dense connective tissue, and this in turn impedes osteogenic cells from growing across the gap to effect a bony union. Likewise, if the parenchyma of the liver is badly damaged, with much cell death, the reticular and connective tissue framework supporting lobules and sinusoids collapses. Regeneration of hepatocytes may begin in isolated areas where healthy cells remain. However, the nodules of new liver parenchyma that develop may be divorced from proper connections with the portal circulation, and hence lack the proper organization of sinusoids. Meanwhile, fibroblasts in the partly collapsed framework may proliferate and form inappropriate amounts of new connective tissue that in turn may interfere with new normal connections being established between regenerating nodules of parenchyma and the system of bile ducts. Furthermore, this connective tissue may also interfere with the development of proper connections between the sinusoids in the regenerating parenchyma and the afferent venous and arterial vessels. Moreover, the increased amount of connective tissue prevents the liver as a whole from expanding as nodules of parenchyma become larger and, indeed, the connective tissue itself may shrink as it matures. This irreversible and serious condition is termed *cirrhosis*.

As the student will learn if he studies pathology, degeneration of hepatocytes can occur from many different causes (for instance, virus infection and consuming alcohol in quantity) and can begin in different sites within lobules. As a consequence the cirrhotic process can begin in different parts of the liver lobule.

THE GALLBLADDER

Microscopic Structure. A side branch (the *cystic duct*) extends from the hepatic duct to a somewhat elongated pear-shaped sac, the *gallbladder* (Fig. 22-26). The gallbladder is lined by a mucous membrane thrown into so many folds when the bladder is contracted (Figs. 22-27 and 22-28) that a student, on seeing a section of the wall of the organ, might think its mucosa riddled with glands (Fig. 22-27). Actually, there are no glands in the mucosa of the gallbladder except near its neck, and if the organ is distended, most (but not all) of its mucosal folds disappear.

The epithelium of the *mucous membrane* of the gallbladder is high columnar (Fig. 22-28). Each cell in the membrane resembles the one beside it; in this respect the lining membrane resembles the epithelium of the stom-

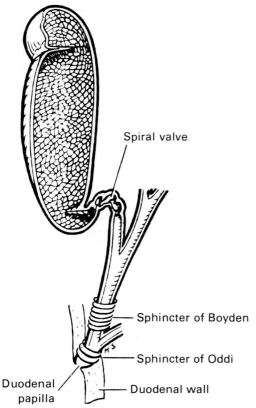

Fig. 22-26. Diagram of the gallbladder (cut open to show its corrugated inner surface), cystic duct, bile duct, and sphincters of Boyden and Oddi. (Grant, J. C. B., and Basmajian, J. V.: Grant's Method of Anatomy. ed. 7. Baltimore, Williams & Wilkins, 1965)

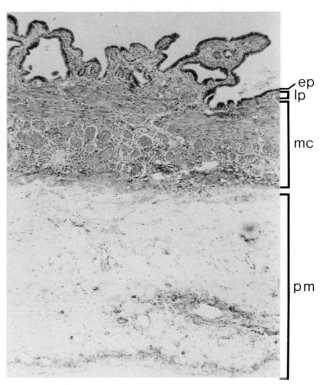

Fig. 22-27. Low-power photomicrograph of human gallbladder. The layers in its walls are: simple columnar epithelium (ep); lamina propria (lp); muscular coat (mc), consisting of smooth muscle and equivalent to muscularis externa; and perimuscular (subserosal) coat (pm) of connective tissue, containing blood vessels and fat cells.

ach. But the cells themselves are not like those lining the stomach. They resemble more closely the absorptive cells of the small intestine and, like them, are provided with microvilli. Secretory granules have been described in the more superficial parts of the cytoplasm of the cells, but the primary function of the lining cells is absorptive rather than secretory.

The epithelium rests on a *lamina propria* of loose connective tissue (Fig. 22-28). There is *no muscularis mucosae* in the gallbladder; hence the mucous membrane rests on a skimpy layer of smooth muscle comparable in position, but not in thickness, with the *muscularis externa* of the intestine (Fig. 22-27). Some of the smooth muscle fibers of which the muscularis externa is composed run circularly and longitudinally, but most run obliquely. Many elastic fibers are present in the connective tissue filling the interstices between the smooth muscle bundles of this coat.

Outside the muscle coat is a well-developed *perimuscular (subserosal) coat* (Fig. 22-27). This con-

sists of loose connective tissue, and may contain groups of fat cells. It conveys arteries, veins, lymphatics and nerves to the organ. Along the side of the gallbladder attached to the liver, the connective tissue of its perimuscular coat (which here cannot be termed properly its subserosal coat) is continuous with the connective tissue of the liver.

The neck of the gallbladder is twisted in such a fashion that its mucosa is thrown into a spiral fold (Fig. 22-26). Somewhat similar crescentic folds of mucosa are present in the lining of the cystic duct. More muscle appears in the wall of the gallbladder at its neck, and in the wall of the cystic duct, than is present in the remainder of the gallbladder.

The Bile Duct and the Sphincter of Oddi. The duct that extends from the point of junction of the cystic and hepatic ducts to the duodenum was, in the past, generally termed the *common bile duct*. There is now a tendency to omit "common" from the term. This duct penetrates the outer coats of the duodenum, close to the point of entry of the pancreatic duct. Part way through the

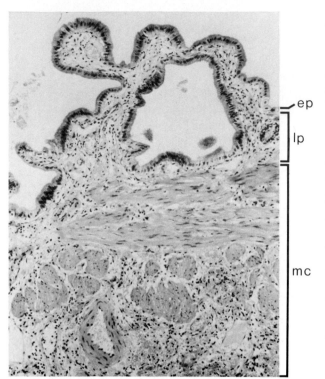

Fig. 22-28. Medium-power photomicrograph of the inner part of the wall of human gallbladder, showing its lining epithelium (ep), which consists of tall columnar cells, all of which are alike and have apical microvilli; the loose connective tissue of the lamina propria (lp) with its abundant capillaries; and most of its muscle coat (mc), with larger blood vessels in it. The bundles of smooth muscle near the lumen are cut longitudinally, the deeper ones in cross section. Note that the mucous membrane of the gallbladder shows folds, not villi, and that there is no muscularis mucosae. The muscle coat corresponds to muscularis externa.

duodenal wall the 2 ducts fuse, and the lumen of the fused duct is sufficiently expanded to be called the *ampulla of Vater*. The ampulla pursues an oblique course through the inner layers of the duodenal wall to open on the summit of a papilla that projects into the duodenal lumen, the *duodenal papilla*.

In the past, the muscle associated with the ampulla and the ends of the 2 ducts that enter the ampulla were said to constitute, collectively, the *sphincter of Oddi*. However, this muscle develops independently and hence is not part of the muscle of the intestinal wall proper. The muscle around the preampullary part of the bile duct becomes strong and serves as a sphincter at the outlet of the bile duct; it is sometimes referred to as the *sphincter of Boyden* (Fig. 22-26). The muscle that develops around the ampulla itself and the preampullary part of the pancreatic duct is not substantial enough to be considered a true sphincter (except in a minority of individuals). The closure of the strong sphincter of Boyden, surrounding the preampullary part of the bile duct, prevents the secretion of the liver from entering the intestine and as a result bile formed during its closure is bypassed, by way of the cystic duct, to the gallbladder, where it is stored and concentrated. There are also smooth muscle fibers disposed parallel

with the preampullary parts of the bile and pancreatic ducts; their contraction shortens (and presumably broadens) the ducts so as to encourage flow through them.

Functions of the Gallbladder. The gallbladder stores and concentrates bile. Concentration is effected by absorption of water and inorganic salts through the epithelium into the vessels of the lamina propria of its mucosa. This results in increased concentration of bile pigment, bile salts, and cholesterol. Radiopaque substances excreted by the liver appear in the bile, and if the gallbladder is concentrating normally, these become sufficiently concentrated in the gallbladder to allow that organ to be outlined by x-rays. In this way, gallbladder function can be checked. The absorption of inorganic salts from bile in the gallbladder results in its becoming less alkaline.

A hormonal mechanism is concerned in causing gallbladder contraction. Eating fat is particularly effective in causing the gallbladder to contract. Boyden showed that if blood of a recently fed animal is injected into another animal, it causes the gallbladder of the recipient to empty. It is believed that a hormone is made by the intestinal mucosa under the influence of digesting food, and that this travels to the gallbladder by the bloodstream to cause its contraction. This hormone is known as *cholecystokinin*. Peristaltic waves in the intestine probably affect the opening and closing of the sphincter that lets bile enter the intestine, so that bile enters the intestine in squirts.

The muscle of the wall of the gallbladder is so thin that some investigators have doubted that its contraction could be an important factor in emptying it. However, experimental work provides little ground for these doubts.

The Development of the Bile Ducts, Gallbladder, and Liver

The liver originates from endoderm-derived epithelium of the developing duodenum; the epithelium here first bulges outward to form what is termed the *hepatic diverticulum*. One branch of this forms the cystic duct and gallbladder. The epithelial cells of another part project into the splanchnic mesoderm and split it up. Branches from what will become the portal vein grow into the area and the spaces between the developing epithelial projections become richly vascularized. The whole mass grows rapidly. The mesoderm provides a capsule for the organ and also the tree of connective tissue that forms in the interior of the organ.

In the usual development of exocrine glands, the terminal epithelial outgrowths become secretory units, and the epithelial cells that connect these with the site of origin form ducts. However, there is a difference in the way the cells of the outgrowth differentiate in forming the liver. The cells closer to the site of origin begin to differentiate to form tubules, whereas farther away from the origin the cells become arranged into thick irregular clumps. At this time there is no difference in appearance of cells that form tubules or clumps. Later, however, their appearance changes, and the cells forming tubules become cells of bile ducts (*duct cells*), whereas those forming clumps become cells of secretory units, that is, *hepatocytes*. The thick plates in which future hepatocytes are at first arranged become split up to form the trabeculae of the parenchyma, with blood vessels between them; the latter become the *sinusoids*.

REFERENCES AND OTHER READING

PANCREAS

Caro, L. G., and Palade, G. E.: Protein synthesis, storage and discharge in the pancreatic exocrine cell. An autoradiographic study. J. Cell Biol., *20:*473, 1964.

Ciba Foundation Symposium on the Exocrine Pancreas. Boston, Little, Brown, 1962.

Ekholm, R., and Edlund, Y.: Ultrastructure of the human exocrine pancreas. J. Ultrastruct. Res., *2:*453, 1959.

Farquhar, M. G., and Palade, G. F.: Junctional complexes in various epithelia. J. Cell Biol., *17:*375, 1963.

Jamieson, J. D., and Palade, G. E.: Condensing vacuole conversion and zymogen granule discharge in pancreatic exocrine cells: metabolic studies. J. Cell Biol., *48:*503, 1971.

Munger, B. L.: A phase and electron microscopic study of cellular differentiation in pancreatic acinar cells of the mouse. Am. J. Anat., *103:*1, 1958.

For further references on the fine structure of, and mechanism of secretion in, acinar cells, *see* Chapter 7.

For islets of Langerhans, *see* Chapter 27.

LIVER

Babcock, M. B., and Cardell, R. R., Jr.: Hepatic glycogen patterns in fasted and fed rats. Am. J. Anat., *140:*299, 1974.

Bergeron, J. J. M., Levine, G., Sikstrom, R., O'Shaughnessy, D., Kopriwa, B., Nadler, N. J., and Posner, B. I.: Polypeptide hormone binding sites *in vivo:* initial localization of ^{125}I-labeled insulin to hepatocyte plasmalemma as visualized by electron microscope radioautography. Proc. Natl. Acad. Sci. U.S.A., *74:*5051, 1977.

Blouin, A., Bolender, R. P., and Weibel, E. R.: Distribution of organelles and membranes between hepatocytes and nonhepatocytes in the rat liver parenchyma. A stereological study. J. Cell Biol., *72:*441, 1977.

Bollman, J. L.: Studies of hepatic lymphatics. *In* Trans. of 9th Conf. on Liver Injury. p. 91. New York, Macy, 1950.

Brooks, S. E. H., and Haggis, G. H.: Scanning electron microscopy of rat's liver. Lab. Invest., *29.*60, 1973.

Bruni, C., and Porter, K. R.: The fine structure of the parenchymal cell of the normal rat liver. 1. General Observations. Am. J. Pathol., *46:*691, 1965.

Bucher, N. L. R.: Regeneration of mammalian liver. Int. Rev. Cytol., *15:*245, 1963.

————: Experimental aspects of hepatic regeneration. N. Engl. J. Med., *277:*686, 1967.

Burkel, W. E.: The fine structure of the terminal branches of the hepatic arterial system of the rat. Anat. Rec., *167:*329, 1970.

Cardell, R. R., Jr.: Action of metabolic hormones on the fine structure of liver cells III. Effects of adrenalectomy and administration of cortisone. Anat. Rec., *180:*309, 1974.

————: Smooth endoplasmic reticulum in rat hepatocytes during glycogen deposition and depletion. Int. Rev. Cytol., *48:*221, 1977.

Carruthers, J. S., and Steiner, J. W.: Fine structure of terminal branches of the biliary tree. Arch. Pathol., *74:*117, 1962.

Doljanski, F.: The growth of the liver with special reference to mammals. Int. Rev. Cytol., *10,* 1960.

Ehrenreich, J. H., Bergeron, J. J. M., Siekevitz, P., and Palade, G. E.: Golgi fractions prepared from rat liver homogenates. J. Cell Biol., *59:*45, 1973.

Elias, H.: A re-examination of the structure of the mammalian liver: I. Parenchymal architecture. Am. J. Anat., *84:*311, 1949.

————: A re-examination of the structure of the mammalian liver: II. Hepatic lobule and its relation to vascular and biliary systems. Am. J. Anat., *85:*379, 1949.

Farquhar, M. G., Bergeron, J. J. M., and Palade, G. E.: Cytochemistry of Golgi fractions prepared from rat liver. J. Cell Biol., *60:*8, 1974.

Fawcett, D. W.: Observations on the cytology and electron microscopy of hepatic cells. J. Natl. Cancer Inst., *15:*1475, 1955.

Frank, B. W., and Kern, F.: Intestinal and liver lymph and lymphatics. Gastroenterology, *55:*408, 1967.

Hamilton, R. L., Regen, D. M., Gray, M. E., and LeQuire, V. S.: Lipid transport in liver. I. Electron microscopic identification of very low density lipoprotein in perfused rat liver. Lab. Invest., *16:*305, 1967.

Howard, J. G.: The origin and immunological significance of Kuppfer cells. *In* van Furth, R. (ed.): Mononuclear Phagocytes. Oxford, Blackwell Scientific Publications, 1970.

Hruban, Z., and Swift, H.: Uricase, localization in hepatic microbodies. Science, *146:*1316, 1964.

Ito, T.: Recent advances in the study of the fine structure of the hepatic sinusoidal wall: a review. Gunma Rep. Med. Sci., *6:*119, 1973.

Jézéquel, A., Arakawa, K., and Steiner, J. W.: The fine structure of the normal neonatal mouse liver. Lab. Invest., *14:*1894, 1965.

Jones, A. L., and Fawcett, D. W.: Hypertrophy of the agranular endoplasmic reticulum in hamster liver induced by phenobarbital. J. Histochem. Cytochem., *14:*215, 1966.

LeBouton, A. V., and Marchand, R.: Changes in the distribution of thymidine-^{3}H labeled cells in the growing liver acinus of neonatal rats. Dev. Biol., *23:*524, 1970.

Ma, M. H., and Biempica, L.: The normal human liver cell. Am. J. Pathol., *62:*353, 1971.

Matter, A., Orci, L., and Rouiller, C.: A study on the permeability barriers between Disse's space and the bile canaliculus. J. Ultrastruct. Res., *11*(Suppl.), 1969.

Mosbaugh, M. M., and Ham, A. W.: Stimulation of bile secretion in chick embryos by cortisone. Nature, *168:*789, 1951.

Novikoff, A. B., and Essner, E.: The liver cell. Am. J. Med., *29:*102, 1960.

Porta, E. A., Hartroft, W. S., Gomez-Dumm, C. L. A., and Koch, O. R.: Dietary factors in the progression and regression of hepatic alterations associated with experimental chronic alcoholism. Fed. Proc., *26:*1449, 1967.

Rappaport, A. M.: The structural and functional acinar unit of the liver; some histopathological considerations (Monograph). Int. Symp. Hepatitis Frontiers. Boston, Little, Brown, 1957.

————: The structural and functional unit in the human liver (liver acinus). Anat. Rec., *130:*673, 1958.

————: Acinar units and the pathophysiology of the liver. *In* Rouiller, C. (ed.): The Liver; Morphology, Biochemistry, Physiology. vol. 1. New York, Academic Press, 1963.

————: The microcirculatory hepatic unit. Microvasc. Res., *6:*212, 1973.

————: The microcirculatory acinar concept of normal and

pathological hepatic structure. Beitr. Pathol. Bd., *157:*215, 1976.

Rappaport, A. M., Black, R. G., Lucas, C. C., Ridout, J. H., and Best, C. H.: Normal and pathologic microcirculation of the living mammalian liver. Rev. Int. Pathol., *16*(4):813, 1966.

Rappaport, A. M., Borowy, Z. J., Lougheed, W. M., and Lotto, W. N.: Subdivision of hexagonal liver lobules into a structural and functional unit; role in hepatic physiology and pathology. Anat. Rec., *119:*11, 1954.

Rappaport, A. M., and Hiraki, G. Y.: The anatomical pattern of lesions in the liver. Acta Anat., *32:*126, 1958.

———: Histopathologic changes in the structural and functional unit of the human liver. Acta Anat., *32:*240, 1958.

Rappaport, A. M., and Knoblauch, M.: The hepatic artery, its structural, circulatory and metabolic functions. 3rd Int. Symp. Int. Assoc. Study of Liver, Kyoto, 1966. T. Gastorent. p. 116, 1967.

Rhodin, J. A. G.: Ultrastructure and function of liver sinusoids. Proceedings IVth International Symposium of R.E.S., May 29-June 1, 1964, Kyoto, Japan.

Rouiller, C. (ed.): The Liver; Morphology, Biochemistry, Physiology. 2 vols. New York, Academic Press, 1963-64.

Stein, O., and Stein, Y.: The role of the liver in the metabolism of chylomicrons, studied by electron microscope autoradiography. Lab. Invest., *17:*436, 1967.

Steiner, J. W., and Carruthers, J. S.: Studies on the fine structure of the terminal branches of the biliary tree. I. The morphology of normal bile canaliculi, bile pre-ductules (ducts of Hering) and bile ductules. Am J. Pathol., *38:*639, 1961.

Steiner, J. W., Carruthers, J. S., and Kalifat, S. R.: The ductular cell reaction of rat liver in extrahepatic cholestasis. I. Proliferated biliary epithelial cells. Exp. Mol. Pathol., *1:*162, 1962.

Steiner, J. W., Jézéquel, A.-M., Phillips, M. J., Miyai, K., and Arakawa, K.: Some aspects of the ultrastructural pathology of the liver. Prog. Liver Dis., *2:*303, 1965.

Steiner, J. W., Phillips, M. J., and Miyai, K.: Ultrastructural and subcellular pathology of the liver. Int. Rev. Exp. Pathol., *3:*65, 1964.

Trump, B. F., Goldblatt, P. J., and Stowell, R. E.: An electron microscope study of early cytoplasmic alterations in hepatic parenchymal cells of mouse liver during necrosis in vitro (autolysis). Lab. Invest., *11:*986, 1962.

Wisse, E.: An electron microscope study of the fenestrated endothelial lining of rat liver sinusoids. J. Ultrastruct. Res., *31:*125, 1970.

———: An ultrastructural characterization of the endothelial cell in the rat liver sinusoid under normal and various experimental conditions, as a contribution to the distinction between endothelial and Kupffer cells. J. Ultrastr. Res., *38:*528, 1972.

———: Observations on the fine structure and peroxidase cytochemistry of normal rat liver Kupffer cells. J. Ultrastruct. Res., *46:*393, 1974.

Wisse, E., and Daems, W. Th.: Fine structural studies on the sinusoidal lining cells of rat liver. *In* van Furth, R. (ed.): Mononuclear Phagocytes. Oxford, Blackwell Scientific Publications, 1970.

GALLBLADDER

Chapman, G. B., Chiardo, A. J., Coffey, R. J., and Weineke, K.: The fine structure of the human gallbladder. Anat. Rec., *154:*579, 1966.

Hayward, A. F.: Aspects of the fine structure of gallbladder epithelium of the mouse. J. Anat., *96:*227, 1962.

———: The structure of gallbladder epithelium. Int. Rev. Gen. Exp. Zool., *3:*205, 1968.

Jit, I.: The development of the unstriped musculature of the gallbladder and the cystic duct. J. Anat. Soc. (India), *8:*15, 1959.

Kay, G. I., Wheeler, H. O., Whitlock, R. T., and Lane, N.: Fluid transport in rabbit gallbladder. A combined physiological and electron microscope study. J. Cell Biol., *30:*237, 1966.

Mueller, J. C., Jones, A. L., and Long, J. A.: Topographical and subcellular anatomy of the guinea pig gallbladder. Gastroenterology, *63:*856, 1972.

Ralph, P. H.: The surface structure of the gallbladder and intestinal epithelium of man and monkey. Anat. Rec., *108:*217, 1950.

Yamada, E.: The fine structure of the gallbladder epithelium of the mouse. J. Biophys. Biochem. Cytol., *1:*445, 1955.

23 The Respiratory System

General Function of the System. Blood leaves the capillaries of the systemic circulatory system with a diminished oxygen and an increased carbon dioxide content. This blood is emptied into the right heart, from which it is pumped via the pulmonary circuit through the lungs. The latter are two large organs, spongy because they contain innumerable little pockets of air and a vast number of capillaries which abut on the air pockets. Carbon dioxide diffuses from the blood in the pulmonary capillaries into the air pockets, and oxygen diffuses in the reverse direction. The air in the pockets would, of course, quickly become highly charged with carbon dioxide and depleted of oxygen if there were no provision for changing it. This is accomplished by respiratory movements: *inspiration,* by which fresh air is drawn into the lungs; and *expiration,* by which vitiated air is expelled from the lungs.

The Lungs, Thoracic Cavity, and Pleural Cavities. The two lungs are contained in the thorax (Fig. 23-1). This has a cage-like framework comprising the vertebral column, ribs, costal cartilages, and sternum. The bottom of the cage is a dome-shaped musculotendinous sheet, the *diaphragm.*

Each lung fills a large compartment in the thoracic cavity lined with a fibroelastic membrane, the *parietal pleura* (Fig. 23-1), the surface of which consists of squamous mesothelial cells. Likewise, each lung is covered with a similar membrane, the *visceral pleura* (Fig. 23-1), the outermost layer of which also consists of squamous mesothelial cells. A film of fluid is present between the parietal pleura (that lines each cavity) and the visceral pleura (that covers each lung); this fluid has lubricating properties so that it allows the visceral pleura covering the lungs (and hence the lungs themselves) to slide during respiratory movements along the parietal pleura lining the cavities.

Except at its hilus, the root of the lung where a bronchus and blood vessels enter (Fig. 23-1), each lung by virtue of its slippery pleural surfaces is freely movable within its cavity. Around its point of attachment at the hilus, the visceral pleura covering each lung becomes continuous with the parietal pleura lining each cavity (Fig. 23-1). The space between the two layers of pleura contains only a film of fluid; hence it is only a *potential space* (*cavity*). Under certain abnormal conditions, however, the amount of fluid becomes increased; this converts the potential cavity into a real one. The potential (or real) space between the two layers of pleura is known as the *pleural cavity.* It should be understood that, although a lung occupies a cavity in the thorax, it does not lie inside the pleural cavity but outside it, just as the intestines occupy the abdominal cavity but lie outside the peritoneal cavity.

RESPIRATORY MOVEMENTS

Inspiration. The arrangement of the ribs with respect to the vertebral column and sternum is such that contraction of the muscles attached to the ribs not only deepens the thoracic cage in the anteroposterior plane but also widens it. Moreover, contraction of the diaphragm (with simultaneous relaxation of the muscles of the abdominal wall, permitting the diaphragm to descend) elongates the cage. Hence, by contraction of certain muscles and relaxation of others, the thoracic cage can be made larger by becoming deeper, wider, and longer. This is what occurs in inspiration.

In order for the thoracic cage to become larger on inspiration, something has to be drawn into it for the same reason that one cannot open bellows if the inlet is closed. Inspiratory movements are not powerful enough to create a vacuum in the thoracic cage.

Normally, the thoracic cage can be enlarged by inspiratory movements only to the extent to which air can be drawn into its air spaces, which therefore expand, and blood can be drawn into blood vessels to increase the amount they contain. Under normal conditions, air is drawn only into the lungs, but extra blood is drawn into the vessels of the lungs and also into thoracic vessels outside the lungs. Air is not drawn into any other part of the thoracic cavity except the lungs because there is no opening to the surface from the other parts of the thorax through which it can be drawn. If, however, an opening is made in the chest—for example by a deep knife wound—

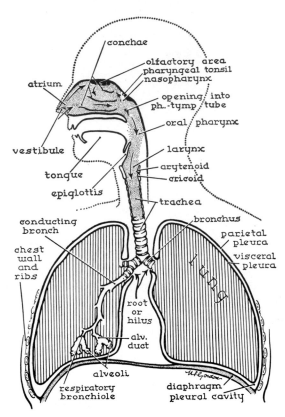

Fig. 23-1. Diagram of the parts of the respiratory system. (After Grant, J. C. B.: A Method of Anatomy. ed. 4. Baltimore, Williams & Wilkins, 1948)

air can be drawn by inspiratory movements into parts of the thorax other than the lungs, as explained in the following section.

The lungs consist essentially of: (*1*) spongy respiratory tissue in which gaseous exchange occurs between blood and air, and (*2*) a branching system of air tubes called *bronchioles* and *bronchi* which "pipe" air into and out of the pockets and passageways of the spongy respiratory tissue. The main bronchus from each lung connects with the *trachea* (Fig. 23-1), and this, in turn, by means of the larynx in conjunction with the nasopharynx and nose (or mouth if need be), connects with the outside air. Hence, on inspiration air is drawn through the nose, down the trachea, and into the bronchial tree to its end branches. From there it reaches the passageways and pockets of the spongy, capillary-rich respiratory tissue, where there is gaseous exchange (Fig. 23-1, alveolar duct and alveoli).

The Role of Elastin. Before briefly considering the mechanism of expiration, it is necessary to point out that the lungs would not be large enough to fill the cavities in which they lie unless they were considerably *stretched* in

all directions. A large amount of elastin is present in the visceral pleura that covers them, in the partitions between the air pockets, and in the walls of the bronchial tree. Since the lungs fill their respective cavities when they develop in embryonic life, and since there is no easy way for fluid to be drawn into the pleural cavity during fetal life, the lungs are gradually stretched as the thoracic cavity increases in size. The same process continues in the postnatal growing period. As a result, the elastic tissue of the lungs, under normal conditions, is always stretched (even at the end of expiration), and the lung is always tending, as it were, to collapse and retract to the point where it is attached (its root or hilus). Hence, if a hollow needle is inserted through the chest wall into the pleural cavity (between the parietal and the visceral layers of pleura), air immediately rushes through it into the pleural cavity, which thereupon, as the lung retracts toward its hilus, becomes a real (air-filled) cavity instead of only a potential cavity. Letting air into the pleural cavity is a procedure sometimes used to put a lung at rest in the treatment of tuberculosis. The condition in which there is air in the pleural cavity is called a *pneumothorax*. In certain diseases the fluid in the pleural cavity, which normally constitutes no more than a film, becomes greatly increased in amount. This, too, permits the lung to retract. This condition is known as a *hydrothorax*.

Expiration. Since the elastic tissue of the lungs remains stretched even at the end of expiration, and becomes still more stretched on inspiration, it is scarcely necessary for an individual at rest to exert muscular contractions to expel air. The elastic recoil of the lungs is almost enough in itself to expel air through the bronchial tree and draw in the sides and bottom of the thoracic cage. But during exercise expiration is facilitated—and probably also to some extent even in quiet breathing—by contractions of the abdominal muscles, which force the abdominal viscera against the undersurface of the diaphragm and so push it up into the thorax.

The descent and expansion of the lungs on inspiration require that the bronchial tree itself be elastic. Bronchi, for example, become longer and wider on inspiration. The root of the lung also descends on inspiration. On expiration, the various parts of the lung return to their original positions due to the recoil of the elastin in the bronchial tree.

The Two Parts of the System: the Conducting and the Respiratory Portions. The system of cavities and tubes that conducts air from outside the body to all parts of the lungs constitutes the *conducting portion* of the respiratory system; the pockets and passageways of the respiratory tissue of the lung (the only sites where gaseous exchange occurs) constitute the *respiratory portion* of the system. The conducting part of the system consists of the nose, nasopharynx, larynx, trachea, bronchi, and bronchioles (Fig.

23-1). It is to be noted that some of these structures lie outside the lung and others (some bronchi and all the bronchioles) within it. It should be realized that those parts of the conducting system that lie outside the lung must be provided with reasonably rigid walls; otherwise, a strong inspiratory act might collapse them, as in sucking a drink through a wet straw. Rigidity is provided by cartilage or bone. Moreover, it should be kept in mind that the conducting part of the respiratory system performs functions other than conducting air to and from the lungs. The mucous membrane lining the conducting passageways strains, washes, warms or cools, and humidifies the air passing through it toward the respiratory portion of the system. In other words, the conducting portion of the respiratory system is an excellent air-conditioning unit. Its different parts and their microscopic structure will now be described.

THE NASAL CAVITIES

The nose contains two *nasal cavities,* one on each side and separated by the *nasal septum.* Each cavity opens anteriorly at a *naris* or *nostril* and posteriorly into the *nasopharynx* (Fig. 23-1).

Bone, cartilage, and, to a small degree, dense connective tissue provide rigidity to the walls, floor, and roof of the nasal cavities and so prevent their collapse on inspiration.

Each nasal cavity is divided into two parts: (*1*) a *vestibule,* the widened part just behind the naris, and (*2*) the remainder of the cavity, called its *respiratory portion.*

The *epidermis* covering the nose extends into each naris to line the anterior part of each vestibule. It is provided with many hair follicles and some sebaceous and sweat glands. Conceivably the hairs strain very coarse particles from air being drawn through the nostrils. Farther back in the vestibule the *stratified squamous epithelium* is not keratinized, and still farther back it becomes *pseudostratified ciliated columnar* with goblet cells. From here on the epithelium becomes part of a mucous membrane lining the remainder of each nasal cavity (its respiratory portion). The epithelial component of this mucous membrane is pseudostratified columnar ciliated epithelium with goblet cells. The lamina propria component of the mucous membrane contains mucous and serous glands and is adherent to the periosteum of the bone, or the perichondrium of the cartilage, beneath it. The basement membrane separating the respiratory epithelium from the lamina propria is thicker than that of most epithelia.

The epithelial surface is normally covered with mucus provided by its goblet cells and the glands of its lamina propria. Probably over a pint of fluid is normally pro-

duced by the nasal mucous membrane each day. The mucus, together with the particles of dust and dirt it picks up, is moved posteriorly through the nasopharynx to the oral pharynx by the action of the cilia with which the epithelial lining cells (except the goblet cells) are provided. Each cell has between 15 and 20 cilia about 7 μm in height. Drainage of the nose depends to a great extent on orderly ciliary action, and loss of cilia due to trauma or disease can interfere with its proper drainage.

The *lamina propria* contains collagenic and elastic fibers. In some sites, and evidently by no means regularly, the lamina propria reveals a well-developed basement membrane with elastic properties. Lymphocytes, plasma cells, macrophages, and even granular leukocytes may be seen in the lamina propria. In general, it is a very vascular membrane, and in cold weather it helps to warm the air drawn into the lungs. In some sites lymphatic nodules appear; these are most numerous near the entrance to the nasopharynx.

The mucous membrane of the respiratory portion of the nose has special characteristics in two places. The lining of the upper parts of the sides, and also the roof, of the posterior part of each cavity constitutes the organ of smell (the *olfactory organ*), and its special microscopic structure will now be described. The other unusual part of the mucous membrane of the nose will be described after this.

THE OLFACTORY ORGAN

General Features. In Chapter 17 we explained how the first neurons to evolve represented specializations of surface ectodermal cells (Fig. 17-3). As evolution proceeded, the nerve cell bodies of most afferent neurons migrated to a more central and better-protected position in cerebrospinal ganglia. However, the olfactory organ represents an exception to this general rule, because in olfactory areas the cell bodies of afferent neurons are at the body surface.

There are two olfactory areas, one in each of the two nasal cavities. The mucous membrane lining the nasal cavities in the two olfactory areas constitutes the *olfactory organ.* The nerve cell bodies present in the epithelium of the mucous membrane at this site are stimulated by odors of different kinds. It should be kept in mind that the presence of nerve cell bodies at the body surface is a more hazardous arrangement than having them more deeply situated, with afferent fibers extending to the surface, for when this mucous membrane containing nerve cell bodies is injured by a disease process or trauma, the nerve cell bodies also can be destroyed. So, as might be expected, the sense of smell often becomes impaired and probably the functional input of about 1 per cent of the fibers of the olfactory nerves (which lead from the receptors to the brain) is lost each year of life. Virtually all function of the olfactory receptors can be lost at a comparatively early age as a result of destruction of the olfactory epithelium by the infections to which the nasal mucous membrane is so susceptible.

Gross Characteristics. The mucous membrane of the olfactory areas is yellowish in color, due to pigment, and lines most of the roof of each nasal cavity (Fig. 23-1). It begins in front of the anterior end of the superior concha (the conchae are curved shelves of bone, covered with mucous membrane, that extend inward from the lateral wall of each nasal cavity as shown in Figure 23-1). From here the olfactory area extends posteriorly for about 1 cm. From the roof it also extends down both sides of each nasal cavity; on the lateral side it extends over most of the superior concha, and on the medial side it extends about 1 cm. down the nasal septum.

THE MICROSCOPIC STRUCTURE OF THE OLFACTORY AREAS

The mucous membrane of the olfactory organ consists of a thick *pseudostratified epithelium* (Fig. 23-2) and a thick *lamina propria.*

The *epithelium* consists of three kinds of cells: (*1*) olfactory receptor cells, (*2*) sustentacular (supporting) cells, and (*3*) basal cells.

The Olfactory Receptor Cells. These are modified bipolar nerve cells, each having a cell body with a dendrite extending from its superficial end to the surface of the epithelium and an axon extending from its deeper end into the lamina propria (Fig. 23-2, OC). Like the sustentacular cells supporting them, the receptor cells lie perpendicular to the surface of the membrane, with their cell bodies fitted in between the sustentacular cells so that their nuclei constitute a broad zone of rounded nuclei in the lower half of the membrane (Fig. 23-2). The dendritic process of each bipolar cell ascends in a crevice between sustentacular cells toward the surface, where it terminates as a swelling termed an *olfactory vesicle* (OV in Fig. 23-2); this is a bulb-like mass of cytoplasm that bulges out through the surface. Just below the surface the olfactory vesicle is connected to the adjacent sustentacular cells by a junctional complex, and at the level of the zonula adherens of the complex, which lies just deep to a very tight zonula occludens, the sustentacular cells exhibit a well-developed terminal web (TW in Fig. 23-3). In some sites the superficial parts of nearby dendritic processes lie close to one another. The olfactory vesicles bear clusters of long *olfactory cilia* (Fig. 23-3). The cytoplasm of the vesicles contains mitochondria, microtubules, some sER, and the basal bodies of the olfactory cilia (these are seen in cross and longitudinal section in Fig. 23-3, labeled BB).

The proximal portions of the cilia (and the basal bodies) have the usual arrangements of microtubules. However, farther out the cilia become narrower (Fig. 23-3), with generally only two microtubules extending into their narrow distal portions. Moreover, these long cilia lie along the surface of the membrane so as to form a tousled layer covering the microvilli on the apical surface of the sustentacular cells (Fig. 23-3). This layer is kept moist by the secretion of underlying glands.

The unmyelinated axon from each receptor cell extends down into the lamina propria beneath the olfactory epithelium and joins with others to constitute bundles of *olfactory nerve* fibers. These reach the olfactory bulbs (ovoid structures developing as anterior extensions of the olfactory area of the brain) via foramina in the cribriform plate of the ethmoid bone.

The Sustentacular Cells. The word *sustentacular* (L. *sustentaculum,* a prop) is commonly used with reference to sensory organs to denote supporting cells. The supporting cells of olfactory epithelium are tall and for the most part cylindrical except that they are irregularly tapered toward their bases (Fig. 23-2, SC). The free surface of these cells is covered with microvilli (Fig. 23-2). In between the sustentacular cells, the dendritic processes of the olfactory receptors reach to the surface (Fig. 23-2). A brownish yellow pigment similar to lipofuscin is present in the cytoplasm of the supporting cells and it is this that gives the olfactory area its yellow color in the gross. The nuclei of the sustentacular cells stain lightly and are ovoid in shape. They lie more or less in one row that extends parallel to the surface and lies superficial to a broader zone of rounded nuclei belonging to the receptor cells (Fig. 23-2). Deep to its nucleus, each sustentacular cell tapers somewhat, reaching down to the basement membrane except where prevented from doing so by the presence of a basal cell (Fig. 23-2).

The Basal Cells. These are roughly conical cells lying at intervals along the basement membrane (Fig. 23-2, BC). The intensity of staining of the nucleus is intermediate between that in sustentacular cells and that in receptor cells. These basal cells are generally regarded as relatively undifferentiated reserve cells that form new sustentacular cells when the need arises. However, in at least some species there are indications that basal cells are able to give rise to new olfactory receptor cells, and that these can even establish synaptic connections with the olfactory bulbs (Graziadei). This is suggestive that there may also be a replacement mechanism for the olfactory receptor cells, and indeed such a mechanism is warranted in view of the vulnerable position of these receptors at the body surface. However, since no other mechanism for postnatal replacement of nerve cells is known, this would constitute a very exceptional case to the general rule that neurons are not formed in postnatal life.

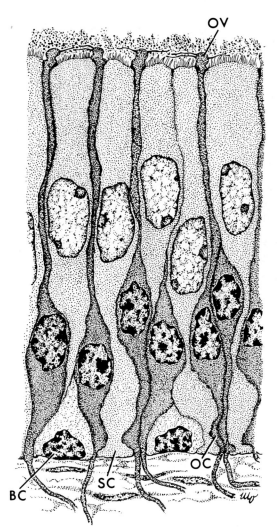

Fig. 23-2. Drawing of a section of olfactory epithelium as seen with the LM. OV, olfactory vesicle; BC, basal cell; SC, sustentacular cell; and OC, olfactory cell.

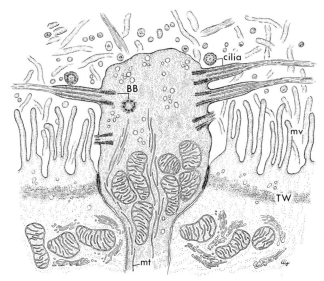

Fig. 23-3. Drawing illustrating the fine structure of an olfactory vesicle and the adjacent areas of olfactory epithelium. BB, basal bodies; mv, microvilli; TW, terminal web; and mt, microtubule. (Based on Frisch, D.: Am. J. Anat., *121*:87, 1967)

continuously freshen the thin layer of fluid bathing the olfactory cilia; since these are chemoreceptive, the substances responsible for odors have to dissolve in this layer.

The way odors are perceived is not understood. Individual olfactory receptors respond to a wide range of odoriferous substances. Odor discrimination undoubtedly requires recognition by the CNS of particular patterns of afferent impulses, relayed through the olfactory bulbs, from very large numbers of olfactory receptors.

THE MUCOUS MEMBRANE OF THE NASAL CONCHAE

General Features. As noted before we described the olfactory organ, the mucous membrane of the nose in two sites is of a special character. We have described the first site where it is unusual (the olfactory area) and will now describe the other site where it has a special character, which is over the middle and inferior conchae.

Three plates of bone, arranged one above the other like shelves, lie along the lateral wall of each nasal cavity. However, they are not flat like useful shelves; they are more like unsupported shelves that have had to bear too much weight, for they all curve downward. Since this makes them look something like shells, they are called the *superior, middle,* and *inferior conchae* (*concha* is Latin for shell), respectively (Figs. 23-1 and 23-4A). They are

The Lamina Propria. The deeper layers of the fibroelastic connective tissue comprising the lamina propria contain many veins and in some places resemble erectile tissue, which is discussed in the next section.

The lamina propria also contains tubuloalveolar glands called the *glands of Bowman*. These seem to be confined to olfactory areas, so that if found elsewhere it implies that such sites were once olfactory areas and that these lost their olfactory function due to injury. The principal secretory cell type contains abundant sER in its cytoplasm. The thin, watery secretion, which is delivered by ducts to the surface of the epithelium, has some of the characteristics of a watery mucus. Its role seems to be to

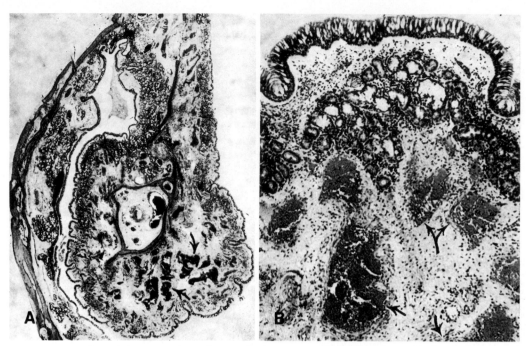

Fig. 23-4. (A) Very low power photomicrograph of a cross section of a concha. Thin bone may be seen *below center* in its central part. The blood in the venous spaces is dark. *(B)* Medium-power photomicrograph of a section of the mucous membrane covering a concha. Glands may be seen in the upper region, and large venous spaces distended with blood (arrows) in the lower region.

also often referred to as the *superior, middle,* and *inferior turbinate* (L. *turbineus,* shaped like a top) bones.

Microscopic Structure. Although the lamina propria of the mucous membrane of the nasal cavities is very vascular, containing many arteries, capillaries, and veins, that covering the middle and inferior conchae has, in addition, a large number of venous structures that under normal conditions are collapsed. However, under certain circumstances they can become distended with blood (Fig. 23-4B, arrows), and this increases the thickness of the mucosa. In some individuals the mucous membrane encroaches on the airway to such an extent that nose breathing is made difficult and these people complain about having a stuffed-up nose.

The term *erectile tissue* is usually used to designate any tissue with a large number of endothelial-lined cavities that, although on the circuit of the bloodstream, are usually collapsed and only become distended with blood to increase greatly the volume of the tissue in which they lie, as a result of special nervous stimulation. Most of the substance of the penis, for example, is erectile tissue; this accounts for the changes associated with its erection under conditions of erotic stimulation. The lamina propria of the nasal mucosa of the conchae is not such a typical erectile tissue as that of the penis, and some observers do not consider it true erectile tissue at all. Perhaps it is better described as possessing a great many thin-walled veins along which smooth muscle fibers are

circularly and longitudinally disposed (Fig. 23-4B). Nevertheless, it reacts like erectile tissue in that it can rapidly become turgid with blood. Furthermore, in certain individuals the mucosa covering the conchae is affected by erotic stimuli. Many years ago, Mackenzie described individuals encountered in his own practice in whom erotic stimulation was associated with sneezing, engorgement of the nasal mucosa covering the conchae, and even nosebleeds. Indeed, he quotes one 16th century report of a youth who sneezed whenever he saw a pretty girl. In attempting to understand the purpose served by having the function of the erectile tissue of the nose linked with that of the genital system, it should be borne in mind that sex stimulation is very dependent on olfactory stimuli in a great many animal species.

PARANASAL AIR SINUSES OF THE NOSE

The air *sinuses* (L. *sinus,* a hollow) are spaces in bones. There are four associated with each nasal cavity. They are named after the bones that contain them and hence are called the *frontal, ethmoidal, sphenoidal,* and *maxillary* sinuses, respectively. The maxillary sinus is the largest and is sometimes called the *antrum* (Gr. *antron,* cave) *of Highmore.*

The four sinuses on each side all communicate with the nasal cavity of that side. They are all lined by mucous membrane continuous with that lining the nasal cavity. The ciliated epithelium in the sinuses is not as thick as that in the nasal cavity itself, and does not contain nearly as many goblet cells. The lamina propria is relatively thin and is continuous with the periosteum of the underlying bone. It consists chiefly of collagenic fibers and contains eosinophils, plasma cells, and many lymphocytes, in addition to fibroblasts. It has relatively few glands embedded in it.

The openings by which the sinuses communicate with the nasal cavities are not large enough to prevent their becoming closed if the mucosa around these openings becomes inflamed or swollen for other reasons. Normally, the mucus formed in the sinuses is moved to the nasal cavities by ciliary action. If the openings of the sinuses become obstructed, however, the sinuses may fill with mucus or, under conditions of infection, with pus. Drugs acting similarly to hormones of the adrenal medulla, that cause contraction of the blood vessels of the part, are often used locally to lessen congestion around the openings of inflamed sinuses and so permit them to drain.

THE PHARYNGEAL TONSIL

This consists of an unpaired median mass of lymphatic tissue in the lamina propria of the mucous membrane lining the dorsal wall of the nasopharynx (Fig. 23-1). A child with an enlarged pharyngeal tonsil is said to have *adenoids* (Gr. *aden,* gland) because the enlarged lymphatic follicles of the tonsil give it a gland-like appearance. Adenoids may obstruct the respiratory passageway and lead to persistent mouth breathing. The muscular actions entailed in keeping the mouth always open, by changing the lines of force to which the facial bones are normally subjected, may prevent these bones from developing as they should. For this reason, and also because an enlarged pharyngeal tonsil is usually more or less persistently infected, removal of adenoids is a relatively common operation.

The pharyngeal tonsil resembles the palatine tonsil in microscopic structure except that: (*1*) it is more diffuse, (*2*) its covering epithelium dips down into it as folds rather than crypts, and (*3*) its epithelium may be pseudostratified, at least in some areas, instead of being stratified squamous nonkeratinized epithelium.

THE LARYNX

General Features. The larynx is the segment of the respiratory tube that connects the pharynx with the trachea (Fig. 23-1). Its walls are kept from collapsing on inspira-

tion by a number of cartilages contained in its wall and bound together with connective tissue. Muscles that pull on the cartilages are present both outside them (*extrinsic muscles* of the larynx) and between them and the mucous membrane (*intrinsic muscles* of the larynx). The larynx has many functions. It plays the most important part in phonation; however, this is phylogenetically a late development. A more fundamental function of the larynx is that of preventing anything but air from gaining entrance to the lower respiratory passages. It is said to be the watchdog for the lung and if, in spite of its efforts, anything but air enters it a cough reflex is set in motion immediately. It is of interest in this connection to note that some of the individuals that apparently died from drowning are found at autopsy to have very little water in their lungs; they probably died from asphyxiation due to a laryngeal spasm induced by water gaining entrance to and irritating this organ.

The Epiglottis. This is a flap-like structure that projects upward and slightly posteriorly from the top of the larynx, to which it is attached anteriorly (Fig. 23-1). It is now thought that the epiglottis plays a subsidiary and passive role in keeping food and fluid out of the larynx during swallowing. The main factor responsible for achieving this is the larynx being brought upward and forward in the act of swallowing, so that the upper end of its tubular part is pressed against the posterior aspect of the epiglottis, under the root of the tongue. Individuals who have had their epiglottis removed for some reason can still swallow without food entering their larynx.

The epiglottis is supported internally by a plate of *elastic cartilage*. The perichondrium of this is continuous with the lamina propria of the mucous membrane that covers both its surfaces. The type of epithelium of the mucous membrane varies in relation to the function of the different parts of the epiglottis. On the anterior surface, where the epiglottis comes into contact with the root of the tongue in the act of swallowing, the epithelium is of the *stratified squamous nonkeratinizing* type (Fig. 23-5) so well adapted for wet surfaces subjected to wear and tear. The epithelium covering the upper part of the posterior surface comes into contact with whatever is being swallowed and so is also subjected to wear and tear. It, too, is of the stratified squamous nonkeratinizing type. Taste buds are occasionally present in it. However, the epithelium covering the lower part of the posterior surface does not come into contact with food, and, since it constitutes the lining of part of the respiratory tube, it is lined with *pseudostratified columnar ciliated* epithelium with goblet cells (Fig. 23-5, *bottom*). The cilia beat toward the pharynx and move mucus and particles picked up by it in that direction. Mucous *glands* with some serous secretory units are present in the lamina propria under the posterior surface. They are said to be present

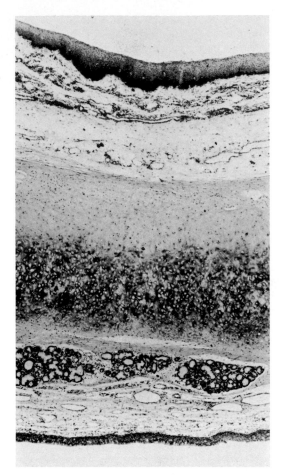

Fig. 23-5. Low-power photomicrograph of the full thickness of the epiglottis. The anterior surface is at *top,* the posterior at *bottom.* For details, *see* text.

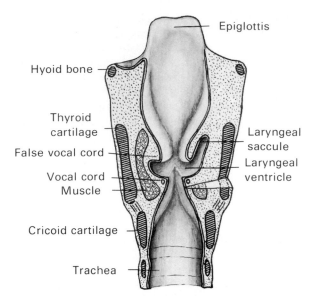

Fig. 23-6. Drawing of the posterior aspect of the anterior half of the larynx after being cut in coronal section. The cut is farther forward at the upper right side of the illustration so that the saccule is disclosed. (After Schaeffer, E. A.: Textbook of Microscopic Anatomy. Quain's Elements of Anatomy. ed. 11, vol. 2, part I. New York, Longmans, 1909)

also under the anterior surface. Glands are more numerous toward the attached margin of the epiglottis.

The Vocal Cords. The lumen of the larynx is narrowed and made more or less slit-like (the slit being in an anteroposterior direction) in two sites by folds of mucous membrane projecting into the lumen from each side. The upper pair of folds constitute the *false vocal cords* (Fig. 23-6). The second pair of folds lie below the first pair, and their cordlike free margins constitute the *true vocal cords* (Fig. 23-6). The opening between the two true vocal cords is termed the *rima glottidis.* It is slit-like when the vocal cords are close together but somewhat triangular in shape, with the apex of the triangle directed forward, when the vocal cords are farther apart. The expansion of the lumen of the larynx between the two sets of folds is called the *sinus* or *ventricle* of the larynx (Fig. 23-6). Anteriorly, the sinus of each side is prolonged upward. Each

cul-de-sac, so formed, is called a *laryngeal saccule* ((Fig. 23-6). The cores of the false vocal cords are composed chiefly of loose lamina propria with glands. The cores of the lower pair of folds consist of connective tissue and muscle, with the cores of the vocal cords themselves (the parts of the folds nearest their free edges) consisting of connective tissue composed chiefly of elastic fibers. The aperture between the true vocal cords, and the tension under which the cords are held, are affected by muscles that act on the cords directly and by muscles that affect the cords indirectly by shifting the tissues to which they are anchored.

The type of epithelium on the mucous membrane of the larynx varies in relation to the functions performed by its different parts. That covering the true vocal cords, which are subjected to considerable wear and tear, is of the stratified squamous nonkeratinizing type. All the epithelium lining the larynx below the true vocal cords is of the pseudostratified columnar ciliated type with goblet cells. Most of that lining the larynx above the true vocal cords is also of this type, although patches of stratified squamous nonkeratinizing epithelium may be present. The cilia beat toward the pharynx. Except over the true vocal cords, the lamina propria of the mucous membrane contains mucous glands. Lymphatic nodules occur in the lamina propria of the mucous membrane, especially in the region of the ventricle and false vocal cords.

The larynx is responsible for *phonation,* the ability to utter vocal sounds. It is due to vibration occurring in the vocal cords. Vibrations are generated by air currents in a somewhat complex manner and the pitch of the sound depends on the extent to which the vocal cords are stretched or relaxed, and also on functional changes in the arrangement of their edges. Vocalization is a further complex matter. Lips, tongue, soft palate, and the various cavities with which these structures are associated are all involved.

THE TRACHEA

General Features. The trachea is a tube continuous with the larynx above and ending below by dividing into two primary bronchi, which pass toward the right and the left lung, respectively (Fig. 23-1).

The trachea is prevented from collapsing by about twenty U- or horseshoe-shaped *cartilages* that are set in its wall one above the other so that each almost encircles the lumen. The open ends of these incomplete cartilaginous rings are directed posteriorly (Fig. 23-7), and the gap between the two ends of each ring is bridged by connective tissue and smooth muscle (Fig. 23-7).

If a *longitudinal section* is cut from the wall of the trachea, the cartilaginous rings that encircle its wall are cut in *cross section.* The cross-sectional appearance of each ring is roughly ovoid (Fig. 23-8), with a greatest superoinferior diameter of 3 or 4 mm. and a greatest mediolateral diameter of 1 mm. or thereabouts. The inner surface of each ring is convex and its outer surface relatively flat (Fig. 23-8). The space between adjacent rings is considerably less than the superoinferior diameters of the rings themselves and is filled with dense connective tissue continuous with that of the perichondrium of each ring (Fig. 23-8). The bundles of collagenic fibers constituting

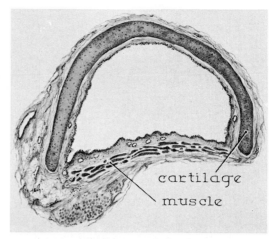

Fig. 23-7. Drawing of a cross section of the trachea of an adult (very low power). The anterior side is at *top.*

this connective tissue are woven in such a way that some degree of elasticity is imparted to the tracheal wall. Some elastic fibers, distributed among the bundles of collagenic fibers, may also be of some importance in this respect.

The Mucous Membrane of the Trachea. The epithelial lining of the trachea and bronchi is of the *pseudostratified ciliated* type, with goblet cells. It appears in an H and E section as shown in Figure 5-48. Its fine structure is shown in Figure 23-9. Since the fine structure of *ciliated cells* was described in detail on page 151 and illustrated in Figures 5-49 to 5-54, it will not be discussed further here. The *goblet cells,* also called *mucous cells,* have also been described (pp. 131 and 191). However, in connection with the tracheobronchial epithelium it appears that goblet cells may secrete in a cyclical fashion, so that when they empty their contents onto the surface of the membrane, they appear as neither ciliated nor mucous cells.

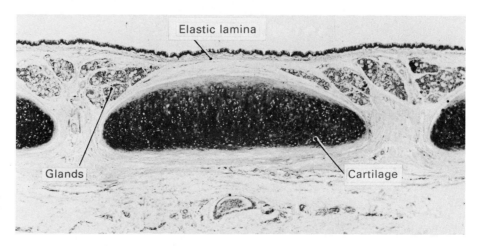

Fig. 23-8. Very low power photomicrograph of a longitudinal section of the anterior wall of the trachea of an adult. The lumen extends across the *top.*

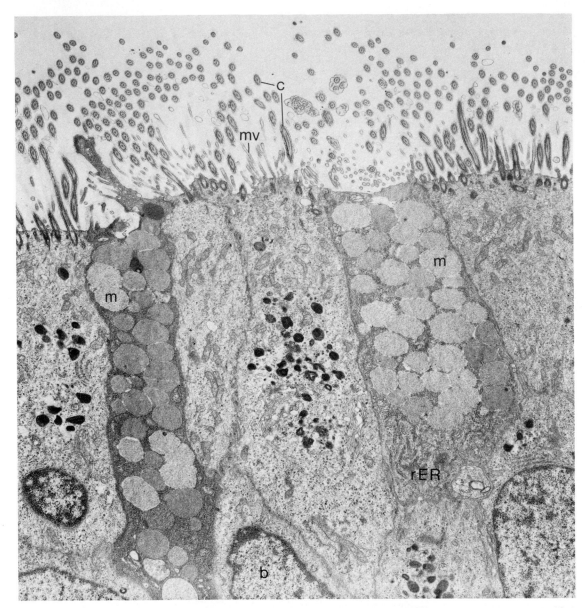

Fig. 23-9. Electron micrograph (×7,500) of pseudostratified ciliated columnar epithelium, containing mucous (goblet) cells. This type of epithelium is characteristic of the trachea and bronchi; that illustrated here is the lining of a bronchus (human). Two slightly darker-staining mucous cells are seen among the pale-staining, ciliated columnar cells; their apical cytoplasm contains large spherical secretory vesicles of mucus (m), and below these some rER is visible. On the apical surface of the columnar cells there are cilia (c) and microvilli (mv). Note also the basal cells (b) lying deeper in the membrane. (Courtesy of J. M. Sturgess)

Since in this condition they develop regularly arranged microvilli on their free surface, they have been termed *brush cells* (Fig. 23-10, bc), presumably because of the microvilli (mv in Fig. 23-10) appearing like the bristles of a brush. In view of there being disagreement as to whether what was described as the brush border of the osteoclast (where the term *brush border* originated) is no more than freed collagen fibrils of a bone surface that is being resorbed by the osteoclast (p. 415), it might be less confusing to refer to the "brush" cells as nonciliated cells with striated borders. The term *striated border* denotes regularly disposed microvilli on the free surface of cells as

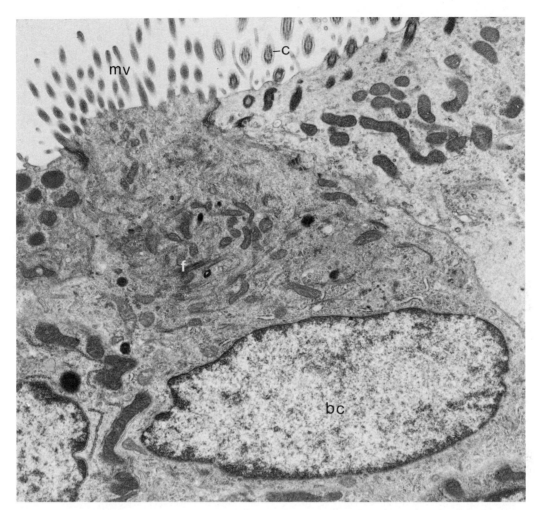

Fig. 23-10. Electron micrograph (×12,000) of a brush cell (bc) of pseudostratified ciliated columnar epithelium. This is a cell type found in tracheobronchial epithelium; the cell illustrated here is in a rat bronchiole. Note that there are microvilli (mv) on its apical surface instead of cilia. In its cytoplasm filaments (f), a few small round apical vesicles, mitochondria, and some rER (just above the nucleus) may be seen. The portion of the pale-staining ciliated cell at *upper right* has surface cilia (c), and prominent mitochondria. (Courtesy of B. Meyrick and L. Reid)

in Figure 5-7. Cells of a fourth type observed in the tracheobronchial epithelium are termed *basal cells* (labeled b in Fig. 23-9). It is generally believed that these are sufficiently undifferentiated to be able to form both ciliated and mucous (goblet) cells.

Afferent nerve fibers are said to end on and synapse with the base of some of the epithelial cells. Neuroendocrine cells analogous to enteroendocrine cells of the gastrointestinal tract have also been described as being present in the epithelial membrane.

The *lamina propria* on which the tracheal epithelium rests is condensed to contribute to a moderately distinct basement membrane. The remainder of the lamina pro-

pria contains a fairly high proportion of elastic fibers. A tendency toward a lymphatic character is indicated by the presence of lymphocytes and occasional lymphatic nodules. The deep border of the lamina propria is marked by a dense lamina of elastin (Fig. 23-8). The tissue just deep to this is termed *submucosa*. The secretory portions of many mucous *glands*, with some serous secretory units, are embedded in the submucosa. In longitudinal sections of the trachea the secretory portions of these glands are seen to be disposed chiefly in the submucosa that fills in the triangular spaces between adjacent cartilages (Fig. 23-8). The ducts from these glands pierce the elastic lamina of the lamina propria to empty on the inner surface of the trachea. Some secretory units may be present also in the lamina propria.

The posterior wall of the trachea is composed of interlacing bundles of smooth muscle fibers, arranged chiefly in the transverse plane and knitted together by connective tissue (Fig. 23-7). The inner surface of the posterior wall of the trachea is lined with a mucous membrane similar to that lining the remainder of its wall. The secretory units of glands are present in the mucous membrane, and outside the mucous membrane in the interstices between the bundles of smooth muscle, and even outside the smooth muscle, in the connective tissue of the outer layers of the wall.

THE BRONCHIAL TREE

The trachea ends by dividing into two branches, the two *primary bronchi,* that pass to the roots of the lungs (Fig. 23-1). The microscopic structure of these is the same as that of the trachea.

Usually the right lung is made up of three lobes and the left lung of two. Each primary bronchus, in a sense, continues into the lower lobe of the particular lung to which it passes. The right primary bronchus, before doing so, gives off two branches to supply the middle and the upper lobes, respectively, of that lung. Likewise, the left primary bronchus, before continuing into the lower lobe of the left lung, gives off a branch to supply the upper lobe of that lung. At the hilus of each lung the primary bronchus and its main branches become closely associated with the arteries that also enter the lung at this site and the veins and lymphatics that leave the lung, and all these tubular structures become invested in dense connective tissue. This complex of tubes invested in dense connective tissue is termed the *root* of the lung.

As noted, a large bronchus enters each of the lobes of the two lungs. Within the lobes these bronchi branch to give rise to progressively smaller bronchi. Although there is variation, particular parts of each lobe tend to be supplied by certain main branches of the bronchus that enters the lobe.

THE MICROSCOPIC STUDY OF THE CONDUCTING PORTION OF THE LUNG

THE INTRAPULMONARY BRONCHI

Although the bronchi within the lung (*intrapulmonary bronchi*) have a microscopic structure basically similar to the trachea and extrapulmonary portions of the two primary bronchi, they differ in a few respects, as will now be described.

(*1*) The U- or horseshoe-shaped cartilages of the trachea and the extrapulmonary parts of the primary bronchi are replaced in the intrapulmonary bronchi by *cartilage plates* of irregular shape. In a cross section of an intrapulmonary bronchus these may appear as crescents or ovals (Fig. 23-11). The impression that several are required to encircle the tube is deceptive, for what seem several cartilages in a section are commonly various prolongations of a single cartilage of irregular shape. Some of the irregular cartilages encircle the lumen completely. Since there are cartilages around all parts of the walls of these bronchi, the latter are not flattened on one surface like the trachea and extrapulmonary bronchi. At sites of branching saddle-shaped cartilages commonly support the two branches where they make an acute angle with one another. The spaces between cartilages and parts of the same cartilage that would otherwise be weak spots in the bronchial wall are filled with collagenic connective tissue continuous with the perichondrium of the cartilages concerned.

(*2*) In the intrapulmonary bronchi, the smooth muscle, which is present only in the posterior part of the trachea and extrapulmonary bronchi, constitutes a layer that completely encircles the lumen. This layer of muscle lies between the mucous membrane and the cartilages (Fig. 23-11). It does not appear as a complete layer in every section because it is composed of two sets of smooth muscle fibers that wind down the bronchial tree in a left- and a right-hand spiral, respectively. The arrangement of muscle can be demonstrated by winding two shoelaces down a broomstick in fairly close spirals, one clockwise and the other counterclockwise.

(*3*) The contraction of the smooth muscle after death, and perhaps to some extent during life, throws the mucous membrane into the longitudinal folds characteristic of intrapulmonary bronchi seen in cross sections (Fig. 23-11).

(*4*) The elastic lamina that marks the outer limit of the mucous membrane of the trachea is not present as such in the intrapulmonary bronchi, but instead elastic fibers are distributed in a way that will now be described. In the bronchi, the cartilages are bound together by coarse elastic fibers. Finer elastic fibers are present in the adventitia, in between the muscle fibers, and in the lamina propria. The most remarkable feature, however, is the presence of several strong stripes of elastic tissue situated in the lamina propria and running parallel to each other the full length of the bronchial tree. The stripes may easily be seen with the naked eye on inspection of the mucosa. They branch with successive bronchial branches and are continuous with the elastic components of the terminal air passages.

The intrapulmonary bronchi are lined with ciliated pseudostratified columnar epithelium, and the secretion

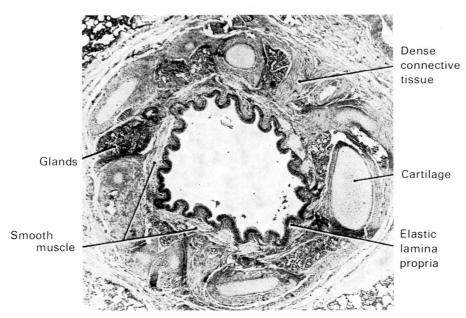

Fig. 23-11. Very low power photomicrograph of an intrapulmonary bronchus.

of the goblet cells disposed in this membrane is augmented by that of glands. The secretory portions of these lie, for the most part, outside the muscular layer and in between cartilages (Fig. 23-11).

Both lymph nodes and lymphatic nodules are scattered along the bronchi in the outermost fibrous parts of their walls.

Type of Branching. In general, branching in the bronchial tree is *dichotomous* (Gr. *dicha,* in two; *tome,* a cutting), with the total cross-sectional area of the lumina of every pair of branches being *greater* than the cross-sectional area of the lumen of the parent tube. This has implications with regard to the relative speeds at which air travels in the smaller and larger branches of the bronchial tree. Since the same volume of air (per unit of time) can pass through a parent tube as can pass through its two branches (which together have a greater total cross-sectional area) only if it moves faster in the parent tube, it follows that air moves slowest in the smallest tubes of the bronchial tree and fastest in the largest. This must be kept in mind in interpreting the breath sounds heard with a stethoscope.

The Differences Between Bronchi and Bronchioles. Continued branching of the bronchial tree results in formation of successively narrower bronchi. The smaller ones differ from the larger ones chiefly in that their cartilages are not as large and do not extend as far around their walls.

As will be explained later, the lung develops like a gland, and as a result its substance in made up of *lobules.* The bronchi of the lung are the equivalent of extralobular

ducts of glands because they are outside lobules. The branches of the bronchial tree that enter lobules, generally at their apices, are termed *bronchioles* (Fig. 23-12); hence they are counterparts of the intralobular ducts of glands. They differ in structure from bronchi in being smaller (generally bronchioles are less than 1 mm. in diameter), having ciliated columnar epithelium instead of pseudostratified columnar ciliated epithelium, and also by *not* having any cartilages in their walls (Fig. 23-12). As will also be explained later, bronchioles do not require cartilages in their walls to keep them from collapsing on inspiratory movements because they are inside the substance of the lung, which is opened up and hence expanded by inspiratory movements.

As is true for intralobular ducts, some connective tissue from interlobular septa extends along bronchioles to provide particularly the larger ones with support (Fig. 23-12).

Lung Lobules. Likening bronchioles to intralobular ducts is helpful because each of the bronchioles that arises from the branching of smaller bronchi enters what is called a *lobule* of the lung to course thereafter, like an intralobular duct, through the substance of a lobule and branch within it. Before discussing how bronchioles connect with the air spaces where interchange of gases between blood and air occurs, we shall discuss the structure of lobules in more detail.

Lung *lobules,* like pyramids, have an apex and a base. But here their resemblance to pyramids ends, for lobules are very irregular in shape. They vary greatly in size;

Elastic lamina propria

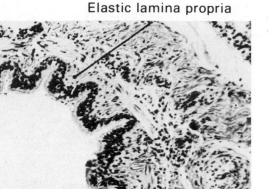

Fig. 23-12. Low-power photomicrograph of a large bronchiole in the lung of a child.

Smooth muscle

Dense connective tissue

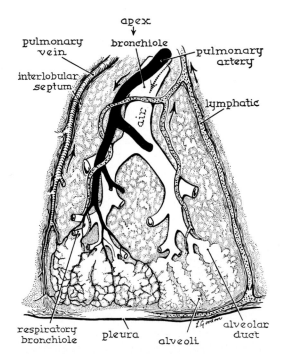

Fig. 23-13. Diagram of a lobule of the lung with its base abutting on the pleura. The sizes of the bronchioles and air passages, as well as those of the blood vessels and lymphatics, have been exaggerated for clarity. To make it easier to follow the course of the blood vessels and lymphatics, the former have been omitted from the *right* side, and the latter from the *left* side.

their base varies from less than 1 cm. to more than 2 cm. in diameter, and their height varies even more. Before considering how they are arranged within lobes, it may be helpful to compare each main bronchus to the trunk of a tree in that the bronchus "grows" from the root of the lung toward the central part of a lobe, and even beyond this point, branching as it grows. The smaller branches of the tree that are going to enter lobules, and so become bronchioles, mostly point outward toward the periphery of the lobe, but some point inward, toward the middle of the lobe. The lobules fill the space available to them, and this affects their shape. The peripheral lobules tend to have the shape of elongated pyramids, as is illustrated in Figure 23-13, but the more central lobules may be of irregular shapes and have angular contours. However, all the lobules are so arranged that their apices receive bronchioles (Fig. 23-13). This means that the bases of some lobules face the periphery of the lobe and those of others face its interior.

The bases of the peripheral lobules are visible as polygonal areas beneath the pleura. They are separated from one another by fibrous septa, which in man extend for only a short distance (as complete septa) into the lung. In certain other species, however—for example, the pig—the lobules are completely separated from each other by interlobular septa of dense connective tissue. This is continuous with the connective tissue of the visceral pleura at the base of the lobule and with the dense connective tis-

Fig. 23-14. Low-power electron micrograph (×6,000) of cells in the mucous membrane of a small bronchiole of mouse lung. In among the ciliated epithelial cells (cc) there is a nonciliated Clara cell (ncc). Note its numerous mitochondria and abundant sER, especially under its apical surface. The asterisks indicate the basal lamina of the epithelium. Smooth muscle cells (mc) and fibroblasts of connective tissue (ct) are present in the underlying lamina propria. The white space at *upper left* is the lumen of the bronchiole. (Courtesy of A. Collet)

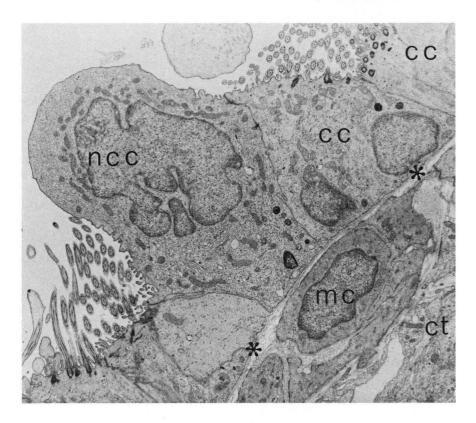

sue that ensheathes the bronchi at the apex of the lobule. However, in other animals—for example, the rabbit—the lobules are not separated from one another by septa. In man the septa are incomplete.

THE BRONCHIOLES

A bronchiole on entering a lobule gives rise to many branches, and these extend in tree-like fashion to all parts of the lobule. Since bronchioles, like intralobular ducts, lie within the substance of lobules, they are attached on all sides to the elastic spongework of tissue that contains the air spaces where gaseous exchange occurs (Fig. 23-15). There is, then, no tendency for them to collapse on inspiratory movements; indeed, on an inspiratory movement they are "pulled on," all around their circumference, as the elastic fibers of the respiratory spongework are stretched. Hence, there is no need for the walls of bronchioles to be held open by cartilaginous rings or plates, and they have none in their walls. They differ from bronchi also in not having any glands in their walls; indeed they are so close to the respiratory spaces that if they were to deliver secretions from glands, these might be sucked into the respiratory spaces. Moreover, their epithelial lining is not as thick as that of bronchi. In the larger branches, ciliated columnar cells are in the majority but nonciliated cells are scattered between them (Fig. 23-

14). These are tall and are sometimes termed *Clara cells.* They are unusual in being very rich in mitochondria (in some species), and between the nucleus and the surface through which they secrete there is a great abundance of sER. They have a high metabolic rate. The precise function of their serous secretion, however, has not yet been clearly established. In the final branches, nonciliated cells of a high cuboidal type are present. In summary, the walls of bronchioles (Fig. 23-12) consist of *epithelium* that rests on a thin elastic *lamina propria,* and this layer, in turn, is surrounded by the *muscular coat* previously described for bronchi. The muscle is supported by connective tissue (Fig. 23-12).

The Orders of Bronchioles. Once inside a lobule, the bronchiole entering it, a *preterminal bronchiole,* gives off branches known as *terminal* bronchioles, the number of which varies according to the size of the lobule. There are usually three to seven terminal bronchioles.

The next order of bronchioles arising from terminal bronchioles are called *respiratory* bronchioles (Figs. 23-13 and 23-15). The reason for their name is that as they branch and extend into lung substance they exhibit an increasing number of delicate air-containing outpouchings from their walls. These small pouches are limited by capillary networks ensconced in delicate frameworks that will be described presently. The point to be made here is that *gaseous exchange* occurs between the blood in the

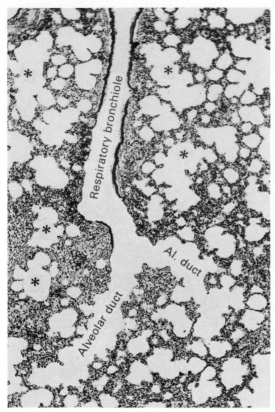

Fig. 23-15. Very low power photomicrograph of lung of a very young child. A respiratory bronchiole is cut longitudinally and may be seen opening into two alveolar ducts. The asterisks indicate alveolar sacs. These in turn open into rounded air spaces called alveoli.

capillaries in the walls of the outpouchings and the air within these pouches. Because exchange occurs in the outpouchings from these bronchioles, the latter are called *respiratory bronchioles.* The free terminations of the respiratory bronchioles flare out to some extent and open into what are called *alveolar ducts.*

THE RESPIRATORY PORTION OF THE LOBULE; ALVEOLAR DUCTS, ALVEOLAR SACS (SACCULES), AND ALVEOLI

Before commenting on alveolar ducts, into which the respiratory bronchioles open, it may be helpful to emphasize that the bronchi and bronchioles are tubes *with walls of their own,* and that they serve primarily to conduct air back and forth to the respiratory portions of the lobules. The terms that we shall now use to describe how air is conducted into all parts of the respiratory portion of the lobule (alveolar ducts, alveolar sacs or saccules, and alveoli) do not refer to structures with walls of their own,

but to *spaces of various orders and shapes* that exist in a huge elastic sponge-like arrangement of capillary beds (Figs. 23-13 and 23-15). Alveolar ducts, alveolar sacs, and alveoli all contain air that is repeatedly changed. The air in all these spaces is in close contact with capillaries in the walls of the spongework that divides this portion of the lung into spaces, and since air and blood are separated only by thin films of tissue through which diffusion occurs readily, there is an efficient working arrangement permitting blood to lose carbon dioxide and take up oxygen as it passes through the capillary beds of this portion of the lung.

Alveolar Ducts, Alveolar Sacs (Saccules), and Alveoli. The spaces into which the respiratory bronchioles directly open have the shape of long branching *hallways* along which there are many *open doors* of two general sizes. The hallways are termed *alveolar ducts* (Fig. 23-15). The larger open doors communicate with rotunda-like spaces termed *alveolar sacs* (*saccules*), marked by asterisks in Figure 23-15. Projecting inward from the periphery of the rotunda-like saccules, spur-like partitions divide the peripheral zone of each saccule into a series of cubicles that open into the central part of the saccule. The cubicles are *alveoli.* It has been estimated that there are about 300 million alveoli in the adult lungs, which would present a total surface area of 70 to 80 square meters to the air they contain.

Before describing the histological structure of the walls that separate the air spaces from one another, we shall comment briefly on units of respiratory structure smaller than lobules; these are of importance in understanding certain pathological conditions of the lung.

Units of Structure Within the Lobule. As already noted, bronchi branch to finally form bronchioles that enter units of lung structure called *lobules.* However, there never have been any generally agreed on terms for the units supplied by the succeeding divisions of the bronchiole that enters a lobule, except that the unit of lung served by a *terminal bronchiole* is now often termed an *acinus.* Millard suggests this is the most practical unit of structure for dealing with pathological conditions. There are no standard names for the more distal units, but Barrie suggested they should be designated according to the channel that supplies them. Thus the unit supplied by a respiratory bronchiole could be termed a *respiratory bronchiolar unit,* and the unit supplied by an alveolar duct, a *ductal unit.*

THE MICROSCOPIC STUDY OF THE RESPIRATORY PORTION OF THE LUNG

The elastic fibers present in the spongework of the lung are stretched to enable a lung to fill the cavity in which it lies. Hence, when the pleural cavities are opened at autopsy the lungs collapse toward their roots. Sections cut from collapsed lungs do not give a representative picture of the structure of the respiratory spongework during life because the spaces in the spongework become smaller and the partitions between them thicker. A better impression of lung structure during life can be obtained by studying sections cut from lungs that have been redistended to their original size immediately after death (by injecting fixative through a cannula into a bronchus and tying off the latter so that the lung cannot collapse again).

Alveolar Walls (Septa) vs. Interalveolar Walls (Septa). As shown in Figure 23-15, most partitions seen in the sponge-work of the lung separate adjacent alveoli from one another. Some partitions, of course, separate the passageways of alveolar ducts from alveolar spaces that lie just outside the duct but that may nevertheless communicate with some other duct. All these partitions are generally called *alveolar septa (walls).* However, it should be understood that the word *alveolus* has two meanings; it can mean either a little *space* or a little *structure.* In the instance of the postnatal lung this term is used to depict a *space.* The structure often referred to as an *alveolar wall* is more correctly regarded as an *interalveolar wall* or *septum* since it lies *between alveoli.*

THE STRUCTURE OF THE INTERALVEOLAR WALLS

The Use of Thick Sections. In the usual thin sections of distended lungs, interalveolar walls are always cut in cross or oblique sections. The reason for this is that in distended lungs these interalveolar partitions are as thin as the sections themselves, and since they are never perfectly flat (as sections are), it is impossible for a whole interalveolar wall to be present in a thin section so that its full face may be examined. To see a partition in full face, it is necessary to cut sections that are about as thick as the diameter of alveoli. In such sections, sites may be found where the top of one alveolus has been sliced away together with the bottom of the alveolus immediately below it. One may then look down into an alveolus as one looks into a cup to inspect its bottom. In this instance the bottom of the cup is represented by the inter-alveolar partition between the alveolus into which one is looking and the alveolus that was immediately below it (Fig. 23-16), and on looking into it one can sometimes see that the bottom of the "cup" has a hole in it, which we shall discuss presently.

The Capillaries of the Walls. It is not easy to identify the various cells and structures in interalveolar walls seen this way. Many nuclei are visible; the various cells that contain these will soon be described. The extent of the capillary network in an interalveolar septum can only be realized if thick sections of lungs with their blood vessels injected with opaque material are studied. Seen in full

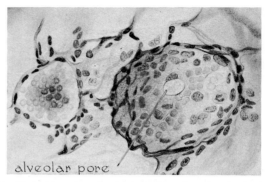

Fig. 23-16. Drawing of a thick section of an alveolus in the respiratory portion of a lung of a rabbit. A venule lies at *left.* The floor of an alveolus is seen at *right*; the blood cells in the floor lie in capillaries. Note the alveolar pore in the floor of the alveolus.

face, the networks of capillaries in the interalveolar walls in such preparations are of very close mesh (Fig. 23-17).

Alveolar Pores and Lambert Channels (Sinuses). Some interalveolar walls studied in full face in thick sections reveal little round or oval holes termed *alveolar pores* (Fig. 23-16). Where present, these permit air to pass from one alveolus to another. They also facilitate interchange of air between alveolar sacs whose own supply routes have become obstructed. Additional intercommunicating channels were discovered by Lambert: short channels from the walls of preterminal bronchioles provide passageways for air to pass into alveolar sacs belonging to the same or a neighboring unit. They thus provide an alternative (collateral) route for air to enter, or escape from,

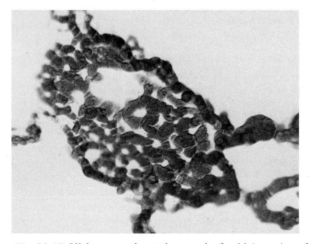

Fig. 23-17. High-power photomicrograph of a thick section of lung with the blood vessels injected with opaque material. In the floor of this alveolus the extensive and close mesh of the alveolar capillaries is readily seen.

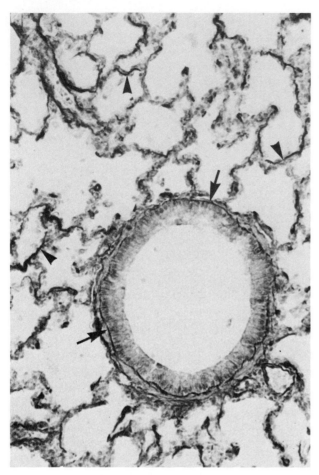

Fig. 23-18. Photomicrograph of respiratory portion of lung, stained with orcein to demonstrate its elastin. Elastic fibers are evident, particularly in the wall of the bronchiole seen at *lower right* (the fibers are indicated by arrows) and in interalveolar walls (fibers indicated by arrowheads).

terminal units and probably play an important role when parts of the lungs become fibrotic.

The Internal Support of Interalveolar Walls. The capillary networks comprising the chief components of interalveolar walls have little tensile strength. If the walls did not possess internal support, alveoli might become so expanded with air that their capillaries would be torn. But the support given to interalveolar walls cannot be too rigid lest it interfere with the normal expansion of alveoli. It is therefore not surprising that the basic support of interalveolar walls is provided by elastic fibers (Fig. 23-18). But since these are too coarse and widely spaced to provide intimate support for the many capillaries, there is also intimate support for these, as will be described presently. However, elastic fibers provide a backbone that resists overexpansion. In addition to the occasional

elastic fibers that course along interalveolar walls, there are, according to Short, elastic fibers around the free margins of alveoli (where they open into alveolar sacs or ducts). The elastic fibers in interalveolar walls, according to Collett and DesBiens, are produced by fibroblasts. These cells are derived during embryological development from a kind of progenitor cell that also gives rise to smooth muscle cells. Both the smooth muscle cells developing in relation to the bronchial tree and the fibroblasts of alveolar structures were found to be able to produce elastin. Fibroblasts of interalveolar walls assume various shapes; some may be greatly elongated, while others, like the cell labeled connective tissue cell in Figure 23-19, have a more or less rounded form.

The intimate support for the capillaries is provided by delicate fibrils of the reticular or collagenic variety and by basement membranes, as will now be described. Some smooth muscle fibers may be seen along alveolar ducts, particularly around their doorways.

THE COMPONENTS OF THE BARRIER BETWEEN BLOOD AND AIR IN THE INTERALVEOLAR WALLS

Development of Knowledge. First, studies with the EM, beginning with the pioneer studies of Low, showed clearly that alveoli are lined with a continuous layer of epithelium that, except in sites where nuclei are present, is so thin it cannot be resolved with the LM. Second, the use of the PAS technic made it possible, as shown by Leblond, Bertalanffy, and associates, to demonstrate the existence and distribution of the basement membranes in the lung. With the knowledge gained from the EM and from the PAS technic with the LM, it became possible to indicate in a diagram the sites of the basement membranes that underlie the epithelium and cover the capillaries in interalveolar walls (Fig. 23-19). Since experience with the basement membrane of the lens of the eye indicates that it has some rigidity, it is likely that the basement membranes of the surface epithelium and the capillaries constitute important intimate supportive elements in the interalveolar walls. As shown in Figure 23-19, air in the alveoli is separated from blood in the capillaries by: (*1*) the cytoplasm of the epithelial cells that line alveoli; (*2*) the basement membrane of the epithelium, which in sites where it is contiguous with the third component blends with it; (*3*) the basement membrane surrounding the endothelium of the capillaries (the two basement membranes if fused together are referred to as the alveolocapillary membrane); and (*4*) the cytoplasm of the endothelial cells of capillaries. In certain sites there are tissue spaces between the basement membrane of the epithelium and that of the capillaries, and some of these spaces contain fine reticular fibrils and/or elastic fibers (Fig. 23-19, *top right*), and, sometimes, cells.

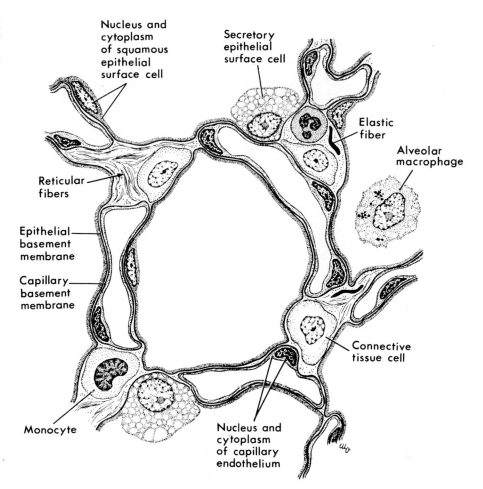

Nucleus and cytoplasm of squamous epithelial surface cell

Secretory epithelial surface cell

Elastic fiber

Alveolar macrophage

Reticular fibers

Epithelial basement membrane

Capillary basement membrane

Connective tissue cell

Monocyte

Nucleus and cytoplasm of capillary endothelium

The epithelium lining the respiratory portion of the lung forms a continuous membrane, with its contiguous cells all being connected by tight junctions, as will be described presently. Moreover, the membrane has been shown to be composed of two types of epithelial cells. The more numerous ones are squamous and termed *Type I pneumocytes*. Interspersed among these are less numerous but larger secretory cells termed *Type II pneumocytes*. The squamous cells are responsible for permitting diffusion of gases through their cytoplasm whereas the Type II pneumocytes perform an essential secretory function. Details follow.

The Squamous Cells, Type I Pneumocytes. A portion of one is shown in Figure 23-20. This is the portion that contains it nucleus. However, at *lower left* the thin cytoplasm through which gases would diffuse between the capillary beneath and the alveolus above is also shown, and it can be seen that the cytoplasm of the squamous cell (labeled squamous surface epithelium in Fig. 23-20) is extremely thin. (This epithelium is so thin it is beyond the limit of

resolution of the LM and before the advent of the EM there was a school of thought that subscribed to the view that alveoli in postnatal life were not lined with epithelium. However, studies with the EM provided convincing evidence that a continuous epithelium does indeed exist.) Low estimated that the thickness of this sheet (except where there are nuclei) is approximately 0.2 μm. in man and 0.1 μm. in the rat (*see lower left* in Fig. 23-20). Beneath the epithelium there is a basement membrane (seen clearly at *upper right* in Fig. 23-20) that fuses with the basement membrane of the capillary beneath it to become a single membrane, the *alveolocapillary membrane* (acm in Fig. 23-21).

The Secretory Cells, Type II Pneumocytes. The LM showed there are occasional fairly large, rounded cells projecting from the surface of alveoli into their lumina (Fig. 23-19, secretory epithelial surface cell). With the EM it can be seen (Fig. 23-21) that these are epithelial cells and that they form part of the membrane because they are connected on either side to adjacent squamous

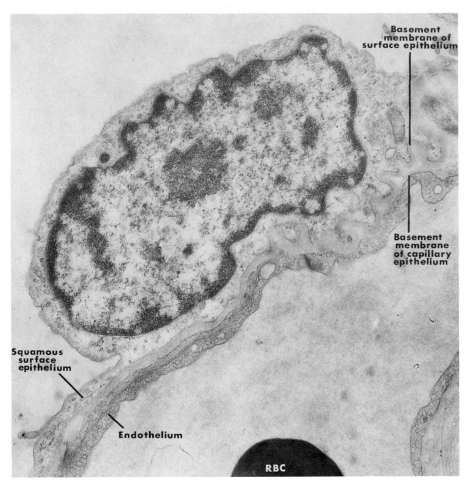

Basement
membrane of
surface epithelium

Basement
membrane
of capillary
epithelium

Squamous
surface
epithelium

Endothelium

RBC

Fig. 23-20. Electron micrograph (×11,900) of interalveolar wall of lung of cat, showing the nucleus and cytoplasm of a squamous epithelial cell, now often referred to as a Type I pneumocyte (*above*) and a capillary (*below*). Note the basement membranes of the squamous epithelium and the endothelial cells of the capillary, and that in some sites they remain separate to enclose a space and in other sites they fuse to form what is known as an alveolocapillary membrane. (Collet, A.: Arch. Ital. Anat. Istol. Pathol., *39:*119, 1965)

cells by tight junctions. This is shown in Figure 23-21, *upper right,* where a capillary is covered above and below with squamous epithelium that connects on both sides of the capillary with the Type II secretory cell by tight junctions (labeled tj). Connection of the Type II pneumocyte with a squamous epithelial cell on its other side is shown at *lower right* (labeled tj). Type II pneumocytes have microvilli and their cytoplasm is rich in rER, mitochondria, and peroxidase-containing microbodies. It also reveals *multivesicular bodies* (p. 142) and what have been termed *composite bodies,* which contain both tiny vesicles and electron-dense lamellae. However, the most prominent feature of the cytoplasm is its content of *lamellar bodies* (1b in Fig. 23-21). These are globules (granules) of electron-dense laminated material rich in phospholipid and surrounded by membrane. By means of radioautography, using tritiated choline as a precursor of phospholipids and labeled leucine and galactose as precursors of protein and carbohydrate, respectively, Chevalier and Collett traced the basic components of these

lamellar bodies back as far as the ER or the Golgi apparatus. In general, the formation of lamellar bodies follows the typical pattern by which secretory vesicles (granules) are formed in cells, although the precise pathway by which the protein, carbohydrate, and lipid components of the lamellar bodies are assembled to leave the Golgi as membrane-enclosed granules is not entirely clear. Composite bodies would seem to be involved. The lamellar bodies are extruded from the cell by exocytosis. The secretory product, the chief component of which is dipalmitoyl phosphatidylcholine, then spreads as a thin film over the entire surface of the squamous epithelium lining the alveoli. The role of this secretory product will now be explained.

The Pulmonary Surfactant. Because there are powerful intermolecular forces between the water molecules in thin films of aqueous solutions, such films exhibit a high surface tension. The film of tissue fluid covering the exposed surface of the squamous alveolar cells could exert a surface tension great enough to cause closely apposing sur-

Fig. 23-21. Electron micrograph (×15,000) of part of an interalveolar wall of mouse lung, illustrating a Type II pneumocyte (secretory epithelial cell). This micrograph shows the position of the cell in the wall in relation to three alveolar air spaces (a) and the neighbouring Type I pneumocytes (squamous epithelial cells), to which cells it is joined by tight junctions (tj) (for further details, *see* text). Note the lamellar bodies (lb), mitochondria (m), and rER in this secretory cell, which also has microvilli (mv) on its surface; its nucleus is labeled n. A blood capillary (bc), containing an erythrocyte (rbc) in this section, is seen at *upper right*. Its basal lamina is fused with that of the overlying squamous epithelium to form an alveolocapillary membrane where indicated (acm). (Collet, A. J., and Chevalier, G.: Am. J. Anat., *148:*275, 1977)

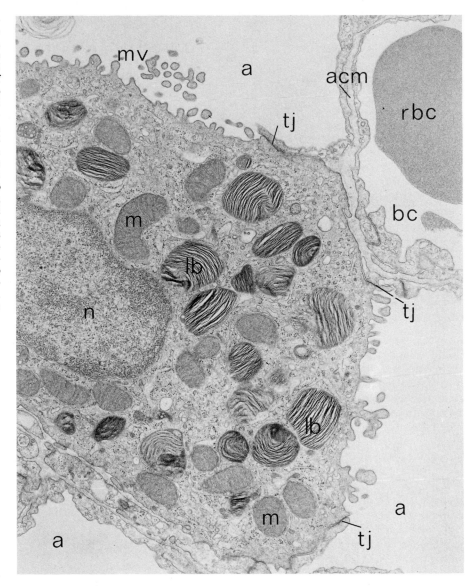

faces of the smaller alveoli to adhere to each other during inspiration were it not for the presence of the secretory product of the secretory epithelial cells (Type II pneumocytes), which has detergent-like *surfactant* activity. The effect of this surfactant is to diminish the intermolecular forces between the water molecules of the tissue fluid, reducing its surface tension and thereby making it much easier for air, on inspiration, to spread adherent interalveolar walls apart; thus it permits the alveolus to become inflated. As we shall see, it is of extreme importance to the newborn infant to have enough surfactant in the lungs when air first gains access to the alveoli that previously contained fluid during fetal life.

Pulmonary surfactant is a complex mixture of phospholipids, the principal one of which is *dipalmitoyl phosphatidylcholine,* which appears to be complexed with both protein and carbohydrate.

Alveolar Phagocytes. It is usual with the LM to see some fairly large, rounded cells, different from Type II pneumocytes, bulging from alveolar walls into the alveolar space. The same kinds of large cells are also seen free in the alveolar space (Fig. 23-19, *upper right*). These cells often contain carbon pigment that they have phagocytosed from smoke-containing air drawn into the alveoli on inspiration (Fig. 23-22). Because of their pronounced phagocytic properties, these cells have long been termed

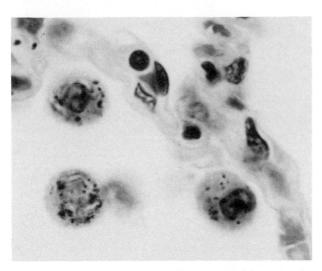

Fig. 23-22. Photomicrograph of lung, showing three alveolar phagocytes free in an alveolar space. Each contains phagocytosed carbon in its cytoplasm. (Courtesy of Y. Clermont)

alveolar phagocytes. Their origin was disputed for many decades, in particular as to whether they originated from the epithelial cells lining alveoli or from monocytes that migrate through the walls of alveolar capillaries. The current view is that alveolar phagocytes develop from *monocytes* that come to the alveolar wall by way of the bloodstream, leave a capillary (Fig. 23-19, *lower left*), and migrate out through the epithelial lining to enter the lumen of an alveolus. Two lines of evidence support this view. First, when mice are given supralethal total body irradiation and then are kept alive by giving them bone marrow cells from a mouse whose marrow cells bear a marker, washings from the lungs subsequently reveal cells (presumably alveolar phagocytes) bearing the marker. Osmond labeled cells developing in the bone marrow of the hind legs of guinea pigs. Later, labeled cells appeared within the interalveolar walls and in alveolar lumina. It would therefore seem that monocytes arising from bone marrow migrate to the interalveolar wall and, from there, break through to the alveolar space to become alveolar phagocytes, which are therefore *macrophages.*

The role of alveolar macrophages is to serve as phagocytes and remove any dust particles or other types of debris that gain entrance to alveolar spaces (Fig. 23-22). Eventually, they move along the air passages to reach bronchioles and then the bronchi, where their future progress is aided by cilia. They may be lost to the outside in sputum or be swallowed.

When lungs are congested with blood because of an incompetent heart, blood commonly escapes into alveoli, where alveolar phagocytes engulf erythrocytes and form iron pigment from the hemoglobin they contain. The pig-ment-containing cells can be coughed up in large numbers under these conditions, and they give positive histochemical reactions for iron. Such cells are called *heart-failure cells.*

THE LUNGS DURING FETAL AND EARLY POSTNATAL LIFE

THE EARLY DEVELOPMENT OF THE LUNGS

The early development of the lungs is much like that of exocrine glands. The outgrowth responsible for them arises from the epithelium of the anterior wall of the foregut and first assumes the form of a longitudinal bulge. This becomes pinched off from the foregut except at its cephalic end. The tube thus formed is the forerunner of the larynx and the trachea. Its caudal end is closed, but cell proliferation at this site soon results in two hollow epithelial bulges forking out from it, one directed to the left, the other to the right. These bulges are termed *primary bronchial buds* because they are the forerunners of the two primary bronchi.

The two primary bronchial buds advance toward the sites at which lungs will develop. Bulges appear on these advancing tubes and they subsequently grow and elongate to give rise to the secondary bronchi. These, in turn, usually by pairs of bulges which appear at their blind ends, continue to branch and grow to give rise to the smaller bronchi (Fig. 23-23). The branching then be-

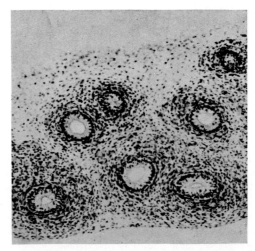

Fig. 23-23. Low-power photomicrograph of lung of a pig embryo in early stage of development. Epithelial tubules (future bronchi) are growing and branching into mesenchyme. (Ham, A. W., and Baldwin, K. W.: Anat. Rec., *81:*363, 1941)

comes more irregular but continues to give rise to the forerunners of bronchioles.

Although it simplifies matters to say that the growing, branching, hollow epithelial tree that develops originally from the epithelium of the foregut gives rise to the bronchi and bronchioles of the lungs, and that these are comparable with interlobular and intralobular ducts of exocrine glands, this is not the whole truth, for the epithelial outgrowth gives rise to only the epithelial lining and glands of the bronchi and bronchioles. The connective tissue and smooth muscle of the walls of bronchi and bronchioles, and the cartilages of bronchi, develop from the mesenchyme invaded by the branching, hollow epithelial tree. The mesenchyme, as it is invaded, becomes condensed around the epithelial tubes (Fig. 23-23) and there differentiates into the connective tissue and smooth muscle cells of their walls.

It is believed that all the orders of bronchioles that will form in a human lung are present by the end of the 16th week in man. The number of orders of bronchi and bronchioles differs in different species and is greater in the lower lobes than in the upper lobes of the lungs of man. From the time all the bronchioles have formed until around the 24th week of development the epithelium of the bronchioles grows into the mesenchyme to form what would be the counterparts of secretory units if one thinks of the lung at this time of development as a gland.

THE LATER DEVELOPMENT AND GROWTH OF THE LUNGS

Up to this point, increase in the size of the lungs and thoracic cage is explained by continuing growth of the epithelial and mesenchymal components of the lung and the tissues comprising the thoracic cage. But from here on *we have to take dynamics into account* in explaining both the microscopic structure and the growth of the lungs. We shall comment first on what happens immediately after birth and then on how the fetus prepares for this throughout the last trimester (3-month period) of fetal life.

First, when a baby is born it almost immediately draws air into its lungs by means of inspiratory movements. These depend on muscular action enlarging the thoracic cage. The latter effect would suck in air (or anything else not fixed in position that had access to the thoracic cage). Normally, the only components with access to the thoracic cage are air and blood. Air is drawn through the nose or mouth down through the trachea, bronchi, and bronchioles into the respiratory portion of the lung, and this allows the lungs to enlarge so the thoracic cage can expand. It is of interest that these inspiratory movements not only draw air into the lungs but also more blood. This may explain why a newborn baby will *increase its weight*

by several ounces if the umbilical cord is not cut immediately upon delivery. Every effort is made by the doctor delivering a baby to remove all the fluid that he can from the upper respiratory tract and so assist its displacement by air. However, only about one third of the fluid in the air spaces of the lung is drained away through the upper respiratory tract after birth (Avery et al.), so most of it must be resorbed.

The Importance of Surfactant at Birth. It is very important that the secretory cells be adequately developed in the lung *before a baby is born* because the surfactant they produce is necessary for reducing the surface tension that might otherwise hold interalveolar walls together at the end of expiration and prevent them from separating on inspiration.

Avery and Fletcher have contributed much valuable information on this matter. Synthesis and secretion of surfactant begins by the 24th week of human fetal life and corresponds to formation of the enzymes necessary for phospholipid synthesis in the cell. Production of surfactant marks the full differentiation (maturation) of the Type II alveolar cells. This maturation can be assessed in pregnant women by tests that evaluate by physicochemical methods the amount of surfactant in the amniotic fluid before birth.

The maturation of the Type II pneumocytes is accelerated by steroids such as cortisol (Avery et al.). Thyroid hormone could also play a role. Furthermore, both the pituitary and the adrenal glands must be intact for normal maturation of the cells that secrete surfactant.

At birth, the forces required for the first breath are strong; they must overcome mainly surface tension forces. This permits introduction of air into the respiratory tract, and surface-active phospholipids (surfactant) help the air penetration. When surfactant is less than normal at birth (a defect of maturation of Type II pneumocytes), the deficiency of surface-active substances could explain why premature infants, and even some full-term babies, can suffer a condition known as the *respiratory distress syndrome*, which is characterized by difficulty in breathing and cyanosis. This is due to widespread failure of alveoli to open or remain open as a result of inadequate amounts of surfactant being produced in the lungs. When a newborn baby takes its first strong breath of air, the alveoli become expanded and are normally prevented from collapsing by the surfactant. If, however, the infant has been born before sufficient surfactant was produced, the alveoli can collapse again on expiration, and respiration may be so difficult and inefficient that the infant may die within the first two days of life.

The Airproof Barrier in the Lung. Now that we have made the point that the thoracic cage is only able to enlarge because it can suck something into it, and furthermore that in the newborn the only two things that can be sucked into it are air and blood, with the lungs becoming enlarged on inspiration only because the cage into which they fit becomes enlarged, we can go on to deal with another matter.

When the lungs are expanded, their elastic components are further stretched. The lungs, therefore, must be surrounded by a totally airproof membrane, because otherwise expansion of the thoracic cage could suck air right through the relatively weak walls of the superficial alveoli into the pleural cavity. The *visceral pleura* covering the lung serves this purpose. If a leak were to develop in this membrane, the delicate wall of any alveolus beside the leak would rupture through it and allow air to enter the pleural cavity, which would thereupon expand, allowing the stretched elastic lung to collapse back to the hilus. This can happen, but fortunately only rarely.

Similar airproof protection is required for the lymphatics of the lung (the distribution of which will soon be described). They, too, need a covering that prevents air from being sucked into them, for if air leaked into the lymphatics of the lung, expiratory movements of the cage could force this air along the lymphatics to other parts of the body. This also sometimes happens, but again only rarely.

The barrier that prevents air from entering the pleural cavity or lung lymphatics, though thin, is composed of dense ordinary connective tissue which, of course, contains few cells and consists chiefly of strong fibrous intercellular substance. This connective tissue has a different mesenchymal origin from that immediately surrounding the epithelial components of the developing lung (Ham and Baldwin). The mesenchyme surrounding all epithelial structures as they develop is soft and very cellular (Fig. 23-23), whereas the mesenchyme that will differentiate into the tissue responsible for protecting the lung against air leakage and that forms the visceral pleura and interlobular septa is relatively noncellular, consisting chiefly of intercellular substance.

This situation raises two questions: (*1*) whether the soft cellular tissue developing in association with the epithelial components of the lung (and which is rich in capillaries) would be strong enough to prevent air from being drawn into its substance if it were stretched; and (*2*) whether this is really the way new alveolar spaces develop in the last trimester of fetal life and subsequently, as will be discussed presently. But first we must describe and comment on interstitial emphysema.

Interstitial Emphysema. If the lungs are punctured, as sometimes happens as a result of a knife wound or a fractured rib piercing the pleura and lung tissue, expiratory movements of the thoracic cage can force air through the inflicted wound into the soft connective tissues of the chest wall, through which tissue the air moves fairly readily. There are examples of it spreading, for example, through the loose connective tissue of the body to the scrotum, enlarging it to such a size that incisions have to be made in it to let the air escape. This condition of air gaining access to soft tissue and spreading through is called *interstitial emphysema* (Gr. for inflation with air). (It should be noted here that the word *emphysema,* when used by itself, relates not to the relatively uncommon interstitial type, but to a condition in which there is enlargement of lung alveoli associated with destructive changes in interalveolar walls.)

The Development of the Lung in the Third Trimester. The reason for all the foregoing is that it is pertinent back-

ground for considering (*1*) whether the lung, in its third phase of prenatal development, would continue to develop like a gland as it did before, so that the alveoli present at birth would all be preformed as epithelial buds and become expanded from within to become thin-walled alveoli, or (*2*) whether physical forces would not by now have become the dominant factor in determining what changes were to occur in its microscopic structure in this its final phase of fetal development, and also during continued growth in postnatal life, as will now be discussed.

In the last trimester of fetal life, the bronchi, bronchioles, and alveoli are all filled with fluid. This consists of amniotic fluid mixed with tissue fluid formed from capillary beds in the lungs. Aspiration of some amniotic fluid into the lungs would, of course, be caused by their expansion due to growth and enlargement of the thoracic cage. However, more substantial entry of amniotic fluid into the future air spaces would result if there were active respiratory movements during the latter part of fetal life. Recently with ultrasonic technics it has become possible to delineate organs and structures within the body and watch changes in their shape and position as they occur. These methods have revealed that the fetus does indeed execute some respiratory movements. The occurrence of these before birth would also help explain what happens to the microscopic structure of the lung during this period. The change that takes place will now be described.

The transition from a glandlike structure, in which alveoli appear as rounded structures composed of cuboidal or columnar epithelium, to a structure in which alveoli are often of irregular shape (Fig. 23-24A) starts around the beginning of the last third of fetal life. The alveoli now acquire the kind of shape they will have following their expansion with air after birth (Fig. 23-24B and C). Furthermore, the acquisition of this kind of shape *before birth* has medicolegal implications. There used to be confusion about whether microscopic examination of the lungs of a dead baby would show whether it had died before or after birth. It was sometimes argued that if its lungs were not glandlike but opened up, it must have breathed air. But as shown in Figure 23-24A, the lungs are opened up long before birth—not by air but by fluid, which as explained above would be mostly amniotic fluid, at least in the later stages of development. As Shapiro points out, a much better way to determine if a dead baby ever breathed air before it died is to see if its lungs will float in water.

Another event that occurs in the third trimester of pregnancy is extensive development of the capillary beds of the interalveolar walls. Respiratory movements before birth could help in drawing blood into these beds and so facilitate their expansion. Numerous investigators, including Ham and Baldwin, have reported seeing capillary

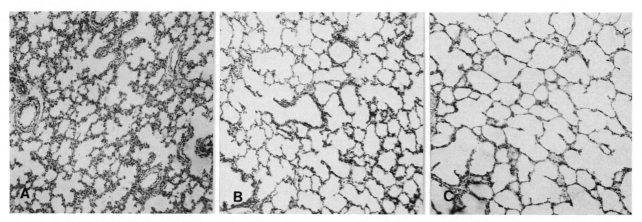

Fig. 23-24. (*A*) Low-power photomicrograph of a lung of a pig about two thirds of the way through prenatal development. It is no longer gland-like, and the developing alveoli are somewhat angular in shape. (*B*) Lung of a pig 3 hours after birth. These alveoli are larger. (*C*) Another area of the lung of a pig 3 hours after birth. The alveoli here are greatly expanded. (Ham, A. W., and Baldwin, K. W.: Anat. Rec., *81*:363, 1941)

loops seemingly sucked partway into air spaces during this period. The establishment of sufficiently extensive capillary beds in interalveolar walls is a *primary prerequisite for viability* should birth occur before its normal time.

HOW ALVEOLI FORM IN LATER FETAL LIFE AND INCREASE IN NUMBER IN EARLY POSTNATAL LIFE

Although there is agreement about alveoli developing in the first two thirds of fetal life as rounded structures with walls of cuboidal or columnar epithelium that bud from the ends of the developing bronchial tree, there does not seem to be any generally accepted concept of how alveoli continue to increase in numbers in the final third of prenatal life and during the first eight years or so of postnatal life. It is unlikely that they would form in the same way as in earlier fetal life because not enough rounded alveoli consisting of cuboidal or columnar cells are seen to justify such an explanation. Indeed, the epithelium of alveoli in the later stages of prenatal life has become mostly squamous in form.

There would seem to be only two possible ways for new alveoli equipped with squamous epithelium to develop in the last part of fetal life and the early years of childhood. First, squamous epithelium from preexisting alveolar epithelium might invade the soft connective tissue of interalveolar walls to form new alveoli, and do so with no air leaks occurring through the epithelium participating in the invasion. But the second and perhaps more likely possibility is that if the stroma of an interalveolar wall were indeed thick and soft enough to be invaded by a growth of squamous epithelium, it would probably also be stretched sufficiently by an inspiratory act for air to be sucked into it and split

it open, thereby creating a new space in the stroma that the squamous epithelium could then proceed to line so as to create a new alveolus. As already mentioned, whenever air in postnatal life (or fluid in prenatal life) is sucked into a lung, something has to expand. If there were more resistance offered to expansion by the elastic fibers that enclose existing alveolar spaces than by new crevices being opened up in the thicker interalveolar walls, the latter process would predominate. The sides of such crevices could then be quickly lined by the squamous epithelium, the continuity of which would of course have been broken by the crevices opening up due to stretching. The size characteristics of the alveoli forming in this manner presumably would be determined by the spacings in the three-dimensional network of intercellular fibers within the stroma of their walls.

The latter of the two hypotheses of how new alveoli develop during the last three prenatal months and early postnatal life requires that the process of *interstitial emphysema* be considered a normal occurrence in connection with new alveoli forming in postnatal life. Actually, there would be no need for the alveolar epithelium to constitute an airproof barrier, because by this stage the capacity of the interalveolar walls for being opened up would be limited in the following way. Every so often a stage would be attained at which expansion of those alveoli already formed would become easier than opening up new air spaces. But this situation would then become reversed on further growth. Hence the development of new alveoli would always occur in relation to growth as a whole, and furthermore it would be limited to meeting increasing functional demands. Finally, it should be pointed out that there would be no danger of the air (and by this mechanism some air would enter the interalveolar walls) escaping from the lungs into the remainder of the body, because of the existence of the airproof barrier already described.

THE BLOOD SUPPLY OF THE LUNGS

Blood from the right ventricle is delivered by the *pulmonary artery* and its branches to the capillary beds of the respiratory tissue of the lung to be oxygenated. Fully

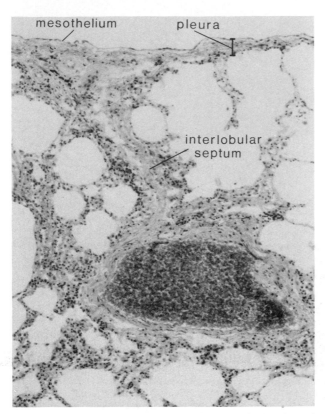

mesothelium   pleura

interlobular
septum

Fig. 23-25. Photomicrograph of adult lung showing its visceral pleura and an interlobular septum extending from the pleura into the substance of the lung. This figure (turned upside down) should be compared with the diagram in Figure 23-13. Note the thin squamous mesothelium covering the pleural surface. Some of the narrow white spaces just deep to this mesothelium, extending parallel with it, are probably lymphatics. The interlobular septum contains dense connective tissue and, in the lower part of the figure, a branch of a pulmonary vein is evident.

oxygenated blood is collected from these capillary beds by the branches of the pulmonary vein and delivered to the left atrium of the heart. It is to be kept in mind that in the pulmonary circulation, the arteries carry what is ordinarily called venous blood, and the veins contain arterial blood.

The pulmonary artery to each lung enters it at its root and branches along with the bronchial tree so that each branch of the tree is accompanied by a branch of the pulmonary artery. The small branches reaching the respiratory bronchioles supply terminal branches that deliver blood to the capillary beds of the alveolar ducts and sacs and the alveoli (Fig. 23-13, *left*).

Blood from the capillary beds of the respiratory tissue is collected by the smallest branches of the pulmonary vein. These begin within the substance of lobules and are here supported by thin connective tissue sheaths. They

enter interlobular septa, where they empty into interlobular veins (Fig. 23-13, *left*). These in turn are conducted by the septa to the site where the apices of the lobules concerned meet. Here the veins come into close association with branches of the bronchial tree. From this point to the root of the lung, the veins follow the bronchi. In other words, except within lobules, the branches of the pulmonary artery and pulmonary vein follow the branches of the bronchial tree; but within lobules only the arteries follow the bronchioles.

Oxygenated blood is supplied to parts of the lung by the bronchial arteries. These also travel in close association with the bronchial tree and supply the capillary beds of its walls. They also supply the lymph nodes scattered along the bronchial tree. Moreover, branches of the bronchial arteries travel out along the interlobular septa and supply oxygenated blood to the capillaries of the visceral pleura.

There are, of course, two differences between the blood in the arteries of the pulmonary circulation and the blood in the systemic circulations, for both pressure and oxygen content are lower in the former than in the latter. Hence anastomoses between the two circulations in the lung would present unusual physiological problems. For a consideration of this matter, *see* Lauweryns.

THE LYMPHATIC SUPPLY OF THE LUNGS

Here as elsewhere, general principles are easier to remember than details. A rough general rule about the distribution of lymphatics in the lung is that they are confined to the relatively *dense connective tissue* structures that confine air to the respiratory tissue of the lung. Hence they are present in the visceral pleura (Fig. 23-25), interlobular septa (Figs. 23-13 and 23-25), and the dense connective tissue wrappings of the bronchioles, bronchi, arteries, and veins (Fig. 23-13). They are *not present in the interalveolar walls*. However, Miller has described lymphatics in the tissue bordering the alveolar ducts. Indeed, lymphatic capillaries in alveolar walls might very well constitute a hazard because, if air were sucked into a lymphatic on inspiration, expiratory movements would pump it along the lymphatic so that it could travel for long distances. If it gained access to the bloodstream, it could cause air embolism.

It is customary to describe the lung as having a *superficial* and a *deep* set of lymphatics. The superficial ones are contained in the visceral pleura (Fig. 23-13, *bottom*). In city dwellers these are usually blackened by carbon particles incorporated into their walls. The larger ones follow the lines where interlobular septa join the pleura; hence the bases of those lobules adjacent to the pleura may be outlined by dark lines. Smaller lymphatics in the pleura form a pattern of closer mesh than those surrounding the bases of lobules. The pleural lymphatics join up with one another to form vessels that are conducted by the pleura to reach and empty into the lymph nodes at the hilus of the lung.

The deep set consists of three groups: (*1*) those in the outer layers of the walls of bronchioles and bronchi (Fig. 23-13); (*2*) those that accompany the branches of the pulmonary artery (Fig. 23-13)—these anastomose with those in the branches of the bronchial tree; and (*3*) those that run in the interlobular septa, particularly in association with the interlobular veins (Fig. 23-13, *right*). All three groups drain toward lymph nodes at the hilus of the lungs.

The lymphatics of the interlobular septa (which belong to the deep set) communicate with those of the pleura (which belong to the superficial set) at sites where interlobular septa join the visceral pleura (Fig. 23-13, *lower right corner*). The lymphatics of the interlobular septa have valves close to the pleura (Fig. 23-13, *lower right corner*). In the past it was generally believed that the valves prevented lymph from the pleural lymphatics from draining into lymphatics of the septa. However, these valves (*1*) are not always present; (*2*) if present, are often poorly developed; and (*3*) do not always point toward the pleura. Indeed, Simer showed that India ink injected into lymphatics of the pleura passed into those of interlobular septa and from there into lymphatics vessels associated with the bronchial tree, eventually reaching the nodes at the hilus.

THE NERVE SUPPLY OF THE LUNGS

Innervation of the Smooth Muscle of Bronchi and Bronchioles. Fibers from both divisions of the autonomic nervous system pass to the bronchial tree. The parasympathetic supply is brought by branches of the vagus nerve. Stimulation via the vagal fibers causes the bronchiolar musculature to contract. Conversely, stimulation via the sympathetic fibers causes the bronchiolar musculature to relax. In the condition known as *asthma,* the smooth muscle of the smaller *bronchioles* contracts, and the mucous membrane of the affected tubes swells. This narrows the passages by which air can enter or leave alveolar ducts and makes breathing exceedingly difficult, Adrenalin, or a similarly acting substance, is often given to relax the bronchiolar musculature and so widen the lumen of the bronchioles of an individual suffering an attack. It is of interest that it is more difficult for an individual with asthma to *expel* air from his lungs than it is to draw it in; the reason is that inspiratory movements tend to expand such tubes as lie within lobules and so enlarge their lumina, while powerful expiratory movements (such as occur in asthma) tend when air cannot be forced out freely through the bronchial tree to compress the tubes

lying within lobules, and so make their lumen still narrower.

Innervation of Interalveolar Walls. Axons have been demonstrated in the thicker parts of interalveolar walls. Both afferent and efferent fibers are believed to be present, with the latter type seeming to be relatively frequent in the vicinity of Type II pneumocytes.

NONRESPIRATORY FUNCTIONS OF THE LUNGS

There are several nonrespiratory functions of the lungs, but two in particular deserve mention here. First, the elaboration of IgA (*see* p. 352) into the respiratory secretions requires collaboration between the epithelial cells of the mucous membrane of the bronchial tree and activated B-lymphocytes or plasma cells in the lamina propria of the membrane. Second, several vasoactive substances are modified in the pulmonary circulation. One that will be described in the following chapter is angiotensin I; in passing through the lung capillaries this is converted to angiotensin II. The modification of these vasoactive substances in many instances seems to be mediated by the endothelium lining the pulmonary capillaries.

REFERENCES AND OTHER READING

Avery, M. E., and Fletcher, B. D.: The lung and its disorders in the newborn infant. *In* Schaffer, A. J. (ed.): Major Problems in Clinical Pediatrics. ed. 3, vol. 1. Philadelphia, W. B. Saunders, 1974.

Avery, M. E., Wang, N. S., and Taeusch, H. W., Jr.: The lung of the newborn infant. Sci. Am., *228:*74, April, 1973.

Bertalanffy, F. D.: Dynamics of cellular populations in the lung. *In* The Lung. Int. Acad. Pathol. Monograph No. 8. pp. 19-30. Baltimore, Williams & Wilkins, 1967.

Boyden, E. A.: Development of the human lung. *In* Kelley, V. C. (ed.): Brennemann's Practice of Pediatrics. vol. 4, Chap. 64. New York, Harper & Row, 1971.

Breeze, R. G., and Wheeldon, E. B.: The cells of the pulmonary airways. Am. Rev. Respir. Dis., *116:*705, 1977.

Chevalier, G., and Collet, A. J.: In vivo imcorporation of choline-³H, leucine-³H and galactose-³H in alveolar Type II pneumocytes in relation to surfactant synthesis. A quantitative radioautographic study in mouse by electron microscopy. Anat. Rec., *174:*289, 1972.

Collet, A. J., and Chevalier, G.: Morphological aspects of Type II pneumocytes following treatment with puromycin in vivo. Am. J. Anat., *148:*275, 1977.

Collet, A. J., and Des Biens, G.: Fine structure of myogenesis and elastogenesis in the developing rat lung. Anat. Rec., *179:*343, 1974.

———: Evolution of mesenchymal cells in fetal rat lung. Anat. Embryol., *147:*273, 1975.

Engel, S.: The Child's Lung. London, Arnold, 1947.

Godleski, J. J., and Brain, J. D.: The origin of alveolar macrophages in mouse radiation chimeras. J. Exp. Med., *136:*630, 1972.

Graziadei, P. P.: Cell dynamics in the olfactory mucosa. Tissue and Cell, 5:113, 1973.

Ham, A. W., and Baldwin, K. W.: A histological study of the development of the lung with particular reference to the nature of alveoli. Anat. Rec., 81:363, 1941.

Harding, J., Graziadei, P. P. C., Monti Graziadei, G. A., and Margolis, F. L.: Denervation in the primary olfactory pathway of mice. IV. Biochemical and morphological evidence for neuronal replacement following nerve section. *Brain Res., 132:*11, 1977.

Heinemann, H. O.: The lung as a metabolic organ: an overview. Fed. Proc., 32:1955–1956, 1973.

Heinemann, H. O., and Fishman, A. P.: Nonrespiratory functions of mammalian lung. Physiol. Rev., 49:1–47, 1969.

Hodson, W. (ed.): Development of the Lung. Lung Biology in Health and Disease. vol. 6. New York, Marcel Dekker, 1977.

Hung, K-S., Hertweck, M. S., Hardy, J. D., and Loosli, C. G.: Innervation of pulmonary alveoli of the mouse lung: an electron microscopic study. Am. J. Anat., 135:477, 1972.

Karrer, H. E.: The ultrastructure of mouse lung. J. Biophys. Biochem. Cytol., 2:241, 1956.

———: The ultrastructure of mouse lung. J. Biophys. Biochem. Cytol., 2 (Suppl.):287, 1956.

———: The ultrastructure of mouse lung: the alveolar macrophage. J. Biophys. Biochem. Cytol., 4:693, 1958.

———: The fine structure of connective tissue in the tunica propria of bronchioles. J. Ultrastruct. Res., 2:96, 1958.

———: The experimental production of pulmonary emphysema. Am. Rev. Respir. Dis., 80:158, 1959.

Krahl, V. E.: Anatomy of the mammalian lung. *In* American Physiological Society: Handbook of Physiology. Section 3 (Fenn, W. O., and Rahn, H., eds.), Respiration. vol. 1, p. 213. Baltimore, Williams & Wilkins, 1964.

Lambert, M. W.: Accessory bronchiolo-alveolar communications. J. Pathol. Bact., 70:311, 1955.

———: Accessory bronchiolo-alveolar channels. Anat. Rec., 127:472, 1957.

Lauweryns, J.: The blood and lymphatic microcirculation of the lung. Pathol. Annu., 6:363, 1971.

Loosli, C. G., and Potter, E. L.: Pre- and postnatal development of the respiratory portion of the human lung. Am. Rev. Respir. Dis., 80:5, 1959.

Low, F. N.: The electron microscopy of sectioned lung tissue after varied duration of fixation in buffered osmium tetroxide. Anat. Rec., 120:827, 1954.

———: The pulmonary alveolar epithelium of laboratory mammals and man. Anat. Rec., 117:241, 1953.

Macklin, C. C.: Alveolar pores and their significance in the human lung. Arch. Pathol., 21:202, 1936.

———: The musculature of the bronchi and lungs. Physiol. Rev., 9:1, 1929.

Mavis, R. D., Finkelstein, J. N., and Hall, B. P.: Pulmonary surfactant synthesis. A highly active microsomal phosphatidate phosphohydrolase in the lung. J. Lipid Res., 19:467, 1978.

Miller, W. S.: The Lung. ed. 2. Springfield, Ill., Charles C Thomas, 1947.

Rhodin, J., and Dulhamn, T.: Electron microscopy of the tracheal ciliated mucosa in rat. Z. Zellforsch., 44:345, 1956.

Ryan, J. W., Niemeyer, R. S., and Goodwin, D. W.: Metabolic fates of bradykinin, angiotensin I, adenine nucleotidase and prostaglandins E1 and F1 alpha in the pulmonary circulation. Adv. Exp. Med. Biol., 21:259, 1972.

Shapiro, H. A.: The limited value of microscopy of lung tissue in the diagnosis of live and stillbirth. Clin. Proc., 6:149, 1947.

Short, R. H. D.: Alveolar epithelium in relation to growth of the lung. Philos. Trans. R. Soc. Lond., 235:35, 1950.

Sorokin, S.: The cells of the lungs. *In* Nettesheim, P., Hanna, M. G., Jr., and Deatherage, J. W., Jr. (eds.): Morphology of Experimental Carcinogenesis. p. 3. CONF 700501, Atomic Energy Commission, Oak Ridge, Tenn., 1970.

———: Phagocytes in the lungs; incidence, general behavior and phylogeny. *In* Brain, J. D., Proctor, D. F., and Reid, L. (eds.): Respiratory Defense Mechanisms. Monograph No. 3 of Series Lung Biology in Health and Disease, Lenfant, C. (ed.). New York, Marcel Dekker, *in press.*

Vane, J. R.: The release and fate of vaso-active hormones in the circulation. Br. J. Pharmacol., 35:209, 1969.

Van Golde, L. M. G.: Metabolism of phospholipids in the lung. Am. Rev. Respir. Dis., 114:977, 1976.

24 The Urinary System

Some General Considerations. The metabolism of food by body cells produces energy but it also produces waste products. The latter seep from cells through tissue fluid into the bloodstream. From there, as was described in the previous chapter, one important waste product, carbon dioxide, is eliminated from the lungs. The elimination of certain other waste products, particularly those resulting from the metabolism of proteins, occurs in two organs of substantial size—the *kidneys*—through which more than one fifth of the total blood of the body circulates every minute. In doing so the blood passes into capillaries, and through the walls of these capillaries water and substances in simple solution are forced out into the beginnings of long tubules. Some of the dissolved substances are useful and some are waste products. Most of the water and any useful substances are resorbed into other blood capillaries through the walls of the tubules. The waste products, however, remain in solution in the tubule and are eventually eliminated from each kidney as *urine.* This is drained away by a tube called a *ureter* that empties into the *urinary bladder.*

Other Functions of the Kidneys. The same cellular arrangements that permit the kidney to eliminate waste products from the blood into urine permit it to serve several other important functions. For example, they can vary the amount of water lost from the body in urine. Hence, the kidneys play a very important part in regulating the *fluid balance* of the body. Likewise, the kidneys can vary the amounts and kinds of electrolytes that are eliminated from the body in urine; thus they assist in maintaining a proper *salt balance* in blood and tissue fluid. The kidneys also participate in maintaining a normal acid-base balance in the body. To perform these functions they conserve some things and eliminate others.

THE BASIC MECHANISMS INVOLVED IN THE EXCRETION OF WASTE PRODUCTS BY THE KIDNEY

In simpler animals, in which blood circulatory system are not highly developed, tissue fluid is an all-important fluid. Waste products of metabolism tend to accumulate in it and must be excreted. A relatively simple mechanism for this is seen in the earthworm. Its segments are provided with tubules, both ends of which are open. The proximal end is open to tissue fluid and the distal end is open to the exterior. Tissue fluid enters each tubule and passes slowly along the tubule to be eliminated at the exterior of the worm as a sort of urine.

Since the tubules are long and coiled, it takes some time for tissue fluid to pass along them. This provides an opportunity for the tissue fluid *to be altered as it passes along the tubule,* because the epithelial cells lining the tubule either (1) *absorb* certain valuable constituents of the fluid back into the organism or (2) *excrete* further things into the fluid in the tubule. It would be anticipated, then, that the fluid finally emerging from the distal end of the tubule (for all practical purposes, urine) would contain fewer valuable constituents than the tissue fluid entering the tubule, and also that the fluid leaving the tubule would contain waste products in greater concentration. We shall see that in man, too, *urine is tissue fluid that has been modified* in the above-described fashion by passing along a tubule.

Evolution of the Glomerulus. As animals became more complex, the blood circulatory system came to be of increasing importance in distributing oxygen and food to cells in different parts of the body and in carrying away their waste products. This required some mechanism by which waste products could be removed from the blood on a more or less continuous basis. In the arrangement that evolved in mammals, excretory tubules are retained, but they are all segregated and housed in the kidneys. Furthermore, instead of each tubule being open at both ends, its innermost end is closed. The arrangement that evolved to give the tubules access to the blood was that of having a little cluster of capillaries form in association with the proximal end of each tubule and push, as it were, into this blind end. The thin epithelium constituting the blind end thus became a covering for each of the capillaries that pushed into it. The cluster of capillaries projecting into the blind end of each tubule is called a *glomerulus* (L. for a small ball) (Fig. 24-1), and the tissue fluid formed by the glomerular capillaries passes into the

753

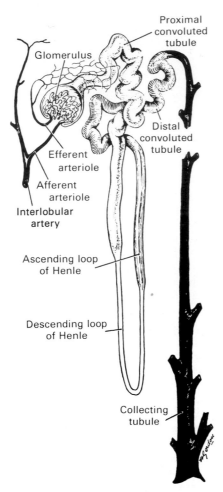

Proximal
convoluted
tubule

Glomerulus

Distal
convoluted
tubule

Efferent
arteriole

Afferent
arteriole

**Interlobular
artery**

Ascending loop
of Henle

Descending loop
of Henle

Collecting
tubule

Fig. 24-1. Diagram of a typical nephron, with its glomerulus at its blind end, and connecting at its distal end with a collecting tubule. In order to simplify the diagram, the normal anatomical relation between the distal convoluted tubule and the root of the glomerulus is not shown. Actually, the tubule returns closer to the glomerulus, fitting into the space at the vascular pole in between the afferent and efferent arterioles, where it forms the macula densa as shown in Figure 24-5.

lumen of the tubule as what is called the *glomerular filtrate.* Due to this arrangement, vast amounts of tissue fluid are delivered into the kidney tubules. As this filtrate passes through the long tubules, valuable substances (including water) are resorbed, so that the fluid emerging from their distal ends as urine to drain via the ureters into the urinary bladder has waste products concentrated in it.

The Nephron. A single kidney tubule, together with the glomerulus pushed into its blind end, is the structural and functional unit of the kidney and is termed a *nephron* (Fig. 24-1). There are over a million of these in each kidney in man. The nephrons drain into a system of *collect-*

ing ducts that in turn drains the fluid (which is now urine) into the expanded funnel-like end of a *ureter.*

Why Glomerular Capillaries Produce More Tissue Fluid Than Ordinary Capillaries. Tissue fluid is formed at the arterial end of capillaries in most parts of the body and resorbed at their venous end (Fig. 8-6). The reasons for this were explained in Chapter 8, and, if still not clear in the reader's mind, the section dealing with formation and absorption of tissue fluid (beginning on p. 218) should be reviewed. The situation in glomerular capillaries is somewhat similar to that existing in ordinary capillaries when outflow at their venous end is obstructed (Fig. 8-7A). This situation causes hydrostatic pressure to remain high along their entire length. Hence tissue fluid is *not resorbed* by such capillaries, it is only produced. In ordinary capillaries this causes edema. In glomerular capillaries, however, it results in *continuous production of glomerular filtrate,* the forerunner of urine.

Another factor that contributes to the production of copious amounts of filtrate is that the endothelial cells of the glomerular capillaries are fenestrated, and it is generally believed that most, if not all, of the fenestrations lack closing diaphragms, so that there are open holes through which the filtrate (but not blood cells) can pass.

As a result of this arrangement, glomerular capillaries produce vast amounts of tissue fluid that pass through the epithelium covering the glomerular capillaries to enter the blind end of the nephron. As soon as the tissue fluid passes through the epithelium covering the capillary, it is referred to as *glomerular filtrate.*

Resorption as the Filtrate Flows Along the Tubular Part of the Nephron. According to Allen, from the 1,700 liters of blood that pass along the glomerular capillaries of the two kidneys every 24 hours, 170 liters of glomerular filtrate are formed. It follows, then, that every 24 hours 170 liters of glomerular filtrate are delivered into the tubular portions of nephrons. As the filtrate passes along the nephrons, over 168 liters of it are resorbed into the bloodstream, so that only about 1.5 liters emerge into the ureters every 24 hours to constitute the daily output of urine. Obviously, there must be as efficient a mechanism for *tubular resorption* of fluid as there is in glomeruli for its production. Resorption involves the activities of the epithelial cells that form the walls of the tubular part of a nephron and also the absorptive function of the extensive low-pressure capillary bed in which the tubules lie, as will be described later.

The various specialized resorptive and excretory functions carried out by the nephron are not performed with equal facility along its whole length. The tubular portion of each nephron (Fig. 24-1) exhibits three consecutive segments that reveal somewhat different structural features and arrangements and perform somewhat different functions. These are termed the *proximal convoluted seg-*

ment, *the loop of Henle,* and the *distal convoluted segment,* respectively (Fig. 24-1). Their particular structure and functions will be described in detail later when the nephron of the human kidney is considered.

THE UNILOBAR KIDNEY

In beginning a laboratory study of the histology of the kidney there are some advantages to starting with the kidney of a rat or rabbit. This is because the unit of gross structure of the kidney is the *lobe.* The kidney of man contains many lobes, whereas the kidney of the rat or rabbit consists of only one. Next, the kidney of a rat (or even a rabbit) is small enough for a section cut along its long axis through its greatest diameter to fit on a slide, as shown at the top of Figure 24-2. In one such section all parts of a lobe and all its connections with the ureter can be seen. Since the kidney of man is large and multilobar, any one section shows only a small part of it, and generally incomplete parts of more than one lobe, which makes the section difficult to interpret unless the student has first seen a section of a unilobar kidney. We shall therefore deal first with the unilobar kidney, and so as to prevent undue repetition, we shall cover only what can be seen with the low power of the LM.

Inspection of the Section With the Unaided Eye. The unilobar kidney is shaped like a lima bean; hence, if one is laid down on its side, it discloses an extensive convex, and a smaller concave, border. Fat is generally present in its concavity, which is called its *hilus.* The drainage tube of the kidney, the *ureter,* together with the renal artery and vein and a surrounding plexus of fine nerves, reach the kidney through the fat at the hilus.

If such a kidney is laid on its side flat on a table and then cut in half, keeping the knife parallel with the table, the cut surface viewed with the naked eye discloses that the kidney substance consists of two chief parts. The outermost region is called the *cortex* (L. for bark or shell) (Fig. 24-2); it consists of a broad red-brown granular layer that lies immediately beneath the convex border and follows its contours (Fig. 24-2). The remainder of the kidney is referred to as its *medulla* (L. for marrow, meaning the middle) and is shaped like a broad conical pyramid that is upside down. The base of the pyramid is convex rather than flat and is fitted up against the concave inner border of the cortex (Fig. 24-2). The apex of the pyramid points downward in Figure 24-2 and juts into the concavity (hilus) of the kidney. In contrast with the darker granular cortex, the cut surface of the medulla is lighter and has striated appearance, with the striations fanning out from the apex of the pyramid to all parts of its broad base (Fig. 24-2).

A conical pyramid of medullary substance, together with the cap of cortical substance that covers its base, constitutes a *lobe* of kidney tissue, and one lobe comprises the whole kidney of the rat or rabbit. We shall now consider how nephrons are disposed in a lobe of kidney; this will explain why the cut surface of the cortex has a granular appearance and that of the medulla has a striated appearance. It will also show how a kidney lobe is divided into *lobules.*

Disposition of Different Parts of Nephrons in Kidney Substance. Nephrons are so long that they fit into a kidney only by pursuing a devious course. Figure 24-2, *bottom,* shows two complete nephrons in solid black; the remainder of the illustration shows the cortex and medulla as seen in an ordinary section under low power.

The glomeruli of the two nephrons are represented by solid black balls. The other glomeruli in this illustration are shown, as they appear in H and E sections, as tufted structures lying in circular cavities (Fig. 24-2). All the glomeruli lie in the cortex.

As can be seen by following either of the two nephrons depicted in black in Figure 24-2, a tubule, the *proximal convoluted tubule,* leads from the glomerulus and pursues a looped and tortuous course in the cortical tissue close to the glomerulus from which it originated. It then turns down to pursue a fairly straight course toward and into the medulla. This segment of the nephron that passes straight down into the medulla is termed the *descending limb of the loop of Henle.* The reason for the term *loop* is that the tubule, after descending for a certain distance into the medulla, loops back and ascends to the cortex again: the part that ascends is called the *ascending limb of the loop of Henle.* In the lower part of the descending limb, the diameter of the tubule and its epithelial wall, both of which up to this time have been relatively thick, become very thin and then, part way up the ascending limb, they become thick again (Fig. 24-2).

The ascending limb of the loop of Henle, on approaching the glomerulus from which this nephron originated, curves in to touch the *root* of the glomerulus; this lies between the site of entry of the afferent arteriole and the site of exit of the efferent arteriole. The portion of the wall of the tubule that comes into contact with the glomerular root is heavily nucleated, and because it constitutes a *thick spot* it was termed the *macula densa* (Figs. 24-2 and 24-5).

The segment of nephron that continues on from the macula densa is known as the *distal convoluted tubule.* It pursues a mildly tortuous course in the neighboring cortical tissue (Fig. 24-2). It then joins a little side branch of one of the members of a branching system of long straight *collecting tubules* that extend from the cortex down through the medulla (Fig. 24-2) to open through the apex of the pyramidal medulla; this apical part of the pyramidal medulla is called its *papilla* (Fig. 24-2).

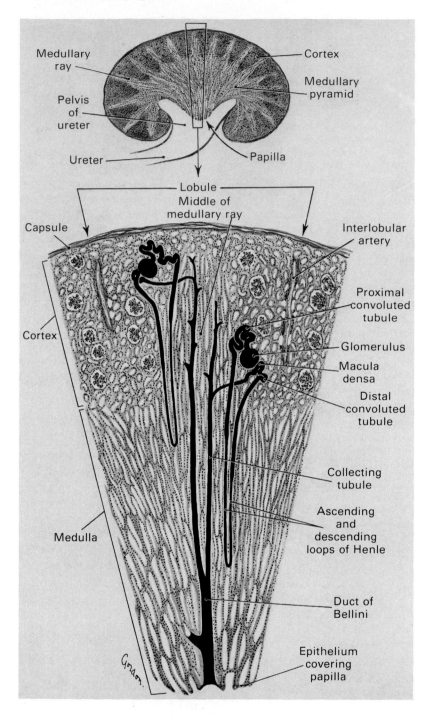

Fig. 24-2. Schematic diagrams of a *unilobar* kidney. Two complete nephrons and the collecting ducts into which they empty (indicated in black) have been included so that their course may be followed. Of course, complete nephrons cannot be seen in any single section.

Collecting Tubules. The collecting tubules are not parts of nephrons. They convey fluid from the nephrons to the renal pelvis and ureter, their relation to nephrons being similar to that between ducts and secretory units of glands. Indeed, they have a different developmental origin. A nephron develops from mesodermal cells that become organized into a tubule; this later becomes associated with blood capillaries that are forming a renal corpuscle in the kidney cortex. On each side of the body a tube grows up from the developing bladder into the developing kidney, where it branches. This tube becomes the ureter and pelvis of the kidney, and each of its many branches becomes a collecting tubule that later connects with a nephron in such a way that the lumina of the two become continuous.

Why the Cortex Is Granular and the Medulla Striated. The cortex contains all the glomeruli and all the convoluted parts of the proximal and distal tubules; hence, except for some straight parts of loops of Henle, the cortex consists of a mixture of glomeruli and convoluted tubules (Fig. 24-2). When the cortex is cut across, the proximal and distal convoluted tubules, being tortuous, are cut in cross and oblique section. Tubules cut this way, with glomeruli scattered among them, give a granular appearance to the cortex when its cut surface is examined with the naked eye.

The part of nephrons that lies in the medulla is the loop of Henle. Since loops of Henle and the collecting tubules mixed with them all run fairly straight courses, the medulla, when sliced roughly parallel with them, has a striated appearance (Fig. 24-2), with the striations fanning out from the apex of the medullary pyramid toward the base of the pyramid, which, as noted, fits into the concave border of the cortex.

The Connection Between the Ureter and the Kidney. It can be seen in a fresh unilobar kidney that the ureter extends from the kidney through the fat at its hilus. If this tube is traced back up into the fat of the hilus, it will be found that it is expanded to form a cap fitting over the papilla of the pyramid (Fig. 24-2). This expanded funnel-shaped end of the ureter is called the *renal pelvis* (L. for basin). Urine formed by nephrons passes into collecting tubules that carry it out through the papilla, and here it is collected by the funnel-like proximal end of the ureter. Urine can only enter the lumen of the expanded end of the ureter because the epithelium that lines the renal pelvis is continuous with the epithelium covering the papilla, and this, in turn, is continuous with that lining the collecting tubules (Fig. 24-2). The papilla is so riddled with the collecting tubules that pass through it that it is sometimes referred to as the *area cribosa* (L. *cribrum,* a sieve). Smooth muscle has been described in the wall of the ureter where it forms the renal pelvis, and it has been suggested that its contraction may exert a milking effect on the papilla, squeezing urine out of the collecting tubules into the renal pelvis.

Lobules and Medullary Rays

It is important not to confuse lobules with lobes.

A *lobe* of kidney tissue is a medullary pyramid with its cap of cortical tissue (Fig. 24-2). Accordingly, a unipyramidal kidney is a unilobar kidney. Each human kidney, however, consists of a dozen or more lobes, so that each lobe resembles a whole unipyramidal kidney.

The Two Definitions of a Lobule. As was explained in connection with liver lobules, a lobule can be defined as a small part of an organ that is separated from other parts by connective tissue partitions or by some other means. However, in glandular tissue the small parts separated from one another by partitions are generally constituted of secretory units that drain into a single common duct that leaves the lobule. Hence the parts that drain into a single common duct came to be called *lobules* in the kidney even though these parts are not separated from one another by partitions. So in the kidney, lobules correspond to the parts of the organ in which the nephrons all drain into the same collecting tubule. Since these areas of tissue (lobules) are not separated from one another by other tissues, it is not easy to find them; it is much easier to locate their central cores, which are known as *medullary rays,* and these will now be described.

Medullary Rays as Cores of Kidney Lobules. The cortex of a freshly cut kidney has a granular appearance. But it is not evenly granular because ray-like extensions of light-colored, striated medullary substance project up into it at intervals from the base of the medullary pyramid (Fig. 24-2). These extensions of medullary substance into the cortex are termed *medullary rays,* and the student must take care to remember that these do not lie, as their name might be thought to imply, in the medulla but in the cortex.

To explain them requires that we amplify our description of the disposition of nephrons in the kidney. A proximal convoluted tubule pursues a tortuous course in the vicinity of its glomerulus and dips down toward the medulla as the descending limb of a loop of Henle. It returns to the cortex as an ascending limb of the loop of Henle, touches the glomerulus again at the macula densa, and becomes the distal convoluted tubule. This pursues a tortuous course and empties, together with many other nephrons, into a *common collecting tubule* that in turn descends into and through the medulla to open through the papilla into the renal pelvis. Hence, *many nephrons drain into each collecting tubule* (Fig. 24-2).

The core of a lobule is a medullary ray, and the core of a medullary ray is the branched collecting tubule into which the distal convoluted segments of the many nephrons that surround it empty. The branched collecting tubule in the kidney cortex is the counterpart of a branched *intralobular* duct of an exocrine gland. In addition to a branched collecting tubule, a medullary ray contains the descending and ascending limbs of the loops of Henle of the nephrons that, in the cortex, empty into the branched collecting tubule that the ray contains. The medullary ray, together with the surrounding glomeruli and proximal and distal convoluted tubules of the nephrons that empty into its branched collecting tubule, constitutes a *lobule* of kidney tissue (Fig. 24-2). However, as noted, kidney lobules are not clearly delineated.

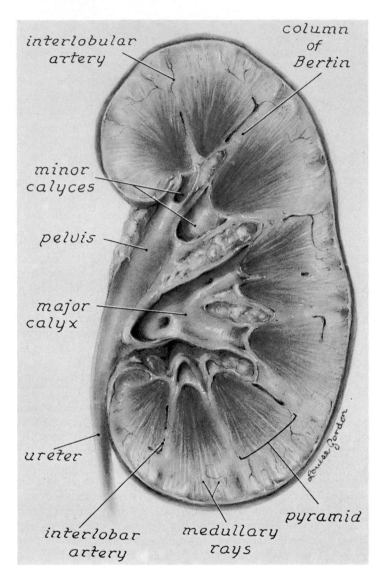

interlobular
artery

column
of
Bertin

minor
calyces

pelvis

major
calyx

ureter

interlobar
artery

medullary
rays

pyramid

Fig. 24-3. Drawing of the cut surface of a human (*multilobar*) kidney. The granular cortex appears streaked with medullary rays.

But when we study the blood supply of the cortex, we shall find that interlobular arteries ascend into the cortex roughly between lobules, and where present in sections these arteries serve as landmarks delineating lobules (Fig. 24-4).

The medullary ray is narrowest where it most closely approaches the capsule of the kidney. The reason is that medullary rays in the outer part of the cortex only contain, in addition to collecting tubules (which narrow as they approach the cortex), the descending and ascending limbs of loops of Henle of the nephrons whose glomeruli are in the outermost zone of the cortex. But as medullary rays descend in the cortex toward the medulla, they are added to by the descending and ascending limbs of loops of Henle of the nephrons whose glomeruli are in the deeper parts of the cortex, and this, of course, makes the rays broader (Fig. 24-2).

A medullary ray, on entering the medulla, is no longer called a ray, because it does not stand out like a ray against a background of different character; the substance of the medullary continuation of the ray is the same as that of medullary substance in general (Fig. 24-2). This may lead to students visualizing kidney lobules as purely cortical structures. However, it should be remembered that the bundle of tubules that enters the medulla from each medullary ray, even though its limits can no longer be identified, is as much a part of the lobule as the bundle that projects into the cortex as the medullary ray. In other words, kidney lobules have medullary as well as cortical components.

Fig. 24-4. Low-power photomicrograph of cortex of human kidney showing two lobules separated by an interlobular artery. The two medullary rays that form the central cores of the two lobules are each surrounded by the glomeruli and convoluted tubules of the nephrons that empty into the collecting ducts of the ray; they comprise what is termed the cortical labyrinth.

Interlobular artery

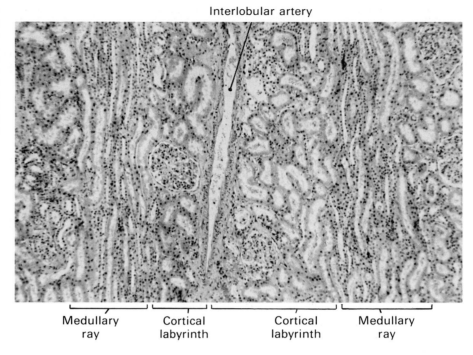

Medullary ray   Cortical labyrinth   Cortical labyrinth   Medullary ray

THE MULTIPYRAMIDAL (MULTILOBAR) KIDNEY OF MAN

Some General Features. The human kidney contains from 6 to 18 *lobes*—individual conical pyramids of medullary tissue capped by cortical tissue. These are arranged so that the tip of each pyramid points toward the renal pelvis (Fig. 24-3). In fetal life, and for at least part of the first year after birth, the lobes are sufficiently distinct for their limits to be seen on the surface of the kidney. This condition occasionally persists into adult life and accounts for what is termed *fetal lobulation.* This term is not apt because *lobes* (not *lobules*) are demarcated. Normally, however, as growth continues the visible delineation between lobes is lost in early childhood, and the cortical tissue that covers each medullary pyramid blends with that covering adjacent ones.

Columns of Bertin. A lobed appearance is nevertheless retained in the medulla, for although some pyramids fuse during development and come to have a common papilla, many remain separated and provide the basis for a multilobar structure. Individual medullary pyramids, curiously enough, are separated from one another to some extent by substantial *partitions of cortical substance* that extend down between them for some distance from the cortex proper. When a kidney is sectioned, these partitions of cortical substance between pyramids appear as columns and are called the *columns of Bertin* (Fig. 24-3).

The Cortical Labyrinth. Medullary rays extend from the base of each pyramid of medullary tissue into cortical substance, as they do in unipyramidal kidneys, to form the cores of *lobules* (Fig. 24-4). In sections of cortex a ray is surrounded by cortical substance composed of the convoluted tubules and glomeruli of the nephrons that empty into its branched collecting tubule (Fig. 24-4). Because convoluted tubules pursue such tortuous courses, the cortical substance that surrounds the medullary rays is termed the *cortical labyrinth* (Gr. *labyrinthos,* maze), illustrated in Figure 24-4, to distinguish it from the substance of the ray.

The Calyces of the Pelvis of the Multilobar Kidney. Since the multilobar kidney has many medullary pyramids, each of which passes urine through the dozen or more collecting tubules that empty through its papilla, the pelvis of the multilobar kidney is more complex than that of the unipyramidal type. The ureter, on approaching the hilus of a multilobar kidney, becomes expanded into a pelvis as it does in the instance of a unipyramidal kidney. But, since there are many papillae from which urine must be collected, the pelvis of the ureter of the multilobar kidney divides into several large primary branches. Each in turn branches into another set so that an individual tube (with an open end) is provided to fit over the papilla of each pyramid. Since these tubular branches from the pelvis fit over the individual papillae like cups, they are termed *calyces* (Gr. *kalyx,* the cup of a flower). Each cup that fits over a papilla is termed a *minor calyx* (Fig. 24-3), and the main (primary) branches of the pelvis, from which the minor calyces arise, are termed *major calyces* (Fig. 24-3). Each papilla is, as it were, inserted for a short distance into the open end of its calyx. Of course, it cannot reach into the open end of the tubular calyx for any great distance because of its pyramidal shape (the tip of a pencil can be pushed into the open end of a smaller tube for only a short distance). The walls of the open end of a calyx come into contact with the sides of the papilla a short distance from its tip, and here the tissues of the wall of the calyx become continuous with those of the papilla. In particular, the epithelium that lines the calyx is reflected back to become the covering of the papilla.

The Nephrons. These in human kidneys average 50 to 55 mm. in length. Their general microscopic structure and disposition within lobules are as in unipyramidal kidneys. Those nephrons with glomeruli situated close to the medulla (the juxtamedullary glomeruli) have longer loops of Henle than those with glomeruli nearer the exterior of the kidney (*see* nephrons in black in Figure 24-2). There are probably about 1.3 million nephrons in each kidney; some estimates run as high as 4 million. Allen estimates that the total length of all the tubules of both kidneys is approximately 75 miles. The nephron of the kidney of man (Fig. 24-1) consists of the four typical parts: (*1*) the *renal (malpighian) corpuscle,* which contains the *glomerulus,* (*2*) the *proximal convoluted tubule,* (*3*) the *loop of Henle,* and (*4*) the *distal convoluted tubule* (Fig. 24-1). The microscopic structure of each of these parts will now be described and related, so far as is practicable, to particular functions.

THE RENAL CORPUSCLE

Definition and Development. A *glomerulus,* as noted, is a tuft of capillaries supplied by an *afferent arteriole* and drained by an *efferent arteriole* — a unique kind of arrangement admirably suited for production of tissue fluid. When, during development, a glomerulus forms in the blind end of an epithelial tubule, the structure formed is known as a *renal (malpighian) corpuscle* (Fig. 24-5). This is a complex structure comprising capillaries, mesangial cells (described later), a special sort of epithelium, and the lumen of the expanded blind end of the epithelial tubule into which the epithelially covered capillaries project. The epithelium covering each capillary is known as the *visceral layer of Bowman's capsule* or, more commonly, *glomerular epithelium* (Fig. 24-5). It is important to appreciate that the epithelium covers the individual capillaries (Fig. 24-5) in such a way that, except in certain sites to be described later, each capillary will be completely covered with *basement membrane,* as will be explained in detail later. The epithelium that forms the outer wall of the corpuscle (the bulged end of the nephron), into which the epithelially covered glomerulus is invaginated, is known as the *parietal layer of Bowman's capsule* or, more com-

monly, *capsular epithelium* (Fig. 24-5). It is continuous with the glomerular epithelium. The lumen of the tubule, which in effect consists of all the spaces between the epithelially covered capillaries and the parietal layer of Bowman's capsule, constitutes *Bowman's* or the *capsular space* (shown but not labeled in Fig. 24-5).

Renal corpuscles range from about 150 to 250 μm. in diameter. They are ovoid rather than spherical. The juxtamedullary corpuscles are generally larger than those nearer the capsule, probably because juxtamedullary ones are the first to form during development and hence are the oldest.

The Course and Character of the Larger Glomerular Blood Vessels. The overall diameter of the afferent arteriole of a glomerulus is generally about twice that of the efferent arteriole. However, the size of the *lumen* of the afferent arteriole of most glomeruli is probably about the *same* as in the efferent one during life (in preparations fixed by injection under pressure, they are of about the same size). Trueta and his associates showed that the lumen of the efferent arteriole in juxtamedullary glomeruli can even become wider than that of the afferent arteriole. Since the overall diameter of the afferent arterioles is so much greater than that of the efferent ones, it is obvious that afferent arterioles must have thicker walls than efferent arterioles. The difference in thickness of the walls of the two vessels is due to the afferent arteriole having a *more substantial muscular media.* Although the muscular media of the efferent vessel is not well developed, Bensley provided definite evidence of contractile cells in the wall of this vessel.

The Glomerular Root, Vascular Pole, and Macula Densa. The afferent and efferent arterioles generally pursue curved diverging courses as they enter or leave glomeruli (as the case may be) close to one another (Fig. 24-5). This site is termed the *vascular pole* of the glomerulus. The ascending limb of the loop of Henle of each nephron returns to the glomerulus of that nephron, and before it continues on as the distal convoluted tubule it bends in between the afferent and efferent arterioles at the vascular pole so that its wall, on one side, comes into close contact with the root of the glomerulus and also with the wall of the afferent arteriole (Fig. 24-5). As noted, the epithelial cells of the wall of the nephron, where it touches the root of the glomerulus and the afferent vessel, exhibit a concentration of nuclei (Fig. 24-5). This heavily nucleated portion of the wall of the nephron constitutes a structure which, although not sharply defined in ordinary sections, was shown very clearly and measured by Oliver. It appears as a group of epithelial cells that are higher than those in other parts of the distal convoluted tubule, and it is termed the *macula densa.* Between it and the glomerulus proper, in the concavity between the afferent and efferent arterioles, is a curious aggregation of small cells with pale-

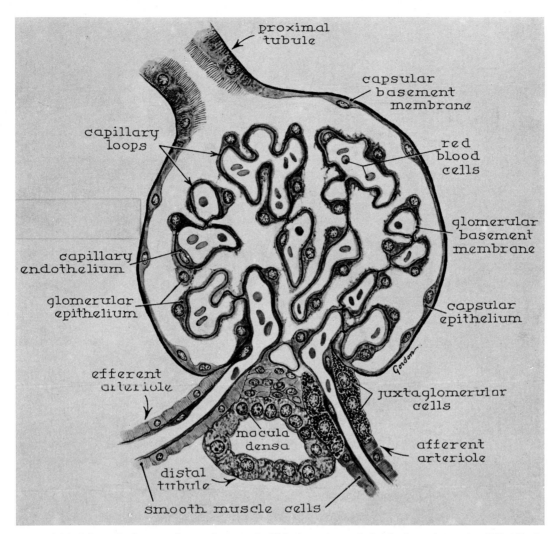

Fig. 24-5. Schematic diagram of a renal corpuscle. This shows in particular the juxtaglomerular (JG) cells. It also gives a cross-sectional view of the ascending loop of Henle, after it becomes the distal convoluted tubule, fitting in between the afferent and efferent arterioles of the corpuscle from which this tubule originated, and there forming the macula densa.

staining nuclei (Fig. 24-5). This little group of cells is termed the *polkissen* (Ger. for pole cushion). There is still uncertainty about the function of these cells. Some consider them equivalent to mesangial cells (soon to be described).

THE JUXTAGLOMERULAR COMPLEX

The cells of the *media* of the *afferent arteriole* of glomeruli, in the region of the glomerular root, are distinctly different from ordinary smooth muscle cells. Their nucleus instead of being elongated is rounded, and their cytoplasm, instead of containing an abundance of fila-

ments, contains granules (Fig. 24-5). The cells are known as *JG (juxtaglomerular) cells.* They have been found in all species examined, including reptiles, birds, and mesonephric fish. The granules of JG cells are not visible with routine staining but can be demonstrated with the PAS technic. However, the best method for their demonstration in the LM is the one evolved by Wilson (*see* References and Other Reading). The granules are clearly seen in the EM.

There are several peculiarities about the position of the JG cells. (*1*) They are found in the walls of afferent arterioles but are seldom seen in the walls of efferent ones. (*2*) The internal elastic lamina of the afferent arteriole is absent where they are present; therefore, they are in very close contact with the endothelium lining the afferent arteriole and hence with the blood in its lumen. (*3*) They are in very close contact with the macula densa (Fig. 24-5) nestling in the depression between the afferent and efferent arterioles. (*4*) The basement membrane that otherwise surrounds the nephron throughout its length is absent at the macula densa (McManus). Hence, the JG cells come into intimate contact with cells of the distal convoluted tubule at this site. Finally, the Golgi apparatus, which in cells of a nephron is generally situated between the nucleus and the lumen, is situated on the other side in most of the cells of the macula densa, between the nucleus and the outer border of its cells—in fact, on the side of the cell that faces the JG cells (McManus). In due course it became established that the JG cells are concerned in the *control of blood pressure,* as will now be described.

The student is doubtless aware that a condition termed *high blood pressure (hypertension)* is by no means uncommon in individuals who have passed the prime of life, and that it may also occur, but less commonly, in younger people. Hypertension is due to the *arterioles* of the body becoming *constricted;* this raises the pressure within the arterial system. This, of course, puts more work on the heart, which therefore tends to become hypertrophied. The arteriolar constriction may be due, at least for a time, to increased tonus or hypertrophy of the muscle cells of the arteriolar walls, with the cells of the wall remaining healthy. But in all too many instances the cells of the arteriolar walls become diseased, and deposits of abnormal materials accumulate in and beside them; these encroach on the lumen of the vessel and narrow it further. This type of hypertension is almost always associated with kidney disease; indeed, the relation between kidney disease and hypertension has been so noticeable through the years that each has been proposed as a cause of the other.

In 1939 Goldblatt made a brilliant discovery that threw some light on the matter; he showed that if the arterial blood supply of the kidneys was diminished but not entirely cut off, the blood pressure of an animal would rise. Moreover, he showed that this was due to the kidneys liberating into the blood, under these ischemic conditions, an enzyme called *renin* (L. *renis,* kidney). In the bloodstream renin acts on a plasma globulin known as *angiotensinogen* to convert it to a decapeptide called *angiotensin I*. This is inactive but when acted on by an enzyme (converting enzyme) it is changed to an octapeptide, *angiotensin II* (previously called *angiotonin*) that causes *arteriolar constriction* and so raises blood pressure. Angiotensin II has, however, only a transient effect, so to cause sustained hypertension it must be formed continuously. (Renin had already been extracted from kidneys before Goldblatt's discovery.)

Relation of JG Cells to Renin. A predictable conjecture was that the JG cells make renin, and that the granules in them (Fig. 24-5) are either renin or its precursor. There are three lines of evidence that JG cells elaborate renin. First, there is a correlation between the amount of renin in the kidneys and the degree of granulation of their JG cells (Pitcock and Hartroft). Second, microdissection technics demonstrated that the concentration of renin is highest in the region of the JG cells. Third, fluorescent-labeled antiserum to renin attached itself chiefly to JG cells (Hartroft and Edelman).

The Functions of JG Cells. It now seems likely that JG cells are involved in two ways in a homeostatic mechanism concerned in the control of blood pressure. If the blood pressure falls, the afferent arterioles of the glomeruli are not stretched as much from within as normally. It has been suggested that the JG cells in the walls of these arterioles are baroceptors sensitive to degree of stretch due to the blood pressure within the arteriole. If not stretched by a normal pressure they respond by secreting more renin; this results in there being more angiotensin II formed in the blood, and this has two effects, both of which would raise the blood pressure.

First, angiotensin II has a direct effect on *arterioles,* stimulating their muscular walls to contract, and hence decreasing the size of their lumina and raising the blood pressure in the circulatory system as a whole.

Second, angiotensin II stimulates the *adrenal cortex* to secrete increased amounts of the hormone *aldosterone* (which will be described in the next chapter). Aldosterone acts on the tubular parts of nephrons, causing them to *conserve more sodium and water.* This increases the fluid content of the circulatory system (and the tissue fluid content of the body as well). Increasing the amount of fluid in the circulatory system contributes to increasing the pressure within the system.

The fundamental role of JG cells would therefore seem to be that of responding to a fall in blood pressure by releasing renin, which by producing angiotensin II would act to bring blood pressure up to normal. The effect would not be permanent because the extra sodium in the blood or in the filtrate passing the macula densa, and also the increased pressure within the arteriole, would act to cause the JG cells to stop releasing renin and perhaps slow down their secretory activity and in due course contain fewer granules. These negative feedback mechanisms would prevent the blood pressure from being maintained at an excessive level.

The JG mechanism can, however, cause sustained hypertension, at least in some animals, if the arterial circulation through one or both kidneys is *chronically* impaired. Even in man disease in one or both kidneys can permanently obstruct the arterial flow. Experimentally, a permanently diminished arterial flow and pressure can be

Fig. 24-6. Diagram illustrating the position of mesangial cells in relation to the surrounding capillaries in a glomerular tuft. Note that whereas the basement membrane of the endothelial cells completely surrounds each capillary in the tuft, the basement membrane beneath the podocyte feet does *not* surround each capillary completely. It is present only where the capillaries in the tuft are covered with epithelium (in the form of podocyte feet), as shown at *lower right.* The podocyte feet would, of course, extend over all the capillary tuft shown in this diagram. The mesangial cells are essentially macrophages immersed in an amorphous intercellular substance that forms the core of a capillary tuft.

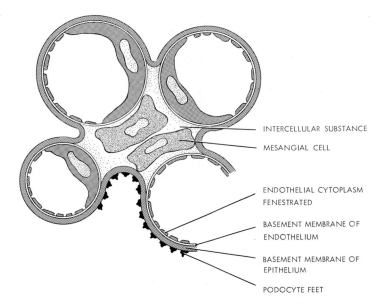

INTERCELLULAR SUBSTANCE

MESANGIAL CELL

ENDOTHELIAL CYTOPLASM FENESTRATED

BASEMENT MEMBRANE OF ENDOTHELIUM

BASEMENT MEMBRANE OF EPITHELIUM

PODOCYTE FEET

achieved, for example by applying the clips to the renal arteries. Under these circumstances, the JG cells of the affected kidney or kidneys try to raise the pressure by releasing renin, but if the highest pressure thus generated in the circulatory system as a whole cannot be transmitted to the arterioles of the two kidneys because of the arterial circulation in even one kidney being impeded, the JG cells of that kidney will continue to release renin, and, as a result, the blood pressure in the body as a whole will remain elevated.

Seen with the EM, the granules of JG cells of mammals are round to oval in shape, large, surrounded with membrane, but not particularly homogeneous. P. Hartroft notes that JG cells of the American bullfrog reveal two types of granules, which, of course, might mean that there are two different types of secretion. This observation is of interest with regard to the possibility that JG cells may also be the source of the renal erythropoietic factor as well as renin. It has been known for some time that the kidneys are the principal source of what becomes erythropoietin in the blood plasma and there is some experimental evidence suggesting that the cellular source of this substance is the JG cells (Hartroft, Bischoff, and Boucci).

It is possible that by discussing this particular histological feature of the kidneys, namely the JG cells and their relation to blood pressure, we might inadvertently create the impression that the usual cause of hypertension in man is excessive and sustained release of renin from these cells. So we should point out that the basis for the usual kind of hypertension is complex; salt and water retention, aldosterone secretion, kidney disease, and even emotional factors all seem to be variously involved with development and continuance of this condition.

THE GLOMERULUS

Glomerular Capillaries. Primary branches of the afferent arteriole give rise to capillaries that drain into primary branches of the efferent arteriole, suggesting that there are what might be termed *lobules* in the glomerulus. A lobule would consist of the capillary loops hanging from one primary branch of the afferent arteriole and draining into one primary branch of the efferent arteriole. Anastomoses occur between the capillaries of a given lobule, and there is some indication they also occur between the capillary loops of adjacent so-called lobules. So glomerular capillaries are essentially arranged in lobules, but there are enough anastomoses between lobules for the capillaries to constitute an anastomosing network.

Mesangial Cells. The glomerulus hangs from the vascular pole of the renal corpuscle. The sites where the afferent arteriole branches to give rise to the capillary loops in its lobules, and where the capillary loops of lobules join the branches of the efferent arteriole, can be considered stalks from which the lobules hang. In the stalk regions the capillaries in many places are in intimate contact with one another. Whereas glomerular epithelium covers all the exposed surfaces of glomerular capillaries that are close together, it does not always penetrate far enough between the capillaries adjacent to one another in a stalk to provide a complete covering for each capillary in that stalk. Instead, the glomerular epithelium surrounds little groups of contiguous capillaries as a whole; this is shown in Figure 24-6.

In such sites, the basement membrane derived from the epithelial cells therefore does not completely surround each capillary (dark gray in Fig. 24-6). Hence, the parts of the walls of the grouped capillaries that are not covered with glomerular epithelium, and therefore its basement membrane, are relatively weak. Some support is provided in these sites, however, because of mesangial cells being disposed between the contiguous capillaries (Fig. 24-6). The mesangial cells make an intercellular substance (Fig. 24-6) that is similar to basement membrane, and this covers the endothelial cells of the capillaries where they are not covered by epithelially derived basement membrane. The endothelial cells of the capillaries too are surrounded with a thin basement membrane (dark line in Fig. 24-6), and this fuses with the epithelially derived basement membrane where there is epithelium. Where there is no epithelial basement membrane, it more or less fuses with the matrix of the mesangial cells.

Mesangial cells have a more or less stellate shape. Sometimes a cytoplasmic process reaches between endothelial cells to abut directly on the lumen of a capillary.

The general nature of the mesangial cell seems to be similar to that of a pericyte or undifferentiated smooth muscle cell. There is also some suggestion that mesangial cells represent a continuation into the glomerulus of a type of cell similar to the JG cells of the afferent arteriole. Granules have been seen in them, and they behave in certain ways like JG cells. However, they possess (or can develop) phagocytic properties and where present are able to cope with any macromolecular materials that enter the intercapillary spaces. Their other role, as noted, is providing support where the usual relatively strong basement membrane provided by the glomerular epithelial cells is not present.

Whether mesangial cells are associated with free capillary loops in a glomerulus is perhaps open to question. If ever present in such sites, they would in effect be pericytes located on the outer surface of the basement membrane produced by the endothelial cells, and hence between this basement membrane and that made by the epithelial cells. Mesangial cells are easier to demonstrate in certain animals—for example, rats and mice—than in man.

The Respective Roles of Epithelium and Endothelium in the Formation of Basement Membranes. As described in Chapter 8 (p. 222), there is evidence that the epithelium plays a major role in forming basement membrane that lies between epithelium and connective tissue. Endothelial cells of capillaries also produce a basement membrane on their outer surface, but it is so thin it can be seen only with the EM.

In examining a PAS-stained section of kidney with the LM, well-defined basement membranes can be seen only where epithelial cells abut on connective tissue cells (including endothelium). Basement membrane can be seen in renal corpuscles in two sites. First, there is a substantial basement membrane between the continuous squamous epithelium that constitutes the parietal layer of Bowman's capsule and the connective tissue that supports this epithelium (Fig. 24-5 and Plate 24-1). Second, there is a continuous basement membrane interposed between the walls of glomerular capillaries (endothelium with some pericytes) and the epithelium (the so-called visceral layer of Bowman's capsule or the glomerular epithelium) that covers the capillaries. An important fact to take into account in attempting to visualize the arrangements of glomerular capillaries in three dimensions is that, except where a mesangial cell lies between two or three contiguous capillaries, every capillary in cross or oblique section in a PAS preparation is *completely surrounded with basement membrane* (Fig. 24-5).

In other parts of the cortex, basement membrane is not seen with the LM around the capillaries associated with the tubular parts of the nephron because it is too thin. The tubules themselves, however, are each surrounded with a substantial PAS-positive basement membrane that can be seen readily with the LM, as in Plate 24-1.

Accordingly, it seems that epithelium interacting somehow with connective tissue is a requisite for the formation of substantial basement membranes in the kidney.

The Surface Area of Glomerular Capillaries. The total surface area of the capillaries of a glomerulus has been estimated and also measured by making large-scale models of each section cut through an injected glomerulus and measuring the surfaces of the capillaries of the models. The procedure is so laborious and fraught with difficulties that few have attempted it. Book, two of whose preparations are shown in Figure 24-7, injected the blood vessels of a kidney of a child of 6, and calculated that the capillaries of the glomerulus have a surface area of almost 0.4 sq. mm. Kirkman and Stowell measured the capillary surface area of several rat glomeruli and found that it averages almost 0.2 sq. mm., but state that Book's figure is the most reliable one available for the human glomerulus (rat glomeruli are smaller than human glomeruli). Since it has been estimated that there are well over 1 million glomeruli in each human kidney, it seems probable that the total filtration surface of the glomeruli of both kidneys is well over 1 square meter.

It has been estimated that the glomerular capillaries of all the renal corpuscles of the two kidneys produce from 170 to 200 liters of tissue fluid (glomerular filtrate) every 24 hours. By the time the fluid reaches the pelvis of the ureter, almost 99 per cent of it has been resorbed through the walls of the tubules back into the bloodstream.

Pressure Factors Involved in Glomerular Filtration. The first of these to consider is the *net hydrostatic pressure.* As already mentioned, production of glomerular filtrate is similar to tissue fluid formation elsewhere in the body, except that the situation in glomerular capillaries resembles what is seen under conditions of venous obstruction, with a high hydrostatic pressure being maintained along the whole length of the glomerular capillaries. This is due to the resistance offered to their outflow by the efferent arteriole. Measurements made on mutant rats of a special strain characterized in part by having surface glomeruli on their kidneys (the Munich-Wistar strain) indicate the hydrostatic pressure in glomerular capillaries is around 45 mm. Hg.

Next, there is a positive hydrostatic pressure outside the glomerular capillaries because the tissue fluid (glomerular fil-

Fig. 24-7. (*A*) Medium-power photomicrograph of a glomerulus in a kidney after injection of its blood vessels. (*B*) Photograph of a wax plate made from an enlargement of a section of an injected glomerulus (not the same one). (Courtesy of M. Book)

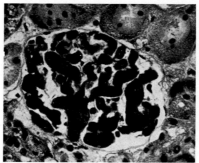
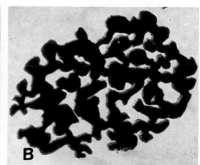

trate) they form is unable to flow away readily. The only escape route available when this tissue fluid is forced into the expanded end of a nephron is for it to flow along the lumen of the nephron for a comparatively long distance. In order to make this journey it needs to be under a hydrostatic pressure of around 10 mm. Hg. So to calculate the *net hydrostatic pressure* in the glomerular capillaries, the hydrostatic pressure outside the capillaries has to be subtracted from that inside them, which means that the net hydrostatic pressure is around $45 - 10 = 35$ mm. Hg.

Next, to determine the *net filtration pressure* (which is different from the net hydrostatic pressure), we have to take into account the fact that protein macromolecules, which confer (colloid) osmotic pressure on blood plasma, remain in the blood as it passes through the glomerular capillaries. As a consequence, the osmotic pressure due to these macromolecules acts so as to draw fluid back into the glomerular capillaries from the glomerular filtrate. Hence, to calculate the *net filtration pressure*, the osmotic pressure within the capillaries has in turn to be subtracted from their net hydrostatic pressure. However, this is complicated by the fact that as glomerular filtrate is produced along the course of a glomerular capillary, the concentration of protein increases in the plasma left behind in the capillary. So whereas the osmotic pressure at the beginnings of these capillaries is only about 20 mm. Hg, it rises along the length of the capillaries to become around 35 mm. Hg. Since the net hydrostatic pressure is only around 35 mm. Hg at the beginnings of glomerular capillaries, the net filtration pressure would only be $35 - 20 = 15$ mm. Hg at their beginnings. But at their ends, where the osmotic pressure has risen to 35 mm. Hg, the net filtration pressure would be reduced to zero. Hence glomerular filtrate is formed in decreasing amounts from the beginnings of glomerular capillaries to their ends, where none is formed.

Plasma flow rate in glomerular capillaries would seem to be a very important factor in filtrate production. For a review of all the factors concerned in glomerular filtration, *see* Brenner et al.

THE FILTRATION BARRIER OF THE GLOMERULUS—ITS FINE STRUCTURE AND FUNCTION

There are three layers in this barrier to consider: (*1*) the endothelium of the glomerular capillaries, (*2*) the basement membrane between the endothelium of these capillaries and the epithelium on their outer aspect, and (*3*) the epithelium covering the capillaries (the visceral layer of Bowman's capsule). Before discussing their respective roles in the filtration process, we shall describe each layer.

The Endothelium of Glomerular Capillaries

The cytoplasm of the endothelial cells of glomerular capillaries, in all but the perinuclear region containing most of the organelles, is very attenuated and also *fenestrated* (Figs. 24-9 and 24-10). The diameter of the fenestrae is rather variable (60 to 100 nm.), and it is generally accepted that most fenestrae are not closed over by diaphragms. However, it is said that a few of the fenestrae are in fact spanned by diaphragms; if true, the purpose of this would seem obscure.

The Glomerular Basement Membrane

This is about 320 to 340 nm. thick, which is over three times the usual thickness of basement membranes found elsewhere in the body. In electron micrographs it appears as an amorphous material with an extremely fine filamentous component embedded in it. It is also unusual in comprising three layers, each roughly 100 nm. thick. Its central layer is relatively electron-dense and hence termed the *lamina densa*. (This is the one that is obvious in micrographs, for example Fig. 24-10, where it is labeled bm.) On either side of this there is a more electron-lucent layer—the *lamina rara interna* to the inside and the *lamina rara externa* to the outside (Fig. 24-10).

Because of the endothelial cells being weak and the glomerular epithelium discontinuous (this will be explained shortly), the construction of glomerular capillaries is such that the strongest structure supporting them is their basement membrane. Moreover, since this structure possesses tensile strength (it contains Type IV collagen), it serves also to resist stretching of these capillaries by the unusually high pressure (for a capillary) of the blood within them. The important role of the basement membrane in filtration will be dealt with below.

Turnover of Basement Membrane Substance. It was found by giving experimental animals silver salts that became deposited in their glomerular basement membranes that new basement membrane substance became added to the epithelial side of the membrane so as to

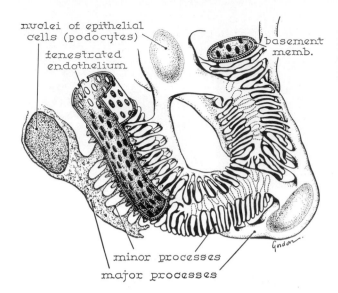

nuclei of epithelial cells (podocytes)

fenestrated endothelium

basement memb.

minor processes

major processes

Fig. 24-8. Schematic diagram illustrating in three dimensions part of a capillary loop of a glomerulus, with its covering of podocytes and its fenestrated endothelium. A portion of a podocyte and part of a capillary have been cut away to show the components of the filtration barrier. (After Pease, D. C.: J. Histochem., *3:*295, 1955)

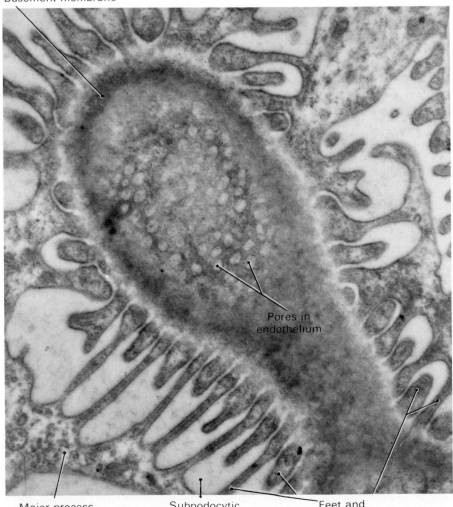

Basement membrane

Pores in endothelium

Major process of podocyte

Subpodocytic space

Feet and minor processes of podocyte

Fig. 24-9. Electron micrograph (×30,000) of a tangential section through a glomerular capillary, showing the pores in the endothelium and the interdigitating processes and feet of podocytes. (Pease, D. C.: J. Histochem., *3:*295, 1955)

Color Plate
24–1

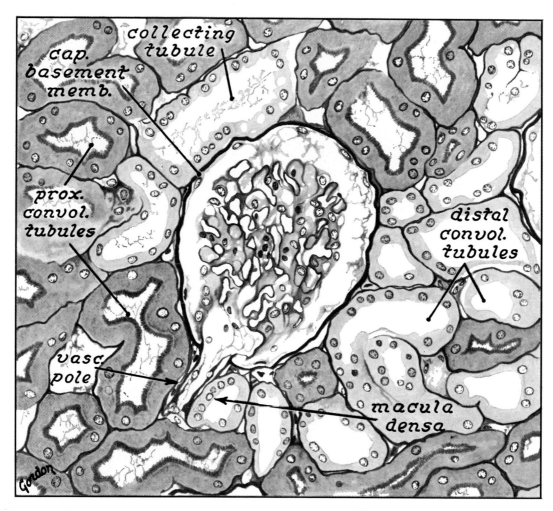

Plate 24-1. Illustration of cortex of human kidney stained with PAS and hematoxylin. Note the PAS-positive brush borders of the proximal convoluted tubules, and that the cytoplasm of the cells of these tubules stains more deeply than that of cells of the distal convoluted or collecting tubules. Note the PAS-positive basement membranes that surround the tubules. Basement membrane is also present under both the visceral and the parietal layers of Bowman's capsule. The numerous capillaries that lie between adjacent tubules are collapsed and hence not seen in this preparation. (The vascular pole of the glomerulus is cut obliquely and is not as prominent as it would be in a less oblique section.)

cover the surface on which the salts were deposited. Hence it seems probable that the epithelial cells are active in forming new basement membrane material throughout life.

If new material is continuously added to the exterior of the basement membrane by the epithelial cells, it seems reasonable to assume that equal amounts are lost from its inner surface to prevent it becoming unduly thick. Mesangial cells, where present, probably aid in disposing of the inner part of the basement membrane and removing accumulations of debris or old altered membrane by phagocytosis. Thus there is probably a maintenance mechanism operating here similar to that seen in appositional growth of bone, with formation of new layers on one surface and removal of old layers from the other surface. Indeed, Walker has shown that new basement membrane is formed continuously on the epithelial side of the membrane and that in the rat the basement membrane is thus replaced every year.

The Epithelial Cells of the Visceral Layer of Bowman's Capsule (the Glomerular Epithelium) — Podocytes

Although several histologists studying the kidney over the years with the LM suggested that the epithelial cells comprising the visceral layer of Bowman's capsule were unusual in form, with many processes attached to the glomerular basement membranes, not much attention was paid to their views, and there was a general belief that these cells were typically squamous in shape and that they formed a continuous covering over the capillaries. With the EM, however, it became evident that this view was incorrect on both counts, for the cells are not squamous in type nor do they provide a continuous covering for the capillaries. Indeed, they have a most unusual form and, because they have feet, are termed *podocytes* (Gr. *podos,* foot) (*see* Figs. 24-8 and 24-9).

The main *cell body* of a podocyte (which contains its nucleus) is separated from the capillary over which it lies by what was originally termed the *subpodocytic space* (Fig. 24-9); it is, of course, filled with glomerular filtrate. Numerous arms of cytoplasm, which we shall call *major processes,* extend from the cell body (Figs. 24-8 and 24-9). These run roughly parallel with the long axis or circumference of the capillary (Fig. 24-8) and for the most part are also separated from the capillary by spaces (Figs. 24-8 and 24-9). The spaces are also filled with glomerular filtrate and are continuous with the *glomerular space* proper (as in Fig. 24-10). From the major processes, delicate minor processes extend in orderly array to the capillary; these are labeled in Figures 24-8 and 24-9. The minor processes terminate in *feet* (labeled in Fig. 24-9 and seen to advantage in Figs. 24-8 and 24-10, pf). The soles of the feet are firmly planted on the lamina rara ex-

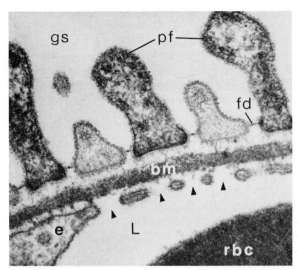

Fig. 24-10. Electron micrograph (×60,000) of the glomerular filtration barrier. This is a portion of a glomerulus of rat kidney fixed with glutaraldehyde containing tannic acid. The white space at the bottom of the micrograph (L) is the lumen of a glomerular capillary containing an erythrocyte (rbc). From the lumen of such a capillary, plasma would pass through the pores (indicated by arrowheads) of the fenestrated endothelium (e) and then through the glomerular basement membrane. This is a thick structure comprising a lamina densa (the dark layer indicated by bm) and a lamina rara on each side of it. Note that the lamina rara portions are characterized by showing much lighter, fuzzy staining, and that their outer limits are indistinct. Lodged on the lamina rara externa is a row of podocyte feet (pf), between which filtration slit diaphragms (fd) are seen to extend across the filtration slits. Each slit diaphragm shows a central dense spot. The glomerular filtrate, after passing through the basement membrane, filters through the slit diaphragms and enters the glomerular space (gs) in the upper part of the micrograph. (Tisher, C. C.: Anatomy of the kidney. *In* Brenner, B. M., and Rector, F. C. (eds.): The Kidney. vol. 1. Philadelphia, W. B. Saunders, 1976)

terna of the basement membrane of the capillary (Fig. 24-10) and follow its curvature (Figs 24-8 and 24-9). The minor processes and feet that interdigitate with one another many be derived from two or more major processes of the same podocyte or from major processes of two or more podocytes (Fig. 24-8). There is some evidence that a given podocyte is able to send processes to two capillaries but generally they supply only one.

As may be seen in Figures 24-8, 24-9, and particularly 24-10, the interdigitating feet do not come into contact with each other; there are always slits between them. These are about 20 to 30 nm. wide and are termed *filtration slits.* With special fixation, such as that used in obtaining the micrograph shown in Figure 24-10, it can be seen that every filtration slit is spanned by a shelf-like filtration *slit diaphragm,* 5 to 7 nm. thick, that extends across the potential gap between podocyte feet, much as a diaphragm closes over a fenestra in the usual kind of fenestrated capillary found in sites other than the kidneys. This filtration slit diaphragm (fd in Fig. 24-10) has a central dense spot (visible in Fig. 24-10) that represents an axial thickening extending along the middle of the slit membrane midway between the podocyte feet on either side.

The Respective Roles of the Three Layers of the Filtration Barrier of the Glomerulus

Since the glomerular endothelium is fenestrated and its pores are up to 100 nm. in diameter (Figs. 24-9 and 24-10), with few (if any) of these pores being closed over with diaphragms, the endothelial component of the barrier would be unable to hold back anything smaller than blood cells and platelets. Hence it acts as a sieve for large particulate components (larger than 100 nm. in diameter) and serves as a prefilter. So we must look to the basement membrane and/or the filtration slit membrane between the podocyte feet lodged on the basement membrane for permeability characteristics that would allow them to hold back macromolecular substances such as proteins in the plasma.

How Pore Sizes in the Glomerular Filtration Barrier and Other Factors Involved in Filtration Were Investigated. The size of protein molecules is reflected by their molecular weights. Therefore, one way of investigating the permeability characteristics of the glomerular filter would be to inject proteins of various molecular weights into the bloodstream of experimental animals and then determine with the EM whether they were held back by the glomerular filter and, if so, the site where this occurred. However, to do this the proteins would have to be recognizable in the EM. Ferritin is one substance that can be used for this purpose because it is a protein combined with iron. It has a molecular weight of around 480,000 and a molecular diameter of 12.2 nm. Studies with it showed that it is arrested by the basement membrane. But the molecular weights of the proteins in the blood plasma are for the most part considerably smaller than that of ferritin. For example, albumin has a molecular weight of 69,000 while the immunoglobulins have molecular weights around 160,000, with the macroglobulins having a molecular weight of 930,000.

Graham and Karnovsky employed a histochemical method by which they could observe in the EM how far two different peroxidases (one of higher and the other of lower molecular weight) penetrated the filtration barrier. Whereas the one of molecular weight 40,000 seemed capable of passing through all three layers of the barrier to reach the urinary spaces, the one with a molecular weight of 160,000 after passing through the endothelium and basement membrane was held up at the slit diaphragms. This showed first that there is no effective barrier to the passage of a protein of relatively low molecular weight (40,000 or less) and second that the slit diaphragm can filter out a protein with a molecular weight of 160,000. It had already been established by using ferritin that the basement membrane itself acts as a barrier to the passage of proteins of high molecular weight.

When the passage of catalase, an enzyme with a molecular weight of 240,000 was investigated using a modification of the same histochemical method, it was found that it too penetrated

the basement membrane but was held up at the slit diaphragms. Lower concentrations of the peroxidase of molecular weight 40,000 were also investigated in this study (Venkatachalam et al.); it was found under these conditions that although the protein permeated the full thickness of the basement membrane, there were gradients of staining, suggesting that a limited amount of filtration might have been taking place.

The results of these tracer studies indicate that the basement membrane has the property of restraining the passage of macromolecular substances over a considerable range of molecular weights, with its filtering effect increasing in relation to *molecular size,* and that the slit diaphragms achieve filtration of the macromolecules of slightly smaller size range that are not filtered out by the basement membrane. The peroxidase that has molecules small enough to pass through the basement membrane has an effective molecular diameter of 6 nm., whereas the peroxidase with molecules large enough to be retained by the slit diaphragms has an effective molecular diameter of 9 nm. Hence it would seem that the pore size of the slit diaphragms is somewhere in the neighborhood of 6 to 9 nm. However, the precise size limits of the molecules that can pass both effective barriers of the glomerular filter (the basement membrane and the slit diaphragms) have been difficult to establish. Certainly at least a little protein from blood plasma passes the filter under normal conditions, and so it remained uncertain as to where the very important plasma protein albumin, with a molecular weight of 69,000 and which passes into the urine so commonly in kidney disease, is normally held back by the filter.

Before reading further it should be realized that in the above-described experiments tissue would be removed and fixed in the standard way suitable for electron microscopy.

Next, the finding and breeding of a mutant strain of rats (the Munich-Wistar strain, already mentioned), in which there are glomeruli exposed on the kidney surface, not only enabled direct measurements to be made on blood flow in glomerular capillaries and facilitated elucidation of factors affecting it, but also permitted almost instantaneous fixation of glomeruli in experiments. This could be accomplished, for example, by dropping some gluteraldehyde on functioning glomeruli in living animals. Ryan et al. took advantage of this to study the permeability of the glomerular filter to certain macromolecules that could subsequently be detected with the EM. The first important observation made was that the degree to which macromolecular tracers employed in previous experiments penetrated the barrier was not the same as in these earlier experiments in which instantaneous fixation was not feasible. It would, therefore, appear that a good deal of the penetration of the glomerular filter by macromolecules of various molecular weights previously observed could have occurred in the tissue after circulation ceased and before fixative penetrated the specimen. Next, other experiments indicated that the glomerular barrier constitutes a much more effective barrier with the glomerular circulation functioning normally, which suggests that the *effectiveness* of the barrier would depend on *blood flowing along its inner surface* in the proper fashion.

Next, as already mentioned, the albumin molecule has a molecular weight of 69,000; its effective molecular diameter is 7.1 nm. Blatt et al. found that in the absence of other proteins of greater molecular weight, albumin molecules pass readily through a filter with a pore size of 11 nm. They showed moreover that mixing albumin with larger protein molecules dramatically decreased the passage of albumin molecules through such a filter. This observation, of course, suggests the possibility that whereas albumin macromolecules are small enough to be able to pass through the glomerular filtration barrier, that in health, and with the normal flow of blood through glomerular capillaries, the openings through which it might otherwise pass would be hidden by macromolecules of larger size present in the plasma. A rough conclusion would be that under conditions of a normal circulation the pores that might permit albumin to pass are occupied, as it were, by larger macromolecules.

Another factor that seems to be involved besides *size* with regard to macromolecules passing through the filter is the *electrostatic charge* they carry. Albumin, for example, is polyanionic and hence could be held up by negative charges in the filter through which it might otherwise pass. Ryan et al. point out that negative charges would be associated in particular with the cell coat covering the foot processes and slit diaphragms of the epithelial portion of the filtration barrier.

Summary. From all the foregoing it is apparent that the permeability characteristics of the glomerular barrier depend first on its being a part of a functioning glomerulus. Next, there seem to be several factors besides pore size that determine whether any given kind of macromolecule will pass through it, such as (*1*) whether this particular type of macromolecule is associated with larger ones and (*2*) the numbers and kinds of electrostatic charges this kind of macromolecule carries.

Antigen-Antibody Complexes. A question that might come to mind would be why the glomerular filters would not become permanently plugged or otherwise damaged by straining out macromolecules and other particulates too large to pass through them. In connection with this it should be mentioned that antigen-antibody complexes that form in other parts of the bloodstream or gain entrance to it may be filtered out by the glomerular filter and form irregular deposits underneath the podocyte feet where the latter are lodged on the basement membrane. It is important to realize that it is uncommon for the antibody component of these complexes to be directed against any component of the basement membrane itself. Usually complexes formed elsewhere are merely trapped here as they attempt, as it were, to pass through the filter. However, such antigen-antibody complexes may activate the complement system which can then attract polymorphs to the site. The lysosomal activity of these can damage the glomerulus. (It should be mentioned also that there is a less common type of damage to glomeruli due to antibodies directed against antigens of the basement membrane itself; this is therefore of the nature of an autoimmune reaction. The complement system can be activated by this type of reaction also, with resulting inflammatory disease.)

THE PROXIMAL CONVOLUTED TUBULE

The *proximal convoluted tubule* is about 14 mm. in length and has an overall diameter of about 60 μm. The initial part of it, which leads from the glomerulus, is suf-

ficiently narrow and straight in some species to constitute a neck for the tubule. But in man this portion differs little from the remainder of the proximal tubule. Proximal convoluted tubules pursue looped and tortuous courses in the immediate vicinity of the renal corpuscles from which they originate (Fig. 24-1). They then enter medullary rays (Fig. 24-2) and descend in these as the upper thick parts of descending limbs of loops of Henle. The descending limbs enter the medulla and extend into it for different distances before looping back as ascending limbs (Fig. 24-2). The character of the proximal convoluted tubule does not change much as it becomes the first part of the descending loop of Henle. Only where it becomes thin will its character and functions change. Hence, the thick segment of the descending loop of Henle, though straight, has the same character and presumably performs the same functions as the convoluted part of the tubule proper, and so should be considered part of the proximal tubule.

Some Aids to Recognizing and Studying Proximal Convoluted Tubules With the LM

These may be itemized as follows. (*1*) For the most part, proximal tubules are seen in sections of cortex as oblique cuts through curved tubes (Plate 24-1). (*2*) Oblique and cross sections of proximal convoluted tubules are the most common component visible in a section of kidney cortex (Plate 24-1), and indeed they are the only component seen between the outermost glomeruli and the capsule of the kidney. (*3*) The cells of proximal convoluted tubules become altered very rapidly as a result of postmortem degeneration. However, even if fixation has not been prompt, their cytoplasm is generally more acidophilic and more granular than that of the other kinds of tubules. Accordingly, proximal convoluted tubules are not only the most numerous tubules seen in kidney cortex, but also the pinkest (Plate 24-1). (*4*) Finally on their free surface, the cells of proximal tubules have a striated border (Plate 24-1).

The Epithelial Cells of Proximal Convoluted Tubules. These are broader at their base where they lie against a basement membrane than at their free margins abutting on the lumen. In good preparations a *striated border* can be seen on the free surface of each cell (Plate 24-1). The boundaries between adjacent cells cannot be seen to advantage because they interdigitate extensively. In tissue fixed immediately after death and suitably stained, the appearance of proximal convoluted tubules varies between two extremes. At one extreme the epithelium is low and the lumen wide and round; at the other, the epithelium is high and the lumen small and triangular. These extreme appearances (as well as intermediate ones) are attributable to two factors: (*1*) the state of functional activity of the epithelial cells of the tubule, and (*2*) the degree to

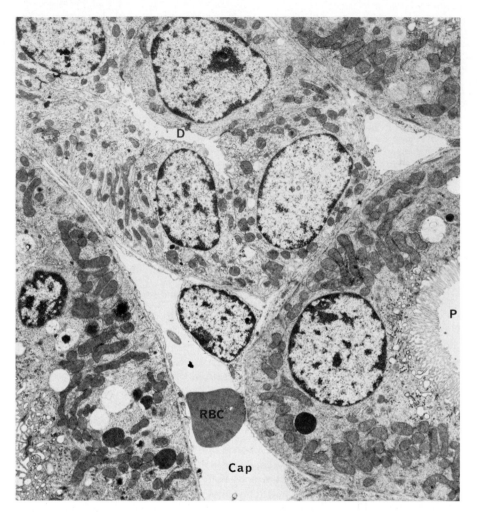

Fig. 24-11. Electron micrograph (×7,100) of cortex of kidney (rat). At *top left* is a distal tubule (D) with a narrow lumen. Portions of several proximal tubules (P) are also seen, particularly at *bottom right*. Capillaries (Cap) are present in the spaces between the tubules. Note the microvilli lining the proximal tubule at *right*, just below *middle*, and the abundant mitochondria in the more basal parts of the cells. (Courtesy of E. Rau)

which the lumen of the tubule was distended by glomerular filtrate; the latter is affected by whether the glomerulus of the nephron was producing much or little filtrate. It is believed that a low epithelium and wide round lumen are associated with production of much filtrate.

The nucleus in cells of proximal convoluted tubules is disposed toward the base of the cell.

Proximal convoluted tubules are ensheathed in a substantial basement membrane, which is beautifully demonstrated by the PAS technic (Plate 24-1).

The cell surface that faces the lumen is covered with thin microvilli about 1 μm. long and in many respects similar to those of the lining cells of the small intestine (Fig. 24-11, *right,* just below *middle*); these, of course, account for the striated border seen with the LM in Plate 24-1. They are associated with so much cell coat material that the border is PAS-positive (Plate 24-1). The microvilli are very numerous and increase the surface greatly, so

that the total surface area available in the proximal tubules of both kidneys is enormous.

Mechanisms of Resorption

The Resorption of Sodium and Water. The proximal convoluted tubules resorb 85 per cent or so of the water and sodium that pass along them. This is due to the action of two kinds of sodium pumps (one kind, the sodium-potassium pump, was described on p. 111) that are particularly active along the lateral regions of the cell membrane. These drive sodium ions out into the intercellular spaces around the sides and bases of the epithelial cells. The sodium ions pumped out into these spaces accumulate in the tissue fluid there and, together with chloride ions that follow them passively, draw water osmotically from the cytoplasm of the epithelial cells, mainly from their basal parts. But this water does not accumulate in the intercellular spaces because it passes continuously into the capillaries that form an extensive network in this region. Thus the remarkable degrees of resorption of sodium ions and water occurring in this portion of the nephron are both attributable to the action of the sodium pumps.

The operation of the sodium pumps requires expenditure of energy. It is therefore not surprising to find the mitochondria are long and abundant in the cytoplasm at the base of these cells (Fig. 24-12). To provide abundant cell membrane for effective pumping there are also what seem to be numerous infoldings of the cell membrane into the base of these cells (Fig 24-12). However, much of this infolding is due to the cell membranes at the *lateral* borders of adjacent cells (in both proximal and distal tubules) interdigitating in complex fashion so that the sides of these cells are thrown into many ridges and grooves. Moreover, near the base of the cells, the infoldings of the lateral and basal membranes split the basal aspect of these cells up further into root-like *basal processes*. These are so extensive that the basal processes of contiguous cells may interdigitate to some extent. Hence, a basal process that in a section might seem to belong to the cell whose cytoplasm surrounds it may actually belong to a contiguous cell.

The Resorption of Glucose and Amino Acids. Active transport mechanisms, which are fully dealt with in biochemistry textbooks, operate in the cells to resorb many useful substances. However, the resorption of protein involves histological considerations and so will now be described.

The Resorption of Proteins. A not inconsiderable amount of plasma protein leaks through the glomeruli every 24 hours, and this is normally resorbed by the proximal convoluted tubule. Protein is absorbed at the free surface by pinocytosis (that is, by means of little membranous vesicles containing protein being pinched off from the cell membrane between microvilli). The protein-filled vesicles pass into the cytoplasm where they fuse with lysosomes. The enzymes of the lysosomes digest the protein and the products of digestion (amino acids) are freed in the cytoplasm.

Excretory Role

The cells of the proximal convoluted tubules also perform certain *excretory* functions. Among the various substances excreted here are certain metabolites, dyes, and drugs, including penicillin.

THE LOOP OF HENLE

Although glucose and amino acids, and also calcium, phosphate, and some other ions, are resorbed in the proximal tubule, so much water and sodium are resorbed in approximately the

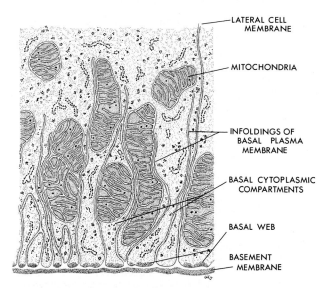

LATERAL CELL MEMBRANE

MITOCHONDRIA

INFOLDINGS OF BASAL PLASMA MEMBRANE

BASAL CYTOPLASMIC COMPARTMENTS

BASAL WEB

BASEMENT MEMBRANE

Fig. 24-12. Drawing illustrating the basal portion of the cells of a proximal convoluted tubule as seen in the EM. (Courtesy of E. Rau)

same proportions that the fluid remaining to enter the thin descending limb of the loop of Henle has approximately the same osmotic pressure as the glomerular filtrate entering the proximal tubule. In other words, the fluid in the proximal tubule remains isosmotic (*isotonic*) with blood plasma. Although the total volume of fluid that enters descending limbs of loops of Henle is only about 15 per cent of that of the glomerular filtrate, it still would constitute an enormous amount of urine unless it were reduced further as follows.

Mechanisms Involved in Concentrating Urine. Many years ago Crane observed that only animals with a loop of Henle in their nephrons excrete urine that is hypertonic to blood. It was at first incorrectly thought that water might be resorbed along the course of the loops, with the result that sodium and chloride would become more concentrated as the fluid passed along them; hence the fluid delivered into distal convoluted tubules would be expected to be hypertonic. But it was found that the fluid entering the distal convoluted tubule has an even *lower* osmotic pressure than that leaving the proximal tubules.

Before describing what really happens in the loop of Henle, we shall deal briefly with what happens in the distal convoluted tubule and the collecting tubules. As fluid passes along the distal convoluted tubule, more water than salt is resorbed from its contents, and so in this tubule the fluid once more becomes *isotonic*. The resorption of fluid in the distal convoluted tubules (and collecting tubules) is regulated by the *antidiuretic hormone* (ADH) secreted by the posterior lobe of the pituitary. If the pituitary gland is removed, this resorption does not occur and great quantities of dilute urine are passed. This will be explained in connection with diabetes insipidus in the next chapter.

Since the fluid normally becomes isotonic again in the distal convoluted tubule, the concentration of urine that results in its finally becoming *hypertonic* must occur as the fluid passes along the collecting tubules. In order to account for this, we now have to consider what happens in the loops of Henle, for what happens in the loops of Henle is indirectly responsible for what happens in the collecting tubules.

The role of the loops of Henle is to *create a hypertonic environment* in the tissue fluid that surrounds them, so that the collecting tubules that pass through the same environment (consult Fig. 24-2) will have water drawn out of them into the tissue fluid surrounding them. This extra water in due course passes into the capillaries and so is taken back into the circulation. It is easiest to describe what happens in the loops of Henle if we begin with what happens as fluid passes back up the ascending limb of the loop.

The lining cells of the ascending loops allow sodium to pass from the fluid in the lumen out into the tissue fluid in which they and the descending loops are bathed. Moreover, the walls of the ascending loops hold back water in the lumen. As a consequence, the fluid contained in the ascending loops, since it is losing sodium (and with it chloride), becomes increasingly *hypotonic* as it ascends toward the distal convoluted tubule; hence, the fluid delivered into the distal convoluted tubules is hypotonic. However, what happens in the ascending tubule has another and more important effect, as follows.

As a result of the ascending limb of the loop of Henle contributing sodium to the tissue fluid, but at the same time holding back water, the *tissue fluid in the surrounding region becomes hypertonic.* The walls of the thin descending limbs of the loops of Henle, unlike those of the ascending limbs, do let water pass from their lumina out into the tissue fluid. Accordingly, the extra sodium chloride in this tissue fluid withdraws water from the fluid in the descending limb of the loop of Henle and as a result the fluid in the descending limb of the loop becomes increasingly hypertonic as it approaches and reaches the bottom of the loop. But, as already noted, as the fluid begins once more to ascend, the cells of the tubule pump out sodium, and so the fluid first becomes isotonic and then, as it reaches the distal convoluted tubule, it becomes hypotonic.

The whole purpose of these elaborate activities in the thin loops of Henle, and in particular in loops of nephrons beginning at juxtamedullary glomeruli (whose loops descend deep toward the apex of a medullary pyramid), is to render the tissue fluid surrounding them in the part of the medullary pyramid toward its apex more salty (hypertonic). Since the collecting tubules pass through this same hypertonic environment (*see* Fig. 24-2), the hypertonic tissue fluid draws water osmotically from the previously isotonic fluid in the lumina of the collecting tubules, with the result that by the time the fluid in the collecting tubules has passed down through this hypertonic region, it, too *has become hypertonic.* Hence the urine delivered into the pelvis of the kidney by the collecting tubules is hypertonic. The *antidiuretic hormone,* as well as acting on distal convoluted tubules controls the permeability of the cells of collecting tubules, and hence influences the extent to which they permit the hypertonic tissue fluid to draw water through their walls into the tissue fluid.

All the capillary loops present in this area contain blood that has passed through glomeruli (Fig. 24-15). As blood passes along capillaries (Fig. 24-15) toward the tip of the pyramid it gains sodium but as it passes up again toward the cortex it loses sodium, thus more or less duplicating what happens in the descending and ascending arms of the loop of Henle.

A more precise and detailed account of the *countercurrent mechanism* will be found in textbooks of physiology; what we have explained here is intended to provide some background that may be of assistance later in assimilating more detailed physiological information.

The Microscopic Appearance of Loops of Henle. The loops are either short or long. The majority of nephrons

extending from glomeruli in the outer part of the cortex have short loops that do not extend for any great distance into the medulla; perhaps the reason is that they were the last nephrons to develop, and their loops had to accommodate themselves to such space as was available. The nephrons that arise from glomeruli near the medulla, the *juxtamedullary glomeruli,* have long loops that extend well down toward the apex of the medulla (Fig. 24-2).

The first part of the descending loop is the straight continuation of the proximal convoluted tubule (Fig. 24-1). As it passes down into the medulla its lumen rather abruptly becomes narrower, and the cells of its walls squamous (Figs. 7-4 and 24-2). The tubule from here on is known as the *thin segment of the descending limb of the loop of Henle.* The thin segments of nephrons that arise from juxtamedullary glomeruli are much longer than those that arise from glomeruli in the outer part of the cortex (Fig. 24-2).

The appearance of a thin loop of Henle is so similar to that of a large capillary the student may find it difficult to distinguish these tubules in the medulla from the capillaries that run between them (Fig. 24-13). The tubules are wider than capillaries, but they may be partly collapsed. The nuclei of the squamous cells of the tubules are somewhat closer together than the nuclei of the endothelial cells of capillaries. The presence of red blood cells in the capillaries may also be helpful for identifying them, but artifact can lead to red blood cells being present in the tubules to compound confusion.

In the instance of long loops, the first portion of the ascending limb may be similar to the thin portion of the descending limb. But this soon gives way, in the ascending limb, to a wider tubule with thicker walls; this is known as the *thick segment of the ascending limb of the loop of Henle* (Fig. 24-13B). The character of the thick segment is very similar to that of the distal convoluted tubule, next to be described. In the instance of nephrons with short loops of Henle, the epithelium may change from the thin squamous type to the thick type even before the nephron has looped back to begin its ascending arm.

Munkacsi and Palkovits provided evidence that the ability of animals to live in a desert environment is related to the degree to which their juxtamedullary nephrons, with long thin loops of Henle, are developed. The better developed they are (and they are well developed in desert rats), the more able they are to conserve water.

THE DISTAL CONVOLUTED TUBULE

The thick segment of the ascending loop of Henle, as noted, returns to the root of the glomerulus from which the nephron takes origin, and there the part of its wall which comes into contact with the glomerular root becomes heavily nucleated and forms a thick spot, the *macula densa* (Fig. 24-5 and Plate 24-1).

Some authorities define the *distal convoluted tubule* as only that part of the nephron extending from the macula densa to a collecting tubule. However, most classify the thick ascending arm of the loop of Henle as part of it. Distal convoluted tubules differ from proximal convoluted ones in several respects, as follows.

(*1*) They are not as long; hence, cross and oblique sections of them are not as commonly seen in a section of kidney cortex (Plate 24-1).

(*2*) Their diameters are generally not quite as big, but since the cells of their walls are commonly lower, their lumina tend to be larger (Plate 24-1).

(*3*) The cells of their walls are smaller; hence a cross section through a distal tubule reveals many more nuclei than one of a proximal convoluted tubule (Plate 24-1).

(*4*) The cells of their walls have no striated border on their free surfaces, and their cytoplasm is not nearly so acidophilic (Plate 24-1).

(*5*) Since the borders between contiguous cells do not interdigitate quite as extensively as those of cells of the proximal tubules, cell borders can be distinguished more clearly than in proximal tubules.

Like proximal convoluted tubules, the distal ones have a pronounced basement membrane encircling them (Plate 24-1).

Fine Structure and Relation to Function. The luminal surface bears a few microvilli (Fig. 24-11D). The basal part of the cell shows infoldings of the cell membrane that are even more highly developed than in cells of proximal convoluted tubules; these more or less divide this portion of the cytoplasm into basal processes containing large long mitochondria. Here also sodium passes out of the tubular cells into the tissue fluid. As already noted, the withdrawal of water from the tubule is regulated by the antidiuretic hormone of the posterior pituitary.

OTHER FEATURES OF THE KIDNEYS

Collecting Tubules. These are not parts of nephrons, even though they too absorb water under the influence of the antidiuretic hormone. They comprise a system of drainage ducts into which urine is delivered by distal convoluted tubules; this is conducted to medullary papillae, where it is emptied into the calyces of the ureter (Figs. 24-1 and 24-2).

Collecting tubules form a branched system. The largest are known as *ducts of Bellini*. These are easily seen in the apical part of a medullary pyramid, where they empty through its papilla. They are large ducts with wide lumina and thick walls composed of pale-staining, high columnar

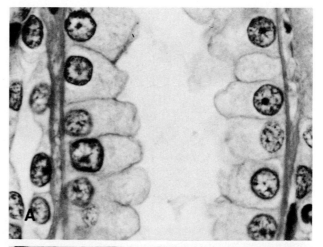

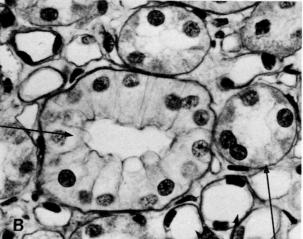

Fig. 24-13. (*A*) Photomicrograph of a portion of a collecting tubule from medulla of monkey kidney in longitudinal section. To the left of the collecting tubule there is a thin portion of a loop of Henle. (*B*) Cross-sectional view of a collecting tubule (long arrow at *middle left*), from medulla of dog kidney. Note also the thin- and thick-walled portions of loops of Henle (both parts of the loop are indicated by the arrows at *bottom right*).

cells. In contrast with the cells of the walls of tubules of nephrons, the borders between the cells of ducts of Bellini and smaller collecting tubules emptying into them are distinct in ordinary sections. The pale-staining cytoplasm of these cells is illustrated in Figure 24-13. With the EM, the cells of collecting tubules show only moderately deep infoldings of the cell membrane at their base.

In the medulla the ducts of Bellini branch at very acute angles (Fig. 24-2). Several generations of branches arise to provide enough collecting ducts to supply each medullary ray. In the rays the ducts give off side branches. There each pursues a short arched course before becoming continuous with the termination of a distal convoluted tubule (Fig. 24-1).

Although each nephron is provided with an individual collecting tubule, several of these initial arched tubules empty into a single straight collecting tubule. Hence there are not nearly as many straight collecting tubules as nephrons in the kidney.

Casts. When used with regard to kidneys, the term *cast* means impacted cellular debris or coagulated protein in the lumina of the more distal parts of nephrons and collecting tubules. Casts are not seen in the strictly normal kidney. But material obtained at autopsy and used for teaching histology may not always be perfectly normal, so casts are sometimes seen in the lumina of kidney tubules.

The Connective Tissue Component of the Kidneys. Each kidney is covered with a thin translucent *capsule* of fibrous connective tissue; the intercellular substance in it is chiefly collagen, but a few elastic fibers may be present. In health the capsule is smooth and glistening and at autopsy can be stripped easily from the cortex. In certain kinds of kidney disease, fibrous connective tissue forms in the parenchyma of the cortex and extends out to the capsule to bind it firmly to the organ. Under these conditions the capsule cannot be stripped readily from the organ, and this is noted at autopsy as an indication that the kidney has become diseased.

The basement membranes that surround the tubules are supported on their outer surface by delicate reticular fibers. More substantial connective tissue fibers are found in association with the larger vessels of the kidney. But, all in all, the fibrous connective tissue of the kidney parenchyma (except between the ducts of Bellini in the papilla, where there is some connective tissue) is extraordinarily scanty. Increased fibrous tissue in the kidney is a manifestation of past disease and in itself can interfere with function by impeding diffusion.

THE CIRCULATION OF BLOOD THROUGH THE KIDNEY

Each kidney is supplied by a *renal artery*. These are large vessels that arise from the aorta, so each kidney receives large amounts of blood. The renal artery divides close to the hilus into two large branches. From these branches five end arteries originate; these are called *segmental arteries* and each supplies a particular part of the kidney. From the five segmental arteries further branches arise that ascend toward the cortex as *interlobar arteries* (Fig. 24-14).

Arcuate Arteries. Some of the interlobar arteries divide into main branches as they ascend in the columns of Bertin, but most of them do so only when they have almost reached the corticomedullary border. Here their branches

are given off at wide angles and in all directions, but more or less in the same plane. These main branches of the interlobar arteries arch over the bases of the medullary pyramids and so are called *arcuate* (L. *arcuatus,* arched) *arteries* (Fig. 24-14). Just as there is no continuity between the branches of adjacent trees, there is no continuity between the arcuate arteries that arise from adjacent interlobar arteries. In other words, there are no anastomoses between interlobar arteries through arcuate arteries (Fig. 24-14). Accordingly, if an interlobar artery becomes plugged with a thrombus, a pyramidal-shaped segment of kidney tissue dies (the area supplied by the arcuate arteries from that particular interlobar artery); such an area of dead tissue is called an *infarct.*

Interlobular Arteries. The arcuate arteries give off branches that ascend into the cortex (Fig. 24-14). These vessels run *between lobules* and so are termed *interlobular arteries.* They mark the boundaries between lobules and therefore alternate with the medullary rays that form the central cores of lobules (Fig. 24-4).

The interlobular arteries give off branches at wide angles on every side. Since these immediately *enter* the substance of surrounding lobules (the cortical labyrinth), they are called *intralobular arteries* (Fig. 24-15). These give rise to the afferent vessels of glomeruli. However, the terminal branches of the interlobular arteries continue on to the capsule to supply its capillary bed.

How the Capillary Beds of the Cortex and Medulla Are Supplied. The efferent arterioles of glomeruli in different parts of the cortex deliver blood into different capillary beds. As may be seen in Figure 24-15, which is based on the study of Morison, the efferent arterioles from glomeruli in the outer part of the cortex (Fig. 24-15) empty their blood into the capillary beds that surround the proximal and distal convoluted tubules in the cortex. Those from glomeruli somewhat deeper in the cortex contribute to the capillary bed of the cortex but also to long straight capillary-like vessels that descend into the medulla and are called *false straight arterioles (arteriole rectae spuriae)* for reasons that will become obvious later. The efferent vessels from the deepest glomeruli in the cortex, some of which are below the level of the arcuate arteries, deliver most or all of their blood into the arteriolae rectae spuriae (Fig. 24-15).

The return of blood from the capillary beds of the cortex and medulla is illustrated on the right side of Figure 24-15. In general, the veins correspond to the arteries already described. It is to be noted that at the surface of the kidney little veins arise from the capillary beds of the capsule and the superficial part of the cortex to pass in converging fashion to *interlobular veins.* Since these end branches radiate out in star-like fashion from the ends of the interlobular veins, they are called *stellate veins* (Fig. 24-15).

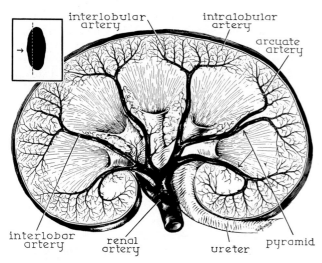

Fig. 24-14. Schematic diagram illustrating the arterial supply of the kidney, simplified for clarity.

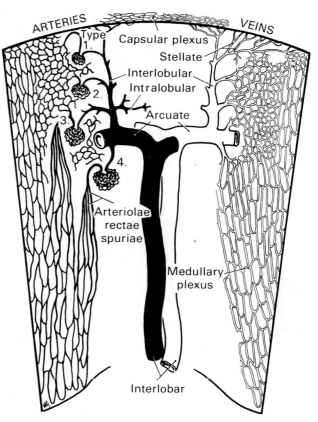

Fig. 24-15. Schematic diagram illustrating the blood supply to the capillary beds of the cortex and medulla. (After Morison, D. M.: Am. J. Anat., *37*:53, 1926)

Since the arteriole rectae spuriae, which supply the capillary beds of the medulla, are all supplied by the efferent vessels of glomeruli in the deeper part of the cortex (Fig. 24-15), it follows that all the blood delivered into the capillary beds of the medulla, like that delivered into those of the cortex, has just passed through glomeruli. However, this concept has been contested from time to time. It has been claimed by some that arterioles arise directly from the arcuate and interlobular arteries to pass directly to the capillary beds of the medulla. To distinguish these from the false straight arterioles, they are called *true straight arterioles (arteriolae rectae verae)*. If these exist, it would mean the medulla is supplied with some blood that has not passed through glomeruli. However, most consider that there are not enough of these vessels to be of any functional significance and the general opinion is that for all practical purposes the blood in the capillary beds of the medulla has passed through glomeruli.

It is possible that a small amount of blood that has not passed through glomeruli may be delivered to the capillary beds of the cortex by means of branches of afferent arterioles known as *Ludwig's arterioles.*

The Two Circulatory Pathways in the Kidneys. During World War II, some individuals were partly buried by rubble when buildings collapsed from bombing. In some instances an individual whose legs had been crushed would, some days after the event, fail to excrete urine. Many injured in this fashion died after a short period of apparent recovery, not from their primary injuries, but from kidney failure. This condition, termed *crush syndrome,* led Trueta (a surgeon) to investigate how the route taken by blood through the kidney may be altered in what is generally termed *shock.*

To understand this the student should refer back to Figure 24-15. This shows that the efferent vessels of the glomeruli in the outer part of the cortex (labeled 1 and 2) empty into the capillary bed of the cortical labyrinth, whereas those of the glomeruli near the border of the medulla, which Trueta terms *juxtamedullary glomeruli* (labeled 3 and 4), empty almost entirely into the arteriolae rectae spuriae that supply the capillary beds of the medulla (the capillary beds of both the cortex and the medulla

are, of course, continuous) (Fig. 24-15). Furthermore, the juxtamedullary glomeruli are larger than those nearer the surface of the kidney and, as noted, the lumina of their efferent vessels may be larger than the lumina of their afferent vessels.

Trueta and his associates found that severe crush injuries of the limbs can cause a reflex spasm of certain blood vessels in the kidneys. The chief effect is on the peripheral two thirds of the interlobular arteries, which become constricted. Another factor that can have much the same effect as spasm of these vessels is a loss of plasma from the circulatory system, for the volume of fluid in the circulatory system is an important factor in keeping blood vessels open. Accordingly, it is easy to visualize that spasm in the smaller arterial vessels in the kidney and a lack of fluid in the circulatory system (as can occur in untreated shock) could result in the smaller arterioles becoming pinched off, and this could lead to impaired function or even death of kidney tissue. Since the greatest effect would be exerted on the smaller arterial vessels, the impairment of circulation would be greatest toward the periphery of the kidney. Conditions can arise, therefore, in which it is possible for blood to continue to circulate through the juxtamedullary glomeruli while ceasing to circulate through the glomeruli in the outer part of the kidney. Under these conditions the whole outer part of the cortex becomes relatively pale and bloodless. Thus, all the blood that circulates through the kidney passes through the more deeply disposed glomeruli (the juxtamedullary ones), and since the efferent vessels of these empty almost entirely into the arteriolae rectae spuriae, the blood from them is conducted to the capillary beds of the medulla rather than to those of the cortex; thus the proximal and distal convoluted tubules would have little or no blood supply. If severe, this causes renal failure, resulting in death.

THE LYMPHATICS OF THE KIDNEYS

Pierce found that the only lymphatics in the kidneys were those accompanying blood vessels, with the periarterial plexuses being richer in lymphatics than the perivenous ones. The lymphatics of the plexuses could be traced from the renal artery and vein along the interlobar, arcuate, and interlobular vessels to the capsule of the kidney, where they communicated with capsular lymphatics. However, they did not seem to extend into the parenchyma from these vessels. Valves were found in the larger lymphatics in the hilus of the kidney.

Rawson studied the lymphatics of a kidney invaded by cancer cells and used their presence for mapping out the lymphatics (cancer cells spread readily through lymphatics). In general, he found lymphatics in the sites described by Peirce; but he also found evidence of some lymphatic capillaries that began beneath the epithelium of the tip of the medullary pyramid and extended toward the base of the medullary pyramid, where they emptied into the lymphatics associated with the arcuate vessels. However, no lymphatics were found in the parenchyma of the cortex.

THE POSTNATAL DEVELOPMENT AND GROWTH OF NEPHRONS

Growth of the kidney in early postnatal life has been investigated more extensively in the rat than in any other species; hence, most of the information given here relates to studies in rats.

Only about one third of the glomeruli in the adult are present at birth. Glomeruli continue to be formed for 3 months or so after birth, but the majority are formed in the first 3 to 4 weeks.

The first-formed glomeruli are in the region close to the medulla; many of these undergo *physiological atrophy* and disappear (Hartroft). However, in some instances their afferent and efferent vessels may remain and fuse to constitute a few arteriolae rectae verae. The oldest glomeruli, which are also the largest, lie near the arcuate vessels. At birth, the outer part of the cortex of the kidney is undifferentiated, and it is here that new nephrons and their renal corpuscles are formed after birth. The tubule of each new nephron then becomes connected to the duct

system. The youngest nephrons are those situated in the outer cortex immediately beneath the capsule, and these do not become fully differentiated until about 3 months after birth. The glomeruli of these nephrons are the smallest in the kidney. The renal corpuscle develops more or less as a unit and not by capillaries invaginating the blind end of a previously formed tubule. In the renal cortex a clump of cells is associated with the end of a developing tubule. Some of these cells become the parietal and visceral epithelial cells of Bowman's capsule, and others become endothelial cells. The capillaries so formed later connect with the vascular system.

The size of the kidneys in postnatal life is affected both by diet and hormones. High protein diets make the kidneys become larger. Injections of male sex hormone also make the kidneys of experimental animals become larger. The increase in size that occurs with high protein diets or male hormone treatment is brought about by nephrons increasing in size and not in number.

If one kidney is removed from an adult animal, the remaining kidney becomes larger. The increase in size is due to the nephrons becoming larger (*compensatory hypertrophy*) and not more numerous. However, in individual nephrons there is an increase in the number of cells of which they are composed, and mitotic figures can be seen in the nephrons of the remaining kidney for a period following the removal of the other. The kidneys also become larger during pregnancy; this is termed *physiological hypertrophy,* and mitotic figures have been found in the nephrons as they enlarge in this condition.

THE URETER

The wall of the ureter has three coats: (*1*) a mucous membrane, (*2*) a muscle coat, and (*3*) a fibroelastic adventitia.

Mucous Membrane. This consists of only two layers, an epithelial lining and a lamina propria. The *epithelium* is of the *transitional* type (Fig. 7-10) and is from four to five cells in thickness, except in the renal pelvis, where it is somewhat thinner. The general features of transitional epithelium were described on page 193. The *lamina propria* consists of fairly dense connective tissue, except in its deepest part, next to the muscular coat, where it is of somewhat looser texture. Some elastic fibers are mixed with the abundant collagenic ones. Occasional lymphatic nodules are encountered in it.

The mucous membrane of the ureter, except in the renal pelvis, is thrown into longitudinal folds, giving its lumen a stellate appearance in cross sections (Fig. 24-16). The combination of transitional epithelium (which can stretch without rupturing) and longitudinal folds makes it possible for the lumen of the ureter to become considerably expanded without the mucous membrane rupturing. This is an asset should renal calculi (L. *calculus,* pebble) —commonly known as kidney stones—form in the pelvis, as they do under various abnormal conditions. These are sometimes "passed" by way of the ureter, bladder, and urethra.

Muscle Coat. In approximately the upper two thirds of the ureter the smooth muscle coat consists of two layers: an inner one of longitudinal fibers and an outer one of circularly disposed fibers (Fig. 24-16). It may be helpful to remember that this is the *reverse arrangement* of that seen in the intestine. Moreover, the layers of smooth muscle in the ureter are infiltrated by connective tissue from the lamina propria and adventitia; hence they are not nearly as distinct as those in the intestine. The amount of smooth muscle in the wall of the renal pelvis is less than that in the remainder of the ureter, except where the calyces are attached to the pyramids. At this site the circularly disposed fibers are prominent, and it could be assumed that if this muscle contracted, the papilla it surrounds would be squeezed. A sustained, pronounced contraction of this muscle conceivably could shut off the flow of urine from the papilla concerned. Occasional contractions could have a "milking" effect on a papilla and squeeze urine out of the ducts of Bellini into the calyx concerned.

In approximately its lower third, a third coat of muscle fibers is present in the ureter. This forms the outermost layer of the muscle coat, and its fibers are longitudinally disposed.

The ureters pierce the bladder wall obliquely. This, together with little valve-like folds of bladder mucosa that guard their entrances into the bladder, prevents contractions of the bladder wall from forcing urine back up the ureters (the contraction of muscle fibers arranged in a thick sheet as they are in the urinary bladder tends to close the lumen of tubes that pass through the sheet obliquely). As each ureter enters the bladder wall, it loses its circularly arranged fibers. However, its longitudinal fibers continue through the wall to the mucous membrane of the bladder, where they are attached.

Urine does not drain from the kidneys to the bladder because of gravity as might be thought; this is convenient for astronauts traveling through weightless space. Peristaltic waves of contraction sweep down the muscle of the ureters and force urine into the bladder. The contraction of the longitudinal smooth muscle fibers in the part of the ureter that passes through the wall of the bladder helps open the lumen of that segment of the tube so as to permit urine to be delivered into the bladder.

Adventitia. This, the outermost coat of the ureter, consists of fibroelastic connective tissue. At its periphery it merges into adjacent loose connective tissue that is in turn connected to other structures.

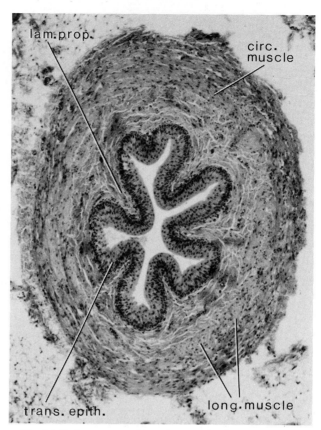

Fig. 24-16. Low-power photomicrograph of a ureter, showing the layers in its walls. From the lumen outward, note: transitional epithelium, lamina propria, longitudinal smooth muscle, circular layer of smooth muscle, and, on the outside, adventitia.

THE URINARY BLADDER

General Features. The wall of the urinary bladder (Fig. 24-17) must accommodate itself to great changes in the size of the cavity it encloses; this cavity is very much larger when the bladder is distended with urine than when emptied. It is easy to understand how the muscular coat of the bladder could accommodate itself to these changes, and also how the more or less elastic lamina propria together with its lining of transitional epithelium could be thrown into folds in a contracted bladder and then be stretched out flat as the bladder became distended with urine. But it is not so easy to understand how the transitional epithelium lining the bladder that becomes stretched as the bladder becomes distended remains intact so that urine cannot leak through it. Furthermore, since transitional epithelium is not keratinized, it is difficult to understand why the surface epithelial cells exposed to urine do not absorb urine as such, or fluid from it.

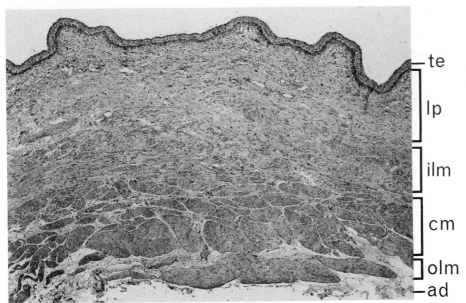

Fig. 24-17. Low-power photomicrograph of the wall of the
urinary bladder (monkey). From
the lumen down, the layers seen
are: transitional epithelium (te);
lamina propria (lp) merging into
submucosa; the muscle coat comprising a poorly defined inner longitudinal layer (ilm), a well-
developed middle, circular layer
(cm), and an outer longitudinal
layer (olm); and adventitia (ad).
(Courtesy of C. P. Leblond)

te

lp

ilm

cm

olm

ad

It should be mentioned in this connection that whereas
the large surface cells of the epithelium in a relaxed bladder are rounded and large (Fig. 7-10), they become
squamous in shape when the bladder is distended. For a
round cell to assume a squamous shape requires its cell
membrane to stretch just as the rubber wall of an inflated
balloon must stretch if someone happens to sit on it to
make it squamous in shape. However, the surface cells of
the bladder do not burst when they are stretched; their
surrounding membrane can accommodate to this change
and still remain intact.

***The Fine Structure of the Transitional Epithelium Lining
the Urinary Bladder.*** The EM has disclosed a further feature of the surface cells of the epithelial lining of the bladder that would help them withstand being stretched and
perhaps also restrict movement of fluid across their luminal plasma membrane. This part of the cell membrane,
which shows irregular contours and recesses in the relaxed bladder (Fig. 24-18B), is reinforced by what have
been termed *plaques* (PL in Fig. 24-18), which are
regions where the cell membrane is to some extent thickened on the outside (the luminal surface). The plaques occupy about three quarters of the surface area of this part
of the cell membrane and are characterized by containing
closely packed hexagonal subunits arranged along the
membrane surface. In between the plaques, however, the
cell membrane is not unusual (the typical regions are indicated by IN in Fig. 24-18). Filaments (F in Fig. 24-18)
are apparently anchored in these plaques. So it seems that
when the bladder is distended and the luminal plasma
membrane of the surface cells is stretched out flat (Fig.
24-18A), undue stretching would be restrained by the filaments anchored in the plaques being pulled taut. When
the bladder is relaxed, however, the luminal surface
membrane would become folded, with bends forming in
the hinge-like regions of cell membrane between the
plaques, as shown in Figure 24-18B. The luminal cell
membrane would thus fold up like an accordion (but not
as evenly). Indeed, relatively extensive profiles of luminal

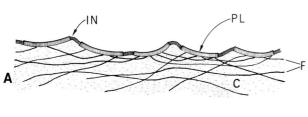

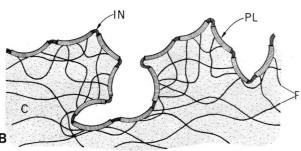

Fig. 24-18. Diagrams of the luminal surface of a superficial
cell of urinary bladder epithelium, as it would be seen in a distended bladder (*A*), and a relaxed bladder (*B*). C, cytoplasm; F,
filaments; PL, plaques; IN, interplaque regions. (Staehelin, L.
A., Chlapowski, F. J., and Bonneville, M. A.: J. Cell Biol.,
53:73, 1972)

cell membrane have been described as extending down into the superficial cytoplasm.

A few desmosomes hold the cells in the epithelium together and tight junctions have been described between the superficial cells. The latter would be important in helping prevent passage of fluid across the wall of the bladder due to osmotic or hydrostatic pressure differences.

The Other Layers of the Wall. The transitional epithelium rests on a *lamina propria* (lp in Fig. 24-17) that is collagenic in character and has only a few elastic fibers in it. Its deepest layer is somewhat looser in texture and has more elastic fibers; this is sometimes termed the *submucosal layer* of the bladder. This extends up into folds forming in the lining when the bladder is relaxed. The *muscular coat* consists of three layers, but these cannot be readily distinguished from one another. Their respective thicknesses vary in different parts of the bladder. In general, the middle coat is the most prominent one, and its fibers are mostly circularly disposed (cm in Fig. 24-17). Around the opening of the urethra, muscle fibers usually form an *internal sphincter.* The *adventitia* is fibroelastic in nature. Over part of the bladder is it covered with peritoneum so that it forms a *serosa.* Over the remainder it blends into adjacent loose connective tissue.

THE URETHRA

The *urethra* is a tube that extends from the bladder to an external orifice and so permits urine contained in the bladder to be evacuated from the body. In the *male,* the urethra courses through the penis, so it will be described when we deal with this part of the body in Chapter 27. However, the urethra of the female serves no genital function but only a urinary one, so its structure will be described here.

The *female urethra* varies in length from 2 to 6 cm. It is a fairly straight muscular tube lined by mucous membrane. The musculature of its walls consists of two coats of smooth muscle fibers, the inner one longitudinal, the outer one circular. At its external orifice, striated muscle fibers reinforce the smooth ones to form an *external sphincter.*

In cross section the lumen of the urethra is roughly crescentic. The mucous membrane is thrown into longitudinal folds. The *epithelium* of most of the urethra is stratified or pseudostratified columnar. However, transitional epithelium is present near the bladder and stratified squamous near the external orifice. The relatively thick connective tissue *lamina propria,* particularly in its deeper part, which is sometimes called the *submucosa,* is rich in elastic fibers and plexuses of veins; the latter are sufficiently extensive to give the deeper portions of the lamina propria a resemblance to erectile tissue.

In many sites the epithelium extends into the lamina propria to form little pockets. These gland-like structures commonly contain mucous cells. In the aged, concretions may form in them. True glands open by ducts into the lumen of the urethra, particularly in its upper part.

THE INNERVATION OF THE URINARY SYSTEM

Nerve fibers reach the kidney by way of the renal plexus. This is a network of nerve fibers that extends along the renal artery from the aorta to the kidney. The bodies of ganglion cells also may be present in the renal plexus; if so, they are regarded as outlying cells of diffuse celiac and aortic ganglia. Most of the fibers in the renal plexus belong to the *sympathetic* division of the autonomic system and are derived from the cells of the celiac and aortic ganglia. *Parasympathetic* fibers are present in the renal plexus in smaller numbers. These are derived from the vagus nerve, whose fibers course through the celiac plexus without interruption to reach the renal plexus.

The nerve fibers from the renal plexus, as noted, follow the arteries into the substance of the kidney. They penetrate glomeruli to form extensive perivascular networks and supply the epithelium of convoluted tubules, the transitional epithelium of the renal pelvis, and the walls of arteries and veins.

Since transplanted kidneys (which are necessarily removed from a nerve supply) and kidneys left in situ, but with their nerve supply cut, function fairly normally, kidney function is not totally dependent on nervous control. However, nervous mechanisms do control kidney function to some extent. It seems likely that most control is mediated by way of the sympathetic fibers that terminate in the blood vessels. The way this nervous regulation can operate to cause blood to circulate chiefly through juxtamedullary glomeruli, as in crush syndrome, has already been described. The part played by the parasympathetic (vagus-derived) fibers in the kidney is obscure.

Afferent impulses travel via nerves in the renal plexus, for cutting fibers of the plexus abolishes pain of renal origin.

Both sympathetic and parasympathetic fibers course along the ureter. But they do not seem particularly concerned with normal peristaltic movements that sweep down this tube, for these continue if the nerves are cut. Some of the nerves here carry afferent impulses.

The bladder is supplied by fibers from both sympathetic and parasympathetic divisions. The parasympathetic fibers are derived from the sacral outflow. The terminal ganglia to which they lead are present in the bladder wall; hence, in sections of bladder the student may occasionally observe ganglion cells.

REFERENCES AND OTHER READING

GENERAL REFERENCES ON THE KIDNEY

Brenner, B. M., and Rector, F. C. (eds.): The Kidney. vol 1. Philadelphia, W. B. Saunders, 1976.

Chapman, W. H., Bulger, R. E., Cutler, R. E., and Striker, G. E.: The Urinary System—an Integrated Approach. Philadelphia, W. B. Saunders, 1973.

Dalton, A. J., and Haguenau, F. (eds.): Ultrastructure of the Kidney. New York, Academic Press, 1967.

Moffat, D. B.: The Mammalian Kidney. Cambridge, Cambridge University Press, 1975.

Rouiller, C., and Muller, A. F. (eds.): The Kidney: Morphology, Biochemistry, Physiology. vols. 1 and 2. New York, Academic Press, 1969.

Smith, H. W.: The Kidney—Structure and Function in Health and Disease. ed. 2. New York, Oxford University Press, 1956.

———: Principles of Renal Physiology. New York, Oxford University Press, 1956.

SPECIAL REFERENCES

The Glomerulus

Blatt, W. F., Dravid, A., Michaels, A. S., and Nelsen, L.: Solute polarization and cake formation in membrane ultrafiltration: causes, consequences and control techniques. *In* Flinn, J. E. (ed.): Membrane Science and Technology. Industrial, Biological and Waste Treatment Processes. p. 47. New York, Plenum Press, 1970.

Boyer, C. C.: The vascular pattern of the renal glomerulus as revealed by plastic reconstruction from serial sections. Anat. Rec., *125:*433, 1956.

Brenner, B. M., Baylis, C., and Deen, W. M.: Transport of molecules across renal glomerular capillaries. Physiol. Rev., *56:*502, 1976.

Elias, H.: The structure of the renal glomerulus. Anat. Rec., *127:*288, 1957.

Farquhar, M. G., and Palade, G. E.: Glomerular permeability. II. Ferritin transfer across the glomerular capillary wall in nephrotic rats. J. Exp. Med., *114:*699, 1961.

———: Functional evidence for the existence of a third cell type in the renal glomerulus. Phagocytosis of filtration residues by a distinctive "third" cell. J. Cell Biol., *13:*55, 1962.

Farquhar, M. G., Wissig, S. L., and Palade, G. E.: Glomerular permeability. I. Ferritin transfer across the normal glomerular capillary wall. J. Exp. Med., *113:*47, 1961.

Graham, R. C., and Karnovsky, M. J.: Glomerular permeability: ultrastructural cytochemical studies using peroxidases as protein tracers. J. Exp. Med., *124:*1123, 1966.

Hall, B. V.: Further studies of the normal structure of the renal glomerulus. Proc. Sixth Ann. Conf. Nephrotic Syndrome p. 1. New York, National Nephrosis Foundation, 1964.

Karnovsky, M. J., and Ryan, G. B.: Substructure of the glomerular slit diaphragm in freeze-fractured normal rat kidney. J. Cell Biol., *65:*233, 1975.

Latta, H., Johnston, W. H., and Stanley, T. M.: Sialoglycoproteins and filtration barriers in the glomerular capillary wall. J. Ultrastruct. Res., *51:*354, 1975.

Menefee, M. G., and Mueller, C. B.: Some morphological considerations of transport in the glomerulus. *In* Ultrastructure of the Kidney (*see* General References). p. 73, 1967.

Michielsen, P., and Creemers, J.: The structure of function of the glomerular mesangium. *In* Ultrastructure of the Kidney (*see* General References). p. 57, 1967.

Ryan, G. B., Hein, S. J., and Karnovsky, M. J.: Glomerular permeability to proteins. Lab. Invest., *34:*415, 1976.

Suzuki, Y., Churg, J., Grishman, E., Mautner, W., and Dachs, S.: The mesangium of the renal glomerulus. Electron microscope studies of pathologic alterations. Am. J. Pathol., *43:*555, 1963.

Trump, B. F., and Benditt, E. P.: Electron microscopic studies of human renal disease. Observations on normal visceral glomerular epithelium and its modifications in disease. Lab. Invest., *11:*753, 1962.

Venkatachalam, M. A., Karnovsky, M. J., Fahimi, H. D., and Cotran, R. S.: An ultrastructural study of glomerular permeability using catalase and peroxidase as tracer proteins. J. Exp. Med., *132:*1153, 1970.

Walker, F.: The origin, turnover, and removal of glomerular basement membrane. J. Pathol., *110:*233, 1973.

The Vascular Pole of Glomeruli and JG Cells

Bing, J., and Kazimierczak, J.: Renin content of different parts of the periglomerular circumferences. Acta Pathol. Microbiol. Scand., *50:*1, 1960.

Evan, A. P., and Dail, W. G.: Efferent arterioles in the cortex of the rat kidney. Am. J. Anat., *187:*135, 1977.

Garber, B. G., McCoy, F. W., Marks, B. H., and Hayes, E. R.: Factors that affect the granulation of the juxtaglomerular apparatus. Anat. Rec., *130:*303, 1958.

Goldblatt, H.: Experimental hypertension induced by renal ischemia. Harvey Lect., *33:*237, 1937–38.

Hartroft, P. M.: Juxtaglomerular cells of the American bullfrog as seen by light and electron microscopy. Fed. Proc., *25:*238, 1966.

———: The juxtaglomerular complex as an endocrine gland. *In* Bloodworth, J. B. (ed.): Endocrine Pathology. p. 641. Baltimore, Williams & Wilkins, 1968.

Hartroft, P. M., Bischoff, M. B., and Boucci, T. J.: Effects of chronic exposure to high altitudes on the JG complex and the adrenal cortex in dogs, rabbits and rats. Fed. Proc., *28:*1234, 1969.

Hartroft, P. M., and Edelman, R.: Renal juxtaglomerular cells in sodium deficiency. *In* Moyer, J. H., and Fuchs, M. (eds.): Edema. pp. 63–68. Philadelphia, W. B. Saunders, 1960.

Hartroft, P. M., and Hartroft, W. S.: Studies on renal juxtaglomerular cells. J. Exp. Med., *102:*205, 1955.

Hatt, P.-Y.: The juxtaglomerular apparatus. *In* Ultrastructure of the Kidney (*see* General References). p. 101, 1967.

McManus, J. F. A.: Further observations on the glomerular root of the vertebrate kidney. Quart. J. Micr. Sci., *88:*39, 1947.

Pitcock, J. A., Hartroft, P. M., and Newmark, L. N.: Increased renal pressor activity (renin) in sodium deficient rats and correlation with juxtaglomerular cell granulation. Proc. Soc. Exp. Biol. Med., *100:*868, 1959.

Tobian, L., Janecek, J., and Tomboulian, A.: Correlation between granulation of juxtaglomerular cells and extractable renin in rats with experimental hypertension. Proc. Soc. Exp. Biol. Med., *100:*94, 1959.

Wilson, W.: A new staining method for demonstrating the granules of the juxtaglomerular complex. Anat. Rec., *112:*497, 1952.

The Tubular Parts of the Nephron

Gottschalk, C. W.: Micropuncture studies of tubular function in the mammalian kidney. Physiologist, *4:*35, 1961.

Latta, H., Maunsbach, A. B., and Osvaldo, L.: The fine structure of renal tubules in cortex and medulla. *In* Ultrastructure of the Kidney (*see* General References). p. 2, 1967.

Munkácsi, I., and Palkovits, M.: Study of the renal pyramid, loops of Henle, and percentage distribution of their thin segments in animals living in desert, semidesert and water-rich environment. Acta Biol. Hung., *17:*89, 1966.

Pease, D. C.: Electron microscopy of the tubular cells of the kidney cortex. Anat. Rec., *121:*723, 1955.

————: Fine structures of the kidney seen by electron microscopy. J. Histochem., *3:*295, 1955.

Rhodin, J.: Anatomy of the kidney tubules. Int. Rev. Cytol., *7:*485, 1958.

Ruska, H., Moore, D. H., and Weinstock, J.: The base of the proximal convoluted tubule cells of rat kidney. J. Biophys. Biochem. Cytol., *3:*249, 1957.

Sjöstrand, F. S., and Rhodin, J.: The ultrastructure of the proximal convoluted tubules of the mouse kidney as revealed by high resolution electron microscopy. Exp. Cell Res., *4:*426, 1953.

Tisher, C. G.: Functional anatomy of the kidney. Hosp. Practice, p. 53, May, 1978.

Wirz, H.:Introduction—Tubular transport mechanism with special reference to the hairpin countercurrent. *In* Duyff, J. W., et al. (eds.): XXII International Congress of Physiological Sciences, Symposium VII. vol. 1, p. 359. New York, Excerpta Medica Foundation, 1962.

The Renal Circulation

Barclay, A. E., Daniel, P., Franklin, J. K., Prichard, M. M. L., and Trueta, J.: Records and findings obtained during studies of the renal circulation in the rabbit, with special reference to vascular short-circuiting and functional cortical ischaemia. J. Physiol., *105:*27, 1946.

Baringer, J. R.: The dynamic anatomy of the microcirculation in the amphibian and mammalian kidney. Anat. Rec., *130:*266, 1958.

Bialestock, D.: The extra-glomerular arterial circulation of the renal tubules. Anat. Rec., *129:*53, 1957.

Brenner, B. M., and Beeuwkes, R.: The renal circulations. Hosp. Practice, p. 35, July, 1978.

Daniel, P. M., Peabody, C. N., and Prichard, M. M. L.: Cortical ischaemia of the kidney with maintained blood flow through the medulla. Quart. J. Exp. Physiol., *37:*11, 1952.

————: Observations on the circulation through the cortex and the medulla of the kidney. Q. J. Exp. Physiol., *36:*199, 1951.

Daniel, P. M., Prichard, M. M. L., and Ward-McQuaid, J. N.: The renal circulation in experimental hypertension. Br. J. Surg., *42:*81, 1954.

Graves, F. T.: The anatomy of the intrarenal arteries and its application to segmental resection of the kidney. Br. J. Surg., *42:*132, 1954.

————: The anatomy of the intrarenal arteries in health and disease. Br. J. Surg., *43:*605, 1956.

MacCallum, D. B.: The arterial blood supply of the mammalian kidney. Am. J. Anat., *38:*153, 1926.

More, R. H., and Duff, G. L.: The renal arterial vasculature in man. Am. J. Pathol., *27:*95, 1950.

Morison, D. M.: A study of the renal circulation, with special reference to its finer distribution. Am. J. Anat., *37:*53, 1926.

Pease, D. C.: Electron microscopy of the vascular bed of the kidney cortex. Anat. Rec., *121:*701, 1955.

Sykes, D.: Some aspects of the blood supply of the human kidney. Symp. Zool. Soc. London, *11:*49, 1964.

————: The correlation between renal vascularization and lobulation of the kidney. Br. J. Urol., *36:*549, 1964.

Trueta, J., Barclay, A. E., Daniel, P., Franklin, K. J., and Prichard, M. M. L.: Studies of the Renal Circulation. Oxford, Blackwell Scientific Publications, 1947.

The Connective Tissue, Lymphatics, and Nerves of the Kidney and Other Parts of the Urinary System

Gruber, C. M.: The autonomic innervation of the genitourinary system. Physiol. Rev., *13:*497, 1933.

Harman, P. J., and Davies, H.: Intrinsic nerves in the kidney of the cat and the rat. Anat. Rec., *100:*671, 1948.

Leeson, T. S.: An electron microscopic study of the postnatal development of the hamster kidney, with particular reference to intertubular tissue. Lab. Invest., *10:*466, 1961.

Peirce, E. C.: Renal lymphatics. Anat. Rec., *90:*315, 1944.

Rawson, A. J.: Distribution of the lymphatics of the human kidney as shown in a case of carcinomatous permeation. Arch. Pathol., *47:*283, 1949.

The Development and Growth of the Kidney

Arataki, M.. On the postnatal growth of the kidney, with special reference to the number and size of the glomeruli. Am. J. Anat., *36:*399, 1926.

Clark, S. L., Jr.: Cellular differentiation in the kidneys of newborn mice studied with the electron microscope. J. Biophys. Biochem. Cytol., *3:*349, 1957.

Hartroft, W. S.: The vascular development of the kidney of the pig. Trans. Roy. Soc. Canada, Sec. V (Biol. Sci.), *35:*67, 1949.

Kurtz, S. M.: The electron microscopy of the developing human renal glomerulus. Exp. Cell Res., *14:*355, 1958.

Leeson, T. S.: Electron microscopy of the developing kidney: an investigation into the fine structure of the mesonephros and metanephros of the rabbit. J. Anat., *94:*100, 1960.

MacDonald, M. S., and Emery, J. L.: The late intrauterine and postnatal development of human renal glomeruli. J. Anat., *93:*331, 1959.

Sulkin, N. N.: Cytologic study of the remaining kidney following unilateral nephrectomy in the rat. Anat. Rec., *105:*95, 1949.

The Urinary Bladder

Hicks, R. M., and Ketterer, B.: Isolation of the plasma membrane of the luminal surface of rat bladder epithelium, and the occurrence of a hexagonal lattice of subunits both in negatively stained whole mounts and in sectional membranes. J. Cell Biol., *45:*542, 1970.

Staehelin, A., Chlapowski, F. J., and Bonneville, M. A.: Lumenal plasma membrane of the urinary bladder. I. Three-dimensional reconstruction from freeze-etch images. J. Cell Biol., *53:*73, 1972.

Strum, J. M., and Danon, D.: Fine structure of the urinary bladder of the bullfrog. Anat. Rec., *178:*15, 1974.

25 The Endocrine System

Development of Knowledge About Endocrine Glands

The finding of glands that secrete into ducts was the basis for the concept of their producing what were termed *exocrine secretions.* When it was discovered that some glands do not have ducts, but instead deliver their secretion into the bloodstream, such glands were called *ductless* or *endocrine glands* (Fig. 6-2). Moreover, the secretions of these glands were found to exert noticeable and generally specific effects on certain cells that were usually located in particular organs. In general they *aroused* activity, so the secretions of endocrine glands came to be known as *hormones* (Gr. *hormaein,* to set in motion or spur on). This concept is still useful, but we now know that not all hormones spur on activity, for some depress it. Furthermore, some hormones are produced by body cells that are not parts of endocrine glands. So this particular branch of medical science, called *endocrinology,* has now expanded into an extraordinarily complex and important subject.

What Led to the Development of Endocrinology and the Advances in Knowledge That Followed. Endocrinology really developed as a result of autopsies that involved carrying out both gross and microscopic studies on tissues of people who had manifested particular and unusual physical changes and symptoms before they died. For example, around the middle of the last century, Thomas Addison, an English physician, described a condition in which a patient became progressively weaker, at the same time showing increased pigmentation of the skin. When such an individual died, autopsy showed that his adrenal glands were diseased. It took a long time, however, before it was established that the manifestations of this disease were due to inadequate production of an essential hormone by the adrenal glands.

Certain other clinical conditions were in due course recognized at autopsy as being linked with what we now know to be endocrine glands. This led to a plethora of animal experimentation, from which it was learned that removal of a particular gland could cause an animal to manifest the sorts of changes observed in people that had diseased glands of this type. The concept of body func-

tions being dependent on the internal secretions of endocrine glands soon followed. Further, it was discovered that extracts made from such glands, when administered to animals from which the same glands had been removed, could substitute for their function. It was also found that excessive levels of such extracts could simulate conditions seen in people who at autopsy showed enlargement of a gland or a tumor of that gland. Then, with improving biochemical methods, isolation of the active principle (or principles) in pure form from extracts of these glands was attempted. Over the years considerable success has been obtained not only in this but also in the next step, that of determining the chemical structure of the hormone involved. A subsequent step would of course be to attempt to synthesize particular hormones, and this too has been accomplished in some instances. The final step is to determine how and where hormones act on or in cells. We shall comment on this shortly.

The Chemical Composition of Hormones

This is a subject dealt with in depth in textbooks of physiology, pharmacology, biochemistry, and endocrinology. We merely note that one group, which could be referred to as an *amino acid* group, consists of hormones ranging from modified amino acids through small and large peptides, to fully fledged proteins.

Second, a few hormones are *glycoproteins.*

Third, another and very different group of hormones is derived from cholesterol; these hormones are termed *steroids.* They are fat-soluble and hence can readily pass through the cell membrane of their target cells.

The Basis for Hormones Affecting Specific Cells

It is usual to say that a given hormone exerts its effect on only a certian cell type, which is commonly referred to as its *target cell.* There are specific target cells for each hormone. This is because only the target cell type possesses the specific receptors for that particular hormone on or in its cell membrane, and the hormone has to bind to specific receptors to exert its effect. However, certain hormones (for example, thyroid hormone) affect not just one kind of cell but many, so they all must be regarded as target cells.

How Hormones Are Thought to Exert Their Effects

Research in this general area has been exciting and has had an important side effect in that many new and valuable drugs have become available to the medical, dental, and veterinary professions. For studying histology, no more than an introductory account is required.

There are several chemically different kinds of hormones, so it could be expected that they might exert different kinds of effects on cells and do this in different ways.

Since in the chapters on nervous and muscle tissue we have already discussed epinephrine (one of the smallest hormones of the amino acid group), we shall begin with it. As already described, it causes contraction of smooth muscle in some sites and relaxation in others. This is now generally ascribed to there being two different types of receptors on smooth muscle cells, termed alpha and beta receptors, respectively. For example, smooth muscle cells in the terminal vascular bed of the skin are considered to manifest an alpha receptor response to epinephrine in that they contract under the influence of the hormone (which is why people pale with fear). However, epinephrine relaxes the smooth muscle of the bronchioles of the lungs, which is why epinephrine is given to patients going into anaphylactic shock (p. 248). So it is thought that smooth muscle cells of the bronchioles manifest a beta receptor response to epinephrine.

Epinephrine, moreover, increases the heart rate; it causes the cell membrane of pacemaker cells (p. 584) to depolarize more frequently than 70 times per minute. This would suggest that epinephrine has a primary effect on the cell membrane of pacemaker cells. Acceleration of the heart rate is a beta response elicited by epinephrine and also by norepinephrine. Both substances decrease the potassium permeability of the cell membrane of these cells, thereby limiting outward diffusion of potassium ions from the cells. This effect accelerates the rate at which their resting potential declines (p. 584) and hence it increases the rate at which they undergo spontaneous depolarization.

One of the more interesting things about epinephrine is that under restful conditions it is not secreted in the bloodstream in sufficient quantities to exert much effect. However, increased and effective amounts of it are secreted into the blood under conditions of fear or rage. This has led to the idea of this particular hormonal mechanism having survival value. It would have helped animals (including *Homo sapiens*) to run away faster or fight harder when these particular emotions were aroused, because epinephrine exerts physiological effects enabling an individual to run faster or fight harder. For example, depending on whether it elicits an alpha or a beta response, it causes the heart to beat faster, the blood pressure to increase, more blood to be diverted to muscles and less to the intestines, and so on. It also causes glycogen in liver cells to be broken down to glucose, which enters the bloodstream, so that muscles have more fuel for flight or fight. For many decades the way it caused glycogen to be broken down to glucose was not understood. The solving of the mystery was of such great importance that it led to Sutherland's receiving the Nobel prize for physiology and medicine in 1971; it led to the discovery of *cyclic AMP*, a substance now known to be involved in mediating the effects of many hormones on their target cells.

Cyclic AMP. Cyclic AMP (cAMP) is the short form for *cyclic 3',5'-adenosine monophosphate*. It is a small molecule formed from ATP in small quantities by an enzyme called *adenylate cyclase,* located in the cell membrane. When epinephrine in the bloodstream becomes attached to receptors on the membrane of a liver cell, it activates the adenylate cyclase in its cell membrane and this in turn causes increased amounts of cyclic AMP to be formed from ATP. The cyclic AMP diffuses throughout the cell. In the instance of liver cells affected by epinephrine, the increased content of cyclic AMP activates an enzyme that triggers further the conversion of glycogen into glucose. This is how epinephrine causes more glucose to be released into the blood when an individual experiences a profound emotional reaction such as fear or rage.

Hormones can be regarded as *primary messengers* sent via the bloodstream that in general activate their target cells. If they act by causing the formation of cyclic AMP as described above, the latter is sometimes termed the *secondary messenger*. This second link in the chain is formed and acts *intracellularly* in the target cell itself.

Hormones That Affect Gene Expression

Several hormones are thought to act this way. It would seem obvious that if the effect of any hormone is to increase protein synthesis, it must either directly or indirectly act at the level of genes, because they control protein synthesis.

Steroid Hormones. These are lipid-soluble and hence pass from their cell membrane receptors on through the membrane. (It is believed the hormone of the thyroid as well as steroid hormones can also *enter the cytoplasm*.) In the cytosol such a hormone combines with a specific *receptor protein* (which is made in very small amounts in certain cells) so as to form a *hormone-receptor complex,* which, after undergoing a few changes, reaches the nucleus. For those who have read in Chapter 6 about regulation of gene activity in prokaryotic cells, it should be mentioned here that the nucleus of eukaryotic cells is different in many respects from the genetic material in prokaryotic cells. First, in eukaryotic cells the chromosomes are enclosed during interphase by a nuclear membrane, and for this and other reasons it is thought unlikely that repressors of gene function in eukaryotic cells would be proteins alone, as they are in prokaryotic cells. Moreover, there is an abundance of RNA in the nucleus of eukaryotic cells which is neither mRNA or rRNA; this is termed *heterogeneous RNA* and there is reason to believe that part of this, termed *activator RNA*, may be concerned in the regulation of gene function. It has been suggested that hormone-receptor complexes move to and combine with specific sensor sites that lie adjacent to what have been termed *integrator genes* along chromosomes. When the sensor site is activated, it causes the adjacent integrator gene to transcribe *activator RNA*, which moves about in the nucleus and is recognized by specific receptor sites, probably along several different chromosomes. In places where activator RNA binds to its receptor sites, which are located beside structural genes, the latter transcribe mRNA. For example, by such a mechanism sex hormones (which are steroids) could be visualized as increasing the protein synthesis required for proliferation and differentiation of cells in connection with the functioning and maintenance of the organs of the reproductive system. A demonstrable example of gene expression being affected by a steroid hormone is that of ovalbumin synthesis being instituted in a chicken's egg, with the transcription of mRNA for ovalbumin synthesis appearing in response to a type of female sex hormone.

Even though steroid hormones enter the cytoplasm and nucleus of their target cells, it appears that for some of their actions they may require mediation by cyclic AMP.

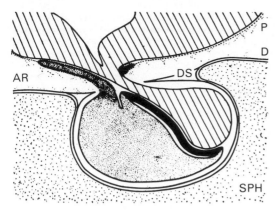

Fig. 25-1. Diagram of the pituitary gland, in sagittal section, showing the relation of the pars tuberalis to the meninges. *Cross hatched,* hypothalamus floor and pars nervosa; *fine stipple,* pars anterior; *coarse stipple,* pars tuberalis; *solid black,* pars intermedia; SPH, sphenoid bone; P, pia mater; D, dura mater; DS, diaphragma sellae; AR, arachnoid spaces. (Atwell, W. J.: Am. J. Anat., *37:*159, 1926)

Polypeptide and Protein Hormones. These in many instances also promote protein synthesis. However, they are not lipid-soluble and so *do not enter the cytosol* of their target cells. Their action is mediated through cyclic AMP. For this to stimulate protein synthesis suggests that the cyclic AMP produced is somehow concerned in facilitating gene transcription.

The Regulation of Secretion by Endocrine Glands

This cannot be explained in any detail until we have described and discussed individual glands. But to prepare for this it can be said that in general the secretory activities of the various glands is controlled by feedback mechanisms of the negative type, and that what is fed back is something produced as a result of the action of the hormone. What makes this somewhat complicated, however, is that feedback mechanisms may operate through a pathway involving more than one gland, so that one hormone may cause another to be produced and the latter then may feed back to the first to control its secretion.

We shall now describe the endocrine glands in the following order:

(*1*) The pituitary gland
(*2*) The thyroid gland
(*3*) The parathyroid glands
(*4*) The adrenal glands
(*5*) The islets of Langerhans of the pancreas
(*6*) The pineal body

The sex glands will be described in the following two chapters.

We begin with the pituitary, since it controls the activity of many of the other endocrine glands.

THE PITUITARY GLAND (BODY) (HYPOPHYSIS CEREBRI)

Gross Features. This gland is ovoid and measures about 1.5 cm. in the transverse plane and about 1 cm. in the sagittal plane. It becomes larger during pregnancy. It lies immediately below the base of the brain, to which it is attached by the pituitary stalk (Fig. 25-1). It rests in a depression in a bony prominence on the upper surface of the sphenoid bone. This bony prominence is shaped something like a Turkish saddle with a high back and a high front, and for this reason is termed the *sella turcica.* The pituitary gland sits, as it were, in the saddle and so has bony protection in front, below, and behind. The dura mater dips down to line the seat of the saddle and so envelop the pituitary gland. Furthermore, a shelf of dura mater, the *diaphragma sellae,* extends over most of the top of the gland to complete its enclosure (Fig. 25-1, DS). The degree of protection afforded the pituitary is in relation to its importance.

The Four Anatomical Parts of the Gland. In many animals a cleft runs downward and posteriorly from near the attachment of the stalk (Fig. 25-1) to separate the gland into an anterior and posterior part. Such a cleft may be seen in the pituitary gland of a young child, but in the adult it is replaced by a row of follicles. There are four parts of the gland. (*1*) The main part anterior to the cleft or row of follicles is termed its *pars anterior* (Fig. 25-1, *fine stipple*) or *pars distalis.* (*2*) A projection from this, the *pars tuberalis* (Fig. 25-1, *coarse stipple*), extends up along the anterior and lateral aspects of the pituitary stalk. (*3*) A rather narrow band of poorly developed glandular tissue along the posterior border of the cleft or row of vesicles comprises the *pars intermedia* (Fig. 25-1, *solid black*). (*4*) The remainder (all that is posterior to the narrow pars intermedia) is called its *pars posterior* or *pars nervosa* (Fig. 25-1, *cross hatched*). The pars nervosa is not so wide as the pars anterior and more or less fits into a concavity on the posterior aspect of the pars anterior, from which it is separated by the pars intermedia.

Development. The pars nervosa develops as a downgrowth from the base of the brain (Fig. 25-2). The other parts of the gland develop from an epithelial membrane, as do endocrine glands in general, as follows.

The anterior part of the mouth results from the inward bulging of ectoderm to form the oral fossa. Very early in development, before the bones of the skull have formed, the ectodermal lining of the roof of the oral fossa is in very close contact with the floor of the developing brain (which at this stage has a tubular form), and indeed the ectoderm of the roof of the oral fossa soon becomes adherent to the lower surface of the developing brain. This connection does not break as mesenchyme proliferates and gradually separates the developing brain from the developing mouth. As a consequence, the gradual separation of the brain and the mouth causes both the lining of the oral cavity and the floor of the brain to be drawn out into funnel-shaped structures with their tips in contact. The funnel-shaped extension of the roof of the oral fossa that points toward the brain is called *Rathke's pouch.* By the end of the second month of development this pouch breaks away from the oral ectoderm and thereupon becomes a hollow island of epithelium surrounded by mesenchyme except at its uppermost part, where a peninsula is attached to the downward extension of the floor of the brain (Fig. 25-2). The main body of the hollow island of epithelium becomes more or less flattened around the anterior surface of the downgrowth of the brain. The cells of the anterior wall of the hollow epithelial island proliferate so that its anterior walls become greatly thickened. This becomes the pars anterior of the pituitary gland, and an upward extension of it becomes the pars tuberalis. The posterior wall of the island becomes the pars intermedia. The central cavity of the epithelial island between the pars anterior and the pars intermedia becomes flattened to form the cleft previously described, and the downward extension from the floor of the brain becomes the pars nervosa.

A residuum of cells similar to those of the pars anterior may be present in the pharynx at the site from which the anterior lobe develops (Fig. 25-2). If so, these cells are said to constitute the *pharyngeal hypophysis.*

The part of the pituitary gland that develops from the epithelium of the pharynx (pars anterior, intermedia, and tuberalis) is often referred to as the *adenohypophysis,* and the part that develops from the brain, the *neurohypophysis.*

THE HYPOTHALAMUS AND ITS RELATION TO PITUITARY GLAND FUNCTION

The possibility of there being some significance in the way the anterior lobe of the pituitary develops from an epithelial membrane, as do other endocrine glands, with the posterior pituitary remaining part of the nervous system and the two parts remaining in juxtaposition throughout life, has intrigued scientists over the years. The reason for this anatomical arrangement has only become apparent relatively recently. It was found, as the anterior lobe was studied, that it produced several important hormones—for example, the hormones required for growth of the body, lactation in females, and the trophic hormones that control the functions of the thyroid gland, cortex of the adrenal gland, and the sex glands. Indeed, its central role in endocrinology has inspired musically inclined lectures to refer to the anterior pituitary gland as the conductor of the endocrine orchestra.

In recent years, however, this expression has fallen

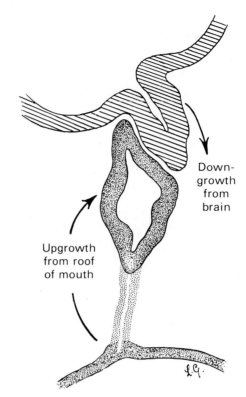

Down-growth from brain

Upgrowth from roof of mouth

Fig. 25-2. Diagram illustrating the development of the pituitary gland from its two main sources.

into disuse because it has become apparent that all this time the real conductor of the endocrine orchestra was, as it were, hiding in the wings—in the *hypothalamus,* a part of the brain that lies just above and a little posterior to the pituitary. Many observations had to be made before it was realized that it was important for the pituitary gland to have a dual origin, from epithelium and nervous tissue respectively, and why the anterior lobe should occupy the position it does. Some will now be described.

Establishing That Nerve Cells Could Produce and Liberate Hormones. It was known for a long time that two hormones, oxytocin and vasopressin, could be extracted from the posterior lobe of the pituitary gland and it was at first assumed that this is where they were made. However, in due course it was shown that these hormones were produced in the cell bodies of neurons located in the hypothalamus, as shown in Figure 25-14. The reason for their presence in the posterior lobe of the pituitary was that the axons of these nerve cells passed down the pituitary stalk to reach the posterior lobe, where they ended in association with capillaries into which the hormones made in these cell bodies were liberated (Fig. 25–16, *bottom right*). Since the hormones sometimes accumulated

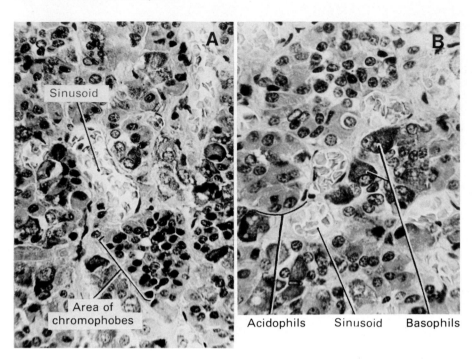

Fig. 25-3. High-power photomicrographs of the anterior lobe of the pituitary gland. (*A*) An area of chromophobes, with their nuclei close together. A sinusoid and some chromophils may be seen also. (*B*) Acidophils, basophils and sinusoids.

near the endings of the axons, the hormones could, of course, be extracted from the posterior lobe. As a result of these findings it became obvious that nerve cells could produce what were called *neurosecretions* and that these could be delivered to the bloodstream and act as hormones at the various sites to which they were carried.

The Role of the Portal Circulation of the Pituitary Gland. In the meantime, some findings were made about the anterior pituitary that were puzzling. It was found, for example, that if it was transplanted to some other site it did not function properly. If, however, it was removed and then placed back in its normal environment it would function. It seemed as if it had to be close to the nervous part of the pituitary if it were to operate properly. An idea that was explored was that its cells must be innervated by nerve fibers for it to work properly. But no nerve fibers were found extending into it from the nervous tissue that could explain how its hormone-producing cells were stimulated. During this time it was pointed out that the blood coursing through the wide capillaries of the anterior lobe had already passed through capillary tufts in nervous tissue (Fig. 25-13, capillary clusters). It was then found that certain nerve cell bodies in the hypothalamus (not the same ones that make the posterior lobe hormones but others, not far away) had short axons and made neurosecretions also, and these moved along their short axons to their endings around the capillaries that drained into the capillaries of the anterior lobe. These neurosecretions that reached the anterior lobe *by way of the bloodstream*

were found to be the hormones that controlled the secretory activities of the various cells of the anterior lobe. These neurohormones were thus called *hormone-releasing* or *hormone-regulating factors,* because they controlled the release of hormones from the cells of the anterior lobe.

Following this introduction on the role of the hypothalamus we shall now comment on the hormones produced by the anterior lobe and the cells that produce them, after which we shall discuss the hormone-regulating factors and describe the elaborate circulation in the pituitary gland which enables such factors to reach the hormone-secreting cells in this part of the gland.

THE ANTERIOR LOBE OF THE PITUITARY (THE PARS DISTALIS)

Microscopic Structure. An H and E section shows that the anterior lobe is composed of thick branching cords of cells (Fig. 25-3). Between these there are capillaries that are wide enough to have been called sinusoids; they are so labeled in Figure 25-3. With the EM it can be seen that the endothelial walls of the capillaries are surrounded by a basement membrane (Fig. 25-6) and that between the borders of the epithelial cells of the cords and the basement membranes of capillaries there is at least a potential pericapillary space which would contain tissue fluid. The secretion of the epithelial cells passes through this space, the basement membrane and the endothelial walls of capillaries to enter the bloodstream.

Classification of the Cells of the Anterior Lobe

There are at least six and probably seven different hormones produced by the cells of the anterior lobe. The first question about their source was whether or not all the cells of the anterior lobe were hormone producers or whether some served some other purpose. So at first they were divided into two types, those that were secreting and those that were not. The cytoplasm of one type was seen to be relatively abundant and to have an affinity for some, but not necessarily the same, kind of stain. Cells of this kind were called *chromophils* because their cytoplasm "liked" color, and the cells whose cytoplasm did not stain were called *chromophobes* because they "disliked" color. Because the chromophils had abundant cytoplasm the impression was gained that the chromophils were the cells that secreted hormones and the chromophobes, which had little cytoplasm, did not. It was proposed, however, that chromophobes had the ability to *become chromophils* and that chromophils could *revert back* to being chromophobes. In other words, chromophobes and chromophils were the same kinds of cells but in different states of functional activity. This view received support from EM studies.

The cells classed as chromophobes with the LM are considerably smaller than chromophils. Indeed, the easiest way for a student to identify chromophobes is to look for a group of cells in which the nuclei are close together — which means, of course, that they have little cytoplasm (Fig. 25-3, Area of chromophobes).

Acidophils and Basophils. The first way that chromophils were classified depended on whether the granules they contained had an affinity for basic or acidic stains. Hence the chromophils were divided into *basophils* and *acidophils;* this terminology is still used to some extent. The next problem was to see if acidophils and basophils made different kinds of hormones and ultimately to find out if each hormone was made by a separate kind of cell that could be identified histologically. Tracing the various hormones to different cell types was first attempted by utilizing special staining methods. While much success was obtained, this method led to confusing nomenclature, partly due to the same staining methods not giving the same results in different species. Two further methods that have subsequently been employed with considerable success in distinguishing the different kinds of chromophils are (*1*) electron microscopy and (*2*) immunofluorescence technics. (The latter were described on p. 245). Thus when sections of pituitary are flooded with fluorescent antibody to a given hormone, it attaches to the type of cell that contains the hormone so that cells making this hormone can be identified. With all the technics now available it is generally conceded that each hormone, with perhaps one exception mentioned later, is made by a *separate* type of cell.

Development of Knowledge About the Hormones Produced in the Anterior Lobe

Learning about the hormones produced by the anterior lobe of the pituitary was much more difficult than learning about those produced by other endocrine glands, for several reasons. First, because of its location, it was difficult to remove the pituitary gland from experimental animals to learn what effects this would have. It took time to develop technics making hypophysectomies possible on animals such as rats so that the effects of loss of anterior lobe hormones could be precisely determined. Furthermore, because the anterior lobe produces so many hormones, extracts made from anterior lobes were initially cocktails containing many different hormones. It took a great deal of time before pure extracts of hormones could be obtained so that the specific effects of each could be ascertained.

When it was realized that the anterior lobe produced and secreted several hormones another problem arose; this related to which particular cells in the anterior lobe produced them. At present it is conceded that there are seven different hormones made by cells of the pars distalis. It seems also that these are produced by at least six different cell types. However, some of the cell types seem not to be absolutely specific, for there are some examples of one cell type being able to make not only its specific hormone but also at least a little of some closely related hormone. The hormones produced by the anterior lobe are:

(*1*) Growth Hormone (GH), also called Somatotrophin (STH)

(*2*) Lactogenic Hormone, also called Prolactin or Mammotrophin

(*3*) Thyrotrophin (TSH)

(*4*) Follicle-Stimulating Hormone (FSH)

(*5*) Luteinizing Hormone (LH)

(*6*) Adrenocorticotrophin (ACTH), also called Corticotrophin or Adrenocorticotrophic Hormone

(*7*) Melanocyte-Stimulating Hormone (MSH)

These will be discussed briefly in turn before we go on to describe specific cell types.

The Hormones Secreted By the Anterior Lobe

Growth Hormone (GH) (Somatotrophin — STH). A young animal stops growing after its pituitary gland is removed and thereafter remains a dwarf unless extracts of pars anterior are given to it. The most striking cessation of

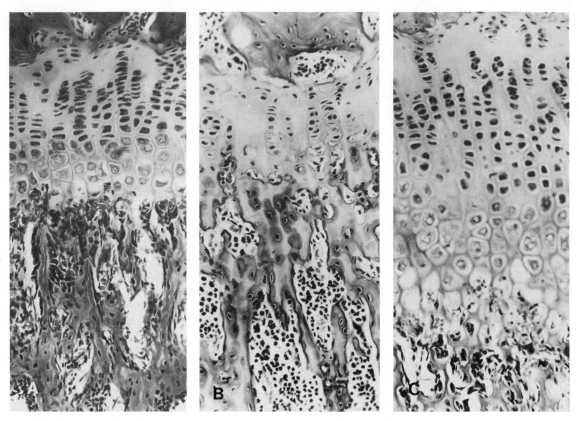

Fig. 25-4. Photomicrographs illustrating the effects of (*B*) suppression and (*C*) administration of growth hormone on the growth of the epiphyseal plate, as compared with growth in (*A*) an untreated control. (*A*) Metaphysis of tibia of a rat nearing full growth. (*B*) Metaphysis of a rat of the same age after injections of female sex hormone, which suppressed secretion of growth hormone. The epiphyseal disk is thinner and lacks a zone of maturing cells. (*C*) Metaphysis of a rat of the same age after injections of anterior pituitary extract containing growth hormone. The epiphyseal disk here is thicker than in (*A*).

growth is observed in the cartilage cells of the epiphyseal disks of the long bones. When the young cells in the zone of proliferation stop dividing, no new cells are produced to mature and so add to the thickness of the disk. Since calcification does not cease, the zone of calcification continues to advance into the zone of maturation, and as a result the zone of maturing cells becomes greatly thinned. (Compare part A of Fig. 25-4, which is normal, with part B of the same figure.) Since this zone is an important factor in the thickness of the disk, a reduction in thickness of this zone makes the disk, as a whole, thinner.

In a normal person, secretion of growth hormone either decreases somewhat or the amount secreted becomes less effective toward the end of adolescence, so that at that time the individual stops growing. The cells of certain rare tumors that may develop in the anterior lobe keep on secreting beyond the time when the cells of normal pars anterior would stop secreting enough hormone to cause

more growth. A person so afflicted keeps on growing and the condition is termed *giantism*.

If growth hormone-producing tumors develop after the epiphyseal disks of long bones have become replaced by bone — that is, after normal growth is over — or if growth hormone is given to a normal animal after its growth is over, no further growth in stature occurs. However, although cartilage would seem to be the primary target for the growth-stimulating effect of growth hormone, some growth of bone is stimulated because the bones, particularly those of the hands and feet, tend to become thicker, and there is great overgrowth of the mandible and lesser growth of certain other bones in the face. Other tissues, for example the skin, are affected as well; the condition as a whole is termed *acromegaly* (Gr. *akron*, extremity; *megas*, large) because the growth of the bones in the head, the hands, and the feet makes these extremities large.

The epiphyseal disks of some laboratory animals are unusual in that they do not ordinarily become replaced by bone when normal growth is over. For example, the epiphyseal disks persist for a long time in the female rat; hence, if female rats that have stopped growing are given growth hormone, they begin to grow again (Fig. 25-4, compare parts A and C). It has also been shown that growth hormone causes a rapid uptake of radioactive sulfur in cartilage.

Growth hormone prepared from pituitary glands of cattle and pigs produces growth and other metabolic effects in laboratory animals, but it is virtually ineffective in man and monkeys. It has now been shown that growth hormone prepared from pituitary glands of monkeys and from human pituitary glands obtained at autopsy is effective metabolically in man and monkeys.

It should be mentioned that growth in fetal life, and for a brief period after birth, is not dependent to any great extent on the hormone.

Although the most evident effect of growth hormone is on cartilage growth in the epiphyseal plates, this hormone also has a widespread effect on almost all kinds of cells, so that in this case the concept of specific target cells seems scarcely applicable. At least some of its effects appear to be mediated by growth-promoting peptides referred to as *somatomedins*.

Lactogenic Hormone (Prolactin). During pregnancy several hormones are required to cause the mammary glands of the female to grow and develop, as will be described in the next chapter. When a baby is born, the mother's mammary glands are large enough to supply it with adequate milk. However, a particular stimulus is required for the glands to begin secreting milk and to continue performing this function. This stimulus is provided by a hormone called *lactogenic hormone*, or *prolactin*, which is made by the pars anterior of the pituitary gland by cells that are believed to secrete large amounts of it at the termination of pregnancy. Thereafter they continue to secrete this hormone in quantities as long as the offspring is fed at the breast. Lesser amounts are secreted during pregnancy; this probably assists in causing the breasts to develop.

Lactogenic hormone has been prepared in crystalline form by White and his associates. In addition to stimulating milk secretion, it arouses maternal behavior in the individual exposed to its action; it will even do this if it is injected into males. It induces broodiness in hens.

In fowl, where the young are fed in part with the epithelial debris that desquamates from the lining of the crop gland of the mother, administration of lactogenic hormone has been found to increase greatly the rate of epithelial proliferation of the thick lining epithelium of the gland. Indeed, the effect of lactogenic hormone on the crop gland of the pigeon constitutes an assay method for this hormone.

The lactogenic hormone will be discussed further in the next chapter in connection with the mammary gland.

The Trophic Hormones. In addition to growth hormone and lactogenic hormone, the pars anterior secretes other hormones, each of which stimulates the growth and function of one particular endocrine gland; for this reason they are termed *trophic* (Gr. *trophe,* to nourish) hormones. (Some authors substitute the less appropriate spelling *tropic* for *trophic*.)

Four trophic hormones have been identified and are named according to the particular gland they affect: (*1*) thyrotrophin (TSH for thyroid-stimulating hormone), which affects the thyroid gland; (*2*) adrenocorticotrophin (ACTH), also called corticotrophin, which affects the cortex of the suprarenal (adrenal) glands; and (*3*) and (*4*) two gonadotrophins, follicle-stimulating hormone (FSH) and luteinizing hormone (LH). Both gonadotrophins are produced in females and also in males, and discussion of their actions on the gonads of the two sexes will be postponed to the next two chapters. The endocrine gland affected by a particular trophic hormone is referred to as its *target gland*. Thus the thyroid gland is the target gland for TSH (thyrotrophic hormone), and so forth.

In order to describe how trophic hormones control growth and secretory activities of cells of their respective target glands, and how the concentrations of the hormones of the target glands control the secretory activities of the respective cells of the anterior lobe of the pituitary that secrete trophic hormones, we must now explain *feedback inhibition*.

A simple type of feedback inhibitory mechanism operating to control the secretion of an endocrine gland was described in Chapter 15, where it was pointed out that it is the level of calcium ions in the blood plasma that controls the secretory activity of cells of the parathyroid gland. If there is too little calcium in the blood, cells of the parathyroid gland secrete more parathyroid hormone and this acts to raise the blood calcium level. If there is too much calcium in the blood, the activity of the parathyroid gland is suppressed (feedback inhibition).

With regard to at least some of the trophic hormones, the secretory activity of the cells secreting them is suppressed if the amount of the hormone of the target gland with which they are concerned rises above its normal level in the blood. Likewise, if there is not enough of the target hormone in the blood, the cells that produce the trophic hormone stimulating that target gland secrete more trophic hormone. For example, secretion of female sex hormone by the ovaries of women decreases very substantially after they reach menopause. The cells of the anterior pituitary secreting the trophic hormone that stimulates female sex hormone secretion in the ovaries immediately respond to this by secreting more trophic hormone. There is so much of this trophic hormone in the

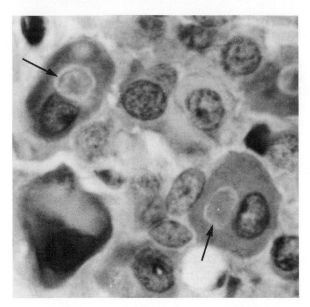

Fig. 25-5. Photomicrograph of cells in anterior pituitary (rat), stained with PAS and hematoxylin. The cytoplasm of the cells that secrete glycoprotein hormones is deeply stained by the PAS reaction. Negative Golgi images are indicated by arrows. (Courtesy of Y. Clermont)

blood that it escapes into the urine. Hence, if one injects some urine from an older woman into an immature female mouse it will cause the mouse to prematurely produce female sex hormone.

It was at first thought that interaction between target hormone and the cells that make the trophic hormone concerned was direct. But with increasing knowledge about hormone-releasing factors from the hypothalamus it appears that the negative feedback mechanisms may act via the hypothalamus, or at least in cooperation with it. In other words, it may be that too much hormone from a target gland decreases release of the hormone-releasing factor that controls secretion of the trophic hormone concerned. However, the situation is complicated, because feedback mechanisms are not always negative and also some releasing factors are inhibitory instead of stimulatory. Furthermore, the secretion of releasing factors is influenced and in some cases controlled by afferent nerve impulses reaching the hypothalamus. We shall deal with this topic later.

The Melanocyte-Stimulating Hormone (MSH). Whether this should be classed as a true anterior lobe hormone is unsettled. In certain fish and amphibia it is undoubtedly produced in the pars intermedia. But the pars intermedia is not very well developed in man and so it has been suggested that the cells of the pars intermedia that produce MSH may have migrated into the pars anterior.

In man MSH has been shown to stimulate formation of melanin pigment and its dispersion in melanocytes. Molecules of MSH and ACTH contain some similar amino acid sequences and it seems probable that both hormones are made by the same cell type in man. It has been established that both ACTH and MSH can cause increased pigmentation in man, but as yet the respective roles of these two hormones in patients with increased pigmentation is not clearly established.

Having named and described some effects of the anterior lobe hormones, we shall now turn our attention to the cells that produce them.

How Different Hormones Were Traced to Different Cells by Light Microscopy

After it became known that giantism or acromegaly was due to the anterior pituitary secreting extra growth hormone, and that this was often due to a tumor in that gland, the anterior pituitary of those afflicted in this way was studied histologically. The anterior lobe commonly showed overgrowth of acidophils, strongly suggesting that acidophils secrete growth hormone.

Next, acromegaly in women is occasionally associated with persistent lactation; this is termed *galactorrhea* (Gr. *galaktos,* milk; *rhoia,* flow). This at first suggested that the cells producing growth hormone may also produce lactogenic hormone. Furthermore, the pituitary glands of women during later stages of pregnancy and in the several weeks following childbirth contain increased numbers of lightly granulated acidophils (these were originally termed *pregnancy cells*).

The Types of Acidophils. The question then arose whether the same acidophils secrete both growth and lactogenic hormones, or whether there are two separate types of acidophils secreting two different hormones (with the reason for two hormones being secreted by acidophil tumors being that differentiation into both types may occur in tumors). When this was investigated by means of staining methods, it was found that erythrosin and orange G would distinguish between the two cell types clearly (the granules of cells that produce prolactin stain with erythrosin and those of cells that produce growth hormone stain lightly with orange G). The EM has permitted a distinction to be made between the two types of acidophils according to the size and variation of size of the granules they contain, as will be described shortly. Hence the type of acidophil that secretes growth hormone is termed a *somatotroph* and that secreting lactogenic hormone, a *mammotroph.*

The Types of Basophils. The problem of distinguishing different kinds of basophils and correlating the various types with different functions has been even more difficult.

First, it became established from chemical studies that whereas growth hormone and lactogenic hormone are *proteins,* the trophic hormones—TSH, FSH and LH—are *glycoproteins.* Accordingly, since the PA-Schiff method specifically stains certain reactive carbohydrate groups present in glycoproteins, it could be expected to stain the granules of any of the basophils producing these three types of glycoprotein hormones, and indeed it was found that it does (Fig. 25-5). The Gomori method also distinguishes clearly between acidophils and basophils (see Plate 25-1, *bottom left*).

Further attempts were then made at using stains to distinguish subtypes of basophils, but there always was the problem of relating particular hormones to the stained cells. Information had to be gathered from clinical and a variety of experimental sources and fitted together with what could be determined by special staining, immunofluorescence technics, and electron microscopy to arrive at our present state of knowledge.

It is now considered that the kind of basophil that makes TSH, and which is therefore termed a *thyrotroph,* is a large cell of irregular shape which, after PA-Schiff staining combined with aldehyde thionin, reveals blue-purple granules. The cells that make FSH and LH are rounded rather than angular, and their granules with the combined PA-Schiff and aldehyde thionin technic are roughly intermediate between red and blue, while the cell that makes ACTH and MSH retains the red color and does not take up any blue. As already noted, there are similarities in amino acid sequence between MSH and ACTH, and this makes it less certain that there are two distinct cell types producing these two hormones. Indeed, there is some uncertainty as to whether FSH or LH can be made by the same cell. It is difficult to distinguish two distinct types of gonadotrophs.

In the foregoing we have explained what special staining and light microscopy achieved in tracing different anterior pituitary hormones to different cell types. We shall now describe how studies with the EM provided further information.

THE FINE STRUCTURE OF CHROMOPHILS AND THEIR MECHANISM OF SECRETION

These subjects have been investigated in depth by Farquhar, on whose findings most of the following account is based; her papers should be read for further information.

Distinguishing Different Types of Chromophils

The EM permits the size and shape of various cells of the anterior lobe to be ascertained more accurately than does the LM. Furthermore, the size and shape of the granules they contain are revealed so clearly that different types of chromophils can be recognized, at least by experts, by the kind of granules they contain. For those who wish to have the details, which are included here for reference only, the granules of mammotrophs (the chromophils believed to secrete lactogenic hormone) have a maximum diameter of around 400 to 700 nm. and are somewhat irregular in shape (Fig. 25-7); those of somatotrophs (which secrete growth hormone), 300 to 400 nm. (Fig. 25-9); those of gonadotrophs, 200 to 250 nm. (Fig. 25-10); those of thyrotrophs, 140 to 200 nm. (Fig. 25-11); and those of corticotrophs (the cells that secrete ACTH), 100 to 200 nm. Comment on the size and shape of the cells that synthesize and secrete these different types of granules will be given later.

Mechanism of Secretion in Mammotrophs

The mammotroph is favorable for studying secretion because its secretory activity can be manipulated readily. Furthermore, the formation and secretion of its granules can be followed easily because of their distinctive features. As shown in Figure 25-7 they are large and dense and often of irregular shape. This is in contrast to the granules of certain other chromophils—for example, those of somatotrophs, which are somewhat smaller and more evenly spherical (Fig. 25-9).

As shown in Figure 25-6, the process of synthesis and mechanism of secretion of granules of mammotrophs are similar to those of zymogen granules described in detail in Chapter 5 and illustrated in Figure 5-21. Prolactin is a protein hormone. Its synthesis begins as shown in Figure 25-6 (*1*) by amino acids being linked by polyribosomes of the rER so that the assembled product enters cisternae of rER as indicated by (*2*) in Figure 25-6. By means of transfer vesicles the assembled product is carried to the forming face of a Golgi stack and, when this saccule has reached the maturing face of the stack, a vesicle containing mature protein hormone buds off from the saccule (Fig. 25-6, *3*). Small secretory vesicles of this type fuse with one another to make larger vesicles (Fig. 25-6, *4* and *5*). A larger secretory vesicle approaches the cell membrane, whereupon its surrounding membrane fuses with the cell membrane as described in Chapter 5 and illustrated in Figure 5-32. The membrane then opens to the surface at the site where the two membranes fused so that the naked granule is discharged by *exocytosis* (Figs. 25-6 and 25-7).

As shown in the diagram (Fig. 25-6), the granule enters an ill-defined pericapillary space between the cell border and the basement membrane of the capillary. The granule or its substance penetrates the basement membrane and capillary wall so that the hormone gains entrance to the circulation.

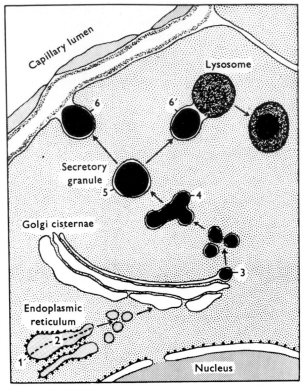

Fig. 25-6. Schematic diagram of the process of hormone secretion by mammotrophs of the anterior pituitary (rat). Prolactin is synthesized on ribosomes (1), segregated and transported by rER (2), and concentrated into granules in the Golgi. Small granules arising from the Golgi (3) aggregate (4) to comprise the mature secretory granule (5). During active secretion, the latter fuse with the cell membrane (6) and their contents are discharged into a perivascular space by exocytosis. When secretory activity is suppressed and the cell must dispose of excess hormone, granules fuse with lysosomes (6′) and are degraded as depicted in Figure 25-8. (Farquhar, M. G.: Mem. Soc. Endocrinol., *19:*79, 1971)

Suppression of Secretion. When the infant ceases to breast feed the stimulus for continued mammatroph function no longer exists. Farquhar found that although secretory granules continued to accumulate over the first 12 to 18 hours, their numbers soon began to decrease. Furthermore, lysosomes became apparent and could be seen fusing with and hence destroying granules (Figs. 25-6 and 25-8). The latter figure shows two lysosomes, the upper a multivesicular body and the lower a dense body, which contain remnants of secretory granules.

Somatotrophs

The fine structure of a somatotroph is illustrated in Figure 25-9, which shows its parallel cisternae of rER, Golgi saccules, some mitochondria, and an abundance of specific granules somewhat smaller and much more regularly rounded than those of mammotrophs. The mechanism of synthesis and secretion of granules is the same as in mammotrophs and the granules similarly enter a pericapillary space.

The effect of suppression is not so easily studied as in mammotrophs but here, too, it seems that lysosomes dispose of excess granules. Farquhar notes that in somatotrophs, removal of excess granules by lysosomes results in the formation of myelin figures, which were illustrated in Figure 5-41. It is not known what components of somatotroph granules could lead to their formation.

Gonadotrophs

As noted, the functions of gonadotrophs will be considered in the next two chapters. In contrast to mammotrophs and somatotrophs, which synthesize and secrete protein hormones, the granules synthesized and secreted by gonadotrophs are glycoprotein. The functioning gona-

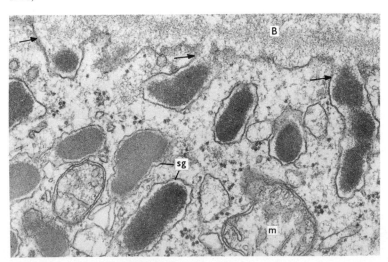

Fig. 25-7. Electron micrograph (×42,000) of a portion of a mammotroph in the anterior pituitary of a lactating rat, showing secretory granules (sg) facing a perivascular space and undergoing discharge by exocytosis. The membranes of several granules is in continuity with the cell membrane where indicated by arrows. B, basal lamina of capillary endothelium. (Farquhar, M. G.: Mem. Soc. Endocrinol., *19:*89, 1971)

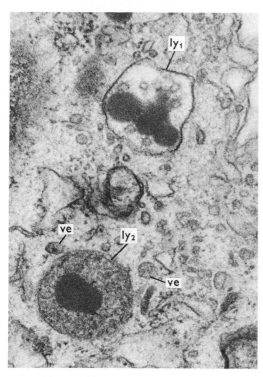

Fig. 25-8. Electron micrograph of a portion of a mammotroph in the anterior pituitary of a lactating rat, 1 day after separation from its suckling young, showing secondary lysosomes. A multivesicular body (ly₁) is seen as well as a dense body (ly₂). The small vesicles (labeled ve) that have a finely granular content are probably primary lysosomes. (Farquhar, M. G.: Mem. Soc. Endocrinol., *19*:91, 1971)

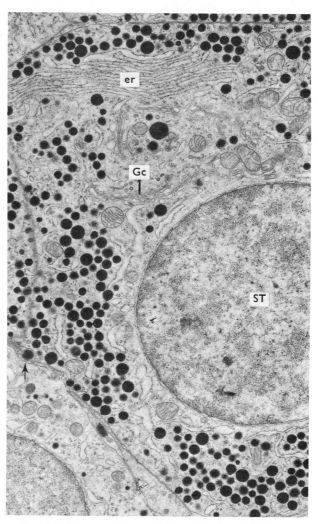

Fig. 25-9. Electron micrograph (×6,900) of part of a somatotroph (ST), or growth hormone-producing cell, in the anterior pituitary of a growing rat. As well as abundant round secretory granules (diameter 300 to 400 nm.), the cell shows a Golgi region (Gc) and cisternae of rER (er). (Farquhar, M. G.: Mem. Soc. Endocrinol., *19*:97, 1971)

dotroph of the female rat is a rounded cell with some rER and a centrally disposed Golgi apparatus (Fig. 25-10). The granules are rounded and vary somewhat in size with the largest being somewhat smaller than those of mammotrophs or somatotrophs. Moreover, gonadotrophs may contain larger dense droplets of glycoprotein (dr in Fig. 25-10) in addition to granules.

There are probably two types of gonadotrophs, one secreting follicle-stimulating hormone (FSH) and another secreting luteinizing hormone (LH). The mechanism of secretion in gonadotrophs is similar to that in other basophils but, in the nonpregnant female, as will be described in detail in the next chapter, the secretory activity of both types of gonadotrophs follows a cyclical rhythm during the years between puberty and menopause.

Effects of Castration. The functions of the gonadotrophic hormones (FSH and LH) are to stimulate the sex glands so as to bring about development and maturation of germ cells and secretion of sex hormones. Under ordinary cir-

cumstances there is a negative feedback arrangement whereby increased levels of sex hormones in the blood prevent the gonadotrophs from oversecreting. However, if the sex glands are removed so that they can no longer produce sex hormone, this inhibitory effect on gonadotrophs is lost and, as a consequence, they work harder and oversecrete. This is usually studied by castrating female animals and if this is done the gonadotrophs become considerably larger. Studies with the EM have shown that this is due largely to a great development of the rER, the cisternae of which become dilated. The Golgi also be-

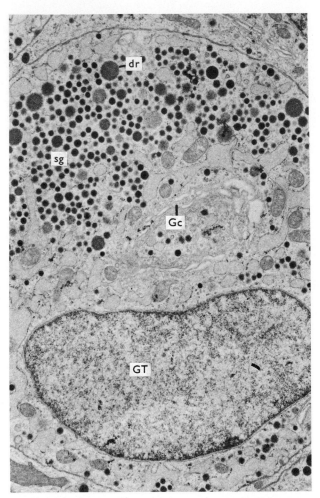

Fig. 25-10. Electron micrograph (×5,450) of a portion of a gonadotroph (GT) in the anterior pituitary of a female rat. Note its rounded contours, rER, Golgi region (Gc), and content of secretory granules (diameter 200 to 250 nm.). The cell also contains a few dense droplets (dr). (Farquhar, M. G.: Mem. Soc. Endocrinol., *19*:101, 1971)

comes more prominent and the number of granules in the cytoplasm increased.

Thyrotrophs

The secretion of thyrotrophs is a glycoprotein hormone (TSH) that controls the activity of the follicular cells of the thyroid gland which, in turn, secrete the thyroid hormones, to be described shortly.

With the EM thyrotrophs present angular contours (Fig. 25-11) and the granules they contain are of a smaller size range than in any of the other chromophils considered, having a maximum diameter of from 150 to 200 nm.

The mechanism of secretion of these granules seems to be the same as that described for other chromophils.

The secretion of TSH is normally controlled by the level of thyroid hormone in the blood through the negative feedback mechanism already described. Hence it is relatively easy to study stimulation or suppression of secretion in thyrotrophs, the former by removing the thyroid and the latter by administering thyroid hormone to the animal involved.

When the thyroid gland is removed, thyrotrophs become greatly enlarged and Farquhar describes this as being due chiefly to a ballooning of the cisternae of rER with material of moderate electron density. However, this increased synthesis is not reflected in an increase of granules for reasons not yet understood.

As noted, secretion by thyrotrophs is easily suppressed by giving an animal extraneous thyroid hormone. Suppression is due to a negative feedback mechanism for if thyroid hormone is given an animal from which the thyroid gland has been removed, the factor stimulating the thyrotrophs is removed and the thyrotrophs revert to their normal appearance, with the product of the rER being increasingly processed by the Golgi and normal granules being formed.

THE PARS TUBERALIS

Although this is an upward extension of the pars anterior, it has a different microscopic structure. The cells it contains are roughly cuboidal and contain no cytoplasmic granules. Their cytoplasm is diffusely and mildly basophilic. The pars tuberalis is fairly vascular. Its function, if any, is unknown.

THE PARS INTERMEDIA

This is not nearly as well developed in man as in many animals. In man, what is often interpreted as the pars intermedia consists chiefly of (*1*) an irregular row of follicles that contain a pale-staining colloidal material and are made of pale cells (Fig. 25-12) and (*2*) a few rows of moderate-sized cells with strongly basophilic granular cytoplasm (Fig. 25-12, *middle*). (The granules disappear very quickly unless fixation is prompt.) These cells may extend into the pars nervosa (Fig. 25-12, *upper right*).

In certain species (for example, fish and amphibia) the cells of the pars intermedia produce the *melanocyte-stimulating hormone* (MSH), also known as *intermedin*. As noted, it is not clear in man whether MSH is made by the same cells that make ACTH. Furthermore, it appears that the cell or cells making these hormones in man are basophils of the anterior lobe. The suggestion that in man

Fig. 25-11. Electron micrograph (×6,400) of a thyrotroph from the anterior pituitary of a rat. Note its angular contours and secretory granules (diameter 150 to 200 nm.), smaller than those of the surrounding somatotrophs (ST). It contains a small Golgi apparatus (Gc) and relatively little rER (er). Secretory granules (sg) arise from Golgi saccules (arrows, *top right inset*), and are released by exocytosis (*inset, bottom left*). (*Bottom left inset*) Several secretory granules are being discharged by exocytosis at the arrows. B indicates the basal lamina. (Farquhar, M. G.: Mem. Soc. Endocrinol., *19:*105, 1971)

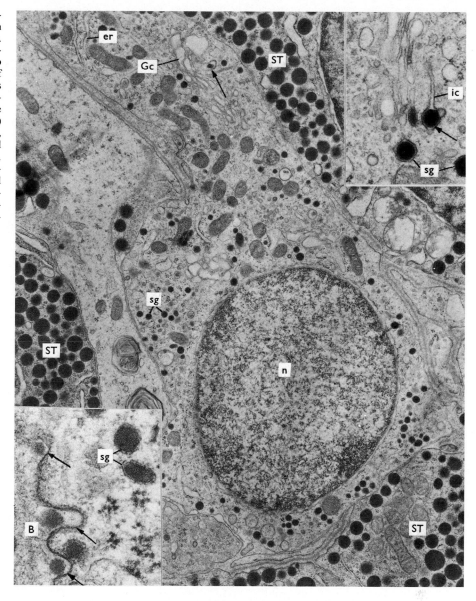

these cells may have migrated from the pars intermedia into the anterior lobe seems reasonable.

HOW HORMONE-REGULATING FACTORS MADE BY HYPOTHALAMIC NEURONS REACH SECRETORY CELLS OF THE ANTERIOR LOBE TO REGULATE THEIR SECRETORY ACTIVITIES

Regulation of secretory cell activity in the anterior lobe by nerve cells of the hypothalamus is made possible by the anterior lobe receiving some of its blood by way of what is termed the *hypophysioportal* (or *hypothalamo-hypophysioportal*) *circulation*. To describe this regulation further we must describe the blood supply of this region, which is derived from the superior hypophyseal arteries.

The superior hypophyseal arteries, of which there are several, originate from the circle of Willis. They approach the gland both as an anterior group and as a posterior group of vessels (Fig. 25-13).

The arteries of the *anterior* group penetrate the upper part of the pars tuberalis (Fig. 25-13) and, in general, turn downward. As they pass downward toward the anterior lobe, they give off numerous branches. The uppermost of

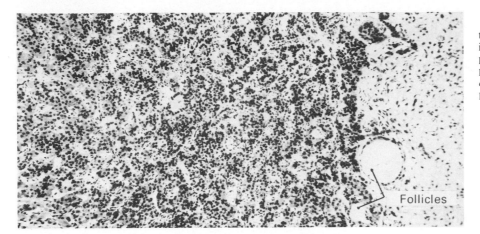

Fig. 25-12. Low-power photomicrograph of a part of the pituitary gland extending from the pars anterior (*left*) through the pars intermedia (*middle* and *middle right*) into the pale-staining pars nervosa (*right*).

Follicles

Pars anterior   Pars intermedia   Pars nervosa

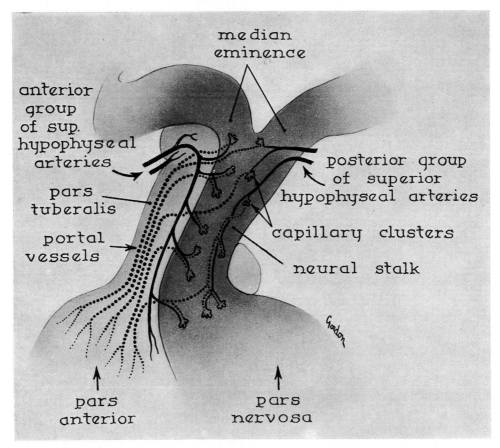

Fig. 25-13. Diagram of the blood supply of the hypophyseal stalk. The course of arterial blood is indicated by solid lines and that of venous blood by dotted lines. (After Green, J. D.: Anat. Rec., *100:*273, 1948)

these pass into the region of the median eminence (Fig. 25-13), and the ones at lower levels pass into the neural stalk (Fig. 25-13). All of these vessels end in clusters of tortuous wide capillaries. Green describes the arterial vessels and the capillary clusters in which they terminate as being enclosed in a curious connective sheath. The capillary clusters empty into venules that run back in the same sheaths toward the pars tuberalis (Fig. 25-13, dotted lines), where they join with one another to form larger venules (Fig. 25-13, dotted lines). These then pass down to empty into the sinusoidal capillaries of the anterior lobe of the gland. Since the venules that drain the capillary clusters of the median eminence and the stalk contain venous blood that then empties into a second capillary bed, they constitute a *portal* system, a term with which the student should already be familiar from studying the portal circulation in the liver.

The *posterior* group of superior hypophyseal arteries penetrates the posterior aspect of the stalk (Fig. 25-13). The upper branches from these supply the median eminence, and the lower branches supply lower levels of the stalk. Here again the branches end in clusters of tortuous wide capillaries that, together with the vessels that supply and drain them, lie in a connective tissue sheath. The venules from these capillary clusters pass anteriorly to the pars tuberalis (Fig. 25-13, dotted lines) to drain down into the pars anterior: hence these venules also constitute a part of the hypophysioportal system.

There appear to be no connections other than capillary anastomoses between the median eminence and the remainder of the hypothalamus. Therefore, the hypophysioportal circulation is concerned not with delivering blood from the bulk of the hypothalamus to the pars anterior but with delivering blood from the median eminence and the neural stalk into the pars anterior. According to Green, the portal circulation is not involved in draining blood from the pars nervosa into the pars anterior.

Hormone-regulating factors are produced by nerve cell bodies in *different parts* of the hypothalamus. The axons of these nerve cells end in the median eminence or possibly the neural stalk, where the regulating factors *enter the capillaries* that drain into the anterior lobe. However, not all the blood that reaches the pars anterior from the superior hypophyseal arteries has to pass through capillary clusters in the median eminence and/or stalk because some arterial branches pass directly down the pars tuberalis to the pars anterior (Fig. 25-13).

The pituitary gland also receives blood from the inferior hypophyseal arteries. This provides the chief blood supply for the posterior lobe and also arterial blood for the pars anterior. However, there is no evidence that blood from this source enters the hypophysioportal system so we need not describe it in any more detail here.

HORMONE-REGULATING FACTORS

Lest confusion arise we should make it clear at the outset that the term *hormone-regulating factor* is used here with specific reference to factors that regulate the secretory activities of cells of the *anterior lobe* of the pituitary gland. Furthermore, it has been shown that these factors are synthesized in the bodies of neurons and pass down their axons to be liberated beside capillary clusters (just described), where they are absorbed. They are then carried to the anterior lobe by the bloodstream where, in passing along the sinusoidal capillaries of the anterior lobe, they exert their effects on the secretory cells. However, this was not all learned immediately. Two important findings helped establish that there are hormone-regulating factors acting on the anterior lobe, as will now be described.

Development of Knowledge. It has already been noted that the pituitary consists of two lobes and we shall shortly go on to consider the posterior lobe. It was known long ago that two hormones could be extracted from the posterior lobe: these are called *vasopressin* and *oxytocin* and their roles in the body will be described presently. What is relevant here is that it was at first thought that the hormones of the posterior lobe were actually made *in* the posterior lobe. But in due course it was found that they were formed in neurons with cell bodies in the supraoptic and paraventricular groups of neurons (neuroanatomists refer to such groups of neuronal cell bodies as *nuclei*); the position of these nuclei is indicated in Figure 25-14. From the cell body of such neurons the hormone travels down the axon to the posterior lobe, where arrangements exist for it to be absorbed into capillaries.

Next, the cells in the hypothalamus that produce *neurosecretions* are also fully functional nerve cells. They synapse with other neurons and their axon propagates nerve impulses. Since they are not only nerve cells but also secretory cells, they are termed *neurosecretory* cells.

Meanwhile observations had been made that suggested that secretory cells of the anterior pituitary were to some extent under nervous control. Since no nerve fibers could be found leading to them that would explain this control, some other explanation had to be found. For example, one of the trophic hormones produced by gonadotrophs of the anterior lobe is luteinizing hormone (LH) and, as will be described in the next chapter, one effect of LH is to cause any ripe ovarian follicles in the ovary to rupture and so release their ova into the oviducts, where they would be available for fertilization should the female at that time mate (in women usually only one ovum is released). It was observed that during summer a female virgin rabbit generally is in a continuous state in which there are several ripe follicles available for rupture in its ovaries. However, they require LH to make them rupture. It was next noted that if such a female mated, even with a sterile male, the follicles ruptured. It was therefore evident that afferent nerve impulses set up from the act of coitus must somehow have stimulated the secretion of LH by cells of the anterior pituitary gland and in due course it was shown that this was due to afferent nerve impulses being relayed to the hypothalamus and causing secretion of a regulating factor. What is perhaps even more interesting is that some virgin female rabbits will ovulate if there is a male rabbit in their immediate vicinity. Furthermore, an LH surge (a prerequisite for ovulation) can be elicited by electrically stimulating the hypothalamus. It is becoming clear that many derangements of the menstrual cycle in women (to be described in the next chapter) result not from ovarian or pituitary failure, but rather from malfunction of hypothalamic nerve circuits that, in part, determine the patterns of secretory activity of the neurosecretory cells concerned.

Another example of pituitary function being affected by mental activity is provided by stress. Psychological situations in which people may find themselves may cause mental stress. It has already been mentioned that in certain situations an individual may experience the emotions of rage or fear and that under these conditions the body becomes geared for fight or flight; this is due to the sympathetic division of the autonomic nervous system being stimulated. Sympathetic stimulation brings about many functional changes in the body that may indeed be of temporary help for fighting or running away but, if long continued, eventually cause undesirable symptoms. However, in addition to activating the sympathetic division of the autonomic nervous system, stress can also cause the hypothalamus to liberate more of the releasing factor that causes the cells making the trophic hormone ACTH to liberate more of it and this, in turn, causes the cortex of the adrenal gland to liberate more hydrocortisone. As we shall see later, this has a variety of metabolic effects. This is an example of how stress can cause changes in the function of certain endocrine glands. With continued stress the histological picture in many endocrine glands becomes altered; as a matter of fact, this is one reason why many endocrine glands obtained from autopsies of persons who have died after long illnesses are not suitable for students needing to study them so as to learn about their normal histological structure.

Releasing and Inhibiting Factors (Hormones)

It is now conceded that hormone-regulating factors produced in the hypothalamus and released into the capillaries of the hypophysioportal system affect the various secretory cells of the anterior lobe as follows. The secretory cells of the anterior lobe are: mammotrophs, somatotrophs, gonadotrophs, thyrotrophs, corticotrophs, and, in some species at least, melanotrophs. The hormone-regulating factors (often called hormones) that stimulate or inhibit release of their respective hormones are generally designated by initials: PRF for *prolactin-releasing factor,* and PIF for *prolactin-inhibiting factor;* GRF for *growth hormone-releasing factor,* and GIF for *growth hormone-inhibiting factor* (which is also called *somatostatin*); FRF for *follicle-stimulating hormone-releasing factor;* LRF for *luteinizing hormone-releasing factor;* TRF for *thyrotrophin-releasing factor;* CRF for *corticotrophin-releasing factor;* MRF for *melanocyte-stimulating hormone-releasing factor,* and MIF for *melanocyte-stimulating hormone-inhibiting factor.* (Where these factors are referred to as hormones, the letter H is used in place of F, as, for example, in CRH, for *corticotrophin-releasing hormone.* The terms *factor* and *hormone* are used interchangeably with regard to hormone-regulating factors.)

The effects of the trophic hormones and their hormone-regulating factors will be dealt with in the remainder of this chapter in connection with the thyroid and adrenal glands, and in the following two chapters in connection with the reproductive systems of the female and the male.

Where Are Hormone-Regulating Factors Formed?

Whereas the locations of the cell bodies of the neurosecretory cells that produce the two hormones liberated by the posterior lobe of the pituitary gland are well known, as shown in Figure 25-14, those that elaborate the regulating factors for the cells of the anterior lobe are not easy to localize and the axonal pathways from these cells to the capillaries of the median eminence remain ill defined. As mentioned, the neurosecretory cells controlling the secretory activities of the anterior lobe release regulating factors from their axon terminals into perivascular areas of the median eminence and the pituitary stalk, and these vessels then carry the factors to the anterior pituitary. The neurosecretory cells producing hormone-regulating factors appear to extend throughout the periventricular hypothalamus and even into nonhypothalamic regions of the brain, such as the parolfactory area and septum pellucidum. In contrast to the neurosecretory cells of the supraoptic and paraventricular nuclei, which produce the two posterior lobe hormones, the hypothalamic cells suspected of producing the hormone-regulating factors are usually small, do not exhibit specific membrane-bound granules, and do not form distinct groups; instead they are dispersed among other cell types. This is well illustrated in the case of the cells elaborating luteinizing hormone-releasing factor (LRF), as will now be described.

Now that some of the hormone-regulating factors have been isolated and purified, specific antisera can be raised against them that are suitable for localizing the hypothalamic cells that make these factors. By this means it was found that in man and monkeys the neurosecretory cell bodies producing LRF form a loose continuum extending right from the anterior limits to the posterior limits of the hypothalamus, but more concentrated in the preoptic area (anterior) and medial basal hypothalamus. Thus the neurosecretory cells elaborating LRF appear to be interspersed with other types of neurons throughout the hypothalamus. Furthermore, there is overlap between the distributions of LRF-secreting neurons and neurosecretory cells making other regulating factors, for example, growth hormone-inhibiting factor (somatostatin). Thus at least some of the neurosecretory cells interspersed among LRF-secreting neurons constitute other components of what is known as the *hypophysiotrophic neurosecretory system,* meaning the entire system of neurosecretory cells that produces the various factors regulating anterior pituitary function. But the matter is even more complex.

Color Plate
25–1

Plate 25-1. Illustrations of some representative parts of the pituitary gland. (*Top, left*) Neurosecretory cell of paraventricular nucleus of hypothalamus, showing neurosecretory granules and Nissl substance in its cell body (stained with luxol fast blue and cresyl violet). (*Center, left*) Anterior pituitary (stained by the method of Ezrin and Wilson). Acidophils are a yellow-orange color. Two types of basophils are seen, red and purple. The distinction between chromophobes and chromophils is not as distinct as with most stains. (*Bottom, left*) Anterior pituitary (Gomori stain). Acidophils are red, basophils light blue-purple. (*Top, right*) Posterior lobe of pituitary (Gomori stain). Note the terminal branchings of an axon, with neurosecretory material around them. A Herring body is also present. (*Bottom, right*) Posterior lobe of pituitary (Gomori stain). The termination of an axon, with an accumulation of neurosecretory material around it, is seen beside a capillary (into which the neurosecretion would pass).

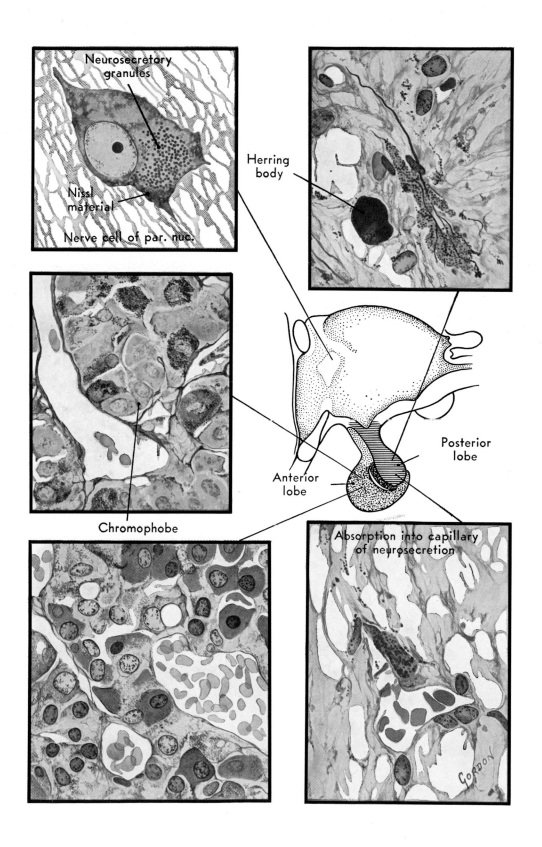

Neurosecretory granules

Nissl material

Nerve cell of par. nuc.

Herring body

Chromophobe

Anterior lobe

Posterior lobe

Absorption into capillary of neurosecretion

GORDON

Further Putative Roles of Hormone-Regulating Factors

The LRF cells located more anteriorly in the preoptic region appear to send their axons to a cluster of capillaries in the vicinity of the lamina terminalis (organum vasculosum of the lamina terminalis). It is not clear, however, whether this neurovascular structure has anything to do with the regulation of LH secretion by the anterior pituitary gland. In fact, some of the hormone-regulating factors may actually be involved in activities other than hypophysiotrophic regulation. For instance, there is evidence that TSH-releasing factor (TRF), which has been found in many regions of the brain, may function as a neurotransmitter in addition to its role in regulating TSH. Conversely, other substances such as dopamine, which is known to function as a neurotransmitter, may also serve as hypophysiotrophic factors. Dopamine is released from perivascular axon terminals in the median eminence and there is good evidence that it inhibits prolactin secretion at the level of the anterior pituitary gland. In fact, many neuroendocrinologists now equate dopamine with the previously identified prolactin-inhibiting factor (PIF). Moreover, hypophysiotrophic factors have been isolated from cerebrospinal fluid (CSF), and the ependymal epithelium lining the median eminence and stalk has been shown to transport a variety of substances injected into CSF to the hypophysioportal blood. Hence it is thought that hormone-regulating factors may pass through the ependymal epithelial cells lining the roof of the median eminence to enter the primary capillary plexus of the portal system of the pituitary gland. It is evident, therefore, that the hypophysiotrophic neurosecretory system is complex and, thus far, difficult to define.

Some of the hormone-regulating factors have been isolated and characterized as small peptides. LRF, for example, is a decapeptide of known amino acid sequence. Synthetic preparations of this factor are now in wide use both in the research laboratory and in the clinic. Almost nothing is known, however, about certain other regulating factors, such as corticotrophin-releasing factor (CRF).

Conclusion

The foregoing account provides insight as to why the anterior lobe of the pituitary gland develops, and remains, so closely associated with the hypothalamus. It also explains how the nervous and endocrine systems, both of which are concerned with drives and emotions, are intimately linked together and hence able and likely to affect one another's functions.

THE PARS NERVOSA (NEUROHYPOPHYSIS)

The pars nervosa of the pituitary gland is involved in the endocrine system in an unusual way, for it does not contain the cell bodies of the nerve cells whose hormones enter the blood passing through it. Their cell bodies, as noted, are located in *supraoptic* and *paraventricular nuclei* (groups of nerve cell bodies) in the hypothalamus (Fig. 25-14). Hence the hormones are synthesized in these nuclei. There are two posterior lobe hormones produced in the cell bodies of these nerve cells, antidiuretic hormone (ADH, also known as *vasopressin*) and *oxytocin*. Antidiuretic hormone is elaborated by neurosecretory cells in the supraoptic nuclei and oxytocin by

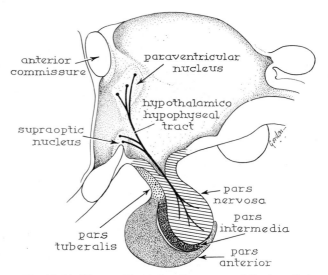

Fig. 25-14. Diagram illustrating the course of the hypothalamo-hypophyseal tract. This tract of fibers is involved in the secretion of ADH and oxytocin by neurosecretory cells with cell bodies in the supraoptic and paraventricular nuclei of the hypothalamus. The hormones are released from the axons of these cells into the pars nervosa of the pituitary gland. The cells secreting hormone-regulating factors are also present in the hypothalamus, but their location is diffuse and their axons are intermingled.

cells of the paraventricular nuclei. However, it seems that in each of these nuclei there are some cells making the other hormone. Nevertheless, none of the cells makes both hormones. From the cell bodies the hormones pass down axons in the hypothalamo-hypophyseal tract into the pars nervosa (Fig. 25-14), where the axons terminate in association with capillaries (Plate 25-1, *top right* and *bottom right*).

Development of Knowledge About Its Endocrine Functions. It was known for a long time that a disease, *diabetes insipidus,* could result from lesions of the pars nervosa. (This is a very different disease from "sugar" diabetes, which will be described later in this chapter.) Diabetes insipidus is characterized by copious production of urine of low specific gravity. For many years it was believed that this disease was due to failure of the pars nervosa to make a hormone called *antidiuretic hormone.* If this is not produced in sufficient quantities, the distal convoluted and collecting tubules of the kidney do not absorb their proper share of glomerular filtrate; hence the volume of urine is many times greater than normal.

However, there were some puzzling aspects about the condition. It was known, for example, that the disease could be caused by injuries to the hypothalamus and also by interrupting the nerve tract that leads from the hypothalamic nuclei to the pars nervosa (Fig. 25-14). Never-

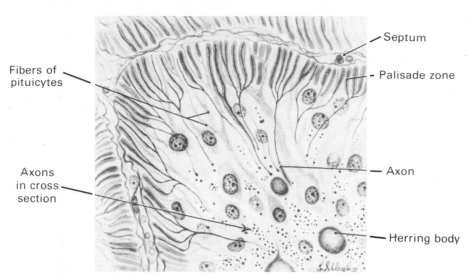

Fibers of
pituicytes

Axons
in cross
section

— Septum

- Palisade zone

— Axon

— Herring body

Fig. 25-15. Diagram of the organization of the pars nervosa in the pituitary gland of the opossum. (Bodian, D.: Bull. Johns Hopkins Hosp., *89*:354, 1951)

theless, the disease could be alleviated by means of extracts prepared from pars nervosa. Hence it was incorrectly assumed that the antidiuretic hormone was made by the pars nervosa and that the pars nervosa required proper innervation from the hypothalamic region to make its hormone.

Next, when extracts of pars nervosa were injected into animals, they were found to cause smooth muscle to contract or develop increased tonus. The hormone causing these effects was termed *oxytocin* (Gr. *oxys*, swift; *tosos*, labor) or *pitocin*, and, as its name implies, it acts chiefly on the smooth muscle of the wall of the uterus where its action facilitates childbirth. Oxytocin is also released under the stimulus of nursing (or milking), and acts by causing the myoepithelial cells surrounding milk-secreting alveoli of the mammary glands to contract; this causes them to express the milk they contain into the duct system of the breast. Both hormones are peptides.

Although both hormones could be extracted from the pars nervosa, it was puzzling that its microscopic structure was not typical of an endocrine gland. However, in due course it became established that the hormones extracted from the pars nervosa are not made there, but in the bodies of nerve cells in the paraventricular and supraoptic nuclei, and reach the pars nervosa by passing down axons in the hypothalamo-hypophyseal tract (Fig. 25-14), in the form of granules containing proteins known as *neurophysins* as well as the hormone. Hence, if the hypothalamo-hypophyseal tract is interrupted, the neurosecretion cannot reach the pars nervosa to enter the bloodstream and reach the kidneys, and diabetes insipidus may develop.

By means of chrome alum hematoxylin staining, neurosecretory granules have been observed in hypothalamic nuclei in every species studied, including man. In mammals they are very small granules (Plate 25-1, *top, left*). The nerve cells that produce them possess all the ordinary features of nerve cells, including Nissl bodies in their cytoplasm (Plate 25-1, *top, left*).

Microscopic Structure of the Pars Nervosa. In most species this lobe of the pituitary does not exhibit well-organized structure. However, in the opossum Bodian has shown that the pars nervosa is divided into lobules by septa; the latter contain many small blood vessels, and it is into these that most of the neurosecretion is delivered (Fig. 25-15). The more central part of each lobule is made up chiefly of bundles of fibers of the hypothalamo-hypophyseal tract. With suitable staining, fine granules of neurosecretion can be seen in these nerve fibers. From the middle of each lobule the fibers approach the septum surrounding the lobule. Near their termination each is coated with a cylindrical wrapping of neurosecretory substance that is absorbed from the end of the cylinder into the blood vessels of the septa. Bodian terms the zone of cylinders that abuts on the septa the *palisade zone* (Fig. 25-15).

In the middle of each lobule the nuclei of *pituicytes* can be seen (Fig. 25-15). Pituicytes are a type of neuroglial cell and serve a supporting function. Their cytoplasmic processes extend out between the cylinders of neurosecretory material in the palisade zone (Fig. 25-15).

Granules that stain darkly with the Gomori technic, known as *Herring bodies*, are seen in the pars nervosa (Plate 25-1, *top right*, and Fig. 25-15). These are probably terminal bulb formations of axons of the hypothalamo-hypophyseal tract that end within the substance of the pars nervosa, and in which there are accumulations of neurosecretory material.

Fig. 25-16. Electron micrograph (×30,000) showing, in the upper part of the micrograph, several bulbous neurosecretory axon terminals (at) in the pars nervosa of the pituitary gland of a rat. Note their abundant neurosecretory granules (sg); small smooth-surfaced vesicles (sv) and mitochondria (m) are also present. Processes of pituicytes (Pp) are seen closely associated with the axon terminals and also with a capillary at *lower left;* one process abuts on a basal lamina (B) lying between the axon terminals above and a perivascular space (pvs) below. On the other side of this space lies another basal lamina (B₁) surrounding the endothelium (E) of a capillary (which is fenestrated). The white space seen at *bottom left* is the lumen of the capillary. (Paterson, J. A., and Leblond, C. P.: J. Comp. Neurol., *175*:373, 1977)

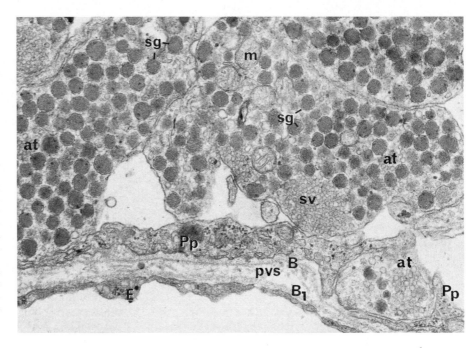

It seems probable that the microscopic structure of the pars nervosa of other species is basically similar to that in the opossum, but not organized so clearly into lobules. Neurosecretory material from axon terminals is absorbed into blood vessels that are more irregularly disposed (Plate 25-1, *bottom, right*).

In the EM, expanded axon terminals in the pars nervosa of hypothalamic neurosecretory cells appear as illustrated in Figure 25-16. When such cells are stimulated in the hypothalamus, stored granules of neurosecretion (sg in Fig. 25-16) are released from their axon terminals and the secretory product passes through the perivascular space (pvs in Fig. 25-16) to enter the lumen of a capillary (seen at *bottom left* in Fig. 25-16). The cell body of a neurosecretory cell in the supraoptic nucleus was illustrated in Figure 17-13.

THE THYROID GLAND

Gross Features. This gland was called *thyroid* (Gr. *thyreos,* an oblong shield; *eidos,* form) because it is shaped like a shield (Fig. 25-17). It has two lobes of highly vascular glandular tissue joined together by an *isthmus* (Fig. 25-17). The isthmus lies over the second and the third cartilaginous rings of the trachea. The two lobes, for the most part, lie anterior and lateral to the trachea, just below the larynx, but their upper parts extend for a short distance up its sides (Fig. 25-17).

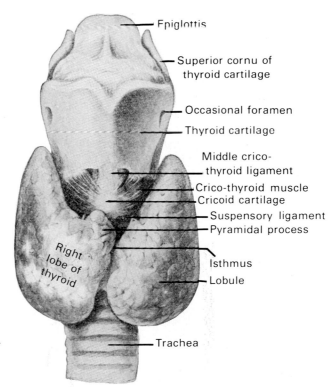

Epiglottis

Superior cornu of thyroid cartilage

Occasional foramen

Thyroid cartilage

Middle crico-thyroid ligament

Crico-thyroid muscle

Cricoid cartilage

Suspensory ligament

Pyramidal process

Isthmus

Lobule

Right lobe of thyroid

Trachea

Fig. 25-17. Drawing illustrating the anatomical relation of the thyroid gland to the trachea and larynx (anterior view). (Huber, G. C.: Piersol's Human Anatomy. ed. 9. Philadelphia, J. B. Lippincott, 1930)

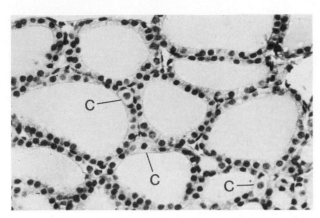

Fig. 25-18. Low-power photomicrograph of a portion of the thyroid gland of a normal dog. Note the low cuboidal follicular cells and the three larger C cells (also know as parafollicular or light cells).

MICROSCOPIC STRUCTURE OF THE THYROID GLAND AS SEEN WITH THE LM

The gland is covered with two capsules. The outer one is continuous with and is part of the pretracheal fascia, which in turn is part of the deep cervical fascia. The inner capsule is to be regarded as the true capsule of the gland. It consists of fibroelastic connective tissue and sends septa into the gland, providing internal support and carrying blood vessels, lymphatics, and nerves into its substance. The septa divide the gland into lobules, the limits of which may be dimly apparent on the surface of the gland (Fig. 25-17). However, the septa do not join with one another so as to delimit entirely separate lobules of tissue; hence the thyroid is not truly lobulated but pseudolobulated.

The Follicles of the Gland. Figure 7-29 illustrates how a clump of cells in an endocrine gland can become a follicle, with secretion stored in its lumen. Follicles are the units of structure of the thyroid gland, and the secretion they contain is called *colloid.* Each follicle is therefore not only a structural unit but also a functional unit. In the thyroid there are no cords of secretory cells, as there are in many endocrine glands.

In a normal thyroid gland the follicles vary from being irregularly rounded to tubular in shape, measuring from 0.05 to 0.5 mm. in diameter. In a section they appear to vary even more in size, due to the fact that in cutting a section the knife passes through the centers of some follicles, the edges of others, and so forth. Follicles whose edges are merely shaved by the knife appear as solid circles of cells.

There are probably about 30 million follicles in the human thyroid, packed together in a delicate reticular network that contains an extensive capillary bed. How-

ever, this does not appear to advantage in ordinary sections because the blood is squeezed out of most of the capillaries.

Each follicle is surrounded by a basement membrane. However, there are apertures in the basement membranes of adjacent follicles where the neighboring follicles are in contact. This feature makes it difficult to outline follicles and count them accurately.

Colloid. The material contained within the follicles, after fixation, appears as a structureless, acidophilic material (Fig. 25-18). However, in sections of fixed tissue, the colloid often shrinks away from the follicular epithelium and presents a scalloped outline. This is particularly true when the gland is very active (Fig. 25-22). Furthermore, the colloid, when hardened by fixative, shows a tendency to break up into even strips when sections are cut. Colloid before fixation is a viscous homogeneous fluid. It consists of a glycoprotein called *thyroglobulin.* Because of the carbohydrate content of the thyroglobulin, colloid, like the basement membrane around the follicle, is PAS-positive.

Thyroglobulin is synthesized by the ordinary cells of follicles and secreted into the lumina of follicles. Its further fate and iodination will be described presently.

The Two Types of Hormone-Secreting Cells in the Thyroid Gland

(*1*) The great majority (about 98 per cent in the rat, for example) are follicular epithelial cells; normally, these form a low cuboidal epithelium. These cells produce and resorb the colloid (thyroglobulin) in the follicle. They are usually called *follicular cells.*

(*2*) The other cells of the thyroid are known as *light, parafollicular* or *C cells.* They are larger and have paler cytoplasm than the low cuboidal epithelial cells.

Light cells are seen in the low-power illustration, Figure 25-18. Despite their appearance in this low-power photomicrograph, as may be seen in Figure 25-24, these cells are actually situated on the outer aspect of the wall of a follicle so that they do not abut on its lumen. Hence they are always separated from colloid by follicular cells. These cells have nothing to do with producing or absorbing the constituents of colloid. As will be described later, they secrete a completely different hormone and develop from a different source.

DEVELOPMENT OF KNOWLEDGE ABOUT THE HORMONES MADE BY FOLLICULAR CELLS OF THE THYROID

The first clue about the function of the thyroid was that a small number of people developed what was called *myxedema* because their connective tissues—for example, that of their skin—become thickened with a firm type of edema (*myxo* refers to the edema fluid being mucoid). Such individuals would become somewhat obese, tend to lose their hair, become slow of speech and mentally and physically sluggish. When they died, it was found at autopsy that their thyroid glands had either atrophied or were absent or destroyed for some reason. Subsequently, it was found that babies born without a thyroid or with an incompetent thyroid became dwarfs and did not develop mentally. This latter condition is termed *cretinism.* So it was recognized that thyroid secretion affects the general metabolism of the body, and it became possible to treat both myxedema and cretinism with extracts of thyroid glands. Later, Kendall extracted from thyroid glands an iodine compound in crystalline form which he termed *thyroxine,* and subsequently Harington and Barger determined its composition and accomplished its synthesis.

Throughout recorded history people have developed greatly enlarged thyroids, called *goiters.* The fact that thyroxine (the hormone of the gland) contains iodine indicated that a basic cause of goiter might be a deficiency of iodine in the food and water in many parts of the world. Surveys of the iodine content of water and the distribution of goiter supported this view. For example, some of the areas close to the Great Lakes in North America proved to be iodine-deficient. Eventually it became customary to add iodide to common salt. That people do not now so commonly develop goiters is an example of one of the many advances in medical knowledge that everyone now takes for granted.

The work of Gross led to the discovery of a second hormone secreted by the thyroid follicular cells that in general has the same kind of action as thyroxine but is more potent. It is termed *triiodothyronine.*

One of the first effects learned about the thyroid hormone was that it played an important role in determining the rate of metabolism in body cells. However, ascertaining the basal metabolic rate of a person gives only indirect information about the functioning of his thyroid gland. As will be explained presently, there are more direct methods for establishing this.

Hypothyroidism and Hyperthyroidism. Disorders of thyroid function may result in under- or overproduction of thyroid hormone. These conditions are termed *hypothyroidism* and *hyperthyroidism,* respectively. Both can vary in severity. These terms apply only to the metabolism-affecting hormones, thyroxine and triiodothyronine.

STEPS IN THE SYNTHESIS AND RELEASE OF THYROID HORMONES STUDIED BY THE EM AND RADIOAUTOGRAPHY

Two important components in thyroid hormones are (*1*) the amino acid tyrosine and (*2*) iodine. However, the formation of the hormone is not brought about by a one-step process whereby tyrosine is linked directly to iodine. Tyrosine is first incorporated into glycoprotein molecules as *tyrosyl* radicals. Iodide brought to cells also has to be altered. First we shall deal with the process whereby thyroglobulin is formed in follicular cells and secreted into the lumina of follicles. To study this process Nadler and his associates used labeled leucine, an amino acid that, like tyrosine, is incorporated into glycoprotein molecules.

(1) Formation of Thyroglobulin. This process, as described by the above-mentioned investigators, is typical of the synthesis and secretion of glycoproteins in that the amino acids are incorporated into polypeptide at cisternae of rER (Fig. 25-19). The polypeptide portion of thyroglobulin is synthesized as subunits and these combine to form the whole protein. Meanwhile, carbohydrate side chains are added in stepwise fashion. The mannose component is added to the subunits soon after their synthesis, probably within the rER. Galactose is added in the Golgi apparatus (Fig. 25-19, G) at about the time the subunits combine to form thyroglobulin. Finally, the glycoprotein is packaged into small secretory vesicles (sg in Fig. 25-19) and transported to the luminal surface of the cell, where the content of the vesicles (now termed apical vesicles, av in Fig. 25-19A) is discharged into, and so becomes part of, the colloid.

(2) Uptake of Iodine by Follicular Cells and Iodination of Tyrosyl Radicals in Thyroglobulin Molecules. The cells of thyroid follicles have a unique ability to trap iodide. As noted, the thyroid gland has an extremely rich capillary blood supply, and hence much blood courses by follicular cells, which manifest a remarkable ability to extract iodine from it. If radioactive iodine, for example, is injected into an individual, it is picked up and concentrated in the thyroid very quickly.

Perhaps through the action of a peroxidase enzyme, the iodide taken up by follicular cells from the blood is converted to *iodine,* which becomes bound to the *tyrosyl* radicals of the glycoprotein molecules (thyroglobulin). The place where iodination of tyrosyl radicals of thyroglobulin molecules occurs can be explored by giving animals radioactive iodine and examining radioautographs made at different times after it was given. Studies with the LM and EM show that silver grains, which of course indicate incorporation of labeled iodine, are first seen not in cells but *in the colloid,* near the luminal border of the follicular cells (Fig. 25-20A). Soon after, they are found *throughout the colloid* (Fig. 25-20B). So the *iodination* step in the formation of thyroid hormone occurs *in the colloid.*

(3) Breakdown of Thyroglobulin and Release of Thyroid Hormones. The next and final step in the formation of thyroid hormones involves proteolysis of thyroglobulin molecules with the release of its component amino acids. The mechanism by which the breakdown of thyroglobulin occurs is as follows.

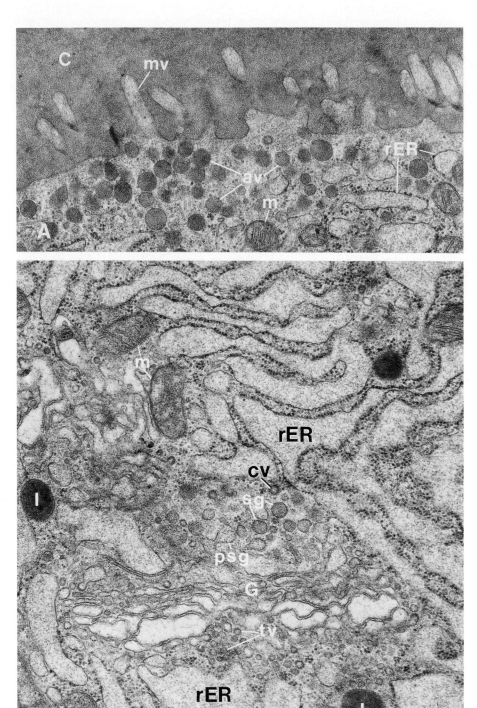

Fig. 25-19. Electron micrographs of two representative regions of a follicular cell of the thyroid. (*A*) The apical surface of the cell, which borders the colloid (C); this surface has microvilli (mv) on it. Note also the apical vesicles (av) containing material with the same electron density as the colloid. (*B*) The organelles involved in the secretion of thyroglobulin. Distended cisternae of rER, where newly synthesized protein is being segregated, are prominent, particularly at *top*. This protein is being transported by transfer vesicles (tv) to the Golgi (G), where most of the carbohydrate groups are being added to the glycoprotein secretion. Prosecretory granules (psg) that bud from the last Golgi saccule go on to become secretory granules (sg) and eventually apical vesicles (as seen in part *A*). A coated vesicle (cv), some dense bodies that are probably lysosomes (l), and some mitochondria (m) are also present. (Haddad, A., Smith, M. D., Herscovics, A., Nadler, N. J., and Leblond, C. P.: J. Cell Biol., *49:*856, 1971)

The luminal surface of follicular cells in contact with the colloid sends out narrow pseudopodia to enclose small amounts of colloid; the colloid droplets thus formed are brought into the cytoplasm (Fig. 25-21A) by phagocytosis. Within the cytoplasm the membrane-surrounded droplets fuse with lysosomes, and after digestion by their enzymes the droplets break down and release thyroid hormones. This sequence of events is readily seen shortly after a single injection of TSH (the thyrotrophic hormone secreted by the anterior pituitary), which enhances *thyroglobulin breakdown* and therefore hormone release (*see* below).

We should emphasize that all the processes involved in synthesis and secretion of thyroid hormones take place continuously and simultaneously; that is, at the same time as synthesis of glycoprotein is going on in the follicular cells, there is also its secretion into the colloid, its iodination there, and finally intracellular breakdown of the iodinated thyroglobulin. The net result is a continuous release of thyroid hormone. By chance, some newly formed thyroglobulin molecules in the lumen may break down as soon as they are formed, while others may survive longer. The faster the gland is working, the less is the turnover time of the thyroglobulin molecules in the follicles.

FACTORS AFFECTING THE HISTOLOGY OF THE THYROID GLAND

In the embryo, thyroid follicles are small because they have little colloid in their lumina. During growth, the thyroid gland increases in size because all the components of its follicles increase in size and also because of occasional formation of new follicles. In the young, when the follicles are small, the gland has a uniform appearance. However, with age, *considerable variation* appears in the size of follicles. In old age, previously spherical follicles often take on an irregular shape.

The Effects of TSH

The histological appearance of the thyroid gland is profoundly affected by TSH. After hypophysectomy, for example, the follicular cells become less active and change in appearance. Without the stimulus of TSH the cells gradually change from cuboidal to squamous, and their nucleus flattens.

These changes are reversed by giving TSH. The effects of this hormone are to (*1*) augment the iodide-accumulating ability of follicular cells, (*2*) increase the rate of synthesis and secretion of glycoprotein into the colloid, (*3*) increase the rate of iodination of glycoprotein in the colloid, and (*4*) increase the rate of breakdown of thyro-

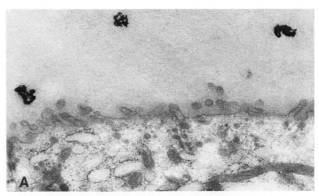

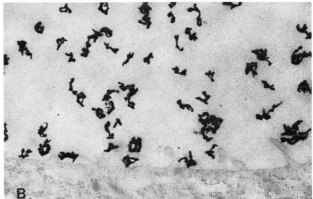

Fig. 25-20. Electron micrographs of parts of the apical surfaces of thyroid follicular cells after radioautography; the thyroid glands were obtained from two animals injected with radioactive iodine. (*A*) From a follicle 2 minutes after injection. The few silver grains (black squiggles) lie over the colloid and hence indicate that iodination of thyroglobulin is commencing in the colloid fairly close to the apical border of the cell. (*B*) From a follicle 12 hours after injection. Note that the grains are now more numerous and distributed widely throughout the colloid. (Courtesy of H. van Heyningen)

globulin and the liberation of thyroid hormones. Morphologically, the effect of TSH is to (*1*) increase the size of the follicular cells, (*2*) decrease the volume of colloid, and (*3*) increase the number of intracellular colloid droplets.

How Dietary Iodine Intake Can Affect the Histology of the Thyroid — Parenchymatous and Colloid Goiter

A low iodine diet provides too little iodine for the thyroid to make adequate amounts of hormone. As a result of decreased thyroid hormone in the blood, the anterior pituitary begins to secrete increased levels of TSH. This stimulates the cells of the thyroid follicles so that they secrete and grow in the ways just described. As a result of increased activity, including thyroglobulin breakdown to form thyroid hormone, the colloid content of

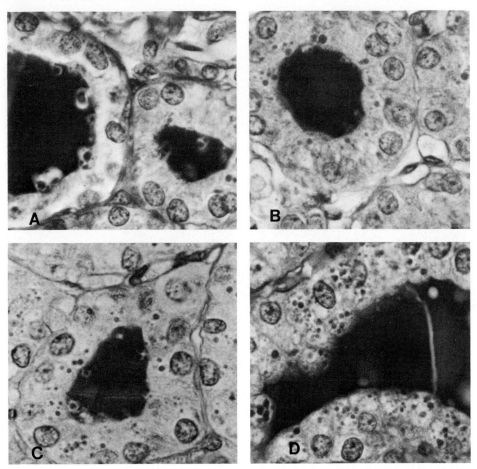

Fig. 25-21. Photomicrographs (×1,000) of representative follicles of the thyroid gland (stained PAS), taken at various times after giving an animal TSH. (*A*) After 8 minutes. Note colloid droplets (dark) being taken up from the lumen by pseudopodia of follicular cells. (*B*) After 12 minutes. Colloid droplets are now evident in the apical cytoplasm of the cells. (*C* and *D*) After 30 minutes and 4 hours, respectively. Droplets of colloid have now reached the basal parts of the cells, and are disintegrating. (Nadler, N. J., Sarkar, S. K., and Leblond, C. P.: Endocrinology, *71:*120, 1962)

the follicle becomes reduced, and the colloid itself becomes thin and pale-staining (Fig. 25-22). As a result of stimulation of growth, the epithelial cells of the follicles become taller and increase in number by division, that is, undergo both hypertrophy and hyperplasia. The follicles thus have thicker walls and are composed of far more cells than before (Fig. 25-22); this is reflected in an increase in the size of the gland as a whole, although as the follicles grow they lose most of their colloid, there being little within them to keep them distended. As a consequence, their walls become collapsed and infolded to a considerable extent. Since enlargement of the gland is due chiefly to an increase in number and size of follicular epithelial cells (the parenchymatous cells of the gland) and not to an increased amount of colloid, the enlarged gland that results from thyrotrophic stimulation is termed a *parenchymatous goiter.* Before the days of iodized salt such goiters were common in many regions. Probably because the body's demands for thyroid hormones are greater at certain times, such as at puberty and during

pregnancy, parenchymatous goiters are more likely to develop at those times than others.

Parenchymatous goiter can be thought of as a physiological response to a lack of iodine. It is not a spontaneous disease state of the thyroid and not in itself a cause of hyperthyroidism (described below).

From a Parenchymatous to a Colloid Goiter. On the assumption that a parenchymatous change has developed to some degree in an individual at a time when supplies of iodine were not adequate for the amount of hormone needed—for example, at puberty—and that subsequently either the needs for thyroid hormone became less, or more iodine was taken in the diet, the microscopic appearance of the thyroid would change once more. With lessened demand for hormone, or with more iodine with which to make hormone, the gland would be able gradually to raise the concentration of thyroid hormone in the bloodstream. As the concentration of hormone rises, secretion of TSH by the pars anterior is gradually suppressed. With lessened thyrotrophic stimu-

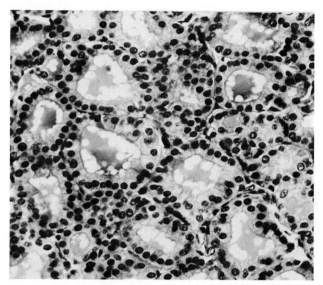

Fig. 25-22. Low-power photomicrograph of a portion of the thyroid gland of a dog given injections of anterior pituitary extract containing TSH. This is the typical appearance of a *parenchymatous goiter.*

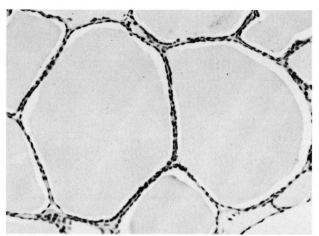

Fig. 25-23. Medium-power photomicrograph of a small area of the thyroid gland in a case of simple *colloid goiter.*

lation, the follicular cells would then revert to their former state; instead of being high cuboidal or columnar, they would become low cuboidal again (Fig. 25-23). Since the follicles would no longer be stimulated to secrete so much hormone into the bloodstream, they would be able to make and store more thyroglobulin within their follicles, and as a result the follicles would increase in size (Fig. 25-23). Further, since follicles, as a result of preceding proliferation, would have more cells in their walls than before, they would become much larger than before when they were distended with colloid. As a result, the gland as a whole would become larger than when it was primarily a parenchymatous goiter. Further, since its increased size would now be due primarily to its large content of colloid (instead of parenchyma as previously), it would now be termed a *colloid goiter* rather than a parenchymatous goiter (compare Figs. 25-22 and 25-23).

Hyperthyroidism. Excessive secretion of thyroid hormones (*thyrotoxicosis*) occurs mostly in a disease called *exophthalmic goiter* (*Graves' disease*) or as a result of the development of little (generally benign) tumors called *toxic adenomas* in the thyroid gland. Hyperthyroidism is associated with clinical signs and symptoms that will be learned about in later courses. We should note here, however, that hyperthyroidism is hardly ever caused by excessive TSH stimulation. In exophthalmic goiter, so called because the eyes protrude, the thyroid has a histological appearance similar to parenchymatous goiter without excessive TSH secretion. In this condition there is a factor in the blood with an effect similar to TSH except that it acts more slowly and is more long lasting. It is termed LATS for *long-acting thyroid stimulator* and has been identified as an antibody. However, some doubt has been cast on its being the actual cause of the great activity in the thyroid. In thyroid adenomas, which are secreting tumors of the gland, the neoplastic follicular cells do not respond properly to hypothalamic-pituitary regulation and hence may secrete abnormally high levels of thyroid hormone, causing hyperthyroidism.

Drugs That Interfere With the Formation of Thyroid Hormones. It is now possible to treat patients with certain kinds of hyperthyroidism with drugs, most notably thiouracil, that prevent the thyroid gland from properly synthesizing thyroid hormone even if the diet contains adequate amounts of iodine. Therefore administration of thiouracil can cut down production of hormone by the gland and allay hyperthyroidism. It is of interest that thiouracil administered to a normal animal with adequate iodine intake will soon cause its thyroid gland to assume the microscopic appearance of a parenchymatous goiter. The explanation is self-evident.

Testing Thyroid Function. Thyroid hormones for the most part become linked to globulins in the blood. The iodine attached to protein (serum protein-bound iodine, abbreviated to PBI) can be measured, and its level gives an indication of the activity of the thyroid gland. However, there are conditions under which this can be misleading and methods enabling direct measurement of the levels of the two thyroid hormones in blood are becoming available. Furthermore, thyroid function can now be tested by measuring a patient's TSH response to thyrotrophin-releasing factor (TRF).

THE CASE OF THE SECLUDED ANTIGEN—AUTOIMMUNE DISEASE

This is described here, not just because of its medical interest but because it is, in our opinion at least, of general biological significance. As was explained on pages 333 to 335, immunological tolerance develops toward macromolecules to which a fetus (or, in many species, a newborn) is appropriately exposed.

However, if a fetus is to become tolerant to macromolecules that develop within it during fetal life, these macromolecules must gain entrance to the tissue fluid, lymph, or blood of the fetus, so that premature contact with precursors of B- and T-lymphocytes can bring about clonal abortion of any programmed to react to these macromolecules. As already explained, the period during which immunological tolerance can be induced ter-

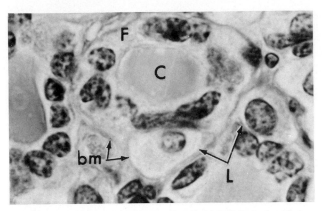

Fig. 25-24. Photomicrograph of a thyroid follicle (rat) with two light (or parafollicular) cells (L), one situated just *below center* and the other *right of center*. Note that the basement membrane (bm) of the follicle extends around the outside of the light cell *below center* so as to include this cell in the same follicle. Note also that the light cells are effectively separated from the colloid (C) by adjacent follicular cells. (Follicular cells are labeled F). Masson's trichome stain. (Young, B. A., and Leblond, C. P.: Endocrinology, *73:*669, 1963)

minates close to the time of birth. Accordingly, if any potential antigen forms in the fetus but is kept hidden from the tissue fluid, lymph, or blood, so that it does not come into premature contact with precursor cells of B- and T-lymphocytes, some will develop that are programmed to react against this antigen. Hence, if previously *secluded antigens* were to gain entrance to one of the fluids of the body and so make their presence known to cells of the lymphocyte series for the first time in postnatal life, it could be expected that lymphocytes would react against them as against any foreign antigen.

The colloid of the thyroid gland provides an example of a secluded antigen. Thyroglobulin is a glycoprotein secreted by follicular cells into the lumina of follicles, and under normal conditions this glycoprotein does not (as such) enter any of the fluids of the body. Accordingly, the body is unlikely to be immunologically tolerant to the glycoprotein in the follicles of its thyroid gland. An animal injected with an extract prepared from its own thyroid gland will react immunologically against it.

There is reason to believe that the development of autoimmunity against thyroglobulin (or its precursor) is a contributing factor to the development of a disease called *Hashimoto's disease.* In this disease the thyroid becomes enlarged, due primarily to its stroma becoming increased in amount and heavily infiltrated with lymphocytes and plasma cells, and even containing lymphatic nodules. The thyroid follicles become atrophic and contain little colloid, and thyroid function is generally impaired. Antibodies to thyroid proteins have been demonstrated in the blood of patients with this disease. Experimentally, it has been shown that if part of the thyroid of an animal is excised, disease can be produced in the remaining part by immunizing the animal with extracts prepared from the excised portion. Therefore Hashimoto's disease seems to have its origin in thyroglobulin (or its precursor) somehow gaining access to the stroma of the thyroid gland. It is not clear whether autoimmune disease of the thyroid is due primarily to humoral antibodies or whether it is cell-mediated, or both.

There are other examples of secluded antigens and autoimmune conditions arising from other causes.

CALCITONIN AND THE C CELLS OF THE THYROID

As noted at the beginning of this section, thyroid follicles contain two types of cells. The ordinary follicular cells and their activities have been described, so we can now discuss what have been variously termed *light, parafollicular,* or *C cells.*

The light cells are larger than the ordinary follicular cells (Figs. 25-18 and 25-24). As noted, they do not abut against the lumen of follicles, but are always separated from the lumen by follicular cells; this is why they were termed *parafollicular* cells. However, like ordinary follicular cells, they are situated on the inner aspect of the basement membrane that surrounds the follicle (Fig. 25-24). With the LM, clear cells in ordinary sections have pale cytoplasm. After suitable fixation the EM shows that the cytoplasm contains large numbers of secretory vesicles, the contents of which stain intensely, as seen in Figure 25-25. The content is considered to be *calcitonin,* a hormone that we shall now describe.

Development of Knowledge About Calcitonin

It has been known for a long time that blood calcium levels are controlled by a feedback mechanism operating between blood calcium and the cells of the parathyroid gland that secrete parathyroid hormone. If the blood calcium level begins to fall, the parathyroid gland is directly stimulated to secrete more parathyroid hormone, which probably acts almost immediately by stimulating resorptive activity of osteoclasts. The resulting bone resorption would liberate calcium to the blood.

It was assumed, probably correctly, that as soon as blood calcium reached normal levels the parathyroid gland would cease secreting hormone in extra amounts, so that the blood calcium level would not rise above normal limits. However, there can be other factors besides parathyroid hormone secretion that can cause the blood calcium level to rise, and furthermore substantial increase in blood calcium level can be harmful because it can cause calcium salts to precipitate into normal tissues. However, it was not ascertained until the 1960s that there is also a hormone that *lowers* blood calcium levels when they exceed normal limits, as will now be described.

One of the main reasons this second hormone took so long to be discovered is that the thyroid and parathyroid glands of most animals are anatomically very closely associated with each other, so as to form a complex. Indeed, they are supplied by the same arteries. So in experiments requiring removal of the parathyroids (particularly in rats, in which the parathyroids lie liter-ally buried in the thyroid) it was customary to remove the entire complex and to compensate for lost thyroid function in long-term experiments by administering thyroxine. Moreover, perfusion (through arteries) perfused both the thyroid and the parathyroid glands simultaneously.

The story of how calcitonin was discovered began with Copp and his associates finding from their experiments that when they raised the blood calcium levels, these levels fell again more rap-idly in animals in which the thyroid-parathyroid complex was kept *intact* than in animals from which the complex was re-moved. This suggested that a humoral factor was released from the complex that brought the blood calcium level down when it exceeded normal limits. Next, when a fluid with a high calcium content was used to perfuse the complex, the *blood calcium level* fell; but it did not fall if the complex was immediately removed. This indicated that when blood (or perfusing fluid) flowing through the gland complex had an elevated calcium content, the complex secreted a humoral factor that lowered the blood cal-cium level. This factor is now known to be the hormone *calci-tonin*.

At this time, of course, it was assumed that the thyroid gland was concerned only with producing iodine-containing hormones that affect the metabolic rate, and that the parathyroid glands were concerned with secreting a hormone that controlled cal-cium metabolism. It was natural enough for it to be assumed that calcitonin, since it affected calcium metabolism, was a second secretion of the parathyroid glands. But in the 1960s evidence was forthcoming that the hormone was in fact produced by cells in the *thyroid* gland, and, as a result, it became fashionable to refer to it as *thyrocalcitonin* instead of *calcitonin*. When it was realized that calcitonin was produced by the thyroid, it was at first assumed that it was made along with thyroxine and triio-dothyronine by the ordinary follicular cells. Then it was suggested that it might be the light cells that produced it and in 1967 Bussolati and Pearse demonstrated that fluorescent an-tibody to calcitonin stained light cells but not ordinary thyroid follicular cells. Pearse suggested that these cells, previously termed *clear* or *parafollicular* cells, should hereafter be termed *C cells* to indicate that they produce calcitonin.

The Embryological Origin of the C Cells of the Thyroid Gland

The thyroid gland develops from a downgrowth of en-dodermal cells from the floor of the pharynx into the neck. The cells that mark the course of the downgrowth constitute the thyroglossal duct. In man this normally atrophies and becomes obliterated, but some of its cells may remain, and these later in life may give rise to cysts.

The downgrowth of cells destined to form the bulk of the thyroid comes into contact with cells derived from certain of the five paired pharyngeal pouches that develop along each side of the pharynx. In man, the third pharyngeal pouches give rise to the epithelial component of the thymus and also to the inferior parathyroid glands, and the fourth pouches give rise to the superior parathy-roid glands. In man the parathyroid glands are associated closely with the thyroid and in certain animals (for ex-ample, rats) they are buried within its substance.

The cells of the fifth pharyngeal pouch (which is often

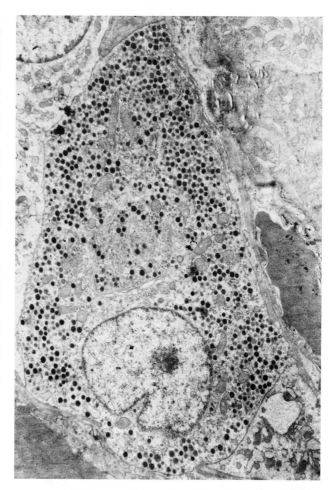

Fig. 25-25. Electron micrograph (×6,000) of a C cell (parafollic-ular or light cell) in the thyroid gland of a dog. Note its numerous dense calcitonin-containing secretory vesicles. The gray areas at *bottom left* and *middle right* are the lumina of capil-laries. Small portions of follicular cells lie at *top left*. (Courtesy of B. Young)

considered to be part of the fourth pouch) give rise to what is termed the *ultimobranchial body*. In fish, am-phibia, reptiles, and birds, the ultimobranchial bodies are separate glands. But in mammals the cells that grow out from the fifth pharyngeal pouch become intimately asso-ciated with the developing thyroid gland. It was suggested many years ago that these cells were the forerunners of the light cells of the thyroid gland. That this is indeed the origin of C cells was confirmed by Pearse and Cavalheira. So attention has been paid to obtaining ultimobranchial glands from large birds and fish, in which they are sepa-rate from the thyroid, and extracting calcitonin from them. There are indications that substantial amounts of calcitonin can be obtained this way.

Ways in Which Calcitonin Could Reduce High Blood Calcium Levels

It must always be remembered that in order to achieve any action whatsoever, a hormone must act on living cells of some type and affect their behavior in some way. Although calcitonin has been shown to exert many effects, its primary effect in causing elevated blood calcium levels to fall to normal limits would seem to be exerted on *osteoclasts*. For example, under conditions of increased levels of parathyroid hormone the numbers and activity of osteoclasts resorbing bone and thus elevating blood calcium levels are well known. Calcitonin acts to reduce the numbers and resorptive activity of osteoclasts under these conditions. It has been shown moreover that ruffled borders of osteoclasts are enlarged by parathyroid hormone and such borders are reduced to normal size by calcitonin (*see* Holtrop et al.).

The possibility of calcitonin stimulating the formation of bone has also been suggested. Calcium of course would be required for calcification of new bone, so if calcitonin did stimulate new bone formation this effect could slowly tend to lower blood calcium levels. However, a direct effect of calcitonin in stimulating new bone formation, which would require a specific effect on osteogenic cells and osteoblasts, has not been well established. It would be natural for new bone formation to follow after excessive stimulation of osteoclastic activity had ceased.

THE PARATHYROID GLANDS

Gross Features. There are usually four parathyroid glands in each person, but there may be more. They are so named because they lie *beside* the thyroid. More precisely, they are usually arranged two on each side, on the posterior side of the lobes of the thyroid gland, immediately outside the true capsule of the thyroid but inside its outer capsule of fascia. The upper parathyroids are about midway along the lobes, while the lower ones lie near the lower ends of the lobes. The upper ones are of a flattened ovoid shape, the lower ones roughly that of a flattened sphere. Their greatest diameter is slightly more than 0.5 cm. and they are yellow-brown when seen in the fresh state. Both upper and lower parathyroids are supplied from the inferior thyroid artery and these small glands can sometimes be found conveniently by tracing the arterial branches arising from the inferior thyroid artery to their terminations.

The numbers and sites of parathyroid glands vary with species. In the rat there are only two, and these lie buried in the substance of the thyroid gland, one in each lobe. In the dog parathyroid glands may sometimes be found as far down as the bifurcation of the trachea. Even in man, aberrant parathyroid glands are not uncommon, and if a tumor develops in one of these, it may be difficult to find.

Microscopic Structure as Seen With the LM. Each parathyroid gland is covered by a delicate connective tissue *capsule*. Septa from it penetrate the gland to carry blood vessels and a few vasomotor nerve fibers into its substance. The septa do not divide the gland into distinct lobules. Until a few years before puberty, only one type of secretory cell is found in the gland. This is termed the *chief (principal)* cell. It is smaller than the secretory cells of most endocrine glands; hence in the parathyroid glands the nuclei of the parenchymal cells are generally very close (*right* in Fig. 25-26). Granules are not seen in the cytoplasm of chief cells in H and E preparations, but some can be demonstrated by special staining. Although their cytoplasm is never very dark-staining, that of some chief cells is darker than that of others. Those with darker cytoplasm are called *dark chief* cells; and those with very pale cytoplasm, *light chief* cells. Some light chief cells have so little stainable substance in their cytoplasm that they are called *clear* cells. Part of the clear appearance of the light cells in H and E sections is due to their content of glycogen, which, of course, is not stained.

Although chief cells are smaller than cells of most endocrine glands, they are arranged in clumps and irregular cords that are wider than those of most endocrine glands. The cells within cords and clumps are supported by reticular fibers. Large capillaries are also present.

A few years before puberty, clumps of cells with much larger amounts of cytoplasm than chief cells make their appearance in the gland. In contrast to that of chief cells, the cytoplasm of these cells is acidophilic; hence the cells are termed *oxyphil* (Gr. *oxys*, acid) cells (Fig. 25-26, *left*). The easiest way for the student to find clumps of these is to look for sites where nuclei are more widely separated from each other than they are in areas of chief cells (Fig. 25-26). Such areas are more common in the periphery of the gland. Oxyphil cells are not nearly as numerous as chief cells, and they are not present at all in the parathyroid glands of most animals. In man, transitions between chief and oxyphil cells are commonly seen; since chief cells appear in the gland first, this suggests that oxyphil cells probably arise from chief cells. However, the function of oxyphil cells, if any, is unknown. One interesting feature is that they have very large numbers of mitochondria.

In the parathyroid glands of older people, occasional clumps of chief cells may form follicles and there may be considerable amounts of fat.

The Fine Structure of Chief Cells. The chief cells produce *parathyroid hormone*. Their cytoplasm, as shown in Figure 25-27, contains the usual content of mitochondria, as well as some rER. The Golgi apparatus is well developed (Fig. 25-27). The secretory granules have dense material in their middle and a pale rim between this and the surrounding membrane (Fig. 25-27); they are few in number. The chief cells do not seem to store granules of secretion to any extent.

DEVELOPMENT OF KNOWLEDGE ABOUT PARATHYROID GLANDS AND PARATHYROID HORMONE

Tetany. In the early 1920s it was found that if the parathyroid glands were removed from an animal, the animal would develop a condition called *tetany* (not to be confused with *tetanus,* which is an infection). Tetany is characterized by prolonged or convulsive contractile spasms of certain muscles. When it is very severe, spasms of muscles of the larynx or of those responsible for respiratory movements may cause death. Next, it became known that the immediate cause of tetany was inadequate concentration of calcium ions in the blood. Since the blood calcium level fell when the parathyroid glands were removed, it seemed obvious that the parathyroid glands were in some way helping to maintain a proper level of calcium in the blood. That the glands do this by producing a hormone, however, was not established until 1925, when Collip succeeded in making an extract of parathyroid glands that would raise the level of blood calcium in dogs from which the parathyroid glands had been removed, and so prevent tetany from developing in them.

Effects on Bone. The other classic way of investigating the action of a hormone is to observe what happens when abnormalities of the endocrine gland secreting it occur in man. It was found that at least some people developing nonmalignant tumors of the parathyroid glands (that it could be assumed would produce too much hormone) also developed a bone disease called *generalized*

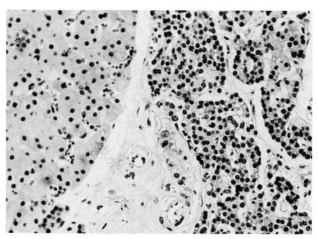

Fig. 25-26. Medium-power photomicrograph of a representative portion of a parathyroid gland. An area of oxyphil cells is seen at *left,* chief cells at *right.*

osteitis fibrosa in which there was an increased blood calcium level and widespread resorption of bone. The resorption was associated with the formation of much new intercellular substance of bone of poor quality and fibrous tissue, and the presence of many osteoclasts. Such bones were fragile, and indeed the presence of a parathyroid tumor, even though it was not obvious as a swelling, could be suspected if a patient had suffered one or two fractures with the degree of trauma involved not seeming sufficient to break a normal bone.

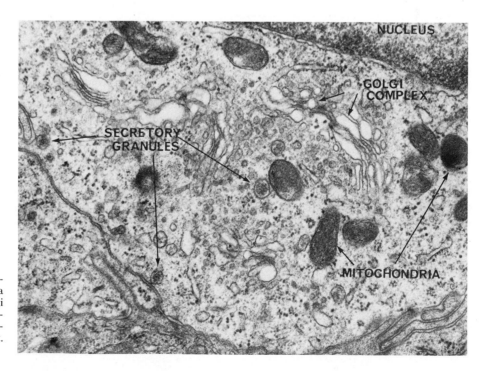

Fig. 25-27. Electron micrograph (×35,000) of a chief cell of a rat parathyroid gland. The Golgi is well developed, and a few secretory granules with dense material in their middle are present. (Courtesy of Dr. Nakagami)

From all the foregoing it was obvious that parathyroid hormone (PTH) had the effect of raising the level of the blood calcium. But it was difficult to establish whether this was a direct or indirect effect. This problem arose because there is an inverse relation between the levels of calcium and phosphate in the blood. Since it was shown that PTH, administered to normal animals, increased excretion of phosphate by the kidney, it could be argued that this was its primary effect and that a rise in blood calcium level resulted from the lowered phosphate level. It was also known that parathyroid glands tended to become enlarged in rickets. Moreover, it was shown that enlarged parathyroid glands could be produced in animals either by a low-calcium diet or by giving them injections of phosphate. So a case could be made for the parathyroid glands becoming enlarged in response to a low blood calcium level or to a high blood phosphorus level, and both views were entertained. In 1940, Ham et al. showed that (*1*) parathyroid enlargement did not occur in low-phosphorus rickets, but only in low-calcium rickets, and (*2*) it was possible to devise a diet to produce a relatively high blood phosphorus level while at the same time keeping the blood calcium at a normal level, and under these conditions parathyroid hyperplasia did not occur. The fact that the parathyroid glands proved to be responsive only to calcium and not to phosphorus suggested that PTH acts primarily on *calcium* and not on phosphorus metabolism.

It was, however, also argued that PTH became ineffective in raising blood calcium levels if the kidneys of an animal were removed, and that this showed that its primary action was on the kidneys, where it causes increased phosphate excretion. However, it was eventually shown by Grollman that if animals from which the kidneys had been removed were kept alive by peritoneal lavage, PTH would indeed raise their blood calcium levels.

Effects on Osteoclasts. With the general acceptance that the hormone had at least a *primary effect on blood calcium levels,* the next problem was to determine how and where PTH acted so as to cause calcium to be liberated into the blood. To investigate whether it had a direct effect on bone and somehow caused its resorption with the liberation of calcium, two experiments were done that threw light on this matter. In 1948 Barnicott, and in 1951 Chang, studied the effects of transplanting parathyroid glands in animals so that gland tissue would lie against the inner surface of a skull bone. For controls, they transplanted other glandular tissues to similar sites. Both investigations showed that parathyroid tissue, and only parathyroid tissue, exerted a local effect that resulted in marked resorption of the bone beside it. They both noticed, moreover, that *osteoclasts* appeared at the scene of the resorption. Although at that time there was uncertainty about whether the gathering of osteoclasts was the cause or an effect of bone resorption, Barnicott concluded from his experiment that parathyroid hormone was capable of stimulating osteoclastic resorption by direct action. A few years later the EM became available for histological studies and Scott and Pease described the ruffled cytoplasmic border of osteoclasts that thereafter became accepted as the means by which osteoclasts resorbed bone.

Moreover, further experiments revealed that PTH increased both the activity and number of osteoclasts engaged in resorbing bone. It was also shown with the EM that PTH increased the extent of the ruffled border of an osteoclast.

Other Concepts. It might be thought from all the above that the way PTH causes calcium to be liberated from bones into blood would be well established and generally accepted. But complications arose. First, many of the early experiments with PTH indicated it might have some effect on the cells that normally form bone. Next, it was thought that the increase in blood calcium level observed after administration of PTH was too rapid for it to be explained by PTH stimulating the resorptive activity and formation of osteoclasts. It is now evident that this concept is not necessarily true (*see* p. 406). Third, some histological studies seemed to suggest that after administration of PTH there were changes in osteocytes and in the intercellular substance that directly borders on them. As a result there was wide acceptance of a concept to the effect that PTH could cause calcium to be removed from bone, and do this quickly, by acting on *osteocytes* and causing them to exert a lytic effect on their adjacent intercellular substance. It was postulated that this effect liberated calcium that would pass out through canaliculi to some surface and gain entrance to capillaries, and so raise the blood calcium level. This view, which of course also hinges on bone being regarded as a storehouse for calcium, is still widely entertained (*see* p. 406).

Summary. We conclude first that for PTH to cause release of calcium from bone it must act on some type of cell. Second, for that cell to liberate calcium from bone matrix it must destroy calcified intercellular substance. Third, it is clear that this is what happens in the instance of osteoclasts since they have special equipment (ruffled borders) for performing this function. Fourth, it has been shown that they can perform this function quickly enough after PTH administration to account for the fairly rapid rise in blood calcium levels that follows. Fifth, when new bone is formed after an osteoclast has eroded bone, the new layer of bone can be distinguished from the old bone on which it is deposited by a cementing line. Successive rings of cementing lines are not seen around individual osteocytes to suggest they alternately resorb bone and then cover it with new bone. Finally, it is now accepted that osteoclasts are derived from a different cell lineage than are osteocytes — that they represent fusions of cells of the monocyte-macrophage series and hence have a very different origin than osteocytes. Although PTH may exert effects on osteogenic cells, osteoblasts, and osteocytes, it seems to us that they would be effects related to the normal functions of these cells in producing and maintaining bone intercellular substance, and that bone resorption ac-

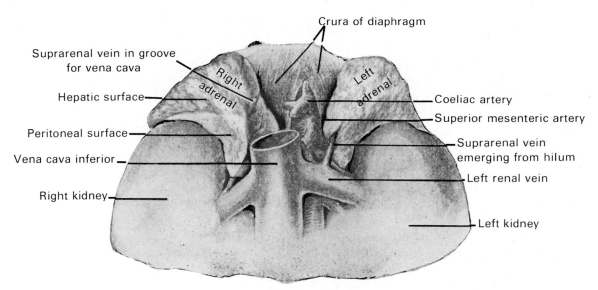

Fig. 25-28. Drawing of the anterior view of the paired adrenal glands. (Huber, G. C.: Piersol's Human Anatomy. ed. 9. Philadelphia, J. B. Lippincott, 1930)

tivated by PTH is mediated by osteoclasts, as described in Chapter 15.

NORMAL FUNCTION OF THE PARATHYROID GLANDS

The role of PTH amounts to promoting cellular activities that ensure the blood calcium is kept up only to normal levels. However, the usual way of ascertaining how the hormone does this is to study the effects of abnormally high levels of it in animals. A complication involved in this approach is that as soon as the blood calcium rises beyond normal levels, the C cells of the thyroid start secreting calcitonin so that the observer sees the combined effects of both hormones.

With regard to the normal role of the parathyroid, the extra PTH secreted in response to declining blood calcium levels can probably act in four different ways to restore calcium to normal levels. (*1*) It affects the kidneys so as to reduce loss of calcium to the urine. (*2*) It increases phosphate excretion by the kidneys; the reduction in blood phosphate tends to raise the blood calcium level. (*3*) Probably through interaction with vitamin D metabolites, it enhances calcium absorption from the intestine. (*4*) It stimulates the formation and resorptive activity of osteoclasts, inducing them to resorb bone matrix and thereby release its calcium to the blood.

In investigating the structure of the PTH molecule in relation to its biological effects, it seems that different fragments of the polypeptide molecule exert different kinds of effects.

THE ADRENAL (SUPRARENAL) GLANDS

Gross Features. The adrenal glands are paired, flattened yellow masses that lie, as their name implies, in contact with the upper surface of the kidneys (Fig. 25-28). The right gland—sometimes described as having the shape of a cocked hat—is wedged between the upper surface of the right kidney and the inferior vena cava; the left gland— roughly crescentic—occupies the medial border of the left kidney from top to hilum. Each gland is about 5 cm. long, 3 to 4 cm. wide, and somewhat less than 1 cm. in thickness. In many animals the adrenal glands, although situated close to the kidneys, do not lie above them; hence the term *adrenal* (L. *ad,* to) has more general application than *suprarenal.*

Each gland consists of a *cortex* and *medulla.* These two parts have different origins, characters, and functions. In some animals cortical and medullary tissue form separate bodies no more related to one another anatomically than they are functionally.

Development. The first intimation of development of the cortex of the glands is a thickening in the mesoderm near the root of the dorsal mesentery. Two masses of cells, one on each side, form in this region and come to lie close to the developing kidneys. As development proceeds, the original mass of cells making up the cortex becomes sur-

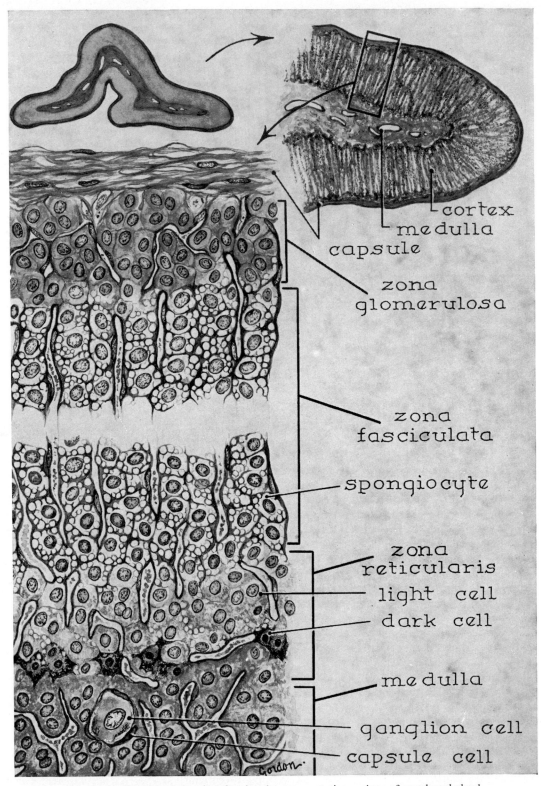

cortex

medulla

capsule

zona
glomerulosa

zona
fasciculata

spongiocyte

zona
reticularis

light cell

dark cell

medulla

ganglion cell

capsule cell

Fig. 25-29. Composite drawing showing the representative regions of an adrenal gland.

rounded by a second mass of cells derived approximately from the same site as the first. The original (inner) mass forms what is called the *provisional* or *fetal cortex of the gland,* and the second (outer) mass that covers it, the *permanent cortex.*

In the meantime, ectodermal cells have migrated from the neural crests to form the celiac ganglia. However, some of the cells, instead of developing into ganglion cells at this site, migrate into the cortical tissue to take up a position in its central part. A continuous migration of cells from the developing celiac ganglia proceeds until about the time of birth, so that substantial numbers of cells come to occupy the central part of the adrenal gland to comprise its *medulla.* Thus the cells of the medulla are the same kind as those that become ganglion cells of the sympathetic nervous system.

The provisional or fetal cortex — derived from the first group of mesodermal cells to separate from the coelomic epithelium — becomes arranged into cords separated by blood vessels, and the structure as a whole reaches a high state of development during fetal life. Not only do the cells of the provisional cortex comprise the bulk of cortical tissue that exists at this time, they are so numerous that they make each adrenal cortex of the human fetus an organ of impressive size. The cells of the permanent cortex do not develop to any great extent during this time. However, after birth the provisional cortex, so highly developed during fetal life, undergoes rapid involution. As this occurs, the cells of the permanent cortex begin to differentiate, but for a few years they do not become organized into the three zones characteristic of the adult cortex.

The fact that the provisional cortex has a somewhat different origin from the permanent cortex, and in man is enormously developed in fetal life but involutes after birth, strongly suggests that it should be regarded as an endocrine gland that, like the placenta, has a special function in fetal life. It is now believed to cooperate functionally with the placenta in producing sex hormones during fetal life. Since comparable development of the provisional cortex does not occur in fetuses of common experimental animals, experimental study of the provisional cortex of the human fetus is somewhat limited.

GENERAL MICROSCOPIC APPEARANCE

Inspection of a section of the adrenal gland with the low-power objective establishes certain prominent landmarks. First, the gland has a relatively thick *capsule* of connective tissue (Fig. 25-29). Next, in the central part of the gland large veins may be seen (Fig. 25-29, *top*). These are the veins of the *medulla,* and a moderate amount of connective tissue is associated with them. Between this

connective tissue and that of the capsule is the parenchyma of the gland. Most of this is *cortex,* which consists of epithelial secretory cells (despite their origin from mesoderm) that are arranged so as to secrete into wide capillaries. Although the medulla occupies the more central part of the gland and so is surrounded by cortex, the gland is so flattened that the medulla generally appears in a section as a rather thin "filling" in a sandwich of cortex (Fig. 25-29, *top, right*). Moreover, the medulla is not sharply demarcated from the cortex. However, the cytoplasm of the cells of the medulla is more basophilic than that of the cortical cells; hence, even in a casual low-power inspection of an H and E section, the medulla may generally be identified as a muddly blue layer between two light layers of cortex.

With more detailed study it will be observed that the parenchymal cells of both cortex and medulla follow the general plan seen in endocrine glands; that is, they are arranged in clumps or cords with blood passageways between them (Fig. 25-29).

The vessels in the cortex have been described by some authorities as capillaries and by others as sinusoids. Yet others sit on the fence and call them sinusoidal capillaries. In the medulla both narrow capillaries and wider venous channels are found between the clumps and the cords of cells; these drain into the large veins mentioned previously.

The EM has shown that the endothelium of the cortical and medullary capillaries is fenestrated (Fig. 19-21).

THE ADRENAL CORTEX

Microscopic Structure as Seen With the LM

The parenchymal cells of the cortex between the capsule and medulla reveal three different types of arrangements called *zones.* Immediately beneath the capsule, in the *zona glomerulosa,* the cells are grouped into little, irregular clusters with capillaries between them (labeled in Fig. 25-29). Beneath this is a thick layer, the *zona fasciculata,* in which the cells are radially arranged in fairly straight cords one or two cells wide perpendicular to the surface, with straight capillaries between them (labeled in Fig. 25-29). Between the zona fasciculata and the medulla is a relatively thin layer, the *zona reticularis,* in which the cells are disposed in cords that run in various directions and anastomose with one another (Fig. 25-29). Wide capillaries occupy the interstices between the cords. The three zones described usually are not sharply defined from one another.

The parenchymal cells of the zona glomerulosa tend to be columnar. Their nuclei are somewhat smaller and darker than those of the next zone; likewise their cyto-

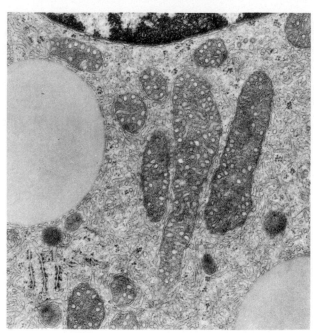

Fig. 25-30. Electron micrograph (×28,600) of a portion of a cell of the zona fasciculata of human adrenal cortex. The large pale circular areas at *upper left* and *bottom right* are lipid droplets; these store cholesterol esters that serve as a precursor of steroid hormones. Three flattened vesicles of rER may be seen at *lower left*. What appear as little holes in the large dark mitochondria are tubular cristae cut in cross or oblique section. Note in particular that the cytoplasm is packed with tubules of sER. The enzymes of the mitochondria and sER are concerned in the synthesis of steroid hormones. A small portion of the nucleus is seen at *top.* (Courtesy of J. Long)

plasm is of a more even texture, but contains some lipid droplets.

The cells of the zona fasciculata are roughly polyhedral. Their nuclei are larger and less dense than those of the zona glomerulosa. Their cytoplasm appears extensively vacuolated, because in life it contains large numbers of lipid droplets (Fig. 25-29). Indeed, this feature of the cells of this zone is so pronounced that the cells here are sometimes referred to as *spongiocytes.* Cholesterol is said to be more concentrated in these cells than in any other part of the body. The cholesterol esters in their lipid droplets serve as precursors of the steroid hormones made by these cells. These cells can also be shown to contain considerable quantities of ascorbic acid (vitamin C). The adrenocorticotrophic hormone (ACTH), if given in sufficient amounts, rapidly depletes these cells of much of their cholesterol and ascorbic acid. Both effects—depletion of ascorbic acid or cholesterol—have been used in experimental animals to assay ACTH. The cells are rich in mitochondria; these differ from mitochondria in

most cells in that their cristae tend to be tubular (Fig. 25-30) instead of flat shelves.

The cells of the zona glomerulosa and zona fasciculata contain large amounts of sER concerned in the production of steroid hormones. They also contain cisternae of rER as well as a few lysosomes. These can be seen in Figure 25-30.

The cells of the zona reticularis vary in appearance. Some have a small dark nucleus and acidophilic cytoplasm and appear to be degenerating. Others have a lighter nucleus and cytoplasm. Some cells here contain considerable quantities of lipofuscin pigment (Fig. 25-29). Like the cells in the two other zones, they contain abundant sER (Fig. 5-44).

THE HORMONES OF THE CORTEX AND THEIR EFFECTS

The adrenal cortex (or substitution therapy with adrenocorticoids) is essential to life because of the vital importance of its hormones in regulating the metabolism of the body. (The hormones made by the adrenal medulla, on the other hand, are not essential.)

Unlike the hormones we have considered in the preceding pages, which are peptides, polypeptides, proteins, or glycoproteins, the hormones produced by the adrenal cortex to be described here, together with the hormones produced by sex glands (described in the next two chapters), are what are termed *steroids.* They are all derived from cholesterol and all have a basic four-ring structure, but differ from one another in certain other respects.

The two major classes of hormones produced by the cortex are termed *glucocorticoids* and *mineralocorticoids.* In addition the cortex produces, in a minor way, some *sex hormones.* We shall briefly describe these hormones and their biological effects.

The Glucocorticoids

The most important of the glucocorticoids is *cortisol,* also called *hydrocortisone.* Cortisol exerts a great many effects in the body, as follows.

Effects of Cortisol on Protein and Carbohydrate Metabolism. With regard to protein, in general cortisol acts as a catabolic hormone. Thus in the liver it stimulates conversion of protein into carbohydrate. However, to do this it must stimulate the synthesis of the protein enzymes that have this effect. This effect is associated with the increased synthesis of RNA so it is believed that cortisol acts at the level of genes, turning on the appropriate ones to bring about its effects.

Since both cortisol and insulin cause liver cells to accumulate glycogen, it should be explained that the ways in which these two hormones exert this effect are quite different. Insulin causes liver cells to take up glucose from the blood and to store it as glycogen; in other words, the glycogen that appears in liver cells as a result of insulin activity *lowers* the blood sugar level. On the other hand, cortisol causes production of carbohydrate from protein or protein precursors; hence cortisol can promote glycogen synthesis in liver cells without taking glucose from the blood and so lowering the blood sugar level; indeed, its action in causing formation of carbohydrate from protein provides extra sugar for the blood and tends to *raise* the level of blood sugar. Insulin, therefore, has an antidiabetogenic effect in that it tends to lower the blood sugar level, and cortisol has a diabetogenic effect in that is tends to raise the blood sugar level. Normally, of course, these two effects are nicely balanced, but in the absence of either hormone the effects of the other are manifested.

Effect of Cortisol on Lymphatic Tissue and Immune Responses. The catabolic effect of cortisol is manifested by its effect on lymphatic tissue also; administration of the hormone leads to rapid reduction in the size of the thymus, spleen, and other lymphatic tissue. Since its effect is to inhibit DNA synthesis, and hence mitosis, the reduction in size of lymphocyte depots is to be explained by rapid turnover of cells in these depots. Because of its effect on cellular proliferation and protein synthesis, cortisol inhibits the formation of killer and plasma cells and antibody production, and thus has a potent *immunosuppressive* effect.

Suppression of Growth. In addition to affecting lymphatic tissue, cortisol affects other connective tissues. Its administration while fractured bones are healing leads to the formation of less callus tissue than usual. Cortisol also inhibits proliferation of fibroblasts in the healing of wounds. Given in sufficient amounts, it slows the growth of the epiphyseal disks of young rats; this effect, however, could be explained if it were to inhibit secretion of growth hormone by somatotrophs.

Anti-inflammatory Effect. Cortisol has a capacity for suppressing allergic and inflammatory responses. It is not clear how it suppresses inflammation. However, it does not act on its cause, but on inflammation from any cause. Cortisol or synthetic steroids can therefore be harmful if used to allay inflammation essential for overcoming infections. An observable effect of administering cortisol is that of causing eosinophils to leave the vascular system to enter loose connective tissue; so it produces an *eosinopenia.* In many species it also causes lymphocytes to leave the bloodstream.

The Control of Secretion of Cortisol. Cortisol is secreted mainly by the *zona fasciculata;* however, some is also produced and released from the *zona reticularis.* The secretion of cortisol is kept under control by a negative feedback mechanism that acts between it and the corticotrophs of the anterior pituitary. Thus when the level of cortisol tends to fall in the blood, more ACTH is secreted and this stimulates the adrenal cortex to produce more cortisol. As the blood level of cortisol increases, the secretion of ACTH is slowed and by this means cortisol levels are maintained at normal levels. However, the normal level of cortisol does not seem to be static, for it appears that ACTH secretion is greater in the early morning hours so that in the afternoon the level of cortisol in the blood falls to about half that attained in the morning. It appears that this normal diurnal rhythm is due to rhythmic secretion of corticotrophin-releasing factor. It is also believed that corticotrophin-releasing factor is the important factor in causing excessive ACTH and hence excessive cortisol secretion in stress situations.

Cortisol secretion is controlled by feedback arrangements operating at both the pituitary and the hypothalamic levels. Thus the neurosecretory cells of the hypothalamus that produce corticotrophin-releasing factor respond to elevated cortisol levels by secreting less of the factor, and to reduced levels of the hormone by releasing more of the factor.

The Mineralocorticoids

These help maintain the sodium and potassium balance in the body by increasing the capacity of the kidney tubules for resorbing sodium into the blood. The most potent mineralocorticoid is *aldosterone.* The role of aldosterone is thus to conserve body sodium. In Addison's disease (adrenocortical insufficiency), or in adrenalectomized animals, sodium is lost from the body into the urine, and potassium accumulates in the blood. Some amelioration can be accomplished by administration of extra sodium chloride; for example, adrenalectomized rats can be kept alive for long periods of time by putting sodium chloride in their drinking water. Giving mineralocorticoids to such animals will, of course, restore their ability to retain sodium.

Control and Site of Secretion. There is convincing evidence that mineralocorticoids are secreted only by the cells of the *zona glomerulosa.* Furthermore, the secretory functions of these cells is almost entirely *independent of ACTH.* The main factor controlling the secretion of aldosterone is the concentration of angiotensin II in the bloodstream. As was described in the previous chapter, this is formed from angiotensin I, which in turn is formed by the action of renin on a substrate, with the renin being secreted by the JG cells of the kidney. The secretory activity of JG cells, in turn, is stimulated by fall in blood pressure or lowered sodium levels in blood. Hence increased granulation of JG cells occurs under conditions of adrenalectomy or low sodium intake.

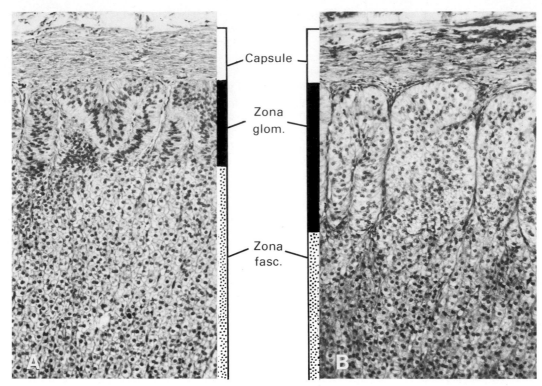

Fig. 25-31. (*A*) Low-power photomicrograph of outer part of the cortex of the adrenal gland of a normal dog. (*B*) Photomicrograph (same magnification) of the adrenal cortex of a dog that has received anterior pituitary extract containing ACTH. Note the great thickening of the zona glomerulosa. High-power examination shows many mitotic figures in this zone under these conditions.

Sex Hormones

The steroid hormones of the third group made by the adrenal cortex are sex hormones, chiefly weak androgens. Such sex hormones as are made by the adrenal cortex are produced by the cells of the zona fasciculata and probably also the zona reticularis. The ability of the adrenal cortex to produce sex hormones becomes important in understanding how certain disorders of the adrenal gland can be responsible for pseudohermaphrodites—for example, chromosomal females developing masculine sex characteristics.

CELL RENEWAL IN THE ADRENAL CORTEX AND THE EFFECTS OF ACTH

The effects of ACTH on the adrenal cortex are of two kinds. First, ACTH is essential for maintaining proper mass of the cortex. In hypophysectomized animals the cortex becomes much smaller, due primarily to substantial reduction in the zona fasciculata. Giving such animals ACTH restores proper size to this zone and adequate

function in terms of producing cortisol. However, it seems that it is sometimes assumed that restoration to normal size of the zona fasciculata is due to ACTH stimulating mitosis in this zone, and moreover that the zona glomerulosa is not affected in the process because sections taken from the adrenal cortex of a hypophysectomized animal being given ACTH show a zona glomerulosa of normal thickness.

There is, however, evidence to the effect that the zona glomerulosa represents what might be termed the *germinative zone* of the adrenal cortex. First, as is shown in Figure 25-31, the adrenals of dogs given anterior pituitary extract for a few days show a greatly thickened zona glomerulosa with many mitotic figures. This would be a relatively early response. Second, if the capsules of adrenal glands, to which some glomerulosa cells remain adherent and from which the remainder of the gland has been expressed through an opening made in the capsule, are transplanted back into the rats from which they were removed, the cortex regenerates. However, the contents of the capsules transplanted into the animals from which the glands were removed do not regenerate. Finally, it has been found that in cell cultures zona glomerulosa cells are transformed by ACTH into the fasciculata type of cells. The fact that the zona glomerulosa remains relatively unchanged in a hypophysectomized animal given ACTH, while the zona fasciculata becomes much thicker, could be easily explained by the ACTH causing both growth in the zona glomerulosa and differentiation of the deepest cells of the zone into cells of the fasciculata type.

With regard to stimulating secretion, the second kind of effect of ACTH, there is some evidence suggesting that ACTH can stimulate secretion of aldosterone under certain conditions, but this is generally regarded as being only a permissive type of action. As noted, the secretion of aldosterone from the zona glomerulosa is controlled primarily by angiotensin II. However, ACTH does have a profound effect on the secretory activity of the zona fasciculata (and to a lesser extent that of the zona reticularis) in promoting the secretion of cortisol.

Thus it would seem that ACTH is responsible for maintaining the cell population of the adrenal cortex by instituting growth in the zona glomerulosa and differentiation of glomerulosa cells into those of the fasciculata type. Whether it is concerned in causing further differentiation of fasciculata cells into cells of the reticularis type is problematical.

The status of the zona reticularis (other than its forming small amounts of glucocorticoids and sex hormones) is not clear. If it is assumed that the zona glomerulosa is the germinative zone of the cortex and maintains its cell population, it could be assumed that cells formed in the glomerulosa slowly move down the cords of the fasciculata and finally die in the reticularis. This is the "graveyard" concept of this zone.

THE ADRENAL MEDULLA

Microscopic Structure. The cells of the adrenal medulla are large and ovoid and are commonly grouped together in clumps and irregular cords arranged around blood vessels (Fig. 25-32). Many contain fine granules that are colored brown with chromium salts. This is called the *chromaffin reaction,* and can be observed in the gross by exposing the freshly cut surface of the gland to a weak solution of chromium salts or chromic acid, whereupon the medulla of the gland stains brown. This reaction is due to the presence in the cells of granules of hormone destined for secretion.

Development of Knowledge About the Adrenal Medullary Hormones

The adrenal medulla has the distinction of being the first gland from which a pure crystalline hormone was obtained in 1901. The hormone was named epinephrine. A

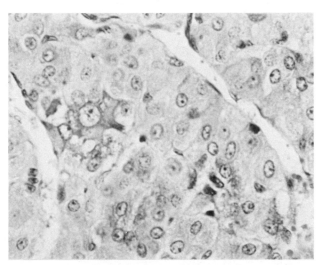

Fig. 25-32. Photomicrograph of a representative portion of adrenal medulla. Note the ganglion cell *left of center.* The secretory cells appear pale and ovoid. Note the wide fenestrated capillaries extending diagonally across the field at *lower left* and *upper right.*

proprietary name for it is *Adrenalin.* More than half a century later it was shown that what were believed to be pure extracts of the gland actually contain two closely related substances: *epinephrine* and *norepinephrine* (noradrenaline). The two substances have somewhat different effects.

The medulla secretes its two hormones in amounts that produce no major physiological effects under ordinary conditions. But these hormones are released in quantity under extraordinary conditions. We shall elaborate.

How Secretion of Medullary Cells Is Affected by Emotional and Physical Stress. As was explained in describing the development of the gland, the parenchymal cells of the adrenal medulla are derived from the same group of cells as those that become the sympathetic ganglion cells of the celiac plexus. However, after migrating into the central region of the adrenal cortex, only a few of them develop into ganglion cells (Figs. 25-29 and 25-32). Most differentiate into secretory cells arranged along blood vessels (Fig. 25-32). Nevertheless, it is important to appreciate that they occupy the same position of a two-neuron sympathetic chain as do the ganglion cells themselves; therefore, they are innervated by cholinergic *preganglionic fibers* (instead of postganglionic fibers, as are the other types of secretory cells in the body).

From the foregoing it is obvious that developmentally the secretory cells of the adrenal medulla are counterparts of the postganglionic neurons of the sympathetic division of the autonomic nervous system, so it is not surprising that they function similarly.

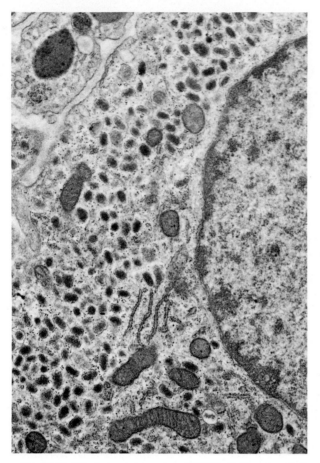

Fig. 25-33. Electron micrograph (×18,000) of adrenal medulla (rat), showing a portion of the cell type believed to secrete epinephrine. The granules here are less dense than those of the cell type considered to secrete norepinephrine. Moreover, epinephrine fills the rounded vesicles more completely. A few cisternae of rER are evident just *below center.* Part of the nucleus is seen at *right,* and some mitochondria are present. (Courtesy of W. Lockwood)

Since norepinephrine is secreted at the endings of almost all postganglionic sympathetic fibers, it is clear that if there were a sudden secretion of medullary hormones (in man, mostly epinephrine) into the circulation from the secretory cells of the adrenal medulla, the action of the neurotransmitter (norepinephrine) released at most terminations of axons of postganglionic fibers of the sympathetic system would be reinforced, and hence would temporarily dominate the activity of the parasympathetic division. As we began to explain at the beginning of this chapter, if an individual suffers severe frustration—for example, if he is kept from obtaining something he wants very badly, or prevented from running away from a situation he considers very dangerous—he may experience an emotional reaction (rage or fear). The development of rage or fear is associated with an increase of sympathetic activity over parasympathetic. The increased sympathetic activity results not only in more norepinephrine being produced at most postganglionic sympathetic nerve endings, but also in the parenchymal cells of the adrenal medulla, with their very direct sympathetic connections, being stimulated to produce their hormones more rapidly than usual. Enough norepinephrine and epinephrine enter the bloodstream to reinforce the norepinephrine effect at sympathetic nerve endings all over the body. As already mentioned, the result of this is that the heart beats faster and stronger, blood pressure becomes increased, the spleen contracts and adds more blood in the circulatory system, more blood is diverted to striated muscles and less to the viscera, and glycogen in the liver is converted to glucose and liberated into the bloodstream. There are also effects on heat production. (The two medullary hormones have somewhat different effects with regard to causing these changes.)

Effective secretion of norepinephrine and epinephrine by the cells of the medulla occurs not only in association with emotional states but also reflexly as a result of the afferent stimulation involved in severe cold, pain, and other stress conditions.

Characteristics of the Medullary Hormones. Chemically, the two hormones of the adrenal medulla, epinephrine (adrenaline) and norepinephrine (noradrenaline), are *catecholamines* because they are amines with a catechol group in their molecular structure. Both act as reducing agents, but norepinephrine forms a darker product than epinephrine when sections are treated with oxidizing agents, and this has led to the finding that the product formed in response to oxidizing agents is darker in some cells than in others and hence to the concept that some cells produce norepinephrine and others epinephrine.

The chemical building block of both hormones is tyrosine. This first is converted to dopa (dihydroxyphenylalanine), then to dopamine, and finally to norepinephrine. The formation of epinephrine involves methylation of norepinephrine.

Fine Structure of Adrenal Medullary Cells

The most striking feature of the medullary cells is their content of dark granules (Figs. 25-33 and 25-34), each enclosed by a membrane (Fig. 25-34) and denser in its core than in its periphery. The number of granules varies with secretory activity. As noted, there are two types of cells, one specialized to secrete norepinephrine and the other, epinephrine. The formation of granules is different from that associated with the synthesis of a protein, for granule formation involves bringing about successive changes in an amino acid. The fact that the granules are enclosed by a membrane would suggest that a packaging process at least occurs in the Golgi apparatus. Membrane-enclosed granules move to the surface of the cell, where their contents are discharged. Empty membranous shells left behind have been seen at the cell membrane. The other features of the cytoplasm are not remarkable. The medullary cells do not have the abundance of rER that would be expected if the cell synthesized protein for secretion. However, they do contain a moderate content of free ribosomes.

Blood Vessels, Lymphatics, and Nerves

Usually, each adrenal gland is supplied by three arteries from different sources; these branch as they approach the gland. Some branches supply the capillary beds of the capsule. Others penetrate directly into the medulla to supply the capillary bed of that region with arterial blood. However, the majority empty into the capillaries that run from the zona glomerulosa to the zona reticularis, where they empty into medullary venules. The medullary cells therefore have access to two types of vessels: capillaries, which are supplied with fresh blood; and venules containing blood that has passed along the capillaries of the cortex. Both the capillaries and the venules of the medulla have fenestrated endothelium. It is said that in the zona fasciculata most cells abut on two capillaries, one at each of their ends. In ordinary sections, the capillaries of the cortex are often collapsed and hence do not show to advantage.

The capillaries of the medulla empty into venules that unite to form a large central vein that emerges from the hilus of the gland; the central vein has numerous longitudinally disposed smooth muscle fibers in its wall. Veins also arise from the capsule. Lymphatics have been described only where substantial amounts of connective tissue are present in the gland, that is, in association with the larger veins and in the capsule.

Fibers from the parasympathetic system also reach the adrenal glands, but their function (if any) is unknown. Furthermore, little is known about the functions of the sympathetic fibers distributed in the capsule and cortex. The significant innervation of the gland is provided by the preganglionic sympathetic fibers that run directly to the parenchymal cells of the medulla; the chemical mediator here, as noted, is acetylcholine. True ganglion cells are also present in the medulla (Figs. 25-29 and 25-32).

PARAGANGLIA

It has been explained how the cells of the adrenal medulla are the result of migration of forerunners of sympathetic ganglion cells from the developing celiac ganglia

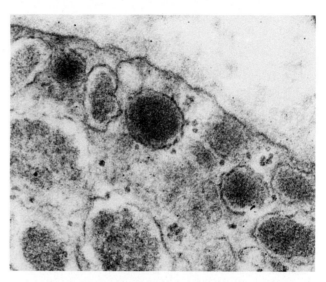

Fig. 25-34. High-power electron micrograph showing what are believed to be membrane-enclosed epinephrine granules about to be discharged from the cytoplasm of a cell of the adrenal medulla. (Courtesy of W. Lockwood)

to the developing adrenals. This is probably not the only example of migration of these cells that occurs, for many little clusters of cells that probably originate the same way are found under the peritoneum in various sites. The cells are arranged in clumps and cords and are provided with an extensive blood supply. Since these little bodies are associated with ganglia, they are said to constitute the *paraganglia* of the body. Furthermore, since the cells in these bodies give chromaffin reactions, the medullary tissue of the adrenal glands and the paraganglia together are often said to constitute the *chromaffin system*.

THE ISLETS OF LANGERHANS

The general features of the islets of Langerhans of the pancreas were described in Chapter 22. Here we shall discuss their cells in relation to the hormones they make.

Development of Knowledge

Diabetes (Gr. diabetes, a syphon, or running through) was the name used by the Greeks to designate diseases characterized by a great production of urine *(polyuria)*. In the 18th century it was proved that the urine in most cases of diabetes contained sugar; hence this kind of diabetes was called *diabetes mellitus* (L. *mellitus,* sweetened with honey) to distinguish it from the other kind *(diabetes insipidus,* described earlier in this chapter) in which polyuria is not associated with glycosuria and urine is tasteless (insipid). It was also realized at this time that it was an ill omen for anyone to begin passing large quantities of sugar-containing urine, for, almost invariably, their health would decline steadily from then on. Many so afflicted literally wasted away, being particularly susceptible while doing so to the development of a great variety of infections and degenerative diseases. Research-minded students may be interested in how progressive steps in the development of knowledge about this condition culminated in replacement therapy that has now saved an incalculable number of lives all over the world.

In 1869 Langerhans, while still a medical student, discovered the islets in the pancreas that now bear his name. Figure 22-1 is a low-power picture of a section of pancreas showing two of these islets (labeled) lying in the exocrine tissue. However, Langerhans did not suspect that these islets were little organs of internal secretion. Soon afterward, it was pointed out that they contained extensive capillary networks; this was to help later in leading other investigators to suspect that they had an endocrine function.

Although Cowley, an English physician, had suggested a full century before that there was some relation between diabetes and the pancreas, it was not until 1889 that this was positively established. At this time, von Mering and Minkowski removed the pancreas from dogs and found that they passed increased amounts of urine, containing sugar. (It has been said that someone noticed that the urine from these dogs attracted large numbers of flies; if so, he made an important contribution to research because he or someone else asked "why".)

This finding could be interpreted as indicating that a lack of some pancreatic function is responsible for diabetes. But what function? The obvious function known at that time was that of making an external secretion. Nevertheless, the concept of Claude Bernard—that certain bodily functions depend on internal secretions—had by this time made a considerable impression on the scientific world, so further work was done in an attempt to discover whether diabetes results from the pancreas failing to make a proper external or internal secretion. To determine this point, Hedon performed an ingenious experiment. He found that a piece of pancreas grafted back into a depancreatized animal would keep the animal free from diabetes even though the graft had no duct connections. In other words, he showed that the anti-diabetic principle made by the pancreas was absorbed into the blood—that is, it was an internal secretion.

At this time, however, it was not at all clear whether acinar or islet cells produced the internal secretion. Indeed, it was not even clear whether islet cells were fundamentally different from acinar cells. However, this matter was settled soon afterward by Ssobolew and Schultze, who tied off the pancreatic ducts of experimental animals and found that after a time the acinar tissue of the pancreas all became atrophied and that only islet tissue was left. Animals so treated, although they suffered from impaired digestion and certain other complaints, did not develop diabetes.

Only one thing more, it appeared, had to be established for universal acceptance of the islet theory of diabetes: proof that the islets were diseased in those dying of the disease. Evidence was first provided by Opie, a distinguished pathologist who around the turn of the century noted that those who died from diabetes in most instances either lacked islets or showed degenerative changes in such islets as were present. So it became generally believed that diabetes mellitus was due to failure of islets to make a hormone, and the as yet undiscovered hormone was even given the name *insulin*.

Two Kinds of Islet Cells are Discovered. In 1908, Lane established not only that the granules of islet cells had histochemical properties different from those of zymogen granules (and hence that islet cells were fundamentally dif-

ferent from acinar cells), but also that two kinds of islet cells could be distinguished. He found that certain alcoholic fixatives dissolved the granules from the majority of cells in the islets but preserved granules in a minority of the cells. Conversely, fixatives made up with water instead of alcohol preserved granules in the majority of the cells but dissolved those from the minority. The numerous cells with alcohol-soluble granules he termed *beta cells,* the scarcer ones with alcohol-resistant, water-soluble granules, *alpha cells.* This led to various staining technics being devised for coloring alpha and beta cells differently (Fig. 25-35).

Next, although not so common as certain other types of degenerative lesions observed in islets of diabetics, a type of islet lesion called hydropic degeneration was sometimes seen. The islet cells showing this change appeared swollen with watery fluid and contained little stainable substance (Fig. 25-36). Later it was shown that the clear fluid contains glycogen. Both Homans and Allen found that if most of the pancreas was removed, and the animal was fed carbohydrate or protein liberally, (*1*) hydropic degeneration occurred in the islets of the part of the pancreas left intact, and (*2*) diabetes developed. However, if the animal was given a minimal diet, the islet cells showed no disease, and the animal remained healthy. Furthermore, they showed that hydropic degeneration occurred only in the *beta cells* of the islets, and that this change was preceded by degranulation of the cells concerned.

These experiments and others led to development of what is called the *overwork hypothesis*. Allen showed that if from 80 to 90 per cent of the pancreas were removed from a dog, the remaining portion had enough islets to keep the animal free from diabetes, provided the dog's diet was restricted. However, if such an animal were fed additional carbohydrate, the beta cells in the fragment of pancreas still remaining would become degranulated and hydropic. He considered that the extra carbohydrate fed the animals placed increased secretory demands on the beta cells, and their degranulation and hydropic degeneration were evidence of exhaustion through overwork. With continued additional food intake, he found that the islet lesions became permanent, with no evidence of recovery.

Allen's findings still have great implications with regard to the *treatment of diabetes*. In particular, they apply to those in danger of *developing* diabetes, for they show that if an individual overstrains his beta cell capacity, for example by eating too much carbohydrate, beta cells will be destroyed from overwork and this, of course, will decrease the individual's beta cell capacity and make those remaining more susceptible to overstrain than before.

Although the overwork hypothesis led to better treatment, diabetes remained a widespread and usually fatal disease. It could be expected that many investigators would attempt to extract the beta cell hormone from the

Fig. 25-35. Oil-immersion photomicrograph of an islet of Langerhans in guinea pig pancreas, stained by Gomori's method. Alpha cells, with pink-staining cytoplasm, appear darker than the blue-staining beta cells, and they occupy the periphery of the islet. Most of the interior of the islet contains beta cells situated along capillaries. (Courtesy of W. Wilson)

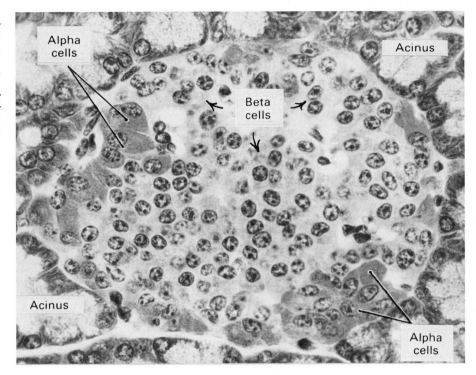

pancreas of animals so that substitution therapy could be employed in man. Some of these earlier attempts to extract the antidiabetic hormone gave tantalizing promising results, but this was about as far as they went, and the world remained without substitution therapy for diabetes until the time of Banting and Best.

The Discovery of Insulin. On the afternoon of October 30, 1920, Banting, then a young medical graduate, read in a medical journal an article in which the findings of Ssobolew and others who had tied off the ducts of the pancreas were described. Banting was very much impressed with the fact that the acinar tissue atrophied after duct ligation, and it is generally believed that he began to suspect that previous attempts to obtain an active extract of islet tissue had failed because the digestive enzymes of the acinar tissue destroyed the islet hormone before it could be extracted. In any event, before going to bed that night he had decided to try making extracts from pancreases after their ducts had been tied off for 6 to 8 weeks, so that they presumably would contain only islet and not acinar tissue. The events that occurred between the inception of the idea and the isolation of insulin, the collaboration of Best and later of Collip, the inevitable succession of encouraging and discouraging results, the lack of funds and above all the dogged persistence of Banting and finally the emergence of insulin as an effective treatment for diabetes make an inspiring story.

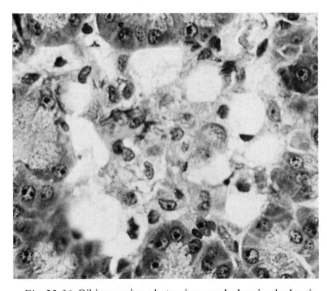

Fig. 25-36. Oil-immersion photomicrograph showing hydropic degeneration in an islet of Langerhans in the pancreas of a dog injected with anterior pituitary extract with diabetogenic effect. The beta cells have degenerated and exhibit large droplets of fluid. This hydropic degeneration is an indication of severe overwork by beta cells. (Ham, A. W., and Haist, R. E.: Am. J. Pathol., *17*:787, 1941)

Relation of Other Hormones to Insulin

In 1930, Houssay and Biasotti showed that diabetes produced in animals by removing the pancreas could be ameliorated by removing the pituitary gland as well, and that such animals, instead of declining steadily in health like those from which the pancreas only is removed, would live free from diabetes for long periods. Some intimation that the pars anterior of the pituitary gland can exert a diabetogenic effect had, of course, been obtained in finding that individuals with certain types of anterior lobe tumors tended to develop diabetes. Furthermore, in 1927, Johns et al. had produced signs of diabetes in dogs by giving them injections of anterior pituitary extract. Other investigators also later observed this phenomenon. However, Evans and his collaborators noted something additional. Whereas all the others had noted signs of diabetes only while injections were continued, Evans observed that two animals continued to have diabetes after the course of injections of anterior pituitary had been finished. One animal was still diabetic 4 months after the last injection. The importance of this finding was not realized until Young, in 1937, showed that a sufficiently prolonged course of injections of anterior pituitary extract would make dogs *permanently diabetic*. Richardson and Young made histological studies of the islets of these dogs. In some islets they found histological appearances similar to those observed in long-standing cases of diabetes in man; in others they found degranulation and hydropic degeneration of beta cells and, in some, mitotic figures. Subsequently, Ham and Haist showed that anterior pituitary extracts injected daily caused progressive degranulation of beta cells; this was followed by hydropic degeneration (Fig. 26-36). The similarity between the findings with anterior pituitary extracts and those observed by Allen after partial pancreatectomy and liberal feeding was so obvious it was realized that *anterior pituitary extracts somehow cause beta cells to overwork* to the point of exhaustion and death.

The relatively crude extracts of anterior pituitary gland used at that time contained several trophic hormones as well as growth hormone. Anterior pituitary extracts containing ACTH stimulate the adrenal cortex to make more cortisol, which furthers conversion of protein and protein precursors into sugar in the liver. The administration of cortisol alone can cause diabetes. However, it seems most probable that the chief diabetogenic factor made by the anterior pituitary gland is growth hormone.

Diabetes Mellitus

It seems that anterior pituitary extracts activate beta cells in a direct way so that they become exhausted more easily than in the absence of anterior pituitary stimulation. In any event it is now generally accepted that *many diabetogenic influences* are present in the body; however, they do not produce diabetes because they are opposed successfully by adequate levels of the *antidiabetogenic hormone,* insulin. Those unfortunate individuals who develop diabetes mellitus do so because the total mass of their beta cell population becomes inadequate to provide enough insulin to combat the diabetogenic influences also operating in them. The reason for their functional beta cell mass being inadequate is that beta cell proliferation in their islets does not keep pace with beta cell loss and, as

already explained, beta cell loss is accelerated when the surviving beta cell population is overstrained. Hence a key issue in diabetes research is trying to learn more about the control of beta cell proliferation and why cell production does not keep up with cell loss. We shall mention this again when we deal with the origin and differentiation of the cells of islets. But first we should mention a few more points about diabetes.

BLOOD SUGAR LEVELS AND GLYCOSURIA

In a normal individual on a normal diet, the amount of sugar in the blood remains at a fairly constant level, varing between 0.08 and 0.11 per cent. Since it is dissolved in the blood plasma, sugar in this concentration is present in the glomerular filtrate. However, at this concentration all the sugar in the filtrate can be resorbed as the filtrate passes along the nephron. Hence, in such a normal individual sugar does not appear in the urine. However, in an untreated diabetic the blood sugar rises above the normal level (*hyperglycemia*), to the point at which increased amounts in the glomerular filtrate cannot all be resorbed by the kidneys; hence sugar appears in the urine (*glycosuria*). The concentration above which the kidney cannot resorb all the sugar filtered through its glomeruli is called its *threshold* for sugar.

The Effects of Insulin

The most obvious action of insulin is that it *lowers the blood sugar (glucose) level*. It will, of course do this whether it is injected into a normal person or a diabetic. A dose of insulin greater than required can so diminish the blood sugar level that an individual may have convulsions or become unconscious; this is called *insulin shock*. Too much insulin can lower the blood sugar to the point at which death ensues because the blood sugar is below the minimum required to sustain life. Occasionally secreting islet cell tumors occur; if beta cells are involved this may lead to hyperinsulinism and even lethal hypoglycemia, since the insulin released is not controlled by the blood sugar level.

Insulin acts in the normal person to lower the blood sugar level by affecting the metabolism of several kinds of tissues throughout the body, as follows. (*1*) The sugar absorbed from a hearty meal would be enough to raise the blood sugar substantially were it not for the fact that some sugar becomes stored as glycogen in hepatocytes and muscle cells; insulin facilitates the *conversion of sugar into glycogen*. (*2*) Excess sugar is also removed from the blood by *converting it into fat,* which is stored in the various fat depots; insulin facilitates this also. (*3*) In addition to promoting storage of sugar as glycogen, insulin facilitates the metabolism of carbohydrate in muscle cells; by speeding up utilization of carbohydrate in muscle it again acts to lower the blood sugar level. (*4*) As noted, the action of insulin opposes the catabolic action of cortisol.

THE CELLS OF ISLETS

In early studies (as described above) two kinds of islet cells, *alpha* and *beta,* were distinguished by the staining and other features of their cytoplasmic granules. It was at first shown that the *beta cells* secrete *insulin* or its immediate precursor and later that the *alpha cells* secrete the hormone *glucagon,* the function of which will be described briefly a little later. Continued studies on islets suggested that a third type of cell was present in islets, which was termed a *delta* or *D cell.* Later, definitive proof of a third cell type was provided first by silver impregnation methods and afterward by the immunofluorescence technic, which showed that this third cell type contains *somatostatin (GIF),* the hypothalamic hormone-regulating factor that suppresses secretion of growth hormone (*see* Hellerstrom). This cell type is now generally termed the A_1 *cell* and the alpha cell is often referred to as the A_2 *cell*. A fourth type of cell has also been distinguished by staining technics, electron microscopy, and immunocytochemical means. The four types of cells all appear to make their own type of peptide but the function of only the alpha and beta cells is as yet well established.

Beta cells are the most numerous in the mammalian pancreas, comprising about 60 to 80 per cent of the islet population. Alpha cells make up around 10 to 30 per cent of the islet cells. A_1 cells, according to Hellerstrom, usually comprise less than 10 per cent of the islet cells in laboratory animals, but it is thought they are more numerous in human islets.

The Development of Islets

As described in connection with the exocrine pancreas (p. 694), exocrine and endocrine components of the pancreas both develop from the same outgrowth of endoderm. The common progenitor cells, however, differentiate along different pathways to form acinar secretory units, ducts, or islets. It has, however, been suggested that the islet cells may arise from cells of the neural crest that migrate to the pancreas very early in its development. There is reason to believe that beta cells can develop independently of the neural crest, but it is possible that at least some other types of islet cells might originate from a neural crest. There is no indication that acinar cells are transformed into islet cells; both cell types, however, can develop from the same source.

The order in which islet cells first appear in fetal life has been much investigated in laboratory animals. Alpha cells appear first, A_1 cells next, and beta cells a day or two later. Furthermore, it appears that secretion of insulin by the fetal pancreas is not regulated by the blood sugar level; this happens only after birth.

The Growth and Maintenance of Beta Cells

There are several methods for determining the number of islets in a pancreas and for determining the total mass of the islets. Whereas in fetal life islets may grow because of progenitor cells dividing and differentiating into islet cells, it appears that the increase in islet cell mass that occurs during the postnatal growth period is due to mitosis occurring in islet cells themselves. In adulthood it is believed that there is a slow turnover of the beta cell population and that in diabetes the production of new cells is not enough to compensate for the loss of beta cells. The turnover of beta cells has been studied by using labeled thymidine in experimental animals. It is very slow, but the studies show that beta cells undoubtedly divide and hence under normal conditions would be able to maintain a population of beta cells sufficient to meet the insulin needs of the body. In the type of diabetes that manifests itself in people of mature age, it is suspected that the beta cells of the individual's pancreas are no longer able to reproduce themselves at a rate commensurate with that at which their beta cells are wearing out, so there comes a time when those that remain are no longer able to supply all the insulin needs of the body. Whereas it is easy to suggest that this is comparable to what happens when fibroblasts, for example, cultivated continuously in cultures, seem unable to pass through more than a given number of divisions, the problem of beta cell regeneration could be different. This is because although they are highly differentiated cells of an endocrine gland, it might be expected that they would be of the Category 3 type (*see* p. 44), and that they could reproduce as, for example, do the cells of the thyroid parenchyma. However, like the cells of the parathyroid glands, there is no specific trophic hormone to control their function and proliferation. As in parathyroid glands, secretory and perhaps growth activities depend on the concentration of a particular substance in the blood: glucose in this case and calcium in the case of parathyroid cells. Growth hormone may, however, be able to stimulate mitosis in both kinds of cells, for Ham and Haist observed mitotic figures in the parathyroid glands of dogs given diabetogenic anterior pituitary extracts. It has also been shown that when diabetogenic extracts of the anterior pituitary are given to dogs along with enough insulin to prevent hyperglycemia, mitotic figures are found in the islets (Fig. 25-37).

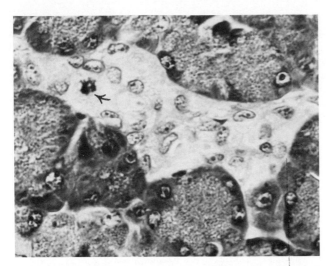

Fig. 25-37. High-power photomicrograph of an islet of Langerhans in the pancreas of a dog injected with a diabetogenic anterior pituitary extract and, in addition, enough insulin to protect the beta cells from becoming hydropic from overwork. Note the mitotic figure in a beta cell (*arrow*).

The Control of Insulin Production and Secretion

There is now much evidence to show that insulin secretion varies in relation to blood sugar level and that an *elevated blood sugar level stimulates insulin secretion.* There is also evidence that insulin production by beta cells depends on the demands made on beta cells by the glucose level of the blood. Furthermore, it would seem that up to a point the demand for more insulin is readily met by increased insulin production. It is conceivable that physiological demands could stimulate division of beta cells in individuals with normal beta potential.

Under normal conditions, only about a 1- to 2-day supply of insulin is stored in the cytoplasm of beta cells. However, this is an amount sufficient, or almost so, to cause death if it were all discharged into the bloodstream at once. Indeed, a phenomenon much like this actually occurs if an animal is given suitable amounts of alloxan. This chemical exerts a rapid lethal effect on the beta cells of the islets (Fig. 4-17). As soon as they are destroyed, their content of stored insulin almost immediately washes into the bloodstream, and unless sugar is given the animals at this time, they may die of hypoglycemia. If the animals survive this preliminary hypoglycemia, they of course go on to develop hyperglycemia.

Granule Content of Beta Cells as Seen With the LM

The cytoplasmic granules appear as very fine blue granules in sections stained by Bowie's neutral ethyl violet-Biebrich scarlet stain, in numbers representative of the insulin content of the cell. With Haist, Ham observed that the number of beta granules revealed by this method is reduced if animals are starved, given insulin, or fed a high proportion of fat. Obviously, the reduction in number of granules under these circumstances is not the result of degranulation from overwork but instead due to lack of synthesis as a result of lack of work stimulus. Therefore, reduction in granule content of beta cells can be caused either by overwork or underwork.

Fine Structure of Beta Cells

The mitochondria of both beta and alpha cells appear fine in contrast with the coarser ones of acinar cells. Golgi saccules are present between the nucleus and the surfaces through which secretion takes place. Well-defined negative Golgi images can be seen with the LM in cells that are actively secreting.

The capillaries of islets are of the fenestrated type. There is a basement membrane around each capillary, but a minimum of connective tissue, so that it does not impede secretion into the capillaries. There is reason to believe that increase in pericapillary connective tissue as a result of injury, at least in certain experimental conditions, hinders delivery of insulin into the capillaries.

The granules of beta cells differ in appearance, depending on species. In the rat and mouse, they are round and homogeneous and enclosed in membranous vesicles. In contrast with granules of alpha cells, they generally do not fill the membranous vesicles in which they lie; hence, a space can be seen between the granules and the membranous vesicles that contain them. In the dog, beta granules often appear as rectangular crystalloid structures. The plate-like granules do not fill the rounded membranous vesicles containing them; hence a comparatively large space can be seen between the surfaces of the granules and the rounded vesicles in which they lie. In the cat also, beta granules have a crystalloid appearance; but in this species the central part of each granule contains a dense rhomboidal or prismatic structure. In the guinea pig, the beta granules have a rounded shape (Fig. 25-38). In man, the beta granules vary from being round to crystalloid in appearance. Here again, the beta granules, whatever their shape, tend to be withdrawn from the membranous vesicles in which they are contained.

Since insulin is a protein it might be expected that the beta cells that synthesize and secrete it would have a well-developed rER and Golgi apparatus. However, rER does not appear to advantage in beta cells well filled with granules. On the other hand, some cells in islets have a great content of rER and few granules (Fig. 25-38). Beta cells may therefore pass through two stages, one in which there is much rER during which insulin is being synthesized, and a second stage in which secretion is delivered into the bloodstream.

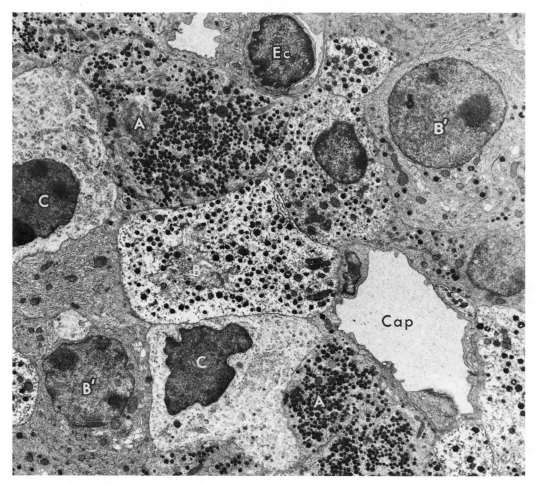

Fig. 25-38. Electron micrograph (×3,000) of cells in an islet of Langerhans in the pancreas of a guinea pig. Note the alpha cells containing alpha granules (A), beta cells filled with granules (B), beta cells in the stage of synthesizing insulin (B'), a chromophobe (C), a capillary (Cap), and another capillary (*top center*) showing the nucleus of an endothelial cell (Ec). (Courtesy of L. Herman)

The protein synthesized in the rER is probably *proinsulin,* which acts more slowly than insulin in lowering blood sugar levels. Normally this is packaged and modified in the Golgi, from which it buds off in the form of secretory vesicles that under normal conditions contain *insulin.* These vesicles correspond to the granules seen in sections. The way they are released is probably the same as that described for the secretory cells of the anterior pituitary. Under certain conditions beta cells may secrete proinsulin as such.

Alpha Cells

Appearance With the LM. The granules of alpha cells are larger than those of beta cells. Alpha cells can be distinguished from beta cells by several staining methods;

Gomori's method is excellent for this purpose (Fig. 25-35).

In some species (for example, the rat) the alpha cells tend to have a peripheral distribution in islets. In other species (including man and dog) the alpha cells are scattered throughout the islets but show a general tendency to form little groups toward the middle of islets.

Except in a few species (such as the guinea pig) alpha and beta cells cannot be distinguished from one another by the morphology of their nuclei.

Fine Structure of Granules. The granules of alpha cells are similar in different species, being round, dense, and homogeneous, and filling the membranous vesicles in which they lie (Fig. 25-38, labeled A).

Function. Alpha cells appear unaffected when diabetes is artifically produced. Islets composed only of alpha cells

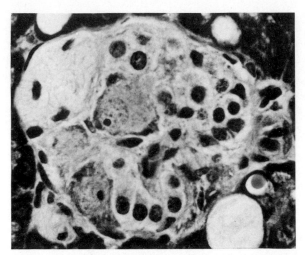

Fig. 25-39. High-power photomicrograph of a neuro-insular complex in the pancreas of a rat. Note the large ganglion cells at *center* and *bottom left* in association with islet cells. (Courtesy of W. S. Hartroft)

trophs of the anterior pituitary. Since growth hormone can exert such profound effects on the beta cells of the islets, it is tempting to speculate that the D cells may serve some role in connection with the "pseudotrophic" effect that growth hormone has on beta cells.

Nervous Control of Islet Cells

Whether islet cell secretion is affected by autonomic impulses as, for example, in severe emotional states, has not been worked out as satisfactorily as might be wished, but there is some indication that the autonomic system may indeed be involved. It has been shown that there are intimate associations between islet cells and ganglion cells in the pancreas. These little aggregates, termed *neuro-insular complexes* (Fig. 25-39), have been studied by Simard. Perhaps the discovery that some islet cells produce a hypothalamic hormone-regulating factor will stimulate new interest in neuro-insular complexes.

THE PINEAL BODY

Gross Features. The pineal body (epiphysis) is a cone-shaped gland about 0.5 to 1 cm. in length, resembling a pine cone in shape (L. *pineus,* relating to the pine). It develops from, and remains connected to, the posterior end of the roof of the third ventricle, projecting posteriorly so that it lies dorsal to the midbrain.

Development. Posterior to the site of origin of the choroid plexus of the third ventricle, the roof of the diencephalon bulges dorsally to form a diverticulum, the walls of which thicken so as to gradually obliterate its lumen. In postnatal life there is a lumen only at the base of the pineal body, called the *pineal recess* of the third ventricle.

There are two kinds of cells in the outgrowth. The diverticulum of the roof itself contains neuroectodermal cells; the pia mater covering the outgrowth contains mesenchymal cells. Both kinds participate in forming the pineal body. The neuro-ectodermal cells in turn give rise to two further cell types: (*1*) parenchymal secretory cells called *pinealocytes,* and (*2*) *neuroglial* cells. The mesenchymal cells form *fibroblasts* and the connective tissue components of the pineal: the *capsule, trabeculae,* and incomplete *septa* that more or less subdivide the gland into lobules.

Microscopic Structure as Seen With the LM

The appearance of the pineal body varies considerably from one individual to another. Lobules consisting of pinealocytes and glial cells are incompletely separated by irregular *trabeculae* and incomplete *septa* of connective tissue that extend into the substance of the gland from its *capsule,* conveying blood vessels and nerves along with

may be encountered in the pancreas of diabetics. However, it was noticed that sometimes the insulin requirement of an animal in which the beta cells had been destroyed seemed to be greater than that of an animal from which the entire pancreas had been removed. This finding suggested that the pancreas makes a hormone that has an action opposite to that of insulin in that it *raises the blood sugar level.* A polypeptide hormone called *glucagon* with this effect was then found in pancreatic extracts. Much evidence has now been obtained to indicate that alpha cells produce glucagon; for example, Bencosme found it was not present in extracts made from pancreas lacking alpha cells. Glucagon has been shown to cause glucose release from the liver into the blood; its secretion is *stimulated by low blood sugar levels.* It also affects protein and fat metabolism.

Delta (D or A₁) Cells

In addition to alpha and beta cells, which have been well characterized, a third type of cell was often noticed, particularly in human islets, that did not seem to fit into either the alpha or the beta category. For a time it was thought that it might be one or the other kind in a state of function that did not permit its proper identification. Granules were seen in it but they were not nearly as dense as those seen in alpha or beta cells. However, more recently it became possible to demonstrate this cell by means of Hellerstrom-Hellman silver impregnation procedure. Later it was shown by immunochemical technics to contain *somatostatin,* the hypothalamic hormone that inhibits the release of growth hormone by the somato-

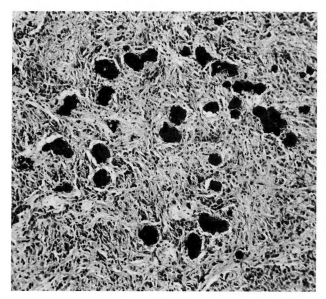

Fig. 25-40. Low-power photomicrograph of a portion of the pineal body, showing brain sand. (Courtesy of E. Anderson)

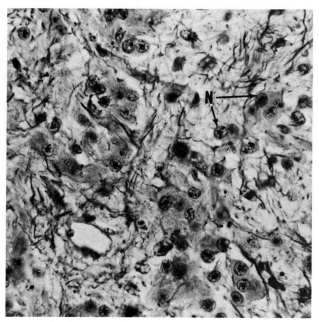

Fig. 25-41. Photomicrograph (×500) of a representative part of the pineal body (stained with Heidenhain's iron hematoxylin). Pinealocytes have relatively large nuclei (N) and prominent nucleoli. The many densely stained processes belong to the pinealocytes and glial cells. (Anderson, E.: J. Ultrastruct. Res., Suppl. 8, 1965)

them; some of these irregular partitions may be seen at the periphery of Figure 25-40. Like all endocrine organs, the pineal has a very rich capillary blood supply; this is derived from the posterior choroid arteries. In the rat and mouse these capillaries are fenestrated to facilitate the release of secretions from pinealocytes into the bloodstream.

The pineal body in man reaches its greatest development in childhood and then progressively involutes but nevertheless is believed to continue functioning. Concretions of calcified material, often called *brain sand,* accumulate in it and this is regarded by some authors as indicating a degenerative change. The appearance of these calcareous granules, which can be of assistance in identifying the position of the pineal body in x-ray films, is illustrated in Figure 25-40.

Pinealocytes

Most of the cells in the pineal body are pinealocytes. They are relatively large cells, commonly grouped in clumps. Their nuclei are large and their nucleoli prominent (Fig. 25-41). Clumps of basophilic material (RNA) are seen in their cytoplasm and they have extensive processes extending from their cell body. The substance of the pineal body consists to a large degree of an entanglement of cell bodies and intertwining processes of pinealocytes and glial cells, which also have extensive processes. The processes seen in Figure 25-41 cannot be distinguished as belonging to the one kind of cell or the other.

With the EM, the cytoplasm of pinealocytes reveals numerous mitochondria, a well-developed Golgi apparatus, dense bodies (probably lysosomes), sER, ribosomes, and polysomes. There are also numerous microtubules (Fig. 25-42).

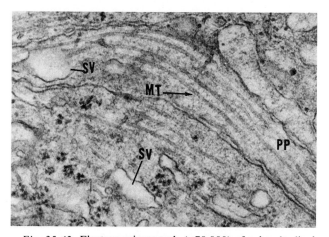

Fig. 25-42. Electron micrograph (×70,000) of a longitudinal section of a process of a pinealocyte, showing microtubules (MT) and smooth-surfaced vesicles (SV). Polysomes are present at *lower left.* (Anderson, E.: J. Ultrastruct. Res., Suppl. 8, 1965)

Neuroglial Cells

These are recognizable by their nuclei, which are more flattened and have more of their chromatin condensed than in pinealocytes. Some have a more or less triangular shape and often two or three are seen close together. Their cytoplasm is more basophilic than that of pinealocytes.

With the EM, the glial cells reveal the usual organelles, including microtubules, but not so many as in pinealocytes. The most striking feature of their cytoplasm, however, is its extensive content of filaments described as being 5 to 6 nm. in diameter and commonly arranged in bundles. Filaments in the processes of glial cells run parallel to their axis and insert in attachment plaques at the cell membrane. Another way cytoplasmic organelles of pinealocytes and glial cells differ is that the mitochondria of the glial cells have a much denser matrix than those of pinealocytes. The processes of the glial cells end mostly as bulbous expansions on pinealocytes, other glial cells, or on the cells lining perivascular spaces. Their endings sometimes contain much glycogen.

Nerve Supply

Although the pineal body develops from the brain, it seems to lose all original functional nerve connections with it soon after birth. Instead, it becomes invaded by postganglionic sympathetic fibers extending from the superior cervical (sympathetic) ganglion to enter the gland by way of its connective tissue trabeculae and septa. Efferent nerve endings have been described in association with the pinealocytes and even with the glial cells, and synapses have been observed between adrenergic fibers and pinealocytes in the cat and also in the rat. Some of the adrenergic sympathetic fibers, however, end in association with capillaries in the pericapillary spaces.

The Functions of the Pineal Body

Before considering the possible role of the pineal in man, it is useful to describe what has been learned about its functions in experimental animals.

There is reason to believe that the secretory cells of the pineal body (pinealocytes) represent counterparts of photoreceptive secretory cells, since photoreceptive cells not very different from those found in the retina (Chap. 28) are present in the pineal body of certain lower vertebrates. However, in higher vertebrates the pinealocytes do not respond directly to light stimuli, but only indirectly, as will now be explained.

Metabolically, pinealocytes are very active, secreting two humoral substances, *melatonin* and *serotonin,* into the bloodstream. However, they do not secrete both substances at the same time. Melatonin is made only at night, whereas during the daylight hours serotonin, but not melatonin, is formed. The diurnal rhythm directing secretion seems to be generated within the hypothalamus in relation to the time periods during which light is entering the eyes. The secretory activities of the pineal gland are thought to be regulated and coordinated through the nerve impulses that reach the pinealocytes from the adrenergic postganglionic sympathetic fibers supplying them from the superior cervical ganglion. Light, it would seem, constitutes a stimulus that inhibits the formation of melatonin, which would account for why release of this hormone occurs only during the normal hours of darkness. Thus, animals kept in the dark have a large, active pineal, producing a relatively high level of melatonin, whereas those kept in continuous light possess only a small and rather inactive pineal. The effect of light is to decrease levels of melatonin-forming enzymes in the gland.

Role of Melatonin. Removal of the pineal gland from rats has been found to cause them to undergo precocious sexual development; pineal extracts, on the other hand, reverse this effect. There is now much evidence to support the contention that an important role of melatonin is to hold back reproductive development until a suitable age has been reached, and this is probably done by this hormone inhibiting the secretion (or release) of gonadotrophic hormones or their releasing hormones. The role of melatonin therefore seems to be to modify certain neuroendocrine functions, in particular those relating to secretion of gonadotrophins.

Pineal Secretion in Man. The role and importance of pineal secretion in man are not easy to establish and much of our understanding is necessarily based on what has been learned from experimental animals, as outlined above.

The pineal body in man is generally regarded as a neuroendocrine gland that regulates gonadal function. Indeed, there is some direct evidence for this. For example, some boys that develop certain nonsecreting pineal tumors, in which there are enough tumor cells to crowd out functional (secreting) pinealocytes, show precocious puberty. Nevertheless, the casual relation between pineal secretion and the regulation of gonadal development in man is poorly understood. But melatonin probably acts as the intermediary, with environmental lighting conditions (certainly a complex and variable factor in modern societies) somehow acting by way of the eyes and hypothalamus to influence the secretory activity of the pineal via the sympathetic nervous system. Humans are no different from experimental animals in making melatonin at night and serotonin by day. The main effect of this nocturnal hormone would seem to be to regulate normal sexual development. In man, melatonin does not exert its other known effect, which is on skin pigmentation; in amphibian tadpoles, however, it aggregates the melanin in certain epidermal cells (melanophores) to render the skin lighter in color–an effect opposite to that of MSH, which hormone causes their melanin to disperse and thus darken the skin.

A commonly held view is that the pineal body is probably less important in humans than in some other vertebrates. However, there is renewed interest in this poorly understood endocrine organ because of the possibility that melatonin might not be the only hormone made in it. Some of the peptides and proteins also made by the gland are now under scrutiny for potential hormonal effects.

REFERENCES AND OTHER READING

COMPREHENSIVE GENERAL REFERENCE

Martin, C. R.: Textbook of Endocrine Physiology. Baltimore, Williams & Wilkins, 1976.

GENERAL

Kahn, C. R.: Membrane receptors for hormones and neurotransmitters. J. Cell Biol., *70*:261, 1976.
McEwen, B. S.: Interactions between hormones and nerve tissue. Sci. Am., *235*:48, July, 1976.
O'Malley, B. W., and Schrader, W. T.: The receptors of steroid hormones. Sci. Am., *234*:32, Feb., 1976.

THE PITUITARY GLAND AS A WHOLE

Daniel, P. M.: The anatomy of the hypothalamus and pituitary gland. *In* Martini, L., and Ganong, W. F. (eds.): Neuroendocrinology. vol. 1, p. 15. New York, Academic Press, 1966.
Ezrin, C.: Chapters 1-4. *In* Ezrin, C., Godden, J. O., Volpé, R., and Wilson, R. (eds.): Systemic Endocrinology. Hagerstown, Md., Harper & Row, 1973.
Green, J. D.: The comparative anatomy of the portal vascular system and of the innervation of the hypophysis. *In* Harris, G. W., and Donovan, B. T. (eds.): The Pituitary Gland. vol. 1, p. 127. Berkeley, University of California Press, 1966.
Green, J. D., and Harris, G. W.: Observation of the hypophysioportal vessels of the living rat. J. Physiol., *108*:359, 1949.
Holmes, R. L., and Ball, J. N.: The Pituitary Gland. A Comparative Account. Biological Structure and Function Series. vol. 4. London, Cambridge University Press, 1974.
von Lawzewitsch, I., and Sarrat, R.: Comparative anatomy and the evolution of the neurosecretory hypothalamic-hypophyseal system. Acta Anat., *81*:13, 1972.

THE ANTERIOR LOBE OF THE PITUITARY AND ITS RELATION TO THE HYPOTHALAMUS

Bain, J., and Ezrin, C.: Immunofluorescent localization of the LH cell of the human adenohypophysis. J. Clin. Endocrinol., *30*:181, 1970.

Burgers, A. C. J.: Melanophore-stimulating hormones in vertebrates. Ann. N.Y. Acad. Sci., *100*:669, 1963.
Ezrin, C.: The Hypophysis, the Pineal Gland. *In* Netter, F. H. (ed.): The Ciba Collection of Medical Illustrations. vol. 4, Endocrine System and Selected Metabolic Diseases. p. 3. Summit, N.J., Ciba, 1965.
Farquhar, M. G.: Fine structure and function in capillaries of the anterior pituitary gland. Angiology, *12*:270, 1961.
———: Processing of secretory products by cells of the anterior pituitary gland. Mem. Soc. Endocrinol., 19, Subcellular Organization and Function. *In* Heller, H., and Lederis, K. (eds.): Endocrine Tissues. London, Cambridge University Press, 1971.
Guillemin, R., and Burgus, R.: The hormones of the hypothalamus. Sci. Am., *227*:24, Nov., 1972
Halmi, N. S., McCormick, W. F., and Decker, D. A., Jr.: The natural history of hyalinization of ACTH-MSH cells in man. Arch. Pathol., *91*:318, 1971.
Herlant, M.: The cells of the adenohypophysis and their functional significance. Int. Rev. Cytol., *17*, 1964.
von Lawzewitsch, I., Dickmann, G. H., Amezúa, L., and Pardal, C.: Cytological and ultrastructural characterization of the human pituitary. Acta Anat., *81*:286, 1972.
Lerner, A. B., and Takahashi, Y.: Hormonal control of melanin pigmentation. Recent Progr. Hormone Res., *12*:203, 1956.
McCann, S. M.: Luteinizing-hormone-releasing hormone. N. Engl. J. Med., *296*:797, 1977.
Purves, H. D.: Cytology of the adenohypophysis. *In* Harris, G. W., and Donovan, B. T. (eds.): The Pituitary Gland. vol. 1, p. 147. Berkeley, University of California Press, 1966.
Salazar, H., and Peterson, R. R.: Morphologic observations concerning the release and transport of secretory products in the adenohypophysis. Am. J. Anat., *115*:199, 1964.

THE POSTERIOR LOBE OF THE PITUITARY (NEUROHYPOPHYSIS)

Bargmann, W.: Neurosecretion. Int. Rev. Cytol., *19*:183, 1966.
Bodian, D.: Nerve endings, neurosecretory substance and lobular organization of the neurohypophysis. Bull. Johns Hopkins Hosp., *33*:354, 1951.
———: Herring bodies and neuroapocrine secretion in the monkey. An electron microscope study of the fate of the neurosecretory product. Bull. Johns Hopkins Hosp., *118*:282, 1966.
Palay, S. L.: The fine structure of the neurohypophysis. *In* Waelsch, H. (ed.): Progress in Neurobiology. II. Ultrastructure and Cellular Chemistry of Neural Tissue. p. 31. New York, Paul B. Hoeber, 1957.
Paterson, J. A., and Leblond, C. P. L.: Increased proliferation of neuroglia and endothelial cells in the supraoptic nucleus and hypophysial neural lobe of young rats drinking hypertonic sodium chloride solution. J. Comp. Neurol., *175*:373, 1977.
Sawyer, W. H.: Neurohypophyseal hormones. Pharmacol. Rev., *13*:225, 1961.

THE THYROID GLAND: FOLLICULAR CELLS

General

Werner, S. C., and Ingbar, S. (eds.): The Thyroid, A Fundamental and Clinical Text. ed. 3. New York, Harper & Row, 1971.

Special

Bowers, C. Y., Schally, A. V., Reynolds, G. A., and Hawley, W. D.: Interactions of L-thyroxine of L-triiodothyronine and thyrotrophin-releasing factor on the release and synthesis of thyrotrophin from the anterior pituitary gland of mice. Endocrinology, *81:*741, 1967.

Nadler, N. J.: Anatomy of the thyroid gland. *In* Werner, S. (ed.): The Thyroid. ed. 3. New York, Harper & Row, 1969.

Nadler, N. J., Young, B. A., Leblond, C. P., and Mitmaker, B.: Elaboration of thyroglobulin in the thyroid follicle. Endocrinology, *74:*333, 1964.

Studer, H., and Greer, M. A.: The Regulation of Thyroid Function in Iodine Deficiency. Bern, Huber, 1968.

Wayne, E. J., Koutras, D. A., and Alexander, W. D.: Clinical Aspects of Iodine Metabolism. Oxford, Blackwell, 1964.

THE LIGHT CELLS OF THE THYROID: CALCITONIN

Bussolati, G., and Pearse, A. G. E.: Immunofluorescent localization of calcitonin in the "C" cells of pig and dog thyroid. J. Endocrinol., *37:*205, 1967.

Copp, D. H.: *In* Bourne, G. H. (ed.): The Biochemistry and Physiology of Bone. vol. 2, p. 337. New York. Academic Press, 1972.

Copp, D. H., Cockcroft, D. W., and Kyett, Y.: Ultimobranchial origin of calcitonin, hypocalcemic effect of extracts from chicken glands. Can. J. Physiol. Pharmacol., *45:*1095, 1967.

Copp, D. H.: Historic development of the calcitonin concept. Am. J. Med., *43:*648, 1967.

Foster, G. V., MacIntyre, I., and Pearse, A. G. E.: Calcitonin production and the mitochondrion-rich cells of the dog thyroid. Nature, *203:*1029, 1964.

Hirsch, P. F., and Munson, P. L.: Thyrocalcitonin. Physiol. Rev., *49:*548, 1968.

Holtrop, M. E., Raisz, L. G., and Simmons, H.: The effects of parathyroid hormone, colchicine and calcitonin on the ultrastructure and activity of osteoclasts in organ culture. J. Cell Biol., *60:*346, 1974.

MacIntyre, I.: Calcitonin: a general review. Calcif. Tissue Res., *1:*173, 1967.

Marks, S. C.: The thyroid parafollicular cell as the source of a potent osteoblast-stimulating factor: evidence from osteopetrotic mice. J. Bone Joint Surg., *51A:*875, 1969.

Nonidez, J. F.: The origin of the "parafollicular" cells, a second epithelial component of the thyroid gland of the dog. Am. J. Anat., *49:*479, 1932.

Nunez, E. A., and Gershon, M. D.: Cytophysiology of thyroid parafollicular cells. Int. Rev. Cytol., *52:*1, 1978.

Pearse, A. G. E.: The cytochemistry of the thyroid "C" cells and their relationship to calcitonin. Proc. R. Soc. Biol., *164:*478, 1966.

Pearse, A. G. E., and Carvalheira, A. F.: Cytochemical evidence for an ultimobranchial origin of rodent thyroid C cells. Nature, *214:*929, 1967.

Rasmussen, H., and Pechet, M. A.: Calcitonin. Sci. Am., *223:*42; Oct., 1970.

Taylor, S. (ed.): Calcitonin. Proc. Symp. Thyrocalcitonin and the C Cells. London, Heinemann, 1968.

Young, B. A., and Leblond, C. P.: The light cells as compared to the follicular cell in the thyroid gland of the rat. Endocrinology, *73:*669, 1963.

See also references under Osteoclasts at the end of Chapter 15.

THE PARATHYROID GLANDS

Barnicot, N. A.: The local action of the parathyroid and other tissues on bone in intracerebral grafts. J. Anat., *82:*233, 1948.

Chang, H.: Grafts of parathyroid and other tissues to bone. Anat. Rec., *111:*23, 1951.

Copp, D. H., and Talmage, R. V. (eds.): Endocrinology of calcium metabolism. Proc. 6th Parathyroid Conf., 1977. Amsterdam, Excerpta Medica, 1978.

Greep, R. O., and Talmadge, R. V. (eds.): The Parathyroids. Springfield, Ill., Charles C Thomas, 1961.

Ham, A. W., Littner, N., Drake, T. G. H., Robertson, E. C., and Tisdall, F. F.: Physiological hypertrophy of the parathyroids, its cause and its relation to rickets. Am. J. Pathol., *16:*277, 1940.

Holtrop, M. E., King, G. J., Cox, K. A., and Reit, B.: Time related changes in the ultrastructure of osteoclasts after injection of parathyroid hormone in young rats. Calcif. Tissue Res., *in press.*

Howard, J. E., and Thomas, W. C.: The biological mechanisms of transport and storage of calcium. Can. Med. Assoc. J., *104:*699, 1971.

King, G. J., Holtrop, M. E., and Raisz, L. G.: The relation of ultrastructural changes in osteoclasts to resorption in bone cultures stimulated with parathyroid hormone. Metabolic Bone Disease and Related Research, *1:*67, 1978.

Mundy, G. R., Varani, J., Orr, W., Gondek, M. D., and Ward, P. A.: Resorbing bone is chemotactic for monocytes. Nature, *275:*132, 1978.

Munger, B. L., and Roth, S. I.: The cytology of the normal parathyroid glands of man and Virginia deer. A light and electron microscopic study with morphologic evidence of secretory activity. J. Cell Biol., *16:*379, 1963.

Talmage, R. V., Owens, M., and Parsons, J. A. (eds.): Calcium-regulating Hormones. Proc. 5th Parathyroid Conf., Amsterdam, Excerpta Medica, 1975.

See also references under Osteoclasts at the end of Chapter 15.

THE ADRENAL GLAND: CORTEX AND MEDULLA

Currie, A. R., Symington, T., and Grant, J. K. (eds.): The Human Adrenal Cortex. Baltimore, Williams & Wilkins, 1962.

Eisenstein, A. B. (ed.): The Adrenal Cortex. Boston, Little Brown & Co., 1967.

Hewer, E. E., and Keene, M. F. L.: Observations on the development of the human suprarenal gland. J. Anat., *61:*302, 1927.

Idelman, S.: Ultrastructure of the mammalian adrenal cortex. Int. Rev. Cytol., *27:*181, 1970.

Long, C. N. H.: Pituitary-adrenal relationships. Ann. Rev. Physiol., *18:*409, 1956.

Long, J. A., and Jones, A. L.: Observations on the fine structure of the adrenal cortex of man. Lab. Invest., *17:*355, 1967.

Moon, H. D. (ed.): The Adrenal Cortex. New York, Hoeber, 1961.

Prunty, F. T. G. (ed.): The adrenal cortex. Br. Med. Bull., *18:*89, 1962.

Ryan, U. S., Ryan, J. W., Smith, D. S., and Winkler, H.: Fenestrated endothelium of the adrenal gland: freeze-fracture studies. Tissue and Cell, *7:*181, 1975.

Selye, H.: Physiology and Pathology of Exposure to Stress. Montreal, Acta, 1950.

Symington, T.: Functional Pathology of the Human Adrenal Gland. Baltimore, Williams & Wilkins, 1969.

Tepperman, J.: Metabolic and Endocrine Physiology. Chicago, Year Book Medical Publishers, 1962.

Vane, J. R., Wolstenholme, G. E. W., and O'Connor, M.: Adrenergic Mechanisms. Ciba Foundation Symposium. Boston, Little, Brown & Co., 1960.

Yates, R. D.: A light and electron microscope study correlating the chromaffin reaction and granule ultrastructure in the adrenal medulla of the Syrian hamster. Anat. Rec., *149:*237, 1964.

THE ISLETS OF LANGERHANS

Allen, F. M.: Pathology of diabetes: I. Hydropic degeneration of islands of Langerhans after partial pancreatectomy. J. Metabolic Res., *1:*5, 1922.

Banting, F. G., and Best, C. H.: The internal secretion of the pancreas. J. Lab. Clin. Med., *7:*251, 1922.

Bencosme, S. A., Mariz, S., and Frei, J.: Studies on the function of the alpha cells of the pancreas. Am. J. Clin. Pathol., *28:*594, 1957.

Best, C. H., Campbell, J., Haist, R. E., and Ham, A. W.: The effect of insulin and anterior pituitary extract on the insulin content of the pancreas and the histology of the islets. J. Physiol., *101:*17, 1942.

Campbell, J., Haist, R. E., Ham, A. W., and Best, C. H.: The insulin content of the pancreas as influenced by anterior pituitary extract and insulin. Am. J. Physiol., *129:*328, 1940.

Gomez-Acebo, J., Parrilla, R., and R-Candela, J. L.: Fine structure of the A and D cells of the rabbit endocrine pancreas in vivo and incubated in vitro. I. Mechanism of secretion of the A cells. J. Cell Biol., *36:*33, 1968.

Ham, A. W., and Haist, R. E.: Histological effects of anterior pituitary extracts. Nature, *144:*835, 1939.

———: Histological studies of trophic effects of diabetogenic anterior pituitary extracts and their relation to the pathogenesis of diabetes. Am. J. Pathol., *17:*787, 1941.

Hellerström, C.: Growth pattern of pancreatic islets in animals. *In* Volk, B. W., and Wellmann, K. F. (eds.): The Diabetic Pancreas. New York, Plenum Press, 1977.

Hellerström, C., and Andersson, A.: Aspects of the structure and function of the pancreas B-cell in diabetes mellitus. Acta Paediatr. Scand. [Suppl.], *270:*7, 1977.

Lacy, P. E.: The pancreatic beta cell: structure and function. N. Engl. J. Med., *276:*187, 1967.

von Mering, J., and Minkowski, O.: Diabetes mellitus nach Pankreasextirpation. Arch. exp. Path. Pharmakol., *26:*371, 1889.

Ssobolew, L. W.: Zur normalen und pathologischen Morphologie der inneren Secretion der Bauchspeicheldrüse. Virchows Arch. path. Anat., *168:*91, 1902.

Volk, B. W., and Wellmann, K. F. (eds.): The Diabetic Pancreas. New York, Plenum Press, 1977.

For further papers of historical importance, *see* references for Chapter 25 of the 7th edition of this textbook (1974).

THE PINEAL BODY

Anderson, E.: The anatomy of bovine and ovine pineals: light and electron microscope studies. J. Ultrastruct. Res., Suppl. 8, May, 1965.

Kelly, D. E.: Pineal organs: photoreception, secretion and development. Am. Sci., *50:*597, 1962.

Møller, M.: The ultrastructure of the human fetal pineal gland. Cell Tiss. Res., *151:*13, 1974.

Møller, M.: Presence of a pineal nerve (nervus pinealis) in the human fetus; a light and electron microscopical study of the innervation of the pineal gland. Brain Res., *154:*1, 1978.

Quay, W. B.: Cytologic and metabolic parameters of pineal inhibition by continuous light in the rat. Z. Zellforsch., *60:*479, 1963.

Reiter, R. J., and Fraschini, F.: Endocrine aspects of the mammalian pineal gland: a review. Neuroendocrinology, *5:*219, 1969.

Relkin, R.: The Pineal. Montreal, Eden Press, 1976.

Wolstenholme, G. E. W., and Knight, J. (eds.): The Pineal Gland. Ciba Foundation Symposium. Edinburgh, Churchill-Livingstone, 1971.

Wurtman, R. J., and Axelrod, J.: The pineal gland. Sci. Am., *213:*50, July, 1965.

26 The Female Reproductive System

INTRODUCTORY ACCOUNT OF THE PARTS OF THE FEMALE REPRODUCTIVE SYSTEM AND THEIR FUNCTIONS

The female reproductive system consists of two *ovaries*, two *oviducts* (also called *uterine* or *fallopian tubes*), a *uterus*, a *vagina*, *external genitalia*, and two *mammary glands* (breasts). All but the latter are illustrated in Figures 26-1 and 26-2.

The Ovaries. In the sexually mature woman the ovaries are somewhat flattened, ovoid bodies, 2.5 to 5.0 cm. long, 1.5 to 3 cm. wide, and 0.6 to 1.5 cm. thick (Fig. 26-1). The anterior wall of each is attached to the broad ligament (Fig. 26-1), close to the lateral wall of the true pelvis, by means of a short fold of peritoneum called the *mesovarium* (Fig. 26-9), which conducts vessels and nerves to and from the hilum of the ovary. A rounded ligament, *the ligament of the ovary,* connects the medial end of each ovary with the uterus (Fig. 26-1). The ovary itself is unusual in being covered not with typical peritoneum, but with *epithelium* (Fig. 26-9) that ranges from columnar to flattened cuboidal. The cut surface of the ovary shows a *cortex* and *medulla;* the latter contains many blood vessels.

Ovulation and How It Causes Scars on the Surface of the Ovary. The surface of a mature ovary is scarred and pitted; this is due to it having shed many germ cells. As we shall see, these are contained within the cortex in epithelial vesicles called *follicles.* In a nonpregnant, sexually mature woman a follicle in either of the ovaries matures and ruptures through the surface (and in doing so liberates a secondary oocyte) approximately every 28 days. This is known as *ovulation.* Since each time ovulation occurs an oocyte, surrounded by some epithelial cells (plus some fluid), has to burst through the surface of the ovary, each ovulation results in a break on the surface that has to heal. The remaining cells of the follicle from which the oocyte was liberated become transformed into a body called a *corpus luteum,* the endocrine function of which will be described presently. If pregnancy does not occur, the corpus luteum functions for only about 10 to 12 days, after which it degenerates and is replaced by a gradually contracting scar. The scars forming from repeated ovula-

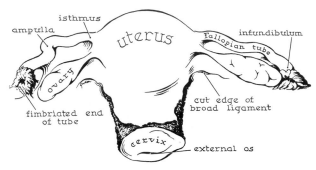

Fig. 26-1. Diagram of the posterior aspect of the uterus, oviducts, and ovaries.

tion result in the surface of the ovary becoming increasingly wrinkled and pitted. As we shall see, the fact that the covering epithelium of the ovary dips down in the crevices that form in this way is important, for the epithelium at the bottom of a crevice may become pinched off from the surface and form a small inclusion cyst.

If pregnancy occurs after an ovulation, the corpus luteum that forms at the ovulation site continues to develop and function for several months, and by the time it finally degenerates, it has become large enough to leave a relatively large scar in the ovary.

The Path of the Ovum. When a follicle ruptures through the surface of an ovary, its oocyte, surrounded by some of the cells of the follicle that still adhere to it, is extruded directly into the peritoneal cavity. As is illustrated in Figure 26-1, the open end of each oviduct is funnel-shaped, and the wide end of the funnel is more or less fitted over the aspect of the ovary from which ova are liberated. Figure 26-1 also shows that the expanded open end of the oviduct is *fimbriated* (L. *fimbriae,* fringe); this arrangement permits much of the ovarian surface to be encompassed in such a way that a liberated oocyte is led into what is labeled the *infundibulum* (L. for funnel) of the oviduct (labeled Fallopian tube) in Figure 26-1, *right,* and as a result it enters the lumen of the oviduct.

The *oviducts* (labeled *Fallopian tubes* in Fig. 26-1) are the tubes that connect the ovaries to the uterus. Each is covered with peritoneum (the broad ligament is its mesen-

834

tery). Each oviduct has a muscular wall and is lined with a mucous membrane equipped with ciliated epithelium, which will be described later. Unlike male germs cells (spermatozoa), an ovum cannot move by its own efforts; hence an ovum, delivered (as a secondary oocyte) into the open end of the oviduct, must be moved to the cavity of the uterus by actions performed by the walls of the oviduct. It is probable that peristalic contractions sweeping from the proximal end of the oviduct toward the uterus are chiefly responsible for moving an ovum to the uterus, although some believe the action of the cilia of the epithelial lining of the tubes may somehow assist.

The Usual Site of Fertilization. The mucous membrane of the oviduct is thrown into an extraordinary arrangement of longitudinal folds (Fig. 26-15A). Each fold has a core of lamina propria. These folds probably ensure that an ovum that enters the open end of the tube is kept in close contact on almost all sides with living cells and compatible fluids as it passes along the tube. These folds probably also provide similar protection for male germ cells, should these have been introduced into the vagina (Fig. 26-2), for spermatozoa swim up the cervical canal into the cavity of the body of the uterus (Fig. 26-2) and then enter the oviducts. It is in the maze created by the folds of mucous membrane in the oviduct that fertilization occurs (Fig. 26-12). It is therefore not surprising that fertilization can occur in what is generally described by the media as a test tube, because in vivo it actually occurs in fluid that is outside the body substance in a fallopian tube.

The Uterus. This is a hollow muscular organ with thick walls. It occupies a central position in the pelvis (Fig. 26-2). In shape it resembles an inverted pear that is somewhat flattened. Its narrower part is the *body*. The uppermost part of the body—that part above the level of the entrance of the oviducts—is the *fundus*. Since the body of the uterus is somewhat flattened, its central cavity is slit-like, with its anterior and posterior walls in apposition. In its upper part, this slit-like cavity is continuous at each side with the lumen of an oviduct. The cavity of the body narrows below and is continuous with the canal of the *cervix*, which is the lowermost part of the uterus (Fig. 26-2). The cervical canal, in turn, opens into the *vagina* (Fig. 26-2).

The Endometrium and Menstruation. The body of the uterus is lined by a special kind of mucous membrane termed *endometrium* (Gr. *metra*, womb) that is pitted with simple tubular glands. In the sexually mature, but not old, nonpregnant woman the innermost (thicker) part of this layer breaks down and is exfoliated into the cavity of the uterus approximately every 28 days. The process of exfoliation takes about 4 days, during which time the raw surface created by continuing exfoliation bleeds. The mixture of blood, glandular secretion, and broken-down endometrium delivered into the cavity of the uterus and passed out through the cervical canal and vagina consti-

tutes the *menstrual* (L. *mensis*, monthly) *flow*, and the process is called *menstruation*. Following menstruation the endometrium *regenerates*. Ovulation also occurs every 28 days. Although there is much variation, ovulation does not coincide with menstruation but occurs about halfway between menstrual periods. Both ovulation and menstruation are results of cyclical secretion of hormones, as will be described later.

Pregnancy. The liberation of an ovum (as a secondary oocyte) from an ovary, its fertilization in the oviduct, the changes that occur in it as it passes along the oviduct to the uterus, and its implantation into the endometrium—and this marks the beginning of pregnancy—are all illustrated diagrammatically in Figure 26-12. Details will be given later.

The further development of the fertilized, embedded ovum into an embryo constitutes the subject matter of *embryology*. The formation of the *placenta,* the organ responsible for interchange of dissolved substances between the bloodstreams of mother and embryo, is described later in this chapter.

Menstruation becomes interrupted once a fertilized ovum implants in the endometrium; hence, a "missed" menstrual period is a time-honored, though by no means conclusive, sign of pregnancy. Menstruation does not occur throughout pregnancy.

Parturition. When the fetus has reached full term, parturition (L. *parturire*, to be in labor) occurs so that a baby is born. The muscle wall of the uterus, which has become very thick during pregnancy, contracts, and the cervix

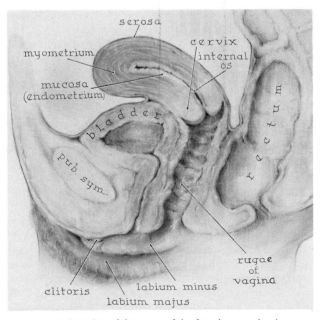

Fig. 26-2. Drawing of the parts of the female reproductive system, as seen in sagittal section.

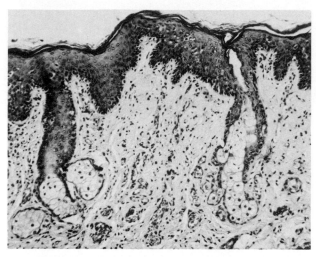

Fig. 26-3. Low-power photomicrograph of a labium minus. Note that only rudimentary hair follicles are present; these produce no hairs but are associated with sebaceous glands, which are seen as islands of large, pale-staining cells at *lower left* and *lower right.*

present. The cores of the folds contain fat and some smooth muscle.

Near the anterior end of the cleft between the labia majora is a small body of erectile tissue, the *clitoris* (Fig. 26-2). This is the homologue of the penis of the male. Two delicate folds of skin, the *labia minora,* arise just anterior to it. After investing part of the clitoris between them they pass posteriorly, following much the same course as the labia majora to which they lie medial. The labia minora consist of thin folds of skin but possess no hairs (Fig. 26-3). Sebaceous and sweat glands are found on both their surfaces (Fig. 26-3). Although the inner surface of each fold consists of skin, it exhibits the pink color of a mucous membrane.

The Hymen. The labia minora enclose the vestibule of the vagina. In the virgin, an incomplete membranous fold, the *hymen* (Fig. 26-4), projects centrally from the rim of the vestibule and partially occludes the vaginal entrance. Two small glands, the *glands of Bartholin,* which are tubulo-alveolar in type and secrete mucus, are present,

(Fig. 26-2) – the outlet of the uterus – dilates, whereupon the fetus, usually head foremost, slips through the dilated cervix and vagina to reach the outside world. The placenta then separates, and the baby begins an independent existence.

The Vagina. The vagina (L. for sheath) is a flattened tube; it serves as a sheath for the male organ in sexual intercourse. Its walls consist chiefly of smooth muscle and fibroelastic connective tissue, lined with a mucous membrane thrown into transverse folds known as *rugae* (Fig. 26-2). The epithelium is of the stratified squamous nonkeratinizing type. This type of epithelium also covers the region of the cervix that projects into the vagina.

The External Genitalia. The external genitalia consist of several structures (Fig. 26-2). A collection of fat deep to the skin that covers the symphysis pubis causes the skin to be raised here in the form of a rounded eminence; this is called the *mons pubis* or *mons veneris.* At puberty this eminence becomes covered with hair. Two folds of skin, the *labia majora* (Fig. 26-2), originate just below the mons pubis. They separate from one another as they pass posteriorly and approach one another again (but do not actually meet) a short distance posterior to the external opening of the vagina; hence, the vagina opens into the cleft which they enclose. Each of these folds has two surfaces covered with skin. The epidermis covering the outer surface of each tends to be pigmented and is equipped with many large hair follicles and sebaceous glands. That of the inner surface also has hair follicles and sebaceous glands, but the hairs are delicate. Sweat glands are also

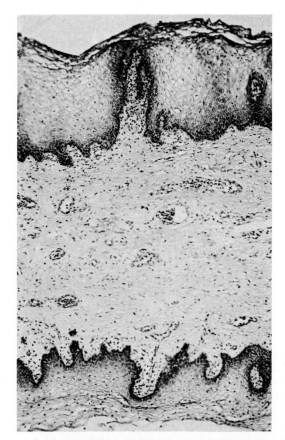

Fig. 26-4. Low-power photomicrograph of the full thickness of the hymen. Both surfaces are covered with stratified squamous nonkeratinizing epithelium and have high papillae.

one on each side of the vestibule. Each drains into a duct that empties into the groove between the hymen and the labium minus on the side on which the gland is situated. Two elongated masses of erectile tissue, constituting the bulb of the vestibule, lie beneath the surface along each side of the vestibule. Anteriorly, these two masses approximate each other. Many mucous glands are present beneath the surface around the vestibule. The urethral orifice is in the midline between the labia minora and between the clitoris and the opening of the vagina (Fig. 26-2).

The external genitalia are richly provided with sensory nerve endings.

THE OVARIES

Basic Microscopic Features. Each ovary consists of a *cortex* and *medulla.* The surface of the cortex is covered with a single layer of epithelium. In young women this is cuboidal (Fig. 26-9), but later in life it becomes flattened over parts of the ovary, though it remains cuboidal in the surface pits and crevices.

The connective tissue substance of the cortex is called its *stroma.* It consists of spindle-shaped cells that in most respects resemble fibroblasts, and intercellular substance. Most of the cortex contains a high proportion of cells to intercellular substance; hence in sections it appears heavily nucleated (Fig. 26-5). Moreover, the bundles of cells and fibers run in various directions; hence in sections the stroma of the cortex has a characteristic "swirly" appearance (Fig. 26-5). However, the layer of cortex immediately beneath the epithelium differs in having a higher proportion of intercellular substance, and its fiber bundles and cells are arranged more or less parallel to the surface. This layer is called the *tunica albuginea,* the white appearance that its name suggests being due to its great content of intercellular substance and lack of vascularity.

The medulla is small compared to the cortex, and its connective tissue is loosely arranged. It differs further in containing more elastic fibers, some smooth muscle cells, spiral arteries, and extensive convolutions of veins. The veins may be so large and contain so many blood cells that in a section the student may mistake one for an area of hemorrhage or a hemangioma (blood vessel tumor). Small blood vessels extend from the medulla into the cortex.

The Development of the Ovaries and the Origin of Follicles. The ovaries develop from ridges, termed *gonadal* (*genital*) *ridges,* bulging from the surface of the coelomic cavity. The ridges are located one on each side of the midline between the dorsal mesentery and mesonephros. Eventually the tissue of these two ridges forms the two almond-shaped ovaries.

First, the mesodermal cells at the surface of the devel-

oping ovary differentiate into a layer of epithelial cells covering the organ. In other sites in the coelomic cavity surface cells differentiate into the thinner mesothelial cells that line the periotoneal cavity.

Second, beneath the covering epithelium, cords of cells similar to the covering cells appear among the stromal cells. This is reminiscent of the development of epithelial glands, and a commonly held view is that the cords of cells that appear in the cortex represent downgrowths from the surface epithelium.

Third, about the time when developing cords of cells are seen, *primordial* (original) *germ cells* make their appearance in the cortex along with the cells of the cords. It was once incorrectly thought that the primordial germ cells develop from cells of these epithelial cords. However, it became established that the primordial germ cells originate in the *endoderm of the yolk sac,* from which they migrate to the developing ovary and move into its substance at about the time the cords are forming in the cortex. Hence, the epithelium of the ovary, which is still commonly referred to as a *germinal* epithelium, is *not* germinal in giving rise to the primordial germ cells.

Next, it is questionable whether the covering epithelium is even germinal with regard to giving rise to the cords and/or cells that surround the primordial germ cells. If the covering epithelium of the ovary is ever germinal in this respect, it subsequently loses potentiality, for cysts or tumors developing from covering epithelial cells (pinched off in crevices following the repair of a ruptured follicle) are of a different character from cysts or tumors developing from the granulosa (epithelial) cells that surround the germ cells to constitute the follicles. An alternative source of both the cords and the cells that surround the germ cells could be stroma cells which, at that time, could be expected to possess a great deal of potentiality.

Moreover, in the study of pathology, conceiving of the covering epithelium of the ovary as a germinal epithelium is a handicap in understanding certain lesions that may develop in the ovary. The term *germinal epithelium* is nevertheless so firmly entrenched in the literature that it unfortunately continues to be used.

The female germ cells that migrate to the ovaries and gain entrance to their stroma are called *oogonia* (Gr. *oon,* egg; *gone,* generation). Early in the development of the ovaries they proliferate by mitosis so as to increase greatly in numbers. However, as prenatal development proceeds, most of these germ cells die. There are roughly 2 million in the two ovaries at birth, but by puberty large numbers have already degenerated so that only 40,000 or thereabouts remain. Beginning at puberty, a germ cell is liberated from one or the other of the ovaries every 28 days or so; this process is called *ovulation.* Normally, ovulation is interrupted only if a pregnancy occurs. It ceases at the menopause.

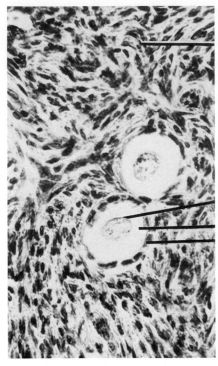

stroma

oocyte:
nucleus

cytoplasm
follicular
epithelium

Fig. 26-5. High-power photomicrograph of an ovary of a sexually mature woman, showing its characteristically "swirly" stroma and two primary follicles. Note that the follicular epithelium is only one cell thick and consists of low cuboidal cells. These follicles have not yet responded to FSH.

The continued development of a germ cell and its coverings (*see* below) is associated with secretion of two hormones, *estrogen* and *progesterone*. The initiation of puberty in girls is due primarily to estrogen being secreted by the succession of follicles beginning to develop in the ovaries at this time. Estrogen is responsible for the development of the secondary female characteristics that appear at puberty.

We shall now go on to described how the follicles develop and liberate their germ cells.

Primary (Primordial) Follicles. When in the developing ovary a primordial germ cell becomes enclosed by a single layer of epithelial cells, the little body thus formed is called a *primordial* or *primary follicle* (Fig. 26-5). At about the end of the third month of fetal life the covered oogonia have begun to develop into larger cells, each termed a *primary oocyte.* The cells of the single layer that surrounds each oocyte are termed *follicular epithelial cells* or, more commonly, *granulosa cells* (why they should be termed granulosa cells is not clear, but this is nevertheless the common term used for them in pathological and clinical circles).

As was described in Chapter 3 on page 76 in connection with meiosis and chromosome anomalies, a germ cell

possesses only the haploid number of chromosomes and for this to be achieved primary oocytes have to undergo *meiosis.* The first meiotic (reduction) division begins during prenatal life.

Soon after primary oocytes are formed from the oogonia, they enter the prophase of their first meiotic division but do not complete it at this time. So by the time of birth they are still in the prophase of their first meiotic division, resting in that stage. They complete the first meiotic division only after puberty and in follicles about to rupture at the surface of the ovary (Fig. 26-9).

The Prepubertal Ovary and Its Endocrine Functions. From birth until puberty the ovary increases in size, but individual follicles only occasionally begin to grow and develop as they do after puberty. It is believed, however, that enough follicles undergo development to lead to formation of cells that secrete a little estrogen (the generic term for the female sex hormone). It is also believed that almost up until the time of puberty, the hypothalamic neurosecretory cells with the function of secreting FSH-releasing factor are very sensitive to estrogen and hence the small amounts made by a girl's ovaries up to the time of puberty are enough to keep them from secreting FSH-releasing factor. However, as puberty nears, these cells become less sensitive to estrogen, so that the small amounts made no longer keep them suppressed. They therefore secrete FSH-releasing factor and this stimulates production of FSH by the gonadotrophs of the anterior pituitary gland. The FSH in turn stimulates the development of follicles and the secretion of enough estrogen to initiate puberty.

The Ovary at Puberty — the Beginning of Cyclical Changes. The changes that occur in a woman at puberty are due to her ovaries beginning to come into full function. This is because they are stimulated by gonadotrophs of the anterior pituitary beginning to secrete the two gonadotrophic hormones: the follicle-stimulating hormone (FSH) and the luteinizing hormone (LH), also called the interstitial cell stimulating hormone (ICSH). To describe how these hormones affect follicles and stroma requires that we first describe primary follicles in more detail.

The Primary Follicles in the Postpubertal Ovary. Each of the several thousand *primary follicles* present in the cortical stroma of the ovaries at puberty consists of a primary oocyte around 25 to 30 μm. in diameter (Fig. 26-5) enclosed by a single layer of flattened follicular epithelium (Fig. 26-5), which gives the follicle as a whole a diameter of about 40 μm. The nucleus of the primary oocyte is large and pale and its chromatin fine and dispersed apart from that associated with its prominent nucleolus. Since the nucleus is resting in the prophase of its first meiotic division, it might be thought that it would have the appearance of a mitotic figure, instead of that of an interphase cell in which the chromatin is extended and dispersed. However, after prophase begins and before it is resumed much later in life, the prophase chromosomes become sufficiently extended to lose the appearance of prophase chromosomes. They stay this way until meiosis is resumed years later.

At the level of the LM, the cytoplasm of an oocyte is pale (Fig. 26-5) and can be shown to possess yolk granules. The EM shows that the cytoplasm contains a representation of the usual organelles.

THE DEVELOPMENT OF OVARIAN FOLLICLES UNDER HORMONAL STIMULATION

THE EFFECTS OF GONADOTROPHINS ON THE OVARY

Every 28 days or so in a sexually mature, nonpregnant woman, these cause several follicles in an ovary to develop, enlarge, and approach the surface. However, usually only one develops to its full extent (ripens fully) and ruptures through the surface, releasing its secondary oocyte into the open end of an oviduct.

The earliest sign of development of a follicle is manifested by the follicular epithelial cells. At first these become cuboidal, then columnar, and then, as a result of proliferation, stratified (Figs. 26-6 and 26-9); when the follicle has more than one layer of cells in its walls, it is known as a *secondary follicle*. In the meantime, the primary oocyte it contains increases in size, but its growth is not proportional to that of the follicular epithelium; hence follicular cells soon come to constitute the bulk of the follicle. When the primary oocyte has become about twice as big, a thick darker-staining membrane called the *zona pellucida* (Fig. 26-8) develops around it. Probably both the oocyte and the innermost follicular epithelial cells contribute to its formation.

During this period in which the oocyte grows in size it must of course receive nutrients from its exterior. The EM shows that its membrane extends into the zona pellucida in the form of microvilli and, furthermore, the follicular cells extend cytoplasmic processes into and through the zona pellucida to achieve contact with the cell membrane of the oocyte. It is thus via the follicular cells that the oocyte is provided with food. Furthermore, the oocyte contains many coated vesicles, indicating that it absorbs protein from its surface.

After the follicular cells have undergone continued division and become many cells thick, fluid begins to accumulate in little pools between them (Fig. 26-9). The precise origin of this fluid, which is called *follicular fluid,* is not known; its composition suggests that it is something more than tissue fluid and, hence, that it must be at least modified by the follicular cells among which it accumulates. The follicle enlarges because the follicular epithelial cells continue to proliferate, and fluid accumulates between them. The smaller pools fuse and this

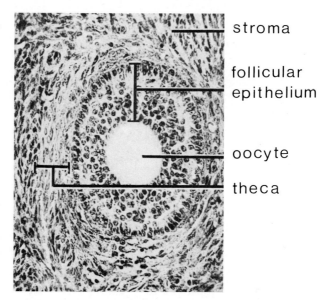

stroma

follicular epithelium

oocyte

theca

Fig. 26-6. Low-power photomicrograph of a secondary follicle in an ovary of a sexually mature woman. The follicular epithelium has begun to respond to FSH by becoming stratified but has not yet started to secrete fluid. The plane of section is such that it does not include the nucleus of the primary oocyte in the follicle. At this stage the theca can be discerned, indistinctly demarcated from the ovarian stroma.

leads to the bulk of the follicle comprising a large pool of fluid with the primary oocyte, together with the follicular cells that cover it, projecting into it from one side (Fig. 26-7). The little hill of follicular cells that contains the ovum is known as the *cumulus oophorus* (L. *cumulus,* heap; Gr. *oon,* egg, *phorus,* bearer).

While the follicle is developing as described above, the ovarian stroma that immediately surrounds the follicle becomes organized into a cellular wall called the *theca* (Gr. *theke,* a box).

The cells of this ensheath the epithelial follicle closely and soon become differentiated into two layers. The innermost layer, the *theca interna,* is relatively cellular and provided with many capillaries (Fig. 26-8). The outer layer, the *theca externa,* is more fibrous and not so vascular (Fig. 26-8). However, the line of demarcation between the two layers is not very distinct.

A fully developed follicle is so large in relation to the thickness of the cortex that it causes a bulge on the surface of the ovary (Fig. 26-9). Moreover, as the follicle grows, the width of the cortex between it and the ovary surface becomes thin.

For the changes thus far described, which amount to ripening of a follicle, both FSH and LH are necessary; however, the primary stimulus for growth and development of the follicle is considered to be FSH. A fully mature follicle is illustrated at extreme *right* in Figure 26-9.

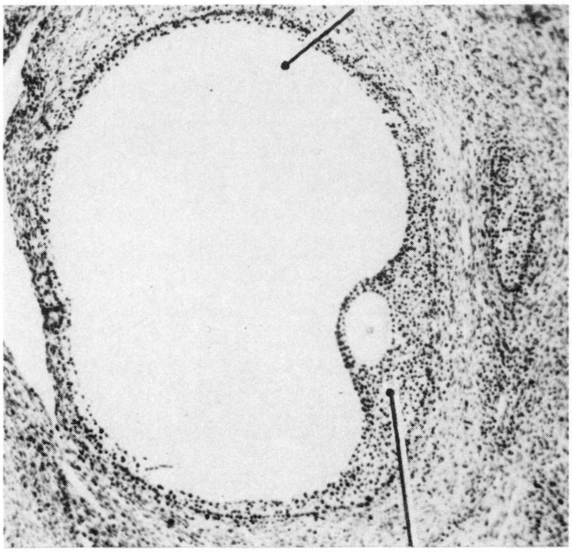

Follicular fluid

Fig. 26-7. Very low power photomicrograph of a developing follicle distended with follicular fluid, with its oocyte contained in a cumulus oophorus, in an ovary of a woman.

Cumulus oophorus

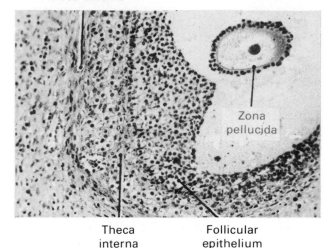

Theca externa

Zona pellucida

Theca interna   Follicular epithelium

Fig. 26-8. Low-power photomicrograph of a developing follicle in an ovary of a woman. The oocyte, with some surrounding follicular epithelial cells, appears free in the follicle, an appearance due to the plane of section. The oocyte shows an evident zona pellucida, and the two layers of the theca are now apparent.

There is at this time a surge in the secretion of LH and this has two effects. First, it causes the maturing follicle to grow further and burst. This action is not fully understood but seems to involve an increase in the vascularity of the theca interna, resulting in greater production of tissue fluid. When the follicle (several follicles in multiparous animals) bursts, the secondary oocyte it contains, still surrounded by the neighboring follicular cells that form what is termed its *corona radiata,* is liberated close to the proximal end of an oviduct (Figs. 26-9 and 26-12).

Before we go on to consider the second effect of the surge in LH we shall briefly review some changes occurring during the formation and liberation of the secondary oocyte at ovulation. The primary oocyte, which was in the late prophase of its first meiotic division, rapidly passes through the remaining stages of division. The apportionment of cytoplasm in this first meiotic division is very unequal, since one daughter cell, the *secondary oocyte,* retains almost all the cytoplasm and the other, the *first polar body,* receives almost none (Fig. 3-15A). The second meiotic division, which amounts to a mitotic division, is associated with further uneven distribution of cytoplasm since it involves the formation of an *ovum* and a small *second polar body* (Fig. 3-15B). The second meiotic division is also unique in two important respects. First, the secondary oocyte goes into division *without there being any S phase (DNA duplication) in the interphase* (this was dealt with more fully in Chap. 3 on p.

78). Second, the division does not reach completion unless *fertilization has taken place,* and this normally does not happen until the secondary oocyte is traveling along the oviduct (Fig. 26-12). Because the chromosome number is reduced to one half by the first meiotic division, the secondary oocyte and hence the ovum receive only the *haploid* number of chromosomes (Fig. 3-15).

Further to its effect in causing the mature follicle to burst and liberate its secondary oocyte, continuing secretion of LH by the gonadotrophs of the anterior pituitary causes a body termed a *corpus luteum* (L. *luteus,* yellow) to develop in the remains of the follicle, as will now be described.

The Development of a Corpus Luteum

After the secondary oocyte and some follicular fluid have been extruded at ovulation, the follicle collapses and its edges form a seal on the surface of the ovary (*lower right* in Fig. 26-9). The reduction in size of the follicle causes remaining follicular cells and theca interna to be thrown into folds (Fig. 26-9); only the theca externa retains its original shape. Rupture and collapse of the follicle usually results in a slight amount of hemorrhage so that a blood clot (*corpus hemorrhagicum*) forms in the ruptured follicle.

An early step in the development of the corpus luteum is that the remaining follicular epithelial cells enlarge greatly (Fig. 26-10) to become what are called *follicular*

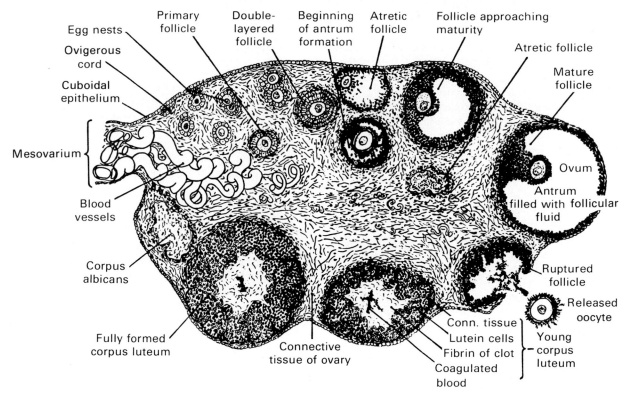

Fig. 26-9. Schematic diagram of an ovary, showing the sequence of events in the development, growth, and rupture of an ovarian follicle, and the formation and involution of a corpus luteum (following clockwise around the ovary, starting at *top left*). (Patten, B. M.: Human Embryology. New York, Blakiston Division of McGraw-Hill, 1946)

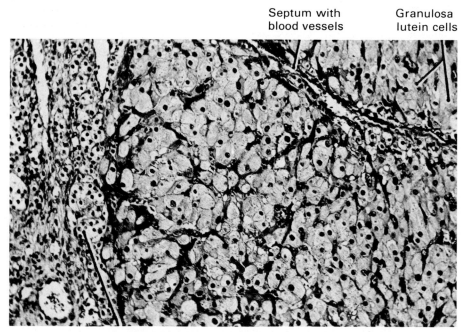

Fig. 26-10. High-power photomicrograph of part of a corpus luteum of pregnancy. Note the large, pale granulosa lutein cells with vacuoles in their cytoplasm. The theca lutein cells at *left* are smaller.

(granulosa) lutein cells. Their cytoplasm becomes abundant as a result of its accumulating lipid. Lutein pigment also forms somewhat later, and when enough accumulates, it imparts a yellow color to the corpus luteum.

The cells of the theca interna, which before ovulation had become enlarged, also become lutein cells. These are called *theca lutein* cells (Fig. 26-10) and, although of connective tissue origin, develop many of the characteristics of granulosa lutein cells.

Capillaries from the theca interna grow in among the cords and clumps of lutein cells as these develop. Hence the corpus luteum acquires the appearance of a typical *endocrine gland* (Fig. 26-10) and begins to secrete the hormone *progesterone,* which acts on the endometrium of the uterus (soon to be described) to make it a suitable implantation site for a fertilized ovum, should one come along. Fibroblasts from the theca interna grow into the more central part of the corpus luteum and there form an undifferentiated type of connective tissue with a high proportion of amorphous intercellular substance. This connective tissue surrounds remains of follicular fluid and clotted blood that are still present in the central part of the corpus luteum (Fig. 26-9).

Following ovulation the corpus luteum grows to a diameter of 1.5 to 2 cm. (Fig. 26-9). The growth it manifests is probably due to hypertrophy (and not hyperplasia) of its lutein cells. Unless the ovum (liberated as a secondary oocyte from the follicle before it becomes a corpus luteum) is fertilized, the corpus luteum grows and secretes progesterone only for about 10 to 12 days, after which it begins to involute; this is associated with its vessels collapsing. Moreover, as will be described later, the corpus luteum no longer continues to secrete enough progesterone to maintain the endometrium in luxuriant condition, so that it begins to show signs of impending disintegration, and is soon mostly cast off (in menstruation).

THE OVARIAN HORMONES: THE FINE STRUCTURE OF THE CELLS THAT PRODUCE THEM AND THE CONTROL OF THEIR SECRETION

The primary hormone made by the ovary is an *estrogen* (estradiol). In the following discussion, we shall use the generic term *estrogen* for female sex hormone. On being produced in effective amounts at puberty, estrogen is chiefly responsible for causing development of the secondary sex characteristics of the female. The other ovarian hormone is progesterone. Both are steroid hormones.

Estrogen Secretion in the Ovarian Cycle

Estrogen is in all likelihood secreted by the cells of the *theca interna* of the developing follicle. These are spindle-shaped cells, well supplied with capillaries. They reveal the usual organelles, rER, well-developed sER, a Golgi, free ribosomes, and some lysosomes. The cytoplasm also contains lipid droplets. Their mitochondria differ from those of most cells in often having tubular cristae. After ovulation these cells become *theca lutein* cells, to be described later.

In most mammals estrogen secretion reaches its peak when the follicle reaches the surface of the ovary and is ready to rupture, and this is generally the only time the female will copulate with a male. This, of course, is the very time that coitus is most likely to result in pregnancy. In women, estrogen secretion persists throughout the whole cycle but is somewhat greater at the time of ovulation. As estrogen secretion reaches it peak it exerts a negative feedback on the hypothalamic neurosecretory cells that secrete FSH-releasing factor so that further secretion of FSH and hence further follicular growth is inhibited. However, the estrogen peak has the reverse effect on the hypothalamic cells making LH-releasing factor, for at this time these are stimulated so that there is a surge of secretion of LH, the effects of which have been described in the preceding section.

It should be mentioned that women differ from the females of most mammalian species in that estrogen secretion does not go through wide swings, and as a consequence there is no exclusive time in their 28-day cycles when women will engage in coitus. In the human, psychological factors play important roles.

As already described, a surge in secretion of LH by the anterior pituitary roughly midway through the cycle triggers a corpus luteum to develop from what is left of the ruptured follicle. The corpus luteum, while its theca lutein cells (derived from the theca interna) continue to secrete estrogen, now also begins to secrete *progesterone*.

Progesterone Secretion and Its Control

The cells considered to secrete progesterone are the epithelial granulosa cells, once they have become transformed into *granulosa lutein cells* by LH. Prior to ovulation, these cells are in general cuboidal in shape. Their nucleus is large and their cytoplasm contains the usual organelles of epithelial cells plus a few lipid droplets. As noted, in the growth phase of the follicle they probably provide nutrients to the oocyte through the zona pellucida via cellular contacts with the oocyte.

After ovulation the granulosa cells that remain in the

follicle change considerably. They enlarge and become transformed into lutein cells. These are characterized particularly by possessing large amounts of sER; in this respect they are like other types of secretory cells involved in synthesizing and secreting steroid hormones. They also have some rER and prominent Golgi stacks and contain a good many lipid droplets.

Fate of the Corpus Luteum. Unless pregnancy occurs, the corpus luteum does not persist for more than 10 to 12 days; thus, unlike estrogen, progesterone is not made continuously in the nonpregnant female. The chief function of progesterone is to prepare the uterus for reception of a fertilized ovum. It does this anew each month, even in a virgin. Preparation entails making the endometrium (the lining of the uterus) grow thick and succulent so that a fertilized ovum, on reaching it from the oviduct, may become embedded and be nourished adequately. However, unless implantation occurs, the corpus luteum regresses, so that progesterone production ceases. As a result, the endometrium, brought to a high state of development by this hormone, disintegrates, desquamates, and bleeds; this constitutes menstruation. A new 28-day cycle then begins, with a new follicle beginning to develop.

Why the Corpus Luteum Fails. While the *formation* of the corpus luteum is triggered by the surge of LH secretion at around the midpoint of the cycle, its development for 12 days or so afterward is not dependent on high levels of LH being maintained in the blood. Although some LH may be present, it seems that unless there is a pregnancy the life of the corpus luteum is inherently determined. However, if fertilization occurs, the ovum becomes implanted in the lining of the uterus and pregnancy begins. This interferes with the ovarian cycle. Under these circumstances, for some reason the corpus luteum that formed does not regress after 12 days or so, but continues to develop and secrete progesterone, which is required to support the pregnancy (the reason for its persistence will be described presently). It does this for a few months, after which hormones produced by the placenta, to be described in due course, take over its function.

The hormonal and morphological changes that follow one another during the ovarian cycle in women are easier to understand —that is, they make more sense—if the reader is familiar with sex cycles in other mammals. Moreover, it was by studying these that knowledge developed about what happens in humans.

SEX CYCLES IN MAMMALS

The Estrous Cycle. In animals the mating instinct in the female becomes aroused only at certain seasons and she is said to have come into *heat* or *estrus* (Gr. *oistros,* mad desire); only at these times will a female mate. In some animals that live in the far north, estrus (like Christmas) occurs only once a year, whereas in rats and mice it happens every few days.

It took a long time to find out the cause of estrus. First, Stockard discovered that the stratified epithelium that lines the vagina of guinea pigs became keratinized at the time of estrus. Next, the finding that female mice from which ovaries had been removed did not go into estrus and that their vaginal epithelium did not become keratinized suggested that both estrus and keratinization of the vaginal epithelium were caused by a hormone produced by the ovary at the time of estrus.

In 1923, Allen and Doisy succeeded in preparing an extract from hog ovaries that, when injected into ovariectomized animals, caused their vaginal epithelium to become keratinized. Subsequently, the hormone itself (estrogen) was isolated and its chemical nature determined.

As noted, estrus as such does not occur in women. However, its counterpart does occur at about the time of ovulation, because at that time FSH (in the presence of low levels of LH) has acted on the ovary to make it secrete estrogen and bring a ripe follicle to its surface. But, although the amount of estrogen made is somewhat greater at this time, the *proportional increase* is not nearly as great as in animals at estrus.

Progesterone and Pseudopregnancy

The action of estrogen in itself was not enough to explain all the changes observed during the menstrual cycle of women. For example, it did not explain the histological changes in the lining of the uterus after ovulation (which will be described later in this chapter). It was natural that another ovarian hormone should be sought that would be capable of bringing about these changes, and soon *progesterone* was discovered. Studies using laboratory animals were again of the greatest assistance not only in elucidating the role of progesterone but also in ascertaining the factors involved in producing and maintaining the corpus luteum that secretes it, as will now be described.

It was noted in the preceding chapter that ovulation in the isolated female rabbit does not proceed automatically when she comes into estrus. Instead, she remains in a prolonged state of estrus until she mates. Under ordinary conditions, only on mating does ovulation occur. The explanation for this seems to be that afferent impulses set up as a result of coitus are relayed to the hypothalamus, where they stimulate neurosecretory cells to discharge into the hypophysio-portal circulation the releasing factor that causes secretion of LH. It is to be noted, however, that this mechanism is operative when the rabbit is in estrus and therefore has a relatively high blood level of estrogen. Accordingly, a high blood level of estrogen may be a prerequisite for this releasing factor to be secreted. The females of animals mate only when they are in estrus and have a high blood estrogen level.

Human females are apt to engage in intercourse at almost any time in the cycle, and there is no evidence to indicate that coitus early in the cycle automatically causes ovulation. It is, however, conceivable that, at about the time when ovulation might occur in any event, coitus could modify the time of ovulation slightly because of afferent impulses affecting secretion of LH-releasing factor.

There is evidence from studies on laboratory rats that effective secretion of LH-releasing factor at the appropriate time is dependent on there being relatively high levels of estrogen present, which in turn is due to there being ripened follicles in the ovary. Moreover, it has been suggested that the estrogen facilitates ovulation not only through triggering prepared LRF-secreting cells to liberate their LRF at this time, but also by raising the sensitivity of anterior pituitary gonadotrophs to LRF.

Pseudopregnancy in Animals. In a female rabbit mated with a sterile male not only does multiple ovulation occur but, in addition, corpora lutea develop. These for a time grow, develop, and secrete progesterone, and as a result the animal begins to exhibit all the signs of pregnancy except that its uterus does not contain any embryos. This false pregnancy is called *pseudopregnancy*. It continues for a considerable time, though not as long as true pregnancy. Its maintenance is due to the anterior pituitary continuing to secrete LH. However, after a time the corpora lutea in the ovaries involute, and the pseudopregnancy comes to an end. Before discussing why a false pregnancy terminates, we should consider a few other common animals.

The estrus cycle of that rat is different from that of the rabbit, for the isolated female rat remains in estrus for only a few hours and then begins a new estrous cycle. A new cycle is repeated approximately every 4 days. The rat ovulates spontaneously at the time of estrus. Nevertheless, if it does not mate, functional corpora lutea do not develop; hence, no estrogen and progesterone are made by corpora lutea to inhibit the anterior pituitary from secreting FSH, and so after estrus the anterior pituitary immediately begins again to secrete FSH. This brings a new crop of follicles to the surface of one of the ovaries in 4 days' time and stimulates the production of enough estrogen to put the rat into estrus by the time the follicles mature. The rat, therefore, illustrates that the *hormones made by the corpora lutea* are necessary if the secretion of FSH is to be *inhibited* immediately after estrus. If, however, a female rat mates with a sterile male at the time of estrus, functional corpora lutea do develop and these are maintained for a while. They secrete enough estrogen and progesterone into the bloodstream to cause pseudopregnancy and prevent the anterior pituitary from secreting FSH, which would cause a new estrous cycle to begin immediately. Therefore, the mating of a female rat with a sterile male interrupts her estrous cycle. When the pseudopregnancy has run a course of several days, it terminates. As the corpora lutea involute and cease making their hormones, the anterior pituitary thereupon is permitted once again to secrete FSH, and so a new estrous cycle begins.

The estrous cycle of the female dog is different still. An isolated bitch normally comes into estrus twice a year. Ovulation occurs spontaneously at estrus; evidently the high level of estrogen in the blood at the time of estrus triggers liberation of LRF from suitably prepared neurosecretory cells of the hypothalamus and leads to the surge of LH that causes ovulation. Moreover, the anterior pituitary, following ovulation, continues to secrete LH and/or prolactin for a considerable time and, as a result, pseudopregnancy automatically follows estrus in the isolated bitch. This continues approximately half as long as a real pregnancy. Under the influence of the hormones from the corpora lutea, the uterus enlarges, the belly droops, and the mammary glands begins to enlarge. When they notice these signs, owners not familiar with pseudopregnancy often wonder if the isolation they imposed on their pets at the time of estrus was as effective as they thought. But then pseudopregnancy terminates. The endometrium, previously built up by the action of progesterone, reverts to normal thickness; slight hemorrhages into the substance of the endometrium may occur at this time.

Relevance to the Human Female. It should be clear from the foregoing that menstruation in women is the counterpart of termination of pseudopregnancy in animals, and that it is precipitated by *failure of a corpus luteum to continue secretion of its hormones, particularly progesterone.* The reason for termination of pseudopregnancy in

women being associated with such a severe and prolonged event as menstruation, with pseudopregnancy terminating in animals with almost no disturbance, is related to the special pattern of blood vessels supplying the lining of the uterus in human females, which will be described in due course.

SUMMARY OF THE HORMONAL FACTORS IN THE SEX CYCLE OF NONPREGNANT WOMEN

Following failure of the corpus luteum there is not enough of the ovarian hormones in the blood to suppress secretion of FSH-releasing factor by the hypothalamus. As a consequence, FSH-releasing factor (FRF) is secreted and it stimulates gonadotrophs of the anterior pituitary to secrete FSH. This hormone, together with the low levels of LH, causes follicles to develop and approach the surface of the ovary as they mature. Usually only one follicle matures fully. Meanwhile, the cells of the theca interna of the developing follicle (or follicles) produce estrogen, so that the blood level of estrogen rises. This hormone then promotes liberation of LH-releasing factor (LRF) when the latter is secreted at the appropriate time by neurosecretory cells of the hypothalamus; it perhaps also augments the effectiveness of LRF by rendering gonadotrophs more responsive to it. The hypothalamus itself seems to control the timing of LRF release, acting something like an alarm clock. Estrogen is thus clearly implicated in the development of the surge of LH that occurs at this time. The estrogen has by now reached levels sufficient to inhibit further secretion of FSH-releasing factor, so FSH secretion ceases to be effective. LH secreted at this time causes ovulation and triggers development of a corpus luteum in the ruptured follicle. The corpus luteum secretes both estrogen and progesterone. Over the lifetime of that corpus luteum, probably both hormones—but particularly the estrogen—continue inhibiting secretion of the releasing factor for FSH (this inhibition began about the time of ovulation). The progesterone builds up the endometrium to be receptive to a fertilized ovum. However, if pregnancy does not occur, the corpus luteum after about 12 days begins to involute. It seems that the life span of the corpus luteum is predetermined unless pregnancy occurs. However, if pregnancy does occur, as described shortly, another hormone, *chorionic gonadotrophin,* which has many effects like LH, appears in the blood to maintain the corpus luteum. If pregnancy does not occur, the corpus luteum involutes. Since the endometrium was built up by the progesterone secreted by the corpus luteum, the withdrawal of progesterone occurring when the corpus luteum involutes causes menstruation. Since the estrogen (and to some extent the progesterone) produced by the corpus luteum have been inhibiting the anterior pituitary (via the hypothalamus and FRF) from secreting FSH, the failure of the corpus luteum (which results in the cessation of estrogen and progesterone secretion from this source) releases the anterior pituitary from suppression so that it immediately begins to secrete FSH again, and a new ovarian cycle is on its way.

ANOVULATORY CYCLES

Occasionally, women experience bleeding from the endometrium at the time of menstruation without ovulation having occurred, and thus without the development of a corpus luteum in the ovary. These unusual instances of menstrual bleeding without previous ovulation (anovulatory menstruation) are probably due to preceding variations in the level of blood estrogen. We shall elaborate.

If estrogen is withdrawn—for example, by removal of the ovaries from a sexually mature woman—the endometrium may bleed as a consequence. Furthermore, if estrogen is given to a female at a standard rate for a time and then the dosage is considerably reduced, but not entirely stopped, bleeding from the endometrium will occur not immediately but only after an interval of some days. Therefore it is believed that the bleeding that occurs in anovulatory menstruation is a delayed response to the reduction in the estrogen output of the ovary that occurs following the maturation of a follicle.

Anovulatory cycles in women are probably not as rare as was thought; a healthy woman may have three or four anovulatory cycles a year, with a higher proportion near puberty and menopause.

THE CORPUS LUTEUM OF PREGNANCY

If pregnancy does *not* occur, a corpus luteum reaches a diameter of from 1.5 to 2 cm. and begins to involute. Its capillaries collapse and its lutein cells disintegrate. It shrinks and finally becomes a small white scar called a *corpus albicans* (Fig. 26-9 and 26-11).

If pregnancy occurs, however, the corpus luteum continues to grow and function and attains a diameter of about 5 cm. in the third month of pregnancy. At that time, or somewhat later, it begins to involute. However, involution of a corpus luteum of pregnancy at this late date does not cause menstruation, because by this time the *placenta is producing progesterone,* and hence involution of the corpus luteum of pregnancy does not cause progesterone deficiency. Indeed, the placenta after a few months makes enough progesterone to support pregnancy. Involution of a corpus luteum of pregnancy leaves a substantial scar in the ovary since it is so large.

The Cause of Persistence and Growth of the Corpus Luteum in Pregnancy—Chorionic Gonadotrophin. How does pregnancy prevent a corpus luteum from involuting 12

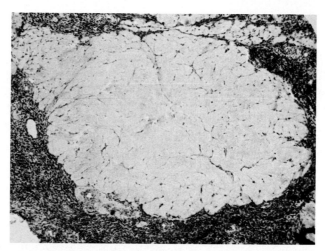

Fig. 26-11. Very low power photomicrograph of a corpus albicans that has formed as a result of involution of a corpus luteum of menstruation, in an ovary of a woman.

days or so after ovulation? The corpus luteum continues to develop because a new hormone that acts very much like LH with regard to the corpus luteum is made by the trophoblastic cells of what will become the placenta, soon after the ovum becomes implanted in the endometrium (Fig. 26-12). This hormone is called *chorionic (placental) gonadotrophin*. It differs from LH chiefly in that it cannot do everything that LH can do in an animal from which the anterior pituitary gland has been removed. However, if such an animal is given some anterior pituitary gonadotrophic hormone, chorionic gonadotrophin then exerts an LH effect. In other words, given a little collaboration by the appropriate hormones of the anterior pituitary, the action of chorionic gonadotrophin is similar to that of LH.

Pregnancy Tests. So much human chorionic gonadotrophin (HCG) is made in pregnancy that it is excreted in the urine. Indeed, if the urine of a pregnant woman is injected into an animal it causes observable physiological effects. This is the basis for pregnancy tests involving the use of animals. An instructive one is known as the Aschheim-Zondek test (Friedman modification), which will now be described briefly because it illustrates some points relevant to the general discussion.

As noted a few pages back, a sexually mature female virgin rabbit remains in estrus, with mature ovarian follicles present (labeled mf in Fig. 26-13) until she mates. At that time, ovulation would occur in response to the excitement and afferent stimulation of mating. However, it would also occur if LH were injected instead, and it would be possible by inspecting her ovaries to tell whether any hemorrhagic follicles (labeled hf in Fig. 26-13, as seen in section at *right*) or corpora lutea had developed as a result of ovulation. Furthermore, if human chorionic gonadotrophin (HCG) were injected instead, the same results could be expected, since HCG acts like LH in animals with an intact pituitary. There is so much HCG in a pregnant woman's urine that an intravenous injection of her urine into a mature virgin rabbit will cause it to ovulate, with the formation of hemorrhagic

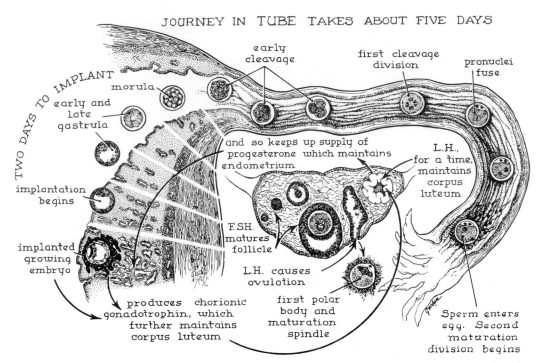

Fig. 26-12. Diagram illustrating the liberation of an oocyte from the ovary (*lower right*), entrance into the oviduct (*lower right*), fertilization, passage through the oviduct, and implantation in the endometrium, presented in an anticlockwise direction. The five segments of uterine wall shown represent, from *top* to *bottom,* the changes that occur in the endometrium from the time of ovulation to the time of implantation. (After Dickenson, R. L.: Human Sex Anatomy. Baltimore, Williams & Wilkins, 1933)

follicles (hf in Fig. 26-13, section at *right*), which, of course, would go on to form corpora lutea. Because there is no HCG in the urine of a woman unless she is pregnant, and never enough LH to cause the injected rabbit to ovulate, the appearance of the rabbit's ovaries (whether the ovaries appear as at *left* or as at *right* in Fig. 26-13) permits a conclusion to be drawn as to whether the woman tested was pregnant. It is not necessary to cut sections to tell the result since the corpora hemorrhagica and lutea can be seen on the ovarian surface.

Immunological Pregnancy Tests. These are quicker and more sensitive than animal pregnancy tests and have the cost benefit of not requiring upkeep of animals; hence they have almost entirely superseded testing in animals. They are based on utilizing antibody to HCG (raised in another species) to detect HCG in urine.

HORMONAL CONTRACEPTION

The development of knowledge about sex hormones over the last few decades has had, to say the least, a profound effect on society in providing a convenient and effective means of contraception for females.

Development of Knowledge. It was observed long ago that a pregnant female did not ovulate during pregnancy. Eventually it was realized that ovulation was suppressed because in pregnancy blood levels of estrogen and progesterone are quickly established that effectively inhibit production of FSH and hence ripening of follicles. Estrogen has a more potent effect than

progesterone in this respect, although in most animals progesterone will prevent ovulation. The source of estrogen early in pregnancy is the corpus luteum of pregnancy, which, of course, also produces progesterone. Later in pregnancy the placenta (in women) also produces estrogen and progesterone.

The next step was to use this knowledge to devise means for preventing ovulation in nonpregnant females. Although various approaches are now used to effect hormonal contraception, the basic one is to prevent ovulation artificially by the same means as occurs naturally during pregnancy.

Oral contraceptives in common use generally contain a synthetic estrogen that maintains a level of estrogenic activity in the blood sufficient to inhibit secretion of the releasing factor for FSH. Without effective amounts of FSH being secreted, follicles do not ripen in the ovary. Substances with progesterone-like activity are, in addition, also used in the preparations. These are not as potent as estrogen in inhibiting secretion of FSH, but they may inhibit to some extent the secretion of LH. At the proper time in the cycle some days are skipped, or a placebo (L. for "I will please," meaning a dummy pill containing only an inert substance) is taken, to cause both estrogen and progesterone withdrawal which, of course, brings on menstruation. On the proper day taking the effective preparation is resumed so that estrogen again becomes available to keep the anterior pituitary from secreting FSH during the next cycle.

It is to be noted that suppression of ovulation by any of these preparations depends on their exerting effects over 24-hour time periods. This is longer than a single dose of a natural hormone would last because natural hormones are soon metabolized.

Hence synthetic agents that have sufficiently long-lasting hormonal effects are used in oral contraceptives.

Certain side effects sometimes result from the use of oral contraceptives.

ATRETIC FOLLICLES

The cortex of the ovary of a sexually mature, nonpregnant woman who has borne children can contain a great variety of structures: primary follicles, follicles in various stages of development, follicles in various stages of degeneration, perhaps a functioning corpus luteum, and scars of corpora lutea, including large ones resulting from corpora lutea of pregnancy. We shall now describe features of some of these structures in more detail to help the student distinguish between them in sections.

Of the several follicles stimulated to develop in a woman in each cycle, usually only one reaches final stages of development and maturation and liberates its oocyte. The other large ones all undergo what is termed *atresia,* which from its derivation means the closing of a hole or opening. They do not, then, remain in a state of suspended animation, waiting for an opportunity to ovulate in a subsequent month, but die. For ovulation to occur in another month, a new set of follicles must develop and approach the surface.

In a given section of ovary, there may be many atretic follicles, and if they are just beginning to undergo atresia, it may be difficult to distinguish them from normal follicles. If atresia has proceeded for any length of time, however, the student's task is easier, for later on in atresia fibroblasts grow into the disintegrating follicle and replace it with connective tissue (Fig. 26-14, *right*). But before

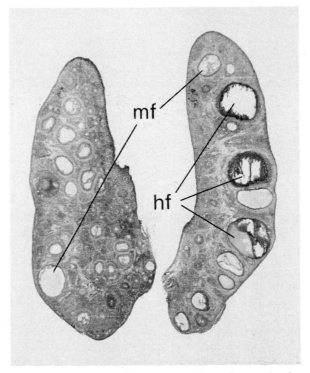

Fig. 26-13. (Left) Very low power photomicrograph of an ovary of a virgin rabbit injected with urine from a nonpregnant woman. Mature unruptured follicles (mf), but no hemorrhagic follicles (hf), are seen near the surface. (*Right*) Very low power photomicrograph of ovary of a virgin rabbit injected with urine from a pregnant woman. Note that three large follicles (labeled hf) are filled with blood as a result of ovulation. On high-power examination, each of these would be seen to have developed a lining of granulosa luteal cells. This is the picture seen in a positive rabbit pregnancy test.

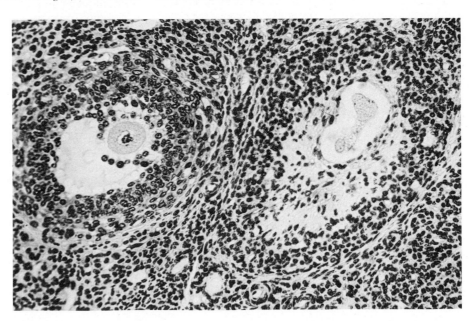

Fig. 26-14. Low-power photomicrograph of ovary of guinea pig, showing a normal developing follicle at *left,* and an atretic follicle at *right*. Note that the oocyte has degenerated in the atretic follicle, and that fibroblasts have grown into the follicle.

this occurs, recognition of atresia requires the use of less obvious criteria. Two early signs are the pulling away of the follicular epithelium from the theca interna (or a break in the follicular epithelium) and the presence of pyknotic nuclei in the follicular cells. Histological signs of cell death may also be visible in the oocyte if it is included in the plane of section.

In distinguishing old atretic follicles from degenerating corpora lutea, it is helpful to keep in mind that the term *atresia* is reserved for follicles that degenerate *before they mature,* and hence there would be no reason for bleeding to have occurred in them. On the other hand, old corpora lutea, whether of menstruation or pregnancy, usually contain blood pigment and sometimes even evidence of a blood clot that remains behind in them to indicate they were once a site of hemorrhage.

THE INTERSTITIAL GLAND

In the ovaries of some species, including man, groups of glandular cells are present scattered about in the stroma. The individual cells have the appearance of luteal cells but they are not organized into corpora lutea. Collectively, these cells are termed the *interstitial gland* of the ovary. Their origin is considered to be from theca interna cells of developing follicles that underwent atresia. In support of this view, evidence of the presence of an interstitial gland is seen in prepubertal ovaries before follicles have matured and ruptured. It has been suggested that at this time the cells of the gland produce the small quantities of estrogen required to bring about the prepubertal development leading to acquisition of secondary female sex characteristics. After puberty, the interstitial gland appears to be an important source of estrogen during the postovulatory part of each ovarian cycle.

THE OVARIES AFTER THE MENOPAUSE

After functioning for 30 years or so in regard to both liberating oocytes and secreting hormones, the ovaries become exhausted, and, after a short period during which they function sporadically, they finally cease liberating oocytes and producing hormones. When they fail to liberate oocytes, there are, of course, no new corpora lutea formed, and as a result the endometrium thereafter neither becomes greatly thickened nor collapses every 28 days. The most obvious sign of ovarian failure, then, is that the *menses* (menstrual flow) cease; indeed, it is for that reason that this time in a woman's life is described as the *menopause* (Gr. *men*, month, *pausis*, cessation). The menopause usually occurs between the ages of 45 and 50 and marks the end of the reproductive life of a woman. Actually, fertility declines during the 10 years or so before menopause. An artifical menopause occurs earlier if the ovaries are removed, or if their function is otherwise ended as, for example, by irradiation or disease.

The onset of the menopause is usually indicated, though not always, by other signs and symptoms. Commonly, the function of vasomotor nerves becomes disturbed, and women suffer what are called "hot flashes." Moreover, for a time they may find it more difficult for both physiological and psychological reasons to maintain their usual adjustment to life; hence some women exhibit a certain degree of emotional instability at this time. Other symptoms, such as headache, insomnia, and alterations in pulse rate, are sometimes experienced. Much can be done to alleviate the more distressing symptoms by judicious administration of estrogen.

It should be understood that the hormonal disturbances that occur at the menopause are due to *ovarian failure,* not to the failure of the anterior pituitary. Indeed, as the estrogen level of the blood falls after the menopause, the negative feedback arrangement between estrogen and FSH leads to FSH being secreted in such increased amounts that fairly large quantities of it appear in the urine (hence, the urine of a postmenopausal woman will stimulate follicular development and estrogen production in young female animals and so bring about precocious puberty). There is no point, then, in giving a woman gonadotrophic hormone at this time to stimulate her ovaries. Substitution therapy with estrogen is all that can be done.

The ovary of a woman who has recently passed the menopause can be distinguished by the relative *absence of:* (*1*) primary follicles, (*2*) follicles in various stages of normal development or atresia, and (*3*) recent corpora lutea. As the years pass, the ovary becomes increasingly shrunken, consisting of little more than fibrous tissue.

It seems probable that the decline in progesterone production is more abrupt at the menopause than the falling-off in estrogen secretion. New corpora lutea are necessary if progesterone production is to be carried on for any length of time. Estrogen production by the ovary, though diminished, may be carried on for some time after the menopause. Estrogen is made by thecal cells. So, as long as thecal elements persist in the ovary, as for example in the form of interstitial gland cells, some estrogen can be produced. Moreover, there are some minor extraovarian sources of estrogen in the body. The inner layers of the adrenal cortex, for example, make minute quantities of it.

The great decrease in estrogen production at menopause may be reflected sooner or later by substantial tissue changes in certain parts of the body. Those parts of the female reproductive tract dependent on this hormone for maintenance of structure tend to become atrophic. For example, the functional capacity of the glands associated with the cervix and external genitalia becomes di-

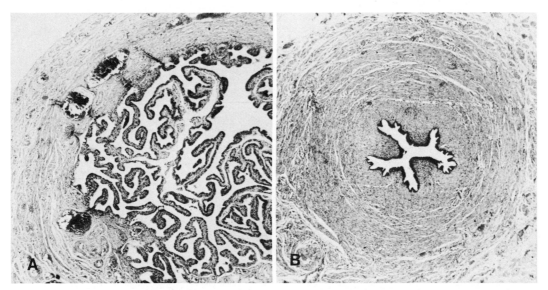

Fig. 26-15. (A) Very low power photomicrograph of part of the ampulla of an oviduct of a sexually mature woman. The dark areas in the muscle coat are congested veins. The complex longitudinal folds are cut in cross section. *(B)* Very low power photomicrograph of the isthmus of an oviduct.

minished; the external genitalia themselves tend to atrophy, and the vaginal lining may become very thin and increasingly susceptible to infection. Substitution therapy can do much to relieve these conditions if and when they occur.

THE OVIDUCTS (UTERINE OR FALLOPIAN TUBES)

Each oviduct (Fig. 26-1) is about 12 cm. long and consists of four parts: *(1)* an *intramural* part—that portion of the tube that extends through the wall of the uterus; *(2)* an *isthmus*—the short narrow part of the tube next to the uterus; *(3)* an *ampulla*—the longest part of the tube, about the diameter of a pencil and extending from the isthmus to *(4)* an *infundibulum*—the flared termination of the tube provided with processes *(fimbriae)*. The wall of the oviduct is made up of three layers, a mucous membrane, a muscular coat, and a serosa (Fig. 26-15).

Mucous Membrane. The epithelium consists of a single layer of columnar cells. There are two types of these, ciliated and secretory, and they alternate irregularly with one another (Fig. 26-16A). Their relative and absolute heights vary in relation to different times in the menstrual cycle. Beginning shortly after menstruation, both kinds increase in height, and at the time of ovulation they are both about 30 μm. high (Fig. 26-16A). Following this, however, the ciliated cells become much shorter, and the nonciliated secretory cells only somewhat shorter, so that they project between the ciliated cells into the lumen of

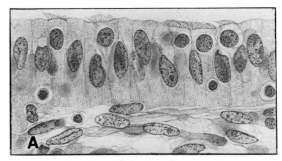

Mid-interval

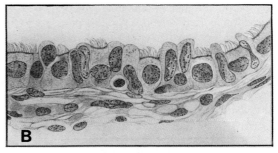

Premenstrual

Fig. 26-16. (A) The epithelium of human oviduct at about midinterval stage. *(B)* The oviduct epithelium at the premenstrual stage. (Camera lucida drawings; ×700) (Snyder, F. F.: Bull. Johns Hopkins Hosp., *35:*141, 1924)

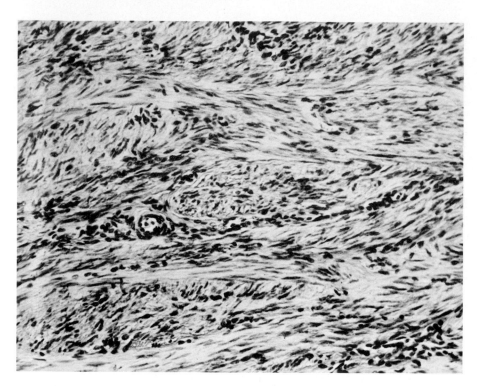

Fig. 26-17. Low-power photomicrograph of myometrium of
uterus, showing its interlacing
bundles of smooth muscle fibers.

the tube, making the surface somewhat irregular (Fig. 26-16B). A few clear cells with a dark-staining nucleus may be scattered about in the epithelial membrane close to the basement membrane. They are probably young secretory cells. In addition, occasional lymphocytes are found in this site. The nonciliated cells do not become ciliated or vice versa. It might be thought that the cilia would beat toward the uterus and be an important factor in moving an ovum along the tube to the uterus. However, some cilia beat in the other direction, so contractile movements of the muscle of the tube appear to be of primary importance in propelling the ovum along. It is probable that the watery secretion in the tube is nutritive or otherwise helpful for the ovum, and that hormonal stimulation of the cells concerned in making secretions occurs at a time when an ovum would be likely to be passing along the tube.

The lamina propria of the mucous membrane is like loose connective tissue except that its cells have potentialities similar to those of the endometrial stroma, for they react similarly if a fertilized ovum inadvertently becomes implanted in the mucosa of the oviduct, as sometimes happens.

As described in the general account of the parts of the reproductive system, the mucous membrane of the oviduct is thrown into extensive longitudinal folds (Fig. 26-15A). These become reduced in size and extend into the isthmus (Fig. 26-15B); they amount to little more than ridges in the intramural portion of the tube.

Muscle Coat. This consists of two layers of smooth muscle fibers: an inner one of circularly or somewhat spirally disposed fibers and an outer longitudinal one. The line of demarcation between the two layers is not clear-cut, and since some connective tissue extends between the bundles of muscle fibers, the muscle coats may be difficult to identify in anything but a general way. The inner coat of circular fibers is thickest in the intramural portion of the tube and least prominent in the infundibulum. Peristaltic movements of the muscle are believed to be accentuated close to the time of ovulation. The tonus and contractions of the muscle are affected by hormones.

The histological structure of the serosa is typical.

THE BODY AND FUNDUS OF THE UTERUS

The wall of the uterus (Fig. 26-2) varies in thickness from 1.5 cm. to slightly less than 1 cm. It consists of three coats: (*1*) a thin external serous coat (*serosa*); (*2*) a thick muscle coat, the *myometrium;* and (*3*) a lining mucous membrane, the *endometrium.*

The serosa (the peritoneal investment of the organ) consists of a single layer of mesothelial cells supported by a thin layer of loose connective tissue; it is continuous at each side of the organ with the peritoneum of the broad ligament but is absent from the lower half of the anterior surface (Fig. 26-2).

Fig. 26-18. (*A*) Very low power photomicrograph of one horn of the uterus of a rat, 1 month after its ovaries were removed. Its uterus has atrophied as a result of estrogen deficiency. (*B*) Photomicrograph (same magnification) of a uterine horn of a rat similarly ovariectomized but also given large doses of estrogen. This shows not only that estrogen stimulates the cells of an atrophied uterus to grow, but also that estrogen causes its epithelial cells to secrete, for this uterus is enormously distended with secretion.

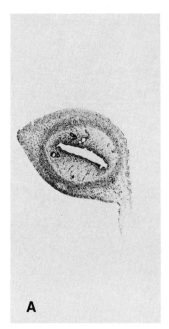

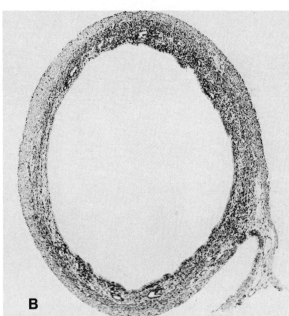

The myometrium consists of bundles of smooth muscle fibers separated from one another by connective tissue (Fig. 26-17). The bundles are arranged so as to form three ill-defined layers. The outermost and innermost layers are thin and consist chiefly of longitudinally and obliquely disposed fibers. The middle layer is much thicker, and its muscle fibers tend to be disposed circularly. The larger blood vessels of the wall of the uterus are mostly contained in this middle layer; hence it is sometimes called the *stratum vasculare*.

Growth of the Uterus During Pregnancy. The smooth muscle cells of the myometrium become 10 times as long and many times as thick during pregnancy. The great increase in thickness of the myometrium in pregnancy is brought about not only by hypertrophy of previously existing fibers but also by increase in the number of fibers, the new ones being derived from division of preexisting fibers and perhaps also from relatively undifferentiated cells, for example, pericytes, in the connective tissue between the bundles.

The Hormonal Basis for Growth of the Myometrium. Since the placenta (in women) produces very large amounts of estrogen during pregnancy, and since estrogens are known to cause pronounced growth of the myometrium if given to ovariectomized animals, as shown in Figure 26-18, it is likely that the great growth of the myometrium in pregnancy is caused primarily by estrogen.

The way in which estrogen causes growth involves its stimulating protein synthesis in the cells to enable them to enlarge and divide. It has been shown by radioau-tography that labeled estrogen becomes bound to the chromatin of uterine smooth muscle cells within two minutes of being made available. Other studies indicate that this results in increased production of RNA and acceleration of the transport of ribosomal precursor particles (associated with mRNA) to the cytoplasm, where new polysomes appear that are different from those present prior to estrogen stimulation. Thus protein synthesis is increased, with the growth effect of estrogen being achieved at the level of genes.

THE ENDOMETRIUM

This, the mucous membrane that lines the body and fundus of the uterus, consists of a layer of epithelium and a connective tissue lamina propria continuous with the myometrium. Customarily, the lamina propria is referred to as the *endometrial stroma.* The stroma is riddled with simple tubular glands that open onto the epithelial surface and whose deepest parts almost reach the myometrium (Fig. 26-19B). The glands represent ingrowths of the surface columnar epithelium.

It is helpful to describe the endometrium as consisting of two layers: a thick superficial one, called the *functional* layer, and a thin deep one, termed the *basilar* layer. The functional layer is so called because its character changes greatly during the menstrual cycle; indeed, at menstruation it is mostly shed (Fig. 26-19A). The character of the basilar layer does not change to any great extent during the menstrual cycle, and it remains through menstruation

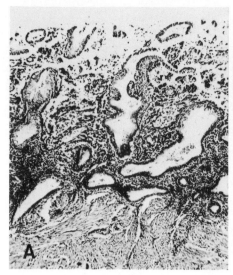
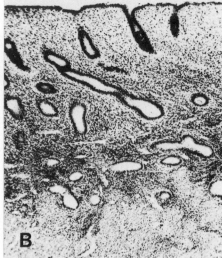

Fig. 26-19. (*A*) Low-power photomicrograph of endometrium and adjacent myometrium, late in menstruation. Note the raw inner surface; all but the deeply situated parts of the glands and stroma are degenerating and being sloughed. (*B*) Low-power photomicrograph of endometrium, in an early proliferative phase. The previously raw surface has become re-covered with epithelium, and the glands are now straight.

to regenerate another functional layer after the menstrual flow ceases.

THE ENDOMETRIUM DURING THE MENSTRUAL CYCLE

The 28-day menstrual cycle is by no means constant in length; it may be a few days shorter or longer. The length of the cycle may even vary in the same individual. It is usual to number the days in the cycle *from the first day of menstruation;* this is a concession to medical practice because the first day of menstruation is a date a patient can set with exactitude. Most commonly, menstruation lasts for 4 days, but periods a day shorter or longer are common.

The endometrium passes through several *phases* in each cycle. From days 1 to 4 it is said to be in its *menstrual phase* (Fig. 26-19A). From day 4 until a day or two after ovulation the endometrium is said to be in its *estrogenic, proliferative, reparative,* or *follicular phase* (Fig. 26-19B). During this time it grows from something less than 1 mm. to 2 or 3 mm. in thickness. Mitosis occurs in both gland and stromal cells. Growth of the endometrium during this period is encouraged by the estrogen being secreted by the ovary as a follicle matures and approaches the surface (hence the terms *estrogenic* and *follicular*). Figure 26-18 illustrates how potently estrogen affects the growth of rat uterus.

The last day of the estrogenic phase cannot be set exactly because of variability in the time of ovulation. Ovulation occurs somewhere between days 8 and 20 and rarely before or after this. The latter (indefinite) part of the estrogenic phase is often termed the *interval phase.* This term is used to denote the time period that ensues after the endometrium has become thoroughly repaired

but has not yet begun to be affected by progesterone. The last phase of the menstrual cycle is called either: (*1*) the *progestational phase,* because the changes that occur in the endometrium during this phase are due to the action of progesterone, or (*2*) the *progravid phase,* (L. *gravida,* heavy) *phase,* because pregnancy, when it occurs, begins in this phase, or (*3*) the *secretory phase,* because the epithelial cells of the glands actively secrete at this time. This phase begins shortly after ovulation. The lifetime of a corpus luteum being about 10 to 12 days is a much more constant feature of the menstrual cycle than the time of ovulation. The last day or two of the progestational phase is sometimes called the *ischemic* (Gr. *ischo,* to keep back; *haima,* blood) *phase* because the vessels that supply the more superficial parts of the functional layer of the endometrium are intermittently shut off for variable periods during this time, and the endometrium suffers a lack of blood supply, as will be described later.

The Microscopic Appearance of the Endometrium in the Different Phases of the Cycle

The Estrogenic (Interval) Phase. The endometrium in the latter part of the estrogenic (that is, the interval) phase is from 2 to 3 mm. thick. The epithelial cells that line the surface and comprise the glands are columnar and often piled up on one another because of active proliferation. The small amount of mucus they secrete at this time is thin and watery. Patches of ciliated columnar cells are scattered about among the secretory cells. The glands in the functional layer of the endometrium tend to be narrow and straight. The stroma consists of star-shaped cells whose cytoplasmic processes connect with each other. The cells are adherent to a network of reticular fibers.

Fig. 26-20. (*A*) Low-power photomicrograph of the superficial part of the endometrium, in early progestational phase. (*B*) High-power photomicrograph of one of its glands. At this stage glycogen is present as indicated.

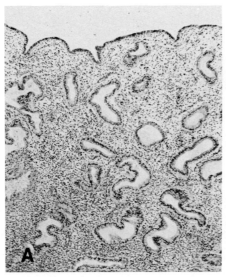 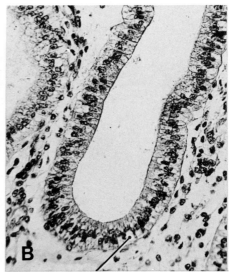

Glycogen

Amorphous intercellular substance is not so abundant at this time as somewhat earlier. Leukocytes are not common in the stroma in this phase.

The Progestational Phase. In this phase the endometrium becomes more than twice as thick as in the interval phase. The increase in thickness is due in part to increased amounts of tissue fluid in the stroma (edema), in part to glands accumulating increased amounts of secretion, and in part to the increase in the size of stromal cells. Except in the more superficial part of the functional layer and in the basal layer, the glands become wide, tortuous, and sacculated (Figs. 26-20A and 26-21). Their cells come to contain considerable amounts of glycogen. At first this accumulates between the nucleus and the base of the cells (Fig. 26-20B), but later it appears between the nucleus and the free border of the cells; the luminal border thereupon becomes ragged in appearance (Fig. 26-21). The secretion in the glands becomes much thicker and more abundant than formerly. The cells of the stroma are enlarged, undergoing what is called a *decidual reaction* (the L. word *deciduus* means a falling off and refers to the membrane into which the functional zone of the endometrium becomes transformed during pregnancy, which is cast off at the time of birth). Stromal cells evidence this reaction by becoming large and pale, and their cytoplasm comes to contain glycogen and lipid droplets. If pregnancy occurs, the decidual reaction is intensified and persists.

The changes that occur in all but the latter part of the progestational phase are due to the action of progesterone, acting in collaboration with such estrogen as is still present in the circulation. In general, these changes seem designed to make the endometrium nutritive for a fertilized ovum; for example, the glycogen that forms may serve as a readily available form of carbohydrate.

The changes that occur toward the end of the progesta-

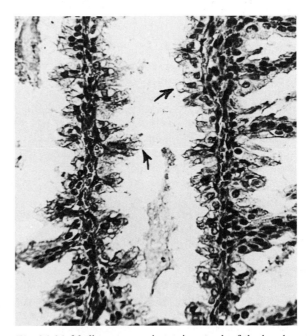

Fig. 26-21. Medium-power photomicrograph of the basal part of an endometrial gland, in late progestational phase. Note its ladder-like appearance and that the free border of its cells appears ragged because there is glycogen stored in these cells (arrows).

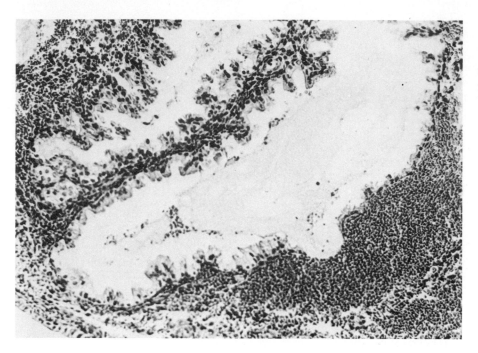

Fig. 26-22. Medium-power photomicrograph of endometrium, at the beginning of menstruation. A pool of blood has formed in the stroma (*bottom right*). The white space is the lumen of an endometrial gland.

tional phase (provided that pregnancy does not occur) have been described by Markee, who studied them by implanting bits of endometrium of monkeys into the anterior chambers of their eyes, where they not only became vascularized but could be observed directly. Toward the end of the progestational phase the endometrium begins to regress (shrink). As regression begins, leukocytes invade the endometrium. Regression, according to Markee, always precedes menstrual bleeding.

To explain how regression of the endometrium (which occurs because of decreasing stimulation by both estrogen and progesterone at this time) institutes bleeding and breakdown of the functional layer of endometrium requires that we first describe the special features of the blood supply of the endometrium.

THE BLOOD SUPPLY OF THE ENDOMETRIUM AND ITS RELATION TO MENSTRUATION

Two types of arteries lead from the stratum vascularis of the myometrium to the endometrium. Those of the first type, on approaching the endometrium, assume a *coiled* (spiral) form and, without branching to any great extent, extend through the endometrium to its superficial part; there they terminate in a fountain-like arrangement of arterioles that supply the capillary beds of this part of the endometrium. The second type of artery extends from the stratum vascularis to end, after pursuing a *straight* course, in the deeper layer of the endometrium. The blood supply of at least the more superficial (inner) part of

the functional layer of the endometrium is therefore derived from the coiled arteries.

The Ischemic and Menstrual Phases. The coiled arteries are of the greatest importance in bringing about menstruation; indeed, menstruation occurs only in those species in which the endometrium is supplied by this particular type of blood vessel. Markee found that, as the endometrium regresses, the coiled arteries become increasingly coiled to accommodate themselves to the thinning endometrium. As the time of menstruation approaches, the circulation in them slows, and beginning on the day before menstruation, the coiled arteries become individually constricted for prolonged periods of time so that the part of the endometrium they supply becomes blanched. After a coiled artery has remained constricted for a time, it dilates, and as blood once more reaches the arterioles and capillaries supplied by the artery (these have suffered a lack of blood supply during the period of vasoconstriction), it escapes through their walls into the stroma. By this means little pools of blood accumulate beneath the endometrial surface (Fig. 26-22). These soon rupture through the the epithelium into the uterine cavity. Meanwhile, the coiled artery concerned has become constricted again, and its terminal portions die. The same sequence of events is repeated in other arteries. As small pieces of endometrium become detached, arterioles may bleed directly onto the surface rather than into the stroma. As deeper parts of the functional layer become involved, veins become opened, and they, too, slowly bleed. The lack of adequate blood supply is considered to be the factor causing progressive disintegration of the endometrium. As the endometrium regresses, the coiled arteries become buckled and this too aggravates the ischemia caused by vasoconstriction and contributes further to necrosis of the endometrium. Eventually, over a few days, most of the functional layer of the endometrium is lost. The basal layer is not seriously affected by the process because of its different kind of blood supply and hence it survives menstruation.

The cause of regression of the endometrium in the latter stages of the progestational phase, and of the vasoconstriction of the coiled arteries that follows in its wake, is hormone deficiency. Although both estrogen and progesterone are deficient at this time, progesterone failure is the more important precipitating factor; indeed, menstruation can be delayed by administration of progesterone. Nevertheless, the reduction in blood estrogen from the level attained in the midpart of the cycle plays some part in the process, for in anovulatory cycles (which are less common in women but occur seasonally in monkeys), bleeding occurs at the regular time for menstruation without ovulation having occurred, without a corpus luteum having formed, without progesterone having been secreted, and without the endometrium having passed through a proper progestational phase. Hence, estrogen withdrawal, as it is often termed, can itself cause regression of the endometrium and bleeding from coiled arteries.

The Early Part of the Estrogenic Phase. As noted, the basal layer of endometrium, with its separate arterial supply, is left intact throughout the cycle (Fig. 26-19A). When the menstrual phase has run its course, the epithelium from the glands, under the influence of newly secreted estrogen, grows out over the denuded surface and rapidly covers it again (Fig. 26-19B). Mitotic figures become numerous both in the gland and in the stroma cells. Amorphous intercellular substance and reticular fibers are formed in the stroma, and repair is so rapid that the interval appearance of endometrium is soon attained.

THE PLACENTA

General Features. The placenta develops during pregnancy in intimate association with the lining of the uterus. When fully developed it has the shape of a rather floppy flat cake (L. *placenta*, cake), approximately 15 cm. in diameter and 3 cm. thick. It is, of course, basically of fetal origin. Its primary function is to permit substances dissolved in the blood of the mother to diffuse into the blood of the fetus and vice versa, and it is designed to facilitate this over a vast area. Under normal conditions the bloodstream of the fetus and that of the mother do not mix with one another. They are always separated by what is termed the *placental barrier;* this, as we shall see, is composed of certain fetal tissues. In the placenta, food and oxygen, dissolved in the mother's blood, diffuse through the placental barrier into the bloodstream of the fetus, and by this means life and growth of the fetus are supported until it is born. Likewise, waste products pass through the barrier from the blood of the fetus to that of the mother and are eliminated by the mother's excretory organs. Humoral antibody (IgG) and hormones are also able to cross the barrier. Fetal blood passes to and fro from the fetus to the placenta by means of vessels in the umbilical cord; the latter structure connects the fetus to the placenta during pregnancy. At birth the fetus is expressed from the uterus, still connected by means of the umbilical cord to the placenta. One task of the attending physician is to tie off the umbilical cord, for soon after delivery the placenta becomes detached and is also expressed from the uterus.

Development

Here we shall describe only enough of the development of the placenta to make its microscopic structure understandable.

Fertilization of the ovum usually occurs in the oviduct (Fig. 26-12). The ovum passes along the tube, taking about 4 days to reach the uterus. By this time several cell divisions have occurred and it consists of a clump of cells resembling a mulberry (Fig. 26-23A) and therefore called a *morula.* A cavity appears in this solid mass of cells, after which it is called a *blastocyst* (*cyst* because it has a cavity, and *blasto* because it will form something) (Fig. 26-23B). The blastocyst remains free in the uterine cavity for only 2 or 3 days (Fig. 26-23B), after which it becomes *implanted* in the wall of the uterus (Fig. 26-23C and D). Usually, therefore, implantation begins about 1 week after fertilization. At this time the endometrium (Fig. 26-20) has been under the influence of progesterone for several days; hence it is "receptive" toward the ovum. The site of implantation may be anywhere on the wall of the uterus but usually is high up on the posterior wall (Fig. 26-23E).

The wall of the hollow blastocyst is thin, consisting of a single layer of cells, the *trophoblast* (Fig. 26-23B) (Gr. *trophein,* to nourish; *blastos,* germ), except where there is an aggregation of cells called the *inner cell mass,* which bulges inward from the wall of the blastocyst into its cavity (Fig. 26-23C and D). The inner cell mass gives rise to the *embryo.* The trophoblast, however, is concerned in the development of the placenta, so we shall now go on to consider this further.

The trophoblast becomes adherent to the luminal surface of the endometrial epithelium. At the point of contact, the cells of the trophoblast proliferate to become several cells thick (Fig. 26-23C). The uterine epithelium breaks down at this point, probably because of enzymatic activity of the trophoblast. This leaves a gap in the uterine lining that permits the blastocyst to sink into the endometrial stroma (Fig. 26-23C and D). The defect in the endometrium is closed temporarily by a plug of fibrin and cellular debris called the *closing coagulum* (Fig. 26-23D). Later, the endometrial epithelium grows over the embedded blastocyst to reconstitute a continuous uterine lining. The blastocyst then lies surrounded by stromal cells in the superficial layer of the endometrium (Fig. 26-23E).

By the 11th day after fertilization the cells of the trophoblast

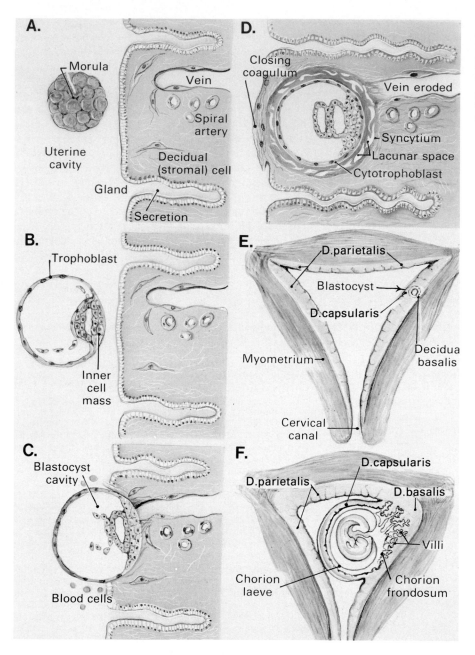

have formed two layers. The cells of the inner layer are well defined; this layer is called the *cytotrophoblast* because it is clearly composed of individual cells (Figs. 26-23D and 26-27A). The outer layer does not consist of individual cells but of a continuous mass of cytoplasm containing many nuclei. Since the cells of this layer are all fused together, this layer constitutes a *syncytium* (labeled in Fig. 26-23D), and the layer itself is called *syncytiotrophoblast* (Figs. 26-24 and 26-27). At this stage there are a few small spaces called *lacunae* in the syncytium (Figs. 26-23D and 26-24). By the 15th day these have increased in size and become confluent. Moreover, they are filled with maternal

blood from the uterine veins and venous sinuses that the trophoblast has eroded. Only later does the trophoblast erode coiled arteries so that these, too, deliver maternal blood into these spaces.

As the lacunae enlarge, extensions of trophoblast left between them are called *primary trophoblastic villi*. Each villus consists of a core of cytotrophoblast covered with an outer irregular layer of syncytiotrophoblast. The villi that extend out from the blastocyst around its whole periphery come into contact with the endometrium in which the blastocyst is buried, and cells from the villi apply themselves to the endometrium to form a lining for the

Fig. 26-24. Photomicrograph of part of a 12-day implantation site. Lacunae are lined by syncytiotrophoblast (labeled), which has eroded a maternal artery and a uterine gland. (Courtesy of J. Boyd and W. Hamilton)

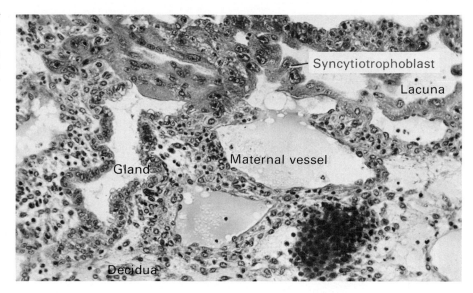

cavity in the endometrium in which the blastocyst lies (Fig. 26-23D). This lining of the cavity is peripheral to the blastocyst, and so it is called the *peripheral syncytium.* Hence, at this time trophoblast cells form a *covering* for the blastocyst and a *lining* for the cavity in which it lies, and between the two there are strands of cells, the villi, that partly separate lacunar spaces (Fig. 26-23D), filled with maternal blood. The cytotrophoblastic component proliferates rapidly at the tips of the villous structures that are forming.

The villi at this stage thus consist of cytotrophoblast covered by syncytiotrophoblast. Mitoses are seen in cytotrophoblast but are not very common in the syncytiotrophoblast. It would seem that the latter grows by cells of the cytotrophoblast fusing to become syncytiotrophoblast.

The structure of the villi begins to change about the 15th day. By this time the different germ layers are forming in the embryo, and mesoderm has grown out from the developing embryo to form a lining for the shell of trophoblast that surrounds the blastocyst. When the trophoblast has gained a lining of mesoderm, it is called the *chorion* (Gr. for membrane). The mesoderm from the chorion then extends into the villi to provide them with mesodermal cores; when this happens, the villi are called *secondary* or *definitive villi.* These grow and branch. Fetal blood vessels develop in the mesoderm in their cores, and later these vessels become connected with the fetal circulation (Fig. 26-27).

So far the changes occurring in the trophoblast have taken place all around the periphery of the blastocyst. From here on, development differs in various sites around the circumference of the blastocyst. To explain these we must introduce some further terms.

The endometrium that lies between the blastocyst and the myometrium is called the *basal plate,* and it is on this side of the blastocyst that the placenta will develop from the chorion. This is accomplished by the villi (with their cores of mesoderm) continuing to grow and branch. In so doing, they continue to destroy and erode endometrium. As they do this, the raw surface of endometrium that is exposed becomes lined with cytotrophoblast cells from the tips of the villi. Since the lacunae between villi are filled with maternal blood, and the capillaries of the villi with fetal blood, diffusion of dissolved substances can occur between the maternal blood in the lacunar spaces and the fetal blood in the capillaries of the villi.

The continuation of the processes described above in the region of the basal plate results in the formation of the placenta; this will be described in more detail presently.

The Deciduae. Since all but the deepest layer of endometrium is destined to be shed when a baby is born, much like leaves of deciduous trees in autumn, it is referred to as the *decidua* (Fig. 26-23E). Various areas of the decidua have different names that designate their positions relative to the site of implantation.

The *decidua parietalis (parietal* means *forming,* or *situated on, a wall*) lines the entire pregnant uterus except where the placenta is forming (Fig. 26-23F).

The *decidua capsularis* is the portion of endometrium superficial to the developing embryo; it forms a *capsule* over it (Fig. 26-23E and F). As the embryo becomes larger, the decidua capsularis has to cover a larger and larger area and becomes very thin and atrophic. After 3 months the size of the chorionic sac that contains the embryo has become so large that the decidua capsularis comes into contact with the decidua parietalis at the opposite surface of the uterus; hence the uterine cavity is obliterated. The decidua capsularis thereupon blends with the decidua parietalis and disappears as a separate layer.

The *decidua basalis* is the zone of endometrium that lies between the chorionic sac (with its contained embryo) and the basal layer of endometrium (Figs. 26-23E, 26-25 and 26-26). The decidua basalis becomes the maternal part of the placenta. This is the only part of the placenta of maternal origin. After the placenta is delivered at term, this layer is visible only as poorly defined bits of membrane.

Until about 12 to 16 weeks, the entire surface of the chorionic sac is covered with chorionic villi. As the sac enlarges, those villi associated with the decidua capsularis degenerate and disappear, so that by 16 weeks the greater part of the surface of the sac is smooth. This large area is called the *chorion laeve* (L. *levis,* smooth) (Figs. 26-23F, 26-25, and 26-26). The remainder of the surface of the sac, that is, the part adjacent to the decidua basalis, continues to be covered with villi which keep growing and branching. This part, which constitutes the fetal part of the placenta, is called the *chorion frondosum* (Fig. 26-23F). By 16

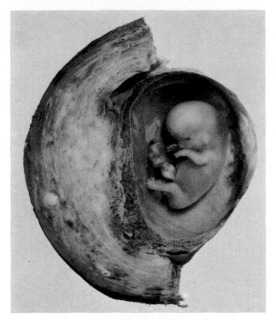

Fig. 26-25. Photograph of part of the uterine wall with attached placenta, fetus, and fetal membranes. At *lower right,* the wall of the chorionic sac (in which the fetus lies) is smooth. This is the chorion laeve. At *center,* the fetal part of the placenta is formed by the chorion frondosum. This embryo was 36 mm. long; compare this photograph with Figure 26-26 (which illustrates an earlier stage). (Courtesy of J. Boyd and W. Hamilton)

weeks the placenta is discoid in shape, consisting of chorion frondosum and associated decidua basalis. At the time of birth it occupies almost one third of the internal surface of the expanded uterus.

THE MICROSCOPIC STRUCTURE OF THE PLACENTA

Chorionic Villi

The basic unit of the placenta is the chorionic villus. The early villus is a compact, bush-like tuft with its base attached to and arising from the chorion and its tip attached to the decidua. By the 2nd month side branches are formed with free tips, some of which later fuse with similar branches of adjacent villi to create a villous spongework. It is doubtful if such fusion permits anastomosis between fetal blood vessels in the cores of the fusing villi. However, the cytotrophoblast at the tips of the main villi fuses to form a continuous placental covering for the eroded surface of the decidua basalis. In the fully formed human placenta, there are usually 8 to 15

large villi, each of which, together with its many branches, forms a *fetal cotyledon* (*lobule*).

Villi are alike histologically. A section of placenta cuts villi in all planes (Fig. 26-26), and between them is maternal blood. From a single section of placenta it is not particularly easy for a student to visualize the fetal and maternal circulations (which will be described later), but the student can readily identify the tissue layers that comprise the placental barrier separating fetal from maternal blood, as follows.

The Components of the Placental Barrier

In each villus there is a fetal capillary lined with endothelium (Fig. 26-27). The capillary is contained in the loose connective tissue core of a villus. In the core there are also some scattered smooth muscle fibers. Larger cells with a large spherical nucleus (cells of Hofbauer) are also present; possibly these are phagocytic. The trophoblast covering each villus consists of two well-defined layers, cytotrophoblast and syncytiotrophoblast, until approximately the middle of the 3rd month of pregnancy, after which cytotrophoblast progressively disappears until at term only isolated clumps of its cells are left (compare parts A and B of Fig. 26-27).

Cytotrophoblast (Langhans' Layer). This consists of large, discrete, pale cells with a relatively large nucleus (Fig. 26-27A); the cells rest on a well-defined basement membrane. Their cytoplasm contains vacuoles and some glycogen but no lipid. Under the EM cytotrophoblast cells reveal glycogen, mitochondria, and ribosomes, but compared with the syncytiotrophoblast they are relatively poorly differentiated.

Syncytiotrophoblast. This is a dark, variably thick layer in which numerous small nuclei are irregularly dispersed (Figs. 26-24 and 26-27A). This layer becomes progressively thinner throughout pregnancy (Fig. 26-27B). Its outer surface has an irregular border with numerous extensions. The EM shows that the outer surface has many microvilli. The cytoplasm contains mitochondria, abundant rER, Golgi saccules, and lipid droplets. The latter may be very large and abundant early in pregnancy, but later they become smaller and less numerous. Glycogen is usually absent, or present in only small amounts. After the cytotrophoblast has disappeared, the syncytiotrophoblast rests on a condensed network of reticular fibers.

By the time of birth the layers comprising the placental barrier between maternal and fetal blood have become very thin (Fig. 26-27B). In the thin syncytiotrophoblast layer a few mitochondria and fat droplets are still visible; the cytotrophoblast cells have all but disappeared. With the EM it can be seen that the five layers comprising the placental barrier close to term are as follows: (*1*) in con-

Fig. 26-26. Low-power photomicrograph of part of a uterus with placenta in situ. The embryo (which was 15 mm. long) has been removed. (Courtesy of J. Boyd and W. Hamilton)

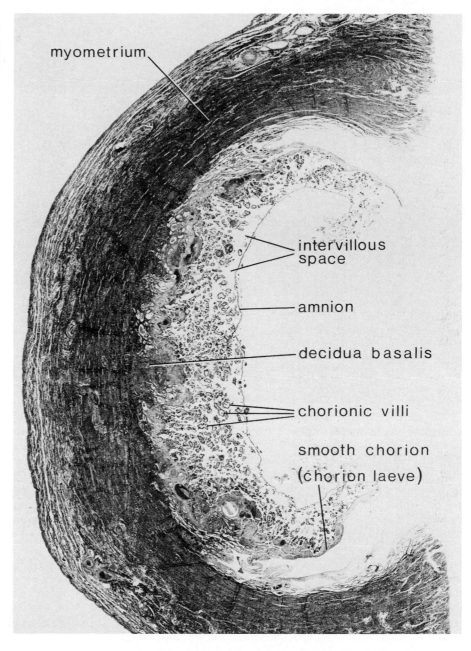

myometrium

intervillous space

amnion

decidua basalis

chorionic villi

smooth chorion (chorion laeve)

tact with the maternal blood lies the thin layer of syncytiotrophoblast with surface microvilli; (*2*) beneath this there is a substantial basement membrane; (*3*) deep to this there is loose connective tissue containing delicate reticular fibers; (*4*) surrounding the fetal capillary there is its basement membrane; and (*5*) the endothelium of the fetal capillary lies in contact with the fetal blood.

At intervals along a villus the syncytotrophoblast is aggregated into protuberances of cytoplasm that contain many nuclei; these protuberances are called *syncytial knots* or *sprouts*. It is known that some of these syncytial sprouts break off to become free in the intervillous space; from here they can pass into the maternal circulation and on to the lungs of the mother, where they are destroyed by local enzymatic action and present no problem.

In the early placenta and becoming increasingly abundant with time are irregular masses of an eosinophilic, homogeneous substance called *fibrinoid*. At term aggrega-

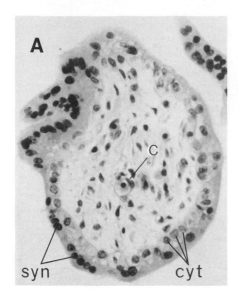
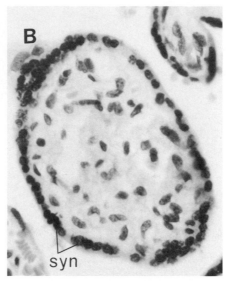

Fig. 26-27. Photomicrographs of placental villi. (*A*) At a stage when the chorionic villi still show both layers of trophoblast, the deeper layer being the cytotrophoblast (cyt) and the superficial layer being the syncytiotrophoblast (syn). Note the capillary (c) in the core of the villus; it contains a nucleated red blood cell. (*B*) Placenta delivered at full term. Note that the villi are now covered only by a layer of syncytiotrophoblast (syn).

tions of it may be visible to the naked eye. The possible significance of this extracellular material will be discussed when we come to consider the immunological implications of pregnancy.

The Maternal Part of the Placenta

The zone where the trophoblastic shell is in contact with the endometrium is variously called the *junctional, composite,* or *penetration zone.* The last of these terms indicates the way the maternal tissue undergoes degeneration and necrosis in this zone as it becomes penetrated by trophoblastic villi. In this zone it is possible to distinguish decidual cells (derived from endometrial stroma) from cytotrophoblastic cells because the former are surrounded with collagenic and reticular fibers, whereas the latter have no such material between them. The endometrial stromal cells of the decidua basalis almost all take on the appearance of *decidual* cells; they become large, polygonal, and rich in glycogen and lipid droplets. The epithelial cells lining the endometrial glands during pregnancy are rich in glycogen and lipid droplets. By the 3rd month these glands in the decidua basalis are stretched and appear as horizontal clefts. The decidua basalis as a whole (the basal plate) consists chiefly of a connective tissue stroma, the cells of which are of the decidual type; endometrial glands, fibrinoid, and small clumps of trophoblast cells are also present. The syncytiotrophoblast may penetrate through all layers of the maternal endometrium and even into the myometrium. Giant cells, believed to be derived from the fetal syncytium, may be present in the basal plate. Passing through the basal plate are coiled arteries that open into the intervillous spaces. They are

lined with endothelium, but near their openings they are lined with cells of the syncytiotrophoblast type. Growth of these cells into the maternal coiled arteries probably reduces the pressure at which maternal blood is delivered into the intervillous spaces.

The decidua is eroded more deeply opposite the main villi than elsewhere, and this leaves projections of decidual tissue between the main villi, extending from the basal plate toward the chorion (Fig. 26-28). Such projections are called *placental septa* (Fig. 26-28), and they divide the placenta into lobules (*cotyledons*). From the 4th month, the tissues of the decidua basalis become composed chiefly of a very dense venous plexus with dilated and distorted uterine glands. The latter have very thin walls, and secretion persists in them until late in pregnancy. Toward the margins of the placenta, the decidua is more compact.

The Intervillous Space. The intervillous space (Figs. 26-26 and 26-28) develops rapidly to become an enormous blood sinus bounded on one side by the chorion (chorionic plate) and on the other by the decidua basalis (Figs. 26-26 and 26-28). The space is labyrinthine in form because the villi in it are connected to each other. The space is incompletely divided into compartments by placental septa. The intervillous space is much expanded toward the embryonic side, where there are only main stems of villi and hence plenty of space for blood. The *marginal sinus* is the circular marginal region of the intervillous space at the periphery of the placenta.

Maternal arterial blood enters the intervillous space from arterial vessels that traverse the decidua basalis, there being many such vessels for each cotyledon (lobule) (Fig. 26-28). Maternal blood pressure drives the arterial blood entering the intervillous space high up toward the chorionic plate. After bathing the villi, blood flows back toward venous orifices in the basal plate.

PLACENTAL HORMONES

As already mentioned in connection with pregnancy tests, HCG (*human chorionic gonadotrophin*) is produced very early in pregnancy and in sufficient quantities to appear quickly in the mother's urine. Its source is believed to be the syncytial trophoblasts. Another hormone that appears in increasing amounts as pregnancy proceeds has been given several names to designate that it has something to do with both growth and lactation. One name for it is the *somatomammotrophic hormone.* Chemically, it bears a considerable resemblance to growth hormone and functionally, to prolactin. The placenta, moreover, can synthesize *progesterone* but cannot by itself produce *estrogen,* although it does so with the cooperation of the adrenal cortex and liver of the fetus. A hormone called *human chorionic thyrotrophin,* similar to TSH, is also secreted by the placenta. Thus the placenta is more or less a hormone factory.

IMMUNOLOGICAL IMPLICATIONS—THE PLACENTA AS A HOMOGRAFT

It might be thought that when a fertilized ovum developed into an embryo, it would incite a maternal homograft reaction against those of its antigens that were specified by paternal genes (since these antigens would be foreign to the mother's body), and that as a result there would be rejection of the early trophoblast-enclosed embryo or, later, of the placenta. Since this is obviously not the case, the explanation why an effective homograft reaction does not develop in an allogeneic pregnancy (the kind that occurs in humans) has been sought. A number of possibilities have been entertained, as follows.

At first, it was thought that the endometrium might act as an immunologically privileged (preferred) site, like the anterior chamber of the eye and also the brain. Homografts transplanted to these sites are able to survive by virtue of their lacking any effective lymphatic drainage (the equivalent of lymphatic drainage from the anterior chamber of the eye occurs directly into veins; lymphatics are altogether lacking in the substance of the CNS). With regard to the uterus, however, there is evidence that at least the lumbar and renal lymph nodes, into which the uterine lymphatics drain, are stimulated immunologically by the antigens of an implanted allogeneic embryo. The content of T cells in these nodes, for example, increases during the latter half of an allogeneic pregnancy. Moreover, in virtually all pregnancies there is limited exchange of blood cells across the placenta, even though the fetal and maternal bloodstreams remain for the most part separated. Clearly, maternal lymphatic tissues can and do become exposed to the paternally derived antigens, by probably more than one route, so that the concept of the endometrium providing an immunologically privileged site for the embryo, in the sense of preventing the embryonic antigens from reaching the mother's

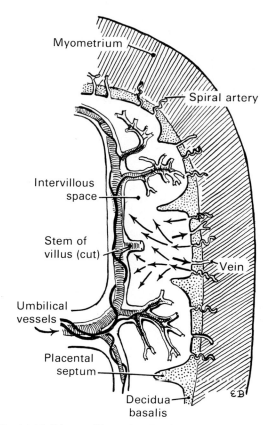

Fig. 26-28. Diagram illustrating the circulation of blood in the placenta. Blood from the fetus reaches the placenta by the two umbilical arteries (*left, solid black*), passes to the villi, and is returned to the fetus by the single umbilical vein (*left, cross-hatched*). Maternal blood enters the intervillous space via numerous coiled arteries and returns to the maternal circulation through many veins. There is no mingling of the two bloodstreams. Placental septa, which subdivide the placenta into cotyledons, are also shown.

lymphatic tissues, is untenable. Indeed, a fertilized ovum will develop in the normal way even if it is implanted experimentally into a body site that has an excellent lymphatic drainage.

The next possibility considered was that trophoblast cells might entirely lack the kinds of paternally derived antigens that would elicit an immune response in the mother. But as matters turned out they do possess histocompatability (HLA) antigens and also other kinds of antigens that, at least under other circumstances, are indeed capable of eliciting an immune response. Whether these antigens are necessarily expressed at the surface of trophoblast cells during a pregnancy, however, is controversial.

The next idea to evolve was that even though present, paternal antigens might be somehow hidden from recognition, much as chondrocytes in a cartilage homograft, for example, are protected from a homograft reaction by the cartilage matrix surrounding them (as was explained on p. 375). Accordingly, there was a great deal of interest when an amorphous, electron-dense coating (0.1 to 2 μm. thick) was demonstrated on the exposed surface of the trophoblast. This layer of extracellular material, called *fibrinoid,* was found to contain sulfated proteoglycans, which led to the suggestion that due to its sulfate content the layer would be negatively charged and hence would repel maternal lymphocytes, because the cell membrane of all cells, including lymphocytes, bears a net negative surface charge. Thus even if killer cells directed against paternally derived antigens were formed, they would be prevented by electrostatic forces from establishing contact with target trophoblast cells in order to kill them. Hence this would constitute an efferent inhibition of potential maternal immune responses. It is possible that the fibrinoid coating would also act as a nonantigenic barrier, masking potentially foreign (paternally derived) foreign antigens on the trophoblast surface so that they would remain nonimmunogenic. Hence the coating could also play a role in afferent inhibition of immune responses directed against the embryo. The concept emerging from this was that the fibrinoid layer constitutes a neutral barrier between trophoblast and decidua that acts (*1*) to hinder the development of transplantation immunity in an allogeneic pregnancy, and (*2*) to protect the embryo (and fetus) from any transplantation immunity that might develop. According to this view, the embryo literally isolates itself from its hostile maternal environment by covering its entire trophoblastic-decidual interface with a layer of fibrinoid. However, another idea is that the fibrinoid is a mutual product of both trophoblast and decidual cells and that its role is to keep trophoblastic invasion of the decidua in check.

More recently, attention has been paid to the possibility of further factors also protecting the embryo (and later the fetus) from rejection. These include (*1*) formation of blocking humoral antibodies that would block the foreign antigens on target embryonic (and fetal) cells and so protect them from recognition by maternal killer cells, should these be formed; (*2*) paralysis (nonreactivity) of the mother's immune system to paternally specified antigens, perhaps involving formation of specific suppressor cells from the mother's T-lymphocytes—and this would amount to the mother's developing tolerance to the antigens of the developing embryo; and (*3*) impairment of the mother's immune responses by the hormones produced during her pregnancy. The relative importance of these three mechanisms remains to be assessed.

It seems unlikely that any one factor could explain why an allogeneic pregnancy reaches term without rejection due to a homograft reaction. Many, if not all, of the factors discussed above are probably involved.

THE CERVIX OF THE UTERUS

The uterine cervix is the relatively narrow inferior segment of the uterus (Fig. 26-2). Since its wall is continuous with the rest of the uterus, it might be thought that its wall would be composed chiefly of smooth muscle. But the amount of smooth muscle and elastic tissue is not great and the wall of the cervix is composed chiefly of dense collagenic connective tissue. Elastic fibers, except in the walls of its blood vessels, are relatively scarce.

The cervix must become widely dilated at parturition to permit passage of the fetus. It does not contain enough smooth muscle to exert a strong sphincter effect. Hence, it seems that the main factor permitting the cervix to dilate at parturition, in response to the mechanical force

exerted upon it, is softening of its intercellular substance. This is associated with an increased blood supply and tissue fluid content, probably due to the hormones of pregnancy. In particular it is believed that a group of peptides collectively referred to as *relaxin* is important in this connection. The ovary would seem to be their primary source.

There is so little elastic tissue in the cervix (except in its blood vessels) that stretched elastic fibers would not be a very important factor in bringing about the slow contraction of the cervix that occurs after parturition. What, then, makes the cervix become constricted again? It seems not unlikely that although the cervix does not contain enough smooth muscle to enable it to act as a true sphincter, it does contain enough to help it contract after birth, particularly since after birth the smooth muscle fibers would be in a stretched state and would be reactive to such oxytocin as is secreted in the posterior lobe of the pituitary at this time. But further return to its original size probably involves reorganization of its fibrous tissue.

The cervical canal is flattened and its mucous membrane consists of epithelium with a connective tissue lamina propria. A longitudinal ridge (raphe) is present on the anterior surface of the canal and another is present on the posterior surface, and from these ridges mucosal folds extend at angles toward each side. The ridges do not directly face one another, so that when the lumen is collapsed they fit alongside one another. In addition to the ridges and folds there are numerous large, branched, tubular glands. In the vaginal end of the canal these mostly slant from the lumen toward the body of the uterus (Fig. 26-29A).

The epithelium of the mucous membrane (including that of the glands) consists of tall *mucus-secreting columnar cells.* In H and E sections their cytoplasm appears pale, and their deeply stained nucleus lies close to their base (Fig. 26-29B). Ciliated cells are sometimes seen. The glands extend deep into the lamina propria and somewhat beyond (Fig. 26-29A). The lamina propria is a cellular type of fibrous connective tissue. The nuclei of the fibroblasts are relatively close together. The cytoplasm of the cells cannot be seen clearly in an H and E section; nor can the small amounts of intercellular substance (Fig. 26-29B).

The *lamina propria* contains no coiled arteries and does not change much during the menstrual cycle. However, secretion of mucus by the cervical glands becomes increased at the time of ovulation; it is stimulated by estrogen. The glands sometimes become closed off, whereupon they may become cysts called *nabothian follicles.* These may cause elevations on the surface of that part of the cervix that projects into the vagina and so be seen or felt on vaginal examination.

The portion of cervix that projects into the vagina is

Fig. 26-29. (*A*) Very low power photomicrograph of a longitudinal section of the uterine cervix, showing the cervical canal and the glands extending out from it. The bottom is the end of the section nearer the vagina. (*B*) Medium-power photomicrograph showing the terminal part of one of the glands. Note the character of the stroma immediately surrounding the gland and that of the general stroma of the cervix.

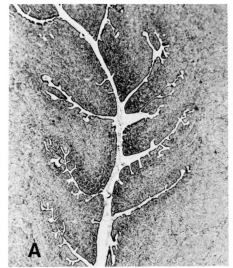
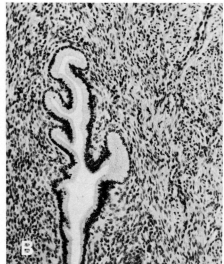

covered by *stratified squamous nonkeratinizing epithelium* similar to that lining the vagina (which will be described presently), and with which it becomes continuous. This type of epithelium extends usually for a very short distance into the cervical canal, where it borders on the epithelium of the columnar type that lines most of the canal (Fig. 26-30). In some instances the narrow zone of transition between the two types of epithelium is farther in; however, in others the columnar epithelium of the canal may continue out from the canal to cover little areas of the vaginal surface of the cervix close to the beginning of the canal; if so, these areas are termed *physiologic erosions.* (The stratified squamous nonkeratinizing epithelium that normally covers the cervix is pink-gray in color: columnar epithelium appears red. Hence the term *erosion.*) A factor in producing this appearance of erosions is that the lips of the canal may become somewhat everted as a result of childbearing; this tends to expose the columnar epithelium.

The portion of the uterus with which the cervix con-

Fig. 26-30. High-power photomicrograph of a longitudinal section of the cervix, near the site where the cervical canal opens into the vagina. The stratified squamous nonkeratinizing epithelium that covers the vaginal portion of the cervix, and extends for a very short distance into the canal, is seen at *left,* and the columnar epithelium that lines the remainder of the canal, at *right.* The somewhat abrupt transition between the two types of epithelium occurs midway between *left* and *center.*

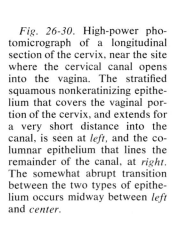
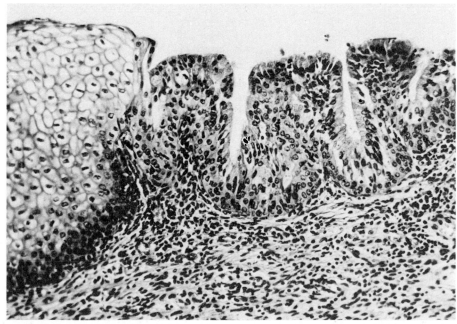

cervical type of mucous membrane and the endometrial type may be gradual and the so-called internal sphincter not at all obvious. The wall of the so-called isthmus is composed chiefly of smooth muscle, and in this respect the isthmus may be regarded as part of the body. When there is a need for more room to accommodate the fetus than can be provided by the body, the isthmus becomes expanded and elongated. Eventually, the more fibrous cervix becomes the only part of the uterus not expanded during pregnancy. The isthmus, then, is best considered not as a separate part of the uterus, but as the lower end of its body.

THE VAGINA

Microscopic Structure

The vagina is a musculofibrous tube lined with a mucous membrane (Fig. 26-31). Under ordinary conditions it is collapsed, with the mucous membranes of its anterior and posterior walls in contact. Except in the upper part of the tube, a longitudinal ridge is present on the mucosal surface of the anterior and posterior walls. From these two primary ridges numerous secondary ridges or *rugae* extend toward the sides of the tube (Fig. 26-2). No glands are present in the mucous membrane of the vagina. The epithelium is of the *stratified squamous* type, and the way its character alters in relation to the level of sex hormones in the bloodstream will be discussed presently. The *lamina propria* on which the epithelium rests is of a dense connective tissue type. It may exhibit lymphatic nodules. Farther out toward the muscle coat, the lamina propria — which in this site is sometimes regarded as a *submucosa* — becomes loose in texture and contains numerous blood vessels, particularly veins. Elastic fibers are numerous in the lamina propria directly under the epithelial lining, and they extend out through the mucous membrane to the *muscular layer*. The latter contains both longitudinally and circularly disposed smooth muscle fibers, but these are not arranged in discernible layers (Fig. 26-31). The longitudinally disposed fibers predominate. A fibrous *adventitia* lies outside the muscular coat and this connects the vagina with adjacent structures. The superior part of the posterior wall of the vagina is covered on its outside with peritoneum in the form of a serosa (Fig. 26-2).

Vaginal Smears. It has become common to study the cells found in the vagina by means of films (smears). Such cells may be derived from: (*1*) the endometrium of the body of the uterus, (*2*) the cervical canal, or (*3*) the vaginal surface of the cervix or the lining of the vagina. Their study may be informative for two reasons. (*1*) Since the appearance of the cells of these various sites is af-

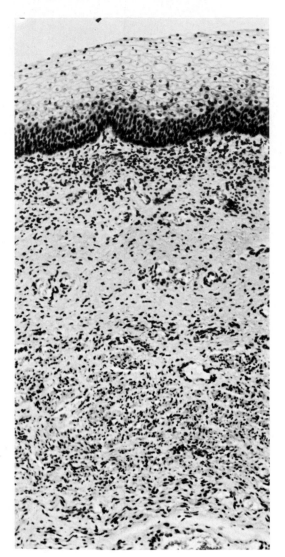

Fig. 26-31. Very low power photomicrograph of the wall of the vagina. Note that the more superficial epithelial cells are large and pale because of their glycogen content. The smooth muscle coats of the wall may be seen in the lower half of the photograph.

nects is sometimes termed the *isthmus* of the uterus. The isthmus is supposed to be the narrowed segment of the organ that begins at its cervical end, where the typical mucous membrane of the cervix begins to change into the endometrial variety. The upper end of the isthmus is supposed to be the site where the lumen becomes constricted (the internal os) before opening out into the wide cavity of the body. However, the landmarks for both the beginning and the end of the isthmus are neither very obvious nor constant in position. The line of transition between the

Fig. 26-32. (*A*) Low-power photomicrograph of a portion of the vagina of a rat from which the ovaries were removed. This shows that, under conditions of estrogen deficiency, the vaginal epithelium becomes thin, and the superficial cells nucleated. (*B*) Preparation from a rat treated similarly, except that it was then injected with estrogen. Note that the epithelium has become greatly thickened, and that the surface layers are now heavily keratinized. This is similar to what is seen in normally occurring estrus.

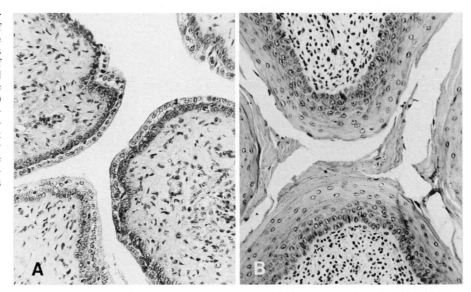

fected by hormone levels, the cells in vaginal smears may give some indication about the hormone balance of the woman at the time they are obtained; and (*2*) cells indicative of having desquamated from an early cancer, growing in the cervix or the body of the uterus, may sometimes be found during an otherwise routine check of a patient and so indicate the need for more detailed examination for cancer. For both reasons it has become common practice to study cells obtained by gently wiping the lining of the vagina or the covering of the cervix and/or cells aspirated or otherwise obtained from the entrance of the cervical canal.

Cyclic Changes in the Vaginal Epithelium

The importance of the discovery that vaginal epithelium of laboratory animals becomes keratinized at the time of estrus has already been acknowledged in connection with the discovery of sex hormones. Mature mice and rats come into estrus spontaneously every 4 days and in between these periods of estrus the epithelium changes its character as will be described presently.

The changes that occur in the vaginal epithelium throughout the 28-day cycle of a woman, however, are not nearly as pronounced. Nevertheless, such changes as do occur are more easily interpreted if the observer knows something about the pronounced changes seen in the estrous cycle of the rat or mouse. These will therefore be described briefly.

The 4-day estrous cycle of the rat and the mouse is divided into four periods: *proestrus, estrus, metaestrus,* and *diestrus.* In proestrus, follicles approach the surface of the ovary, the uterus becomes swollen with secretion, and its blood vessels become engorged. The epithelium of the vagina becomes thick as a result of proliferation in its deeper layers, but its most superficial cells are still nucleated. However, cells with keratohyalin granules appear beneath the superficial nucleated cells. The epithelial membrane thus comes to have a 2-layered appearance. In estrus or

thereabouts, ovulation occurs, and throughout this stage the uterus remains swollen and red. The vaginal epithelium has now become thick and heavily keratinized (Fig. 26-32B), and the mating impulse is aroused. If the animal does not mate it passes into the metaestrus stage. As this progresses, the uterus becomes smaller and the vaginal epithelium much thinner (similar to Fig. 26-32A). The basement membrane disappears, and neutrophils (polymorphs) invade the epithelium and pass through it to appear in great numbers among the epithelial cells seen in vaginal smears (Fig. 26-33A). In diestrus, the uterus is small and pale, and the vaginal epithelium is still thin. However, neutrophils are confined mostly to superficial layers of the epithelium. As proestrus develops, great mitotic activity occurs in the deeper layers of the epithelium so that it becomes thick again.

Since only the superficial cells desquamate, they are the only type seen in vaginal smears. Hence, in estrus, the vaginal smears contain only keratinized cells (Fig. 26-33B). As metaestrus proceeds, vaginal smears contain first keratinized cells and then later nucleated cells and large numbers of the polymorphonuclear leukocytes that are making their way through the epithelium at this stage (Fig. 26-33A). The diestrus stage is characterized by nucleated epithelial cells and leukocytes. In proestrus, the leukocytes have disappeared, so only nucleated epithelial cells are present.

The Microscopic Appearance of the Epithelium of the Human Vagina. The epithelial lining of the human vagina is stratified and substantial (Fig. 26-31). Its deepest stratum consists of a single basal layer of cylindrical cells, each with an oval nucleus. The next stratum is several layers thick. The cells in this stratum are polyhedral in shape and seem to be joined together much like those in the stratum spinosum of the epidermis of thick skin; however, the cells here do not have a prickly appearance. The next stratum consists of a few layers of more flattened cells; these contain glycogen. Hence the cells of this and the more superficial strata appear swollen and empty. The

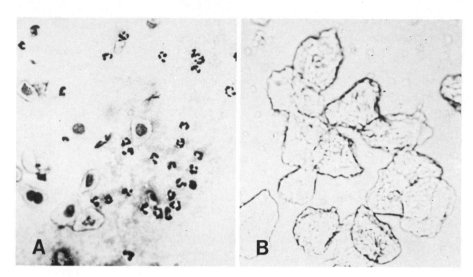

Fig. 26-33. (*A*) High-power photomicrograph of a stained vaginal smear of a rat in the later stages of metaestrus. Note the nucleated epithelial cells at *center* and *lower left* and the characteristic nuclei of polymorphonuclear leukocytes. (*B*) High-power photomicrograph of a stained vaginal smear of a rat in estrus. The smear contains nothing but large pale-staining, non-nucleated squames of keratin.

most superficial stratum consists of several layers of more flattened but somewhat swollen cells, all of which possess nuclei.

The epithelium lining the vagina of a woman differs in two important respects from that lining the vagina of the mouse or the rat. First, since there is no true period of estrus in the human female, there is no time in the menstrual cycle when the epithelium becomes truly keratinized. At the time of ovulation, which is the counterpart of estrus, the epithelium may show a tendency toward keratinization but, unless the epithelium is unduly exposed to air or another unusual environmental factor, it does not proceed all the way to forming keratin; hence, the surface cells always contain a nucleus. Second, the cells of the more superficial layers of the vaginal epithelium tend to accumulate considerable quantities of glycogen in their cytoplasm, particularly at the time of ovulation. This has two possible functions: (*1*) it may serve for nutrition of spermatozoa during their passage through this organ, and (*2*) it is fermented by bacteria in the vagina that convert it to lactic acid, and this acid environment is probably an important factor in maintaining a suitable type of bacterial flora in the vagina.

The appearance of the cells that desquamate from the lining of the vagina and from the covering of the vaginal surface of the cervix has been studied at great length by Papanicolaou by the smear method. Essentially, such progesterone as is secreted during the menstrual cycle appears to be without effect on the vaginal epithelium. The amount of estrogen secreted at the time of ovulation, while not enough to cause keratinization, does, however, have some effect. Papanicolaou considers that there is a relative increase in acidophilic cells with small dark nuclei in the vaginal smear at this time. The development of acidophilic properties by the surface epithelial cells is evidently preliminary to their becoming keratinized, but this is as far as the process usually goes. There are also other criteria that can be employed. The study of desquamated vaginal cells in smears can be helpful in determining the time of ovulation, the effectiveness of estrogen therapy, and in diagnosing atrophic conditions of the vaginal epithelium due to estrogen deficiency.

Advantage is taken of the ability of estrogen to thicken and even keratinize the vaginal epithelium in the treatment of certain vaginal infections, particularly those that occur before puberty, for in young girls the epithelium is thin and vulnerable.

THE MAMMARY GLANDS (BREASTS OR MAMMAE)

Development. The first step in the development of mammary glands in humans occurs near the end of the 6th week of embryonic life when in embryos of either sex the ectoderm becomes thickened along two lines, each of which runs from the axilla to the groin of the same side. These are called the "milk lines," and their epithelial cells have the potentiality to grow down into the underlying mesenchyme at any point along either line to form mammary glands. Usually, in humans, invasion of the underlying mesenchyme by epithelial cells destined to form mammary glands occurs at only one site along each line. However, in most other mammals the mammary glands develop at many sites along each line so that such animals acquire two rows of mammary glands with which to feed their own large families. Occasionally, extra mammary glands develop along the milk line in man (and sometimes elsewhere); if so, they are called *supernumerary nipples (breasts)*. Among civilized peoples, supernumerary breasts are usually removed surgically for cosmetic and other reasons. Aberrant mammary gland tissue in the axilla may not become obvious until pregnancy or lactation causes it to swell.

As the embryo develops, the epithelial cells at the point along the milk line where a breast will develop form a little cluster from which up to 20 or so separate cords of epithelial cells push into the underlying mesenchyme in various directions. Each one of these original cords of cells develops into a separate *compound exocrine gland;* hence, each breast is actually composed of many separate compound glands, each of which empties by a separate duct through the nipple. During fetal life the cords of cells that invade the mesenchyme branch to some extent and tend to become canalized so that at birth a *rudimentary duct system* has formed. At birth there is no obvious difference between the degree to which the glands of the female and male infant are developed. During the first few days of life the glands of a baby may become distended for reasons to be described later, but the condition soon subsides.

Changes at Puberty. As puberty approaches, the breasts of the female, which up to this time have been flat, become enlarged and more or less hemispherical in shape. The nipples become more prominent. The changes in the breasts constitute one of the secondary sex characteristics of the female that appear at this time. Most of the increase in their size is due to *fat* accumulating in the connective tissue between their lobes and lobules. At puberty the epithelial duct system develops beyond a rudimentary stage, but this change is not as striking as the increased amount of fat in the connective tissue. True secretory units do not develop at this time; their formation awaits pregnancy.

In the male, the mammary glands usually experience little or no change at puberty, remaining flat. Uncommonly, considerable enlargement resembling that in the female may occur; this condition is called *gynecomastia* (Gr. *gynaikos,* woman; *mastos,* breast).

Estrogen, probably in conjunction with some lactogenic hormone (the secretion of which would be dependent on estrogen appearing in the circulation), brings about the changes in the female breast described above. The progesterone cyclically secreted from the time of puberty onward may play a contributing role. Estrogen given to males causes their rudimentary mammary glands to begin to develop into the feminine type.

THE MICROSCOPIC STRUCTURE OF THE RESTING BREAST

The breast of a sexually mature nonpregnant female is termed a *resting breast* to distinguish it from one that is in the process of active growth in pregnancy or one that is functioning in lactation.

The Nipple. This part of the breast is a cylindrico-conical structure of pink or brownish-pink color, covered with stratified squamous keratinized epithelium. Numerous papillae of irregular shape extend into the epidermis from the dermis to approach the surface closely; hence, over papillae the epidermis may be very thin (Fig. 26-34). The main duct of each of the many separate glands that make up the breast is called a *lactiferous duct.* These ducts ascend through the nipple (Fig. 26-34) to open by separate orifices on its summit, the orifices being so minute they cannot be seen with the naked eye. The epithelium lining each lactiferous duct, close to its orifice, is similar to that over the nipple. Deeper in the nipple the lactiferous ducts are lined with *2 layers of columnar epithelial cells* that rest on a basement membrane.

The substance of the nipple consists of dense connective tissue and smooth muscle (Fig. 26-34). The fibers of the latter are arranged circularly around the lactiferous ducts and parallel with (and close beside) them as they ascend through the nipple. Many blood vessels and encapsulated nerve endings are also present.

The epidermis of the nipple, like that of the vagina, is sensitive to estrogen. In connection with the problem of "sore nipples"—a condition that results when some women attempt to nurse their babies—it is interesting to note that estrogen may be lacking in a woman shortly after she has given birth. The reason is that estrogen production during pregnancy involves the placenta; hence, when the placenta is delivered following birth, the mother is deprived of what has been her chief source of this hormone. Eventually, of course, her ovaries will produce a sufficiency, but there may be an interval during which the epidermis of the nipples suffers lack of stimulation by estrogen. Indeed, one type of sore nipple can be ascribed to estrogen deficiency. However, there are certain complications (too involved to discuss here) in attempting to use estrogen to thicken the epidermis of nipples of women who have just begun to nurse their babies.

The skin surrounding the nipple, the *areola,* is of a rosy hue. However, it becomes pigmented in pregnancy, and after pregnancy never returns to its original shade; it always retains some pigment. Large modified sweat glands, but not so large or modified as the mammary glands themselves, lie beneath the areola and open onto its surface; these are called the *areolar glands* (of Montgomery). Sebaceous glands and large sweat glands are present around the periphery of the areola. Smooth muscle fibers are disposed, both circularly and perpendicular to the skin surface, beneath the areola.

The Ducts. The lactiferous ducts from the different compound glands of the breast converge under the areola to enter the base of the nipple. As they near this point the

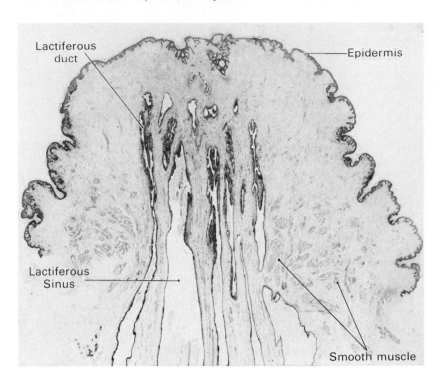

Lactiferous
duct

Epidermis

Lactiferous
Sinus

Smooth muscle

Fig. 26-34. Very low power photomicrograph (lightly retouched) of a section of a nipple, cut perpendicular to the skin surface.

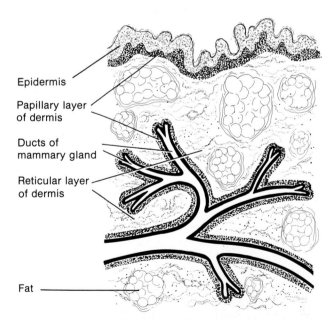

Epidermis

Papillary layer
of dermis

Ducts of
mammary gland

Reticular layer
of dermis

Fat

Fig. 26-35. Diagram illustrating the relation of the layers of the dermis to the connective tissue of the breast. The papillary layer of the dermis and the intralobular connective tissue of the breast are comparable; both are *stippled* in the illustration. The dense connective tissue (reticular layer of the dermis) extends deeply as septa or ligaments that pass between lobules of fat to become continuous with the interlobular connective tissue of the breast.

ducts become somewhat expanded to become what are termed *lactiferous sinuses* (Fig. 26-34). In the lactating breast, these sinuses probably act as little reservoirs for milk.

The many separate compound glands drained by individual lactiferous ducts through the nipple each constitute a *lobe* of the breast. Each lobe in turn consists of many *lobules;* hence, each main lactiferous duct gives rise to many branches that, since they run within lobules, are *intralobular ducts.* The parenchyma of the lobes and lobules of the mammary gland lies in the subcutaneous tissue (the superficial fascia). Nevertheless, this parenchyma (which, it must be remembered, develops from the epidermis of the skin) does not entirely escape the confines of the dermis. It will be recalled that the dermis consists of two layers, and that the *papillary layer* directly adjoining the epidermis is more cellular and of finer texture than the coarser, less cellular *reticular layer* deep to it (Fig. 26-35). When cords of epidermis grow down into mesenchyme to form the duct system of the breast, it seems they carry the developing papillary layer of dermis along with them so that this layer forms a cellular connective tissue wrapping for each duct (Fig. 26-35) or a common wrapping for groups of small adjacent ducts. Then, between the single or grouped ducts so wrapped, substantial bundles and partitions of coarse, less cellular connective tissue extend down from the reticular layer of dermis overlying the breast, to separate lobes and lobules from

Fig. 26-36. Low-power photomicrograph of resting breast.
The ducts are each surrounded by
cellular intralobular connective
tissue, and the two lobules shown
are separated and surrounded by
relatively noncellular interlobular
connective tissue.

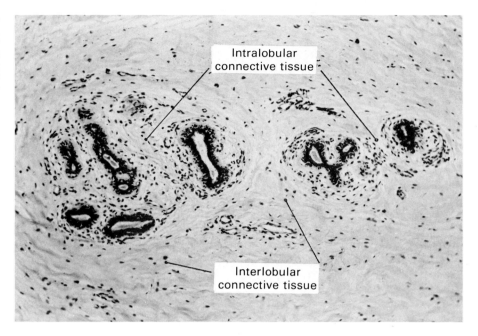

one another and to hold the whole breast parenchyma
tightly to the skin (Fig. 26-35). The larger of these bundles and partitions are termed *suspensory ligaments of
Cooper.* Fat accumulates in them (Fig. 26-35), so that
they hold the fat of the breast in place as well as the
epithelial parenchyma. Fat also accumulates in the connective tissue between the breast parenchyma and (*1*) the
skin overlying it and (*2*) the fascia lying deep to it.

In a section of resting breast, epithelial parenchyma is
scanty, consisting only of single ducts or little clusters of
ducts widely separated from one another by connective
tissue (Fig. 26-36). Most of the ducts seen are cut obliquely or in cross section. Occasionally, a lactiferous
duct may be observed, but almost all the ducts commonly
seen are of the different orders of branches that arise from
lactiferous ducts. Since the branches of the main ducts
run out into the lobules that dangle, as it were, from the
main ducts, most of the ducts seen in a section are inside
lobules and hence *intralobular* ducts (Fig. 26-36). Their
walls are generally composed of two layers of epithelial
cells with pale cytoplasm and a pale-staining oval nucleus. The long diameters of the nuclei in the inner layer
of cells commonly lie radially and those of the outer layer
lie parallel with the duct, but the arrangement of epithelial
cells in these ducts is variable. The epithelial cells of the
ducts rest on a basement membrane.

Each duct is surrounded by a tunic of relatively cellular
connective tissue about as thick as the duct is wide (Fig.
26-36). This layer is the counterpart of the *papillary layer*
of dermis that abuts on epidermis (Fig. 26-35). The
cellular connective tissue that surrounds the individual

ducts in a group of ducts may be confluent. Since this
cellular connective tissue that invests the duct lies inside
lobules, it is termed *intralobular* connective tissue. Fibroblasts are numerous in it and may be easily identified by
their large, oval, pale nucleus (Fig. 26-36). Macrophages,
lymphocytes, and plasma cells are also normal constituents of the intralobular connective tissue.

Single ducts or groups of ducts, invested with intralobular connective tissue, are separated from one another
by thick partitions of coarse and *relatively noncellular*
dense *interlobular* connective tissue. These may be regarded, as is indicated in Figure 26-35, as deep extensions of the *reticular layer* of dermis (the larger partitions
seen correspond to the suspensory ligaments of Cooper).
The interlobular connective tissue characteristically contains lobules of fat within its substance; the fat of the
breast, then, is tied to the skin by the interlobular connective tissue.

CHANGES IN THE BREAST DURING
PREGNANCY

The resting breast consists of little more than its duct
system. As pregnancy proceeds, however, great development of the duct system occurs, and finally secretory alveoli develop at the ends of its smaller branches. By the
end of the 5th month of pregnancy, the lobules are packed
and greatly expanded with alveoli (Fig. 26-37, *left*). The
intralobular connective tissue becomes broken up as al-

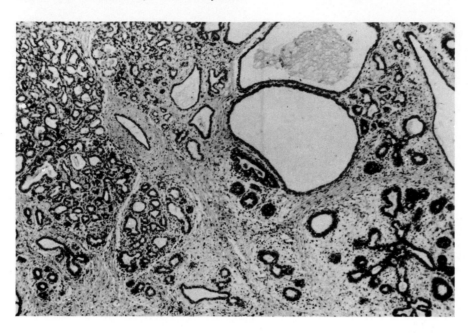

Fig. 26-37. Low-power photomicrograph of breast during the fifth month of a pregnancy. The ducts have proliferated and at *left* have given rise to alveoli.

veoli bud from the ducts, so that eventually it becomes reduced to film-like partitions between adjacent alveoli; however, these contain extensive capillary networks. The alveoli themselves are composed of a single layer of columnar cells. Myoepithelial cells are sometimes seen around their periphery. Because of the great expansion of epithelial elements within the lobules, the partitions of interlobular connective tissue become greatly stretched and thinned (Fig. 26-38).

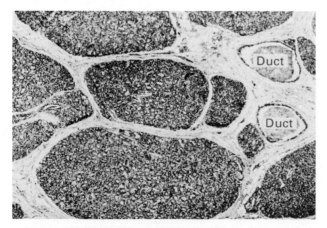

Fig. 26-38. Low-power photomicrograph of lactating breast. The lobules illustrated here, although expanded by a great content of alveoli, are not cut through their widest parts. The interlobular septa are thicker here than in most other sites in the section.

Most epithelial growth in the breast occurs before the end of the 6th month of pregnancy; further growth occurs, but very slowly. However, the breasts continue to enlarge; this is due chiefly to the cells of the alveoli beginning to secrete a fluid that expands them (and therefore the breast) from within. This secretion is not milk; milk appears only after parturition, as will be explained presently.

Factors Causing Growth of Breasts During Pregnancy. Several hormones are involved. It is difficult to be precise about any of their actions because not all species on which experiments are done react the same way. Furthermore, secretion of one hormone affects secretion of others, and this makes it difficult to determine just which hormone does what.

If intact animals are given enough *estrogen,* the mammary glands promptly develop. In some species estrogen by itself seems sufficient to prepare the glands for function. However, in others it seems *progesterone* is also required to bring about full development of secretory alveoli. In any event, estrogen is certainly involved in bringing about the great development of the epithelial component of the breast in pregnancy.

However, estrogen, or a combination of estrogen and progesterone, will not bring about full development of the mammary glands in a hypophysectomized animal. Accordingly, it seems that pituitary hormones, or the hormones of the target glands they control, are also concerned in development of the breasts in pregnancy. There is evidence that *growth hormone* (somatotrophin), *lactogenic hormone* (prolactin), and adrenal *glucocorticoids* all participate with estrogen and progesterone in causing development of the breasts. However, the anterior pituitary is not essential because if the pituitary gland is removed from a pregnant animal, provided the placenta remains intact and functional, the mammary glands will continue to develop. In this connection it should be remembered that the placenta makes a lactogenic-like hormone (*somatomammotrophin*) as well as several other hormones.

When more is learned about how different hormones affect growth and secretory functions of cells, it should be possible to be more specific about the roles of the different hormones in this instance. However, there is no doubt that estrogen is a key hormone in this connection because it can affect the growth of mammary gland tissue even if applied locally.

THE BREASTS DURING LACTATION

As noted, most of the growth of the breasts from the 6th month of pregnancy on is due to secretion accumulating in the alveoli and ducts. As this secretion is made, some appears and escapes from the nipple (in women who have previously borne children, this may occur relatively early in pregnancy). This secretion is not milk but a somewhat different fluid termed *colostrum*. After parturition, colostrum is secreted more abundantly but only for 2 or 3 days, after which the breasts (in women) begin to secrete milk.

Colostrum contains a higher concentration of protein than milk, but very little fat. It also contains fragments of cells and even whole cells of large size. These frequently contain phagocytosed fat and are called *colostrum bodies*. It is probable that these cells are phagocytes that have made their way through the epithelium of the alveoli and so gained entrance to their lumina.

It is now generally accepted that almost no milk is secreted during the nursing of a baby; milk is secreted and accumulated during the intervals between nursings.

Microscopic Structure of the Lactating Breast

The lobules are packed with secretory alveoli, among which intralobular ducts may be seen (Fig. 26-38). In general, the interlobular septa are greatly thinned; those illustrated in Figure 26-38 are wider than most. The alveoli in some parts of the breast have high columnar cells and others have low columnar cells. Some alveoli are distended with secretion, and some contain only a little. It is probable that the alveoli in different parts of the same breast may, at the same time, be in different stages of a secretory cycle.

The Fine Structure of Secretory Cells of the Mammary Gland and Their Process of Secretion

Milk contains protein, fat, sugar, and mineral salts. The EM shows that secretory alveoli of mammary glands have the same equipment (rER) in the more basal parts of their cells for synthesizing protein as other types of cells that secrete proteins. The Golgi apparatus is located on the luminal side of the secretory cells, and it seems that the proteins synthesized in the rER would be delivered via transfer vesicles to saccules on the forming face of the Golgi. Protein destined for secretion leaves the mature face of the Golgi secretory vesicles; these move toward the lumen and are discharged by exocytosis. The same vesicles would contain the lactose of milk, the formation of which component would occur in the Golgi.

The fat in the milk is synthesized in the cytoplasm of the secretory cells, probably in the cytosol in much the same manner as fat is synthesized in fat cells (as described in Chap. 9). Fat droplets move to the luminal surface of the cell, from which they are extruded. In leaving the cell they become enclosed by cell membrane, which they carry with them. During the preparation of paraffin sections the fat droplets in the cytoplasm are extracted so that the spaces they occupied appear as vacuoles. These are particularly numerous between the free border and the nucleus of the alveolar cells (Fig. 26-39).

The Cause of Lactation and Its Maintenance

Lactogenic hormone (prolactin) secreted by mammotrophs of the anterior pituitary is the hormone chiefly

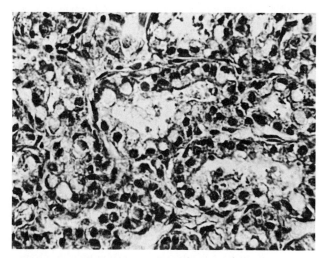

Fig. 26-39. High-power photomicrograph of a small part of a lobule of lactating breast. One alveolus is seen at *center*, another at *lower right*. Fat droplets are evident in the secretory cells of the alveoli, particularly beneath their free borders.

responsible for causing the mammary glands to secrete milk. Under ordinary conditions the activity of mammotrophs is suppressed by the secretion of prolactin-inhibiting factor (PIF) by the hypothalamus. Prolactin is secreted in small quantities by mammotrophs during pregnancy, and a lactogenic-like hormone (somatomammotrophin) is produced by the placenta. These probably collaborate with estrogen is causing the breasts to develop.

The termination of pregnancy, with expulsion of the placenta, has many effects. This is because the placenta has been making several hormones, capable of inhibiting (by negative feedback) the secretion of similar or other hormones by the mother. When the placenta is delivered at parturition, this suppressive effect on hormone production in the mother is removed. One consequence may be that the anterior pituitary begins to secrete increased amounts of lactogenic hormone. Moreover, nursing a baby sets up afferent impulses that act on the hypothalamus to *inhibit* secretion of PIF, the hypothalamic hormone that ordinarily restrains secretory activity in mammotrophs. Hence as long as nursing is continued, the mammotrophs keep on secreting prolactin.

Ovulation and menstruation may be interrupted while a mother is nursing her baby. However, this is by no means universal, and women can become pregnant again during the nursing period. It is of interest that pregnancy does not interfere with well-established lactation, so that a mother can continue nursing one baby after another has been conceived.

Myoepithelial Cells, Oxytocin, and the Milk Ejection Reflex. As in other exocrine glands, secretory alveoli of the mammary glands are each surrounded by a cell having the form of a loose basket, with a cell body from which many processes extend to clasp the alveolus. These surrounding cells are called *myoepithelial cells* because they have an epithelial origin and yet contain cytoplasmic filaments similar to those of smooth muscle cells. Similar myoepithelial cells of secretory alveoli of submaxillary glands are shown in Figure 7-25. Mammary glands continue to secrete between nursings so that milk accumulates in the lumina of their alveoli and ducts. When a baby begins to nurse, afferent impulses reach the paraventricular nuclei of the hypothalamus (Fig. 25-14) and cause the neurosecretory cells they contain to release oxytocin from their axon terminals in the posterior lobe of the pituitary. Oxytocin causes the myoepithelial cells of the mammary gland to contract, and this squeezes the secretion in the alveoli into the lactiferous sinuses; it may even spurt through the nipple. In any event, this *milk ejection reflex* causes milk to be available at the nipple for the nursing baby.

Thorough emptying of the breasts at nursing helps maintain and even increase their functional capacity, not only because the afferent impulses restrain the hypothalamus from secreting PIF, but also because increased demand stimulates further growth to meet the demand.

Maintenance of Lactation. Lactation cannot proceed in the absence of the adrenal cortex, since glucocorticoids are necessary. The thyroid hormone facilitates lactation, and insulin is also required. The breasts must be emptied regularly if their structure is to be maintained and secretion of lactogenic hormone is to be continued.

Regression After Lactation. Discontinuing breast feeding, provided the breasts are not regularly emptied by other means, leads to their gradually regaining almost the same type of microscopic structure they had before pregnancy began. However, they do not return to precisely the same state because a few alveoli persist in them. But most of the alveoli are resorbed, and the lobules shrink. The partitions of interlobular connective tissue again become thick and strong. For esthetic reasons mothers like to preserve the shape of their breasts as much as possible. It is very important that their breasts be properly supported while the interlobular partitions are thin, particularly while alveoli are being resorbed, lobules are shrinking in size, and interlobular partitions are becoming thick again during the 2 to 3 months following cessation of lactation. If the interlobular septa become "set" in a stretched state, the breasts will subsequently sag unduly.

THE BREASTS AFTER THE MENOPAUSE

Various changes occur after the menopause. The general trend is toward atrophy of both epithelial and connective tissue components of the breast. The intercellular substance may undergo a hyalin change. Irregular growth and secretory changes, moreover, may be superimposed on the general atrophic changes; the epithelium of some ducts may proliferate whereas that of others may secrete and convert the ducts concerned into cysts. Estrogen and progesterone deficiency are doubtless chiefly responsible for progressive atrophy following the menopause.

REFERENCES AND OTHER READING

COMPREHENSIVE GENERAL REFERENCES

Austin, C. R., and Short, R. V. (eds.): Reproduction in Mammals. Books 1 to 6. Cambridge, Cambridge University Press, 1972 to 1976.

Greep, R. O.: The female reproductive system. *In* Greep, R. O., Koblinsky, M. A., and Jaffe, F. S. (eds.): Reproduction and Human Welfare: A Challenge to Research. p. 81. Cambridge, Mass., MIT Press, 1976.

Greep, R. O. (ed.): Handbook of Physiology, Section 7: Endocrinology. Vol II: Female Reproductive System. Washington, D.C., Am. Physiol. Soc., 1975.

GENERAL REFERENCE

Martin, C. R.: Hormones and reproduction. *In* Martin, C. R. (ed.): Textbook of Endocrine Physiology. Baltimore, Williams & Wilkins, 1976.

SPECIAL REFERENCES

The Ovaries, Oviducts, Uterus, and Vagina, and the Hormones They Produce or That Affect Them

Anderson, E., and Beams, H. W.: Cytological observations on the fine structure of the guinea pig ovary with special reference to the oogonium, primary oocyte and associated follicle cells. J. Ultrastruct. Res., *3:*432, 1960.

Aron, C., Asch, G., and Roos, J.: Triggering of ovulation by coitus in the rat. Int. Rev. Cytol., *20,* 1966.

Austin, C. R.: The Mammalian Egg. Oxford, Blackwell Scientific Publications, 1961.

Balboni, G. C.: Histology of the ovary. *In* James, V. H. T., Serio, M., and Giusti, G. (eds.): The Endocrine Function of the Human Ovary. Proceedings of the Serono Symposia, vol. 7. London, Academic Press, 1976.

Bartelmez, G. W.: Histological studies of the menstruating mucous membranes of the human uterus. Contrib. Embryol., *24:*141, 1933.

Bertalanffy, F. D., and Lau, C.: Mitotic rates, renewal times, and cytodynamics of the female genital tract epithelia in the rat. Acta Anat., *54:*39, 1963.

Blandau, R. J., and Bergsma, D. (eds.): Morphogenesis and Malformation of the Genital System. Birth Defects: Original Article Series, Vol. 13, No. 2. New York, Liss, 1977.

Cowell, C. A., and Wilson, R.: The Ovary. *In* Ezrin, C., Godden, J. O., Volpé, R., and Wilson, R. (eds.): Systemic Endocrinology. Hagerstown, Md., Harper & Row, 1973.

Crisp, T. M., Dessouky, D. A., and Denys, F. R.: The fine structure of the human corpus luteum of early pregnancy and during the progestational phase of the menstrual cycle. Am. J. Anat., *127:*37, 1970.

Daron, G. H.: The arterial pattern of the tunica mucosa of the uterus in Macacus rhesus. Am. J. Anat., *58:*349, 1936.

de Allende, I. L. C., Shorr, E., and Hartman, C. G.: A comparative study of the vaginal smear cycle of the rhesus monkey and the human. Contrib. Embryol., *31:*1, 1945.

Enders, A. C.: Observations on the fine structure of lutein cells. J. Cell Biol., *12:*101, 1962.

Hafez, E. S. E. (ed.): Scanning Electron Microscopic Atlas of Mammalian Reproduction. New York, Springer-Verlag, 1975.

Hafez, E. S. E., and Blandau, R. J.: The Mammalian Oviduct: Comparative Biology and Methodology. Chicago, University of Chicago Press, 1969.

Hertig, A. T., and Adams, E. C.: Studies on the human oocyte and its follicle. I. Ultrastructural and histochemical observations on the primordial follicle stage. J. Cell Biol., *34:*647, 1967.

Jones, R. E. (ed.): The Vertebrate Ovary. New York, Plenum, 1978.

Ludwig, H., and Metzger, H.: The Human Female Reproductive Tract. A Scanning Electron Microscopic Atlas. New York, Springer-Verlag, 1976.

McCann, S. M.: Luteinizing-hormone-releasing-hormone. N. Engl. J. Med., *296:*797, 1977.

McEwen, B. S.: Interactions between hormones and nerve tissue. Sci. Am., *235:*48, July, 1976.

Markee, J. E.: Menstruation in intraocular endometrial transplants in the rhesus monkey. Contrib. Embryol., *28:*219, 1940.

———: The morphological and endocrine basis for menstrual bleeding. Prog. Gynec., *2:*63, 1950.

Ohno, S., Klinger, H. P., and Atkin, N. B.: Human oogenesis. Cytogenetics, *1:*42, 1962.

Papanicolaou, G. N.: The sexual cycle in the human female as revealed by vaginal smears. Am. J. Anat., *52:*519, 1933.

Pincus, G.: Control of conception by hormonal steroids. Science, *153:*493, 1966.

Richardson, G. S.: Ovarian physiology. N. Engl. J. Med., *294:* May 5, p. 1008; May 12, p. 1064; May 19, p. 1121; and May 26, p. 1183, 1966.

Ryan, K. J., Peters, Z., and Kaiser, J.: Steroid formation by isolated and recombined ovarian granulosa and thecal cells. J. Clin. Endocrinol. Metab., *28:*355, 1968.

Snyder, F. F.: Changes in the human oviduct during the menstrual cycle and pregnancy. Bull. Johns Hopkins Hosp., *35:*141, 1924.

Sotello, J. R., and Porter, K. R.: An electron microscope study of the rat ovum. J. Biophys. Biochem. Cytol., *5:*327, 1959.

Van Blerkom, J., and Motta, P.: Cellular Basis of Mammalian Reproduction. Baltimore, Urban and Schwarzenberg, 1978.

Witschi, E.: Migration of germ cells of human embryos from the yolk sac to the primitive gonadal folds. Carnegie Inst. Contrib. Embryol., *32:*67, 1948.

Wynn, R. M. (ed.): Biology of the Uterus. New York, Plenum Press, 1977.

Young A.: Vascular architecture of the rat uterus. Proc. R. Soc. Edinb., *64:*292, 1952.

Zamboni, L.: Modulations of follicle cell-oocyte association in sequential stages of mammalian follicle development and maturation. *In* Crosignani, P. G., and Mishell, D. R. (eds.): Ovulation in the Human. Proceedings of the Serono Symposia, vol. 8. London, Academic Press, 1976.

Aspects of Pregnancy: Implantation and Development and Structure of the Placenta

Avery, G. B., and Hunt, C. V.: The fetal membranes as a barrier to transplantation immunity. Transplantation, *5:*444, 1967.

Beer, A. E., and Billingham, R. E.: The Immunobiology of Mammalian Reproduction. Englewood Cliffs, N.J., Prentice Hall, 1976.

Blandau, R. J. (ed.): The Biology of the Blastocyst. Chicago, University of Chicago Press, 1971.

Boving, B. G.: Implantation. Ann. N.Y. Acad. Sci., *75:*700, 1959.

Boyd, J. D., and Hamilton, W. J.: The giant cells of the pregnant human uterus. J. Obstet. Gynaecol. Br. Emp., *67:*208, 1960.

———: Development of the human placenta in the first three months of gestation. J. Anat., *94:*297, 1960.

———: The Human Placenta. Cambridge, England, W. Heffer and Sons, 1970.

Edwards, R. G., Howe, C. W. S., and Johnson, M. H. (eds.): Immunobiology of Trophoblast. Cambridge, Cambridge University Press, 1975.

Enders, A. C.: Fine structure of anchoring villi of the human placenta. Am. J. Anat., *122:*419, 1968.

Hamilton, W. J., and Boyd, J. D.: Development of the human placenta in the first three months of gestation. J. Anat., *94:*297, 1960.

King, B. F., and Tibbitts, F. D.: The fine structure of the chinchilla placenta. Am. J. Anat., *145:*33, 1976.

Kirby, D. R. S., and Wood, C.: Embryos and antigens. Science J., *3:*56, December, 1967.

Paine, C. G.: Observations on placental histology in normal and abnormal pregnancy. J. Obstet. Gynaecol. Br. Emp., *64*(5): 668, 1957.

Pierce, G. B., Jr., and Midgley, A. R., Jr.: The origin and function of human syncytiotrophoblastic giant cells. Am. J. Pathol., *43:*153, 1963.

Ramsey, E. M.: Vascular adaptations of the uterus to pregnancy. Ann. N.Y. Acad. Sci., *75:*726, 1959.

Simmons, R. L., Cruse, V., and McKay, D. G.: The immunologic problem of pregnancy. Am. J. Obstet. Gynecol., *97:*218, 1967.

Terzakis, J. A.: The ultrastructure of normal human first trimester placenta. J. Ultrastruct. Res., *9:*268, 1963.

Villee, C. A.: The Placenta and Fetal Membranes. Baltimore, Williams & Wilkins, 1960.

Villee, D. B.: Development of endocrine function in the human placenta and fetus. N. Engl. J. Med., *281:*473, 1969.

The Mammary Glands

Cowie, A. T., and Folley, S. J.: The mammary gland and lactation. *In* Young, W. C. (ed.): Sex and Internal Secretions. ed. 3, p. 590. Baltimore, Williams & Wilkins, 1961.

Dempsey, E. W., Bunting, H., and Wislocki, G. B.: Observations on the chemical cytology of the mammary gland. Am. J. Anat., *81:*309, 1947.

Gardner, W. U., and White, A.: Mammary growth in hypophy-sectomized male mice receiving estrogen and prolactin. Proc. Soc. Exp. Biol. Med., *48:*590, 1941.

Gunther, M.: Sore nipples; causes and prevention. Lancet, *249:*590, 1945.

Jeffers, K. R.: Cytology of the mammary gland of albino rat. Am. J. Anat., *56:*257, 279, 1935.

Linzell, J. L.: The silver staining of myoepithelial cells, particularly in the mammary gland, and their relation to the ejection of milk. J. Anat., *86:*49, 1952.

Petersen, W. E.: Lactation. Physiol. Rev., *24:*340, 1944.

Speert, H.: The normal and experimental development of the mammary gland of the Rhesus monkey with some pathological correlations. Carnegie Inst. Contrib. Embryol., *32:*9, 1948.

Trentin, J. J., DeVita, J., and Gardner, W. U.: Effect of moderate doses of estrogen and progesterone on mammary growth and hair growth in dogs. Anat. Rec., *113:*163, 1952.

Turner, C. D.: General Endocrinology. ed. 4. Philadelphia, W. B. Saunders, 1966.

Vorherr, H.: The Breast. Morphology, Physiology and Lactation. New York, Academic Press, 1974.

Waugh, D., and van der Hoeven, E.: Fine structure of the human adult female breast. Lab. Invest., *11:*220, 1962.

Wellings, S. R., Grunbaum, B. W., and DeOme, K. B.: Electron microscopy of milk secretion in the mammary gland of the C3H/Crgl mouse. J. Natl. Cancer Inst., *25:*423, 1960.

Wellings, S. R., and Philp, J. R.: The function of the Golgi apparatus in lactating cells of the BALB/cCrgl mouse. An electron microscopic and autoradiographic study. Z. Zellforsch., *61:*871, 1964.

27 The Male Reproductive System

THE PARTS OF THE SYSTEM AND THEIR FUNCTIONS

The male reproductive system (Fig. 27-1) consists of: (*1*) two gonads, the *testes,* which produce male germ cells and male sex hormone; (*2*) a copulatory organ, the *penis,* by which the germ cells may be delivered into the vagina of the female; (*3*) a long, complicated set of tubes leading from each testis to the penis that permits the germ cells made in the testes to mature and also stores them before being delivered to the male copulatory organ; and (*4*) certain glands called the male *accessory glands,* with much smooth muscle in their walls. These glands not only provide a fluid vehicle for carrying the germ cells but also, by reflex contraction of the smooth muscle of their walls during sexual intercourse (certain voluntary muscles also participate), cause a mixture of their secretions and male germ cells (the mixture is called *semen*) to be expressed vigorously from the penis, which occurrence is termed *ejaculation.*

The male reproductive system thus consists of four kinds of structures with somewhat different functions. We shall first discuss their main features and their relation to one another.

Some General Features of the Testes. Although the testes develop in the abdomen from the indifferent gonads of the embryo, they migrate so that in postnatal life they are contained in the scrotum. This is a pouch that hangs between the anteromedial borders of the thighs (shown, but not labeled, in Fig. 27-1). Its wall is thin, being composed of skin, an incomplete layer of smooth muscle (the dartos), and some subcutaneous tissue. The wall of the scrotum has a considerable surface area, and this permits its contents to be maintained at a temperature slightly below that of the body as a whole. This lower temperature is an important requisite in man for the production of germ cells. The dartos muscle in the wall of the scrotum contracts in response to cold and certain other stimuli; its contraction makes the scrotum smaller and its wall corrugated.

Like the ovaries, the testes perform the dual functions of producing germ cells and sex hormone. Male germ cells are called *spermatozoa* (Gr. *sperma,* seed; *zoon,* animal). The generic term for substances having male sex hormone activity is *androgen* (Gr. *anēr,* man; *gennan,* to produce).

The testes each have two important functional components. First, tubules with walls many cells in thickness, and with a total length of almost half a mile, are packed into the two testes (Fig. 27-2). These are the *seminiferous tubules.* The cells of the innermost layers constantly turn into spermatozoa and these become free in the lumen of the tubules. The second functional component consists of *interstitial cells.* These are disposed in small groups in the connective tissue stroma between the tubules and produce the androgen made by the testes.

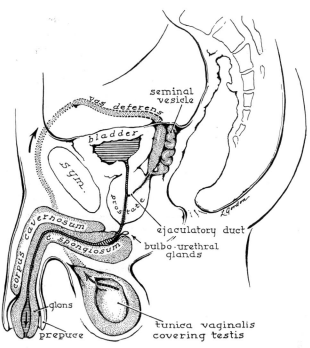

Fig. 27-1. Diagram of the parts of the male reproductive system, showing their connections with one another.

875

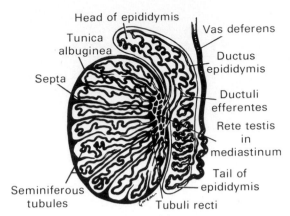

Fig. 27-2. Diagram showing the parts of the testis and epididymis.

The structure and functions of the testes are controlled by the anterior pituitary gland. In males, as in females, this secretes both FSH and LH—but not in cyclical fashion as occurs in females. Puberty in the male results from the anterior pituitary gland beginning to secrete LH. This gonadotrophin stimulates the cells in the testes that produce male hormone; the hormone-secreting cells it stimulates are called *interstitial cells* (Leydig cells), and these will be described later. Because it affects these particular cells, LH is sometimes referred to as *interstitial-cell-stimulating hormone* (ICSH) in the male. Under the influence of LH the interstitial cells secrete the androgen *testosterone*, which is responsible for the development of the secondary sex characteristics of the male that appear at puberty. The role of FSH is not as simple as was first thought (which was that it directly stimulated production of male germ cells, so that their production was under its direct control). It is now evident that it plays a somewhat different role, as will be described later.

Each testis is ovoid, 4 to 5 cm. long. It is covered with a thick capsule called the *tunica albuginea* because it contains so much white fibrous tissue (Fig. 27-2). Along the posterior border of each testis, the capsule becomes greatly thickened and extends into the substance of the gland for a short distance to form an incomplete partition. Since it tends to be in the middle of the gland, this abortive partition and the thickened part of the capsule from which it arises are said to constitute the *mediastinum* (L. for being in the middle) of the testis (Fig. 27-2).

The mediastinum of each testis is riddled with a network of passageways lined with epithelium. These constitute the *rete* (L. *rete*, net) *testis* (Fig. 27-2). The seminiferous tubules of the testis all empty into the spaces of the rete.

General Features of the Set of Conducting Tubes and Tubules. The spermatozoa present in the testis or rete

testis are *not capable of fertilization.* Spermatozoa complete their maturation *outside* the testis in tubules that are enormously long and convoluted. The changes are mostly biochemical, but nevertheless of great importance. The names and general distribution of the tubules through which the spermatozoa must pass will now be given.

The spaces of the *rete testis*, at the upper part of the mediastinium, drain into 15 to 20 tubules called the *ductuli efferentes* (L. *effere*, to bring out) that arise in this region (Fig. 27-2). These penetrate the tunica albuginea of the testis and emerge from its upper part. They thereupon pursue an extraordinarily convoluted course as they pass upward. Each tubule is so wound on itself that each forms a little cone-shaped structure. The cones are bound together by loose connective tissue, and together they constitute most of the head of a narrow crescentic structure that caps the upper pole of the testis and extends down along one of its sides. Since the testes are alike (twins), this narrow structure that caps each of them is termed an *epididymis* (Gr. *epi*, upon; *didymos*, twin).

Each epididymis has a head, body, and tail. The head fits over part of the upper pole of the testis and consists essentially of the cones of convoluted ductuli efferentes (Fig. 27-2). The body extends down along the posterolateral border of the testis and consists chiefly of the *ductus epididymis.* This duct begins in the head, where all the ductuli efferentes empty into it. In the body of the epididymis it pursues an extremely convoluted course (Fig. 27-2). This part of it, if unraveled, would be several yards long. In the tail of the epididymis, which reaches nearly to the lower pole of the testis, the ductus epididymis gradually assumes a less convoluted course and finally emerges from the tail to become the *ductus (vas) deferens* (L. *deferre*, to carry away) as shown in Figure 27-2.

The ductus deferens ascends from the tail of the epididymis along the posterior border of the testis, medial to the epididymis. It becomes associated with blood vessels and nerves and takes on coverings derived from the anterior abdominal wall, whose lowest medial part it traverses in a region known as the *inguinal canal.* The ductus deferens, together with the blood vessels and nerves associated with it and the wrappings it obtains from the tissues of the anterior abdominal wall, constitutes a structure known as the *spermatic cord.* The ductus deferens, in the spermatic cord, traverses the inguinal canal, which leads through the muscles and the fascia of the abdominal wall, to enter the abdominal cavity, although remaining under the peritoneal lining of the cavity. Here the ductus deferens becomes free of its coverings and, after entering and pursuing a course through the pelvis, reaches the posterior aspect of the urinary bladder (Fig. 27-1). Here, an epithelially lined sac called a *seminal vesicle*, which is a blind outpouching of the ductus deferens, lies lateral to each ductus deferens along the posterior aspect of the bladder (Fig. 27-1). Immediately beyond the point at which the seminal vesicle empties into the ductus deferens, the duct—which is now the common duct of the testis and the seminal vesicle—is known as the *ejaculatory duct* (Fig. 27-1). This pierces the upper surface of the *prostate gland,* traverses the substance of the gland, and empties into the *urethra,* which in turn courses through the prostate on its way from the bladder to the penis.

General Features of the Glands Supplying the Fluid Vehicle for Spermatozoa. As noted, the fluid delivered in ejaculation is semen, a composite of spermatozoa and a fluid vehicle, most of which is supplied by the seminal vesicles and the prostate gland. Moreover, these structures, as well as containing epithelial secretory cells that provide the fluid vehicle, have considerable smooth muscle in their walls, and sudden reflex contraction of this during ejaculation provides part of the force required to eject the semen.

The *seminal vesicles* are lined with secretory cells and their lining is thrown into an enormous number of folds (Fig. 27-19). The secretion produced by the lining cells accumulates in the cavity of the vesicle, and the resulting engorgement of the vesicle, together with the filling of the glands of the prostate gland (to be described later), by stimulating afferent nerve endings is probably a very important factor in arousing the sex urge in males.

The *prostate gland*—about the size and shape of a horse chestnut—is essentially a rounded mass of smooth muscle and connective tissue, the substance of which is thoroughly riddled with a great many separate compound tubulo-alveolar glands. The prostate surrounds the proximal portion of the urethra as the latter emerges from the neck of the bladder (Fig. 27-1). The tubulo-alveolar compound glands extending throughout its substance drain through multiple ducts into the prostatic portion of the urethra.

The Penis. The urethra courses through the penis to open through its end. The penis under ordinary conditions is flaccid and in this state could not function as a copulatory organ. However, if a male is subjected to sufficient erotic influence, the penis becomes greatly increased in size and assumes a more or less erect position (*erection*), enabling him to perform the sexual act. Erection is involuntary, controlled by the autonomic nervous system, and is explained by the fact that most of the substance of the penis is erectile tissue. This is disposed in three long cylindrical bodies, arranged two side by side and known as the *corpora cavernosa,* and one situated medially below these, known as the *corpus cavernosum urethrae* because it conducts the urethra from one of its ends to the other (Figs. 27-1 and 27-23). The corpora cavernosa contain a vast number of vascular cavities, all connected with the vascular system. When the penis is flaccid, the cavities are collapsed and contain only a little

blood, because the vascular arrangement is such that blood can drain from the cavities more easily than it can enter them. But under conditions of erotic stimulation, nerve impulses flow to the organ and relax the smooth muscle of the arterial vessels that supply the cavities. This causes greatly increased amounts of blood to enter them, more than is being drained away. As the cavities of the corpora cavernosa become distended with blood, some of the veins ordinarily draining blood away from the cavities become compressed. The net result of the increase in arterial supply and impeded venous drainage is that the cavernous bodies become longer, thicker, wider, and straighter, and, as a consequence, the penis becomes enlarged and erect. Eventually, when the smooth muscle of the arteries that supply the cavities contracts, the rate of drainage of blood from the spaces in the erectile tissue exceeds the rate at which it is delivered into the spaces and as a result the organ becomes flaccid again.

THE TESTES

Development. For details, texts on embryology or the testes should be consulted. The following account is provided only to give some background.

The embryonic development of a testis for the first five weeks is the same as that described for an ovary. The *primordial germ cells* migrate from the yolk sac to a developing testis during the 5th week and become incorporated into *cords* of epithelial-like cells in its stroma. Here the germ cells intermingle with the cells of the cords so that when the latter develop into tubules, primordial germ cells (*gonocytes*) constitute part of their walls. Eventually gonocytes become *spermatogonia* of seminiferous tubules. After puberty these proliferate as stem cells, with many going on to differentiate to produce spermatozoa. The cells of the sex cords themselves give rise to supportive and nutritive cells of the seminiferous tubules termed *Sertoli cells.*

In the 7th week, sex cords become clearly delineated and the mesenchyme beneath the surface epithelium takes on a distinctive appearance, indicating the site where the thick *tunica albuginea* will later form. *Interstitial cells* destined to serve an endocrine function also develop from stromal cells in between the epithelial tubules. The sex cords become continuous with another group of cords of different embryologic origin that become organized somewhat more deeply in the testis; these deeper cords are the forerunners of the *rete testis.*

By the 4th month, the cords of epithelium have become more sharply delimited from the mesoderm-derived stroma between them. Some of the cells of the stroma now constitute clusters of interstitial cells and these produce androgen during fetal life; indeed, the testis is much more active in the fetus than it is from birth until puberty.

In many animals the septa radiating from the mediastinum to the tunica albuginea divide the organ into lobules. However, in human testes the septa are incomplete. Within the imperfectly separated lobules the cords develop lumina in boyhood, at around the seventh year of life. These *seminiferous tubules* become arranged in the form of long convoluted loops (Fig. 27-2). At the point where each loop closely approaches the mediastinum, the tubule becomes continuous by means of relatively straight *tubuli recti* (L. *rectus,* straight) with the rete testis (Fig. 27-2).

Descent and Maldescent of the Testes. Each testis originates deep to the peritoneum on the medial side of each developing kidney. As development proceeds and the testis migrates caudally, the peritoneum bulges out through the anterior abdominal wall, just above the medial end of the inguinal ligament, into the inguinal canal. The elongated tubular pouch of peritoneum so formed is called the *processus vaginalis* (L. for sheath-like extension). The testis, which by this time lies immediately behind the peritoneum, is pulled down into the inguinal canal behind the processus vaginalis. The processus vaginalis traverses the inguinal canal and descends into the scrotum (arriving there at about the 7th month or somewhat later). The testis, pulling the ductus deferens behind it, follows along behind the posterior wall of the processus vaginalis to reach the scrotum shortly before birth. The posterior wall of the processus vaginalis is invaginated by the testis and so covers its lateral and anterior walls as well as its two poles. In this way the testis is provided with visceral peritoneum (visceral layer of tunica vaginalis). The remainder of the processus vaginalis lies in its own half of the inner wall of the scrotum and constitutes the parietal layer of the tunica vaginalis. The canal by which the processus vaginalis communicates with the peritoneal cavity then becomes obliterated (this may occur before birth but usually occurs afterwards).

Occasionally, one or both testes fail to descend into the scrotum during fetal life or immediately after birth. Testes that fail to descend may be held up at almost any point along the course they normally follow. An individual with undescended testes is termed *cryptorchid* (Gr. *kryptos,* concealed; *orchis,* testis). In some instances undescended testes descend spontaneously during infancy, but in the majority of instances they do not, and measures must be taken to get them down into the scrotum. It is important for the testes to descend before the age of 7, because this is when the cords become seminiferous tubules if the testes are in their proper environment. Unless the testes gain entrance to the favorable environment of the scrotum, they *will not produce spermatozoa;* however, the interstitial cells *may still produce androgens.*

It has become apparent that hormones direct normal descent of the testes to a considerable degree. As noted, interstitial cells develop in significant numbers in the 4th month. This development and general growth of the testes at this time suggest that it is being stimulated by some trophic hormone. It seems likely that placental gonadotrophin stimulates growth of the testes early in fetal life; but, as was described in the previous chapter, placental gonadotrophin requires assistance from the anterior pituitary to exert an LH effect, so a pituitary factor would also be involved in stimulating interstitial cell function in fetal life. The androgen thus secreted would bring about changes in the inguinal canal that permit the testis to descend through it more readily. It would also facilitate growth of the scrotum and ductus deferens. It seems very probable that it is the androgen made by the fetal testes that is responsible for bringing about the important changes that permit their descent.

The Microscopic Appearance of the Testes From Birth Until Puberty. The interstitial cells of the testes are not at all prominent during childhood (from birth until 10 years of age). The seminiferous tubules are small and composed of two types of cells: the *gonocytes* that are the precursors of the spermatogonia that will later give rise to spermatozoa, and the supporting cells. The latter, called

Sertoli cells, are numerous and show a small irregular nucleus and poorly delimited cytoplasm. The gonocytes, fewer in number, have a spherical nucleus and a clearly visible periphery. During adolescence (between the ages of 10 and 14 years) the gonocytes—which are now called *spermatogonia*—begin proliferating to eventually go on to produce spermatozoa. Concomitantly, the supporting cells increase in volume, and each comes to have a large, pale-staining irregular nucleus and much cytoplasm that extends inward from the periphery of the tubule, through the many layers of cells concerned with forming spermatozoa, to the lumen of the tubule. These *Sertoli cells* (Fig. 27-4, Ser) have several important functions. They nourish the developing germ cells. They also provide a barrier (to be described later) between tissue fluid and germ cells in the later stages of formation, and they are involved in the production of a highly specialized tubular fluid. Being phagocytic, they dispose of degenerating germ cells and bits and pieces left over during their development (residual bodies). As we shall see, they play an essential role in the process by which spermatozoa are formed.

During this period of active growth, the seminiferous tubules develop a lumen and the interstitial cells become distinguishable again in the stroma of the testes. A section of testis showing seminiferous tubules in which spermatogenesis is already proceeding, and also distinct groups of interstitial cells in the stroma, is illustrated in Figure 27-3.

SPERMATOGENESIS

Terminology. The term *spermatogenesis* refers to the entire process by which spermatogonial stem cells give rise to spermatozoa. The process includes all the stages that occur in a seminiferous tubule as spermatogonia, which lie against the basement membrane of the tubule, give rise to spermatozoa that eventually become free in the lumen of the tubules.

Seminiferous Tubules. The tubules in a section vary in appearance. Their walls are relatively thick because they contain numerous cells in all stages of forming spermatozoa. In a section in which many seminiferous tubules are cut in cross section, the number of cells (as judged by their nuclei) in their walls varies somewhat (Fig. 27-3), which suggests that the process of differentiation leading to formation of spermatozoa is more advanced in some sites than in others. Indeed, the final stage of spermatogenesis (indicated by the presence of spermatozoa in the innermost layer) will be seen only in some of the tubules in a section. So even a casual glance at a section suggests the process of spermatogenesis is at different stages in different sites along seminiferous tubules. The stages will be described in detail shortly.

The Basic Events in Spermatogenesis. The changes that occur in the cells of the walls of the tubules can be thought of as occurring in two broad compartments, a *basal* one next to the limiting membrane of the tubule, and an *adluminal* one toward the lumen (Fawcett).

First, in the basal compartment a spermatogonium undergoes a number of mitotic divisions. Some of each generation of spermatogonia thus produced begin to differentiate into what are termed *spermatocytes.* The others remain as *stem cells.* Soon after their differentiation into spermatocytes begins, the daughter cells become pushed away from the basement membrane and enter the adluminal compartment, where they become cells known as *primary spermatocytes.* (The morphology of the cells involved here will be described shortly.) There, the primary spermatocytes undergo the first meiotic division to give rise to *secondary spermatocytes.* These almost immediately undergo the second division of meiosis to become what are termed *spermatids.* They in turn are transformed into *spermatozoa* by a process called *spermiogenesis.*

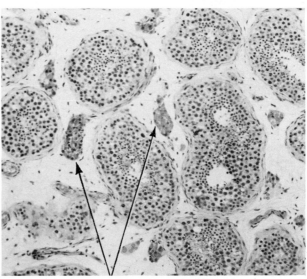

Interstitial cells

Fig. 27-3. Low-power photomicrograph of human testis. Seminiferous tubules, cut in cross and oblique section and separated from one another by a small amount of interstitial connective tissue, may be seen. Note also the groups of interstitial cells.

THE CELLS CONCERNED IN SPERMATOGENESIS

Spermatogonia

Since the cytoplasm of the various cells involved in spermatogenesis does not stain well, distinctions between cells made with the LM are based on the characteristics of their nuclei. Distinguishing particular types of closely related cells in this way can be difficult, because nuclei vary in appearance with the kind of fixative used and with different stages of the cell cycle. They also differ to some extent with species.

Nevertheless, evidence gained from LM studies of sections and by additional methods, including radioautography, indicates that spermatogonia can be classified into two main types, referred to as *type A* and *type B.*

We shall shortly describe the difference in nuclear appearance between these A and B types of spermatogonia. But first it is necessary to point out that the nuclei of type A cells are not all alike; indeed, there are two kinds of them, and these we must describe first.

The nuclei of both kinds of type A cells are characterized by much chromatin being of the extended type, so that it appears as fine granules. However, these granules are so dispersed in the kind termed the *light type of A cell* that the nucleus appears pale; this is seen in Figure 27-4, *top left,* in the left cell labeled A. Farther to the right in the same illustration is a *dark type of A cell;* it also is labeled A. The chromatin of the nucleus of dark A type cells, while of the dispersed type and not condensed enough to form clumps, is sufficiently condensed to cause

some perceptible dark staining of the nucleus. Both the light and dark type of A cells reveal nucleoli and in each instance these lie close to the nuclear membrane.

Type B cells are labeled in the two illustrations at the top of Figure 27-4. Their nuclei appear somewhat larger than those of type A cells, but of greater importance is the fact that their chromatin is not as dispersed as in type A cells; instead it is often aggregated into clumps.

The respective roles of the pale and dark type A cells have not been clarified in man, but may be deduced from what is known of the role of the very similar cells found in the monkey. The pale type A cells in this species are the renewing *stem cells;* they yield new pale type A cells and type B cells in virtually equal numbers. Accordingly, the pale type A cells take up tritiated thymidine before their division. In contrast, the dark type A cells have never been found to take up this label in the healthy adult. Clermont, who made these observations, refers to the dark cells as "reserve cells" that under normal conditions remain dormant. Reserve cells were discovered in rats, where they also remain dormant unless damage to the seminiferous epithelium induces them to divide and thus give rise to renewing stem cells (Clermont). One way of looking at this would be to regard the light type A cells as cycling cells and the dark type A cells as identical cells that do not cycle until the need arises.

Maintenance of the Stem Cell Population in the Testes. On average, half the daughter cells of dividing type A sper-

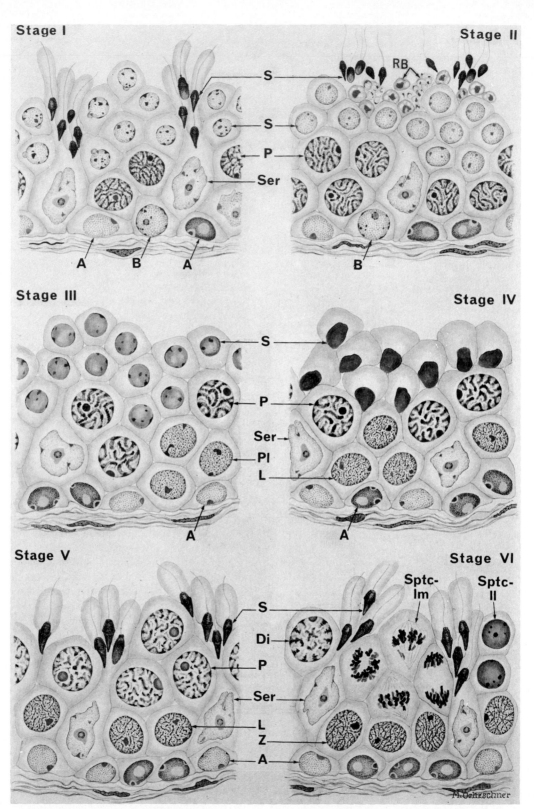

FIGURE 27-4. *(Caption on facing page)*

matogonia in man differentiate to become type B cells, thus losing their potentiality for producing more type A cells. Half persist as stem cells to maintain the stem cell population.

The type B cells undergo mitosis; their daughter cells are called *primary spermatocytes* (Pl in Fig. 27-4).

The Meiotic Divisions of Spermatocytes

The general characteristics of meiosis were described in Chapter 3 (p. 76) and illustrated in Figures 3-14 and 3-15. The account given in Chapter 3 relates specifically to meiosis in the female, but the same stages apply in the male and they achieve the same end—namely, reducing the chromosome number from diploid to *haploid* in the germ cells. To avoid unnecessary repetition we shall confine ourselves to describing the features of meiosis that can be recognized in the seminiferous tubules. Frequent reference to Figures 3-14 and 3-15 while reading the following section may be helpful.

The Prophase of the First Meiotic Division. Primary spermatocytes are most easily recognized when they enter the first meiotic division. The *prophase* of this division is relatively lengthy, but not nearly as long as that of the first meiotic division in the female. It is divided into the five stages described in Chapter 3, and for convenience the important features of these stages will be reviewed briefly here.

The first is called *leptotene*. The d-chromosomes (see p. 46 for the meaning of this term) that become visible are thin and delicate (Fig. 27-4, L). It should be mentioned here that the last duplication of DNA occurring during development of a spermatozoon takes place in the S phase of a primary spermatocyte *before it enters the prophase* of the first meiotic division (Fig. 3-15). The primary spermatocyte, before it begins prophase, is referred to as a *preleptotene spermatocyte* (Fig. 27-4, Pl). DNA duplication is *not* required as a preliminary to the second meiotic division because in this division the DNA of the cells that divide is *halved* in forming haploid cells.

In the second stage of the prophase, *zygotene* (Z in Fig. 27-4), each d-chromosome seeks out its mate to lie beside it (*synapsis*) and form a *bivalent*.

In the third stage, *pachytene*, the d-chromosomes become increasingly condensed and so are thicker and shorter (P in Fig. 27-4).

Before describing the next stage of the prophase of the first meiotic division as seen with the LM, we shall mention a finding made with the EM in connection with synapsis.

Synaptonemal Complexes in Primary Spermatocytes. The EM disclosed that when synapsis occurs in primary spermatocytes and primary oocytes, paired electron-dense and parallel ribbons about 60 nm. wide, separated by a clear space roughly 100 nm. across, extend along the interface between the homologues of each bivalent (Figs. 27-5 and 27-6). These ribbon-like structures are called *synaptonemal complexes* (Gr. *synapsis*, a coming together; *nema*, thread) because they seem to serve in holding the homologous d-chromosome together in a structural complex. Further details such as a narrow medial electron-dense line and fine filaments traversing the space have also been described in the synaptonemal complex. Several are shown in the nucleus at the pachytene stage in Figures 27-5 and 27-6. It is to be noted that the synaptonemal complexes are attached at both ends to the nuclear envelope (Fig. 27-6, A and D).

In man there are 23 synaptonemal complexes at this stage. The X and Y chromosomes of the male become paired over only a very short distance; they remain almost entirely single in what is termed the *XY body* (*sex vesicle*) labeled Sv in Figures 27-5 and 27-6. They, too, are attached at both ends to the nuclear envelope.

Subsequent Stages in Meiosis. In the fourth stage, *diplotene,* the two d-chromosomes of each bivalent separate sufficiently to be visible (Fig. 27-4, Di) and chiasmata can be seen.

In the fifth and final stage of the prophase of the first meiotic division, *diakinesis,* the d-chromosomes are thicker still.

The cell next enters the metaphase of the first meiotic division with the d-chromosomes becoming arranged in the equatorial plane. In the anaphase which follows, the two d-chromosomes in each bivalent separate and move toward the poles of the cell, one chromosome toward each pole (Figs. 27-4, Sptc-Im, and 3-15A). Throughout the first meiotic division the two s-chromosomes of each d-chromosome remained joined at their centromeres so that they do not separate as occurs in mitosis. Instead, in the anaphase of the first meiotic division the two d-chromosomes of each bivalent merely separate from each other (Fig. 3-15A). The result, of course, is that each of

---

Fig. 27-4. (On facing page.) Drawings illustrating the various steps of differentiation seen in seminiferous tubules. The illustrations are arranged to demonstrate the six typical cellular associations found repeatedly in human seminiferous tubules. Some of the terms used in this caption are explained in the text. The six associations (*stages*) are labeled I to VI, respectively. Ser, nucleus of Sertoli cell; A, type A spermatogonia; B, type B spermatogonia; Pl, preleptotene primary spermatocytes; L, leptotene primary spermatocytes; Z, zygotene primary spermatocytes; P, pachytene primary spermatocytes; Di, diplotene primary spermatocytes; Sptc-Im, primary spermatocytes in division; Sptc-II, secondary spermatocytes in interphase; S, spermatids at various steps of spermiogenesis; RB, residual bodies. For further details, *see* caption to Figure 27-7. (Clermont, Y.: Am. J. Anat., *112:*35, 1963)

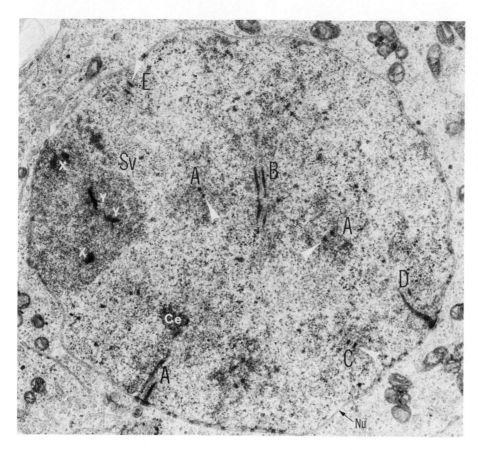

Fig. 27-5. Electron micrograph of the nucleus of a rat spermatocyte at the pachytene stage of meiotic prophase. Note the synaptonemal complexes A, B, C, D, and E, which appear in their entirety if every section of the nucleus is examined (*see* Fig. 27-6). The complexes are attached to the nuclear envelope (Nu). Inside the sex vesicle (Sv) are the cores of the X and Y chromosomes. (Courtesy of A. Hugenholtz)

the two daughter cells forming in the telophase has only 23 instead of 46 chromosomes – the haploid instead of the diploid number.

The daughter cells formed by the first meiotic division are called *secondary spermatocytes* (Fig. 27-4, Sptc-II). They are smaller than primary spermatocytes and are situated in the middle and more superficial layers of the tubules (*bottom right* drawing in Fig. 27-4). Almost immediately, these cells undergo the second division of meiosis and for this reason secondary spermatocytes are seldom seen in interphase. Apart from the fact that secondary spermatocytes possess only the haploid number of chromosomes, the second meiotic division is similar to an ordinary mitosis, involving separation of the two s-chromosomes of each d-chromosome in the anaphase, as shown in Figure 3-15B.

Spermatids

The daughter cells of secondary spermatocytes are called *spermatids* (S in Fig. 27-4). These at first are rather small cells, with a spherical nucleus (S in Fig. 27-4, stages III and IV). But they soon become elongated and their

nucleus takes up a position at the proximal end of the cell (the end nearer the wall of the tubule). The proximal end of the nucleus becomes pointed (S in Fig. 27-4, stages V and VI). Each spermatid develops a flagellum from one of the two centrioles located near the rounded end of its nucleus. Further details of spermatid development will be given when we describe EM studies of spermatogenesis, but first we shall discuss the cycle of seminiferous epithelium and describe the stages of the cycle that can be identified.

The Cycle of the Seminiferous Epithelium

The Term Cycle. In order to understand the meaning of this term, we should comment generally on cyclic changes in tissues. For example, in the previous chapter we dealt with two different tissues that undergo cycles. First, the endometrium of a woman's uterus shows dramatic changes, usually over a 28-day time period, referred to as a menstrual cycle. Second, in animals such as mice and rats, the vaginal epithelium shows a cycle that is repeated approximately every 4 days.

Differences Between Cycles and Cell Turnover. In order to

avoid confusion it should be explained that the time taken by a *cycle* in a membrane may or may not be the same as the *turnover* time of the membrane. The length of the menstrual cycle is about the same as the turnover time of the endometrium because almost the whole thickness of the endometrium is lost at menstruation; so in each menstrual cycle almost all of the endometrium must be regenerated from the little that remains. But the length of a cycle of the seminiferous epithelium is not the same as its turnover time, because only a small fraction of the cells of the membrane are lost in each cycle—those that have become mature spermatozoa.

What then *is* a cycle of the seminiferous epithelium? It could be most easily explained if one could continuously observe the same site in a living seminiferous tubule hour by hour and day by day. If this were possible, the cellular composition of the site would soon be seen to differ, and, after passing through a series of changes, the site would eventually regain the cellular constitution observed when the study began. The epithelium at this site would thus have passed through a *cycle,* and the time taken for this to happen would be the length of a cycle of the seminiferous epithelium. However, since it is impracticable to observe the same site in a living seminiferous tubule over a period of days, knowledge of the cycle had to be obtained by more indirect means, as will now be described.

Cell Associations in the Seminiferous Epithelium and How They Change During a Cycle. This subject was at first intensively investigated in laboratory animals. In many of these it was found that cross sections of seminiferous tubules taken at different sites along the same tubule presented different appearances. For one thing, spermatozoa in their final form were seen only in some sites and not in others, which indicated that spermatogenesis is more advanced at some sites along a tubule than elsewhere. Furthermore, the numbers and state of development of the deeper cells of the wall of the tubule also differed in various sites. Indeed, Leblond and Clermont initially described 14 characteristics and different appearances (*cell associations*) that could be seen in cross sections of the seminiferous tubules of the rat. Other small animals also demonstrate the same phenomenon. These investigators concluded that the various cell associations seen at different sites along a tubule reflected different *stages* in the process by which spermatozoa were developed.

With this knowledge it is easy to understand that a particular cell association seen at a given site at a given time would change, and that sooner or later the same cell association would reappear at this site. The time taken for it to reappear would, of course, be the time taken for a cycle of the seminiferous epithelium.

When the seminiferous epithelium of the tubules of man were studied, however, the cell associations did not

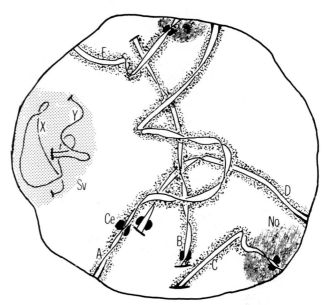

Fig. 27-6. Drawing of an EM reconstruction of the entire nucleus shown in Figure 27-5. There are 20 synaptonemal complexes in the nucleus but only the five visible in Figure 27-5 are shown. These are identified as A, B, C, D, and E. Each complex represents a set of paired d-chromosomes, has a centromere (Ce), and is attached with both ends to the nuclear envelope. A is the longest pair of chromosomes and C and E are nucleolus-bearing (No) chromosomes. The sex vesicle Sv contains the cores of the X- and Y-chromosomes, which have a small paired region. (Courtesy of P. Moens)

seem as clear-cut. The reason for this is that in man the cell associations are not distributed at different sites along the lengths of tubules as they are in laboratory animals; instead, they are present with other associations *in the same cross section* of a tubule, with each association occupying a fairly well-defined sector of the cross section. Furthermore, it was found that only six associations are seen in the tubules of man. These are labeled I to VI in Figure 27-4, which shows the various kinds of cells seen in each. Distinction between different cells was made almost entirely by their nuclear morphology and by determining the stage of meiosis they were in. The six stages are also illustrated in Figure 27-7, in which different stages seen around the circumference of a tubule are marked off from one another. Figure 27-7 contains a description of the cell types seen in each stage. (For microscopic details of the cells in each stage, *see* Fig. 27-4.) Both figures are from the work of Clermont, whose papers should be read for further information.

The fact that spermatogenesis comprises well-defined stages should not suggest that the cell association seen at one stage is instantaneously transformed into that seen in

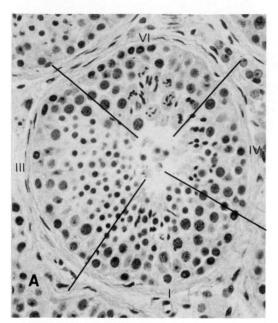

Fig. 27-7. Low-power photomicrographs of human seminiferous tubules cut transversely (*A*) and longitudinally (*B*) to show the distribution of cell associations (*stages*) of the cycle of the seminiferous epithelium. The six stages illustrated in Figure 27-4 can be identified. The details are as follows.

Stage I (seem in *A*): spermatogonia, pachtytene spermatocytes, and two generations of spermatids (one with spherical nuclei, and one with elongated condensed nuclei).

Stage II (seen in *B*): spermatogonia, pachytene spermatocytes, young spermatids with spherical nuclei, and maturing spermatids discarding their residual cytoplasm.

Stage III (*A* and *B*): spermatogonia, preleptotene spermatocytes, pachytene spermatocytes, and spermatids with spherical nuclei.

Stage IV (*A* and *B*): spermatogonia, leptotene and pachytene spermatocytes, and spermatids with slightly elongated nuclei.

Stage V (*B*): spermatogonia, leptotene or zygotene spermatocytes, pachytene spermatocytes, and spermatids with elongated nuclei.

Stage VI (*A*): spermatogonia, early pachytene spermatocytes, maturation divisions of primary spermatocytes, and spermatids with elongated nuclei. Note that the order of stages of the cycle seen around the lumen is variable (not consecutive). (Clermont, Y.: Am. J. Anat., *112*:35, 1963)

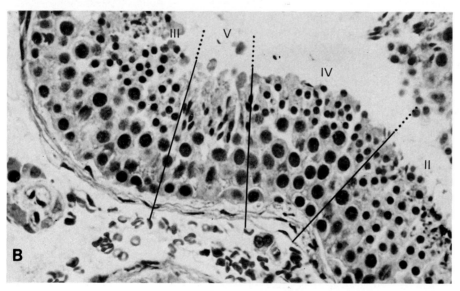

the next, but that changes occur in the seminiferous epithelium in a rhythmic manner.

Determining the Total Duration of Spermatogenesis and the Length of a Cycle. Only a general concept of how this is done need be given here. In the procedures devised by Clermont and Leblond to determine (*1*) the duration of spermatogenesis or (*2*) the length of a cycle of the epithelium, advantage is taken of the fact that the only cells that duplicate their DNA in the seminiferous epithelium are spermatogonia and preleptotene primary spermatocytes. This means that if labeled thymidine is made available to

the seminiferous epithelium for a very brief period, the only cells that will take up label will be those spermatogonia and preleptotene primary spermatocytes that are at that time in the S phase of the cell cycle. So if label is seen in any cell of the sperm cell series following administration of labeled thymidine, it will have been incorporated at the spermatogonium or preleptotene primary spermatocyte stage.

Determing the total *duration of spermatogenesis* is in some ways easier than determining the length of the cycle. For the former, the procedure would be to deter-

Fig. 27-8. Electron micrograph of a preleptotene spermatocyte with four of its five bridges in the plane of section. The bridges are marked by arrows. Nu, nucleus; S, Sertoli cells. (Courtesy of A. Hugenholtz)

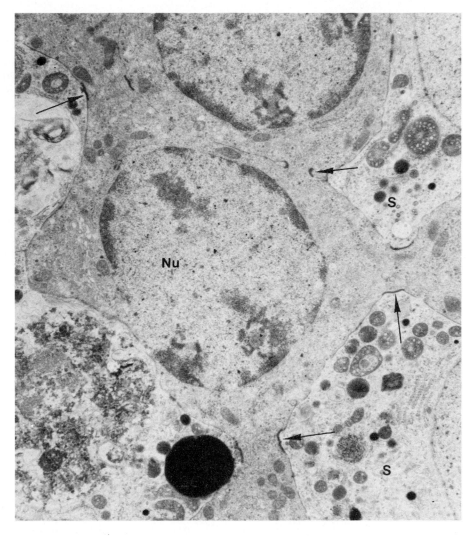

Fig. 27-8. Electron micrograph of a preleptotene spermatocyte with four of its five bridges in the plane of section. The bridges are marked by arrows. Nu, nucleus; S, Sertoli cells. (Courtesy of A. Hugenholtz)

mine the time after labeling when label is seen in mature (testicular) spermatozoa. However, the first labeled spermatozoa seen would have originated from labeled preleptotene primary spermatocytes, because it takes longer for a labeled spermatogonium to give rise to a labeled spermatozoon than it does for a preleptotene primary spermatocyte to do so. This must be taken into account in calculating the *duration* of spermatogenesis, which in man has been estimated to be approximately 64 days.

Determining the *length of a cycle* of the seminiferous epithelium by radioautography is more complex. In general, it depends on finding, immediately after labeling, some preleptotene primary spermatocytes that have not only become labeled but are also in a recognizable cell association. In radioautographs prepared from successive specimens, it could then be reasoned that when labeled cells reappear in an identical cell association, one com-

plete *cycle* will have occurred. However, accurate measurement of the length of a cycle must take into account the fact that the stages of the cycle are not all of equal duration, so that these also have to be determined. Otherwise, it might happen that one labeled cell could be commencing a particular stage when it is seen, while another might be in a late part of that stage. As matters turned out, the stage (Stage III) when preleptotene spermatocytes are in S phase is of short duration.

By means of radioautographic studies it was established that the process of spermatogenesis extends over four cycles, with the length of the cycles being 16 days (plus or minus 1 day). Thus, to progress from the spermatogonium to the spermatozoon stage, it takes 4 × 16 = 64 days, which is the duration of spermatogenesis. For more information, *see* references under Structures and Arrangements in Spermatogenesis.

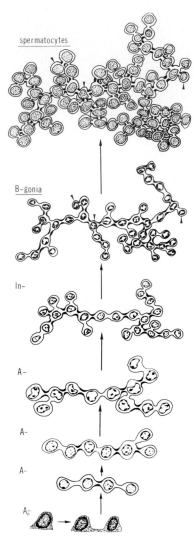

spermatocytes

B-gonia

In-

A-

A-

A-

A₀

Fig. 27-9. Diagram illustrating the syncytial development of spermatocytes. The cells remain connected by cytoplasmic bridges following consecutive mitoses. The early division gives rise to further type A spermatogonia (A), followed by intermediate (In) and type B spermatogonia. Later division produces spermatocytes that then undergo the two meiotic divisions. Although division is synchronous for the cells of the syncytium as a whole, a few (marked by arrowheads) fail to divide. Bridges persisting from previous divisions are heavily outlined. (Courtesy of P. Moens)

EM Studies on the Cells Involved in Spermatogenesis

So far in this account of spermatogenesis as seen with the LM, we have described the various cells involved as is they were separate entities, which of course they seemed to be when examined with the LM. Studies with the EM, however, have shown that they are not separate

but connected to one another by *intercellular bridges,* and this may well explain why they behave as groups instead of as individual cells. The cytoplasmic bridges are the result of the daughter cells produced by each successive division not becoming entirely separated from one another. In the usual kind of telophase, a cleavage furrow appears in the cytoplasm between the daughter nuclei and deepens until the cytoplasm is completely pinched off so as to separate the two daughter cells. In spermatogenesis, however, the pinching-off process is permanently arrested at about the stage illustrated in Figure 2-19, and, as a result, the dividing cells remain connected to one another. Subsequent divisions of connected cells result in all the cells formed being connected to each other. Figure 27-8 shows five cells connected by bridges. The several generations of cells all connected together by cytoplasmic bridges could be regarded as a type of *syncytium* (meaning a multinucleated mass of cytoplasm). However, unlike syncytia that form by adjacent cells fusing together, this kind of syncytium develops from a single cell and hence is a *clone* of unique type.

Because dividing cells remain connected by bridges, it is possible to study the development of spermatogenic cells in relation to the size of groups, as reported in the rat by Moens and Go. The beginning of the process is obscure; it is assumed that single type A spermatogonia cells at some stage (A_0 in Fig. 27-9) divide to produce a doublet (just to the right of A_0 in Fig. 27-9) whose cells further divide to yield chains of type A spermatogonia. In the diagram (Fig. 27-9) bridges already present in a previous chain are drawn with heavy lines, while new bridges are drawn with thinner lines. As spermatogonia become spermatocytes, the syncytium moves away from the basal into the adluminal compartment. The first and second meiotic divisions follow, and it then appears that the syncytium breaks up into smaller segments as some or all of the meiosis I bridges fail to persist.

Divisions in a given syncytium are synchronous, but a few cells do not divide at all. The spermatocyte syncytium illustrated at the top of Figure 27-9 was observed by Moens; the other syncytia in the diagram were deduced from it. The pattern is such that some of the cells—for example, the ones marked by arrowheads in the two upper pictures—could not have divided.

Spermiogenesis—Transformation of Spermatids into Spermatozoa. Spermatids are enveloped by the cytoplasm of Sertoli cells, and, near the lumen of the tubule (as will be described in connection with Sertoli cells), they undergo metamorphosis into spermatozoa. In this process they eventually become detached from one another to become free cells.

A newly formed *spermatid* (Fig. 27-10, a) has a central spherical nucleus, a well-delimited Golgi zone close to the nucleus, numerous granular mitochondria, and a pair

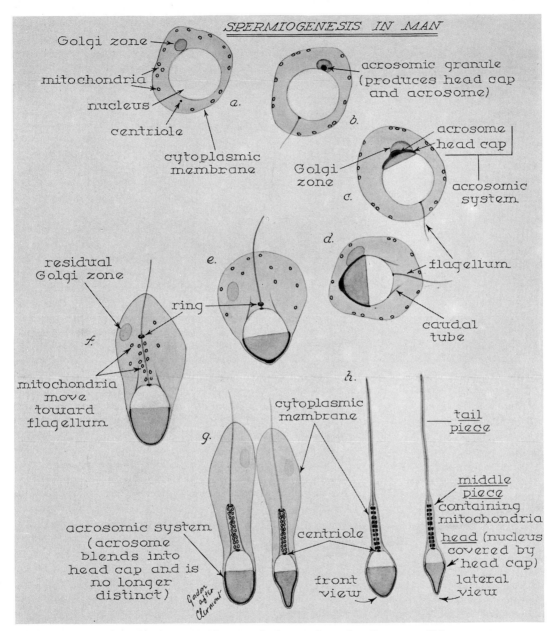

Fig. 27-10. Drawings showing successive steps in the transformation of a spermatid into a spermatozoon. (After Clermont, Y., and Leblond, C. P.: Am. J. Anat., *96:*229, 1955)

of small centrioles. The formation of a spermatozoon involves elaborate changes in all these structures. The first sign of metamorphosis is seen within the Golgi zone; it is indicated by the formation of a dense granule at the surface of the nuclear envelope (Fig. 27-10, b). It is called the *acrosomic granule* because it is formed on the extremity (Gr. *akron,* extremity) of the nucleus. Its deriva-

tives are PAS-positive, indicating the presence of carbohydrates. The growing acrosomic granule differentiates into two parts: (*1*) the *acrosome,* which is a small hemisphere at the anterior end of the nucleus (Fig. 27-10, c, and (*2*) the *head cap,* which is a membrane-like structure growing around the acrosome on the surface of the nuclear membrane (Fig. 27-10), c and d, and Fig. 27-11).

Golgi

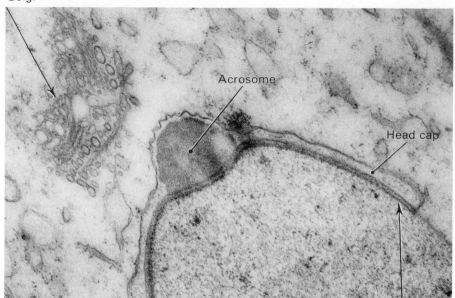

Acrosome

Head cap

Nuclear envelope

Fig. 27-11. Electron micrograph (×20,000) of the head of a human spermatid (corresponding to Fig. 27-10c), showing its nucleus, Golgi zone, and acrosomic system. The acrosomic granule lies inside a vesicular structure, the head cap, on the anterior end of the nuclear membrane. (Fawcett, D. W., and Burgos, M. H.: Ciba Foundation Colloquia on Ageing. vol. 2, p. 86. London, Churchill, 1956)

The head cap eventually covers approximately half the nuclear surface. Once the acrosome and head cap (the acrosomic system) are well developed, the Golgi zone (Fig. 27-11) becomes detached from the head cap and constitutes a "residual Golgi zone" (Fig. 27-10, d and e). As the acrosomic system develops, one centriole (labeled in Fig. 27-10, a) becomes attached to the nuclear membrane in an area opposite the acrosome (Fig. 27-10, b and c) and gives rise to the propulsive organelle of the future spermatozoon, the *flagellum* (labeled in Fig. 27-10, c and d). An additional structure appears and surrounds this flagellum; this is the so-called *caudal tube,* which is made of cytoplasmic filaments attached to the nuclear membrane (Fig. 27-10, d).

The acrosome and the head cap orient themselves toward the basement membrane of the seminiferous tubule. This is accompanied by a displacement of the nucleus within the cytoplasm of the spermatid toward the cell membrane (Fig. 27-10, e). The nucleus then becomes progressively condensed and assumes a flattened elongate shape (Fig. 27-12). Its anterior end is relatively pointed when seen in profile but rounded in full face (Fig. 27-10, g and h). At the surface of the nucleus, the acrosome blends into the head cap from which it becomes indistinguishable (Fig. 27-10). Meanwhile, a small ring appears around the flagellum close to the centriole. This ring, once formed, slides along the flagellum for some distance (Fig. 27-10, e and f). The mitochondria now start moving toward the part of the flagellum between the cen-

triole and the ring (Fig. 27-10, f, g and h). They line up circumferentially along the periphery of the flagellum, close to one another, forming a helical, collar-like *mitochondrial sheath* that characterizes the *middle piece* of the future spermatozoon. As a spermatid completes its development, the cytoplasmic surplus not utilized in forming the spermatozoon is cast off as a *residual body* and this is phagocytosed by a Sertoli cell. All that remains of the cytoplasm is a very thin layer covering the nucleus, middle piece, and tailpiece (except at its extremity).

The basic structure of the flagellum (middle piece and tailpiece) is like that of a cilium in that the number and arrangement of its *microtubules* are the same (Fig. 5-53). However, external to the ring of nine doublet microtubules there are in addition several *coarse fibers* (*outer dense fibers*)— nine in the proximal part of the flagellum — and a *fibrous sheath,* and because of this the flagellum of a spermatozoon has a different structure from an ordinary cilium. The net result of transformation (metamorphosis) of a spermatid is that a spermatozoon, though much smaller than a spermatid, retains the nuclear component in the *head,* part of the Golgi apparatus in the *acrosomic system,* mitochondria in the *middle piece,* and the *centrioles;* the latter are concerned in spindle formation when cell division occurs in the fertilized ovum. The spermatozoon thus contributes cytoplasmic as well as nuclear components to the fertilized ovum. The acrosomic system contains several lysosomal enzymes, hyaluronidase, and a trypsin-like enzyme; these are believed to play a role in penetration of the spermatozoon through the corona radiata and zona pellucida of the ovum. When fully formed, spermatozoa leave the care and nurture of the Sertoli cells and enter the lumen of a seminiferous tubule. Although their flagellum beats, these spermatozoa are probably not very motile and they are moved passively along the system of tubules until they reach the tail end of the epididymis. Then they become actively motile and by lashing their tails can move 2 or 3 mm. a minute. In the past it was thought that this enabled them to swim up the female reproductive tract when introduced into the vagina. But it now seems that their movement through the female tract depends on other factors as well as sperm motility. Segmental and peristaltic contractions in the walls of the oviducts, and perhaps ciliary action in some species, contribute in no small measure to the success of this event.

Spermatozoa were first seen under a microscope by Ham, a young medical doctor who worked with Leeuwenhoek in the 17th century (*see* Muys; Halbertsma) and whom Leeuwenhoek described as a very modest man.

Spermiogenesis as described above occurs in a microenvironment different from that in which spermatogonia proliferate and differentiate into primary spermatocytes. This matter is discussed below.

The Walls of Seminiferous Tubules

Myoid Cells. The cellular walls of seminiferous tubules are surrounded by a basement membrane of the usual type. But immediately outside the basement membrane there is a wrapping of loose connective tissue that contains a single continuous layer of *myoid cells* (Gr. *mys,* muscle; *eidos,* form). In rats and mice these cells are well developed and contractile, so the seminiferous tubules undergo gentle rhythmic contractions. Myoid cells are squamous in shape and in humans bear little (if any) resemblance to smooth muscle cells, which they were at first thought to resemble. They contain actin microfilaments.

Sertoli Cells. The irregularly shaped and typically indented nucleus of Sertoli cells is readily recognized with the LM. With the EM it has been established that the basophilic structures seen on either side of its prominent nucleolus are distinct rounded masses of nucleolus-associated chromatin; these can give the impression that the nucleolus is a triple structure.

The cytoplasm contains the usual organelles and more sER than rER. The Golgi stacks are extensive and form an elaborate interconnected network. Concentric arrangements of smooth-surfaced membrane have been described around some of the lipid droplets that are typically seen in the cytoplasm. Filaments and lipofuscin pigment also are common. Lysosomes, needed for degrading

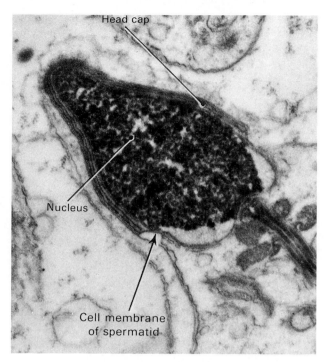

Fig. 27-12. Electron micrograph (×25,000) of the head of a human spermatid at a stage of development corresponding to Figure 27-10g. The nucleus is now more electron-dense and is pressed against the cell membrane. Note that it is assuming an elongate shape. The head cap is still visible, but the acrosome can no longer be identified. A well-developed flagellum extends from the nucleus, at *lower right.* (Fawcett, D. W., and Burgos, M. H.: Ciba Foundation Colloquia on Ageing. vol. 2, p. 86. London, Churchill, 1956)

phagocytosed material such as residual bodies of spermatozoa, and, in human Sertoli cells, crystalloid inclusion bodies are also present.

The Blood-Testis Barrier. Tissue fluid and the substances it contains penetrate the basement membrane to bathe the basal layer of the cellular wall of the tubule. The tissue fluid is, of course, derived from capillaries in the interstitial tissue between tubules.

However, there is not the same free access of tissue fluid (and hence the substances dissolved in it) to cells in subsequent stages of spermatogenesis (leptotene spermatocytes, spermatids, and spermatozoa) which are not in contact with the basement membrane that surrounds the tubules. The reason for this is that the spermatogonia that lie between Sertoli cells along the basement membrane become covered by the much taller Sertoli cells. The cell membranes of adjacent Sertoli cells in this region are joined by *tight (zonula occludens) junctions.* This has important effects. First, the tight junctions separate the *basal compartment* (containing spermatogonia) from the *adluminal compartment* (with dividing spermatocytes and also spermatids). As a result the spermatogonia that abut on the basement membrane have an excellent supply of nutrients, but the cells nearer the lumen of the tubule have no direct access to tissue fluid because the tight junctions prevent tissue fluid from infiltrating between contiguous Sertoli cells to reach them. So dividing spermatocytes, and also spermatids and spermatozoa, must obtain their nutrients indirectly via the cytoplasm of Sertoli cells. The fluid in the lumen of seminiferous tubules is similarly derived from Sertoli cells. Thus, the *tight junctions between Sertoli cells* constitute a *blood-testis barrier* that effectively divides off the microenvironment of the inner part of the wall of the seminiferous tubule from that of its outer part.

There is therefore a very good reason that studies made long ago with the LM stressed a close association between Sertoli cells and the differentiating progeny of spermatogonia, with Sertoli cells being referred to as *nurse cells*. The EM disclosed that these progeny cells (or parts of them) retain their own cell membrane and lie in membrane-lined declivities in the cytoplasm of Sertoli cells. Spermatids, for example, while seeming to lie in Sertoli cell cytoplasm, reveal two cell membranes around them, one belonging to the spermatid, the other to the Sertoli cell. There is an intercellular space between the two membranes.

Functional Considerations of the Blood-Testis Barrier. Maintenance of the blood-testis barrier is complicated by the fact that as successive waves of differentiating germ cells progress from the basal to the adluminal compartment, they have to pass through the zone of tight junctions. This would entail the junctions either opening up and then closing again, or else disappearing and then reforming, in order to maintain the permeability barrier.

The main purposes of having an uninterrupted blood-testis barrier would seem to be as follows. (*1*) It could help maintain the right kind of fluid environment for sperm cell differentiation in terms of nutrients and hormones, and these would not necessarily be the same as those found elsewhere in the body. (*2*) This barrier would isolate and hence serve to protect the differentiating sperm cells from any damaging substances that might enter the bloodstream. (*3*) Keeping the differentiating sperm cells confined to their own special adluminal compartment behind a permeability barrier would prevent their antigens gaining access to the body as a whole. This, of course, would reduce the danger of an autoimmune response developing to any new antigens that might be expressed when spermatozoa begin to be produced after puberty (a male would not be tolerant of these antigens because no spermatozoa are made before this time). (*4*) In the event that antigens of cells of the sperm cell series did enter the body (and this does sometimes happen, for

example, after vasectomy), an effective barrier would serve to protect differentiating sperm cells from any antibodies that might be made against their antigens.

Effects of FSH on Sertoli Cells. As noted at the beginning of this chapter, it was at first thought that since FSH controlled development of ovarian follicles containing the germ cells of females, in the male it would control formation of germ cells in the seminiferous tubules. But it was soon found that spermatogenesis could occur in the absence of FSH if testosterone was available in an animal. Since the more recent discovery of hormone receptors and cyclic AMP, it was found that Sertoli cells bind FSH and this causes the formation of cyclic AMP, which in turn acts in the Sertoli cells to cause formation of a special protein that can bind androgen (androgen-binding protein, ABP). It is this protein that is responsible for Sertoli cells being able to maintain the *high concentration of androgen* required for spermatogenesis. Accordingly FSH acts in an *indirect* way in furthering spermatogenesis.

Negative Feedback Mechanisms in the Male. Because of the feedback mechanisms in the female for controlling the secretion of both FSH and LH, it seemed logical to assume there would be similar feedbacks in the male, and indeed it was established that LH secretion by the anterior pituitary was elevated by lowered blood levels of testosterone and was depressed by high levels. It is now believed that testosterone controls LH secretion by both (*1*) directly acting on the anterior pituitary and (*2*) acting indirectly via the hypothalamus.

The situation with regard to FSH has been more difficult to elucidate. Although there was no established hormone produced in the testes that was known to regulate FSH secretion, evidence obtained from time to time indicated that something could be extracted from the testes that reduced FSH secretion. Interest in the possibility of there being some agent that had this effect was stimulated by the finding that FSH enhanced the uptake of testosterone by Sertoli cells, because it raised the possibility of such an agent having contraceptive effects if administered to males. Such an agent would presumably act by reducing the uptake of testosterone by Sertoli cells, and therefore it might through this action cause the testosterone concentration in Sertoli cells, and hence in the seminiferous tubules, to fall below the minimum level required for spermatogenesis. Moreover, such an agent would not diminish testosterone secretion in the male and hence not diminish masculine characteristics, drives, and behavior, for it would merely have a local effect in connection with the production of spermatozoa. Relatively recently investigators have recovered an agent from testis preparations with the property of diminishing FSH secretion. This agent seems to be formed in the testes and has been termed *inhibin*. It seems probable that it is a polypeptide, but its precise source, actions, and effectiveness in diminishing the production of spermatozoa remain to be established.

OTHER FACTORS AFFECTING SPERMATOGENESIS

It has already been pointed out that spermatogenesis does not proceed normally unless the testes are maintained at a temperature somewhat *lower than that of the body* as a whole.

It will be recalled that the capacity of the ovaries to produce mature germ cells ends more or less suddenly, usually when a woman is between the ages of 45 and 50. However, in the male, with increasing age there is usually only a slow decline in the ability of seminiferous tubules to produce mature germ cells, and there are many authentic cases of men having become fathers at a very advanced age.

Vitamins A and E in particular are required in adequate amounts in the diet if spermatogenesis is to be normal.

FACTORS AFFECTING SPERM MORPHOLOGY

Normal spermatozoa are morphologically a very homogeneous population, each with a well-defined species-dependent structure. The human spermatozoon head, for example, is shaped like a flattened ellipsoid, whereas a mouse sperm head has a hooked shape. Packaged into the head is the haploid chromosome complement of the species. The head is known to be very rigid, of high density, and resistant to a large number of physical and chemical agents—an ideal package for such important contents.

In an ejaculate from a healthy donor, most spermatozoa are of normal morphology. A not insignificant proportion, however, have a noticeably abnormal morphology—about 20 to 25 per cent of spermatozoa in man; in mice, from 1 to 16 per cent, depending upon the strain. In the same donor, however, whether he be man or mouse, the percentage of ejaculate spermatozoa with abnormal shape remains constant over long periods. For causes of temporary variations from the usual pattern, *see* MacLeod.

Certain factors are known to increase the percentage of abnormally shaped sperm that will develop in mice; among these are ionizing radiation, heat, and chemical agents. The list of chemicals includes certain pesticides, certain antitumor drugs and other pharmaceutical agents, as well as known carcinogens and mutagens. Moreover, in man, x-rays, severe allergic reactions, and certain antispermatogenic agents have been reported to show similar effects. Elevated levels of sperm abnormalities have been related to lower fertility in man.

SPERM COUNTS

There are usually more than 100 million spermatozoa per milliliter of semen in fertile men, with 3 to 4 ml. of semen being delivered in an ejaculation. Although there is much variation in individual cases, men whose semen contains only 50 million or so spermatozoa are generally not very fertile and those with 20 million or less per milliliter are usually sterile. Although such an enormous number of spermatozoa is produced by the testes, only 1 spermatozoon actually fertilizes an ovum.

THE ROLE OF INTERSTITIAL CELLS

In discussing this it is necessary to appreciate that there is a profound difference between *fertility* and *potency* in the male. A *fertile* male may be defined as one who can produce at ejaculation, at least on some occasions, enough healthy spermatozoa suspended in a sufficiently normal fluid vehicle to bring about fertilization. A *sterile* male cannot accomplish this. *Potency* refers to another matter—the ability of a male to engage in intercourse. This depends fundamentally on an erection of the penis. A potent but sterile male may be able to ejaculate during intercourse, but the semen expressed will not contain a sufficient number of healthy spermatozoa to bring about fertilization.

A male may be sterilized either by removing the testes or by tying off and cutting the ducti (vasa) deferentes (*vasectomy*). The latter operation prevents egress of spermatozoa from the testes, but the interstitial cells continue to produce androgen, which leaves the testes by way of the bloodstream. The testes of the *cryptorchid* produce androgen, though in less than normal amounts, and usually do not produce spermatozoa. It is possible for a male to be potent but sterile, and it is also possible for an otherwise fertile male to be impotent. In such males, impotency is usually due to emotional factors that interfere with the functioning of the autonomic nervous system in such a way that the blood flow into the cavernous tissue of the penis is insufficient to cause an erection.

The Microscopic Structure of Interstitial (Leydig) Cells

It was mentioned earlier that in fetal life interstial cells develop from mesenchymal cells of the stroma between the developing seminiferous tubules, and that they are much more prominent in the fetal testis (from the 4th month on) than between birth and puberty. In the sexually mature male, interstitial cells are distributed sometimes singly but commonly in clumps in the stroma between the tubules, usually in the angular crevices between the tubules (Fig. 27-3). They are large cells,

Capillaries

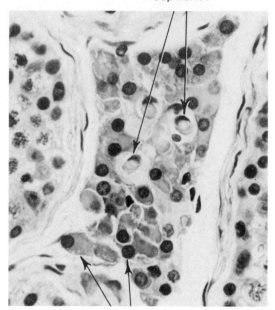

Interstitial cells

Fig. 27-13. High-power photomicrograph of interstitial cells in human testis. Several blood capillaries may be seen in cross section in an island of interstitial cells. This group of cells lies in connective tissue in between the seminiferous tubules. (Courtesy of Y. Clermont)

measuring around 20 μm. in diameter (Fig. 27-13). Their spherical to oval nucleus is pale-staining and contains one or more nucleoli. Some interstitial cells are binucleated. In H and E sections the peripheral cytoplasm may appear vacuolated because lipid droplets have been dissolved in preparation of the section. The cytoplasm immediately surrounding the nucleus may appear granular. Some interstitial cells contain a pigment, probably lipofuscin.

The interstitial cells constitute an unusual type of endocrine gland. They do not develop from an epithelial surface, as do most glands, but from a *mesenchymal* stroma. Since they are scattered about in the stroma, which is abundantly provided with capillaries, they have ready access to the vascular system (Fig. 27-13). All in all, they constitute a very diffuse type of endocrine gland.

Fine Structure. The organelle that characterizes the cytoplasm of interstitial cells is sER which, as already noted, is associated with the production of steroid hormones (Fig. 27-14). This is widely distributed, mostly in the form of branching tubules. In addition, the cytoplasm contains some mitochondria, some rER, a few Golgi stacks, and some inclusions. An interesting type of the latter are crystalloids with a complex but orderly internal structure; when sectioned, these present an appearance not unlike a woven fabric (Fig. 27-15B).

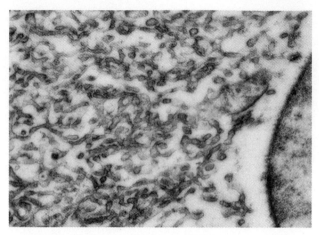

Fig. 27-14. Electron micrograph ($\times$25,000) of part of an interstitial cell of testis of opossum. Part of the nucleus is seen at *right*. Note the interconnected tubules of smooth-surfaced endoplasmic reticulum, a characteristic feature of steroid-synthesizing cells. (Courtesy of A. Christensen and D. Fawcett)

Effects of Androgen on Target Cells. The physiologically important androgen in the male is *testosterone*. This hormone affects, and is also affected by, various kinds of cells in the body. Testosterone is thought to enter most cells, but it may affect them (or be affected by them) only slightly or not at all. In liver cells it can undergo extensive metabolic change. In other cells, termed *androgen-responsive* cells, it is altered and in its changed form stimulates both growth and secretion. In rats and mice the androgen-responsive cells, in a decreasing order of responsiveness, have been found to be in the prostate, seminal vesicles, preputial gland, kidney and skin.

It seems that the reason for certain cells being responsive to its effects is that responsive cells possess the enzyme that converts testosterone to *5α-dihydrotestosterone;* this conversion occurs in both the cytoplasm and the nucleus of responsive cells. In the cytoplasm the dihydrotestosterone is converted into other metabolites. In the nucleus, however, it is not altered but becomes bound, by means of a protein, to euchromatin. The enzyme that in the nucleus converts testosterone to dihydrotestosterone is tightly bound to the euchromatin-protein complex.

The fact that dihydrotestosterone becomes bound to euchromatin suggests that it acts at the level of genes to increase protein synthesis, thereby enlarging cells as well as increasing their secretion. Since many of the androgen-sensitive cells of the prostate and seminal vesicles are secretory, it seems likely that the metabolic processes concerned in producing all components of the secretions of these cells are stimulated.

THE TUBULI RECTI AND RETE TESTIS

Seminiferous tubules, as they approach the mediastinum testis, become straight and are known as *tubuli recti;* they empty into the rete testis of the mediastinum (Fig. 27-2). Spermatogenesis does not occur in the tubuli recti, which are lined by tall Sertoli-like cells. The spaces of the rete are lined by cuboidal epithelium.

Fig. 27-15. (*A*) Electron micrograph (×6,700) of several interstitial cells. Note the densely staining lipid droplets and pigment granules, and the crystalline inclusions (crystalloids of Reinke). (*B*) Electron micrograph (×40,000) showing crystalloid with highly ordered internal structure. (Fawcett, D. W., and Burgos, M. H.: Ciba Foundation Colloquia on Ageing. vol. 2, p. 86. London, Churchill, 1956)

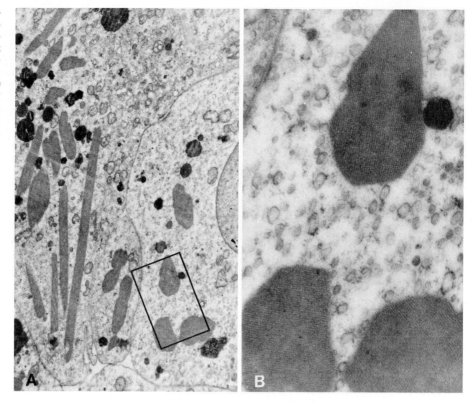

THE EPIDIDYMIS

The general structure of the epididymis was described in the first part of this chapter; further details of its microscopic structure follow.

The epididymis is invested in a fibrous covering similar to the tunica albuginea of the testis, but somewhat thinner.

Ductuli Efferentes. The cone-shaped bodies in which these are arranged are held together by delicate, vascular connective tissue. The ductules themselves consist of an epithelial lining, a basement membrane, and a thin layer of smooth muscle associated with some elastic fibers. The *epithelium* exhibits alternating groups of high columnar cells with typical motile cilia and low columnar cells that usually do not have cilia. The latter cells are probably secretory. Because of this characteristic appearance, the epithelium is often described as looking like a festoon (garland). It seems the combined action of the rete testis, ductuli efferentes, and proximal portion of the ductus epididymis is to remove from the secretory product of the testes not only excess fluid but also extraneous materials carried with this mass. This resorption of fluid in the epididymis would also create negative pressure to facilitate transportation of spermatozoa from seminiferous tubules to the epididymis.

Ductus Epididymis. The convoluted *ductus epididymis*, together with the connective tissue holding its coils together (Fig. 27-16), comprises the body and tail of the epididymis. The duct consists of an epithelial lining, a basement membrane, and thin circular coat of smooth muscle fibers.

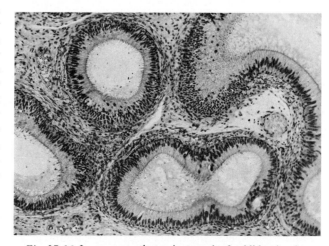

Fig. 27-16. Low-power photomicrograph of epididymis, showing ductus epididymis cut in cross and oblique section.

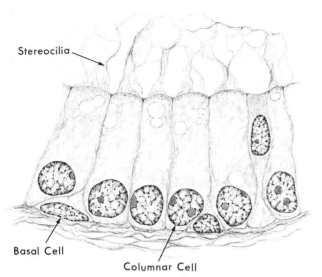

Fig. 27-17. Drawing of the epithelium of ductus epididymis, showing its pseudostratified epithelium and stereocilia. (Courtesy of Y. Clermont)

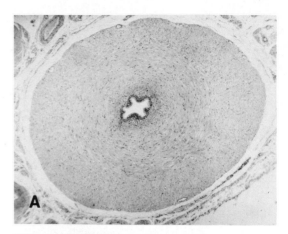

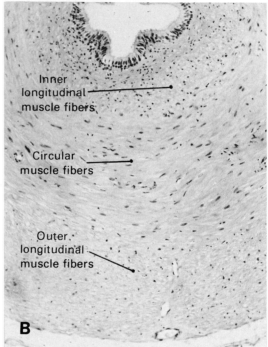

Fig. 27-18. Low-power (*A*), and high-power (*B*) photomicrographs of ductus (vas) deferens, showing the arrangement of the smooth muscle layers in its walls.

The *epithelium* all along the ductus epididymis is pseudostratified columnar because it contains small basal cells and tall columnar ones. The tall cells, however, form a continuous even surface. Tufts of extremely long microvilli project toward the lumen from the free margin of the tall cells (Fig. 27-17). These cytoplasmic processes were called *stereocilia* (Gr. *stereos,* solid) but they do not contain the microtubules characteristic of cilia. Pinocytotic vacuoles are commonly seen in the apical cytoplasm of these tall cells.

It should be borne in mind that the epididymis is the place where spermatozoa mature biochemically and gradually acquire their fertilizing capacity. Even so, when they emerge from the epididymis they still have not attained their full capacity for fertilization and this is only achieved later.

THE DUCTUS (VAS) DEFERENS

This is a sufficiently substantial structure to be palpated through the skin and subcutaneous tissue. Its firm consistency is due to its very thick muscular wall and relatively narrow lumen (Fig. 27-18).

Its mucous membrane consists of an epithelial lining and a lamina propria of connective tissue with a high content of elastic fibers. It is thrown into longitudinal folds of moderate height. As in the ductus epididymis, the *epithelium* is pseudostratified columnar, and here again the tall columnar cells show stereocilia (Fig. 27-17). At the level of the ampulla the columnar cells lose their stereocilia.

The *muscular coat* consists of three layers of smooth muscle (Fig. 27-18B). The inner and outer longitudinal layers are each thinner than the middle circular one. The *adventitia* consists of a loose elastic type of connective tissue and blends with the tissues comprising the *spermatic cord,* which contains arteries, numerous veins, nerves, and some longitudinal striated muscle fibers (*cremaster* muscle). The veins are particularly prominent and form the *pampiniform* (L. *pampinus,* tendril) *plexus;* the plexus is so named because the veins wind around the duct as tendrils of plants wild around supporting structures. This is a common site for veins to become varicosed.

A short distance before the ductus deferens is joined by the seminal vesicle on the same side it becomes dilated to form an *ampulla*. Here the muscular coat, though still thick, is thinner than in the other parts of the duct, and the lumen is considerably larger. The mucous membrane is thrown into very complicated folds similar to those of the seminal vesicle (Fig. 27-19).

THE SEMINAL VESICLES

The size and the function of the seminal vesicles are controlled to a great degree by hormones; hence, the size and shape of these structures vary considerably in relation to age. In the sexually mature male they are elongated bodies, 5 to 7 cm. or more long, the somewhat less than half as wide at their widest point, tapering toward the end at which they join the ductus deferens.

The structure seen on gross dissection and called a *seminal vesicle* is essentially a tube that is much longer and narrower than it looks. Its coils and convolutions, where they touch one another, are connected by connective tissue (Fig. 27-19). This tissue must be dissected if the seminal vesicle is to be unraveled, and if this is done, it will be found to consist of a tube about 15 cm. long. The coils and convolutions are such that if a cross section is cut through the undissected structure, the seminal vesicle will be sectioned in several positions along its length (Fig. 27-19).

The wall of the tube exhibits three coats: an outermost one of fibrous connective tissue with a substantial content of elastic fibers, a middle muscular coat, and a lining mucous membrane.

The *muscular coat* is substantial but not so thick as that of the ductus deferens. It consists of two layers of smooth muscle: an inner circular one and an outer one of longitudinal fibers.

The mucous membrane is thrown into an extraordinary series of folds (Fig. 27-19). These provide the vesicle with an enormous area of secretory epithelium and also permit it to become distended with secretion without undue stretching of the lining membrane of secretory cells. The *epithelial lining* consists essentially of a layer of tall columnar cells, but small cells may be irregularly distributed between these and the lamina propria. The small cells in some instances may form a continuous membrane, deep to the tall cells.

Since the folds of mucous membrane are so very numerous and may branch, the lamina propria of the seminal vesicle (as seen in a section) seems to contain glands. However, the glandular appearance, like that

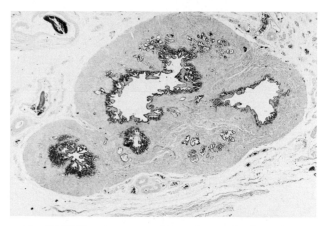

Fig. 27-19. Very low power photomicrograph of a cross section of a seminal vesicle.

presented by the mucous membrane of the gallbladder, is due only to extensive folding of the mucous membrane.

The epithelial cells of the vesicles produce a thick, yellowish secretion. This is delivered into the ejaculatory duct during ejaculation, and hence is one of the fluids present in semen. It provides nutritive materials for the spermatozoa.

The structure and function of the seminal vesicles and prostate glands are similarly affected by hormones and these effects will be described after we have dealt with the microscopic structure of the prostate gland.

THE PROSTATE GLAND

This gland, roughly the size and shape of a horse chestnut, is narrower below than above (Fig. 27-1). It surrounds the urethra as the latter emerges from the bladder. Enlargements of its substance can obstruct the outlet from the bladder, and these are relatively common in men past middle age. Their cause is obviously hormonal, for the reverse of enlargement—atrophy—occurs if the testes are removed. Removal of the prostate gland, or some part of it, to free the urethra from obstruction is a relatively common operation in older men.

The prostate gland is of a firm consistency. It is surrounded by a thin *capsule* that contains both connective tissue and smooth muscle fibers and can be distinguished from the fascia that lies outside it.

As already noted, the substance of the prostate is made up of a *large number of individual glands;* these open by separate *ducts* into the prostatic urethra and are embedded in a *stroma* that is a mixture of smooth muscle and fibrous connective tissue.

A cross section of the prostate shows that the lumen of

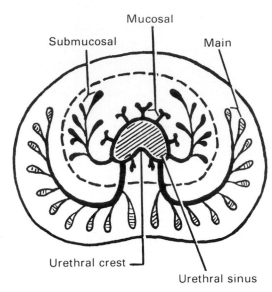

Submucosal   Mucosal   Main

Urethral crest

Urethral sinus

Fig. 27-20. Diagram of a cross section of the prostate gland, showing the distribution of the mucosal, submucosal, and main glands, and where their ducts open. The anterior surface of the gland is shown at the *top.* (After Grant, J. C. B: A Method of Anatomy. ed. 4. Baltimore, Williams & Wilkins, 1948)

the prostatic urethra is V-shaped, with the apex of the V lying anteriorly (Fig. 27-20). The part of the posterior wall in the urethra that bulges forward to make the cross-sectional appearance of its lumen V-shaped is termed the *urethral crest* (Fig. 27-20). The two posterolateral arms of the V constitute the *urethral sinuses* (Fig. 27-20).

The glands embedded in the substance of the prostate are of three different orders of size, and are distributed in three different areas arranged more or less concentrically around the urethra. The *mucosal glands* are the smallest and are disposed in the periurethral tissue (Fig. 27-20). They are of the greatest importance in connection with enlargements of the prostate in older men, for it is these glands that commonly overgrow to form *adenomatous* (Gr. *aden,* gland; *oma,* tumor) *nodules.* The *submucosal glands* are arranged in the ring of tissue surrounding the periurethral tissue (Fig. 27-20). The *main (external* or *proper) prostatic glands*—and these provide the bulk of the secretion of the gland—are situated in the outer and largest portion of the gland (Fig. 27-20). The mucosal glands open at various points around the lumen of the urethra, but the ducts of the submucosal and main prostatic glands open into the posterior margins of the urethral sinuses (Fig. 27-20).

The prostate gland is imperfectly divided into three *lobes* by the passage through it of the ejaculatory ducts. Each lobe is imperfectly subdivided into *lobules.* The ducts that drain the lobules in the bulk of the organ sweep

backward to empty into the urethral sinuses (Fig. 27-20). In the lobules, the ducts branch into *tubulo-alveolar secretory units.* These not only produce secretion but are also adapted to storing it, and as a consequence may be greatly dilated. To accommodate large amounts of stored secretion, the epithelial lining of the gland is greatly folded, and projections of mucous membrane extend into their lumina at many sites (Fig. 27-21). This arrangement, together with the *fibromuscular stroma* between and within the lobules (Fig. 27-21), gives the gland a distinctive microscopic appearance.

In the healthy, sexually mature male, the *epithelium* of the secretory units and ducts (except close to where they enter the urethra) is of a tall columnar type. Smaller flattened or rounded cells may be distributed irregularly beneath these tall columnar cells. The tall cells have a well-developed Golgi between their nucleus and their free border. *Concretions,* which may be calcified to some extent, are not uncommon in the secretion in the secretory units of prostate glands of older men (Fig. 27-21, *left*). The epithelium rests on a fibrous connective tissue *lamina propria* that contains an abundant supply of capillaries.

The secretion of the prostate gland is a thin, somewhat milky fluid. It contains, among other constituents, quantities of acid phosphatase; the role of this enzyme is not known, but its detection in the bloodstream is of use in the diagnosis of malignant tumors that arise from the secretory cells of the prostate gland.

Effects of Hormones on the Seminal Vesicles and Prostate Gland. Androgen produced by the testes is required to bring about full development of the seminal vesicles and

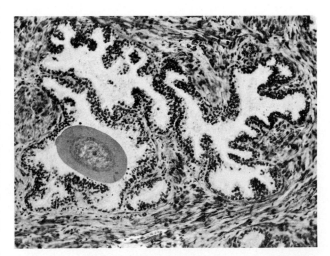

Fig. 27-21. Medium-power photomicrograph of a portion of a lobule of the prostate gland. Note the smooth muscle fibers in the stroma at *upper right* and *bottom,* and the concretion in the lumen of a secretory unit at *left.*

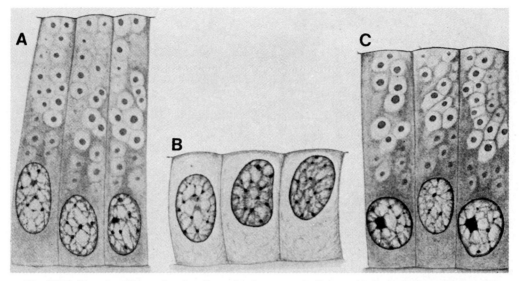

Fig. 27-22. Drawings illustrating the effect of androgen on the lining epithelium of the seminal vesicles. (*A*) Cells from a normal rat. (*B*) Cells from a rat after castration. (*C*) Cells following castration, except that the rat received injections of testis extract. (Moore, C. R., Hughes, W., and Gallagher, T. F.: Am. J. Anat., *45:*109, 1930)

prostate gland. Castration, after these structures have fully developed, causes them to atrophy. The most striking microscopic change brought about by castration occurs in the epithelium.

In a sexually mature male the *epithelial cells* of the seminal vesicles are of the tall columnar type. Their cytoplasm, between their nucleus and free border, contains abundant secretory granules (Fig. 27-22A). If the testes are removed, the epithelial cells shrink, becoming more or less cuboidal (Fig. 27-22B), and secretory granules disappear from their cytoplasm. The height of the epithelial cells of the seminal vesicles and their normal content of secretory granules can be restored by injections of androgen (Fig. 27-22C). The secretory cells of the prostate also shrink if the testes are removed, and their prominent Golgi regions become greatly reduced in size. These effects are reversed by injections of androgen.

As noted, *testosterone* is the physiologically important androgen, and the way in which it exerts it effects in androgen-sensitive cells was described when we dealt with interstitial cells.

Estrogen injected into male animals causes the epithelium of the seminal vesicles and prostate to change from tall secretory into a low nonsecretory type. Moreover, estrogen induces hypertrophy of the fibromuscular stroma of the prostate and walls of the seminal vesicles.

Advantage is taken of the secretory activity of secreting cells of the prostate being dependent on androgen in treating some malignant tumors arising from them. A proportion of cancers of the prostate are benefited by castration.

Being denied androgen, even malignant epithelial cells of the prostate gland may experience diminished function and growth activity. Likewise, in some instances prostatic cancers respond in similar fashion to treatment with estrogen.

The hormonal basis for nonmalignant overgrowths of prostatic tissue that so commonly obstruct the urethra of older men is not thoroughly understood. Both the glandular tissue and the stroma of the prostate participate in these overgrowths.

THE PENIS

The substance of the penis consists essentially of three cylindrical bodies of erectile (cavernous) tissue (Fig. 27-23). Two of these, the *corpora cavernosa,* are arranged side by side in the dorsal part of the organ (Fig. 27-23); this arrangement makes the dorsal surface of the otherwise more or less cylindrical penis somewhat flattened. The third long body of erectile tissue is called the *corpus cavernosum urethrae* because it conducts the urethra in its substance (Fig. 27-23) from one of its ends to the other (Fig. 27-1). It is also termed the *corpus spongiosum.* This cavernous body lies medial and ventral to the paired corpora cavernosa. Moreover, it extends somewhat beyond the corpora cavernosa and becomes expanded distally into a cone-shaped body, the *glans* (Fig. 27-1).

Each cavernous body is surrounded by a stout sheath of connective tissue called a *tunica albuginea* (Figs. 27-23 and 27-24). In the corpora cavernosa, this sheath con-

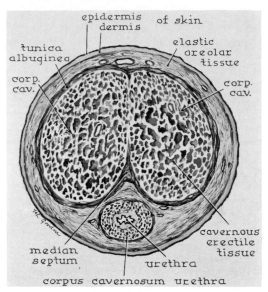

Fig. 27-23. Diagram of a cross section about midway along the penis.

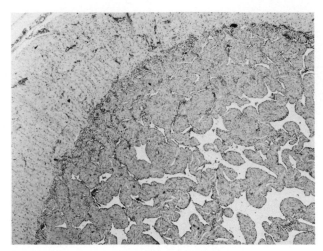

Fig. 27-24. Low-power photomicrograph of part of a cross section of penis, showing the tunica albuginea at *upper left,* with erectile tissue at *lower right.*

sists chiefly of collagenic fibers arranged in an inner circular and an outer longitudinal layer, but it also contains elastic fibers. The tunics covering the paired corpora cavernosa merge with one another along the midline of the penis and fuse to form a median septum (Fig. 27-23); this is thickest and most complete near the root of the penis. The sheath surrounding the corpus cavernosum urethrae is more elastic than that covering the other two bodies. In the glans, a true tunica albuginea is deficient; here the dermis of the skin that covers the glans serves as a tunica albuginea and is continuous with the cavernous tissue deep to it.

The three cavernous bodies (except where the paired corpora cavernosa are fused) are bound together by elastic loose connective tissue (Fig. 27-23) called the *fascia penis.* This also provides a flexible attachment for the skin that covers the penis. The epidermis of the skin of the penis is thin. No terminal hairs are present except near the root of the organ. A circular fold of skin extends forward to cover the glans; this is called the *prepuce* (Fig. 27-1). It is usually sufficiently elastic to permit its being retracted. However, in some instances it is not, and it may fit too tightly over the glans; this condition is called *phimosis.* Modified sebaceous glands are present on the inner surface of the fold; the secretion from these, in a prepuce that cannot be retracted, may accumulate and become an irritant. The common operation by which the prepuce is removed is called *circumcision.*

The substance of the cavernous bodies consists of a three-dimensional network of trabeculae. These are composed of connective tissue and smooth muscle and are covered with endothelium (Fig. 27-24). Between the trabeculae are spaces; since the trabeculae are covered with endothelium, the spaces too are lined with it. These spaces tend to be larger in the more central parts of the cavernous bodies and smaller near their periphery (Fig. 27-23). The substance of the glans is made up of convolutions of large veins rather than of spaces separated by trabeculae.

Blood Supply and the Mechanism of Erection. The arterial supply is of two sorts. Branches from the arteria dorsalis end in capillary beds supplying the tissues of the organ, including those of the cavernous bodies. From the capillaries of the trabeculae, blood drains into the spaces. The spaces communicate in such a fashion that blood emptied into them can make its way to the more peripheral parts of the bodies, where the spaces open into plexuses of veins disposed close to the periphery of each cylindrical body. The blood instrumental in causing erection is derived chiefly from another and larger set of arteries that enters the substance of the bodies and there gives off branches that are conducted to the spaces by way of the trabeculae. These arteries have thick muscular walls, and, in addition, many possess inner thickenings of longitudinal muscle fibers that bulge into their lumina. Many of these arteries disposed along the trabeculae are coiled and twisted when the penis is flaccid; this accounts for their being called *helicine arteries.* Many of the terminal branches of these arteries open directly into the spaces of the cavernous tissue.

The smooth muscle of the arteries and the smooth muscle in the trabeculae are supplied by both sympathetic and parasympathetic fibers. Under conditions of erotic stimulation, the smooth muscle of the trabeculae and helicine arteries relaxes. The arteries tend to straighten, and as a result blood flows freely from them into the spaces. As blood collects in the spaces and dilates them, the venous plexuses in the peripheral parts of the bodies become compressed. With more blood being delivered into the spaces of the cavernous bodies, and with venous drainage from the bodies being impeded, the bodies become enlarged and turgid. The corpus cavernosum urethrae does not become so turgid as its two companions because its sheath is more elastic.

Return of the penis to its flaccid state after erection is termed *detumescence.* This is brought about by the helicine arteries becoming constricted and by the smooth muscle in the trabeculae contracting; this slowly forces blood from the organ.

The penis is richly provided with a great variety of sensory nerve endings.

THE MALE URETHRA

Essentially, this is a tube of mucous membrane. In some sites its lamina propria, which is primarily fibroelastic tissue, contains smooth muscle fibers and, in many sites, glands. Three facts about the urethra, that the medical student will be able to verify when he learns in his clinical years how to pass a catheter, are that it is about 8 inches long, its course is not straight but exhibits a reverse curve (Fig. 27-1), and (noticeable if the catheter employed is of too fine a caliber) its lining forms many small diverticula.

The male urethra is commonly described as consisting of three parts. On leaving the urinary bladder it enters the base of the prostate gland and courses through it to leave its apex. This portion of the urethra is described as its *prostatic part.* It then pierces the fasciae of the urogenital diaphragm. Accordingly, this portion of it is termed its *membranous part.* After this is enters the expanded root (bulb) of the corpus cavernosum urethrae (Fig. 27-1) and extends the entire length of this cavernous body to the apex of the glans (Fig. 27-1), where its *external orifice* is situated. The part of the urethra contained in the corpus cavernosum urethrae is called its *cavernous (spongy) part.* The details are as follows.

The Prostatic Portion. This part of the urethra is more or less V-shaped in cross section. The apex of the V-shaped posterior wall points forward and is called the *urethral crest* (Fig. 27-20). A conical elevation on the crest is termed the *colliculus,* and a small diverticulum (the remains of the fetal Müllerian ducts) opens through it. The slit-like openings of the ejaculatory ducts lie, one on each side of the colliculus, on the urethral crest. The sites of

the openings of the prostatic ducts have already been described.

As noted in Chapter 24, the epithelium of the urinary bladder is of the transitional type, so the epithelium that lines the first part of the prostatic urethra is of the same type. However, in the part of the prostatic urethra nearest the membranous urethra the epithelium changes to the pseudostratified or stratified columnar variety.

The lamina propria of prostatic urethra is composed essentially of fibroelastic connective tissue. It is very vascular, chiefly because of its great content of venules. Indeed, over the urethral crest the lamina propria contains so many venules and veins that it is sometimes described as erectile tissue. Smooth muscle fibers are also present in the mucous membrane of the prostatic urethra. These are disposed in two layers, the innermost one longitudinal and the outer, circular. Those constituting the latter are highly developed at the internal urethral orifice, where they, reinforced by smooth muscle fibers from another source, comprise the *sphincter of the bladder.*

The Membranous Portion. This part of the urethra is the shortest, being about 1 cm. long. The lining cells here are tall columnar in type and stratified. Some smooth muscle is present in the lamina propria, but the fibers of the circular layer in particular are less numerous than in the prostatic portion of the urethra. However, in the membranous urethra, striated muscle fibers of the urogenital diaphragm surround the tube; these comprise the *sphincter muscle of the urethra.* This muscle is sometimes called the *external sphincter of the bladder.* Two small bodies, each about as large as a pea, the *bulbourethral (Cowper's) glands,* are situated on the undersurface of the membranous urethra, close to its midline (Fig. 27-1). Their ducts run anteriorly and medially to open, sometimes by a common opening, on the lower surface of the first part of the cavernous portion of the urethra (Fig. 27-1), to be described next. The glands themselves are of the tubulo-alveolar type, and their secretory cells are mostly of the mucous type. These glands either secrete more copiously, or their secretion is expressed from them due to contraction of smooth muscle fibers in their stroma and voluntary muscle outside them, under conditions of erotic stimulation.

The Cavernous (Spongy) Portion. This part of the urethra is the longest. As noted, the urethra becomes expanded in the bulb of the corpus cavernosum urethrae to form the *bulb of the urethra* (Fig. 27-1). The urethra becomes expanded again in the glans; this expansion of it is termed the *terminal (navicular) fossa* (Fig. 27-1).

The epithelium in the cavernous part of the urethra is of the stratified columnar type, although simple columnar epithelium may be present on the crests of folds. In the proximal part of the terminal fossa some goblet cells may be present. In the distal part of the terminal fossa the epithelium becomes stratified squamous in type. This in turn becomes continuous with the stratified squamous keratinizing epithelium that covers the glans.

In the cavernous portion of the urethra, the smooth muscle of the urethra itself gradually disappears, to be replaced, as it were, by the smooth muscle of the septa of the erectile tissue through which the urethra passes.

Glands. Two groups of these are associated with the urethra. These are often termed the *glands of Littré*. One group, the *intramucosal* glands, consists of small simple glands situated in its lamina propria. Although these are present in all parts of the urethra, they are most numerous in its cavernous part. The second group constitutes the *extramucosal* glands. They are somewhat larger than the intramucosal type. Their ducts commonly pass to the urethra at acute angles. The extramucosal glands are not so widely distributed as the intramucosal glands. Both types secrete mucus. In addition to possessing glands, the lining of the urethra is beset with numerous small outpouchings of its mucous membrane; these are called *lacunae*. The glands described above may open into these.

REFERENCES AND OTHER READING

COMPREHENSIVE GENERAL REFERENCES

Austin, C. R., and Short, R. V. (eds.): Reproduction in Mammals. Books 1 to 6. Cambridge, Cambridge University Press, 1972 to 1976.

Beatty, R. A.: The genetics of the mammalian gamete. Biol. Rev., *45:*73, 1970.

Fawcett, D. W.: The male reproductive system. *In,* Greep, R. O., Koblinsky, M. A., and Jaffe, F. S. (eds.): Reproduction and Human Welfare: a Challenge to Research. p. 165. Cambridge, Mass., MIT Press, 1976.

Hamilton, D. W., and Greep, R. O. (eds.): Handbook of Physiology. vol. 5, Sect. 7. Male Reproductive System. Washington, D.C., American Physiological Society, 1975.

Odell, W. D., and Moyer, D. L.: Physiology of Reproduction. St. Louis, C. V. Mosby, 1971.

GENERAL REFERENCES ON THE TESTIS

Johnson, A. D., Gomes, W. R., and Vandemark, N. L. (eds.): The Testis. vol. 1, Development, Anatomy and Physiology; vol. 2, Biochemistry; vol. 3, Influencing Factors. New York, Academic Press, 1970.

Rosemberg, E., and Paulsen, C. A. (eds.): Advances in Experimental Medicine and Biology. The Human Testis. New York, Plenum Press, 1970.

DEVELOPMENT OF THE TESTIS

Blandau, R. J., and Bergsma, D. (eds.): Morphogenesis and Malformation of the Genital System. Birth Defects. Original Articles Series, vol. 13, No. 2. New York, Liss, 1977.

Gier, H. T., and Marion, G. B.: Development of the mammalian testis. *In* Johnson, A. D., Gomes, W. R., and Vandemark, N. L. (eds.): The Testis. vol. 1. New York, Academic Press, 1970.

Gondos, B., and Conner, L. A.: Ultrastructure of developing germ cells in fetal rabbit testis. Am. J. Anat., *136:*23, 1973.

Lording, D. W., and de Kretser, D. M.: Comparative ultrastructural and histochemical studies of interstitial cells of rat testis during fetal and postnatal development. J. Reprod. Fertil., *29:*261, 1972.

Vilar, O.: Histology of the human testis from neonatal period to adolescence. *In* Rosemberg, E., and Paulsen, C. A. (eds.): Advances in Experimental Medicine and Biology. The Human Testis. New York, Plenum Press, 1970.

HORMONAL INFLUENCES IN THE TESTIS

General

Go, V. L. W., Vernon, R. G., and Fritz, I. B.: Studies on spermatogenesis in rats. III. Effects of hormonal treatment on differentiation kinetics of the spermatogenic cycle in regressed hypophysectomized rats. Can. J. Biochem., *49:*768, 1971.

Gomes, W. R.: Metabolic and regulatory hormones influencing testis function. *In* Johnson, A. D., Gomes, W. R., and Vandemark, N. L. (eds.): The Testis. vol. 3. New York, Academic Press, 1970.

Hall, P. F.: Endocrinology of the testis. *In* Johnson, A. D., Gomes, W. R., and Vandemark, N. L. (eds.): The Testis. vol. 2. New York, Academic Press, 1970.

Odell, W. D., and Moyer, D. L.: Dynamic relationship of the testis to the whole man. *In* Physiology of Reproduction. St. Louis, C. V. Mosby, 1971.

Rosemberg, E., and Paulsen, C. A. (eds.): Regulation of Testicular Function. Role of the hypothalamus. Testicular-pituitary interrelation. Metabolic effects of gonadotropins. Influence of gonadotropins on testicular function. *In* Advances in Experimental Medicine and Biology. The Human Testis. New York, Plenum Press, 1970.

Steinberger, E.: Hormonal control of mammalian spermatogenesis. Physiol. Rev., *51:*1, 1971.

Effects at the Cellular Level

Dorrington, J. H., Vernon, R. G., and Fritz, I. B.: The effect of gonadotrophins on the 3′,5′-AMP levels of seminiferous tubules. Biochem. Biophys. Res. Commun., *46:*1523, 1972.

Lipsett, M. B.: Steroid secretions by the human testis. *In* Rosemberg, E., and Paulsen, C. A. (eds.): Advances in Experimental Medicine and Biology. The Human Testis. New York, Plenum Press, 1970.

Lipsett, M. B., and Savard, K.: Subcellular structure and synthesis of steroids in the testis. *In* Rosemberg, E., and Paulsen, C. A. (eds.): Advances in Experimental Medicine and Biology. The Human Testis. New York, Plenum Press, 1970.

STRUCTURES AND ARRANGEMENTS IN SPERMATOGENESIS

General

Bruce, W. R., and Meistrich, M. L.: Spermatogenesis in the Mouse. Proc. 1st Internat. Conf. on Cell Differentiation. p. 295. Copenhagen, Munksgaard, 1972.

Courot, M., Hochereau-de Reviers, M., and Ortavant, R.: Spermatogenesis. *In* Johnson, A. D., Gomes, W. R., and Vandemark, N. L. (eds.): The Testis. vol. 1. New York, Academic Press, 1970.

Fawcett, D. W., and Bedford, J. M. (eds.): The Spermatozoon: Maturation, Motility and Surface Properties. Baltimore, Urban and Schwarzenberg, 1979.

Roosen-Runge, E. C.: The process of spermatogenesis in mammals. Biol. Rev., *37:*343, 1962.

Odell, W. D., and Moyer, D. L.: The testis and the male sex accessories. *In* Physiology of Reproduction. St. Louis, C. V. Mosby, 1971.

Special

Burgos, M. H., Vitale-Calpe, R., and Aoki, A.: Fine structure of the testis and its functional significance. *In* Johnson, A. D., Gomes, W. R., and Vandemark, N. L. (eds.): The Testis. vol. 1. New York, Academic Press, 1970.

Clermont, Y.: The cycle of the seminiferous epithelium in man. Am. J. Anat., *112:*35, 1963.

———: Spermatogenesis in man. A study of the spermatogonial population. Fertil. Steril., *17:*705, 1966.

Clermont, Y., and Hermo, L.: Spermatogonial stem cells and their behaviour in the seminiferous epithelium of rats and monkeys. *In* Cairnie, A. B., Lala, P. K., and Osmond, D. G. (eds.): Stem Cells of Renewing Cell Populations. New York, Academic Press, 1976.

Clermont, Y., and Trott, M.: Duration of the cycle of the seminiferous epithelium in the mouse and hamster determined by means of radioautography. Fertil. Steril., *20:*805, 1969.

———: Kinetics of spermatogenesis in mammals: seminiferous epithelium cycle and spermatogonial renewal. Physiol. Rev., *52:*198, 1972.

Dym, M.: The mammalian rete testis—a morphological examination. Anat. Rec., *186:*493, 1976.

Dym, M., and Fawcett, D. W.: Further observations on the number of spermatogonia, spermatocytes, and spermatids connected by intercellular bridges in the mammalian testis. Biol. Reprod., *4:*195, 1971.

———: The blood-testis barrier in the rat and the physiological compartment of the seminiferous epithelium. Biol. Reprod., *3:*308, 1970.

Fawcett, D. W.: A comparative view of sperm ultrastructure. Biol. Reprod., *2* (Suppl. 2):90, 1970.

———: The mammalian spermatozoon. Dev. Biol., *44:*395, 1975.

———: Ultrastructure and function of the Sertoli cell. *In* Hamilton, D. W., and Greep, R. O. (eds.): Handbook of Physiology. Endocrinology. vol. 5, Sect. 7. Male Reproductive System. Washington, D.C., American Physiological Society, 1975.

Fawcett, D. W., Eddy, E., and Phillips, D. M.: Observations on the fine structure and relationships of the chromatoid body in mammalian spermatogenesis. Biol. Reprod., *2:*129, 1970.

Fawcett, D. W., Leak, L. V., and Heidger, P. M.: Electron microscopic observations on the structural components of the blood-testis barrier. J. Reprod. Fertil., *10* (Suppl.):105, 1970.

Fawcett, D. W., Neaves, W. B., and Flores, M. N.: Comparative observations on intertubular lymphatics and the organization of the interstitial tissue of the mammalian testis. Biol. Reprod., *9:*500, 1973.

Forer, A., *et al:* Spermatozoan tails. Nature [New Biol.], *243:*128, 1973.

Gilula, N. B., Fawcett, D. W., and Aoki, A.: Ultrastructural and experimental observations on the Sertoli cell junctions of the mammalian testis. Dev. Biol., *50:*142, 1976.

Halbertsma, H.: Ontleedkundige aanteekeningen. VI. Johan Ham van Arnhem, de ontdekker der spermatozoiden. Versl. & Mededeel, d. Kon, Acad. v. Wentensch. (Amsterdam). Afd. Natuurkunde, XIII, 342, 1862.

Hannah-Alava, A.: The premeiotic stages of spermatogenesis. Adv. Genet., *13:*157, 1965.

Heller, C. G., and Clermont, Y.: Kinetics of the germinal epithelium in man. Recent Prog. Horm. Res., *20:*545, 1964.

Huckins, C.: The spermatogonial stem cell population in adult rats. I. Their morphology, proliferation and maturation. Anat. Rec., *169:*533, 1971.

Koehler, J. K.: Human sperm head ultrastructure: a freeze-etching study. J. Ultrastruct. Res., *39:*520, 1972.

Lam, D. M. K., Furrer, R., and Bruce, W. R.: The separation, physical characterization and differential kinetics of spermatogonial cells of the mouse. Proc. Natl. Acad. Sci. U.S.A., *65:*192, 1970.

Leblond, C. P., and Clermont, Y.: Definition of the stages of the cycle of the seminiferous epithelium in the rat. Ann. N.Y. Acad. Sci., *55:*548, 1952.

Loir, M., and Wyrobek, A.: Density separation of mouse spermatid nuclei. Exp. Cell Res., *75:*261, 1972.

Moens, P. B., and Go, V. L. W.: Intercellular bridges and division patterns of rat spermatogonia. Z. Zellforsch., *127:*201, 1971.

Moens, P. B., and Hugenholtz, A. D.: The arrangement of germ cells in the rat seminiferous tubule: an electron microscopic study. J. Cell Sci., *19:*487, 1975.

———: A new approach to stem cell research in spermatogenesis. *In* Cairnie, A. B., Lala, P. K., and Osmond, D. G. (eds.): Stem Cells of Renewing Cell Populations. New York, Academic Press, 1976.

Muys, W. G.: Investigatio Fabricae, quae in partibus musculos componentibus extat. 4º, p. 288 (note 2), Lugd. Bat., 1741.

Percy, B., Clermont, Y., and Leblond, C. P.: The wave of the seminiferous epithelium in the rat. Am. J. Anat., *108:*47, 1961.

Phillips, D. M.: Substructure of the mammalian acrosome. J. Ultrastruct. Res., *38:*591, 1972.

Rattner, J. B.: Observations of centriole formation in male meiosis. J. Cell Biol., *54:*20, 1972.

Rattner, J. B., and Brinkley, B. R.: Ultrastructure of mammalian spermiogenesis. II. Elimination of the nuclear membrane. J. Ultrastruct. Res., *36:*1, 1971.

Rowley, M. J., Berlin, J. D., and Heller, C. G.: The ultrastructure of four types of human spermatogonia. Z. Zellforsch., *112:*139, 1971.

Rowley, M. J., Teshima, F., and Heller, C. G.: Duration of transit of spermatozoa through the human male ductular system. Fertil. Steril., *21:*390, 1970.

Setchel, B. P., and Waites, G. M. H.: The blood-testis barrier. *In* Hamilton, D. W., and Greep, R. O. (eds.): Handbook of Physiology. Endocrinology. vol. 5, Sect. 7. Male Reproductive System. Washington, D.C., American Physiological Society, 1975.

Solari, A. J., and Tres, L. L.: Ultrastructure and histochemistry of the nucleus during male meiotic prophase. *In* Rosemberg, E., and Paulsen, C. A. (eds.): Advances in Experimental Medicine and Biology. The Human Testis. New York, Plenum Press, 1970.

CHROMOSOMES AND MEIOSIS

Dronamraju, K. R.: The function of the Y-chromosome in man, animals, and plants. Adv. Genet., *13:*227, 1965.

Esponda, P., and Stockert, J. C.: Localization of RNA in the synaptonemal complex. J. Ultrastruct. Res., *35*:411, 1971.

Fuge, H., and Muller, W.: Murotubuli contact on anaphase chromosomes in first meiotic division. Exp. Cell Res., *71*:241, 1972.

Moens, P. B.: Mechanisms of chromosome synapsis at meiotic prophase. Internat. Rev. Cytol., *35*:117, 1973.

Ohno, S.: Morphological aspects of meiosis and their genetical significance. *In* Rosemberg, E., and Paulsen, C. A. (eds.): Advances in Experimental Medicine and Biology. The Human Testis. New York, Plenum Press, 1970.

Polani, P. E.: Centromere localization at meiosis and position of chiasmata in male and female mouse. Chromosoma, *36*:343, 1972.

Rimpau, J., and Lelley, T.: Attachment of meiotic chromosomes to nuclear membrane. Z. Pflanzenzuchtung, *67*:197, 1972.

Schnedl, W.: End to end association of X and Y chromosomes in mouse meiosis. Nature [New Biol.], *236*:29, 1972.

INTERSTITIAL CELLS

Christensen, A. K.: Fine structure of testicular interstitial cells in humans. *In* Rosemberg, E., and Paulsen, C. A. (eds.): Advances in Experimental Medicine and Biology. The Human Testis. New York, Plenum Press, 1970.

Hooker, C. W.: The intertubular tissue of the testis. *In* Johnson, A. D., Gomes, W. R., and Vandemark N. L. (eds.): The Testis. vol. 1. New York, Academic Press, 1970.

Reddy, J., and Svobodka, D.: Microbodies (peroxisomes) identification in interstitial cells of testis. J. Histochem. Cytochem., *20*:140, 1972.

Tsang, W. N., Lacy, D., and Collins, P. M.: Leydig cell differentiation, steroid metabolism by interstitium in-vitro and growth of accessory sex organs in rat. J. Reprod. Fertil., *34*:351, 1973.

SEMEN AND METABOLIC ACTIVITIES OF THE TESTES

Amann, R. P.: Sperm production rates. *In* Johnson, A. D., Gomes, W. R., and Vandemark, N. L. (eds.): The Testis. vol. 1. New York, Academic Press, 1970.

Bishop, M. W. H., and Walton, A.: Metabolism and motility of mammalian spermatozoa. *In* Marshall's Physiology of Reproduction. vol. 1, part 2. London, Longmans, Green, 1968.

Lam, D. M. K., and Bruce, W. R.: The biosynthesis of protamine during spermatogenesis of the mouse: extraction, partial characterization and site of synthesis J. Cell Physiol., *78*:13, 1971.

Moresi, V.: Chromosome activities during meiosis and spermatogenesis. J. Reprod. Fertil., *13* (Suppl.):1, 1971.

Nelson, L.: Quantitative evaluation of sperm motility control mechanisms. Biol. Reprod., *6*:319, 1972.

Phillips, D. M.: Comparative analysis of mammalian sperm motility. J. Cell Biol., *53*:561, 1972.

Setchell, B. P.: Testicular blood supply, lymphatic drainage and secretion of fluid. *In* Johnson, A. D., Gomes, W. R., and Vandemark, N. L. (eds.): The Testis. vol. 1. New York, Academic Press, 1970.

———: Characteristics of testicular spermatozoa and the fluid

which transports them into the epididymis. Biol. Reprod., *1* (Suppl. 1):40, 1969.

Suzuki, H.: Effects of Vitamin E-deficiency and high salt supplementation on changes in kidney and testis of rats. Tohoku J. Exp. Med., *106*:329, 1972.

EFFECTS OF MUTAGENS, IONIZING RADIATION AND HEAT ON SPERMATOGENESIS

Bateman, A. J., and Epstein, S. S.: Dominant lethal mutations in mammals. *In* Hollaender, A. (ed.): Chemical Mutagens, Principles and Methods for Their Detection. vol. 2. New York, Plenum Press, 1971.

Bruce, W. R.: Studies of the genetic implications of abnormal spermatozoa. *In* Cairnie, A. B., Lala, P. K., and Osmond, D. G. (eds.): Stem Cells of Renewing Cell Populations. New York, Academic Press, 1976.

Bruce, W. R., Furrer, R., and Wyrobek, A. J.: Abnormalities in the shape of murine sperm after acute testicular X-irradiation. Mutat. Res., *23*:381, 1974.

Carlson, W. D., and Gassmer, F. X. (eds.): Effects of Ionizing Radiation on the Reproductive System. New York, Macmillan, 1964.

Dym, M., and Clermont, Y.: Role of spermatogonia in the repair of the seminiferous epithelium following x-irradiation of the rat testis. Am. J. Anat., *128*:265, 1970.

MacLeod, J.: The significance of deviations in human sperm morphology. *In* Rosemberg, E. R., and Paulsen, C. A. (eds.): The Human Testis. p. 481. New York, Plenum Press, 1970.

Meistrich, M. L., Eng, V. W. S., and Loir, M.: Temperature effects on the kinetics of spermatogenesis in the mouse. Cell Tissue Kinet., *6*:379, 1973.

Röhrborn, G.: The activity of alkylating agents. I. Sensitive mutable stages in spermatogenesis and oogenesis; Röhrborn, G., and Schleiermacher, E.: II. Histological and cytogenetic findings in spermatogenesis. *In* Vogel, F., and Röhrborn, G. (eds.): Chemical Mutagenesis in Mammals and Man. New York, Springer-Verlag, 1970.

Wyrobek, A. J., and Bruce, A. J.: Chemical induction of sperm abnormalities in mice. Proc. Natl. Acad. Sci. U.S.A., *72*:4425, 1975.

RELATED READING

Beer, A. E., and Billingham, R. E.: Immunobiology of mammalian reproduction. Adv. Immunol., *14*:1, 1971.

Brackett, B. G.: Mammalian fertilization in vitro. Fed. Proc., *32*:2065, 1973.

Davajan, V., Nakamura, R. M., and Saga, M.: Role of immunology in the infertile human. Biol. Reprod., *6*:443, 1972.

Gould, K, G.: Application of in vitro fertilization. Fed Proc., *32*:2069, 1973.

Lyon, M., Gleniste, P. H., and Hawker, S. G.: Do H-2 and T-loci of mouse have a function in haploid phase of sperm? Nature, *240*:152, 1972.

Metz, C. B.: Role of specific sperm antigens in fertilization. Fed. Proc., *32*:2057, 1973.

Sherman, J. K.: Synopsis of the use of frozen human semen since 1964: State of the art of human semen banking. Fertil. Steril., *24*:397, 1973.

28 The Eye and the Ear

THE EYE

The eye, except for being rounded, has most of the structural features of an old-fashioned camera, with the *eyelid* being the counterpart of a shutter (Fig. 28-1). The eye has an adjustable diaphragm, termed the *iris* (Gr. *iridos,* a rainbow, colored circle) (Figs. 28-1 and 28-12). Its aperture opens and closes automatically in relation to the amount of light available, a feature of the eye diaphragm now found in many modern cameras. The eye too has a *lens* (Fig. 28-1); this, being composed of altered transparent epithelial cells, is more elastic than the glass lens of a camera. Advantage is taken of its elasticity, for the lens of the eye is suspended in such a way that muscle action can alter its shape and so change its focal length. As a consequence, the eye need not be

shortened or elongated when objects at different distances are brought into focus, as is necessary in a camera with a rigid lens fixed in position. The sides and back of a camera have as their counterpart in the eye a strong connective tissue membrane, the *sclera* (Fig. 28-1). The equivalent in the eye of the light-sensitive film used in a camera is a membrane of living cells of nervous origin, the *retina,* which lines not only the back but the sides of the eye as well (Fig. 28-1). Then, finally, just as black paint is used to blacken the interior surfaces of a camera that might reflect light, black pigment is distributed generously between the retina and the sclera and in other sites where it would be advantageous.

Unlike modern cameras, the lens of the eye is not placed at its very front; in this respect the eye is like the old-fashioned kind of camera, which has its external aperture covered with a glass

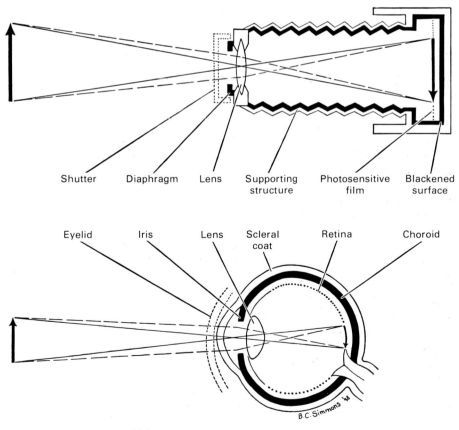

Shutter   Diaphragm   Lens   Supporting structure   Photosensitive film   Blackened surface

Eyelid   Iris   Lens   Scleral coat   Retina   Choroid

B.C. Simmons '84

Fig. 28-1. Diagram illustrating the similarities between the eye and an old-fashioned camera.

903

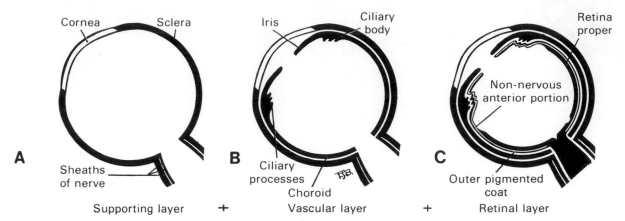

Supporting layer   +   Vascular layer   +   Retinal layer

Fig. 28-2. Schematic diagram illustrating the three layers of the wall of the eye. (*A*) The supporting coat of the eye. (*B*) The vascular coat inside the supporting coat. (*C*) The retinal coat inside the outer two coats.

window to keep out the dust, and its lens inside, a short distance behind the glass window. The transparent window in the central part of the front of the eye is of a curved form and is called the *cornea* (Fig. 28-3); it is composed chiefly of a tough but transparent type of dense connective tissue continuous with the opaque connective tissue of the *sclera* that surrounds and supports the remainder of the eye.

Windows not only permit householders to see out; they also allow the curious to see in. Since the cornea is like a window, the physician by means of an instrument called an *ophthalmoscope* can direct a beam of light into the eye; this enables him to look at the various structures within the eye as they become illuminated. With this instrument much useful information can be obtained not only about the eyes but also about the health of the body as a whole.

GENERAL STRUCTURE

The eye is nearly spherical and about 1 inch in diameter. It is contained in the anterior part of a bony socket, the *orbit;* between the eye and the bony wall of the orbit there are fat, connective tissue, ligaments, muscles, and the glandular tissue that provides the tears. The eye is suspended by the ligaments in such a fashion that voluntary muscles in the orbit (but outside the eye) can move the eye so that one can look up and down and from side to side.

In describing the eye we shall describe first the structure of its *wall,* then its contents (these constitute the *refractive media* of the eye), and finally the *accessory structures* of the eye such as eyelids, tear glands, ducts, and so forth.

The Wall of the Eye. This consists of three layers that form the outside in are designated the (*1*) *supporting* layer, (*2*) *middle* layer, and (*3*) *retinal* layer (Fig. 28-2). Not all three layers are present in all parts of the wall of the eye.

The *supporting layer* consists essentially of a dense connective tissue membrane. Around most of the eye this is called the *sclera* (Gr. *scleros,* hard) (Fig. 28-2). The sclera is white in color; the part of the sclera that shows is the "white" of the eye (Fig. 28-12). The part of the supporting layer covering the central part of the anterior portion of the eye bulges forward slightly and is transparent; this is called the *cornea* (Fig. 28-2). Except where it is penetrated by blood vessels, the supporting layer completely encloses the other layers of the eye but for one site posteriorly where there is an opening to permit the optic nerve to leave the eyeball.

The *middle layer* of the wall is often called the *uveal* (L. *uva,* grape) *layer* or *tract* because when the sclera is dissected away, the exposed middle layer is seen to resemble the skin of a dark grape in that it is pigmented and surrounds the jelly-like contents of the eye. The middle layer of the eye is very vascular; hence it is sometimes called the *vascular layer* of the eye.

Figure 28-2B shows that the middle layer lies on the inner surface of the supporting layer. In the posterior two thirds of the eye, the middle layer consists of only a thin membrane; this thin posterior segment of the middle layer is called the *choroid.* Moreover, in this illustration it will be seen that toward the anterior part of the eye the middle layer becomes thickened to form what is called the *ciliary body.* This, as a thickened rim of tissue, encircles the anterior part of the eye. From it what are termed the *ciliary processes* extend inward (Fig. 28-2B). The middle layer of the eye continues anteriorly to constitute the *iris* (diaphragm) of the eye (Fig. 28-2B). The iris is the pigmented part of the eye that may be seen through the cornea (Fig. 28-12); depending on the pigment content of the iris, the eyes appear blue, brown, or some other color. Indeed, pigment is abundant in all parts of the middle layer; this

Fig. 28-3. Diagram of the eye in longitudinal section.

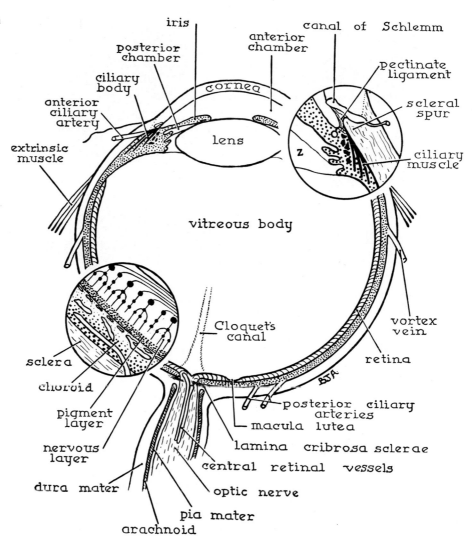

helps to lightproof the wall of the eye and reduce reflection. The middle layer conducts blood vessels and in its anterior part contains smooth muscle. The smooth muscle of the iris controls the diameter of its aperture, the *pupil* of the eye (Fig. 28-12). The smooth muscle of the ciliary body affects the tension of the *zonule* (sometimes called the *suspensory ligament* of the lens), not in the way that might at first be expected, that is, by its contraction pulling the fibers that suspend the lens, but by its contraction easing the tension on them, as will be described in detail later. This is how the eye accommodates its focus for near objects. The muscle of the ciliary body, then, is an important factor in the mechanism of *accommodation.*

The position of the *retinal layer* is illustrated in Figure 28-2C. It consists of two layers; the one that lines the middle coat of the eye is pigmented; the other one that in turn lines the pigmented layer is composed of nervous tissue. The nervous layer of the retina does not extend into the anterior part of the eye (Fig. 28-2C), for there light could not be focused on it. It contains special nerve cells called *rods* and *cones;* these are the *photoreceptors.* In addition, the retina contains the cell bodies of many interneurons and ganglion cells and many nerve fibers. Most of the latter converge on the site at which the optic nerve leaves the eye through the scleral layer (Fig. 28-2C).

Refractive Media of the Eye. Light passes through the following media before it reaches the retina:

(*1*) The substance of the *cornea* (Fig. 28-3).

(*2*) A space between the iris and lens called the *anterior chamber* of the eye (Fig. 28-3); this is filled with a fluid termed *aqueous humor.*

(*3*) The *lens* (Fig. 28-3).

(*4*) A transparent jelly-like material known as the *vitreous body,* which fills the interior of the eye behind the lens (Fig. 28-3).

A beam of light is bent when it passes obliquely from a substance of one refractive index into that of another. The cornea is curved, and the difference between the refractive index of cornea and air is greater than the difference between the refractive indices of any of the media through which light subsequently passes to reach the retina. Hence, with regard to refracting light, the curved anterior surface of the cornea is of the greatest importance. But the lens of the eye has a refractive index only slightly greater than that of the aqueous humor in front of it and that of the vitreous body behind it. Its unique importance lies in the fact that, being elastic, its focal length can be changed by the contraction of muscles attached to the fibers of the zonule suspending it; hence it permits light from objects at different distances to be focused sharply.

On passing through the vitreous body and reaching the retina, light does not immediately strike the photoreceptors, for these are in the deep part of the nervous layer that lies directly against the pigmented layer of the retina (Fig. 28-15). To reach the photoreceptors, light first must pass through the nerve fibers and nerve cells present in the inner layers of the nervous layer of the retina (the layers adjacent to the vitreous body). Then, when the light reaches and affects the photoreceptors in the deep layer of the nervous part of the retina, nerve impulses set up by the stimulus of light must pass in the reverse direction through nerve fibers and nerve cell bodies toward the vitreous body. Here, in the layer of the retina next to the vitreous, the impulses are conducted by nerve fibers that run to the site of exit of the optic nerve, through which nerve they pass to reach the brain (Fig. 28-15).

DEVELOPMENT

The *retina* of the eye develops as an outgrowth from the forebrain, which early in development is hollow. Its anterior wall bulges forward to form the primary *optic vesicle* (Fig. 28-4, 1). The bulge then becomes constricted at its point of origin from the forebrain; the constricted portion is termed the *optic stalk* (Fig. 28-4, 1). While the forebrain is extending anteriorly to form the optic vesicle, the ectoderm immediately in front of it thickens (Fig. 28-4, 1, lens ectoderm). The anterior wall of the optic vesicle then invaginates so that the optic vesicle becomes cup-shaped, with the wall of the cup having two layers (Fig. 28-4, 2 and 3). At the same time the thickened ectoderm in front of the optic vesicle bulges inward to form the *lens vesicle* (Fig. 28-4, 2). The lens vesicle then becomes pinched off from the ectoderm from which it arose (Fig. 28-4, 3). The formation of the lens provides an example of induction as was described in Chapter 6.

Fig. 28-5. (*Left*) Photomicrograph of the cornea. (*Right*) High-power photomicrographs showing representative parts of the cornea: (1) stratified squamous epithelium; (2) Bowman's membrane; (3) substantia propria; (4) Descemet's membrane; (5) Descemet's endothelium.

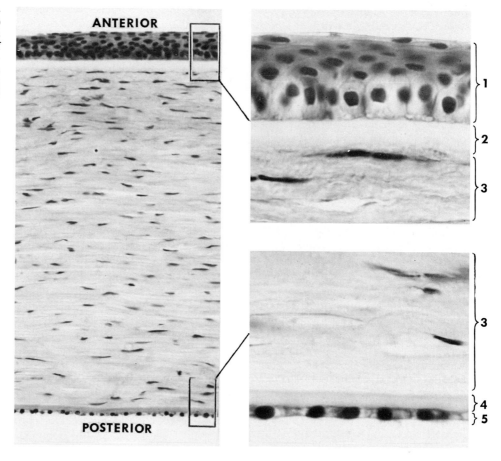

In the meantime the optic vesicle has become a deep cup, and since its original anterior wall is pressed backward, this wall constitutes the inner layer of the cup (Fig. 28-4, 3) and develops into the *nervous layer* of the retina. The outer wall of the vesicle becomes the *pigmented* (outer) *layer* of the retina, shown in black in Figure 28-4, 4.

The actively growing cells in the epithelial elements of the developing eye require a special blood supply and this is provided, as the eye forms, by an artery that enters by way of the optic stalk, called the *hyaloid artery* (Fig. 28-4, 3). This subsequently atrophies as other sources of blood supply develop. The origin of the *vitreous body* is not thoroughly understood; it is a jelly-like amorphous intercellular substance composed mostly of water, held in place by hyaluronic acid. There are also some fine collagenic fibrils in it.

The mesoderm surrounding the developing eye gives rise to both the *middle* and the *supporting layers* of the eye (Fig. 28-4). The *eyelids* develop as a result of two folds of ectoderm with plate-like cores of mesoderm extending over the developing cornea (Fig. 28-4). The substance of the *cornea* forms from mesoderm, but ectoderm persists over its anterior surface to form its epithelial covering (Fig. 28-4). The *anterior chamber* forms as a space in the mesoderm (Fig. 28-4). Epithelium from the optic vesicle continues forward to form a lining for the back of the ciliary body and the iris, both of which form from mesoderm (Fig. 28-4, 4).

THE MICROSCOPIC STRUCTURE OF THE PARTS OF THE EYE AND THEIR RELATION TO FUNCTION

THE CORNEA

The cornea is the anterior part of the supporting layer of the eye (Fig. 28-2A). It is *transparent* and *nonvascular*, and has a smaller radius of curvature than the remainder of the wall of the eye. Since it is exposed, the cornea is subject to cuts, abrasions, and other kinds of trauma. It is important in treating injuries of the cornea to know that it is about 0.5 mm. thick at its middle and somewhat thicker at its periphery.

The Layers of the Cornea. The cornea (Fig. 28-5) consists chiefly of a dense connective tissue called its *substantia propria;* this transmits light freely even though it comprises both intercellular substance and cells (Fig. 28-5, 3). The substantia propria is bordered both anteriorly and posteriorly by membranes of homogeneous intercellular substance (Fig. 28-5, 2 and 4). Anteriorly the cornea is covered with *stratified squamous nonkeratinizing epithelium* (Fig. 28-5, 1), and posteriorly it is lined by a *single layer of endothelial cells* (Fig. 28-5, 5).

The *epithelium* covering the cornea is several layers thick and is replete with *nerve endings,* chiefly of the pain type (Fig. 20-30A). Their stimulation results reflexly in blinking of the eyelids and flowing of tears. The anterior surface of the cornea must be *kept wet* with tears at all times, and mucus from the conjunctival glands may help in this respect. It is probably significant that the free surface of the epithelium on the front of the cornea bears numerous microvilli, similar to those on conjunctival cells (Fig. 28-25) and capable of retaining a film of tears over the corneal surface. If the nerve pathways concerned in the reflexes we have mentioned malfunction or become destroyed by disease, the wiping action of the wet inner surface of the eyelid over the corneal surface (not unlike cleaning a car windshield with the windshield wipers and washing fluid) becomes insufficient to maintain health of the cornea, so that the corneal surface becomes dry and may then ulcerate. The corneal epithelium is a relatively long way from a source of nutrition because the connective tissue beneath it has no capillaries. The diffusion on which its cells depend must nevertheless be effective, because corneal epithelium regenerates rapidly when damaged.

Beneath the corneal epithelium there is a well-developed *basement membrane.* Since corneal epithelium can be readily obtained from eyes of experimental animals, this epithelium has proved suitable for studying basement membrane formation. As mentioned in Chapter 8 in the discussion of how basement membranes are formed, Dodson and Hay have shown that on suitable substrates corneal epithelium is able to produce a basement membrane in vitro even after isolation from the other tissues of the eye, indicating that the basement membrane is a product of the epithelium itself. The epithelium is moreover capable of forming collagenic fibrils just like those seen in the corneal stroma. It is interesting that the epithelium nevertheless seems to require the close proximity of the lens capsule or of the corneal stroma (either dead or alive) for it to achieve its full potential for making basement membrane and collagenic (stromal) fibrils; artificial substrates of collagen alone, however, also support formation of these products to some extent (Dodson and Hay).

The acellular anterior layer of corneal stroma on which the basal lamina of the corneal epithelium rests is referred to as *Bowman's membrane* (Fig. 28-5, 2). This is a transparent homogeneous layer that in the EM is seen to contain collagenic fibrils in random array. It is regarded as constituting a protective barrier resistant to trauma and bacterial invasion; once destroyed it is not regenerated. Bowman's membrane does not extend from the cornea into the sclera; the site where it ends (which is also where the cornea undergoes transition into sclera) is called the *limbus* (L. for border).

The bulk of the corneal stroma, the *substantia propria,* comprises about 90 per cent of the full thickness of the cornea. It contains layers of flattened fibroblasts sandwiched in between something like 25 parallel layers (called *lamellae*) of collagenic fibers. These layers can be seen in the left part of Figure 28-5. The collagenic fibers of the lamellae are arranged parallel with the surface, with those in any given lamella lying at an angle to those in the next; also, fibers extend from some lamellae into adjacent ones so as to bind the layers of the substantia propria together. The collagenic fibers are embedded in a transparent matrix containing sulfated glycosaminoglycans.

Another homogeneous acellular layer, termed *Descemet's membrane* (Fig. 28-5, 4), lies posterior to the substantia propria. This layer is regarded as a highly developed basement membrane and contains collagen in a characteristic array (*see* Jakus). It belongs to the most posterior layer of the cornea, *Descemet's endothelium,* which is a single layer of cells that lines the inner aspect of the cornea (Fig. 28-5, 5). Scanning electron microscopy clearly reveals that its squamous cells have a hexagonal interdigitating outline (Fig. 28-6).

For further details of the fine structure of the cornea, *see* Sheldon and also Jakus.

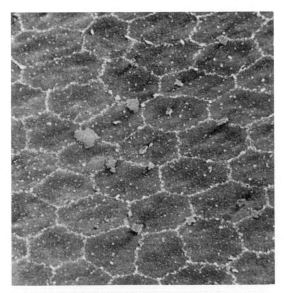

Fig. 28-6. Scanning electron micrograph of the endothelium lining the posterior surface of the cornea of a rabbit's eye. This discloses (in surface view) the regular hexagonal shape and fine lateral interdigitations of its flat cells. (The particles lying on the surface of the membrane are artifact.) (Courtesy of P. Basu)

Corneal Transplantation. Homografts (allografts) of cornea are used with considerable success. The main reason for this would seem to be that the cornea does not contain any blood vessels or typical lymphatics, but rather consists chiefly of intercellular substance. So the antigenicity of the cells that lie in the stroma remains undisclosed and any lymphocytes that might recognize these cells as antigenic are kept by the intercellular substance from having any contact with them. Basu et al., using both sex chromatin (Barr body) as a marker and karyotypic analysis, showed that in experimental animals and also in people the original cells of homografts persist; hence the cells in the stroma of the corneal graft are not replaced by ones from the host. Indeed, they have shown that in one patient the original cells of the graft stroma were still present six years afterward.

THE SCLERA

The sclera is a tough, white, connective tissue layer comprising bundles of collagenic fibers with flattened fibroblasts between the bundles (Fig. 28-7). Some elastic fibers are mixed with the collagenic ones. The fibers are not arranged as regularly as in the substantial propria and the matrix in which they are embedded is of somewhat different composition. The sclera is thick enough to permit its being sutured from the outside without the needle penetrating into the middle layer of the wall of the eye. Moreover, it is strong enough in adults to withstand very high intraocular pressure, should this condition occur, without stretching.

The relative opacity of the sclera, as compared with the cornea, is due to a very important degree to its greater water content. This can be shown very dramatically by blowing a jet of air on an exposed portion of sclera, for this makes it completely transparent. The reason the cornea remains transparent is that water (tissue fluid) is continuously removed from its surfaces, so if either of its surfaces becomes damaged, it may become opaque in that area. For example, if some of the vitreous comes and stays in contact with its posterior surface of any point, the cornea becomes opaque at that point.

It is important in connection with testing the intraocular pressure of the eye by means of a tonometer to know that the scleras of different eyes are rigid to different degrees; hence, if the rigidity of the sclera is extreme, it may give an erroneous pressure reading.

At the posterior part of the eye the outermost part of the sclera is continuous with the dural sheath and usually with the arachnoid sheath also of the optic nerve (Fig. 28-3). Moreover, the innermost layer of the sclera, in the form of a perforated disk, bridges what would otherwise be a gap in the sclera, and through this the optic nerve leaves the eye (Fig. 28-22). The fibers of the optic nerve pass through the perforations of the disk, so this part of the sclera is called the *lamina cribrosa* (L. *cribrum,* sieve).

Blood Supply. The sclera as a whole, being composed of dense connective tissue, is poorly supplied with capillaries. However, many larger vessels pierce it obliquely to gain entrance to the middle layer of the eye. These vessels pass through the sclera in a more or less anterior direction (Fig. 28-3). The anterior ciliary arteries enter beside (or slightly in front of) the ciliary body (Fig. 28-3), and both short and long posterior ciliary arteries pass through the sclera behind the equator (Fig. 28-3). The long posterior ciliary arteries, on entering the middle coat of the eye, take a direct course to the ciliary body; the short ones branch. Four large vortex veins draining most of the blood from the middle coat pass obliquely backward through the sclera near the equator (Fig. 28-3). The ciliary arteries have companion veins.

THE CHOROID

The choroid is that part of the middle layer of the eye behind the ciliary body. It is only 0.1 to 0.2 mm. thick and consists of three layers, as follows.

The Epichoroid. This, its outer layer, consists chiefly of elastic fibers attached to the sclera. Many nerve fibers that terminate on *chromatophores* are present in it. The chromatophores are large pigmented cells seen (though not labeled) in Figure 28-18. Some have irregular shapes with processes like an ameba. Whether this pigment is produced by these cells or taken up from pigment produced in the retina has been questioned. But during a short phase of early fetal life, before pigment is present, the future pigment cells of the choroid have been found to be dopa-positive. This suggests that melanin is produced by the pigment cells of the choroid and thereafter stored *in situ.* It is interesting that melanin pigment recovered from the uveal tract has different antigenic properties from that of other parts of the body.

Through the epichoroid run the two unbranching long posterior ciliary arteries. A few smooth muscle fibers are present in this layer in its anterior part; these represent the beginning of the ciliary muscle.

The Vessel Layer. The choroidal vessels supplied by the short posterior ciliary arteries and drained by the vortex veins lie in this, the middle layer of the choroid (Fig. 28-18). The stroma is similar to that of the epichoroid.

The Choriocapillaris. This, the inner layer of the choroid network (Fig. 28-18), consists of a single layer of capillaries that are among the largest in the body. Some, especially those outside the macula (to be described presently), are as wide as sinusoids; these permit rapid transfer of blood from the arterial to the venous side.

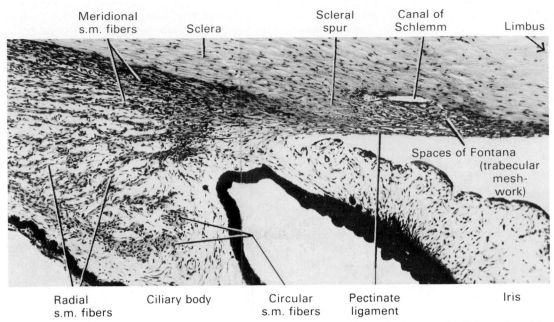

Fig. 28-7. Photomicrograph of the area seen at *left* in Figure 28-14A, illustrating in more detail the region of the angle of the iris. For orientation, Figure 28-14A should first be examined.

Bruch's Membrane. Separating the choriocapillaris from the outer coat of the retina, there is a glassy membrane known as *Bruch's membrane.* This has both elastic and basement membrane components, formed by the choroid and the retina, respectively. Bruch's membrane is semipermeable, and through it and the retinal pigmented epithelium pass the essential metabolites for the photoreceptors.

THE CILIARY BODY

The three strata of the choroid are continuous anteriorly with the ciliary body. This extends forward to a site where a narrow, short flange of sclera, called the *scleral spur,* projects inward (Figs. 28-3 and 28-7). The ciliary body, as a thickening of the middle coat of the eye, forms a ring on the inner surface of the sclera behind the scleral spur (Figs. 28-3 and 28-7). When an eye is cut longitudinally, the ring is cut in cross section. In cross section it appears as a triangle, with its base facing the anterior chamber and its apex passing into the choroid posteriorly (Fig. 28-3). The elastic epichoroid, in the ciliary body, is replaced by fibers of ciliary muscle. These are of the smooth variety and comprise the bulk of the ciliary body (Fig. 28-7).

The smooth muscle fibers of the ciliary body are disposed so as to pull in three different directions. Accordingly, three groups of fibers are distinguished: (*1*) the *meridional fibers* (a meridian of a globe runs from pole to pole, crossing the equator at right angles), which arise in the epichoroid near the ciliary body and pass forward to end in the scleral spur (Fig. 28-7); (*2*) the *radial fibers,* which are farther in than the meridional fibers and fan out posteriorly to make a wide attachment to the connective tissue of the choroid (Fig. 28-7); and (*3*) the *circular* fibers, which lie near the inner edge of the ciliary body near its base and are arranged so as to encircle the eye at this site (Fig. 28-7).

To understand how contraction of smooth muscle fibers in the ciliary body affects the shape of the lens, certain features of the lens and the mechanism by which it is suspended must be described.

THE LENS

Development. The first step in the development of the lens is that the ectoderm overlying the optic vesicle becomes thickened (lens ectoderm, Fig. 28-4, 1). The thickened ectoderm then bulges inward to form the *lens vesicle* (Fig. 28-4, 2). The vesicle then becomes pinched off from the surface ectoderm, and as a result becomes a hollow structure with a posterior wall that is much thicker (being composed of tall columnar cells) than its anterior wall (Fig. 28-4, 3). The cavity within the lens vesicle is more or less crescent-shaped and eventually becomes obliterated. The vesicle after becoming detached from the

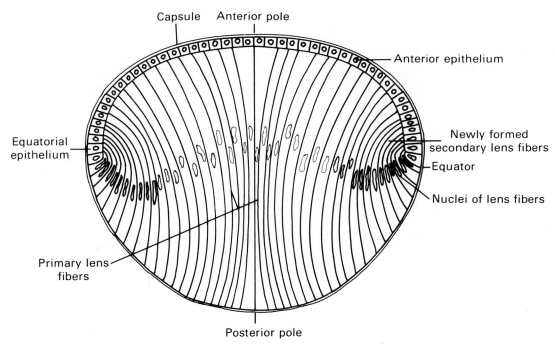

Fig. 28-8. Diagram of developing lens of the eye, in horizontal section. (Courtesy of M. Hollenberg)

ectoderm moves inward and gradually assumes a biconcave form (Fig. 28-4, 4).

Differentiation of Lens Cells Into Fibers. The lens becomes a transparent structure because the epithelial cells of which it is composed differentiate into what are termed *lens fibers;* in this process their nuclei disappear. The first epithelial cells to differentiate are those of the posterior layer of the vesicle; these become *primary lens fibers,* as shown in Figure 28-8). However, the epithelial cells of the anterior wall of the original lens vesicle (these are shown on the upper half of the lens in Fig. 28-8 and labeled *anterior epithelium*) remain intact, and indeed they proliferate, since mitotic figures are seen among them easily during fetal development.

Growth of the Lens. At the equator the columnar cells of the anterior layer provide an appositional growth mechanism. However, at the equator the covering of the lens by columnar cells of the anterior layer terminates (Fig. 28-8, equator). Growth of the lens occurs here because the last (most posterior) cells of the epithelium elongate and becomes transformed into lens fibers; these are called *secondary fibers* to distinguish them from the primary fibers that form from the posterior epithelium (Fig. 28-8). Since the growth process occurs beneath the lens capsule, the epithelial cells can be accommodated as they elongate only by their becoming bent inward, as is shown in Figure 28-8. As each cell in becoming a fiber increases in length,

its bent form subsequently becomes straightened out to some extent, as can be seen in the deeper secondary fibers that have been covered by younger ones (Fig. 28-8).

The lens grows because epithelial cells of the anterior layer at the region of the equator continue to differentiate into lens fibers that are added (beneath the capsule) to the periphery of the lens just posterior to the equator. The cells of the anterior layer, by proliferating and moving to the equator, serve as progenitor cells for the formation of new fibers, but they differentiate into fibers only at the equator. As a result of new fibers being added at this site, the lens increases in diameter.

Lens fibers last a lifetime, which is remarkable because all the epithelial cells that participate in its formation remain. There is no loss of fibers from the lens; hence there is no cell turnover to maintain it. There is only addition of further fibers through life.

Before an epithelial lens cell becomes a fiber, it has a nucleus and most of the usual cytoplasmic organelles. In the transformation of a lens cell into a lens fiber, its nuclear chromatin fades away, nucleoli disappear, and the nuclear envelope develops blebs and apparently dissolves. About the only organelles that persist are a few longitudinally disposed microtubules (Fig. 28-9, MT) and clumps of free ribosomes (Fig. 28-9, R). The remainder of the fiber appears granular of the EM (Fig. 28-9), and contains the characteristic proteins of the fibers, the crys-

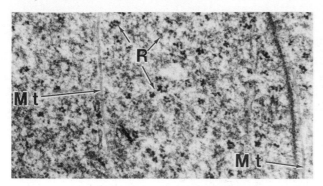

Fig. 28-9. Electron micrograph (×30,000) of part of a lens fiber, from an eye of a rat fetus, in longitudinal section. Microtubules (Mt) lie parallel to the long axis of the fiber. Free ribosomes, single or in aggregates (R), lie scattered about in the substance of the fiber. (Willis, N. R., Hollenberg, M. J., and Braekevelt, C. R.: Can. J. Ophthalmol., *4*:307, 1969)

tallines. However, protein synthesis seems to continue in the newly formed lens fibers. Since the nucleus has gone, continued protein synthesis would require long-lived messenger RNA.

The Lens Capsule. Essentially this is a very thick, well-

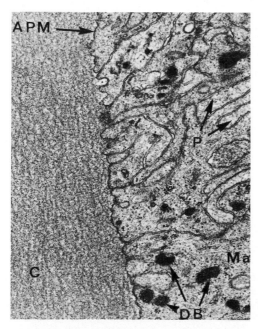

Fig. 28-10. Electron micrograph of lens capsule and adjacent epithelium from an eye of a rat fetus. C, lens capsule; APM, thickened and infolded cell membrane of epithelial cells forming the capsule; P, interdigitating lateral processes of contiguous epithelial cells; DB, dense bodies; and Ma, cytoplasmic matrix. (Willis, N. R., Hollenberg, M. J., and Braekevelt, C. R.: Can. J. Ophthalmol., *4*:307, 1969)

developed basement membrane with an abundance of reticular fibers. It is formed by the epithelial lens cells. In addition to the usual collagen and glycoproteins of basement membranes it contains sulfated glycosaminoglycan. Like basement membranes in general, it is rich in macromolecular carbohydrate components and hence stains brilliantly with the PAS technic.

When the epithelial cells are forming the lens capsule, their cell membranes interdigitate extensively (P in Fig. 28-10) and the membrane on their free surface is thickened (APM in Fig. 28-10). Here delicate laminae of fibrillar material become added successively to the forming capsule (Fig. 28-10).

The lens capsule is under tension forces that tend to make the lens assume a more or less globular form. However, water loss as the lens ages renders it less elastic so that the range of focus achieved by the lens becomes diminished, making spectacles necessary for many for focusing on near objects.

THE ZONULE

The lens is attached to the ciliary body by means of the *zonule* (Fig. 28-3, *upper right,* z). The zonule is composed of filaments, fibers and bundles of fibers (Fig. 28-11). It is sometimes called the *suspensory ligament of the lens.*

The zonule has a broad zone of attachment both to the capsule, at the equator of the lens, and to the ciliary body (Fig. 28-3, *left* side, not labeled, but labeled z in the enlarged view in the *inset*).

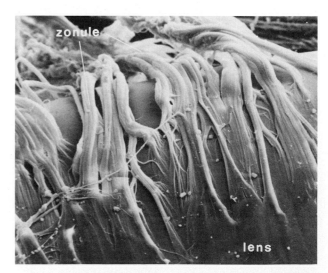

Fig. 28-11. Scanning electron micrograph of a portion of the zonule, attached to the periphery of the lens, from a monkey's eye. Note the large bundles of fibers attached to the capsule of the lens below. (Courtesy of P. Basu)

Mechanism of Accommodation. It might be thought that contraction of smooth muscle of the ciliary body would pull on the zonule and hence on the equator of the lens so that the lens would become flatter and hence accommodated for distant objects. Actually, the contraction has the *opposite* effect. Instead of tensing the zonule, contraction of the muscle of the ciliary body, the muscle fibers of which are firmly attached to the sclera in the region of the scleral spur, pulls the part of the ciliary body to which the zonule is attached *forward* and *inward*. Since the attachment of the zonule to the ciliary body is posterior to its site of attachment to the lens, this action *relaxes the tension in the zonule* and permits the lens, which is itself under tension from its capsule, to assume a more globular shape, and hence become *accommodated* for close objects. It is to be noted, then, that muscular contraction is required for viewing close objects; this is one reason why reading "tires" the eyes more than viewing distant objects.

THE IRIS

The *iris* is a colored disk with a central, variable aperture, the *pupil* (Fig. 28-12). It is not a flat disk, for the lens pushes against its central part (the *pupillary margin*) from behind so that this is more anterior than its periphery (Fig. 28-3).

The space behind the iris, and elsewhere limited by the lens, the vitreous body, and the ciliary body, is called the *posterior chamber* of the eye (Fig. 28-3); the space in front of the iris (and at the pupil, in front of the lens), and otherwise limited by the cornea and the most anterior part of the sclera, is called the *anterior chamber* of the eye (Fig. 28-3). Both the anterior and the posterior chambers are filled with a fluid called *aqueous humor.* A certain amount of circulation takes place in this fluid. In all probability the fluid is formed in the posterior chamber and then passes into the anterior chamber, from which it is resorbed by mechanisms to be described presently. Since the posterior border of the pupillary margin of the iris and the anterior surface of the lens press against each other, the iris acts like a valve in that fluid from the posterior chamber can force the pupillary margin of the iris away from the anterior surface of the lens to enter the anterior chamber, but fluid tending to move in the reverse direction presses the pupillary margin of the iris against the lens and so closes the opening between the two chambers. Posteriorly, the iris is lined by two layers of *pigmented epithelial cells* continuous with the two layers of retinal epithelium that line the ciliary body (Fig. 28-7). Anteriorly, the iris is covered imperfectly with *squamous endothelial cells* comparable and continuous with those of Descemet's endothelium.

The iris (Fig. 28-7) is well supplied with *blood vessels*

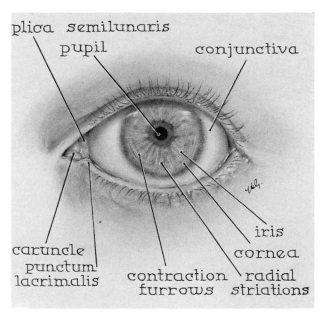

Fig. 28-12. The parts of an eye, as seen from the front.

and networks of *nerve fibers.* The arteries, branches of the major arterial circle, course spirally through its stroma like a corkscrew, so that their lumina are not much affected by changes in the diameter of the iris. They have a thick collagenous adventitia that prevents kinking when the spirals are compressed and also makes the vessels appear as radiating gray lines in pale or blue irises. Throughout the stroma are scattered *chromatophores,* concentrated mostly at the anterior border (Fig. 28-7). The vessels do not extend to this border.

Encircling the pupil, about 1.5 mm. from its margin, is a scalloped line formed by regression of the membrane that extended across the pupil in embryonic life (Fig. 28-12). This line divides the iris into a *pupillary* and a *ciliary portion* (Fig. 28-12). Crypts opening anteriorly are found in the pupillary portion; they form as a result of incomplete atrophy of the pupillary membrane. Shorter crypts are found in the anterior surface of the ciliary portion. The contraction furrows (Fig. 28-12) appear as deeper folds encircling the anterior surface of the iris.

The *muscle fibers* of the iris are derived from the anterior cells of the pigmented epithelial layer, a continuation of the outer retinal layer. The *constrictor of the pupil* is a sphincter-like muscle composed of circularly arranged smooth muscle fibers near the pupillary margin. The force with which the iris is held against the anterior surface of the lens depends on the tone in these fibers. The *dilator of the pupil* is less distinct and consists of a thin sheet of radial fibers near the back of the iris. These fibers are not

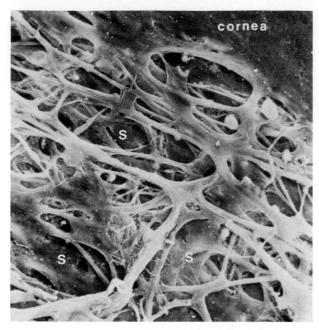

Fig. 28-13. Scanning electron micrograph of the trabecular meshwork of the scleral furrow, from a monkey's eye, as seen from inside the anterior chamber of the eye. The endothelium covering the trabeculae, and hence lining the trabecular spaces (S), becomes continuous at *upper right* with that lining the posterior surface of the cornea. The canal of Schlemm would lie deep to this network. In life the trabecular spaces would contain aqueous humor. (Courtesy of P. Basu)

typical smooth muscle fibers and are considered to be *myoepithelial cells.*

Pupillary size is automatically controlled by a nervous reflex in which the *retina* is the *receptor* organ, and the *muscles of the iris* the *effectors.* When an individual looks at a bright object, the pupil is reflexly constricted, thereby decreasing the amount of light that enters the eye, and vice versa. To anyone familiar with photography the pupillary size has a further significance. A dilated pupil, like a dilated aperture in a camera, results in diminished depth of focus. For this reason, glasses prescribed when the pupil is dilated are likely to be more accurate than those prescribed when the pupil is not.

The *color* of the iris is due to melanin pigment. As noted in discussing the color of skin, melanin pigment, seen through a substantial thickness of tissue, appears blue. Hence, if the melanin pigment in the iris is limited to the epithelial cells that line its posterior surface, the iris (provided that the stroma anterior to the pigment is of usual density) appears blue. If the stroma is somewhat denser than usual, the pigment at the back of the iris gives a gray color to the iris. If sufficient pigment is present in chromatophores in the substance of the stroma as well as

in the epithelium at the back of the iris, the iris appears brown. In the white race the final color of the iris is not necessarily developed at the time of birth.

THE REGION OF THE ANGLE OF THE IRIS

The site at which the sclera becomes continuous with the cornea, as noted, is called the *limbus* (Fig. 28-7). Immediately behind it the internal surface of the sclera is thrown into a ridge, the *scleral spur,* that extends inward and forward (Fig. 28-7) and encircles the eye. Immediately in front of the scleral spur a furrow dips into the inner layer of the sclera; this is called the *scleral furrow* (in Fig. 28-7 this is labeled *spaces of Fontana*) and it, too, encircles the eye. At the bottom of the furrow there is a canal (or group of anastomosing canals) lined by endothelium. This is called the *canal of Schlemm* (Fig. 28-7), and it, too, encircles the eye. In a meridional section, the scleral spur, the scleral furrow, and the canal of Schlemm are all cut in cross section (Fig. 28-7).

The scleral furrow is filled in (over the canal at its bottom) with a loose trabecular meshwork of connective tissue (Fig. 28-13); this extends from the cornea, at the anterior side of the furrow, backward to the anterior border of the sclera spur. The spaces in the meshwork were in the past called *spaces of Fontana* (labeled in Fig. 28-7), and they communicate with the anterior chamber. The spaces are now commonly referred to as *trabecular spaces.* They are lined with endothelium continuous with that lining the cornea (Fig. 28-13) and covering the anterior surface of the iris. Hence, aqueous humor is present in the trabecular spaces. The middle (uveal) coat of the eye extends forward to provide a lining for the wall of the eye between the iris and the scleral spur. In certain species this lining is strong and well developed and called the *pectinate ligament.* Sometimes this name is also used for its relatively undeveloped counterpart in man (Fig. 28-7).

THE CILIARY PROCESSES

About 75 little ridges (each about 2 mm. long, 0.5 mm. wide, and about 1 mm. high) project inward from the ciliary body, immediately behind its junction with the iris, into the posterior chamber of the eye. These are termed the *ciliary processes,* and a few are usually to be seen in a single longitudinal section of an eye (Fig. 28-14A).

As indicated in Figure 28-2B, the cores of ciliary processes are the counterparts of choriocapillaris, since they consist chiefly of capillaries supported by delicate connective tissue (Fig. 28-14B). The processes are covered with two layers of epithelium representing a continuation of the two layers of the retina forward (compare drawings B and C in Fig. 28-2). The cells of the deeper of the two layers are pigmented (Fig. 28-14B). The superficial layer

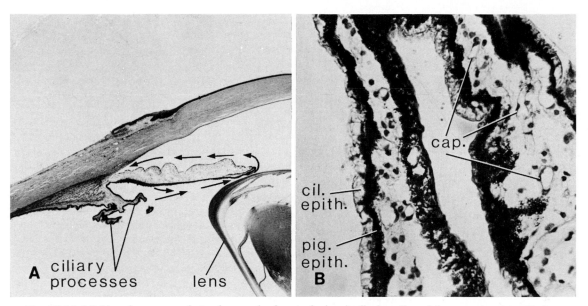

Fig. 28-14. (*A*) Very low power photomicrograph of part of a longitudinal section of the eye, showing ciliary processes. The arrows indicate the course of circulation of the aqueous humor. (*B*) High-power photomicrograph of ciliary processes (in a rabbit's eye). Note the large capillaries (cap.) in the loose connective tissue of the stroma. The superficial layer of the process is known as the ciliary epithelium (cil. epith.), and the layer deep to it, the pigmented layer of the epithelium (pig. epith.).

is called the *ciliary epithelium* (cil. epith. in Fig. 28-14). The epithelial layer, as a whole, rests on a membrane continuous with Bruch's membrane that separates the epithelium from the vascular stroma of the processes.

The ciliary epithelium, which abuts on the aqueous humor, contains many deep folds of cell membrane, and its free surface is covered with a basement membrane, features that conceivably might be involved in the secretion of aqueous humor.

THE AQUEOUS HUMOR

Formation, Circulation, and Absorption. Aqueous humor is a thin watery fluid containing most of the diffusable substances of blood plasma. The albumin to globulin ratio is the same in both aqueous humor and serum, but serum has a protein content of 7 per cent, whereas aqueous humor contains only 0.02 per cent. Like serum, aqueous humor contains no fibrinogen and therefore cannot clot. It has been a matter of controversy whether it should be regarded primarily as a dialysate of blood plasma, comparable with tissue fluid, or as a secretion. For one thing, it is *hypertonic* in relation to blood, and in all probability not only factors concerned in tissue fluid formation and absorption (hydrostatic and osmotic pressure), but specific cellular activities as well, participate in controlling its quality and rate of formation and absorption (*see* Friedenwald).

Although thin and watery, aqueous humor also contains some hyaluronic acid. Studies made on eyes of cattle indicate that the hyaluronic acid is about 95 per cent depolymerized and this is probably the reason why the aqueous humor has such a low viscosity.

Although the general principles of formation and absorption of tissue fluid (explained in Chap. 8) are fundamental to understanding the formation and absorption of aqueous humor, there are certain differences in the mechanism operating in the eye from that in most tissues. These are due to the tissue fluid in the eye being under considerably greater pressure than in most sites in the body. In most sites the tissues surrounding capillaries are not under great tension; hence, a relatively low hydrostatic pressure in the capillaries is sufficient to drive tissue fluid out through their walls at their arterial ends. Correspondingly, the tissue substance in which blood vessels are embedded is under little tension, so that venules are not compressed, even though the hydrostatic pressure within them is extremely low. However, surrounded by a tough, inelastic, fibrous tunic, the contents of the eye are under constant pressure; the usual *intraocular pressure* ranges from about 20 to 25 mm. of mercury. This requires, then, that the blood within the capillaries of the eye be under a considerably greater hydrostatic pressure than the general intraocular pressure if the osmotic pressure of the colloids of the plasma is to be overcome and tissue fluid (aqueous humor) elaborated. Furthermore, it requires that the blood in intraocular veins also be under considerable hydrostatic pressure; otherwise, the veins within the eye would collapse due to the intraocular pressure.

Although it is possible that any capillaries close to the anterior or the posterior chambers could contribute to formation and absorption of aqueous humor, it is highly probable that the capillaries of the *ciliary processes,* and to a much lesser extent those at the back of the iris, elaborate most of it. It is not unlikely that the hyaluronic acid of the aqueous humor is also formed in the delicate connective tissue constituting the cores of the ciliary processes. The most important mechanism for the absorption of aqueous humor is situated in the angle of the iris and will be described presently.

It is to be noted that, since the fibrous tunic of the eye cannot stretch, and since structures within the eye are normally of constant size and incompressible, a normal intraocular pressure depends on a proper balance being maintained between formation and absorption of aqueous humor. If conditions should develop in the anterior part of the eye that in another part of the body would cause edema—for example, interference with the absorption of tissue fluid—the eye cannot swell; instead, the *intraocular pressure becomes increased.* An increase in intraocular pressure sufficient to be incompatible with continued health of the eye constitutes the condition *glaucoma,* and it is obvious that treatment of the condition would be directed toward increasing the absorption of aqueous humor and/or decreasing its production.

Although under certain conditions aqueous humor can be both produced and removed very rapidly, it appears that under normal conditions it is formed and absorbed slowly, probably at about the rate of 2 cu. mm. a minute. After aqueous humor is formed, it passes from the posterior chamber, between the lens and the iris, to enter the anterior chamber (Fig. 28-14). There it moves toward the angle of the iris, where most of it enters the trabecular spaces (Fig. 28-13), from which it is absorbed into the canal of Schlemm.

The *canal of Schlemm* (Fig. 28-7) probably has no direct communication with the trabecular spaces. Hence aqueous humor, to enter the canal, must pass through the endothelium lining the spaces, a thin layer of connective tissue, and the endothelium lining the canal. The canal contains aqueous humor and this drains outward through *collector trunks* in the sclera. These channels pass out under the bulbar conjunctiva, where they are known as *aqueous veins* because they contain aqueous humor; in this position they may be seen with a slit lamp microscope (mentioned again later) during life. The aqueous veins connect with blood-containing veins, so that eventually aqueous humor is emptied into the venous system. Interference with the flow of aqueous humor in the collector trunks and aqueous veins may be a factor in glaucoma. After death, blood may back up into the aqueous and collecting veins and into the canal of Schlemm, so that it may be seen in these sites in sections.

THE VITREOUS BODY

The *vitreous body* is a mass of transparent gelled amorphous intercellular substance sometimes referred to as *vitreous humor;* the cells responsible for its formation are not known with certainty. It is bounded by the internal limiting membrane of the retina (to be described in due course), the lens, and the posterior aspect of the zonule (Fig. 28-3). In addition to transmitting light, its bulk helps, anteriorly, to hold the lens in place and, posteriorly, to keep the inner coat of the retina in apposition with the outer pigmented coat. If any of the vitreous body is lost, as occurs unavoidably in some surgical procedures, the two latter coats of the retina may become separated. The vitreous humor also plays a role in metabolism of the retina, allowing transfer of metabolites through it.

Through the vitreous body runs the *hyaloid canal* (*Cloquet's canal*), the remnant of the hyaloid artery of the embryonic eye (Fig. 28-4, 3). Since it marks the position of the primitive hyaloid artery it is said to represent *primary* vitreous humor (Fig. 28-4, 4). Cloquet's canal runs from the papilla of the optic nerve, described later in this chapter, toward the posterior surface of the lens and is usually inconspicuous in life (Fig. 28-3). In some instances the primitive hyaloid structures persist and may interfere with vision.

The vitreous body is denser at its periphery, where it is adherent to the internal limiting membrane of the retina over all its surface, but it is particularly adherent at the papilla. It is also adherent to the posterior surface of the lens near its edge.

The Composition of the Vitreous Body. The vitreous body is a hydrophilic colloidal system. The dispersed phase of the system probably consists both of a complex protein (*vitrein*), which has marked hygroscopic qualities, and *hyaluronic acid.* It contains the crystalloids normally dissolved in aqueous humor. Under normal conditions the vitreous humor is gelled and transparent. However, it is denatured by fixation, and then exhibits a fibrillar structure when seen in the LM. The gel is seen in the EM to be supported by a loose network of dispersed collagenic fibrils. It was believed that lost vitreous humor was not replaced, but Pirie has shown that it re-forms in rabbits.

THE RETINA

In describing the layers of the retina the terms *inner* and *outer* are used (as they are with regard to the layers of the wall of the eye) with reference to the *center* and the *exterior* of the eye. Hence, the *inner* of any two layers of the wall of the eye, or of any two layers of the retina itself, is the layer *closer to the center* of the eye.

The *retina* develops from the *optic vesicle* (an outgrowth from the brain), and at first consists of two main layers because the anterior wall of the optic vesicle (Fig. 28-4, 1) becomes invaginated backward into its posterior half to make a two-layered *optic cup* (Fig. 28-4, 2, 3, and 4). The outer layer of the cup develops into a layer of *pigmented epithelium* (labeled in Fig. 28-15). The inner and thicker layer becomes adherent to this layer of pigmented epithelium and develops into *nervous tissue* and thereafter becomes responsible for vision.

It is of practical importance to note here that during development there is a cleft between the two layers of the invaginated optic cup. Although the pigmented epithelium (which develops from the outer layer) and the nervous tissue (which develops from the inner layer) of the invaginated cup eventually meet and become adherent to one another, the attachment of the outer layer to the choroid is much stronger than its attachment to the inner nervous layer. Indeed, in postnatal life conditions may develop under which part of the inner (nervous) layer becomes *separated* from the outer pigmented epithelial layer; this is referred to as a *detached retina* (even though it is a separation of the two parts of the retina). Since the nervous portion of the retina depends on nutrients from the choroid diffusing through the pigmented epithelium of the retina, a detached nervous portion undergoes degenerative changes unless it is successfully restored to its normal position, which can be achieved by appropriate surgical procedures.

Of practical importance also is that in preparing sections of the eye for histological study, the lack of strong attachment between the epithelial and nervous parts of the retina can result in the same two layers pulling apart during fixation, as occurred for example in the eye section illustrated in Figure 28-22.

The Basic Histological Components of the Nervous Portion of the Retina. First, since the eye is a sensory organ there must be sensory cells in the retina. Actually there are two kinds, called *rods* and *cones*. Both are long, narrow cells but they were given these names because of the shape of their *long free ends*. These ends extend a short distance into the pigmented epithelium; thus they point *outward* as shown in Figures 28-15, and 28-19, *bottom* (where five rods and one cone are shown). The sensory function of these cells depends on the photoreceptor properties of their free ends, as will be described in detail presently. On the other side of its nucleus, each photoreceptor cell has an axon that passes inward (Fig. 28-15). Here the axons of the rods and cones synapse with dendrites of a second order of nerve cells. Some of these are horizontal cells (H in Fig. 28-16), but the point to make here is that the axons

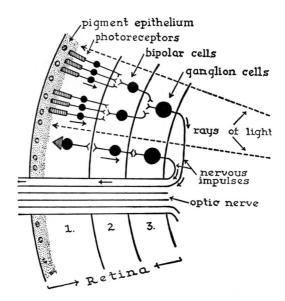

Fig. 28-15. Diagram illustrating the basic arrangement of the three orders of neurons in the nervous portion of the retina. Note that light rays and nerve impulses travel in opposite directions through the retina.

of the rods and cones synapse with the dendrites of a second layer of nerve cells that lies just internal to the rods and cones. These are called *bipolar cells.* (Fig. 28-15) because each has a dendrite that points toward and synapses with the axons of rods or cones and at its other end has an axon that passes inward. These axons in turn synapse with more or less horizontally disposed nerve cells (Fig. 28-16), to be described presently, and also with nerve cells of a third order, termed *ganglion cells* (Fig. 28-15). The latter were given this name not because they are in ganglia but because they superficially resemble the cells seen in ganglia. The ganglion cells have non-myelinated axons that on reaching the inner surface of the retina make a right-angled turn (Fig. 28-15) and pass to the site of exit of the *optic nerve,* the fibers of which are the *unmyelinated axons of the ganglion cells.*

There are some basic points to make from the foregoing preliminary description.

First, to affect the rod- and cone-like processes of the photoreceptors, as shown in Figure 28-15, light from the vitreous body must pass through the inner two layers of nerve cells of the retina (the ganglion cells and bipolar cells) and then through the cell bodies of the photoreceptors themselves to reach their photoreceptive ends. Then, when these are stimulated by light, the excitation set up must travel in the reverse direction, *inward,* through the bipolar and ganglion cells to the innermost part of the retina and from here, along the axons of the ganglion cells, to

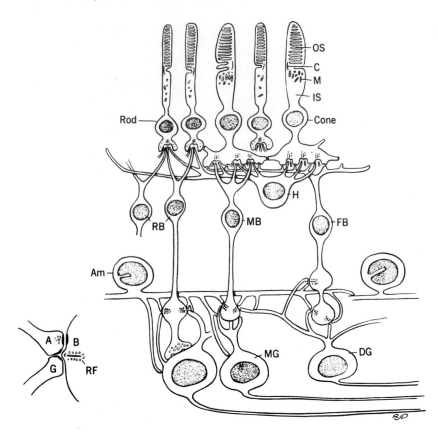

Fig. 28-16. Schematic diagram illustrating the detailed arrangements of nerve cells in the nervous portion of the retina. The photoreceptor outer segments (OS), which face the pigmented epithelium, are shown at the *top* of this drawing; hence light enters the retina from *below*. Representative synaptic arrangements between photoreceptors, interneurons, and ganglion cells in the retina are indicated. For detailed description, *see* text. For the parts of the cone labeled here, *see* the caption to Figure 28-20. The nerve cells illustrated are as follows: rods; cones; rod bipolar cells (RB); midget bipolar cells (MB); flat bipolar cells (FB); horizontal cells (H); amacrine cells (Am); midget ganglion cells (MG); and diffuse ganglion cells (DG). (*Inset, lower left*) Diagram of a ribbon synapse. This kind of synapse is found between (*1*) a bipolar cell (B) and (*2*) an amacrine cell (A) and also a ganglion cell (G). Note its ribbon filament (RF) with associated synaptic vesicles. (From The Human Nervous System, Basic Principles of Neurobiology, ed. 2, by C. R. Noback and R. J. Demarest. Copyright © 1975, McGraw-Hill Book Company. Adapted from Dowling and Boycott, 1966, by Noback, C. R., and Laemle, L. K. *In* The Primate Brain, Appleton-Century-Crofts, Inc., 1970. Used with permission of McGraw-Hill Book Company)

the site of exit of the optic nerve (Fig. 28-15). Obviously, for this arrangement to be functional, the nerve cells and their processes need to allow light to pass freely across them without distortion. Finally, light waves and the nerve impulses from the photoreceptors are transmitted in *opposite directions* through the retina.

Details of the Synaptic Connections Between the Nerve Cells in the Nervous Portion of the Retina. As may be seen in Figure 18-15, there are more rods and cones than bipolar cells, and more bipolar cells than ganglion cells. This provides a basis for summation of the afferent impulses from the photoreceptors before these impulses are relayed by the ganglion cells to the brain. Other aspects of vision also seem to depend on there being direct nervous communication at the retinal level between the different parts of the retina. To serve this purpose there are more or less horizontally arranged interneurons at two levels, which are shown in Figure 28-16. First, at about the level where the axons of the rods and cones synapse with the dendrites of the bipolar cells (labeled **RB, MB,** and **FB** in Fig. 28-16), there are what are termed *horizontal cells* (H, about one third of the way down in Fig. 28-16). As may be seen in this diagram, the axons of rod cells have

synaptic connections with these cells as well as with *rod bipolar cells* (RB). At this same level the axons of cones also have synaptic connections with *horizontal cells* (H) as well as with both *midget bipolar cells* (MB) and *flat bipolar cells* (FB). Then, more or less at the level where the axons of the bipolar cells synapse with the ganglion cells (about two thirds of the way down in Fig. 28-16), there are what are termed *amacrine cells* (Gr. *a,* without; *makros,* long; *inos,* fiber, meaning that they have no long fiber); these cells are generally regarded as having no axon, only dendrites. Amacrine cells (Am) are in synaptic connection with all types of bipolar cells and with ganglion cells, as depicted in the lower third of Figure 28-16. The *ganglion cells* are classified into two groups, *midget* and *diffuse* (MG and DG in Fig. 28-16).

As may be seen by carefully studying Figure 28-16, many of the synaptic contacts in the retina are of a curious type known as a *ribbon synapse.* Their characteristic feature is an electron-dense *synaptic ribbon* (*bar*), which is labeled RF (for ribbon filament) in the enlarged diagram at *bottom left* in Figure 28-16. The synapse illustrated here is a complex one between a presynaptic terminal of a bipolar cell (B) at *right* and postsynaptic terminals belonging to both an amacrine cell (A) at *upper left* and a ganglion cell (G) at *lower left*. The presynaptic terminal in such a synaptic arrangement must divide its synaptic activities so as to stimulate both of these postsynaptic terminals. At the inner ends of the cones (one third of the way down in Fig. 28-16), the synaptic arrangements are even more elaborate. Here, multiple synapses each commonly require presynaptic activity to be distributed to groups of three postsynaptic terminals. The ribbon synapse is regarded as a structural specialization for permitting multiple synaptic transmission. As shown in the enlarged view at *bottom left* in Figures 28-16, the synaptic ribbon is a rod-like structure that lies perpendicular to the presynaptic membrane, directly behind a synaptic ridge between the paired postsynaptic terminals. It is characteristically surrounded by synaptic vesicles and seems to play a part in guiding these vesicles toward both postsynaptic membranes at the same time.

The Supporting Cells of the Nervous Portion of the Retina. As might be expected, not only nerve cells but also glia differentiate in the nervous portion of the retina. The noticeable glial cells here lie perpendicular to the retinal surface and, because first described by Müller, are known as *radial cells of Müller*. These are long and narrow in shape and their elongated nucleus lies more or less at the level of the nuclei of the bipolar cells. Müller cells, which are generally pale-staining (Fig. 28-17), extend outward beyond the photoreceptor nuclei to abut on the photoreceptor cells; here they are connected to the rods and cones by junctional complexes (Fig. 28-17). So much filamentous material is associated with these complexes that the row of them seen at this level (Fig. 28-17) was erroneously interpreted with the LM as being a membrane; indeed, this was termed the *outer limiting membrane* of the retina (labeled in Fig. 28-19). Its true nature was established only when the EM became available. The outer end of Müller cells is further characterized by having large numbers of long microvilli that project down into the intercellular spaces between rods and cones (Fig. 28-17).

The Ten Layers of the Retina. From studies with the LM it became customary to describe the retina as having ten layers. It should be understood, however, that nearly all of these are not true layers that can, for example, be separated from one another; they are more of the nature of zones with different microscopic appearances that can be distinguished from one another when the retina is scrutinized from its outer to its inner surface with the LM. Nevertheless, the classification of the ten "layers" continues to be helpful because the positions of the various microscopic elements of the retina are easy to describe if they can be said to reside in particular layer. The ten layers are numbered in the low-power photomicrograph of the retina in Figure 28-18; interpretation of this illus-

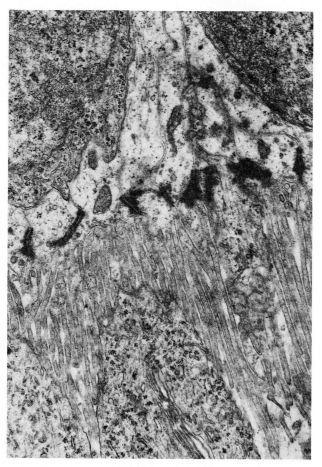

Fig. 28-17. Electron micrograph showing portions of the outer ends of Müller cells in the nervous portion of the retina. This retina is from an eye of a ground squirrel. For orientation, and for a description of the layers, *see* Figure 28-19, which is oriented the same way. The dark interrupted line extending across the middle of the micrograph represents the outer limiting membrane (layer 3). Note that it contains numerous junctional complexes, the filamentous material of which is extremely electron-dense; this is what gives rise to the irregular pattern of intense staining seen at this level. The junctional complexes join the outer ends of the Müller cells, the cytoplasm of which is very light-staining, to the inner segments of the photoreceptor cells (situated below). Part of layer 4 is seen above the level of the junctional complexes; here, nuclei can be seen in two cones (*top left* and *top right*). The pale cytoplasm between these two components of layer 4 (the light triangle above *center*) belongs to Müller cells. Note the numerous long microvilli extending from the outer ends of the Müller cells. These reach below the level of the junctional complexes, so that they extend down between the photoreceptor inner segments lying at *bottom left* and *bottom center*. (Hollenberg, M. J., and Bernstein, M. H.: Am. J. Anat.,*118*:359, 1966)

tration is facilitated by comparing the layers seen in it with the explanatory diagram provided in Figure 28-19. A list and brief description of these layers follow.

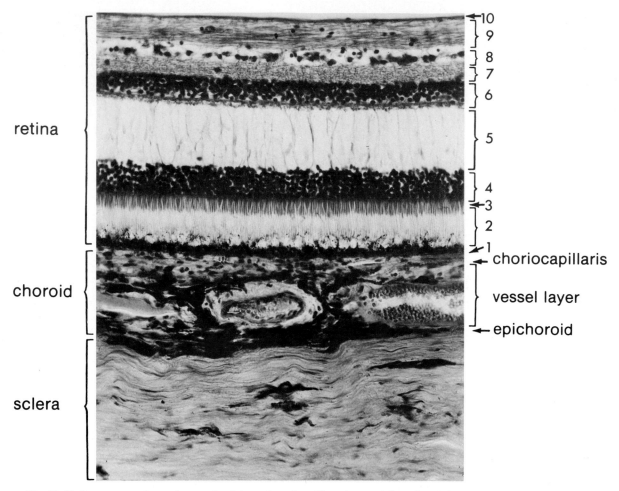

Fig. 28-18. Low-power photomicrograph of the retina, choroid, and part of the sclera. The numbers refer to the layers of the retina described in the text and shown diagrammatically in Figure 28-19.

Layer 1, as shown in Figures 28-18 and 28-19 (where it is labeled 1), is the layer of *pigmented epithelial cells* already described that develops from the outer layer of the optic cup. It is a true layer, having a different origin from the others.

Layer 2, the *layer of rods and cones*, consists of the rod- or cone-shaped light-sensitive processes of the photoreceptors. They are packed closely together and their free ends project slightly into layer 1 (Fig. 28-19).

Layer 3 was named the *external (outer) limiting membrane* from studies of stained sections with the LM. It was initially visualized as a sieve-like membrane through which the outer parts of the photoreceptor projected so that it provided them with support. The EM, however, showed that it represents the numerous junctional complexes between Müller cells and photoreceptors de-

scribed above (Fig. 28-17). The Müller cells project through the "membrane" in the form of microvilli into layer 2 (Fig. 28-17).

Layer 4 is known as the *outer nuclear layer* because it contains the closely packed nuclei of photoreceptors.

Layer 5, designated the *outer plexiform layer*, is the layer in which the axons of rods and cones synapse with bipolar cells and horizontal cells. The fibers involved form such a network that this layer presents a plexiform appearance when suitably stained.

Layer 6 is termed the *inner nuclear layer*. It contains the nuclei of bipolar cells, Müller cells, and horizontal cells.

Layer 7, called the *inner plexiform layer*, is where the axons of bipolar cells synapse with ganglion cells. The latter have extensive dendritic arborizations and these also

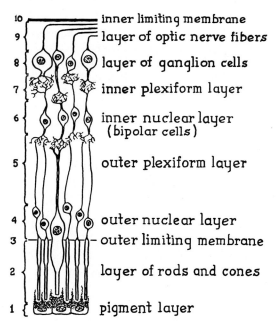

10 ——— inner limiting membrane
9 ——— layer of optic nerve fibers
8 ——— layer of ganglion cells
7 ——— inner plexiform layer
6 ——— inner nuclear layer (bipolar cells)
5 ——— outer plexiform layer
4 ——— outer nuclear layer
3 ——— outer limiting membrane
2 ——— layer of rods and cones
1 ——— pigment layer

Fig. 28-19. Schematic diagram illustrating the layers of the retina. This should be compared carefully with the photomicrograph in Figure 28-18.

give this layer a plexiform appearance when suitably stained.

Layer 8, described as the *ganglion cell layer,* is where the cell bodies and nuclei of the large ganglion cells are disposed, together with some neuroglial cells. Retinal blood vessels are also present in this layer. The amacrine cells would mostly lie along the outer edge of this layer.

Layer 9, the *layer of nerve fibers,* consists of the axons of the ganglion cells; after reaching the innermost part of the retina, these fibers have turned at right angles, to pass thereafter parallel with the inner surface of the retina toward the site of exit of the optic nerve. To aid transparency they possess neither myelin nor sheaths of Schwann. Spider-like neuroglial cells, processes of Müller cells, and blood vessels are also present in this layer.

Layer 10, the *inner limiting membrane,* is a delicate structure composed of the terminations of the processes of Müller cells and their basement membrane.

The Relation of Structure to Function in the Retina

The Respective Roles of Rods and Cones. Schultz, a German anatomist, pointed out over a century ago that the retinas of certain nocturnal animals possessed only rods, while those carrying out activities by day had mostly cones. He therefore concluded that rods were adapted to functioning in dim or negligible light, and cones for bright light. He even surmised that cones were responsible for

color vision. Both his conclusion and his surmise proved to be correct. Cats, for example, have retinas equipped only with rods, and although they see well in dim light they see everything in terms of black and white. Birds, however, have cones and color vision, which is the reason this author (AWH) gave up attempting to grow his own strawberries.

The Fine Structure of Rods. As shown in Fig. 28-20, a rod is divided into two main parts by a constriction (c.s. in Fig. 28-20); these two parts are termed its *outer* and *inner* segments. The *outer segment* (*bottom* in Fig. 28-20) is its light-sensitive portion. It is enclosed by cell membrane and as noted, is rod-shaped. The substance of the outer segment (o.s. in Fig. 28-20) consists of transverse *membranous disks* stacked one above another along its whole length. The disks are very flattened membranous vesicles. Each disk has a narrow space between its two surfaces and there is a narrow space between neighboring disks. The disks of a rod are shown at high magnification in Figure 28-21B. The disk-containing outer segment is connected to the inner segment of the rod by a constricted region representing a *modified cilium,* which is seen at the site labeled c.s. in Figure 28-20.

The *inner segment* consists of two main parts. The first, adjacent to the constriction, is of about the same diameter as the outer segment and contains an abundance of mitochondria, many polyribosomes, a Golgi apparatus, and a little rER and sER. Microtubules are also present (Fig. 28-20). This part of the inner segment is obviously a site for protein synthesis. The innermost part of the inner segment contains the nucleus and, after narrowing considerably, it expands at its termination into a large presynaptic terminal into which postsynaptic terminals are inserted. The latter represent terminations of dendrites of rod bipolar cells (Figs. 28-15 and 28-16) and horizontal cells (Fig. 28-16).

The Relation of Disks to Light Sensitivity. The photosensitive substance responsible for initiating neural activity in rods and cones when they are exposed to light will be described presently. It is contained in the membrane of the disks and its main component is a protein, the continuous synthesis of which will be described in the following.

Turnover of Disks. Throughout this textbook, attention has been paid to how cell populations are maintained in various parts of the body by new cells replacing the old. We noted, however, that (with the possible exception of olfactory receptor cells) there is no provision for turnover of neurons. Rods and cones are, of course, special photoreceptive kinds of nerve cells, but they are nonetheless no exception to this general rule. Young undertook a series of studies that led to an understanding of how functional integrity of visual cells is maintained throughout life. The turnover required for this maintenance is, however, not one of the entire photoreceptor cell but, in the instance of

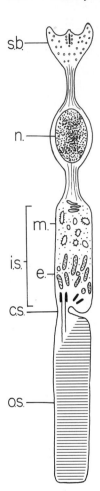

s.b.

n.

m.

i.s.

e.

c.s.

o.s.

Fig. 28-20. Diagram of a retinal rod, showing its component parts and the distribution of its organelles. Its orientation here is the same as in Figures 28-18 and 28-19. Its outer segment (o.s.) contains the disks. The connecting structure between the outer and inner segments is labeled c.s. The inner segment is labeled i.s. In the outermost part of this there is a basal body, from which a modified cilium extends into the inner part of the outer segment. The inner segment is described as consisting of two parts, the ellipsoid portion (e) and the myoid portion (m). The former contains abundant mitochondria. The myoid portion contains rER, free ribosomes, and Golgi saccules. Farther in, the cell is constricted until it bulges to surround the nucleus (n). It then narrows again and ends in an expansion called the synaptic body (s.b.) because here the photoreceptor synapses with other nerve cells. A ribbon synapse (*see inset,* Fig. 28-16, for details) is seen in this part of the rod. (Courtesy of R. Young)

became concentrated in a band across its base, whereupon the band of label moved slowly along the outer segment to reach its free end in about 10 days (in rods of mice and rats); once there, the label disappeared. Next, it was established that the protein migrated in this fashion because it had become incorporated into a disk that moved. This indicated that new disks were being formed repeatedly at the base of the outer segment (by repeated infolding of the cell membrane in this region) and were moving toward its free end as they became displaced by new ones forming beneath them. Then it was found that the reason they disappeared from the end of the outer segment was because they were phagocytosed by the cells of the pigmented epithelium into which the ends of the segments project. Finally, it was found that newly synthesized protein passes through the Golgi before it reaches the outer segment and becomes incorporated into a forming disk, and that a new disk is produced every 40 minutes.

The Cones of the Retina. Young notes that once cones are fully formed they do not produce new disks. However, there is continuous synthesis of protein in their inner segments. This moves to the outer segment but, instead of becoming localized to its base, spreads throughout the outer segment where it is available to replenish the protein of all the disks and so maintain them in good functional condition.

Young suggests that the shape of cones is due to their disks not being replenished. When during development disks are first formed, they are smaller than the ones that form later. Since the disks of cones are not replaced, those formed first are at the outer end of the outer segment, while those formed later are nearer the base of the segment. Since the latter are larger, the outer segment would have a conical shape.

The disks in the distal part of the outer segment of a cone are shown in Figure 28-21A. Farther away toward the base of the outer segment, and not seen in this micrograph, the membranes of the disks are continuous with the cell membrane covering the segment, indicating that the disks were formed here as a result of invagination

rods, replacement of disks, and in cones replacement of important components of the disks. Certain findings led to this conclusion, as will now be described.

By means of radioautography, Droz demonstrated in the 1960s that newly synthesized protein migrated from the inner to the outer segment of rods. Young then showed that labeled protein reaching the outer segment

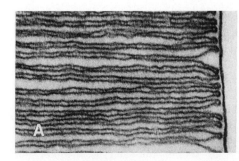

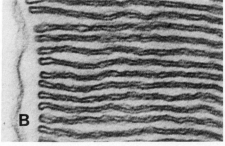

Fig. 28-21. Electron micrographs of disks in photoreceptor cells of retina (×100,000). (*A*) Portion of outer segment of a foveal cone of monkey retina. (*B*) Portion of outer rod segment of monkey retina. For details, *see* text. (Dowling, J. E.: Science, *147*:57, 1965)

of the cell membrane (as in rods). Farther down near the free end of the segment, however, this continuity with the cell membrane is lost (Fig. 28-21A) so that the disks of cones appear much like the free-floating ones seen toward the distal end of the outer segment of rods (Fig. 28-21B).

Color vision is probably to be explained by there being three types of visual pigment found among cones; these would be specially sensitive to yellow and red, or blue or green light. Hence, some cones respond to light of one of these wavelengths and others to one of the others. The various other colors we see depend on the relative numbers of the three kinds of cones stimulated.

Over much of the retina the nuclei of cones, unlike those of rods, tend to be arranged so that with the LM they are seen in a section as a single row.

The inner end of each cone terminates in a club-shaped expansion; this is sometimes called the *synaptic body* or *cone pedicle*. Hollenberg and Bernstein studied the photoreceptors of the retinas of ground squirrels, unique because the photoreceptors are all of the cone type. They found that the pedicles of adjacent cones were often in direct contact with one another, thus providing a basis for interreceptor transmission. Others were separated by processes of Müller cells. The substance of cone pedicles contained numerous synapses with dendrites of cells from the inner nuclear layer, as illustrated in Figure 28-16. This type of basal process is much more complex than that seen in rods (Fig. 28-16).

Since the layer of rods and cones contains no blood vessels whatsoever, all nourishment comes to this layer by diffusion, largely from the choriocapillaris.

How Light Activates Photoreceptors. Only a few introductory comments can be justified here, for this is a matter more properly dealt with in detail in physiology texts. The activation of a photoreceptor depends on its containing a photosensitive pigment in (or on) its transverse disks that on being exposed to light causes a change in the resting potential of the cell. The pigment of rods is *rhodopsin*, which is composed of a protein of the *opsin* type combined with *retinene*, the aldehyde of Vitamin A_1. Since rods are utilized under conditions of low light intensity, it is obvious why adequate intake of this vitamin is essential if one is to see when darkness falls. Indeed, inadequate dietary levels of this vitamin can lead to atrophy of the outer segment of rods. On exposure to light, rhodopsin undergoes a series of changes that results in a change in the potential across the cell membrane of the rod. However, this electrical change is not a depolarization that institutes an action potential, as occurs in other kinds of receptors. The evidence suggests that when a rod is stimulated by light, its membrane becomes *hyperpolarized,* not depolarized. The same electrical change is believed to occur when cones are exposed to light. However, since there are three types of cones, each specialized to react to light of a particular wavelength, it is probable that there are three kinds of photosensitive pigments, one for each type of cone. One kind, *iodopsin,* has been isolated; it is sensitive to red light.

Although it is very difficult to determine transmembrane po-

tentials in the cells of the different layers of the retina, particularly the outermost cells, the evidence available suggests that if hyperpolarization of photoreceptors can be said to initiate impulses, hyperpolarization is also involved in conduction of these impulses to and through the bipolar cells. Only beginning in some amacrine cells and in the ganglion cells of the retina do the impulses received lead to depolarization, with waves of depolarization thereafter being transmitted along the axons of the ganglion cells. These axons, as noted, become the unmyelinated fibers of the optic nerve that deliver the afferent impulses to the visual cortex of the brain.

The Sensitivity of the Retina to Light. The retina is extremely sensitive to light. It has been estimated that a single quantum of light energy is sufficient to stimulate a rod, and that six rods discharging into a common pathway can result in an afferent impulse passing along the path. There are almost 7 million cones in the human retina and 10 to 20 times that number of rods. Since the number of fibers in the optic nerve has been estimated at from 0.5 to 1 million, it would seem that afferent impulses transmitted along a given fiber of the optic nerve to the brain would originate from simultaneous stimulation of at least several and possibly a great many photoreceptors.

The Macula Lutea and Fovea Centralis. Very close to the posterior pole of the eye there is a little depression of the retina. Here the retina is more yellow than elsewhere (after death); hence, it is called the *macula lutea* (L. for yellow spot) (Fig. 28-3). The cells and fibers of the inner layers of the retina diverge from the middle of this area so that the photoreceptors in the central and most depressed part of this area, which is called the *fovea centralis,* are not covered to the same extent as the photoreceptors in other parts of the eye. No blood vessels are present in the retina over this area. The receptors here are all cones. Moreover, these, though longer than usual, are not quite as wide; hence, more are packed into this small area than elsewhere. Therefore this area is specialized in several ways for the greatest degree of visual acuity. Only the image formed in this area is interpreted clearly and sharply by the brain. For example, in reading this page, although the reader is aware of words arranged in lines from top to bottom, he or she can see accurately only a very little at a time. In order that the brain may receive a detailed interpretation of this page, the fovea centralis, like the electron beam originating in a television picture tube, must scan the page, letter by letter, word by word, and line by line, from top to bottom. Fortunately, however, we learn to recognize most words or groups of words from experience merely by their general configuration, thereby saving much time.

Nerve fibers from the macula lutea are provided with more room at the *papilla,* which is the site of exit of the optic nerve (Figs. 28-22 and 28-23) and consequently they are less heaped up and are more securely arranged than the other more converging retinal fibers. Hence, if edema should develop at the papilla, the fibers coming from the macular area are the last to be involved.

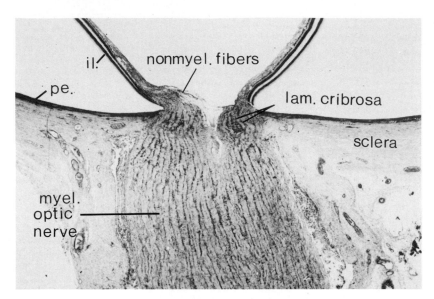

Fig. 28-22. Low-power photomicrograph of part of an eye in longitudinal section, at the site of exit of its optic nerve. Note the way the unmyelinated retinal nerve fibers (nonmyel, fibers) penetrate the scleral coat via the lamina cribrosa, and extend on as the myelinated fibers of the optic nerve (myel, optic nerve). Also passing through the lamina cribrosa is a central retinal blood vessel; this extends down the optic nerve. Note that in this section the inner layer of the retina (il.) has detached from the outer layer, the pigmented epithelium (pe.); separation commonly occurs along this line when eyes are fixed and sectioned. In life, the layer labeled il. would be adherent to the one labeled pe.

The Optic Nerve

Like the nerve fiber layer of the retina, the *optic nerve* at the papilla is composed of *unmyelinated* nerve fibers (nonmyel. fibers in Fig. 28-22), containing glial supporting tissue and some capillaries. At the lamina cribrosa the nerve fibers become *myelinated* (myel. optic nerve in fibrous meshwork extending from the sclera (Fig. 28-22, lam, cribrosa). After piercing the lamina cribrosa, the nerve fibers, become *myelinated* (myel, optic nerve in Fig. 28-22), thus swelling the diameter of the optic nerve. They do not acquire a sheath of Schwann and consequently they resemble the nerve fibers of white matter of the cord or brain. The sheaths covering the nerve have already been described and are illustrated in Figure 28-3.

The Internal Appearance of the Retina

It was already mentioned that the eye is the window of the body, and that structures inside it may be seen from outside. Since many functional and disease changes in the body are reflected by changes in the eye, this is of great importance.

To look within the eye an instrument called an *ophthalmoscope* is used. This provides a bright light that is projected through the cornea into the eye to see the structures in the back (*fundus*) of the eye. With another instrument, the *slit lamp microscope,* the microscopic details of the conjunctiva, cornea, iris, lens, ciliary body, and even the anterior part of the vitreous body can be studied in the living eye.

Figure 28-23 shows the fundus of a living right eye as viewed with an ophthalmoscope. The cup-shaped surface of the retina is red in life because light is reflected back from the red blood cells in the very large capillaries of the choriocapillaris. The whole background has a granular appearance, due in part to irregular distribution of pigment in the retinal epithelium and in part to coarse aggregation of pigment cells in the vascular layer of the choroid.

The unmyelinated fibers of the retina (layer 9) converge at the site of exit of the optic nerve. Here, there is much heaping up of retinal fibers to constitute what is known as the *papilla* (Fig. 28-23). In this region the nerve fibers are loosely arranged. Consequently, accumulation of tissue fluid in the nervous tissue of the retina results in an obvious swelling of the papilla; this is a valuable early clinical sign of certain pathologic conditions. Since the papilla is of disk-like shape, about 1.5 mm. in diameter, it is often called the *optic disk.* It appears much larger when seen through the refracting media of the eye than when exposed. Because the white lamina cribosa (fibrous tissue) is pierced by gray nerve fibers, and is supplied by a capillary network, the papilla has a pale pink color in contrast with the redness of the retina elsewhere. Should the capillaries become atrophied, the papilla appears gray, and the little perforations of the lamina cribrosa, not now so obscured, appear more prominent. Should the nerve fibers atrophy, the papilla becomes chalky white; this appearance may be exaggerated later by the proliferation of glial and fibrous tissue.

The central portion of the papilla, called the *physiologic cup,* is a funnel-shaped space created by the diverging nerve fibers. An increase in intraocular pressure (and other conditions) may displace the lamina cribrosa and its nerve fibers posteriorly. This results in the whole papilla becoming depressed and cup-shaped, a condition referred to as *cupping of the disk.*

The *central retinal artery* and *vein* (labeled in Fig. 28-23) make their appearance at the center of the physiologic cup, and, hugging its medial side, radiate over the inner surface of the retina, branching as they go (Fig. 28-23).

An area at the posterior pole of the eye, the *macula lutea,* is designed to give maximal visual acuity. The depressed middle of this area, the *fovea centralis* (L. for central pit), lies some distance lateral to the margin of the papilla, very slightly inferior to its center (Fig. 28-23). The size of the macula is variable but is usually roughly comparable with that of the papilla.

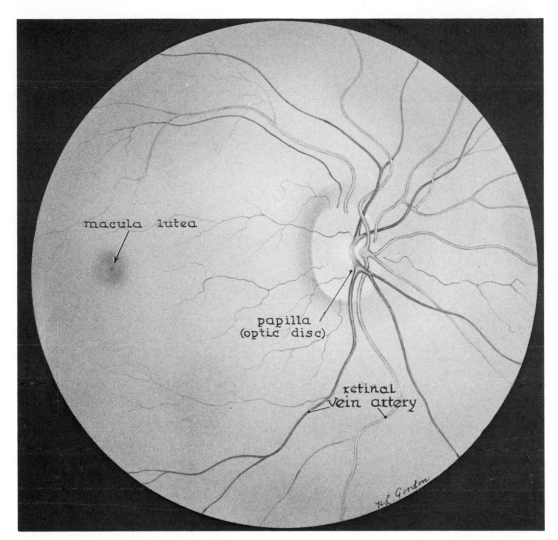

Fig. 28-23. Drawing of the appearance of the fundus of the right eye, as seen through an ophthalmoscope.

Naturally, large retinal vessels that could interfere with vision do not tranverse the macula (Fig. 28-23). Instead, they pass well above and below it in wide curves; this aids the student in locating the macula with the ophthalmoscope. Smaller vessels extend from the curving ones and also from the medial side of the papilla itself into the macular area, but they never quite reach its center, which is left completely nonvascular. Because of yellow pigment in its superficial layers, the macular area appears yellow in the living (in red-free light) or on exposure after death. In ordinary white light is appears darker and redder than the remainder of the retina (Fig. 28-23). Its darker color is due to increased pigmentation of the pigmented epithelium, and its increased redness is due to blood contained in the especially large choroidal capillaries behind this area. The fovea centralis, viewed through the pupil, appears to be a minute bright point because light is reflected, as if by a mirror, from its concave walls.

THE ACCESSORY STRUCTURES OF THE EYE (ADNEXA)

The Conjunctiva. This is a thin transparent mucous membrane that covers the "white" of the eye as the *bulbar conjunctiva* (Fig. 28-12) and lines the eyelid (not seen unless the lid is everted) as the *palpebral conjunctiva* (Fig. 28-24). The space in the angle formed by the palpebral and bulbar conjunctiva is called the *fornix*.

The *epithelium* is characteristically stratified columnar, with three layers of cells: a deep layer of columnar cells, a middle polygonal layer, and a superficial layer of flat or low cuboidal cells. The surface cells studied with the scanning electron microscope reveal a network of microvilli on their free surface (Fig. 28-25). The middle layer is

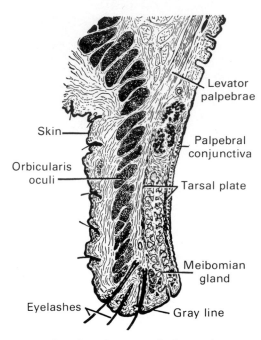

Fig. 28-24. Drawing of a perpendicular section through the upper eyelid. (After Duane, A.: Fuch's Textbook of Ophthalmology. ed. 8 revised. Philadelphia, J. B. Lippincott, 1924)

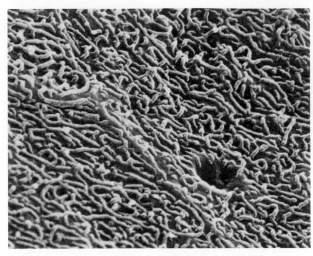

Fig. 28-25. Scanning electron micrograph of the exposed surface of portions of contiguous conjunctival cells, in an eye of a hamster. This shows the surface of the upper tarsal conjunctiva. The opening of a tear duct is evident at *lower right*. Note the numerous microvilli covering the free surface of these cells; the exposed surface of corneal epithelium is similarly supplied with large numbers of microvilli. The microvilli probably aid in retaining a film of tears over the exposed conjunctival and corneal surfaces. (Courtesy of P. Basu and P. Basrur)

absent in most of the palpebral conjunctiva. As the epithelium approaches the lid margin, it changes to stratified squamous; this merges with the epidermis of the skin. Scattered through the conjunctival epithelium are mucus-secreting goblet cells. Near the limbus the epithelium of the bulbar conjunctiva becomes stratified squamous and is provided with deep papillae. It is continuous with the epithelium of the cornea.

The *substantia* (*lamina*) *propria* of the conjunctiva consists of delicate fibrous connective tissue and it is particularly loose over the sclera. In it are scattered accumulations of lymphocytes, which form nodules near the fornices. The substantia propria, except in the lid, merges into a more deeply situated and thicker meshwork of collagenous and elastic connective tissue.

The palpebral fissure is the space between the free margins of the two lids (Fig. 28-12). At the medial end of the palpebral fissure is a little pool of tears, the *lacus lacrimalis*. A free fold of conjunctiva, the concave border of which faces the pupil, is present at the medial end of the palpebral fissure; this is called the *plica semilunaris* (Fig. 28-12), and it is probably homologous to the nictitating membrane of birds. In the very angle of the palpebral fissure at its medial end, a little fleshy mass, the *caruncle* (Fig. 28-12), protrudes; developmentally, this is a detached portion of the marginal part of the lower lid; hence

it contains a few striated muscle fibers as well as a few hair follicles and sebaceous glands.

The Eyelids. Each *eyelid* is covered on its anterior surface with delicate skin; this contains the follicles of very fine hairs and some sebaceous and sweat glands (Fig. 28-24). The dermis is of unusually loose texture, and the subcutaneous tissue deep to it, in members of white races, contains almost no fat. The keratin of the epidermis gradually thins out as the skin approaches the free margin of the eyelid, and here the epidermis becomes continuous with the epithelium of the palpebral conjunctiva, which has already been described as lining the inner (posterior) side of the lid (Fig. 28-24).

Each lid is reinforced with a plate of dense connective tissue, the *tarsal plate*. This is situated in the posterior part of the lid so that the palpebral conjunctiva is apposed to its posterior surface (Fig. 28-24). The secretory portions of long, vertically disposed complex sebaceous glands, called *meibomian glands,* are embedded in the tarsal plate; these open onto the posterior part of the free margin of the lid (Fig. 28-24). Should one of these glands become infected, a painful pea-like swelling develops in the lid.

Deep to the skin covering the anterior surface of the lid are bundles of striated muscle fibers of the *orbicularis oculi* muscle (Fig. 28-24). Some of the collagenic fibers from the aponeurosis of the *levator palpebrae* muscle pass between these bundles to insert into the skin covering the eyelid. Others connect with the tarsal plate, and still others continue toward the margin of the lid in front of the plate. This latter sheet of connective tissue becomes looser in texture as it approaches the margin of the lid, which it reaches to form the *gray line,* a surgical landmark of some importance. Along this gray line the lid may be split surgically, opening up the submuscular space known to the ophthalmologist as the *intermarginal space.*

The hair follicles of the eyelashes slant anteriorly as they pass to the surface. They are arranged in three or four rows, just ahead of the gray line. They are provided with sebaceous glands termed the *glands of Zeis.* Between the follicles, the *sweat glands of Moll* are situated. A *sty* is the result of the infection of either type of gland.

Tear Glands. Tears are produced by the lacrimal gland and several accessory tear glands. The *lacrimal gland* lies in the superolateral corner of the bony orbit. It is divided by the lateral edge of the *levator palebrae* muscle into two lobes: a deep *orbital lobe* and a superficial *palpebral lobe.* Something less than a dozen ducts run from the gland to empty along the superior fornix. Most of the ducts from the orbital lobe, to reach their termination, pass through the palpebral lobe. Small *accessory tear glands,* the *glands of Krause,* are scattered along both fornices, but they are more numerous in the upper one. Still smaller glands are present in the caruncle. It is of interest that the eye may remain healthy in the absence of the lacrimal gland; this suggests that the gland's function is, to some extent, to provide floods of tears on special occasions.

The tear glands develop from the conjunctiva and are of the compound serous tubulo-alveolar type. Their secretory cells contain fat droplets and secretion granules (Fig. 28-26). The secretory units are encircled by myoepithelial cells.

The secretion of the tear glands is slightly alkaline. In addition to various salts, it contains a bactericidal enzyme, *lysozyme.* Tears are spread evenly over the cornea and conjunctiva by blinking the eyelids to keep the surfaces of the cornea and conjunctiva moist; this, as noted, is an essential function. Floods of tears, particularly those elicited by painful stimuli, assist in washing foreign particles from the conjunctival sacs and cornea.

The Drainage of Tears. On the free margin of each lid, near its medial end, is a little papilla called the *lacrimal papilla.* A small opening, which, however, can be seen with the naked eye, exists near the summit of the papilla; this opening is termed the *punctum* and it leads into the *lacrimal canaliculus.* This is a small tube that runs first in the lid and then medially so as to meet its fellow from the adjacent lid in a little ampulla that extends outward from the lateral side of a tubular structure called the *lacrimal sac.* The latter descends as the *nasolacrimal duct,* to open

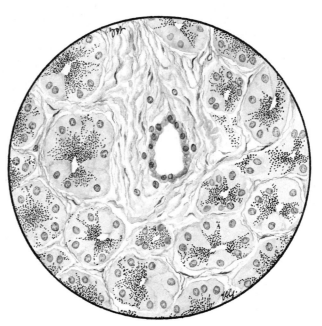

Fig. 28-26. Drawing (high-power) of the lacrimal gland, showing its secretory units and a duct.

through the lateral surface of the inferior meatus of the nose; by means of this mechanism, tears more or less continually drain into the nose. Should any part of this duct system become blocked, tears produced even at an ordinary rate run over onto the side of the face.

The puncta and canaliculi are lined with stratified squamous nonkeratinized epithelium, and the lacrimal sac and nasolacrimal duct with two layers of columnar epithelium containing goblet cells. The lacrimal papilla is rich in elastic fibers.

THE EAR

Each ear consists of three main parts (external, middle, and inner parts), and each part is in itself termed an *ear;* hence each ear is said to consist of an *external ear,* a *middle ear,* and an *inner ear.*

The ear is responsible not only for (*1*) hearing, but also for appreciating (*2*) how the head is oriented in space in relation to gravitational force, and (*3*) whether movement of the head takes place (the overcoming of inertia) or, if steady movement of the head is taking place, whether the rate or direction of movement is altered. It may seem curious that sensory receptors concerned in the maintenance of equilibrium are so closely associated with hearing. In the evolutionary scale, the ear developed as an organ for permitting animals to maintain equilibrium before it also became an organ for hearing.

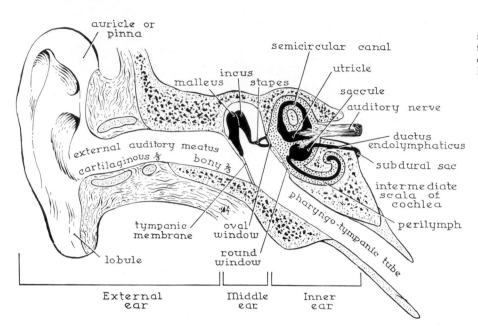

GENERAL STRUCTURE

The *external ear* consists of an obvious appendage, the *auricle,* and a tube, the *external auditory meatus* (L. *meatus,* passage or canal) that extends from the auricle into the substance of the skull (Fig. 28-27) to reach a tiny cavity in the petrous portion of the temporal bone, known as the tympanic cavity or middle ear (Fig. 28-27). The external auditory meatus, however, does not open into the middle ear because the *tympanic membrane* (*eardrum*) extends across the deep end of the external auditory meatus to form a partition between it and the middle ear (Fig. 28-27). This membrane, which thus forms a considerable part of the lateral wall of the middle ear, is of a suitable thickness and is maintained under a suitable tension to vibrate in accordance with sound waves that reach it by way of the auricle and the external auditory meatus.

Before discussing the general structure and function of the middle ear, we shall comment briefly on the inner ear, for here are located the special groups of nerve endings that are selectively stimulated by sound, changes in relation to gravity, or alterations in movement.

The *inner ear* consists of a series of membranous tubes in various arrangements and planes, together with two membranous sacs with which the membranous tubes communicate (Figs. 28-27 and 28-30). This closed system of membranous tubes and sacs is filled with a fluid termed *endolymph,* and at appropriate sites sensory receptors are arranged inside these membranous structures. The whole system of membranous tubes and sacs is said to constitute the *membranous labyrinth* (Gr. *labyrinthos,* a maze) (Fig. 28-30). The membranous labyrinth is loosely fitted into a series of spaces and cavities in the bone; these are of similar pattern to the membranous labyrinth and constitute the *bony labyrinth* (Fig. 28-29). Although in some sites the membranous labyrinth is attached to the periosteum that lines the wall of the bony labyrinth, the bulk of the membranous labyrinth is suspended in a fluid termed *perilymph* that fills all the space in the bony labyrinth not occupied by the membranous labyrinth. To visualize these labyrinths the study of a three-dimensional model is very helpful, if not essential.

The most expanded portion of the bony labyrinth lies deep to the bony medial wall of the middle ear; this part of the bony labyrinth is termed its *vestibule* (Fig. 28-29, Vestibuli) because it is the hallway that would be entered by any microscopic visitor small enough to enter the inner ear from the middle ear. However, there are no doors opening from the middle ear into the vestibule of the bony labyrinth, so the visitor from the middle ear would have to enter by way of a window. There are two of these in the bony wall that separates the air-filled middle ear from the fluid-filled vestibule of the bony labyrinth; the upper one is termed the *oval window* (Fig. 28-29, Vestibuli [ovalis]) and the lower one the *round window* (Fig. 28-29, Cochleae [rotunda]). Both windows normally are closed, but in order to describe how they are closed, we shall digress for a moment.

It has already been noted that sound waves set the eardrum into vibration and that the eardrum constitutes a considerable portion of the lateral wall of the middle ear. A chain of three tiny bones, with joints between them, extends across the *middle ear* from its lateral to its medial wall (Fig. 28-27). The free end of the first bone of the chain is attached to the eardrum, and the free end of the last bone in the chain fits into, so as to close, the oval window in the medial wall of the middle ear (Fig. 28-27). Hence, when sound waves set the eardrum in vibration, the chain of bones transmits the vibrations across the middle ear, and since the free end of the last bone of the chain does not fit rigidly into the window (beyond which is the perilymph of the bony labyrinth) but instead like a piston in a cylinder, the vibrations are transmitted to the perilymph in the vestibule. However, fluid is incompressible; hence, every time fluid is pushed in at the oval window, it must push out somewhere else. This occurs at the round window, for this is closed only by a membrane that has sufficient elasticity for this purpose. Having described the mechanical arrangements that permit sound waves eventually to set up vibrations in the perilymph, we shall leave how these affect nerve endings until later.

Although the *bony labyrinth* (Fig. 28-29) has a complex form, it may be helpful to think of it as having three main parts. The first is the *vestibule;* this has already been described as its most expanded part, situated immediately medial to the middle ear.

The other two main parts of the bony labyrinth may be regarded as two extensions from the vestibule, and in these the bony labyrinth is tubular in form. The more anterior of the two tubular extensions has the form of a flat spiral (Figs. 28-27 and 28-29). Since this coiled part of the bony labyrinth looks something like a snail's shell (Fig. 28-29, *right*), it is called the *cochlea* (L. for snail shell). The more posterior of the two extensions (actually this extension is regarded as part of the vestibule) takes the form of three separate round bony tubes, each of which on leaving the vestibule follows a semicircular path so that it eventually returns to the vestibule (Fig. 28-29, Semicircular canals). Only one could be shown in Figure 28-27, because it is a section. Each bony tube communicates at both of its ends with the vestibule (Fig. 28-29). These bony tubes are referred to as *semicircular canals,* and it is of great significance that they lie in different planes, so that the plane of each is approximately at right angles to the other two (Fig. 28-29).

As noted, the membranous labyrinth (Fig. 28-30) is composed of a system of membranous tubes and sacs fitted loosely into the bony labyrinth. Actually, there are two sacs in the membranous labyrinth, and these are both present in the vestibule of the bony labyrinth. The more anterior and smaller of the two is called the *saccule* (L. *sacculus*, small sac), part of which is shown in black in Figure 28-27, and the larger and more posterior, the *utricle* (L. *utriculus*, little skin bag), part of which is shown in black in Figure 28-27. The two sacs are connected by means of a fine membranous duct.

Now that we have given a general outline of the main parts of the ear, we can discuss the microscopic structure of each part and how this is related to its function.

THE MICROSCOPIC STRUCTURE OF THE PARTS OF THE EXTERNAL AND MIDDLE EAR

The Auricle

In most mammals the pinna of the ear is movable and shaped like a funnel. Hence it can be directed towards a source of sound so as to collect sound waves and conduct them to the middle ear. Burrowing and aquatic animals can close the auricle over the meatus to keep out dirt or water. Although the auricle can be moved only slightly in man, its central area plays an important role in the vertical localization of sound and helps in determining whether this comes from above or below the head.

The shape of the auricle is maintained by its content of elastic fibrocartilage. It is covered with skin on both sides. The subcutaneous tissue on the posteromedial surface is slightly thicker than that on the anterolateral one and contains some fat cells. Hair follicles with associated sebaceous glands are scattered through the dermis on both sides and are most prominent near the entrance to the external auditory meatus. The inferior part of the auricle is termed the *lobule* (Fig. 28-27); this consists of a mass of fat, enclosed in connective tissue septa and covered externally with skin. Its relative paucity of nerve endings and rich capillary bed make the lobule a suitable site for obtaining blood for blood counts.

The External Auditory Meatus

This canal is lined with stratified squamous epithelium continuous with that of the skin. Its walls have rigid support and this keeps them from collapsing. In its outer part the support is provided by elastic cartilage continuous with the cartilage of the auricle; in the inner part of the meatus the support is provided by bone (Fig. 28-27). In the outer one third of the canal there are many short hairs, and associated with their follicles are large sebaceous glands. In the submucosa deep to the sebaceous glands there are clusters of tubular *ceruminous* (L. *cera*, wax) *glands;* the ducts of these open either directly onto the surface of the canal or into sebaceous ducts. Ceruminous glands are considered to be modified sweat glands, and their tubules are lined by tall cuboidal or columnar cells. The combined secretion of the sebaceous and the ceruminous glands, called *cerumen*, may accumulate and keep out sound waves. In the inner two thirds of the canal the ceruminous glands are confined to the roof.

The Tympanic Membrane (Eardrum)

This resembles a sandwich, the filling of which is collagenous connective tissue, and the bread, two epithelial layers (Fig. 28-28). The outer epithelial layer is continuous with the stratified squamous epithelium lining the external auditory meatus (Fig. 28-28); it differs from it in

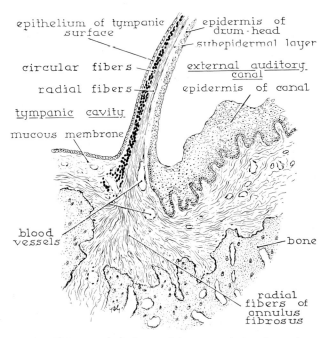

Fig. 28-28. Drawing of part of the tympanic membrane (eardrum) in cross section, showing the relation of the drum membrane to the external auditory canal and tympanic cavity.

having no papillae except short ones near the margin, and also in that over the more central part of the drum it consists of only two layers of cells. Furthermore, mitoses are found only in the periphery, but with time the new cells arising from these mitoses migrate toward the center of the drum. Thus cells lost from the central region of the drum are replaced by new ones from the periphery. The epithelium of the mucous membrane of the middle ear covers the inner side of the drum. It flattens out as a single layer of low cuboidal cells (Fig. 28-28). The middle fibrous filling of the drum consists of two layers of collagen fibers; the outer ones are arranged radially and the inner ones circularly. The upper part of the drum is thin and flaccid because of a lack of collagen filling. Therefore it is known as the *pars flaccida (Schrapnell's membrane)*.

The Middle Ear

Also known as the *tympanic cavity,* this is a tiny epithelially lined cavity in bone, being roughly the shape of a red blood cell set on edge. The tympanic cavity is described as having four walls, a floor, and a roof. It is about as high as it is long, but is very thin. The lateral wall consists largely of the tympanic membrane (Fig. 28-27), and the medial wall is the bone dividing the middle ear from the inner ear. There is a gap between the anterior and medial walls for a canal, called the *eustachian tube,* which extends anteriorly and communicates with the nasopharynx (Fig. 28-27).

The epithelium lining the cavity consists of simple nonciliated cuboidal cells with no basement membrane. The lamina propria is a thin connective tissue layer, closely adherent to bone. In some areas the cuboidal cells may become several layers thick. When infection occurs, the epithelium may become ciliated or may change to stratified squamous epithelium.

The middle ear houses three small bones called *ossicles,* two muscles, and a nerve. Since the middle ear communicates with the pharynx by means of the *pharyngotympanic (eustachian) tube,* the middle ear is an air-containing cavity and offers a direct route for infection to reach it from the upper respiratory tract (Fig. 28-27). Indeed, middle ear infections are sometimes complications of head colds, particularly in children. Posteriorly, the tympanic cavity is continuous with a varying number of alveolar spaces in bone, the *mastoid air cells.* These, too, may become involved in infections that spread up the tube to the middle ear from the nasopharynx.

The Ossicles. The three small bones of the middle ear cavity are the *malleus (hammer),* the *incus (anvil),* and the *stapes (stirrup)* (Fig. 28-27). These bones were doubtless named in the days of the blacksmith shop. The *malleus* is shaped like a crude hammer with a rounded head, a long handle, and a spur in the region of the constricted neck joining the head to the handle. The *incus* is

shaped like a molar tooth with a body or "crown" and a vertical and a horizontal "root." The *stapes,* as its name suggests, is shaped like the stirrup of a riding saddle. It consists of a head, a neck, two limbs, and an oval footplate. The head of the malleus fits into the "crown" of the incus; the vertical "root" of the incus fits against the head of the stapes (Fig. 28-27), and the footplate of the stapes fits into the oval window.

The ossicles transmit vibrations set up in the tympanic membrane by sound waves to the oval window present in the medial wall of the middle ear. The handle of the malleus is firmly attached to the tympanic membrane (Fig. 28-27) and carries vibrations to the incus; this then transfers the vibrations to the stapes, causing the footplate of the stapes, accurately fitted in the oval window, to rock to and fro. This transmits the vibrations to the perilymph of the vestibule, as already explained. During this transfer, the amplitude of vibrations is decreased, but force is increased because the ossicles are arranged to exert leverage. The ossicles are atypical long bones, having no epiphyses and reaching approximately their full size during fetal life. The malleus and the incus have small central marrow cavities, while the stapes has none in the adult. The "ends" of these bones are covered with articular cartilage; they are held together by small ligaments, and the malleus and the incus are suspended by ligaments from the roof of the middle ear. The periosteal surfaces of these bones are covered by the mucous membrane of the middle ear cavity.

The Muscles. The two muscles of the tympanic cavity are the *tensor tympani* and the *stapedius.* The tensor tympani muscle is housed in a bony groove (canal) above the cartilaginous roof of the eustachian tube; its tendon crosses the tympanic cavity mediolaterally and is inserted into the handle of the malleus. The stapedius muscle is housed in the posterior wall of the tympanic cavity, and its tendon, issuing at the summit of a small projection of bone called the pyramid, is inserted into the neck of the stapes. The way in which these muscles affect the transmission of the sound waves by the ossicles is uncertain. The tensor muscle pulls the malleus inward, thus tensing the tympanic membrane and perhaps accentuating high-pitched sounds. The stapedius pulls the footplate of the stapes outward, thus reducing the intralabyrinthine pressure and perhaps making sounds of low frequency more audible. It has been found that reflex contractions of the stapedius occur during exposure to loud noise. Therefore it seems that the stapedius plays a protective role, preventing violent vibrations from injuring the special sense organs in the internal ear.

The Nerves. The chorda tympani nerve traverses the middle ear in contact with the inner surface of the drum. It has no functional concern with the ear. In addition, branches of many other nerves can be found in the mucous membrane and bony walls of the middle ear. The facial nerve runs in a long canal in the medial wall of the middle ear. Its only relation to the ear lies in the fact that it supplies the stapedius muscle. The tympanic branch of the glossopharyngeal (Jacobson's nerve) is the great sensory nerve of the middle ear; the auricular branch of the vagus (Arnold's nerve) supplies the skin of the external auditory meatus. An attack of coughing or vomiting occasionally follows stimulation of the external auditory canal, for example, when a speculum is introduced into it. This is thought to be due to a reflex involving Arnold's nerve as its afferent arm.

The Oval Window. The footplate of the stapes is fitted accurately in the oval window. Its periphery is attached to the cartilaginous rim of the oval window by an *annular ligament* composed of strong collagenous and elastic fibers. The mucous membrane lining the middle ear cavity is reflected from this onto the stapes. Through the oval window, vibrations are conducted to the perilymph of the vestibule.

The Round Window. Since fluid is incompressible, there must be some movable object which the perilymph can displace when it is thrust inward at the oval window. This movable object is a moderately elastic membrane filling in the round window like a flexible windowpane. The membrane has a core of connective tissue and is lined on its middle ear surface by mucous membrane; on its inner side it is lined by the connective tissue of the perilymphatic space of the vestibule.

The Pharyngotympanic (Eustachian) Tube. The simple cuboidal epithelium of the middle ear cavity gives way to respiratory epithelium, namely pseudostratified ciliated columnar epithelium, in the pharyngotympanic (eustachian) tube. There are rugae in the epithelial lining here, and goblet cells can be found in the lining of the cartilaginous part of the tube. Near the pharyngeal end a mixed mucous and serous gland is present in the submucosa. Normally, the mucous surfaces of the tube are in contact, and the tube is open only during swallowing. The pressure in the middle ear can be adjusted rapidly to that of the atmosphere only when this tube is open. Thus, when coming down quickly from heights, one can prevent discomfort by swallowing; this opens the tube and permits the pressure in the middle ear to become equalized with that of the atmosphere.

The Mastoid Air Cells. In early life the mastoid process and all the petrous bone surrounding the inner ear are normally filled with hematopoietic marrow. In the adult, small air pockets continuous with the middle ear cavity have replaced this marrow in the mastoid region. The process whereby the bone is invaded by these air sacs is known as *pneumatization;* it starts as early as the 3rd fetal month, with the greatest extension usually, but not always, occurring between the 3rd year and puberty. The degree of pneumatization of the mastoid area varies greatly from person to person. Heredity seems to play a

more important role than middle-ear infection in determining the extent to which the mastoid and the surrounding petrous temporal bone become pneumatized.

The lining of the mastoid air cells is a thin mucoperiosteum; the cuboidal cells of the middle ear cavity here become flattened to a simple squamous type and lie adjacent to the periosteum of the mastoid air cells.

THE MICROSCOPIC STRUCTURE OF THE PARTS OF THE INNER EAR

The Bony Labyrinth—Space or Structure? The bony labyrinth, in which the membranous labyrinth is contained, is in an intricate maze-like *space* within the substance of the petrous portion of the temporal bone. However, it is commonly visualized as a structure (Fig. 28-29). This is because the layer of bone that is directly apposed to this complicated irregular space in the very young is said to be harder than the bone farther away from the space. Hence the part of the bone that immediately surrounds the irregular space, and that follows the contours of the space, can be dissected away from the temporal bone as a *structure* referred to as the bony lanyrinth. Nevertheless, it is only a part of the petrous portion of the temporal bone that can be artificially separated from it.

The Organ of Hearing—the Cochlea

In describing the *cochlea,* it is convenient to think of it as a bony tube wound in the form of a spiral, with its turns becoming shorter the farther they get from its base (Fig. 28-29). The central axis around which the spiral is wound is a pillar of bone called the *modiolus* (L. for hub).

In the body, the apex of the cochlea is directed anterolaterally (Fig. 28-29). However, in describing its microscopic structure, we shall change its orientation as if it has been laid flat on its base.

As already mentioned, the membranous labyrinth (Fig. 28-30) extends into all parts of the bony labyrinth. The membranous tube extending into the cochlea arises from the saccule (Fig. 28-30). On entering the basal turn of the cochlea it becomes known as the *cochlear duct.* It is not, as might at first be imagined, a round tube; instead, it has more of the shape of a ribbon, particularly that of a thick wide ribbon that has been "ironed down" along one edge so that one side is much thinner than the other. Such a ribbon would thus be somewhat triangular in shape when seen in cross section. The cochlear duct, of course, is not solid like a ribbon but hollow and filled with *endolymph.* A cross-sectional view of it can be seen in Figure 28-34, where it is labeled *scala media* (L. *scala,* staircase). In Figure 28-31 it is labeled *cochlear duct.*

The thicker edge of the ribbon-like cochlear duct is attached to one side of the bony canal of the cochlea by the spiral ligament (labeled in Fig. 28-31). The other, thinner edge of the hollow ribbon-like cochlear duct extends to

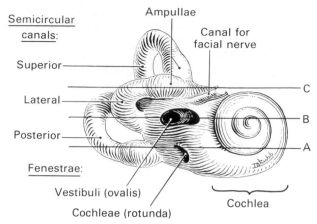

Semicircular
canals:

Superior

Lateral

Posterior

Fenestrae:

Ampullae

Canal for
facial nerve

C

B

A

Vestibuli (ovalis)

Cochleae (rotunda)

Cochlea

Fig. 28-29. The bony labyrinth (anterolateral view). The oval and round windows (labeled fenestrae) open into the vestibule; the cochlea extends from the vestibule at *right,* and the semicircular canals at *left.* Reference lines A, B, and C are provided to aid comparison with Figure 28-30. (After Grant, J. C. B.: Method of Anatomy. ed. 4. Baltimore, Williams & Wilkins, 1948)

spinal fluid and it is in communication with cerebrospinal fluid.) However, the cochlear duct (also termed the *scala media* as in Fig. 28-34) keeps the perilymph in the scala vestibuli separated along the whole course of the cochlea from the perilymph of the scala tympani. (Actually, there is a small opening between the scala vestibuli and the scala tympani at the tip of the cochlea, but this may be disregarded for the time being.)

The Mechanics of Transmission of Sound Waves to the Cochlear Duct. Since the perilymph in the scala vestibuli and that in the scala tympani are not in free communication with each other, any vibrations in the perilymph in the scala vestibuli, to reach the scala tympani, have to be transmitted through the thickness of the ribbon-like, endolymph-containing cochlear duct. The perilymph in the scala vestibuli is continuous with the perilymph that bathes the inner aspect of the oval window. As already described, this perilymph receives vibrations from the eardrum by way of the chain of bones, the last one of which fits into the oval window. Hence vibrations of the eardrum are transmitted up the cochlea by means of the perilymph that extends from the oval window up into the scala vestibuli. However, fluid is incompressible, so that the bone that fits into the oval window cannot push into the window unless the fluid in the body labyrinth can push out somewhere else. Since the perilymph in the other "staircase," the scala tympani, is in free communication with that bathing the inner aspect of the round window, vibrations transmitted into the oval window and through the perilymph of the scala vestibuli *are transmitted through the thickness of the cochlear duct into the perilymph of the scala tympani* and from there to the round window, which "gives" sufficiently to permit the above-described mechanism to operate.

the other side of the bony canal (scala media, Fig. 28-34). Thus the cochlear duct forms a hollow shelf across the bony canal, splitting it into two parts along its whole length. In this fashion the cochlear duct ascends the winding turns of the cochlea; this is why it is called a *scala.* As the *scala media,* the cochlear duct separates the part of the canal below it, which is known as the *scala tympani* (Fig. 28-31), from the *scala vestibuli* (Fig. 28-34) above it. Both the scala vestibuli and the scala tympani are filled with *perilymph.* (This almost is identical with cerebro-

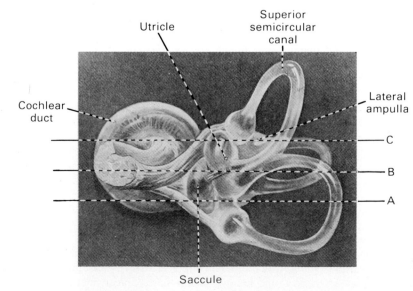

Utricle

Superior
semicircular
canal

Cochlear
duct

Lateral
ampulla

C

B

A

Saccule

Fig. 28-30. Drawing of right membranous labyrinth (posteromedial view), showing the relation between the cochlear duct, utricle, saccule, semicircular canals, and ampullae. Reference lines A, B, and C have been included to facilitate comparison with Figure 28-29. (Spalteholtz, W.: Hand Atlas of Human Anatomy. ed. 14. Philadelphia, J. B. Lippincott, 1939)

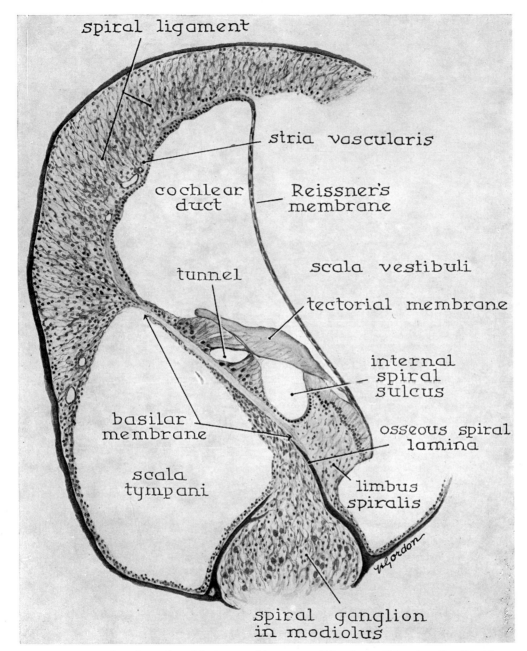

Fig. 28-31. Drawing of a portion of the bony cochlea, cut parallel to the modiolus along line B in Figure 28-29. A section in this plane cuts the bony tube, as it pursues its spiral course, at several different sites. One cross section of the bony tube is illustrated; it shows the cochlear duct extending across the bony canal. The structures in the lower portion of the cochlear duct above the basilar membrane and the adjacent part of the osseous spiral lamina constitute the spiral organ of Corti.

The Microscopic Structure of the Cochlear Duct

A cochlear duct (the scala media) in a cross section has a triangular shape. The base of this triangle is attached to one side of the bony canal by the spiral ligament (Fig. 28-31). One side of the triangle that extends across the bony canal is thicker than the other (Figs. 28-31 and 28-34). This thicker side is referred to as the *floor* of the cochlear duct, and it is on this floor that the spiral *organ of Corti,* which is the sense organ for hearing, rests and ascends up the cochlear duct to its termination.

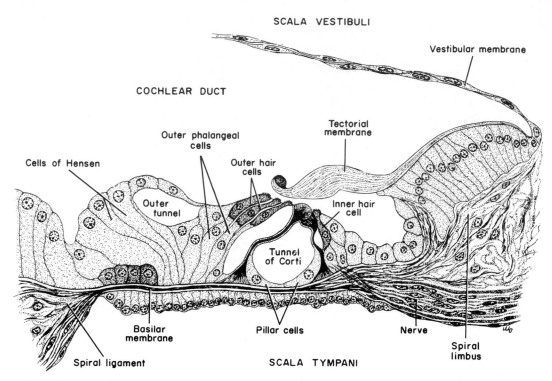

Fig. 28-32. Drawing of the organ of Corti (from a guinea pig). From the *bottom* up, note the following. The epithelium of the scala tympani is columnar under the basilar membrane, but squamous under the spiral ligament at *left* and spiral limbus at *right*. The organ of Corti arises from the epithelium of the cochlear duct, where it lies in contact with the basilar membrane. It includes the large cells of Hensen at *left*, enclosing a space called the outer tunnel; the outer phalangeal cells, which are not prominent in this species and support the outer hair cells; the pillar cells enclosing the tunnel of Corti; the inner hair cell supported by the inner phalangeal cells; and a row of epithelial cells from which the tectorial membrane extends to come close to the two types of hair cells. At *top,* the vestibular membrane separates the cochlear duct from the scala vestibuli. (Courtesy of C. P. Leblond and Y. Clermont)

The floor of the cochlear duct, in order to extend across the bony canal of the cochlea, is not particularly wide because both the outer and the inner walls of the bony canal bulge toward its middle to support the floor and make the distance it must bridge narrower. The bulge from the inner wall is a thin shelf of bone, called the *osseous spiral lamina* (Fig. 28-31) because it winds up the modiolus like the thread on a screw. The bulge from the other side of the bony canal is not bone but a thickening of the periosteum that lines the canal; this line of thickened fibrous periosteum that winds up the turns of the cochlea constitutes the *spiral ligament* (Fig. 28-31). The floor of the cochlear duct is termed the *basilar membrane* (Fig. 28-31), and it bridges the gap between the osseous spiral lamina and the crest of the spiral ligament. The basilar membrane is made up of a dense mat of collagenic and some elastic fibers. The roof of the cochlear duct, in contrast to its floor, is thin, being composed of only two layers of squamous epithelial cells; this is called *Reissner's membrane* (Fig. 28-31). The outer wall of the coch-

lear duct is made up of the spiral ligament already described. The upper and larger part (the part nearer Reissner's membrane) is known as the *stria vascularis* (Fig. 28-31) and is rich in blood vessels; these lie directly below a surface layer of deep-staining cuboidal cells. A small part of the outer wall of the cochlear duct, close to the attachment of the basilar membrane to the crest of the spiral ligament, forms what is known as the *sulcus spiralis externus*. Here, long processes from the surface epithelial cells extend down into the connective tissue of the spiral ligament. Moreover, secretory cells are deeply buried in this area but have access to the surface. They are thought to constitute a secretory mechanism for replenishing endolymph in the cochlear duct.

The General Structure of the Organ of Corti

This exists in the form of a long cellular ribbon that runs from one end of the cochlear duct to the other, resting on the floor of the cochlear duct. Since the floor of the

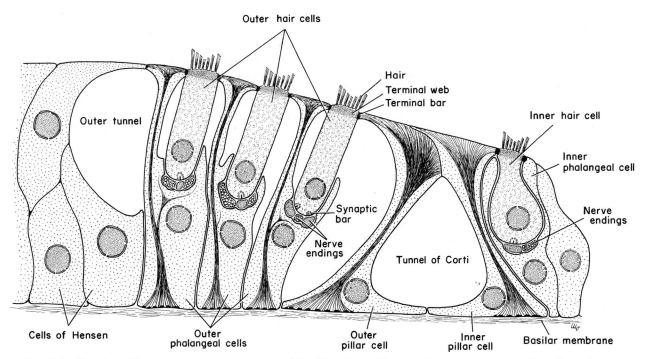

Fig. 28-33. Drawing of the sensory portion of the organ of Corti (based on EM studies in man and monkey). The cells on the basilar membrane include, from *left* to *right:* the cells of Hensen, enclosing the outer tunnel, and then three outer phalangeal cells that contain a thin column of rigid material extending from hemidesmosomes at the base to the apical surface (at *left* of each cell), with a small branch extending to the *right* below the nerve endings and the base of the outer hair cells. The nerve endings come either from afferent or from efferent nerves. The afferent endings (*stippled*) are postsynaptic to ribbon synapses (synaptic bar); the efferent endings contain synaptic vesicles (shown as tiny circles). Next, the tunnel of Corti is enclosed by the outer and inner pillar cells containing prominent columns of rigid material. At *right,* the inner hair cell is supported by the inner phalangeal cell. (Courtesy of C. P. Leblond and Y. Clermont)

duct pursues a spiral course, the organ of hearing is called the *spiral organ of Corti.* (This is not labeled in Fig. 28-31, but it lies directly above the basilar membrane, which is labeled, and it contains a tunnel which is labeled as such in Fig. 28-31). Before giving the details of its structure, we should finish our description of the cochlear duct and its environs.

Except in the area of the organ of Corti, the basilar membrane is lined by low cuboidal cells. To the inner side of the organ of Corti the periosteum of the upper surface of the osseous spiral lamina forms an elevation, the *limbus spiralis* (Fig. 28-31), that bulges into the duct. The outer margin of this limbus presents a groove known as the *internal spiral sulcus* (Fig. 28-31); the edge of the limbus spiralis that overhangs this is called the *vestibular lip.* From the lip a thin, homogeneous, jelly-like membrane extends over and is in contact with the hairs of the hair cells of the organ of Corti (soon to be described). This is the *tectorium* or *tectorial membrane* (Fig. 28-31).

The lining of the scala tympani and scala vestibuli (apart from that provided by the basilar membrane, Reissner's membrane, and the spiral ligament) is composed of

the internal periosteum (endosteum) of the bony cochlear canal.

Detailed Structure. When the cells seen in a section of the organ of Corti are encountered by looking in a medial direction (from *left* to *right* in Fig. 28-32), a group of epithelial cells is first observed, the tallest of which are the *cells of Hensen* (Fig. 28-32); these have no special characteristics. Next are the *outer phalangeal cells* (Figs. 28-32 and 28-33); these are tall columnar cells that serve as support for the outer hair cells (to be described below), and they also provide support for the nerve endings at the bases of the hair cells. The characteristic feature of an outer phalangeal cell is the presence of a column of microtubule-containing fibrillar material which originates from hemidesmosomes on the basal cell membrane (Fig. 28-33); this runs upward through the cytoplasm of the cell, and, just before reaching the bottom of the hair cell it supports, extends on toward the surface beside the hair cell as a thin process called the *phalanx,* which is composed of scanty cytoplasm around the fibrillar column (Fig. 28-33). At the surface of the organ of Corti (that is, on a level with the surface of the hair cells), the phalangeal process, still containing cytoplasm and fibrillar material, expands into a flat plate connected by junctional complexes to the hair cells. Since the free surface of the phalangeal processes is on a level with the free surface of hair cells (which as described below is underlaid by terminal web filaments), they together make up a single plane inadequately named the *reticular lamina.*

The *outer and inner pillar cells* (Fig. 28-33) are located one to either side of the tunnel of Corti. They are modified phalangeal cells. They too extend up to the surface of the organ of Corti. Each cell contains a column of fibrillar material running from base to apex, as indicated in Figure 28-33, but this column is thicker than in phalangeal cells.

The *hair cells* are also classified as *outer* and *inner.* There are from three to five rows of *outer hair cells,* but only one row of *inner hair cells.* They demonstrate many interesting features; a notable one is the way they are supported. Their bases do not rest on the basilar membrane; instead, as shown in Figure 28-33, their bases are cradled in cup-like recesses in phalangeal cells.

Each hair cell has a thick layer of *terminal web* underlying its free surface and around its edges. This web connects with the junctional complexes, which in turn connect with the fibrillar material of the phalangeal processes (Fig. 28-33).

The free surface of a hair cell has *hair-like processes* extending from it; the EM has shown these to be large microvilli. They are often referred to as *stereocilia.* Unlike typical microvilli, they are narrow near their origin and widen out towards their tip. They are arranged in a characteristic pattern, which, when looked at from above, forms a V. At the tip of the V in the young there is a typical cilium. However, in the adult this disappears, though its basal body persists. Another feature of hair cells is that their base has a rounded form with both afferent and efferent nerve endings on it (Fig. 28-33). A *synaptic ribbon (bar)* identical with that described earlier in this chapter in retinal cells is characteristically seen where the base forms afferent synapses (Fig. 28-33, labeled synaptic bar in the middle of the diagram).

Hearing

To understand how the organ of Corti responds to sounds, it should be appreciated that a sound of given frequency, received by the external ear and transmitted through the oval window to the perilymph of the scala tympani, makes the *basilar membrane vibrate.* The vibration predominates in a given region of the organ of Corti vibrating to this particular frequency and it is sensed by hair cells as a result of their hairs (microvilli), which are rigidly supported at their base by the reticular lamina (described above), becoming displaced with respect to the tectorial membrane in which their tips are embedded.

This causes the hair cells to alter the pattern of impulse activity in the afferent branch of the acoustic nerve they contact. (It may be added too that some large efferent nerve endings that contain synaptic vesicles are believed to pass impulses to the hair cells.)

Auditory impulses from the afferent endings on hair cells are carried by fibers that run in the basilar membrane (Fig. 28-32) and then between the two thin plates of bone constituting the osseous spiral lamina (Fig. 28-31, *lower right*) toward nerve cell bodies in the *spiral ganglion,* which is housed in the modiolus (*bottom center* in Fig. 28-31). These afferent fibers are peripheral processes of spiral ganglion cells. A single peripheral process may have many branches and so receive impulses from many hair cells. The bipolar cells of the spiral ganglion send their central processes (as the cochlear division of the auditory nerve) to end synaptically in the cochlear nuclei of the brain stem.

THE ORGAN FOR DETECTING MOTION AND MAINTAINING EQUILIBRIUM

As already noted, there are two sacs of the membranous labyrinth, the *utricle* and *saccule,* filled with *endolymph* and *contained in the perilymph* of the bony vestibule (Fig. 28-30). These two sacs are joined by the short arms of a Y-shaped tube, the *ductus endolymphaticus;* the long arm extends through the petrous bone to the posterior cranial fossa, where it ends in a blind subdural swelling, the *subdural endolymphatic sac.*

Into the utricle open the ends of the three membranous *semicircular canals.* Each canal has one expanded end known as an *ampulla* (Fig. 28-30). The nonexpanded ends of the superior and the posterior canals have a common opening into the utricle, whereas the others open independently. Hence, for the three canals there are five openings into the utricle: one opening adjacent to each of the three ampullae, one opening from the nonampullated end of the horizontal canal, and one opening common to the nonampullated ends of the superior and posterior canals. Since each semicircular canal opens at both its ends into the utricle, the semicircle of endolymph in each canal is *joined into a circle through the utricular endolymph.*

The utricle and the saccule are lined by flattened epithelial cells, usually referred to as a *mesothelium,* resting on a connective tissue membrane. The membranous sacs do not fill the bony vestibular space, nor do they lie free in this space, since fine strands of connective tissue connect them to the endosteum lining the body vestibule. The saccule and the utricle each contains a flat, plaque-like sensory ending, called a *macula* (Fig. 28-34).

The Maculae. A macula is somewhat similar cytologi-

Fig. 28-34. Low-power photomicrograph of a horizontal section of the inner ear of a squirrel monkey. It shows the stapes in the oval window and the saccule with the macula below *center*. Note that the hair cells of the macula are covered by an otolithic membrane. The organ of Corti (not labeled) can be seen in the scala media of the cochlea above *center*. (Courtesy of K. Money and J. Laufer)

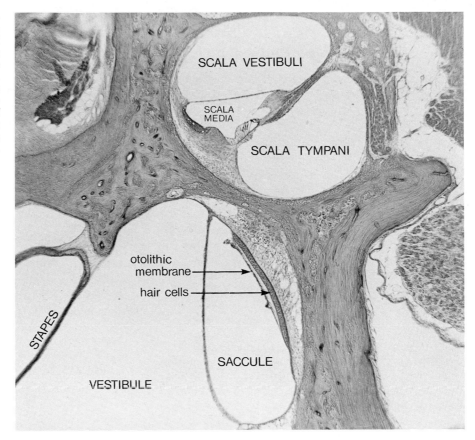

cally to the organ of Corti. It consists of a thickened epithelium, containing neuroepithelial (hair) cells and supporting (sustentacular) cells, separated from a connective tissue layer by a basement membrane.

There are two types of *hair cells* in the maculae: one type is flask-shaped, the other is cylindrical. Both kinds are provided at their free end with a tuft of fine *hairs* similar to those of the organ of Corti (so they also are *microvilli* and often referred to as *stereocilia*) except that they may be much longer; some reach at least 100 μm. in length. In addition to 80 or so stereocilia, each hair cell of the maculae and cristae (to be described shortly) has also a single cilium (*kinocilium*), which has the typical microtubular arrangement of a cilium and is longer than the stereocilia. The hairs of these cells do not float freely in the endolymph but are embedded in a gelatinous membrane called the *otolithic membrane* (Gr. *ous,* ear; *lithos,* stone) (Fig. 28-34). This membrane includes a surface layer of *calcium carbonate crystals* that have a specific gravity of approximately 3, much greater than the specific gravity of the surrounding endolymph.

The otolithic membrane (labeled in Fig. 28-34) lies

upon the macula like a flat stone upon a plate (Fig. 28-34, below *center*). If the head, and therefore the macula (plate), is tilted with respect to gravity, the otolithic membrane (stone) tends to slide downhill. This downhill movement pulls on the hairs and alters the activity in the nerve fibers supplying the macula so that the direction and magnitude of the tilt is reported to the brain. Similarly, if the head is given a linear (straight line) acceleration forward, as during acceleration in an automobile, the otolithic membranes tend to slide posteriorly on the maculae. The utricular otolith organs are thus regarded as sensors of *gravity* and *linear acceleration*. If the otolithic membranes are removed by centrifugation from the maculae of, for example, a guinea pig, the animal loses its sense of gravity and fails to show the usual postural responses to tilting and dropping. It is not known whether the saccular otolith organs are part of the organ of balance as the utricular otolith organs are; the saccules may play a role in the sensing of low-frequency vibration. In man the saccule is probably a sensor of *gravity* and *linear acceleration*.

The Semicircular Canals. The membranous semicircular

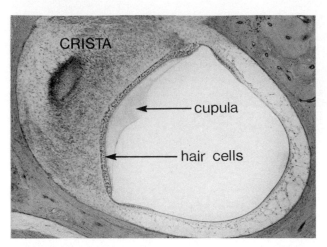

Fig. 28-35. Low-power photomicrograph of the ampulla of a lateral semicircular canal (squirrel monkey), cut in sagittal section. In life, the crista and cupula together form a partition extending all the way across the ampulla in this plane, but the cupula shrinks greatly on fixation. (Courtesy of J. Laufer)

canals (Fig. 28-30) are lined with a *squamous epithelium* (mesothelium) similar to that lining the saccule and the utricle. This also rests on a framework of connective tissue. The membranous tubes take up only a small part of the bony canal and are eccentrically placed, in contact with the cancave wall of the bony canal. Strands of connective tissue fibers join the tubes to the more distant parts of the canal, and *perilymph* fills the interstices.

The Ampullary Cristae. The outer wall (most distant from the center of the rough circle made by each tube) of each ampulla possesses a transverse ridge in its lining called a *crista* (labeled in Fig. 28-35). This is composed of neuroepithelial hair cells, connective tissue, nerve fibers, and capillaries. The surface epithelium of the crista is similar to that of the macula, possessing both flask-shaped and cylindrical *hair cells* with a large, oval, deep-staining nucleus, and supporting (sustentacular) cells, resting on a basement membrane. On the surface of the crista is a structure that closely resembles the tectorial membrane; this is called the *cupula* (L. for a cup) (Fig. 28-35). It is a gelatinous noncellular structure that covers the crista and projects up into the endolymph of the ampulla. The cupula differs from the otolithic membrane in that it contains *no crytals* and has specific gravity equal to that of the surrounding endolymph.

The cupula detects changes in *angular acceleration* (angular acceleration is the rate of change of rotational velocity, whereas linear acceleration is the rate of change of translational [linear] velocity). In life, each cupula extends from the crista right across the ampulla and closes

the lumen of the ampulla like a *flap valve* or swinging door hinged at the crista. When the head is given an angular acceleration, for example, about the spinal axis, the ring of endolymph in the horizontal semicircular canal (completed in the utricular endolymph) tends to remain *stationary* because of its inertia, and the membranous walls move relative to the endolymph. This movement displaces the cupula from its usual position relative to the crista (the swinging door is pushed open) and the displacement pulls on the hairs and changes the activity in the afferent nerve fibers supplying the crista so that information concerning angular movement is reported to the brain. The semicircular canals are therefore regarded as sensors of *angular movement* of the head (and hence of the body as a whole).

If the semicircular canals are put out of commission in the cat by experimental surgery, the animal exhibits angular oscillations of the head and falls down frequently. In man, loss of vestibular function (due, for example, to meningitis) causes postural instability and confers immunity to motion sickness.

REFERENCES AND OTHER READING

THE EYE

Ascher, K. W.: Further observations on aqueous veins. Am. J. Ophthalmol., *29:*1373, 1946.

Ashton, N.: Anatomical study of Schlemm's canal and aqueous veins by means of neoprene casts; aqueous veins. Br. J. Ophthalmol., *35:*291, 1951.

Basu, P. K.: Immune and nonimmune factors involved in the corneal graft reaction. Indian Med. Assoc. J., *66:*229, 1976.

Basu, P. K., and Carré, F.: A study of cells in human corneal grafts. Growth potential in vitro, cellular morphology, and fate of donor cells. Can. J. Ophthalmol., *8:*1, 1973.

Coulombre, A. J.: Cytology of the developing eye. Int. Rev. Cytol., *11:*161, 1961.

DeRobertis, E.: Electron microscope observations on the submicroscopic organization of retinal rods. J. Biophys. Biochem. Cytol., *2:*319, 1956.

————: Morphogenesis of the retinal rods; an electron microscope study. J. Biophys. Biochem. Cytol. (Suppl.), *2:*209, 1956.

Dodson, J. W., and Hay, E. D.: Secretion of collagenous stroma by isolated epithelium grown in vitro. Exp. Cell Res., *65:*215, 1971.

————: Secretion of collagen by corneal epithelium II. Effect of the underlying substratum on secretion and polymerization of epithelial products. J. Exp. Zool., *189:*51, 1972.

Dowling, J. E.: Foveal receptors of the monkey retina: Fine Structure. Science, *147:*57, 1965.

Droz, B.: Dynamic condition of proteins in the visual cells of rats and mice as shown by radioautography with labeled amino acids. Anat. Rec., *145:*157, 1963.

Duke-Elder, W. S., and Davson, H.: The present position of the problem of the intra-ocular fluid and pressure. Br. J. Ophthalmol., *32:*555, 1948.

Friedenwald, J. S.: The formation of the intraocular fluid. Am. J. Ophthalmol., *32:*9, 1949.

————: Recent studies on corneal metabolism and growth. Cancer Res., *10:*461, 1950.

Hollenberg, M. J., and Bernstein, M. H.: Fine structure of the photoreceptor cells of the ground squirrel. Am. J. Anat., *118:*359, 1966.

Holmberg, A.: The fine structure of the inner wall of Schlemm's canal. Arch. Ophthalmol., *62:*956, 1959.

Jakus, M. A.: Studies on the cornea: II. The fine structure of Descemet's membrane. J. Biophys. Biochem. Cytol. (Suppl.), *2:*243, 1956.

MacDonald, A. L., Basu, P. K., and Miller, R. G.: The systemic production of cytotoxic lymphoid cells in corneal allograft reaction. Transplantation, *23:*431, 1977.

MacMillan, J. A.: Disease of the lacrimal gland and ocular complications. J.A.M.A., *138:*801, 1948.

Noback, C. R., and Laemle, L. K.: Structural and functional aspects of the visual pathways of primates. *In* The Primate Brain. Advances in Primatology. vol. 1, p. 55. New York, Appleton-Century-Crofts, 1970.

Oppenheimer, D. R., Palmer, E., and Weddell, G.: Nerve endings in the conjunctiva. J. Anat., *92:*321, 1958.

Richardson, K. C.: The fine structure of the albino rabbit iris with special reference to the identification of adrenergic and cholinergic nerves and nerve endings in the intrinsic muscles. Am. J. Anat., *114:*173, 1964.

Sheldon, H.: An electron microscope study of the epithelium in the normal mature and immature mouse cornea. J. Biophys. Biochem. Cytol., *2:*253, 1956.

Sheldon, H., and Zetterqvist, H.: An electron microscope study of the corneal epithelium in the vitamin A deficient mouse. Bull. Johns Hopkins Hosp., *98:*372, 1956.

Sjostrand, F. S.: The electron microscopy of the retina. *In* Smelser, G. K. (ed.): The Structure of the Eye. New York, Academic Press, 1961.

Tokuyasu, K., and Yamada, R.: The fine structure of the retina studied with the electron microscope. J. Biophys. Biochem. Cytol., *6:*225, 1959.

Wanko, T., and Gavin, M. A.: Electron microscope study of lens fibers. J. Biophys. Biochem. Cytol., *6:*97, 1959.

Willis, N. R., Hollenberg, M. J., and Brackevelt, C. R.: The fine structure of the lens of the fetal rat. Can. J. Ophthalmol., *4:*307, 1969.

Wolken, J. J.: The photoreceptor structures. Int. Rev. Cytol., *11:*195, 1961.

Young, R. W.: The renewal of photoreceptor cell outer segments. J. Cell Biol., *33:*61, 1967.

————: The organization of vertebrate photoreceptor cells. *In* Straatsma, B. R., Hall, M. O., Allen, R. A., and Crescitelli, F. (eds.): The Retina: Morphology, Function and Clinical Characteristics. UCLA Forum in Medical Sciences, No. 8. Berkeley and Los Angeles, University of California Press, 1969.

————: A difference between rods and cones in the renewal of outer segment protein. Invest. Ophthalmol., *8:*222, 1969.

————: Visual cells. Sci. Am., *223:*80, Oct., 1970.

————: The renewal of rod and cone outer segments in the Rhesus monkey. J. Cell Biol., *49:*303, 1971.

————: Visual cells and the concept of renewal. Invest. Ophthalmol., *15:*700, 1976.

Young, R. W., and Bok, D.: Autoradiographic studies on the metabolism of the retinal pigment epithelium. Invest. Ophthalmol., *9:*524, 1970.

THE EAR

Batteau, D. W.: Role of the pinna in localization: theoretical and physiological consequences. *In* Hearing Mechanisms in Vertebrates, A Ciba Foundation Symposium. pp. 234–243. London, J. A. Churchill, 1968.

Davies, D. V.: A note on the articulation of the auditory ossicles and related structures. J. Laryng., *62:*533, 1948.

Duvall, A. J., Flock, Å., and Wersäll, J.: The ultrastructure of the sensory hairs and associated organelles of the cochlear inner hair cell with reference to directional sensitivity. J. Cell Biol., *29:*497, 1966.

Engström, H., and Wersäll, J.: Structure and innervation of the inner ear sensory epithelia. Int. Rev. Cytol., *7:*353, 1958.

Fernandez, C., Goldberg, J. M., and Abend, W. R.: Response to static tilts of peripheral neurons innervating otolith organs of the squirrel monkey. J. Neurophysiol., *35:*978, 1972.

Flock, Å.: The structure of the macula utriculi with special reference to directional interplay of sensory response as revealed by morphological polarization. J. Cell Biol., *22:*413, 1964.

Gulley, R. L., and Reese, T. S.: Freeze fracture studies on the synapses in the organ of Corti. J. Comp. Neurol., *171:*517, 1977.

Hawkins, J. E., Jr.: Cytoarchitectural basis of the cochlear transduct. Cold Spring Harbor. Symp. Quant. Biol., *30:*147, 1965.

Hawkins, J. E., and Johnsson, L.-G.: Light microscopic observations of the inner ear in man and monkey. Ann. Otol., *77:*608, 1968.

Johnsson, L.-G., and Hawkins, J. E., Jr.: Otolithic membranes of the saccule and utricle in man. Science, *157:*1454, 1967.

Kimura, R., Lindquist, P. G., and Wersäll, J.: Secretory epithelial linings in the ampullae of the guinea pig labyrinth. Acta Otolaryngol., *57:*517, 1963.

Lim, D. J.: Formation and fate of the otoconia, scanning and transmission electron microscopy. Ann. Otol. Rhinol. Laryngol., *82:*23, 1973.

Lim, J., and Lane, W. C.: Three-dimensional observations of the inner ear with the scanning electron microscope. Trans. Am. Acad. Ophthalmol. Otolaryngol., 842-872, Sept.-Oct. 1969.

Lundquist, P. G., Kimura, R., and Wersäll, J.: Ultrastructural organization of the epithelial lining in the endolymphatic duct and sac in the guinea pig. Acta Otolaryngol., *57:*65, 1963.

————: Experiments in endolymph circulation. Acta Otolaryngol. (Suppl.), *188:*198, 1964.

Money, K. E., and Friedberg, J.: The role of the semicircular canals in causation of motion sickness and nystagmus in the dog. Can. J. Physiol. Pharmacol., *42:*793, 1964.

Money, K. E., and Scott, J. W.: Functions of separate sensory receptors of nonauditory labyrinth of the cat. Am. J. Physiol., *202:*1211, 1962.

Montagna, W.: The pigment and fatty substances of the ceruminous glands of man. Anat. Rec., *100:*66, 1948.

Nadol, J. B., Mulroy, M. J., Goodenough, D. A., and Weiss, T. F.: Tight and gap junctions in the vertebrate inner ear. Am. J. Anat., *147:*281, 1976.

Potter, A. B.: Function of the stapedius muscle. Ann. Otol., *45:*638, 1936.

Smith, C. A.: Electron microscopy of the inner ear. Ann. Otol., *77:*629, 1968.

Wersäll, J.: Studies on the structure and innervation of the sensory epithelium of the cristae ampullares in the guinea pig; a light and electron microscopic investigation. Acta Otolaryngol. (Suppl.), *126:*1, 1956.

———: Efferent innervation of the inner ear. *In* Von Euler, C., et al. (eds.): Structure and Function of Inhibitory Neuronal Mechanisms. p. 123. Oxford and New York, Pergamon Press, 1968.

Wersäll, J., Flock, Å., and Lundquist, P. G.: Structural basis for directional sensitivity in cochlear and vestibular sensory receptors. Cold Spring Harbor, Symp. Quant. Biol., *30:*115, 1965.

Wiggers, H. C.: The functions of the intra-aural muscles. Am. J. Physiol., *120:*771, 1937.

Index